Textbook of Emergency General Surgery

Federico Coccolini • Fausto Catena
Editors

# Textbook of Emergency General Surgery

Traumatic and Non-traumatic Surgical Emergencies

Volume II

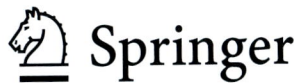

*Editors*
Federico Coccolini
General, Emergency and Trauma
Surgery Dept.
Pisa University Hospital
Pisa, Italy

Fausto Catena
General and Emergency
Surgery Dept.
Bufalini Hospital
Cesena, Italy

ISBN 978-3-031-22598-7  ISBN 978-3-031-22599-4  (eBook)
https://doi.org/10.1007/978-3-031-22599-4

© The Editor(s) (if applicable) and The Author(s), under exclusive license to Springer Nature Switzerland AG 2023
This work is subject to copyright. All rights are solely and exclusively licensed by the Publisher, whether the whole or part of the material is concerned, specifically the rights of translation, reprinting, reuse of illustrations, recitation, broadcasting, reproduction on microfilms or in any other physical way, and transmission or information storage and retrieval, electronic adaptation, computer software, or by similar or dissimilar methodology now known or hereafter developed.
The use of general descriptive names, registered names, trademarks, service marks, etc. in this publication does not imply, even in the absence of a specific statement, that such names are exempt from the relevant protective laws and regulations and therefore free for general use.
The publisher, the authors, and the editors are safe to assume that the advice and information in this book are believed to be true and accurate at the date of publication. Neither the publisher nor the authors or the editors give a warranty, expressed or implied, with respect to the material contained herein or for any errors or omissions that may have been made. The publisher remains neutral with regard to jurisdictional claims in published maps and institutional affiliations.

This Springer imprint is published by the registered company Springer Nature Switzerland AG
The registered company address is: Gewerbestrasse 11, 6330 Cham, Switzerland

# Foreword

The concept of this textbook is very timely with the current existence and the future of general surgery being questioned by many in our current era of super-specialized surgical care. While specialization in elective fields can lead too safe, efficient, and effective care with high levels of patient satisfaction, its feasibility in acute care is questionable. Superspecialist surgeons working within very narrow fields in their daily routine practice are unlikely to be competent to manage all surgical emergencies outside of their expertise. Hospitals providing emergency general surgical service are also unlikely to be prepared to support and maintain dozens of specialist surgical rosters for the management of each individual organ or organ parts. This latter concept of many subspecialist general surgical rosters would also necessitate a second surgical triage system after the emergency department triage, which inadvertently would lead to further delay to definitive care of the acute surgical patients. These facts re-establish the concept of the generalist surgeon in our heavily specialized modern practice. Emergency general surgery practice for a broad spectrum of conditions combined with adequate elective surgical opportunities provides a viable option for surgeons dedicated to public/academic institutions with surgical training programs. This model provides excellent opportunities to maintain surgical skills, cost-effective for healthcare and ideal for resident training programs. The prolific book publishing Professors Catena and Coccolini have produced another Italian masterpiece, probably the most comprehensive one so far. This impressive textbook on emergency general surgery consists of more than 100 chapters with over 300 international contributors from an excess of 40 countries of all continents. After a generous first chapter of overarching concepts, the book covers the key anatomical regions such as head and neck, chest, abdomen, extremities, and soft tissue surgical conditions. Beyond being didactic, this work is also ultra-pragmatic by addressing all aspects of emergency general surgery in different age groups, complications of subspecialties including transplantation, communication principles, and ethical issues, just to mention a few. Considering the topic selection, the exceptional content, the contemporary illustration material, and latest references with evidence-based approach, this work will be an essential companion to all general surgical residents, acute care general surgeons, and subspecialists who occasionally need to deal with general surgical emergencies.

University of Newcastle  
Callaghan, Newcastle NSW Australia  
John Hunter Hospital  
New Lambton Heights NSW Australia

Zsolt J. Balogh

# Foreword

At the beginning of 2020, the challenges raised by the Covid-19 pandemic induced an unprecedented public health crisis. More than 6.2 million people died because of Covid in the last two years, but road traffic injuries caused an estimated 1.3 million deaths worldwide in the last years, and more than 400,000 people die from homicide each year.

The World Society of Emergency Surgery (WSES) has been working on the Emergency General Surgery (EGS) organization since its foundation, collaborating with other societies for training and educational programs throughout the world. Management of emergency surgical patients with traumatic or non-traumatic acute conditions is a challenge and many countries have started a systematic effort in reorganizing EGS systems. Shortage of dedicated trained physicians, unfamiliarity with protocols, absence of dedicated teams, delay in surgery, and overcrowded emergency department and intensive care units may affect patient outcomes in unprepared systems.

In the last years many educational courses were developed and structured worldwide. But this book is a great opportunity to health professionals and undergraduate students learn more about EGS. The editors were very careful and intelligent to bring up various aspects of EGS, such as education, disease physiology, diagnosis, treatment, prognosis, and ethical issues. The authors are well-respected and recognized surgeons in their respective countries with extensive experience in EGS. I am very grateful to be a part of this project and it is an honor to write this preface, without prolonging too much, so that each reader can appreciate each of the chapters. And you can use this very comprehensive book to improve your clinical practice and better assist your patients.

Division of Trauma Surgery  
University of Campinas,  
Campinas, Brazil

Gustavo P. Fraga

# Foreword

*"The future belongs to preventive health care. This science, going hand in hand with curative health care will bring undoubted benefits to mankind."*

N.I. Pirogov (1810–1881)

At present, the problem of diagnosis and treatment of surgical emergencies remain topical. The rapid development of high-tech surgical instruments and the spread of minimally invasive procedures have led to the emergence of unknown postoperative complications and new algorithms for managing such patients.

Gone are the days when S.P. Fedorov's statement "a great surgeon is recognizable by a large incision" was the motto for several generations of emergency surgeons. Today, modern surgeons have many high-tech instruments at their disposal for accurate and quick diagnoses as well as various alternative methods of surgery. In fact, this feature of modern medicine does not always benefit the patient. Indecision, the inability to make quick and correct decisions, lack of knowledge about the latest approaches of evidence-based medicine to treating certain diseases can devalue technological advances and lead to adverse events.

A doctor is the crucial element in the "science—human health" chain. Therefore, even in the era of digital technologies, neural networks, and artificial intelligence, an intelligent mind and skillful hands remain the principal instruments in the fight against illness and death.

I hope that every reader of this book, either a medical student or an experienced specialist, will discover not only something new, but also something useful, for example, a special feature of preoperative patient preparation, subtleties of operations, or equally important issues of postoperative management and rehabilitation of patients.

Sechenov Medical University  Eduard A. Galliamov
Moskow, Russia

# Foreword

The *Textbook of Emergency General Surgery: Traumatic and Non-traumatic Surgical Emergencies* is a comprehensive resource for surgeons throughout the world who provide emergent care for seriously ill and injured patients. The authors are authorities in their respective areas and represent experience and expertise. While the practice domain varies from civilian to military, country to country, and urban to rural, the common objective is to provide as optimal care as possible considering the surgeons' and hospitals' capabilities. Definitive care may require patient transfer to a more experience facility, despite the fact that the surgeon possesses the necessary skills. The first section of the book provides an overview of general principles that apply to initial evaluation and management of the patient requiring urgent care, including triage in mass casualty events. The next section covers the physiologic challenges in the critically ill and injured, including the important differences based on age and comorbidities. Prompt reversal of shock is a common problem in many of these patients that is important to prioritize in operative management. There is also a timely discussion of care during pandemics that we learned painfully during the unprecedented COVID-19 infection, impacting all authors of this text. Palliative and futile care are particularly relevant for emergent surgical challenges because there is frequently limited opportunity to discuss this topic with the patient before their event. The ensuing sections present topics based on anatomic location, literally from head to toe. These anatomic-based sections are complete covering emergent trauma and non-trauma topics, including life-threatening bleeding and infections. I congratulate the editors and authors on a spectacular resource document that highlights the essential role of emergency general surgeons who provide exemplary care 24 h a day/7 days a week throughout the year.

University of Colorado  Ernest E. Moore
Denver, CA, USA

# Foreword

The global burden of emergency surgery is very significant, and several issues need to be addressed in order to promote a global dialogue on what is the most appropriate way to conceive emergency surgery worldwide. Although minimal variations in the spectrum of emergency surgical diseases may be observed among and within countries, "essential" surgery in emergency should be viewed as a core group of services that can be delivered within the context of universal access.

Furthermore, the surgical capabilities required are not only those related to performing operations. Emergency surgical care also involves preoperative assessment, including the decision to operate; provision of safe anesthesia; and postoperative care. Even when patients do not need emergency surgical procedures, surgical providers often provide care and must be prepared to intervene operatively as complications arise or conditions deteriorate.

Finally, many hospitals worldwide continue to have logistic barriers associated with the application of evidence-based practice, leading to an overall poorer adherence to international guidelines and making them impractical to a large part of the world's clinicians.

In this scenario, a *Textbook of Emergency General Surgery* including both traumatic and non-traumatic surgical emergencies, written by experts from all continents can be very useful to promote global standards of care that can drive clinicians around the world by describing "reasonable" approaches to the management of emergency surgery diseases.

General Surgery  
Macerata Hospital  
Macerata, Italy

Massimo Sartelli

# Preface

Emergency General Surgery (EGS) is the most widespread surgical discipline encompassing all traumatic and non-traumatic surgical emergencies. It is widely practiced throughout the entire world. Most general surgeons manage surgical emergencies during their daily activity. The emergency general surgeon may be the last surgeon able to deal with surgical emergencies in almost any region of the body in emergency setting, including traumatic and non-traumatic conditions.

The general emergency surgeon should be ideally trained to manage surgical and physiological derangements in all types of patients, from young and healthy to severely compromised. Currently, notwithstanding the worldwide spread of EGS and its importance along with its public health burdens, comprehensive and reliable textbooks have not been published yet.

This work represents the first in its field and is the result of worldwide participation. More than 250 authors from all continents contributed to the writing process with high-level chapters covering all the different topics. The work covers all aspects necessary for daily practice providing valuable assistance and sure help in handling even those rare and difficult situations.

High-quality photos and images clearly explain concepts giving a quick and effective tool to understand diseases and surgical techniques.

In addition, clear flowcharts will help surgeons around the world to rapidly evaluate and decide on the best strategy.

We devoted the past 2 years to this effort with the goal of improving patient care in a such difficult and widespread field.

This book is aimed at medical school students, residents, and specialists in general surgery, anesthesiology/intensive care, and emergency medicine.

Likewise, all residents and specialists in surgical and medical disciplines seeking to further their skills in the field of acute care surgery may find this textbook a useful guide.

We sincerely hope that it will be of help to all of you.

Enjoy it!

Pisa, Italy  Federico Coccolini
Cesena, Italy  Fausto Catena

# Contents

**Volume I**

**Part I   General Consideration**

1. **History of Emergency General Surgery** .................... 3
   Massimo Chiarugi

2. **General Approach to Emergency General Surgery** .......... 9
   Patricia Correia Sousa Perissé and Antonio Marttos

3. **Evaluation of Traumatic and Nontraumatic Patients** ........ 19
   Vitor F. Kruger and Gustavo P. Fraga

4. **Prioritizing Acute Care Surgery and Trauma Patients** ....... 33
   R. Stephen Smith and Jessica E. Taylor

5. **Triage** ................................................. 39
   Cordoba Mordehay, Ciro Paolillo, Federica Pitoni,
   and Klein Yoram

6. **Mass Casualties** ........................................ 47
   Emmanouil Pikoulis, Anastasia Pikouli, and Athanasios
   Kalogeropoulos

7. **Point-of-Care Ultrasound for Emergency General Surgeons** ... 63
   Bruno M. Pereira

8. **Systemic Response to Injury** ............................. 91
   Philip F. Dobson, Karen Muller, and Zsolt J. Balogh

9. **Coagulation and Thrombosis** ............................. 107
   Jonathan P. Meizoso, Hunter B. Moore, Angela Sauaia,
   and Ernest E. Moore

10. **Septic Shock** .......................................... 127
    Sacha Rozencwajg and Philippe Montravers

11. **Hypovolemic Shock** ..................................... 137
    Tyler J. Jones, Bishwajit Bhattacharya,
    and Kimberly A. Davis

| 12 | **Principles of Perioperative Management in Acute Care Surgery** ................................... 147 |
|---|---|
| | Oreste Romeo, Taylor A. Davidson, and Scott B. Davidson |

| 13 | **Critical Care Medicine** ................................... 159 |
|---|---|
| | Maria Di Matteo and Davide Corbella |

| 14 | **Fluid and Blood Management in Traumatic and Non-traumatic Surgical Emergencies** ................ 183 |
|---|---|
| | Domien Vanhonacker, Michaël Mekeirele, and Manu L. N. G. Malbrain |

| 15 | **Compartment Syndrome** ................................... 197 |
|---|---|
| | Rao R. Ivatury |

| 16 | **Antibiotic and Antimicotic Therapy** ................... 219 |
|---|---|
| | Marcelo A. F. Ribeiro Junior, Gabriela Tebar, and José Lucas Rodrigues Salgueiro |

| 17 | **Pain Management** ................................... 243 |
|---|---|
| | Etrusca Brogi and Francesco Forfori |

| 18 | **Damage Control Surgery** ................................... 265 |
|---|---|
| | Carlo Vallicelli and Federico Coccolini |

| 19 | **Nutritional Support** ................................... 275 |
|---|---|
| | Swathikan Chidambaram, En Lin Goh, and Mansoor Ali Khan |

| 20 | **Palliative Care in the ICU** ................................... 285 |
|---|---|
| | Mayur Narayan and Jeffry Kashuk |

| 21 | **Immunosuppression in Surgical Patients** ................... 313 |
|---|---|
| | Hannah Groenen and Marja A. Boermeester |

| 22 | **Pregnant Women** ................................... 331 |
|---|---|
| | Pintar Tadeja |

| 23 | **Geriatrics: Traumatic and Non-traumatic Surgical Emergencies** ................................... 347 |
|---|---|
| | Kartik Prabhakaran and Rifat Latifi |

| 24 | **Pediatrics** ................................... 367 |
|---|---|
| | Matthew P. Landman and Denis Bensard |

| 25 | **Cirrhotic Patients** ................................... 389 |
|---|---|
| | Greg Padmore and Chad G. Ball |

| 26 | **Management of Animal Bites: A Global Perspective** .......... 401 |
|---|---|
| | Saleh Abdel-Kader, Ihab M. Abbas, and Fikri M. Abu-Zidan |

| 27 | **Burns, Inhalation, and Lightning Injury** ................... 411 |
|---|---|
| | Mariëlle Vehmeijer-Heeman and Edward Tan |

| | | |
|---|---|---|
| 28 | **Blast: Mechanisms of Injury and Implications upon Treatment**........................................... | 427 |
| | Itamar Ashkenazi and Yoram Kluger | |
| 29 | **Major Bleeding Management and REBOA**.................. | 443 |
| | Amelia Pasley, Victoria Sharp, Jason Pasley, and Megan Brenner | |
| 30 | **Robotics**................................................. | 457 |
| | Giorgio Bianchi, Aleix Martínez-Pérez, and Nicola de'Angelis | |
| 31 | **Emergency and Trauma Surgery During Epidemia and Pandemia**............................... | 471 |
| | Belinda De Simone, Elie Chouillard, and Fausto Catena | |
| 32 | **Principles of Management of Surgical Complications**........ | 487 |
| | Nikolaos Pararas, Anastasia Pikouli, Konstantinos Nastos, and Emmanouil Pikoulis | |
| 33 | **Iatrogenic Complications of Digestive Endoscopy**............ | 497 |
| | Aleix Martínez-Pérez, Carmen Payá-Llorente, and Nicola de'Angelis | |
| 34 | **End-of-Life Care, Including the Role of Intensive Care in Tissue and Organ Donation**..................... | 513 |
| | Christopher James Doig and Kevin J. Solverson | |
| 35 | **Futility of Care and Palliative Care**...................... | 523 |
| | Paolo Malacarne and Silvia Pini | |
| 36 | **Communication in Emergency General Surgery**.............. | 531 |
| | Evika Karamagioli | |
| 37 | **Patient Safety and Risk Management**..................... | 539 |
| | Boris E. Sakakushev | |
| 38 | **Quality Evaluation in Emergency General Surgery**.......... | 569 |
| | Michael Sugrue, Randal Parlour, Brendan Skelly, and Angus Watson | |

**Part II  Head, Face and Neck**

| | | |
|---|---|---|
| 39 | **Head and Brain Trauma**................................. | 581 |
| | Giacomo Bertolini, Luca Cattani, Corrado Iaccarino, Anna Fornaciari, and Edoardo Picetti | |
| 40 | **Emergency Surgical Access to the Neck**.................... | 605 |
| | Iván Trostchansky and Fernando Machado | |
| 41 | **Face and Neck Infections**................................ | 623 |
| | Alfons Mogedas, Mireia Pascua, and Xavier Guirao | |

| | | |
|---|---|---|
| 42 | **Trauma to the Face**........................................ 641 | |
| | Kerry P. Latham and Mark W. Bowyer | |

| | | |
|---|---|---|
| 43 | **Traumatic Neck Injuries** ................................. 651 | |
| | Rathnayaka M. Kalpanee D. Gunasingha and Mark W. Bowyer | |

| | | |
|---|---|---|
| 44 | **Management of Neck Surgery Complications** ............... 665 | |
| | Giovanna Di Meo, Alessandro Pasculli, and Mario Testini | |

## Part III  Thorax and Mediastinum

| | | |
|---|---|---|
| 45 | **Emergency Surgical Access to the Thorax** ................. 691 | |
| | Marc de Moya and Rebecca Mitchell | |

| | | |
|---|---|---|
| 46 | **Empyema**................................................ 703 | |
| | Linda C. Qu, Rahul Nayak, and Neil G. Parry | |

| | | |
|---|---|---|
| 47 | **Hemothorax and Pneumothorax**........................... 711 | |
| | David A. Spain, Ara Ko, and Jamie Tung | |

| | | |
|---|---|---|
| 48 | **Chest Trauma** .......................................... 727 | |
| | Joseph M. Galante and Tanya N. Rinderknecht | |

| | | |
|---|---|---|
| 49 | **Thoracic Vascular Trauma**............................... 743 | |
| | G. Janssen, M. Khashram, S. Bhagvan, and I. Civil | |

| | | |
|---|---|---|
| 50 | **Resuscitative Thoracotomy** .............................. 753 | |
| | Ning Lu and Walter L. Biffl | |

| | | |
|---|---|---|
| 51 | **Cardiac Trauma and Tamponade** ......................... 765 | |
| | Lena M. Napolitano | |

| | | |
|---|---|---|
| 52 | **Management of Cardiothoracic Surgery Complications** ...... 783 | |
| | Bernd Niemann, Ursula Vigelius-Rauch, and Andreas Hecker | |

| | | |
|---|---|---|
| 53 | **Acute Congenital and Acquired Heart Disease** .............. 801 | |
| | Alessandro Leone, G. Murana, L. Di Marco, E. Angeli, L. Careddu, G. Gargiulo, and D. Pacini | |

## Volume II

## Part IV  Abdomen

| | | |
|---|---|---|
| 54 | **Principles of Emergency and Trauma Laparotomy**........... 815 | |
| | S. Barbois and C. Arvieux | |

| | | |
|---|---|---|
| 55 | **Principles of Emergency and Trauma Laparoscopy** .......... 833 | |
| | Felipe Vega-Rivera, Ignacio Alvarez-Valero, Fernando Pérez-Galaz, and Alberto Pérez Cantú-Sacal | |

| | | |
|---|---|---|
| 56 | **Esophageal Non-traumatic Emergencies** ................... 855 | |
| | Luigi Bonavina, Emanuele Asti, and Tommaso Panici Tonucci | |

| | | |
|---|---|---|
| 57 | **Esophageal Trauma** .................................. 871 |
| | Michael D. Kelly and Mircea Chirica | |
| 58 | **Caustic Ingestion**..................................... 877 |
| | Mircea Chirica, Helene Corte, and Pierre Cattan | |
| 59 | **Surgical Jaundice and Cholangitis** ..................... 889 |
| | Aleksandar R. Karamarkovic, Jovan T. Juloski, and Vladica V. Cuk | |
| 60 | **Biliary Colic and Acute Cholecystitis** .................. 901 |
| | Paola Fugazzola, Mario Improta, and Luca Ansaloni | |
| 61 | **Hepatic Abscesses** .................................. 911 |
| | Kyra N. Folkert, Sarah Khalil, and Robert Sawyer | |
| 62 | **Spleen Non-traumatic Acute Surgical Conditions** ........... 923 |
| | Marco Ceresoli and Luca Degrate | |
| 63 | **Acute Adrenal Conditions: Pheochromocytoma Emergencies** ..................... 935 |
| | Gabriele Materazzi, Leonardo Rossi, and Piermarco Papini | |
| 64 | **Nontraumatic Liver Hemorrhage** ....................... 949 |
| | Amudan J. Srinivasan and Andrew B. Peitzman | |
| 65 | **Acute Pancreatitis**................................... 969 |
| | Ari Leppäniemi and Matti Tolonen | |
| 66 | **Acute Appendicitis** ................................. 983 |
| | Gaetano Gallo, Mauro Podda, Marta Goglia, and Salomone Di Saverio | |
| 67 | **Acute Left Colonic Diverticulitis**....................... 1001 |
| | Massimo Sartelli | |
| 68 | **Acute Mesenteric Ischemia** ........................... 1007 |
| | Miklosh Bala and Asaf Kedar | |
| 69 | **Upper Gastrointestinal Bleeding**........................ 1017 |
| | Helmut A. Segovia Lohse and Herald R. Segovia Lohse | |
| 70 | **Gastric Outlet Obstruction** ........................... 1035 |
| | Feibo Zheng, Liang Ha, and Yunfeng Cui | |
| 71 | **Acute Lower Gastrointestinal Bleeding** .................. 1049 |
| | Muhammed A. Khalil Ali, Henry Bergman, Salomone Di Saverio, M. Adil Butt, and Ewen A. Griffiths | |
| 72 | **Perforated Peptic Ulcer** .............................. 1067 |
| | Delphina Yeo Boon Xue, Ramkumar Mohan, and Vishal G. Shelat | |
| 73 | **Diagnosis and Management of Acute Small Bowel Obstruction** .......................... 1085 |
| | Pepijn Krielen and Richard ten Broek | |

| 74 | **Small Bowel Perforation**.............................. 1095 |
|---|---|
| | Dimitrios Damaskos, Anne Ewing, and Judith Sayers |
| 75 | **Small Bowel Diverticular Disease** ..................... 1103 |
| | Carlos Yánez Benítez |
| 76 | **Large Bowel Obstruction**.............................. 1117 |
| | Tiffany Paradis, Tarek Razek, and Evan G. Wong |
| 77 | **Large Bowel Perforation** ............................. 1131 |
| | V. Khokha |
| 78 | **Emergency Management of Abdominal Wall Hernia** ........ 1143 |
| | M. M. J. van Rooijen, J. F. Lange, and J. Jeekel |
| 79 | **Emergency Management of Internal Hernia** .............. 1155 |
| | David Czeiger, Julia Vaynshtein, Ivan Kukeev, and Gad Shaked |
| 80 | **Emergency Management Hiatal Hernia and Gastric Volvulus**................................ 1163 |
| | Imtiaz Wani, G. M. Naikoo, and Nisar Hamdani |
| 81 | **Stoma-Related Surgical Emergencies**.................... 1175 |
| | Arda Isik and Rajesh Ramanathan |
| 82 | **Inflammatory Bowel Disease**........................... 1187 |
| | Jeremy Meyer and Justin Davies |
| 83 | **Fulminant/Toxic Colitis** ............................. 1207 |
| | Sanjay Marwah, Rajesh Godara, and Shouvik Das |
| 84 | **Clostridium Infections** .............................. 1227 |
| | Giada Fasani, Angela Pieri, and Leonardo Pagani |
| 85 | **Bowel Parasitic Surgical Emergencies** ................. 1253 |
| | Ibrahima Sall, Magatte Faye, and Ibrahima Diallo |
| 86 | **Anorectal Emergencies**............................... 1263 |
| | Antonio Tarasconi and Gennaro Perrone |
| 87 | **Gynaecological Surgical Emergencies**................... 1283 |
| | Robert Tchounzou, André Gaetan Simo Wambo, and Alain Chichom-Mefire |
| 88 | **Nontraumatic Urologic Emergencies** .................... 1295 |
| | Dyvon Walker, Rodrigo Donalisio da Silva, and Fernando J. Kim |
| 89 | **Non-Obstetric Abdominal Surgical Emergencies in Pregnancy and Puerperium**........................ 1307 |
| | Goran Augustin |
| 90 | **Enterovesical and Enterogenital Fistulae** ................. 1327 |
| | Krishanth Naidu and Francesco Piscioneri |

## Contents

**91 Enterocutaneous and Enteroatmospheric Fistulae** .......... 1337
Ashleigh Phillips, Eu Jhin Loh, and Francesco Amico

**92 Complication of Bariatric Surgery** ...................... 1351
Doron Kopelman and Uri Kaplan

**93 Intra-Abdominal Hypertension and Abdominal Compartment Syndrome** ............................. 1369
Tyler Lamb, Andrew W. Kirkpatrick, and Derek J. Roberts

**94 Open Abdomen Management** ........................... 1397
Pradeep Navsaria, Deidre McPherson, Sorin Edu, and Andrew Nicol

**95 Liver Trauma** ......................................... 1415
Federico Coccolini, Camilla Cremonini, and Massimo Chiarugi

**96 Splenic Trauma** ....................................... 1431
Tian Wei Cheng Brian Anthony, Carlo Vallicelli, and Fausto Catena

**97 Bowel Trauma** ........................................ 1449
Carlos A. Ordoñez, Michael W. Parra, and Yaset Caicedo

**98 Kidney and Urotrauma** ................................ 1461
Federico Coccolini, Camilla Cremonini, and Massimo Chiarugi

**99 Duodeno-Pancreatic and Extrahepatic Biliary Trauma** ...... 1483
Gennaro Perrone, Alfredo Annicchiarico, Elena Bonati, and Fausto Catena

**100 Abdominal Vascular Trauma** ............................ 1499
Franchesca J. Hwang, Jarrett E. Santorelli, Leslie M. Kobayashi, and Raul Coimbra

**101 Genital and Anorectal Trauma** ......................... 1513
Thobekile Nomcebo Shangase, Feroz Ganchi, and Timothy Craig Hardcastle

**102 Pelvic Trauma** ....................................... 1527
Philip F. Stahel and Vincent P. Stahel

**103 Ruptured Abdominal Aortic Aneurysm (rAAA)** ............ 1539
Tal M. Hörer

**104 Visceral Artery Aneurysms** ............................ 1553
Jonathan Parks and George C. Velmahos

**105 Management of Complications Occurring After Pancreas Transplantation** ..................................... 1565
Fabio Vistoli, Emanuele Federico Kauffmann, Niccolò Napoli, Gabriella Amorese, and Ugo Boggi

**106  Liver Transplant Complications Management** .............. 1581
Rami Rhaiem, Raffaele Brustia, Linda Rached,
and Daniele Sommacale

## Part V  Extremities

**107  Emergency Vascular Access to Extremities** ................ 1613
Frank Plani

**108  Extremity Vascular Injuries**........................... 1631
Viktor A. Reva and Adenauer Marinho de Oliveira Góes Junior

**109  Extremities Trauma** .................................. 1653
Ingo Marzi, Cora Rebecca Schindler, and Philipp Störmann

**110  Extremity Compartment Syndrome** ...................... 1663
Dominik A. Jakob, Elizabeth R. Benjamin,
and Demetrios Demetriades

**111  Fasciitis**.................................................. 1679
Yutaka Harima, Norio Sato, and Kaoru Koike

**112  Bone Infections** ........................................ 1689
Luigi Branca Vergano and Mauro Monesi

## Part VI  Soft Tissues

**113  Necrotizing Soft Tissue Infection**......................... 1715
Ashley A. Holly, Therese M. Duane, and Morgan Collom

**114  Cutaneous and Subcutaneous Abscesses**................... 1725
Jan Ulrych

**115  Surgical Site Infections**................................. 1737
A. Walker and M. Wilson

# Part IV

# Abdomen

# Principles of Emergency and Trauma Laparotomy

**54**

S. Barbois and C. Arvieux

## 54.1 Introduction

> **Learning Goals**
> - Identify the indications for emergency laparotomy
> - Explain the principles of peri and post-operative management
> - Identify short- and long-term outcomes after emergency laparotomy

### 54.1.1 Epidemiology

Emergency laparotomy procedures are one of the most frequent procedures in general surgery, with clinical and economic impact. In United Kingdom, for example, the incidence of this procedure in general population was estimated as 1:1100 [1]. It is undoubtedly the procedure that young surgeons learn to performed very early in their training, because of its technical simplicity

S. Barbois
Emergency and General Surgery Department,
Edouard Herriot University Hospital,
Lyon, France

C. Arvieux (✉)
Digestive and Emergency Surgery Department,
Grenoble-Alpes University Hospital,
Grenoble, France
e-mail: carvieux@chu-grenoble.fr

and the very wide range of indications it includes. It allows a large exposure of the abdominal cavity whatever the clinical situation and the hemodynamic status of the patient, and allows a certain diagnosis in most cases and the adapted treatment.

Laparoscopic surgery *(see dedicated chapter "Principles of emergency and trauma laparoscopy" Vega, F.)* has revolutionized the approach to abdominal exploration. It has progressively become the reference technique for an increasing number of surgical procedures, because of better clinical outcomes. This strategy was extensively adopted in elective surgery. Although more and more frequent [2], laparoscopic procedures for emergency situations are still more controversial in emergency procedures, except for some indications with strongest evidence, as appendicitis, cholecystitis, or non-specific abdominal pains [2]. There are still a lot of situations, whether clinical, surgical, or contextual, where exploration by laparotomy remains the gold standard.

It is quite difficult to have a precise idea of the number of emergency laparotomy procedures in a given territory [3]. When it exists, this information is generally collected in databases supplied on the initiative and by some territories, sometimes on the population catchment area of a single hospital [1], or for very specific victim categories such as car crashes for example. It is also possible to question the non-exhaustive nature of data collection, because of the mostly voluntary participation of centers and practitioners. Nevertheless, some national initiatives should be highlighted. For example, the NELA study [4] found that nearly 30,000 laparotomies for non-traumatic indications were performed each year in the United Kingdom. In traumatic situation, one obvious example is the National Trauma Data Bank® (NTDB®) as an important aggregate of US trauma registry data. In Europe, a few national registry and trauma system initiatives have also emerged over the past 10 years [3, 5–8].

Although rather inhomogeneous, these databases nevertheless shed light on specific epidemiological data according to the country. Most studies show a sex ratio in favor of male victims, and most often young, economically active adults. Injuries are the leading cause of death in the first four decades of life [3], raising it to the top of the public health priority list in most industrialized countries. Hemorrhage is still the major cause of early death in trauma patients [4, 5].

## 54.1.2 Etiology

The use of laparotomy exploration is encountered in two main types of situations: traumatic and non-traumatic emergencies.

### 54.1.2.1 Medical or Non-traumatic Situations [9–11]

Sepsis of abdominal origin is a major cause of surgical exploration [12]. Among them are peritonitis due to perforation of hollow organs, such as perforated ulcers, colonic perforations of iatrogenic, diverticular or cancerous origin *(see dedicated chapter « Acute colonic diverticulitis » Sartelli, M.)*, mesenteric ischemia *(see dedicated chapter « Mesenteric ischemia," Bala, M.)* and peritonitis of biliary origin. Indeed, if the cholecystectomy procedure is preferable in laparoscopy because of earlier postoperative recovery, the risk of conversion especially in an emergency situation remains non-negligible and varies between 5 and 40% [10, 13] *(see dedicated chapter "Biliary colic and acute cholecystitis" Ansaloni, L.)*. Acute appendicitis is a very common source of intra-abdominal infection [14] and could be treated either by open or laparoscopic approach [10] *(see dedicated chapter « Acute appendicitis » Di Saverio, S.)*. If the laparoscopic approach is chosen, the conversion rate is estimated at about 2% in a large French series [15], with the main cause being the presence of adhesions. For complicated appendicitis, both open and laparoscopic approach are viable treatment options, according to WSES guidelines, but the open approach is probably the most common approach in the patients with complicated appendicitis worldwide [14].

Indications for acute pancreatitis have evolved recently [16, 17]. A step-up approach is recommended, starting with the least invasive procedures (percutaneous or endoscopic percutaneous drainage, endoscopic necrosectomy…) *(see dedicated chapter "Acute pancreatitis," Leppaniemi, A., Tolonen, M.)*. Surgical debridement by laparotomy still has a place but should be reserved for extreme situations of uncontrollable sepsis or abdominal compartment syndrome (ACS), due to a high morbi-mortality rate *(see dedicated chapter "Abdominal compartment syndrome" Roberts, D., Kirkpatrick, A.)*.

In addition to these de novo etiologies, severe postoperative complications are also a significant cause of repeat surgery, most often due to anastomotic fistulas *(see dedicated chapter "Principles of management of surgical complications," Demko, A)*. Surgical anastomotic breakdowns are actually the most common cause of fecal peritonitis after diverticular disease [18]. Although in the hemodynamically stable patient, laparoscopic revision can be considered in certain indications and under certain conditions, the laparotomy approach must be anticipated.

Acute bowel obstruction is a common reason of laparotomy procedure. The main etiology is certainly adhesions [2], followed by malignancies, hernias, and volvulus. Certain predisposing inflammatory pathologies such as IBD can also cause acute complications, as strictures *(see dedicated chapter « Small bowel obstruction," ten Broek, R.)*.

If occlusions on adhesions are currently treated most often medically [11] with nasogastric and intravenous supplementation with fluids and electrolytes, signs of complications such as clinical or radiological signs of intestinal ischemia are an indication for emergency surgery. Laparoscopic approach is still reserved for selective cases and trained surgeons [13]. Sigmoid volvulus can be treated endoscopically in the absence of signs of digestive ischemia, perforation, or critical distension of the right colon. However, if the endoscopic procedure fails or if any of these signs are present, surgical exploration is necessary. Non-reducible hernial strangulations are a surgical emergency. A median laparotomy approach must always be anticipated to free the digestive segment and to assess its vitality, even in case of an elective inguinal approach.

Recommendations for the treatment of gastrointestinal bleeding have undergone profound changes with the advent of endoscopic and radiological procedures in the last 30 years *(see "Upper gastrointestinal bleeding" Segovia Lohse, H. and « Lower gastrointestinal bleeding », Griffiths, E.).*

The main challenge is to understand where the hemorrhage is located, especially in low hemorrhages where neither endoscopic exploration in unprepared patients nor radiological exploration have great sensitivity. The clinical context may point to one or the other of these etiologies too. In case of failure of medical, radiological, and endoscopic procedures, surgical exploration can sometimes be an option of last resort. The surgeon is most often called upon when less invasive hemostatic procedures fail in a patient who is hemodynamically deteriorating, therefore the laparotomy approach is preferred.

Other non-digestive intra-abdominal emergencies may require an emergency laparotomy procedure, such as ruptured aneurysms including ruptured abdominal aortic aneurysm. Hemorrhages of gynecological origin and in particular due to ectopic pregnancies, although technically accessible to treatment by laparoscopy, may require procedures by laparotomy *(see dedicated chapter "Gynecological surgical emergencies," Chichom-Mefire, A.).*

Abdominal compartment syndrome (ACS), defined as intra-abdominal hyper pressure greater than 20 mmHg associated with the occurrence of at least one organ failure is also an indication for laparotomy without delay, allowing by definition decompression of the abdominal compartment [19] *(see dedicated chapter « Abdominal compartment syndrome," Roberts, D., Kirkpatrick, A.).*

Finally, there are also indications for surgical exploration in cases of uncertain diagnosis and probable abdominal origin, grouped in the literature under the term non-specific abdominal pain (NSAP). If the non-invasive explorations do not allow to confirm or invalidate with certitude any diagnosis, the attitude oscillates between expectation and surgical exploration, according to the repercussion of the symptoms. Exploration by laparoscopy is probably the alternative of choice because of its less aggressive character [13]. Nevertheless, the presence of adhesions, the clinical precariousness of the patient, and the non-exhaustive nature of laparoscopic exploration may prefer exploration by laparotomy.

### 54.1.2.2 Traumatic Situations

The causes of traumatic abdominal injuries are divided into two major etiologies. First, blunt trauma: this is mainly represented by road accidents in industrialized countries, but also by specific trauma related to sports with high kinetics or high risk of falling (motorcycle, winter sports, climbing, paragliding...). By definition, these types of trauma are opposed to penetrating trauma, by stab or fire arms, the proportion of wounds due to one or the other of these wounding agents varying from one country to another, and between civilian [20] and military trauma [21].

Finally, a new issue has emerged recently, owing to the new threat of terrorist attacks. These situations, although fortunately exceptional, represent a medico-surgical challenge due to the massive influx of injured people that they cause compared to the available resources, the multitude of types of injuries found (penetrating wounds, closed trauma, blast, severe burns, poisoning…), and insufficient preparation of civilian teams for damage control procedures [22] comparing to militaries [23].

## 54.2 Classifications

With regard to the etiologies mentioned above, it appears that patients requiring emergency surgical exploration represent a heterogeneous group of patients and clinical situations [24].

The team managing these patients must take into account not only the pathology (suspected or confirmed) but also the clinical condition of the patient. This includes not only the age and history of the patient but also the severity of the clinical picture and its hemodynamic impact.

> **If a laparotomy exploration is decided, two operative strategies can be considered**

- Exploration in the "classic laparotomy" mode: the aim of exploration is to treat the cause in a single step, according to the "see all, repair all" principle. The fascial incision is closed. Drainage may be left in place and subsequently removed. In the case of digestive resection, the anastomoses or stomies are made during the same procedure.
- Exploration in "abbreviated laparotomy" mode or "damage control surgery" *(see dedicated chapter « Damage control strategy », Weber, D.)*: in the event of metabolic and physiological failure, the procedure aims to limit itself to the strict control of lesions that are life-threatening in the short term (bleeding and/or contamination), without attempting to obtain a definitive repair. The procedure is usually limited to 1 h. In the case of digestive resection for example, the digestive segments are left closed in the abdomen. The definitive treatment and the complete closure of the abdominal wall will be carried out in a second procedure during a scheduled reoperation, after a period of resuscitation to restore physiological parameters.

There is currently no randomized study comparing "classic" versus "damage control" procedures in traumatic situations. However, it appears that in this particular case, the benefit in terms of reducing morbidity and mortality of a damage control strategy is no longer in doubt: indeed, the result is a situation where practical applications have outpaced high-level clinical evidence, and randomized trials are difficult to justify for evaluating protocols that are already in place and are legitimized by experience.

However, the debate persists in non-traumatic situations. Widely described and put in evidence in traumatic situations for nearly 20 years, this strategy has been transposed more recently, probably instinctively at first, by emergency surgeons, who have to treat patients concerned by one or other of the situations [25]. For now, the debate persists because the level of evidence remains low, due to retrospective studies generally involving small numbers and varied etiologies.

### 54.2.1 Physiopathology

#### 54.2.1.1 Hemorrhagic Shock: Stop the Bleeding et Limit the Contamination

In traumatic situations, coagulopathy is a complication of hemorrhage with multifactorial origin, related to hypothermia, metabolic acidosis related to tissue hypoperfusion, dilution and consumption of coagulation factors and hypocalcemia *(see dedicated chapter « Hypovolemic shock" Davis, K.)*. These elements are all closely interrelated and mutually supportive, plunging the patient into a potentially fatal "bloody vicious circle" also known as the "lethal diamond" [26] (Fig. 54.1). Therapeutic strategies aim to interrupt this spiral. The surgeon's role is therefore essential: stop the bleeding, as quickly as possible.

The situation is also encountered in cases of hemorrhagic shock of non-traumatic origin, such as duodenal or gastric bleeding on ulcers, postoperative hemorrhages, or even uncontrollable per-operative hemorrhages of delicate repair, as in pancreatic surgery [25]. In these cases, damage control management may be justified too.

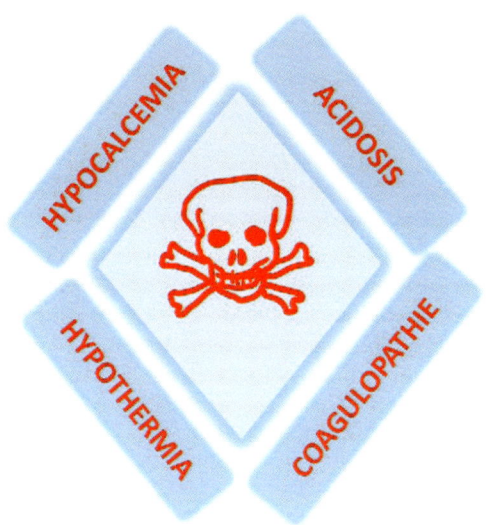

**Fig. 54.1** The lethal diamond (according to Ditzel [22])

### 54.2.1.2 Acute Peritonitis: Control the Sepsis and Prevent Abdominal Hyper Pressure

In the case of septic shock *(see dedicated chapter "Septic shock," Montravers, P., Rozencwajg, s.)*, the systemic inflammatory response causes a cascade of physiological aggressions. The hypothesis supported in recent years is that there is a survival benefit to abbreviated exploration followed by planned surgical resumption also in situations of septic shock: the priority is also given here to the restoration of physiological parameters rather than to immediate organ repair and anatomical reconstruction. However, the physiological mechanisms involved, their consequences, and the impact of resuscitation procedures, both medical and surgical, are not as clear as in the pathophysiology of hemorrhagic shock. In particular, the criteria for deciding on a damage control procedure are not as well defined as in hemorrhagic shock, and they are probably not perfectly adapted to septic shock [25, 27].

Most of the studies conducted to date are retrospective, often with small numbers of patients. One randomized study [28], however, attempted to compare the morbidity and mortality rates in the year after surgery between procedures that systematically included a new surgical exploration at 36–48 h (planned relaparotomy group) versus a new exploration only if necessary (on-demand relaparotomy group). The study did not show a significant difference on these criteria but showed a lower rate of relaparotomy in the on-demand relaparotomy and a lower length of hospital stay.

If the open abdomen technique *(see dedicated chapter "Open abdomen management », Navsaria, P.)* is a rational extension of damage control surgery, mainly for reasons of rapidity, it also appears to be relevant for the prevention of ACS, which can also be observed in traumatic and non-traumatic. Situations. Indeed, visceral edema can become very important in case of ischemia-reperfusion lesions that are encountered in situations of actual or potential digestive ischemia (including complex aortic vascular surgeries), and can be aggravated by aggressive resuscitation [29].

## 54.3 Diagnosis

### 54.3.1 Clinical Presentation

Typically, patients requiring emergency abdominal exploration present with an acute surgical abdomen. The abdomen may be distended by a large hemoperitoneum, by meteorism in case of occlusion, by an abundant effusion, or due to intra-abdominal hyper-pressure. In conscious subjects, signs of peritoneal irritation may be present (rigid abdomen with defense, contracture).

The interpretation of the hemodynamic parameters (tachycardia, hypotension) and their evolution according to the therapeutics engaged from the beginning of the management is very important as it guides the strategy to adopt. A state of hemorrhagic shock will thus be a major contraindication to exploration by laparoscopy. The temperature can be variable depending on the etiology, from hypothermia in situations of severe hemorrhage (especially traumatic) to hyperthermia in severe sepsis.

Of course, specific disease signs should be researched to guide the clinician, as personal medical history, current treatment, digestive symptoms (vomiting, hematemesis, occlusion syndrome...), and also severity clinical signs, as consciousness disorders (Glasgow coma scale) or tachypnea.

According to the traumatic event, the surgeon should also focus on abdominal wall injuries to guide his procedure strategy, watching out for signs of contusion, stab, or gunshot wounds (number, location, entry and exit point), signs of evisceration. Other parameters should be alarming and predictive for the need of damage control procedure, as massive transfusion [exceeding 5 packed red blood cells (RBCs)], and clinical signs of coagulopathy (diffuse bleeding, hemorrhage or hematoma at the puncture sites).

### 54.3.2 Tests

#### 54.3.2.1 Imaging

In case of emergency situation without hemodynamic instability (or after stabilization), computed tomography (CT)-scan remains the best imaging choice [30] (Fig. 54.2a) *(see dedicated chapter « Imaging », Matsumoto, J)* even if it shows some limits in peculiar situation [31]. It would allow a modification of the strategy in almost one case out of two compared to a clinical diagnosis alone in non-traumatic abdominal emergencies [32]. The exam is preferred with intravenous administration of an iodinated contrast medium (contrast-enhanced CT), particularly useful in patients suspected of having mesenteric ischemia or hemorrhage, and perhaps with oral intestinal opacification, particularly in patients with personal history of bariatric surgery [33] *(see dedicated chapter "Complication of bariatric surgery," Kopelman, D., Kaplan, U.).*

CT-scan has an excellent performance and sensitivity near of 100% for the diagnosis of pneumoperitoneum, solid organ injury, presence of an effusion, a 90% accuracy in predicting strangulation and the need for urgent surgery [11], and predicting a site of perforation up to 80% [32, 34]. The accuracy of CT in the diagnosis of mesenteric ischemia is similar to that with conventional angiography [32]. The exam is preferred in elderly and obese subjects [33]. On the other hand, it allows guided gestures to be performed, such as the drainage of abscesses [10].

In situations where X-rays are not recommended, such as in pregnancy (see dedicated chapter « Pregnant women », Pintar, T., Smrkolj, S., Šurlan-Popovič, K.) or in children, the acceptable alternative is the use of ultrasound (see dedicated chapter "Point of care ultrasound," Pereira B.) or even magnetic resonance imaging [14].

In case of life-threatening traumatic condition, complementary examinations must be limited so as not to delay surgical management. Classically, eFAST [35] and X-ray of the thorax and pelvis are helpful in confirming the presence of an abdominal, thoracic, and/or pericardial effusion, identifying pelvic instability, and guiding the strategy and choice of the first compartment to be explored.

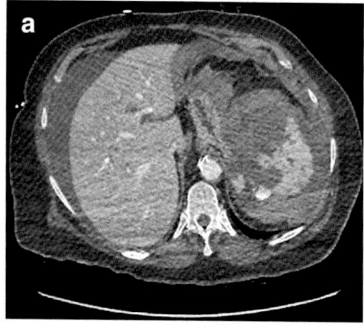
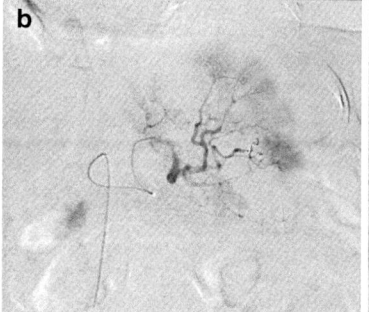
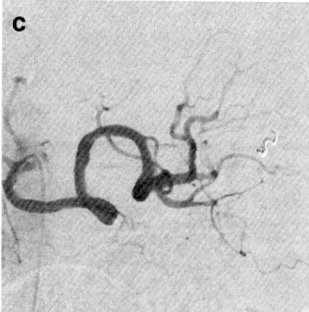

**Fig. 54.2** Female, BMI, age 65; blunt abdominal trauma (fall in a bus). Hypotensive but no shock. (**a**) CT scan at H5: large hemoperitoneum and AIS grade IV splenic trauma with extravasation of contrast agent. (**b**, **c**) Splenic selective arterial embolization H-4

#### 54.3.2.2 Lab Tests

Preoperative blood and others lab tests aim to guide the diagnosis if it is not obvious (blood count, C-reactive protein, search for cholestasis, serum lipase level, blood HCG in women of childbearing age, urinary tests, etc.) and also to explore possible organ failure and impairment of major physiological functions (blood count, coagulation, acid–base balance, kidney function, liver function).

In severe traumatic situations, where every minute counts, means that are much faster than conventional methods can be used to estimate a certain number of parameters that are very important for the management of the patient. Anemia and its depth will be estimated by rapid detection methods (Photometer B-Hemoglobin; HemoCue®). Similarly, the increasing use of thromboelastography (TEG) and thromboelastometry (ROTEM) methods in traumatology to assess total coagulation capacity would be of strategic interest in monitoring the transfusion needs of patients with hemorrhage [36] *(see dedicated chapter "Coagulation and thrombosis," Moore E., Meizoso, J.).*

to change the approach quickly if the first one fails to stabilize the situation *(see dedicated chapter « Resuscitative thoracotomy », Biffl, W., Lu, N.).*

In both cases, the need for surgery may have been overestimated. The term "non-therapeutic laparotomy" is then used if no lesions were found, or if the lesions found did not require surgical treatment.

This is the reason why more and more teams are proposing laparoscopic exploration as a first step [2, 13]. Less invasive, it allows in certain cases to provide precise answers to simple questions such as confirming or invalidating the penetrating nature of a wound, performing simple procedures such as evacuating and draining a collection or freeing a single adhesion, and exploring the abdominal cavity in a minimally invasive manner in case of diagnostic doubt.

> **Differential Diagnosis**
>
> For non-traumatic situations, differential diagnoses are those of each suspected pathology for which a surgical exploration has been proposed.
>
> In traumatic situations, the most common error is to make the mistake of choosing the wrong compartment to explore first (double jeopardy [21]), especially in situations of absolute vital emergency. This is for example the case in thoracoabdominal wounds, where five compartments converge: right and left thoracic cavities, mediastinum, peritoneal and retroperitoneal cavities. Because of the limited preoperative exams, it is possible to start by exploring the thorax when the problem is abdominal, and vice versa. The surgeon, but also the whole team, must be prepared

## 54.4 Treatment

### 54.4.1 Medical Treatment

#### 54.4.1.1 Preoperative Management

According to the situation, several medical measures must be taken to ensure that the surgical procedure is performed under the most appropriate conditions *(see dedicated chapter "Principles of peri-operative management," Romeo, O.).*

In case of hemorrhagic shock, the first measure is not to lose time. Therefore, working as a team, the presence and coordination of all the actors are essential. The surgeon must be notified as soon as possible of the arrival of a seriously injured patient, who will be transported to the operating room as soon as possible. Protocols for direct admission to the operating room already exist in some hospitals to further reduce this delay when the arrival of an unstable penetrating trauma is announced.

Similarly, it is known that delayed management of severe sepsis of abdominal origin is a risk factor for mortality [14, 30].

The patient will then be quickly conditioned. The first thing to be done is to warm him up if necessary. The placement of a nasogastric tube may be useful as limitation of bowel contamination in case of perforation, treatment of an obstruction, securing of the airway, and minimizing the risks of pulmonary aspiration before anesthesia. Two good caliber peripheral venous catheters are immediately necessary to start fluid therapy, a transfusion, some vasopressor drugs temporarily, analgesics, and/or antibiotics. Then, the placement of a central venous catheter will allow the administration and monitoring of catecholamines if necessary. More generally, resuscitation and correction of physiological insults must begin as soon as possible, and continue throughout the therapeutic process [30].

In post-traumatic hemorrhagic shock, hypotension is tolerated, with a systolic blood pressure (BP) goal of 80–90 mmHg in the absence of associated severe head injury [37]. Indeed, attempting to normalize blood pressure before stopping the bleeding (surgically or radiologically) by extensive fluid filling is equivalent to maintaining the blood leak and aggravating the coagulopathy, by cooling the patient and diluting the coagulation factors. Coagulation disorders should be diagnosed as soon as possible in order to start the appropriate treatment. Tranexamic acid is one of the treatments to be administered as soon as possible in polytraumatized patients [38]. Transfusion of RGCs is started, if possible at the same time as the fresh frozen plasma (FFP) transfusion, with a FFP:RGC ratio of between 1:2 and 1:1 [39, 40] *(see dedicated chapter « Fluid and blood management », Malbrain, M.).*

In case of fecal contamination, wide-spectrum antibiotics, which will be secondarily adapted to the results of the intraoperative samples *(see dedicated chapter « Antibiotic and antimycotic therapy," Ribeiro, M).* These antibiotics should be administered as soon as possible [30], although one in five patients actually receives them within the first hour [4]. The germs most frequently found are aerobic gram-negative bacteria (*E. coli*, *K. pneumoniae*), gram-positive bacteria (*E. faecalis*), more rarely anaerobic germs (bacteroides) and fungus (*candida* spp.) [14], with a spectrum of resistance to antibiotics (and in particular to third-generation cephalosporins) that varies according to the region. Local protocols are necessary to adapt antibiotic therapies [10].

### 54.4.1.2 Postoperative Management

After the surgical procedure, a multidisciplinary consensus must be reached on the patient's destination, including the need for intensive care *(see dedicated chapter « Critical care », Corbella, D.).* In all cases, given the situation of hypercatabolism, specific care should be taken to optimize the nutritional status [9, 16] *(see dedicated chapter "Nutritional support," Khan, M.).*

Polytrauma patients, as well as patients operated on in emergency for non-traumatic reasons, have an increased risk of deep vein thrombosis [30] because they represent a state of inflammation and hypercoagulability, associated with venous stasis related to prolonged immobilization. However, there is no clear consensus on the best time to start thromboprophylaxis. The decision must be multidisciplinary and weighed by the secondary hemorrhagic risk.

### 54.4.1.3 Arterial Embolization

Transfemoral arterial embolization is a useful adjunct especially for hemorrhagic patients with pelvic trauma [41]. It has also shown its efficacy (curative or preventive in case of high risk of hemorrhage) in many others traumatic situations as hepatic trauma, splenic trauma [42] (Fig. 54.2b, c). Embolization is also widely used in case of hemorrhagic shock of non-traumatic etiology for example postoperative [43], obstetrical [44] … Resuscitative endovascular balloon occlusion of the aorta (REBOA) could provide a survival benefit as it may improve their initial ability to survive the hemorrhagic shock and its use has expanded worldwide [45, 46]. *(see dedicated chapter: Major Bleedings management and REBOA Pasley, A., Brenner, M.).*

### 54.4.2 Surgical Treatment

Whether for a bleeding emergency or intra-abdominal sepsis, delaying surgical intervention increases the risk of mortality [30, 47].

For an emergency laparotomy, patient is in a supine position, arms in cross. The position of the legs depends on the nature of the suspected lesions. Indeed, in case of perineal damage (blast, impalement) or in the case of a surgical revision after colo-proctectomy, a double approach position can be very useful *(see dedicated chapter "Blast injuries », Kluger, Y.)*. Care should be taken to prepare a wide approach in order to expose oneself correctly and to be able to set up a sloping drainage of the flanks if necessary, that is, a skin preparation that extends as far as the mattress of the table. The chest should also be prepared in case of polytrauma, to allow a supra-diaphragmatic approach if necessary, possibly leaving a supra-clavicular recess for the anesthetists to place a central venous access if this has not been done before. Similarly, in case of imminent peril, the femoral approaches will be included in the operative field, to possibly allow a complementary vascular access, or even the placement of an intraoperative Resuscitative Endovascular Balloon Occlusion of the Aorta (REBOA). This preparation time, although as short as possible, will be used by the scrub nurses to prepare the necessary equipment and set up the instrumentation table. The necessary material is of course a laparotomy equipment set, possibly with a complementary long instrument set. A set of vascular clamps and a thoracotomy set will also be brought to the room. A GIA type linear stapler with refills will also be available. Enough pads and surgical fields will be taken directly on the table in order to consider an effective packing as soon as the incision is made [20–30], as well as sutures to perform vascular ligatures. It is important to check that there is enough warm physiologic serum in reserve (10 L minimum). One or even two aspirations will be installed to anticipate the presence of a possible abundant effusion. The use of a Cell Saver can replace one of the aspirations.

Different types of incision are possible depending on the operative indication (Fig. 54.3). For example, in case of laparotomy cholecystectomy, the subcostal approach gives a satisfactory daylight on the subhepatic region. Nevertheless, the median approach is the incision that allows the most satisfactory access in terms of exposure of the abdominal cavity and is therefore the preferred approach in emergency laparotomies. The latter can be enlarged up to the xiphoid appendix cranially, and up to the pubis caudally. A lateral incision, although rather dilapidating, may be considered in case of difficulties in exposing the hepatic region. In order not to lose the benefit of a complete exposure by this approach, it is impor-

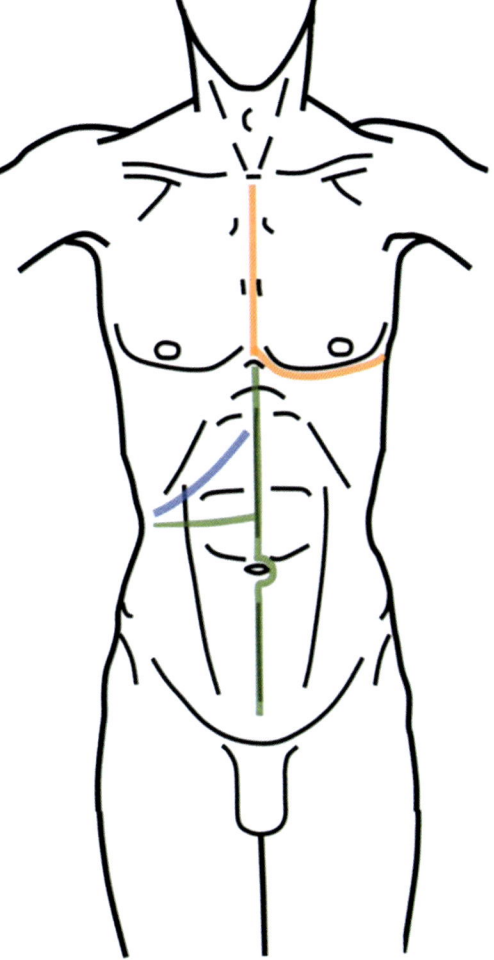

**Fig. 54.3** Abdominal incisions for emergency laparotomies

tant to install retractors or auto static valves as soon as possible. The means of fixing them to the table must be anticipated as soon as the patient enters the operative room.

The surgical procedures performed will then be guided by the intraoperative findings *(see dedicated chapters: "Liver trauma" Coccolini, F., « Spleen trauma » Catena, F., « Bowel trauma » Ordonez, C. « Kidney and urologic trauma » Coccolini, F, « Duodeno-pancreatic and extrahepatic biliary tree trauma », Catena, F., « Abdominal vascular trauma » Coimbra, R.).*

Whatever the strategy initially chosen the observation during the procedure of signs of coagulopathy (biological, clinical with the observation of diffuse, uncontrollable bleeding), the absence of hemodynamic improvement despite (relative) control of the bleeding and/or the source of contamination, the persistence of metabolic acidosis (pH <7. 2), hypothermia (temperature <34 °C), visceral oedema (Fig. 54.4), and/or the absence of possibility of definitive primary repair in a reasonable time are all arguments that should push the team to consider abbreviating the procedure. While the same elements seem relevant to consider in the setting of non-traumatic bleeding emergencies, there is currently no consensus on the pre- and intraoperative factors that predict a possible advantage to this strategy in the management of other types of emergencies [12, 25, 27]. It seems that certain non-traumatic situations are instinctively more amenable to abbreviated procedures [12], for strategical and physiologically relevant reasons. This is the case of explorations for digestive ischemia: after resection of digestive segments in exceeded ischemia, possibly completed with a revascularization procedure, there is a risk of intestinal edema favoring the development of a possible ACS *(see dedicated chapter « Mesenteric ischemia," Bala, M.)*. On the other hand, a second look to check the vitality of the rest of the digestive tract, or even to consider a direct restauration of digestive continuity if the local and general conditions are favorable, may be arguments in favor of an abbreviated initial procedure with abandonment of the stapled digestive segments in the abdomen. Conversely, there are fewer comparable strategic arguments for a procedure as treating an occlusion.

If direct closure is considered, closure follows the same rules as for a conventional laparotomy procedure. It seems preferable to perform continuous sutures, with small catches, and to use a monofilament suture to avoid sinuses, with slow resorption (e.g., polydioxanone type) [48, 49]. In the case of definitive closure, some teams propose the placement of a prosthesis to reduce the risk of incisional hernia, a strategy that is based on the experience of laparotomies in elective sit-

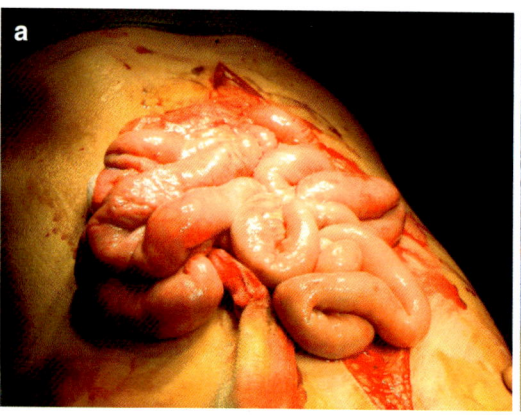
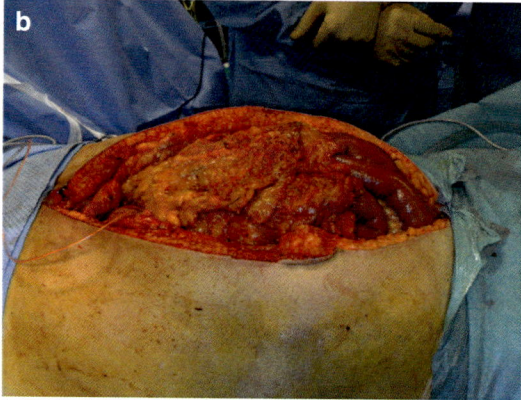

**Fig. 54.4** (**a**) Laparotomy for pelvic packing in a patient with a severe pelvic trauma: intestinal edema due to the hemorrhagic shock. (**b**) Laparotomy in a patient with acute sepsis due to colic perforation that occurred day-6 after acute necrotizing pancreatitis: intestinal edema due to the sepsis

uations. Nevertheless, for emergency situations, there is currently only a low level of evidence to recommend this strategy [50, 51].

If an open abdominal technique is preferred, several temporary closure techniques are available to the surgeon. It is possible to consider skin closure alone, using a continuous suture of non-absorbable material [52] *(see dedicated chapter « Compartment syndrome," Ivatury, R.)*. A device can nevertheless be sutured to the skin edges (Bogotà bag), but this is used less and less because of the high rate of digestive fistula [53]. The application of a vacuum dressing (Negative Pressure Wound Therapy) (Fig. 54.5), associated or not with a continuous fascial traction system (Wittmann patch for example), seems to be the technique that allows the most fascial closure [53, 54]. If possible, direct and definitive closure of the wall should be performed within 8 days [55] (Fig. 54.6). Beyond that, the risk of complications increases. In certain complex situations, complete closure may be impossible. The abdominal cavity will be closed by a cutaneous suture, possibly accelerated by tissue budding under the action of a vacuum dressing.

## 54.5 Prognosis

In general, the 30-day mortality after emergency laparotomy varies from 2 to 15% [9, 56–59], and even 25% for patients over 80 years of age [60]. In traumatic situations, the mortality rate is always around 40% for patients with hypotension [61, 62]. The prognosis of each situation requiring emergency laparotomy depends of course on

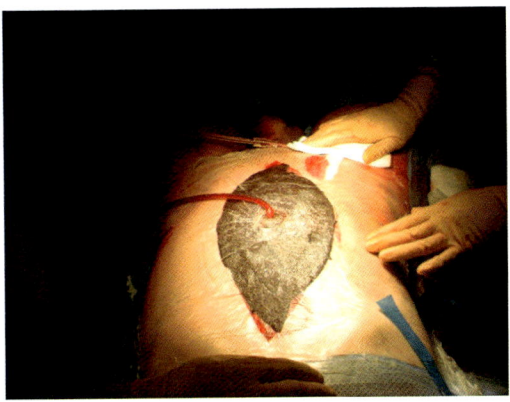

**Fig. 54.5** Laparotomy after damage control laparotomy H4 for a patient with severe pelvic trauma

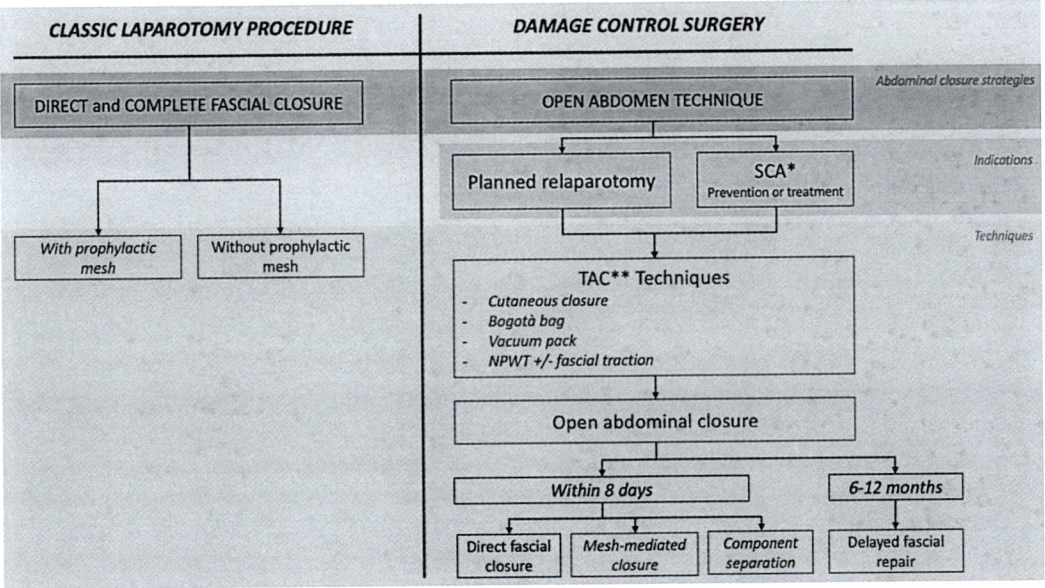

**Fig. 54.6** Strategies for abdominal closure, according to the principles of the first exploration

the situation itself (see corresponding chapter). Tools are available to assess these *risks (see dedicated chapter "Quality evaluation in emergency general surgery," Sugrue, M.)*. In order to reduce the overall mortality of these serious situations, it is necessary to offer individualized intraoperative care, which is based on the identification of populations at risk, and therefore on the assessment of individual risk. For example, the APACHE II (Acute Physiology And Chronic Health Evaluation), ASA-PS (American Society of Anesthesiologists—Physical Status), and P-POSSUM (Portsmouth—Physiologic and Operative Severity Score for the enUmeration of Mortality and Morbidity) scores could be cited as the most frequently studied scores [30, 59].

There are specific scores for trauma situations, built to assess the severity of injury, predict mortality, the need for intensive care hospitalization, or the occurrence of a bleeding syndrome, and are used to monitor the quality of care. The Injury Severity Score (ISS) [63] is calculated from the Abbreviated Injury Score (AIS) thesaurus as the sum of the squares of the highest AIS scores of the 3 most affected regions. It ranges from 0 to 75. A score >15 defines a severe injury. The New Injury Severity Score (NISS) [64] is calculated from the patient's three most severe injuries, regardless of the body region in which they occur and it is most useful for patients whose injuries are concentrated in one system. The Revised Trauma Score (RTS) assesses only respiratory rate, systolic blood pressure, and GCS [65]. Finally, the Trauma Injury Severity Score (TRISS) [66] is a complex logarithmic regression composed of the patient's ISS and RRTS scores and age.

Among the possible complications, several are common and inherent to the laparotomy surgical approach. First of all, there is the risk of revision surgery. In case of complete closure, there is always a risk of unscheduled revision in case of persistent bleeding or a source of contamination (including situations of digestive wounds that went unnoticed during the first exploration), or of the appearance of an abdominal compartment syndrome (Fig. 54.4). In the framework of a damage control strategy, on the other hand, this is not a risk but the logical consequence of a shortened intervention. It is then a planned recovery. If the hemodynamic state of the patient allows it, this recovery will be preceded by a preliminary evaluation by CT scan, which is all the more important if this examination could not be carried out preoperatively [67]. Elderly patients are of course a group at risk [3, 12], and in particular patients suffering from undernutrition and sarcopenia [68] (dedicated chapter « Geriatrics » Latifi, R.).

In the long term, chronic pain is one of the most frequent functional risks, present in almost 20% of cases [60] *(see dedicated chapter "Pain management," Forfori, F., Etrusca, B.)*. The risk of wall dehiscence is significant, in the order of 15–30% of cases [50, 51].

> **Dos and Don'ts**
> - CHOOSE the relevant preoperative examinations, to start the adapted treatments without delay, to reduce the delay of the surgery to a minimum.
> - DON'T lose time with futile examinations.
> - RECOGNIZE situations requiring immediate surgical exploration.
> - DON'T use laparoscopy on unstable patient or with massive ileus.
> - SHORTEN the procedure to the only control of hemorrhagic and potentially contaminating lesions in order to break the vicious circle of coagulation disorders.
> - DON'T do complex surgical procedures in case of a patient with signs of shock.
> - PREFER an open abdominal technique if there is any risk of abdominal compartment syndrome (ACS).
> - ORGANIZE the postoperative care adapted to the individual risks of each patient.

## Take-Home Messages

- Emergency laparotomy procedures are one of the most frequent procedures in general surgery, with major clinical and economic impact.
- On-call and emergency surgeons should know how to recognize situations requiring immediate surgical exploration.
- Essential skills for the emergency surgeon include team management, knowledge of the physiopathology of hemorrhagic and septic shock, ability to read CT scan, and technical expertise of all the damage control procedures.

## MCQ (Good Answer)

1. The incidence of emergency laparotomy procedures in developed country among the population
   A. is estimated as 1:100
   B. **is estimated as 1:1000**
   C. is estimated as 1:10,000
   D. is estimated as 1:100,000
2. Damage control procedures
   A. are legitimated by numerous randomized studies
   B. are applicable only in traumatic situations
   C. are no longer useful since the REBOA
   D. **show numerous applications outside emergency surgery**
3. In case of post-traumatic hemorrhagic shock in the absence of associated severe head injury
   A. the goal is a systolic blood pressure (BP) of 11–12 mmHg
   B. **thromboelastometry (ROTEM) methods are of strategic interest in monitoring the transfusion needs**
   C. coagulation disorders occur lately
   D. The transfusion of RGCs and FFP is prescript with a FFP:RGC ratio of 1:4

*Comment: In post-traumatic hemorrhagic shock, hypotension is tolerated, with a systolic blood pressure (BP) goal of 80–90 mmHg in the absence of associated severe head injury; FFP:RGC ratio is of 1:1*

4. For a trauma patient without hemodynamic instability (or after stabilization), the best imaging choice is:
   A. Ultrasound
   B. **CT-scan**
   C. Ultrasound and CT scan
   D. Ultrasound or CT scan
   E. None of this exam
5. Conditioning for surgery a trauma patient with a severe abdominal and pelvic trauma includes (one wrong answer):
   A. warming the patient up
   B. placement of a nasogastric tube
   C. **placement of a urinary tube**
   D. placement of two good calibers peripheral venous catheter

*Comment: urinary tube can cause severe urethral damage in a patient with a pelvic trauma*

6. For an emergency laparotomy on a patient with a severe abdominal and pelvic trauma includes (one wrong answer):
   A. patient is in a supine position, arms in cross
   B. the chest is included in in the operative field
   C. The femoral approaches will be included in the operative field
   D. **all these propositions are wrong**
7. For an emergency laparotomy on a trauma patient, the necessary material is of course outside a laparotomy equipment set includes (one wrong answer):
   A. a complementary long instrument set
   B. a set of vascular clamps
   C. a thoracotomy set
   D. **2 L 20 °C physiologic serum in reserve**

*Comment: 10 L of warm (37 °C) are necessary*

8. For an emergency laparotomy on a trauma patient, the necessary material is of course outside a laparotomy equipment set includes (one wrong answer):
    A. **One aspiration or a cell saver**
    B. a GIA type linear stapler with refills
    C. sutures to perform vascular ligatures
    D. at least 30 pads and surgical fields

*Comment: two aspirations or one aspiration AND a cell saver are necessary*

9. The abdominal compartment syndrome (ACS) is defined as:
    A. intra-abdominal hyper pressure greater than 10 mmHg associated with the occurrence of at least one organ failure
    B. **intra-abdominal hyper pressure greater than 20 mmHg associated with the occurrence of at least one organ failure**
    C. intra-abdominal hyper pressure greater than 10 mmHg associated with the occurrence of at least two organs failure
    D. intra-abdominal hyper pressure greater than 20 mmHg associated with the occurrence of at least two organs failure

10. Concerning trauma scores which proposition is true?
    A. **The Injury Severity Score (ISS) is calculated from the Abbreviated Injury Score (AIS) thesaurus as the sum of the squares of the highest AIS scores of the 3 most affected regions**
    B. The New Injury Severity Score (NISS) ranges from 0 to 100
    C. A NISS score >30 defines a severe injury
    D. The Revised Trauma Score (RTS) assesses only respiratory rate, systolic and diastolic blood pressures

## 54.5.1 References

1. Shapter SL, Paul MJ, White SM. Incidence and estimated annual cost of emergency laparotomy in England: is there a major funding shortfall? Anaesthesia. 2012;67(5):474–8.
2. Pucher PH, Carter NC, Knight BC, Toh S, Tucker V, Mercer SJ. Impact of laparoscopic approach in emergency major abdominal surgery: single-centre analysis of 748 consecutive cases. Ann R Coll Surg Engl. 2018;100(4):279–84.
3. Alexandrescu R, O'Brien SJ, Lecky FE. A review of injury epidemiology in the UK and Europe: some methodological considerations in constructing rates. BMC Public Health. 2009;10(9):226.
4. NELA Project Team. Fifth patient report of the National Emergency Laparotomy Audit. 2019. https://www.nela.org.uk/downloads/The%20Fifth%20Patient%20Report%20of%20the%20NELA%202019%20-%20Full%20Patient%20Report.pdf.
5. Hietbrink F, Houwert RM, van Wessem KJP, Simmermacher RKJ, Govaert GAM, de Jong MB, et al. The evolution of trauma care in the Netherlands over 20 years. Eur J Trauma Emerg Surg. 2020;46(2):329–35.
6. Gauss T, Balandraud P, Frandon J, Abba J, Ageron FX, Albaladejo P, et al. Strategic proposal for a national trauma system in France. Anaesth Crit Care Pain Med. 2019;38(2):121–30.
7. Cole E, Lecky F, West A, Smith N, Brohi K, Davenport R, et al. The impact of a pan-regional inclusive trauma system on quality of care. Ann Surg. 2016;264(1):188–94.
8. Bège T, Pauly V, Orleans V, Boyer L, Leone M. Epidemiology of trauma in France: mortality and risk factors based on a national medico-administrative database. Anaesth Crit Care Pain Med. 2019;38(5):461–8.
9. Ilyas C, Jones J, Fortey S. Management of the patient presenting for emergency laparotomy. BJA Educ. 2019;19(4):113–8.
10. Sartelli M, Chichom-Mefire A, Labricciosa FM, Hardcastle T, Abu-Zidan FM, Adesunkanmi AK, et al. The management of intra-abdominal infections from a global perspective: 2017 WSES guidelines for management of intra-abdominal infections. World J Emerg Surg. 2017;12:29.
11. Ten Broek RPG, Krielen P, Di Saverio S, Coccolini F, Biffl WL, Ansaloni L, et al. Bologna guidelines for diagnosis and management of adhesive small bowel obstruction (ASBO): 2017 update of the evidence-based guidelines from the world society of emergency surgery ASBO working group. World J Emerg Surg. 2018;13:24.
12. Person B, Dorfman T, Bahouth H, Osman A, Assalia A, Kluger Y. Abbreviated emergency laparotomy in the non-trauma setting. World J Emerg Surg. 2009;4:41.

13. Sauerland S, Agresta F, Bergamaschi R, Borzellino G, Budzynski A, Champault G, et al. Laparoscopy for abdominal emergencies: evidence-based guidelines of the European Association for Endoscopic Surgery. Surg Endosc. 2006;20(1):14–29.
14. Sartelli M, Catena F, Ansaloni L, Coccolini F, Corbella D, Moore EE, et al. Complicated intra-abdominal infections worldwide: the definitive data of the CIAOW Study. World J Emerg Surg. 2014;9:37.
15. Barbois S, Gaget O, Quesada JL, et al. Treatment of acute appendicitis in France by type of hospital: patient profiles are different but practices and results are the same, a prospective cohort study of 1241 patients. Surg Open Dig Adv. 2021;4:100028.
16. Tenner S, Baillie J, DeWitt J, Vege SS, American College of Gastroenterology. American College of Gastroenterology guideline: management of acute pancreatitis. Am J Gastroenterol. 2013;108(9):1400–15.
17. Baron TH, DiMaio CJ, Wang AY, Morgan KA. American Gastroenterological Association clinical practice update: management of pancreatic necrosis. Gastroenterology. 2020;158(1):67–75.e1.
18. Tridente A, Clarke GM, Walden A, McKechnie S, Hutton P, Mills GH, et al. Patients with faecal peritonitis admitted to European intensive care units: an epidemiological survey of the GenOSept cohort. Intensive Care Med. 2014;40(2):202–10.
19. Kirkpatrick AW, Roberts DJ, De Waele J, Jaeschke R, Malbrain MLNG, De Keulenaer B, et al. Intra-abdominal hypertension and the abdominal compartment syndrome: updated consensus definitions and clinical practice guidelines from the World Society of the Abdominal Compartment Syndrome. Intensive Care Med. 2013;39(7):1190–206.
20. Barbois S, Abba J, Guigard S, Quesada JL, Pirvu A, Waroquet PA, et al. Management of penetrating abdominal and thoraco-abdominal wounds: a retrospective study of 186 patients. J Visc Surg. 2016;153(4 Suppl):69–78.
21. Hirshberg A, Mattox KL. Top knife: the art and craft of trauma surgery. Castle Hill Barns: TFM Publishing; 2014.
22. Destan C, De Carbonnière A, Moritz C, Gaudric J, Malgras B, Desterke C, et al. French civilian surgical expertise still inadequately prepared for mass casualties 3 years after major terror attacks in Paris (2015) and Nice (2016). J Trauma Acute Care Surg. 2020;89(2S Suppl 2):S26–31.
23. Falzone E, Pasquier P, Hoffmann C, Barbier O, Boutonnet M, Salvadori A, et al. Triage in military settings. Anaesth Crit Care Pain Med. 2017;36(1):43–51.
24. Boyd-Carson H, Gana T, Lockwood S, Murray D, Tierney GM. A review of surgical and peri-operative factors to consider in emergency laparotomy care. Anaesthesia. 2020;75(Suppl 1):e75–82.
25. Weber DG, Bendinelli C, Balogh ZJ. Damage control surgery for abdominal emergencies. Br J Surg. 2014;101(1):e109–18.
26. Ditzel RM, Anderson JL, Eisenhart WJ, Rankin CJ, DeFeo DR, Oak S, et al. A review of transfusion- and trauma-induced hypocalcemia: is it time to change the lethal triad to the lethal diamond? J Trauma Acute Care Surg. 2020;88(3):434–9.
27. Girard E, Abba J, Boussat B, Trilling B, Mancini A, Bouzat P, et al. Damage control surgery for non-traumatic abdominal emergencies. World J Surg. 2018;42(4):965–73.
28. van Ruler O, Mahler CW, Boer KR, Reuland EA, Gooszen HG, Opmeer BC, et al. Comparison of on-demand vs planned relaparotomy strategy in patients with severe peritonitis: a randomized trial. JAMA. 2007;298(8):865–72.
29. Coccolini F, Montori G, Ceresoli M, Catena F, Moore EE, Ivatury R, et al. The role of open abdomen in non-trauma patient: WSES consensus paper. World J Emerg Surg. 2017;12:39.
30. Peden CJ, Aggarwal G, Aitken RJ, Anderson ID, Bang Foss N, Cooper Z, et al. Guidelines for perioperative care for emergency laparotomy enhanced recovery after surgery (ERAS) society recommendations: part 1-preoperative: diagnosis, rapid assessment and optimization. World J Surg. 2021;45(5):1272–90.
31. Mancini A, Duramé A, Barbois S, Abba J, Ageron F-X, Arvieux C. Relevance of early CT scan diagnosis of blunt diaphragmatic injury: a retrospective analysis from the Northern French Alps Emergency Network. J Visc Surg. 2019;156(1):3–9.
32. Stoker J, van Randen A, Laméris W, Boermeester MA. Imaging patients with acute abdominal pain. Radiology. 2009;253(1):31–46.
33. De Simone B, Ansaloni L, Sartelli M, Kluger Y, Abu-Zidan FM, Biffl WL, et al. The operative management in bariatric acute abdomen (OBA) survey: long-term complications of bariatric surgery and the emergency surgeon's point of view. World J Emerg Surg. 2020;15(1):2.
34. Kim SH, Shin SS, Jeong YY, Heo SH, Kim JW, Kang HK. Gastrointestinal tract perforation: MDCT findings according to the perforation sites. Korean J Radiol. 2009;10(1):63–70.
35. Netherton S, Milenkovic V, Taylor M, Davis PJ. Diagnostic accuracy of eFAST in the trauma patient: a systematic review and meta-analysis. CJEM. 2019;21(6):727–38.
36. Wikkelsø A, Wetterslev J, Møller AM, Afshari A. Thromboelastography (TEG) or thromboelastometry (ROTEM) to monitor haemostatic treatment versus usual care in adults or children with bleeding. Cochrane Database Syst Rev. 2016;8:CD007871.
37. Spahn DR, Bouillon B, Cerny V, Coats TJ, Duranteau J, Fernández-Mondéjar E, et al. Management of bleeding and coagulopathy following major trauma: an updated European guideline. Crit Care. 2013;17(2):R76.
38. CRASH-2 Trial Collaborators, Shakur H, Roberts I, Bautista R, Caballero J, Coats T, et al. Effects of tranexamic acid on death, vascular occlusive events, and blood transfusion in trauma patients with significant haemorrhage (CRASH-2): a randomised, placebo-controlled trial. Lancet. 2010;376(9734):23–32.

39. Bhangu A, Nepogodiev D, Doughty H, Bowley DM. Meta-analysis of plasma to red blood cell ratios and mortality in massive blood transfusions for trauma. Injury. 2013;44(12):1693–9.
40. Borgman MA, Spinella PC, Perkins JG, Grathwohl KW, Repine T, Beekley AC, et al. The ratio of blood products transfused affects mortality in patients receiving massive transfusions at a combat support hospital. J Trauma. 2007;63(4):805–13.
41. Coccolini F, Stahel PF, Montori G, Biffl W, Horer TM, Catena F, et al. Pelvic trauma: WSES classification and guidelines. World J Emerg Surg. 2017;12:5.
42. Arvieux C, Frandon J, Tidadini F, Monnin-Bares V, Foote A, Dubuisson V, et al. Effect of prophylactic embolization on patients with blunt trauma at high risk of splenectomy: a randomized clinical trial. JAMA Surg. 2020;155(12):1102–11.
43. Chatani S, Inoue A, Ohta S, Takaki K, Sato S, Iwai T, et al. Transcatheter arterial embolization for postoperative bleeding following abdominal surgery. Cardiovasc Intervent Radiol. 2018;41(9):1346–55.
44. Hawkins JL. Obstetric hemorrhage. Anesthesiol Clin. 2020;38(4):839–58.
45. Pieper A, Thony F, Brun J, Rodière M, Boussat B, Arvieux C, et al. Resuscitative endovascular balloon occlusion of the aorta for pelvic blunt trauma and life-threatening hemorrhage: a 20-year experience in a level I trauma center. J Trauma Acute Care Surg. 2018;84(3):449–53.
46. on behalf of the AAST-AORTA Investigators and the ABOTrauma Registry Group, Manzano-Nunez R, McGreevy D, Orlas CP, García AF, Hörer TM, et al. Outcomes and management approaches of resuscitative endovascular balloon occlusion of the aorta based on the income of countries. World J Emerg Surg. 2020;15(1):57.
47. Kapan M, Onder A, Oguz A, Taskesen F, Aliosmanoglu I, Gul M, et al. The effective risk factors on mortality in patients undergoing damage control surgery. Eur Rev Med Pharmacol Sci. 2013;17(12):1681–7.
48. Patel SV, Paskar DD, Nelson RL, Vedula SS, Steele SR. Closure methods for laparotomy incisions for preventing incisional hernias and other wound complications. Cochrane Database Syst Rev. 2017;11:CD005661.
49. Henriksen NA, Deerenberg EB, Venclauskas L, Fortelny RH, Miserez M, Muysoms FE. Meta-analysis on materials and techniques for laparotomy closure: the MATCH review. World J Surg. 2018;42(6):1666–78.
50. Burns FA, Heywood EG, Challand CP, Lee MJ. Is there a role for prophylactic mesh in abdominal wall closure after emergency laparotomy? A systematic review and meta-analysis. Hernia. 2020;24(3):441–7.
51. Lima HVG, Rasslan R, Novo FCF, Lima TMA, Damous SHB, Bernini CO, et al. Prevention of fascial dehiscence with Onlay prophylactic mesh in emergency laparotomy: a randomized clinical trial. J Am Coll Surg. 2020;230(1):76–87.
52. Coccolini F, Biffl W, Catena F, Ceresoli M, Chiara O, Cimbanassi S, et al. The open abdomen, indications, management and definitive closure. World J Emerg Surg. 2015;10(1):32.
53. Coccolini F, Roberts D, Ansaloni L, Ivatury R, Gamberini E, Kluger Y, et al. The open abdomen in trauma and non-trauma patients: WSES guidelines. World J Emerg Surg. 2018;13:7.
54. Atema JJ, Gans SL, Boermeester MA. Systematic review and meta-analysis of the open abdomen and temporary abdominal closure techniques in non-trauma patients. World J Surg. 2015;39(4):912–25.
55. Miller RS, Morris JA, Diaz JJ, Herring MB, May AK. Complications after 344 damage-control open celiotomies. J Trauma. 2005;59(6):1365–71.
56. Tan BHL, Mytton J, Al-Khyatt W, Aquina CT, Evison F, Fleming FJ, et al. A comparison of mortality following emergency laparotomy between populations from New York State and England. Ann Surg. 2017;266(2):280–6.
57. Broughton KJ, Aldridge O, Pradhan S, Aitken RJ. The Perth emergency laparotomy audit. ANZ J Surg. 2017;87(11):893–7.
58. Mak M, Hakeem AR, Chitre V. Pre-NELA vs NELA—has anything changed, or is it just an audit exercise? Ann R Coll Surg Engl. 2016;98(8):554–9.
59. Oliver CM, Walker E, Giannaris S, Grocott MPW, Moonesinghe SR. Risk assessment tools validated for patients undergoing emergency laparotomy: a systematic review. Br J Anaesth. 2015;115(6):849–60.
60. Saunders DI, Murray D, Pichel AC, Varley S, Peden CJ, UK Emergency Laparotomy Network. Variations in mortality after emergency laparotomy: the first report of the UK Emergency Laparotomy Network. Br J Anaesth. 2012;109(3):368–75.
61. Harvin JA, Maxim T, Inaba K, Martinez-Aguilar MA, King DR, Choudhry AJ, et al. Mortality after emergent trauma laparotomy: a multicenter, retrospective study. J Trauma Acute Care Surg. 2017;83(3):464–8.
62. Marsden M, Carden R, Navaratne L, Smith IM, Penn-Barwell JG, Kraven LM, et al. Outcomes following trauma laparotomy for hypotensive trauma patients: a UK military and civilian perspective. J Trauma Acute Care Surg. 2018;85(3):620–5.
63. Baker SP, O'Neill B, Haddon W, Long WB. The injury severity score: a method for describing patients with multiple injuries and evaluating emergency care. J Trauma. 1974;14(3):187–96.
64. Osler T, Baker SP, Long W. A modification of the injury severity score that both improves accuracy and simplifies scoring. J Trauma. 1997;43(6):922–6.
65. Champion HR, Sacco WJ, Copes WS, Gann DS, Gennarelli TA, Flanagan ME. A revision of the trauma score. J Trauma. 1989;29(5):623–9.
66. Boyd CR, Tolson MA, Copes WS. Evaluating trauma care: the TRISS method. Trauma score and the injury severity score. J Trauma. 1987;27(4):370–8.

67. Alexander LF, Hanna TN, LeGout JD, Roda MS, Cernigliaro JG, Mittal PK, et al. Multidetector CT findings in the abdomen and pelvis after damage control surgery for acute traumatic injuries. Radiographics. 2019;39(4):1183–202.

68. Rangel EL, Rios-Diaz AJ, Uyeda JW, Castillo-Angeles M, Cooper Z, Olufajo OA, et al. Sarcopenia increases risk of long-term mortality in elderly patients undergoing emergency abdominal surgery. J Trauma Acute Care Surg. 2017;83(6):1179–86.

# Principles of Emergency and Trauma Laparoscopy

**55**

Felipe Vega-Rivera, Ignacio Alvarez-Valero, Fernando Pérez-Galaz, and Alberto Pérez Cantú-Sacal

**Learning Goals**
- Learn the nomenclature on laparoscopy in emergencies
- Understand the indications and contra-indications of laparoscopy for emergencies and trauma
- Recognize the maneuvers of surgical exploration in emergency laparoscopy and trauma

## 55.1 Introduction

Laparoscopy has been positioned over decades as a useful technique in various surgical procedures of different specialties, in some procedures it has come to be considered the gold standard; however, until few years ago it has been given the role in the emergency surgery [1] and trauma [2]; and it is in this last area where it has found an initial role as a diagnostic tool, but its therapeutic usefulness has been questioned. The first description of the use of laparoscopy (coelioscopy) in trauma was in 1925 to diagnose hemoperitoneum due to abdominal contusion [3]. In recent publications there is a tendency to use laparoscopy beyond as only as a superficial visual purpose, and it has been called ***Exploratory Laparoscopy*** [4–6] as a diagnostic tool keeping similarity to the systematic laparotomy of traditional open surgery. It is well known that laparoscopic surgery is associated with reduced pain, earlier discharge, and quicker return to work. It has at the same time reduced complications associated with traditional open surgery, such as wound infections and incisional hernia [7].

Certainly, it will be necessary to specify some terminology concepts for the proper use of the term laparoscopy. According to the British dictionary [8], refers that **laparoscopy**, also called **peritoneoscopy**, is the procedure that allows visual examination of the abdominal cavity with an optical instrument called a laparoscope, which is inserted through a small incision made in the abdominal wall. So, to have a better concept of the use of laparoscopy, we will use the following nomenclature:

F. Vega-Rivera (✉)
Department of Surgery, Hospital Angeles Lomas, Universidad Nacional Autónoma de México, México City, Mexico

I. Alvarez-Valero
General Surgery, Emergency Department, Hospital Angeles Lomas, México City, Mexico

F. Pérez-Galaz
General Surgery, Hospital Angeles Lomas, México City, Mexico

A. P. Cantú-Sacal
General Surgery, Interventional Endoscopy, Hospital Angeles Lomas, México City, Mexico

"Diagnostic laparoscopy" (DL) refers to the diagnosis made by general visualization of the abdominal cavity with the laparoscope. It only requires the introduction of a port for the lens through the navel, the visualization is basically superficial since the mobilization of the structures is passive and only depends on the effect of gravity with the positioning table. In trauma and emergency surgery, it basically allows us to superficially visualize the existence of fluid (blood or intestinal content) or obvious inflammatory processes and in trauma, obvious penetrations, perforations of the liver or anterior abdominal wall. "Exploratory laparoscopy" (EL) is the technique in which the visualization of the organs, structures, and spaces of the abdominal cavity is carried out in a visual and instrumented way. The introduction of auxiliary ports for the manipulation and mobilization of the structures is required for the complete evaluation in places where the only superficial visualization is not enough. Additional terms like "therapeutic," "non-therapeutic," or "assisted therapeutic" are used postoperatively and are defined intraoperatively.

"Therapeutic laparoscopy" refers to the strict performance of another minimally invasive surgical procedure that solves a problem. That is, suture of a perforation, resection by a stapler, placement of a hemostatic agent, compression on a bleeding site, and the cessation of bleeding or aspiration of the hemoperitoneum and surgical lavage of the abdominal cavity, placement of drains or exteriorization of loops, etc. It is clear that "purely diagnostic laparoscopy" could not be possible. This requires advanced surgical skills (intracorporeal suturing, hemostasis, resections, stapling, cannulation, and exteriorization) and other requirements in relation to infrastructure, teamwork, and safety standards to perform it. Instead, "non-therapeutic laparoscopy" is the result of a "negative" exploratory laparoscopy [9], it is a confusing term and not very objective in the surgical nomenclature. The term "non-therapeutic exploratory laparoscopy," on the other hand, does not generate confusion, it is precise and elegant within the surgical nomenclature. It is easy to understand that a formal systematic examination of the entire abdominal cavity (organs, spaces, and structures) was performed without the need for any alternate procedure.

Publications on emergency laparoscopy and good practices [10], as well as the guidelines and consensus [11] they emphasize that any endorsement for a laparoscopic approach is only valid for surgical units with experience and sufficient expertise in minimal access surgery.

## 55.2 Diagnosis

The diagnosis of the different non-traumatic acute inflammatory pathologies includes not only to find the clinical findings, but also uses complementary image studies to establish the possible cause of the acute abdominal pathology. The use of laparoscopy is not only considered a diagnostic surgical technique, but also it is the visualization that also offers and allows us to have the opportunity to expand its use as a therapeutic tool.

In the next paragraphs we will give an overview of the indications and contraindications of laparoscopy in surgical abdominal emergencies and indications of use of laparoscopy in traumatic injuries.

## 55.3 Indications and Contraindications of Laparoscopy in Surgical Emergencies

In 2006, the European Association for Endoscopic Surgery (EAES) developed guidelines to define that subgroups of patients should undergo laparoscopic surgery instead of open surgery for acute abdominal pain [12]. Five years later, these guidelines [13] were reviewed by a group of SICE (Italian Society of Endoscopic Surgery) experts under the auspices of EAES to achieve the following objectives: (1) establish the preferred diagnostic procedures, patient selection, if applicable, and the suitability of the laparoscopic approach responsible for the configuration of acute abdominal disease; (2) evaluate the indication, morbidity, length of hospital stay, costs, and recovery time of laparoscopic treatment for acute abdominal situations; and (3) define optimal laparoscopic practice for each abdominal emergency and provide recommendations that reflect good practice. The indications were the result of key statements each with a grade of recommendation (GoR) followed by a commentary in order to explain the rationale and the level of evidence (LE) behind the statement. The non-traumatic medical pathologies and their level of recommendation are shown below.

### 55.3.1 Acute Appendicitis

Patients with symptoms and diagnostic findings suggestive of acute appendicitis should undergo exploratory laparoscopy (GoR A) and, if the diagnosis is confirmed, laparoscopic appendectomy (GoR A). Complicated appendicitis can be approached laparoscopically, with significant improvement of the surgical site (SS) infection rate. Regarding appendiceal stump closure, stapling has been found to reduce operative time and superficial wound infections [14] (LE 1a) (Fig. 55.1).

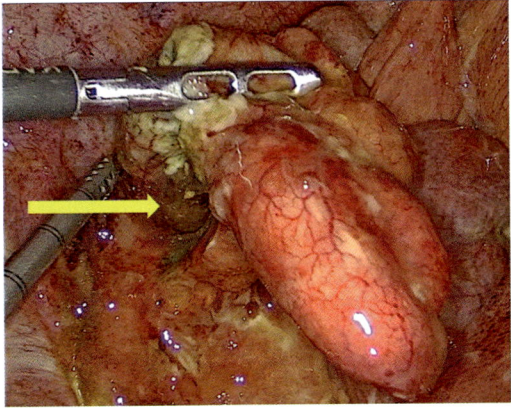

**Fig. 55.1** Acute perforated appendicitis. The yellow arrow shows the perforation site

### 55.3.2 Acute Cholecystitis

Patients should be treated by laparoscopic cholecystectomy (GoR A). Severe cases that include gangrene, empyemic, or perforated cholecystitis and advanced age are not contraindications for laparoscopic cholecystectomy (GoR B) despite a threefold higher conversion rate. Surgery should be performed as soon as possible after the onset of symptoms (GoR A). Early laparoscopic surgery should be offered also to elderly patients (GoR B). In patients with severe comorbidities, conservative treatment or percutaneous cholecystostomy, followed or not by early or delayed surgery, may be alternatives to reduce surgical or anesthetic risks (GoR C). Subtotal cholecystectomy appears to be an acceptable alternative in patients with intense inflammation and increased risk of damage to important structures (LE 2a) [15] (Fig. 55.2a–c).

### 55.3.3 Acute Pancreatitis

Laparoscopic cholecystectomy should be performed as soon as the patient has recovered in mild gallstone-associated acute pancreatitis during the same hospital admission (GoR B). In the other hand, in severe gallstone-associated acute pancreatitis, laparoscopic cholecystectomy should be delayed until there is sufficient resolution of the inflammatory response and clinical recovery (GoR B). In cases of CBD (common bile duct) stones in which an emergency Endoscopic Retrograde Cholangio Pancreatography (ERCP) is indicated, clearance should be obtained by preoperative ERCP or by laparoscopic removal of bile duct stones during cholecystectomy (GoR A) or by combined laparoscopic endoscopic procedure (Transgastric) [16]. When pancreatic necrosis requires surgical treatment (Fig. 55.3) for clinical signs of sepsis or multiorgan failure, necrosectomy (Fig. 55.4) can be performed by laparoscopic debridement through an inframesocolic [17] (Fig. 55.5) or retroperitoneal approach. Open surgery should be reserved to patients not responding to minimally invasive treatment (GoR B). Laparoscopy is

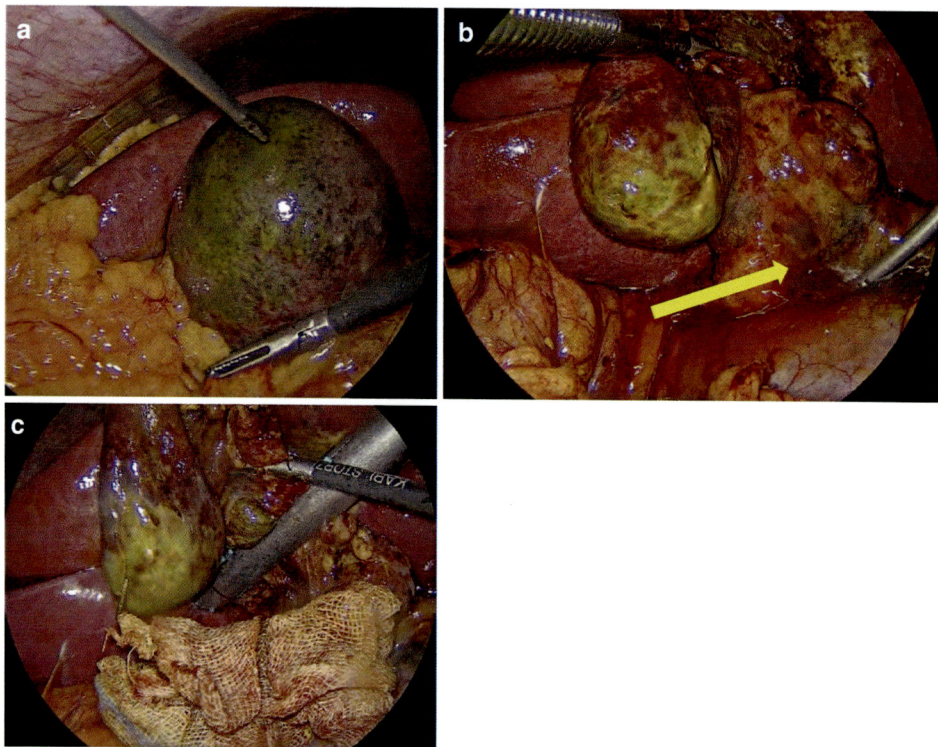

**Fig. 55.2** Acute cholecystitis. (**a**) Gallbladder necrosis, (**b**) Retrograde dissection. Yellow arrow shows the difficult Calot's triangle dissection. (**c**) Stapled cholecystectomy

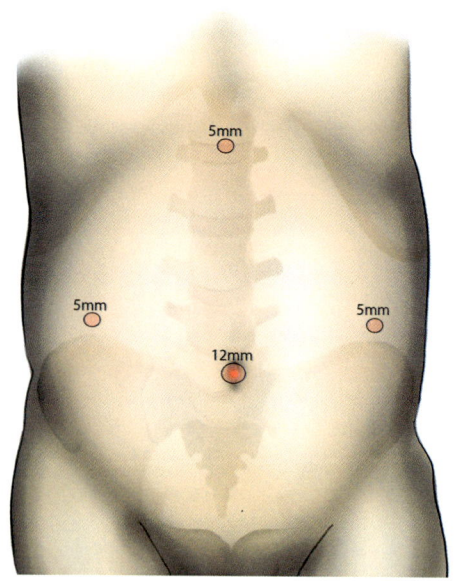

**Fig. 55.3** Trocar placement for pancreatic necrosectomy

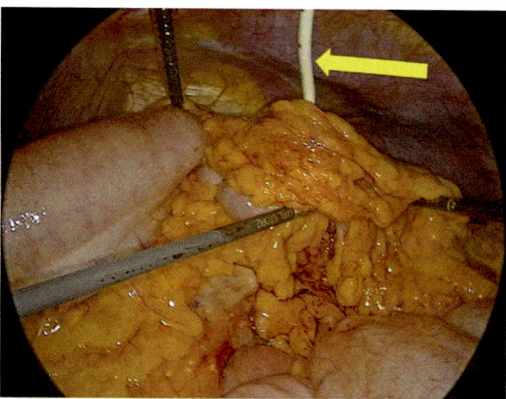

**Fig. 55.4** The yellow arrow shows the failed percutaneous drainage, days before the surgical necrosectomy

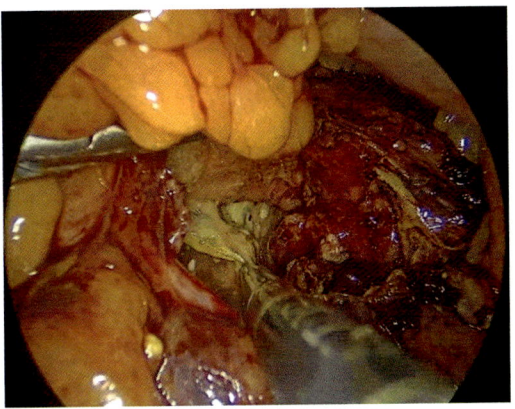

**Fig. 55.5** Transmesocolic (infracolic) pancreatic necrosectomy

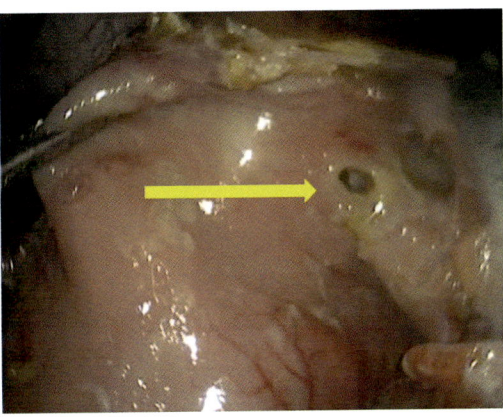

**Fig. 55.6** Perforated peptic ulcer. Yellow arrow shows the 0.8 mm perforation in the posterior face of the stomach

totally contraindicated in cases with abdominal compartment syndrome.

### 55.3.4 Perforated Peptic Ulcer

Laparoscopy is a useful diagnostic tool to detect a perforated peptic ulcer (PPU) when preoperative findings are not conclusive, especially if a laparoscopic treatment is likely (GoR A). Laparoscopy is a possible alternative to open surgery in the treatment of perforated peptic ulcer (GoR B). However, failing to identify a PPU represents one of the most frequent causes of conversion to laparotomy (LE 1a). Decontamination of the peritoneal cavity by washing after treatment of PPU is a fundamental step in the surgical procedure and it can be done by laparoscopy (LE 1a) [18]. A decrease in the incidence of complications has been found with the use of laparoscopic repair compared with open surgery, such as septic abdominal complications, less associated pulmonary infection, complications of the abdominal wall, postoperative ileus, and mortality rate [19] (Fig. 55.6).

### 55.3.5 Acute Mesenteric Ischemia

Acute mesenteric ischemia (AMI) presents a high mortality rate, usually due to arterial occlusion in 50% of cases, in 35% by nonocclusive arterial ischemia and 15% by venous occlusion and prognosis is frequently related to the timeliness of diagnosis. Since laparoscopy does not offer adequate diagnostic accuracy notwithstanding the use of fluorescein and ultraviolet light, it does not offer significant advantages in acute mesenteric ischemia besides a potential role as a bedside and second-look procedure (GoR C) (LE 4) [20]. However, despite the recommendations, some anecdotal cases of severe acute abdominal pain with suspicious of segmentary bowel ischemia can benefit from the laparoscopic procedure (Fig. 55.7).

### 55.3.6 Acute Diverticulitis

There is no role for diagnostic laparoscopy in this condition, because easy diagnosis includes blood count, inflammatory markers, and CT scanning. Laparoscopic approach with lavage and drainage is indicated in complicated diverticulitis when percutaneous drainage failed and when indicated for clinical deterioration (GoR B). Laparoscopic surgery has been utilized in the setting of diverticular perforation with associated peritonitis depending on the general conditions of the patient and on the skill of the operator (GoR C). Elective resection of the ill segment decreases the risk of conversion and increases the rate of primary anastomosis compared to emergency surgery.

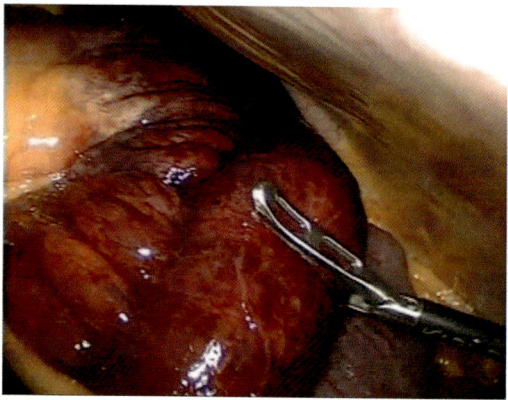

**Fig. 55.7** Acute segmentary mesenteric ischemia. The coloring difference of ischemic and healthy bowel can be observed

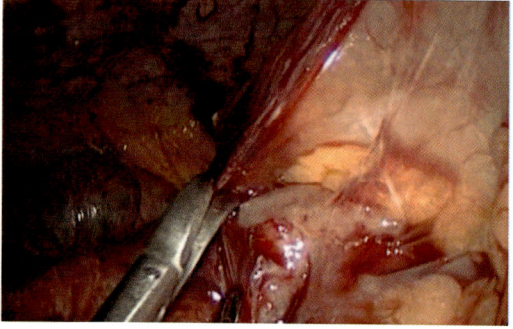

**Fig. 55.8** Small bowel adhesions in the 4 quadrants. The principle of gentle traction and countertraction and cutting without energy sources is essential to resolve multiple bowel adhesions

Associated abscesses can be drained laparoscopically or when the small bowel becomes occluded due to involvement in the diverticular inflammatory process, it can also be resolved in the same way.

### 55.3.7 Small Bowel Obstruction Due to Adhesions

Adhesions are the leading cause of small bowel obstruction (SBO), which account for about 75% of all SBO. Laparoscopic treatment of small bowel obstruction can be successfully accomplished in selected patients (GoR C). The main concern about a laparoscopic approach to SBO is the high conversion rate: complete laparoscopic treatment has been reported possible in only 50–60% of patients. Some reports have tried to define predictive factors for conversion; a history of two or more surgical abdominal operations, late operation (>24 h post-onset), and a bowel diameter exceeding 4 cm [21]. The SAGES guidelines consider laparoscopy contraindicated in patients with a clear indication for surgical intervention such as massive bowel obstruction, perforated viscus, and hemodynamic instability [22]. A systematic review shows a successful therapeutic laparoscopy rate in the range of 40–88% and a conversion rate ranging from 0 to 52%. As for operative technique, the use of atraumatic graspers is essential, adhesiolysis should be proper and cautious, the principle of gentle traction and countertraction and cutting without energy sources are essential and the contents in the defect should be always accurately checked for blood supply, motility, and integrity (Fig. 55.8). If an enterotomy occurs, it can be repaired laparoscopically, trying to isolate the site, and controlling contamination to adjacent structures, always having the suction device prepared. Supposedly benefits of the laparoscopic approach include faster recovery of bowel motility and shorter hospital stay.

### 55.3.8 Incarcerated/Strangulated Hernias

In 2010 a meta-analysis confirmed that the outcome of elective LHR is at least equivalent to that of the open approach [23]. Laparoscopic hernia repair surgery, including TEP or TAPP, may be performed for the treatment of nonreducible or strangulated inguinal hernias (GoR B). The laparoscopic approach, in both techniques, is possible for repairing incarcerated hernia considering the knowledge of anatomy and expertise needed to dissect and reduce the sac (Fig. 55.9). There is a poor evidence that laparoscopic repair of non-inguinal incarcerated hernias may be performed, and further studies are necessary to validate this approach (GoR D).

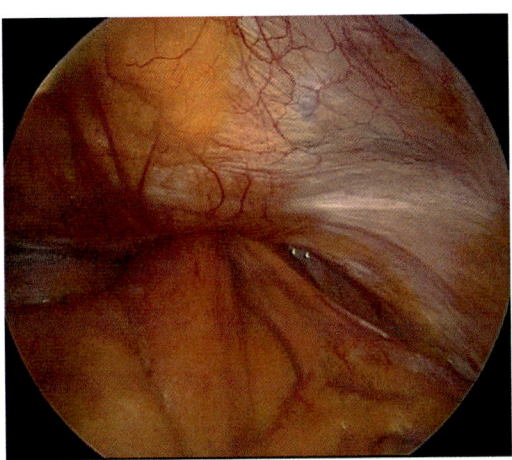

**Fig. 55.9** Incarcerated (nonreductible) inguinal hernia from the small intestine

### 55.3.9 Gynecological Disorders

The most common diagnoses encountered in female patients with acute lower abdominal and/or pelvic pain are ectopic pregnancy (EP), adnexal torsion (AT), endometriosis, pelvic inflammatory disease (PID), and hemorrhagic ovarian cysts. There is a significant amount of high-quality evidence regarding the role of laparoscopic surgery in EP. In the confirmed EP in stable patient laparoscopy should be performed, hospitalization and sick leave times are shorter, and adhesion development reduced when compared to laparotomy. In case of complications with a tubal rupture, salpingectomy can be feasible, and a tube preserving operation can be possible too. When AT, an organ-threatening disease, is suspected, urgent surgical intervention is indicated. Despite the "necrotic" appearance of the twisted ischemic ovary, detorsion is the only procedure that should be performed at surgery. Adnexectomy should be avoided as ovarian function is preserved in 88–100% of cases. Tubo-ovarian abscess is one of the most common types of pelvic abscess. Surgical procedures include laparotomy or laparoscopy with drainage of the abscess, unilateral or bilateral salpingo-oophorectomy, and hysterectomy. However, surgery for tubo-ovarian abscess is often technically difficult and associated with complications [24]. When gynecologic disorders are the suspected cause of abdominal pain, diagnostic laparoscopy (DL) should follow conventional diagnostic investigations, especially US (GoR A), and, if needed, a laparoscopic treatment of the disease should be performed (GoR A). Close cooperation with the gynecologist is strongly recommended (GoR A).

## 55.4 Surgical Imaging and Assistance in Emergency Laparoscopy Setting

### 55.4.1 Indocyanine Green Fluorescence

Indocyanine green is a substance used as a surgical dye requiring special equipment that has many applications nowadays. It was first utilized in critically ill patients to determine cardiac output and cerebral perfusion. It gained more functions later as applications in emergency surgery [25].

In laparoscopy we can use Indocyanine green injected intravenously (in a dose of 0.25–0.5 mg/kg) to the patient following with the use of a compatible light filter, in order to visualize the perfused tissue. For instance, we can use it for viewing bowel ischemia and the possible evaluation of its perfusion (Fig. 55.10). We can actually see the arteries coloring green as we inject the dye within the first 30 s after injection, thus, leading to take decision regarding tissue viability.

Also, in an emergency biliary tract surgery setting [26], we can inject the dye prior to incision, preferably 30 min earlier with the purpose of seeing the biliary tract such as the common bile duct turn green with the light filter (Fig. 55.11) resulting in a much easier identification of anatomical structures and resultingly avoiding injuries to those structures.

In conclusion, Indocyanine green has gained acceptance and usage during laparoscopy because of its simplicity and infrequency of complications. It is important to keep in mind that when emergency arises, a surgeon can have this technique in his pocket in order to identify structures when surgery becomes tricky or is difficult to

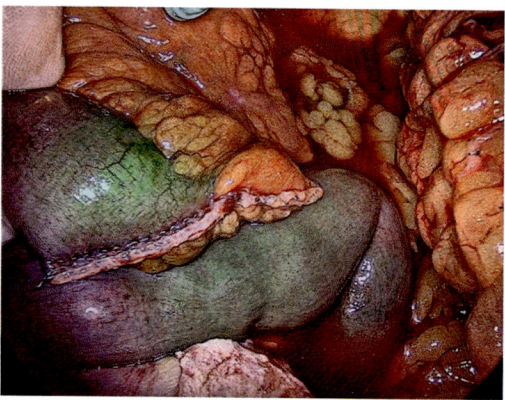

**Fig. 55.10** Indocyanine green can use it for viewing bowel ischemia and the possible evaluation of its perfusion

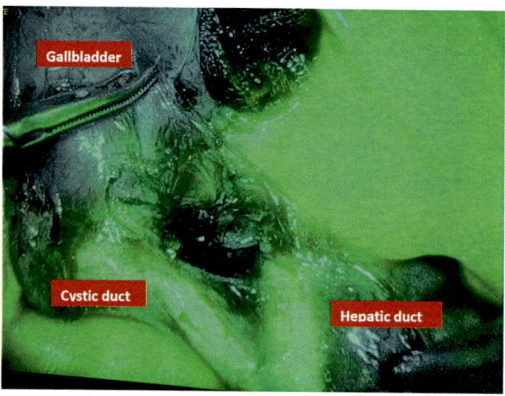

**Fig. 55.11** Biliary tract such as hepatic duct turns green with the light filter

evaluate perfusion by performing a real time arteriography.

## 55.4.2 X-Ray and Fluoroscopy Guidance

The use of X-rays is commonly and widely accepted and routinely used during laparoscopy; more commonly so during biliary tract manipulation and trans-operative cholangiography. As a general principle, when necessary is always beneficial to consider the use of X-rays during surgery. If it is use routinely, we can find associated pathology or intraoperative anatomical findings (Fig. 55.12).

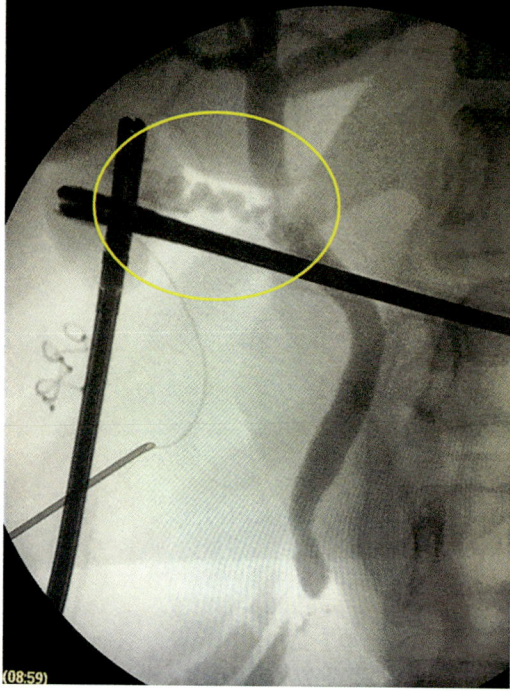

**Fig. 55.12** Note cystic duct corkscrew, and dilation of the biliary tract

## 55.4.3 Endoscopy and Surgery

It is important to keep in mind that when operating on the digestive tract, we always have the endoscopy as a tool, whenever it is available in our hospitals, which in emergency situation (after hours) it is not always available.

**We have three types of endo-visualization that can be used to help us during surgery**
- Esophagogastroduodenoscopy (EGD) includes the visualization of the esophagus, gastric chamber, and duodenum. During surgery it can be a useful tool to have a clear view of the structures from both sides in a real time. It is easily performed, and it can be done simultaneously with the surgical procedure, as the positions do not intervene with each other. It can be used to evaluate anastomosis, review for perforations in difficult zones to expose during laparoscopy, often posterior walls, most commonly in the duodenum and the posterior wall of the

stomach, which is the most common site for inadvertent perforations in trauma scenarios.
- Colonoscopy enable a clear view of the entire colon and in some occasions the last 20 cm of the ileum. Is also used in emergency settings to evaluate anastomoses and hunt for perforations (less often). It is important to remember that this requires previous bowel preparation via laxatives, otherwise, it is hard to obtain good visibility.
- Endoscopic Retrograde Cholangio Pancreatography (ERCP): This procedure allows exploration of the biliary tract, used in emergency setting for one of two scenarios: exploration for injuries in the biliary tract (iatrogenic or otherwise), which can allow a real time treatment for placement of stents or prosthetics. Secondly, the extraction of gallstones from the biliary ducts, which is achievable either by a common ERCP or by a rendezvous technique, includes the passing of a guide wire through the cystic duct in order to find it through the sphincter of Oddi, facilitating access to the biliary tract.

## 55.5 Indications and Contraindications of Laparoscopy in Traumatic Emergencies

Laparotomy for abdominal trauma used to be negative or nontherapeutic in approximately one-third of patients. The major advantage of laparoscopy as identified in these studies was the obviation of unnecessary laparotomy in approximately 60% of cases [27]. However, relevant injuries went undetected in 1% of all laparoscopies, particularly after blunt trauma affecting solid organs or hollow viscus. In hemodynamically unstable patients, emergency surgical exploration of the abdomen may be lifesaving. In this situation, delaying definitive therapy by laparoscopy is contraindicated. Bleeding from minor injuries to the liver or the spleen can be controlled through laparoscopic maneuvers. Diaphragmatic lacerations and perforating stab wounds of the gastrointestinal tract can also be sewn or stapled.

After penetrating abdominal trauma, laparoscopy may be useful in hemodynamically stable patients with documented or equivocal penetration of the anterior fascia (Gor B). Laparoscopy should be considered in hemodynamically stable blunt trauma patients with suspected intra-abdominal injury and equivocal findings on imaging studies or even in patients with negative studies but with a high clinical likelihood for intra-abdominal injury ("unclear abdomen") to exclude relevant injury (GoR C). To optimize results, the procedure should be incorporated in institutional diagnostic and treatment algorithms for trauma patients (Gor D). In 2014 we published [28] these indications and contraindications listed below.

### 55.5.1 Indications for Exploratory Laparoscopy in Abdominal Trauma

1. Diagnosis of low-speed bleeding or doubt of complete hemostasis in case of injury of solid organs (liver and spleen) especially when it has been managed nonoperatively.
2. Probable diaphragmatic rupture or penetration due to clinical suspicion, image, and trajectory.
3. Probable hollow viscus injuries and/or mesenteric injuries, in trauma patients with irrelevant clinical examination and indirect signs on CT (most often free fluid in the peritoneal cavity without solid organ injury) in hemodynamic stable patient.
4. Unfavorable evolution of patients with blunt abdominal trauma with inconclusive imaging results who were managed nonoperatively and with probable diaphragmatic injury, intra-abdominal abscesses, post-traumatic secondary bleeding, mesenteric ischemia, or acute cholecystitis.
5. Contradictions between clinical examination and imaging results, which are inconclusive and are in preparation for general anesthesia for extra-abdominal surgery.
6. Temporary inability to perform a CT scan or FAST, but has the possibility to perform an

exploratory laparoscopy, to avoid a useless laparotomy.
7. Post-traumatic complications: diaphragmatic hernia, delayed evidence of post-traumatic complications, perihepatic biliary or hematic collections, post-traumatic hernias, ureteral injuries.
8. Assistance in the surgical management of intestinal diversion to protect perineal pelvic injuries.

### 55.5.2 Contraindications for the Use of Laparoscopy in Trauma

1. Hemodynamic instability MAP <70 with fluctuations and acidosis and massive transfusion protocol requirements, including septic shock.
2. Multiple injuries.
3. Significant bleeding.
4. Diffuse peritonitis (relative).
5. Immediately life-threatening injuries.
6. Severe head injury (GCS $\leq$12) without intracranial pressure (ICP) monitoring.
7. Severe chest trauma with respiratory failure.
8. Clinically significant blunt cardiac trauma.
9. Uncorrected coagulopathy.
10. Chronic cardiopulmonary disease (relative).
11. Decompensated liver disease.
12. Inability to tolerate pneumoperitoneum.
13. Difficulties of access to the peritoneal cavity.
14. Multiple previous surgeries (relative).
15. Bowel distension (relative).
16. Pregnancy—third trimester (relative).
17. Lack of surgical experience.
18. Lack of multidisciplinary team and surgical conjunction.
19. Equipment limitations and inadequate infrastructure.
20. Lack of a protocol for Exploratory Laparoscopy for Trauma.
21. Lack of laparotomy instruments and equipment for trauma prepared, open and ready.

GCS = Glasgow Coma Scale.
MAP = mean arterial pressure.

## 55.6 Treatment

In the surgical emergencies section, we have been able to review laparoscopic treatment from a simple appendicular resection to complex intestinal resections. This requires training in advanced laparoscopic skills that include intestinal mobilization, intracorporeal suturing, energy use, and staplers. Next, we will review some aspects and principles about the basics of the use of laparoscopy in trauma surgery.

## 55.7 Basics in Laparoscopic Surgery for Trauma

The first two principles to decide to do a full exploratory laparoscopy in surgical emergencies and trauma is the careful selection of patients and have available a highly skilled laparoscopic trauma surgeon. The availability of laparoscopic equipment 24 h a day, 7 days a week (24/7), and adequate support by collaborating and specifically trained surgical nurses and anesthesiologists are another fundamental condition.

### 55.7.1 Basic Equipment

Basic equipment is required to perform a successful procedure in emergency surgery or in a trauma setting like any other surgical procedure. Considering having available some other additional material that may be needed to perform the procedure without delay with the best performance.

### 55.7.2 The Operating Room

It should be noted that in many cases of trauma and emergency surgery, especially in the laparoscopic era, you may need adequate space to house all the equipment you will need from the anesthesia workstation and monitors, space enough for assistance, such as a C-arm or endoscope, among others. Therefore, if an operating room were built from scratch to perform this type of procedures from the user's point of view, the following should be taken into account: Adequate space for proper workflow, for equipment and personnel, with enough space 36–64 square feet (recommended), or adapt it to the equipment it contains, and the most common procedures you perform. Hybrid trauma operating rooms tend to have more space since they harbor larger equipment like angiographic equipment or portable CT-scan machines [29–31]. It is of utmost importance in any operating room to control the environment and patient temperature. The lighting of the operating room ceiling and the lights of the operative field must be cold lights that do not influence the temperature of the patient, they must not cast shadows on the surgical field, or reflections on the monitors, they must be prepared and articulated to be able to convert to open surgery without any problem. The surgical table must be multi-positioning to take advantage of the gravity of the displacement of the organs when mobilizing it, making the surgery more efficient. Remember always that the patient must be strictly restrained to the table.

The monitors must be of very high resolution, preferably 4K, high contrast, commonly 3000:1, since the shadows created within the abdominal cavity give it a perception of depth, with a non-reflective surface and sufficient brightness not to turn off the lights from the ceiling of the operating room. Exploratory laparoscopy for trauma is very dynamic and the surgeon must change sometimes to be able to evaluate the four quadrants and spaces, therefore monitors should be mobile and versatile to adapt to the required visualization and the surgeon's ergonomics to be optimal. The $CO_2$ insufflator must be configured on volume, flow and pressure in the abdominal cavity. It should not be insufflated above 12 mmHg for any procedure. The flow in operative laparoscopy for trauma must be high, ensuring a constant intra-abdominal pressure avoiding fluctuations and delays in reinflation. The anesthesia area must be spacious, so that in addition to the monitoring and ventilation machine, the anesthesiologist can perform additional procedures such as the placement of a central catheter or invasive blood pressure monitoring [32] (Fig. 55.13).

### 55.7.3 Laparoscopic Instruments

The surgeon must use its best option as a method of entry and a second option in case it is not possible with the first. Different methods of entry have been compared, there is no evidence of superiority of one over another. Even though there are several techniques for entering the abdominal cavity such as the open technique, the close technique, direct view trocar entry, Veress needle, Hasson technique and radial expanding trocars (STEP). The surgeon must use the technique that dominates and feels more secure and comfortable [33]. The preferred route for exploratory trauma laparoscopy is the open route through the navel. In our experience, the versatility of having lens of 5 mm and 10 mm with 30° provides an advantage of multiple visions. There is currently no place in exploratory laparoscopy for 0° lenses. It is of the utmost importance to keep the lens with adequate clarity cleaning them continuously with anti-fog or warm water solution. It is important to have the suction/irrigation cannula available from the beginning of the procedure, functioning properly, with a great capacity canister and with the pressure irrigation solution ready for use. The electrosurgery unit and the appropriate devices cannot be missing to make hemostatic vessel control of different diameters. The energy should be used with caution, trying not to have complications to the surrounding tissue during handling.

### 55.7.4 Basic Technique

Within the preparation of the patient for an exploratory laparoscopy, it is imperative to emphasize that before preparation, we have to fasten the pelvis and chest with straps, this allows an active mobilization of the patient during surgery and perform exploration maneuvers helped by the mobilization of organs by gravity. In

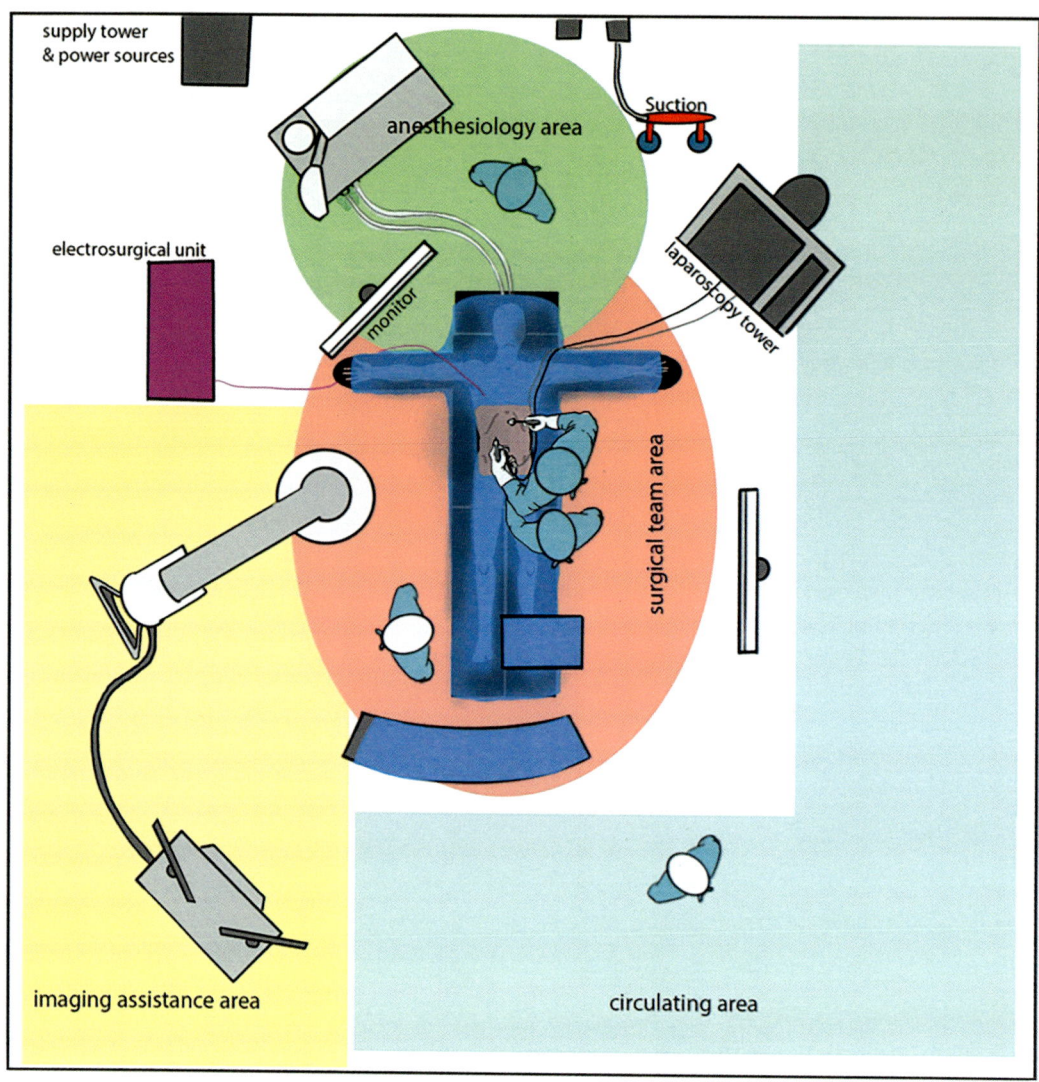

**Fig. 55.13** Example of distribution of the laparoscopic operating room

patients where is possible to place in a French position, holding the legs is also important, being careful of taking care of the bone pressure zones. In trauma patients, the open arms position is recommended, these allow anesthesiologists to be able to have peripheral venous control.

## 55.7.5 Entry Techniques

There are many different entry techniques, and the surgeon should use the technique that feels more comfortable for him. The techniques can be divided into closed and open techniques, the main difference is that in the open technique it carries out an incision in the skin and layers of the abdomen until the peritoneum, and the trocar described by Hasson in 1971 is introduced. In the closed technique, a sharp object is introduced into the abdominal wall thru the peritoneum and subsequently the $CO_2$ is insufflated, a Veress needle is generally used, but a trocar can also be used with or without the laparoscopic lens, or the STEP technique, that uses a Veress needle with a sleeve that allows you to insufflate and create the pneumoperitoneum and then introduce increasingly large trocars that is radially expanded at the access point. Closed maneuvers are time consuming and not recommended in exploratory laparoscopy for trauma. The main risks and complications of any type of entry technique are visceral, vascular, or solid organs injuries, failed access, and gas embolism.

### 55.7.6 Trocar Placement

A good rule of thumb is that the instruments and the lens should create a triangle pointing to the area you wish to work in and the trocars should be spread at least the distance of the handgrip from one to another, so the surgeon could work efficiently and still have an ergonomic position, one way to think about this, is imaging a circle around the area you will be working on the center of the circle will be the vertex of the triangle and you can place the trocars on the radius of the circle. The first access is best achieved at the navel with an open technique using a 10/12 mm trocar. We do not recommend the use of Veress needle in trauma patients, some may have a distended bowel and it may cause misleading iatrogenic bowel or vascular injuries.

## 55.8 Important Issues About Laparoscopy in Trauma Patients

Since the first descriptions of the use of laparoscopy in trauma, its usefulness was valuable in the diagnostic context [34–39] and publications were emerging describing maneuvers for laparoscopic exploration of the abdominal cavity [40, 41] in blunt and penetrating injuries [42].

It is evident that the limitations of monocular vision that existed in the beginning, coupled with poor surgical skills, little technological development, and inexperience in the laparoscopic technique caused that its use was limited. It was not until 1986, when a camera was adapted to the laparoscope, gaving a new dimension to the vision that had existed until then, allowing the sharing of the findings and making the procedures safer. Based on this and with the various technological advances incorporating the 30°- and 45° lens, electrosurgery systems, the variety of instruments and the monitoring and anesthesia techniques that we currently have, they facilitated the procedures and expanded the horizon of laparoscopic possibilities. The benefits of minimally invasive surgery in other surgical areas have encouraged many surgeons to find applications in hemodynamically stable trauma patients, avoiding unnecessary secondary insult with larger wounds and increased morbidity associated with the procedure. In such a way, that exploratory laparoscopy seeks the possibility of being a reliable, feasible procedure that tries to be approved as a tool that allows exploring and repairing the initial injury safely with less morbidity and with a better postoperative recovery.

In recent years the enthusiasm in trauma laparoscopy is less than the post-laparoscopic cholecystectomy era, with fewer publications on laparoscopy in trauma patients. Many factors impact not only in the publications but also in the therapeutic laparoscopy, such as the percutaneous techniques, best imaging systems and protocols that promote the non-operative management, even with the development of laparoscopy techniques and skills in the world. Some examples of these were vision with different graduation angles, versatility of movements, laparoscopes with smaller diameters, cameras with better quality definition, lighting power, constant flow of insufflation without loss of gas, trocars of better quality and bladeless, powerful aspiration systems and more reliable methods of vascular coagulation and sealing with the improvement in electrosurgery systems, methods of better exposure and vascular control with the development and perfection of ultrasonic cutting systems, staplers with articulated movements and number of lines of stapling, various hemostatic agents, adjuvant drugs in the control of bleeding, practical autotransfusion systems and new concepts in relation to the monitoring and management of shock. In this last point, the abandonment of aggressive therapy with intravenous fluids in patients with penetrating trauma and opting for the concept of delayed resuscitation with fluids and the use of vasoactive drugs, allows us to maintain an adequate perfusion, reducing complications due to excess fluid and pulmonary failure up to 30% [43]. When damage control surgery steps were developed in the trauma laparotomy sequence, with quadrant packing, rapid vascular access methods, exposure maneuvers, and management for various types of injuries, it contributed to saving time for the benefit of this type of patients and performed rapid and protocolized surgery; however, the steps and requirements have not been described for systematic exploratory trauma laparoscopy. For this reason, it is particularly important to describe the initial approach site, the characteristics of the pneumoperitoneum that should be used in cases with multisystemic lesions or in cases of head trauma, the number of trocars and their characteristics, the position of the patient for the correct visualization of certain anatomical spaces, as well as the methodology for exposing an organ injury and its repair. Recently, a publication from the University of Sao Paulo [44] by Kawahara et al. standardize and refine their technique, and describe an algorithm for penetrating injuries that is important to consider. Likewise, they graphically represent the trocar placement site, which does not vary from ours. In their report, they refer to the exploration of the small intestine and the possibility of carrying out a complete exploration of this, coinciding with us. They found series of 75 patients injured with sharps and firearms, a general sensitivity of laparoscopy of 97.61%, and specificity of 100%. Positive and negative predictive values with values of 100% and 97.05%, respectively and accurate of 98.66%. Based on this, since 2014 we developed the *Systematic Exploratory Laparoscopy in Trauma (SELT)* technique seeking to standardize the way of performing exploratory laparoscopy in a trauma patient, proposing a way of placing trocars and maneuvers to try to explore practically the entire peritoneal abdomen in hemodynamically stable patients. This includes a checklist for performing the procedure, a list of surgery steps, and specific maneuvers for organ exploration. The surgeon stands on the left to explore the right abdomen (liver, right colon, and small bowel) and on the right to explore the left abdomen (left diaphragm, stomach, spleen, left colon, sigmoid, bladder, and rectum). In the same way, we describe critical points of conversion to traditional trauma laparotomy during laparoscopic exploration.

### 55.8.1 Critical Points to Conversion

If during the laparoscopic exploration the finding is a retroperitoneum Zone I hematoma, is enough reason to convert to laparotomy at once, as well as expanding hematomas in Zone II even when the patient is hemodynamically stable. In expanding hematomas in Zone III, you can have two options, decide to convert to laparotomy, or only perform open preperitoneal packing and assistance with angioembolization. Any hemodynamic decompensation due to bleeding, previously undetected pulmonary or cardiovascular dysfunction, or decompensation due to abdominal hypertension during SELT procedure, is sufficient reason to open the patient. Insufflation should be stopped in case of abrupt rise in respiratory pressure, blood hypotension, or tachycardia; and a low threshold for immediate conversion to open surgery should be kept in mind. A low threshold for open conversion should be maintained if the surgeon is not confident and missing injuries are suspected.

Di Saverio and colleagues mention that they prefer a preliminary exploration by exploratory laparoscopy and seek if there is any indication for the urgent conversion first, and then continue with the rest of the trocars according to the suspicion of identified injury.

## 55.9 Technical Aspects of SELT Procedure

To carry out laparoscopic management of the patient correctly and safely with abdominal trauma, it is necessary to have the equipment, complete instruments, and ready to be used immediately to avoid wasting time that could have an impact on a decrease in the quality of patient care. The preferred laparoscopic equipment should be of high definition and have a light source of at least 300 W, a 20-L insufflator, and a 30°, 5- and 10-mm laparoscope. The instruments should include, in addition to conventional forceps such as graspers and dissectors, atraumatic intestinal forceps, and needle holders. It is essential to have a suction system with conventional and with multiple fenestrations 5- and 10-mm cannulas for a quick and efficient evacuation of the hemoperitoneum. Placement of the first trocar can be performed with open technique. There was not standardized approach to where to place the trocars in the abdominal wall, but any placement must allows functionality, manipulation of practically all the peritoneal organs, options to repair an injury and manipulate the structures, comfort of the team and of course, of the surgeon. At any time, an extra trocar can be placed or one of its positions changed. The abdomen exploration begins with the right upper quadrant like an open approach proceeding clockwise. During the procedure, both hemidiaphragms are required to be explored to rule out injuries that could cause tension pneumothorax, and if present immediately, a pleural tube should be placed [45]. For the evaluation of hemoperitoneum, it is useful to classify it in minimal, moderate, and severe [46] (Table 55.1).

The additional trocars that are necessary according to the findings are placed in an appropriate number and place for the maneuver to be carried out. Preferably, a position contralateral to the injury to be repaired should always be adopted and it is always desirable to have an extra trocar for aspiration. The first maneuver is to exhaustively search for the site or sites that bled, systematizing the search by quadrants. If a large and profusely active bleeding injury is found, there should be no doubt in convert the procedure to open surgery. If the injury is superficial and the bleeding is not profuse, it can be packed with prefabricated roll gauze that allows easy passage through the 10-mm trocars and allows adequate temporary packing and continued exploration of the abdomen searching other bleeding sites and other injuries. The bowel should be entirely and thoroughly explored by run the bowel technique, with two atraumatic intestinal forceps from the ileocecal valve to the duodenal–jejunal flexure, trying to visualize both sides from the intestine and mesenteric and antimesenteric margins.

For the management of intestinal injuries, it is necessary and advisable to have endoscopic staplers. However, it is not mandatory to perform mechanical anastomoses. Depending on the skill of the surgeon, it is possible to perform primary closures and anastomoses manually. Table 55.2 explains the place of the surgeon, the quadrants and the organs that can be explored in each of them, and the positioning of the patient.

### 55.9.1 Ready Check list Description

1. Patient monitoring by anesthesia
2. Open surgery equipment available and open for immediate use if needed (strictly required)
3. Laparoscopic equipment available and working
4. Multi-positioning table functioning
5. Nasogastric tube placed
6. Foley catheter placed
7. Endopleural catheter placed (if needed)
8. Patient restraint to prevent falls and injuries from improper posture
9. Automatic staplers and clips available
10. Hemostats available
11. Electrosurgery unit and devices ready to use

Di Saverio [47] recently published some concepts where the "why" of laparoscopy is ques-

**Table 55.1** Classification of hemoperitoneum

*Minimal* hemoperitoneum: small static amount of blood, including in the parietocolic gutter or between the intestinal loops
*Moderate* hemoperitoneum: obvious 5–10 mm deep blood accumulation in the paracolic gutters and/or pelvis
*Severe* hemoperitoneum—the widespread accumulation of blood throughout the peritoneal cavity including around the intestinal loops floating in or surrounding by a pool of blood

Berci G, Sackier JM, Pas MP. Emergency laparoscopy. Am J Surg. 1991;161:332

**Table 55.2** Surgeon position, organs inspection and surgical table position

| Surgeon side | Quadrant | Organ inspected | Patient position |
|---|---|---|---|
| Left | Right upper quadrant | Liver, gallbladder diaphragm, stomach, lesser sac, ascending colon, right colon flexure, first 2 portions of duodenum and pancreas, [a]right transverse colon | Fowler position and left tilted |
| Right | Left upper quadrant | Stomach great curvature, diaphragm, spleen, left transverse colon, left colon flexure, descending colon | Fowler position and right tilted |
| Left | Right lower quadrant | Cecum, ileocecal valve, and half of small bowel | Trendelenburg and left tilted |
| Right | Left lower quadrant | Half of small bowel to duodenal–jejunal flexure and Treitz ligament, [b]descending colon, sigmoid, and rectum | Trendelenburg and right tilted |

Vega-Rivera F. (2014). Laparoscopia Exploradora Sistematizada para Trauma (LEST). En José de Vinatea (Ed.), Ciencia y práctica en Cirugía Laparoscópica (Primera edición, pp.103–120). Ed. Amolca

[a]The pancreas can be visualized in the first portions, but the body and tail can be explored behind the stomach, cutting the higher omentum

[b]When the small intestine is being explored near the duodenal–jejunal flexure, the mobilization of the patient must be dynamic by changing from the position of Trendelenburg to Fowler to completely visualize the intestine

tioned and refers to certain advantages such as lower inflammation and trauma, high diagnostic accuracy and reduce rate of nontherapeutic laparotomies up to 73% [48], better respiratory management and less postoperative pain, lower rate of adhesions, incisional hernias, and surgical site infection, faster recovery, and less costs [49].

### Dos and Don'ts

- Is laparoscopy indicated?
  - It is very important not to start the wrong way, if a laparoscopic procedure seems like a risky bet in terms of the capacity of the surgical team that will face a complex emergent procedure, consider open surgery from the beginning, since it is of paramount importance, do not waste time.
  - Know the resources in the hospital and in the operating room. Make sure the required technology is at your disposal.
  - Perform night surgery? Every good surgeon should keep in mind that the night shift is often understaffed and that not all resources available during the day are equally available at night. Be aware of the things you can safely count on overnight and use this information when deciding to perform laparoscopic procedures in emergency/trauma situations.
- Beginning of surgery
  - It is often common to see trocars misplaced or placed in sites where there is no possibility of therapeutic maneuver. You should always consider, anatomic variations in patients, previous surgeries/existing scars (beware of adhesions of viscera to the abdominal wall), leaving enough space between them (at least 10 cm) and last but not least, the proper trocar diameter for the proper site (i.e., do not insert a 5 mm trocar where needles or gauzes are likely to be inserted, instead choose a 10–12 mm trocar).
  - It is often seen in less trained surgeons to apply more force than needed to break the tension imposed by the abdominal wall when insert-

ing a trocar, especially in obese patients, therefore it is recommended to grasp the upper part of the trocar with all the palm of the hand and always remember to place the index finger distally to avoid forced entry of the blade/tip and never end up piercing healthy tissue, which can often result in complications.
- NEVER proceed if you are not comfortable with the quality of the image, make sure you view everything with the appropriate resolution, if necessary, make the necessary changes to improve; don't settle for poor image resolution [50].
- During the surgery
  - Whenever possible avoid higher pressures on the pneumoperitoneum, rather work with the least amount of pressure that adequately exposes the surgical site.
  - If you are not a veteran in laparoscopy, consider when alternating instruments (forceps, scissors, needle holders, etc.) that your assistant holding the endoscope visualize the introduction of the instrument into the abdominal cavity to have a safe view of the path that it will take the tip of the instrument to reach the surgical site. Performing this maneuver will result in fewer instrument tips inside the abdominal organs.
  - When using an instrument that carries any type of energy (ultrasonic scalpel, bipolar, monopolar forceps, etc.) always let the instrument do its work before removing or pulling it; By doing so, you will avoid tearing divided or incompletely clotted tissue, resulting in blood loss, or incomplete sealing.
  - If you accidentally open a blood vessel, always keep in mind that the first step is proximal and distal control of the vessel, most often achieved by adequate compression by the quickest means necessary. Do not attempt to use staples when you cannot visualize the vascular ends. If the situation is out of your control, always seek help or convert the procedure to open surgery.
  - Do not be afraid to replace or insert additional trocars when necessary, reconsider repositioning frequently, when you do not have the correct exposure. It is better to place an additional trocar when you have performance problems than to spend too much time with the patient on the surgical table [51].
- After the surgery
  - At the end of the procedure, always remove the trocars with direct endoscopic vision, in this way, you will always avoid postoperative bleeding at the insertion sites. And then, properly evacuate the gas from the abdominal cavity.
  - Trocars larger than 5–8 mm in diameter always require closure of the abdominal wall with suture at the insertion site, regardless of the skin incision.

## 55.10 Summary

Minimally invasive surgery increases in the context of abdominal emergencies in a wide range of acute conditions and nowadays has in our point of view a place in the algorithm of surgical treatment in the trauma patient. The indications and contraindications are clear and the threshold to convert to open surgery is well defined. The surgical expertise, knowledge, and surgical skills are a fundamental piece to improve the experience in trauma laparoscopy. These procedures must be performed by a well-trained surgeon and his team. The Systematic Exploratory Laparoscopic for Trauma (SELT) needs to gain more followers and surgical confidence. The only way to get expertise is to practice, without any risk to the patient. We do not believe that this will be easy, but it is feasible and possible. The availability and surgical facility preparedness are indispensable.

> **Take-Home Messages**
> - Always prepare yourself and discuss with your peers and surgical team to develop an adequate plan execution prior to the first incision.
> - Keep in mind which procedures you are able to perform regarding the equipment available.
> - Previously familiarize yourself with laparoscopic techniques in a simulator prior to attempt four first emergency situation.
> - Whenever possible, evaluate to delay some procedures in order to avoid operate after hours (e.g., cholecystectomy in the middle of the night); surgery at night is more challenging for many reasons.
> - When facing active bleeding, always apply pressure and decide beforehand which hemostatic skills will result for an adequate bleeding control. Every wrong decision becomes the surgery more challenging.
> - If you are not well versed in laparoscopic skills, consider other techniques in vulnerable patients because prolonged surgical times have poor outcomes.
> - When surgery is done, always take time to assess structures and organs involved until you are completely satisfied with what was done before closure.
> - Stick with guidelines and post-operative protocols for patient follow up, in order to detect in early stages when something seems to be wrong.
> - If something goes wrong or seems too overwhelming, always ask for help.
> - If you make a mistake, never make two! Keep calm and think before take action again.

> **Questions and Answers**
> 1. What is the correct term, when you only perform a single trocar laparoscopy to observe the peritoneal cavity?
>    A. Diagnostic laparoscopy
>    B. Exploratory laparoscopy
>    C. Therapeutic laparoscopy
>    D. Non-therapeutic laparoscopy
> Correct Answer: **A**
> 2. What is the correct term, when you perform a laparoscopic procedure with multiple trocars where you able to observe the peritoneal cavity and mobilize the organs to discard any injuries?
>    A. Diagnostic laparoscopy
>    B. Exploratory laparoscopy
>    C. Therapeutic laparoscopy
>    D. Non-therapeutic laparoscopy
> Correct Answer: **B**
> 3. In a routine exploratory laparoscopy, looking to find the cause of an acute abdominal pain, you found an acute appendicitis and perform an appendectomy. What is the correct form to designate the procedure?
>    A. Diagnostic laparoscopy
>    B. Peritoneoscopy
>    C. Exploratory therapeutic laparoscopy
>    D. Exploratory non-therapeutic laparoscopy
> Correct Answer: **C**
> 4. A 32-year-old male patient involved in a motor vehicle collision presents to the Emergency Department with blunt abdominal trauma, no additional injury is identified on primary assessment. There is a well healed surgical scar in the right lower quadrant in the abdomen. Relevant trauma history reveals ethanol halitosis, and GCS 13/15. An initial resuscitation attempt is performed with 0.9% NaCl 2000 mL, rendering MAP to 59 mmHg. The surgeon considers proceed with open surgery. Which of the following is a contraindication to perform an exploratory laparoscopy?
>    A. Severe head injury
>    B. Ethanol halitosis

C. Hemodynamic instability
   D. Difficulty assessment of the peritoneal cavity

   Correct Answer: C

5. A 35-year-old second trimester pregnant female presents to the ER with acute abdominal pain diagnosed by ultrasound as acute cholecystitis, she has a history of thrombophilia, she is with enoxaparin 40 mg subcutaneous once a day, GCS 14/15, MAP 72, normal liver function tests, bowel distension due to intraluminal gas attributed to irritable bowel syndrome. Is there an absolute contraindication for laparoscopic surgery?
   A. Bowel distension
   B. Pregnancy
   C. Thrombophilia treatment
   D. There isn't any

   Correct Answer: D

6. An otherwise healthy 65-year-old male presents to the ER with a single 2 inch (5 cm) knife stabbing wound in the abdomen on the lower left quadrant, with no apparent active bleeding from the wound, the patient has a GCS 15/15, HR 100/m, MAP 75, abdominal pain near the wound, a CT scan shows approximately 200 mL of free liquid in the pelvic region and no free gas. What procedure should be advisable?
   A. Diagnostic laparoscopy
   B. Exploratory laparoscopy
   C. Exploratory laparotomy
   D. Angiography

   Correct Answer: B

7. What is the name of the procedure that we use for abdominal trauma in hemodynamically stable patients that allows us to explore by laparoscopy the entire abdomen in an orderly fashion?
   A. Exploratory laparotomy
   B. Exploratory laparoscopy
   C. Systematic Exploratory Laparoscopy in Trauma (SELT)
   D. Systematic Exploratory Laparotomy in Trauma

   Correct Answer: C

8. Which of the following is an absolute indication for conversion to open laparotomy?
   A. Zone 1 nonexpanding hematoma
   B. Zone 2 nonexpanding hematoma
   C. Zone 3 non expanding hematoma
   D. Zone 3 expanding hematoma

   Correct Answer: A

9. The SELT procedure requires for the surgeon and his team to relocate and adjust the patient position depending on the area they are exploring. Which of the following would be advisable to explore the spleen?
   A. Surgeon on the right side of the patient with Fowler position
   B. Surgeon on the right side of the patient with Trendelenburg position
   C. Surgeon on the left side of the patient with Trendelenburg position
   D. Surgeon on the left side of the patient with Fowler position

   Correct Answer: A

10. Which of the following would be advisable to explore the ileocecal valve?
    A. Surgeon on the right side of the patient with Fowler position
    B. Surgeon on the right side of the patient with Trendelenburg position
    C. Surgeon on the left side of the patient with Trendelenburg position
    D. Surgeon on the left side of the patient with Fowler position

    Correct Answer: C

## References

1. Davis CJ, Filipi CJ. A history of endoscopic surgery. In: Arregui ME, Fitzgibbons RJ, Katkhouda M, Mckernan JE, Reich H, editors. Principles of laparoscopic surgery: basic and advanced techniques. New York: Springer; 1995. p. 3.
2. Cirocchi R, Birindelli A, Inaba K, Mandrioli M, Piccinini A, Tabola R, Carlini L, Tugnoli G, Di Saverio S. Laparoscopy for trauma and the changes in its use from 1990 to 2016: a current systematic review and meta-analysis. Surg Laparosc Endosc Percutan Tech. 2018;28(1):1–12. https://doi.org/10.1097/SLE.0000000000000466.

3. Short AR. The uses of coelioscopy. BMJ. 1925;2:254.
4. Romero Gallego JD, Ramos Durán JM, Saavedra Chacón MJ, Salas Díaz AS. Exploratory laparoscopy in politrauma: knife extraction. Cir Esp. 2017;95(7):403. https://doi.org/10.1016/j.ciresp.2016.10.003.
5. Fuks D, Regimbeau JM. Role of exploratory laparoscopy in hepato-biliary malignancies. J Chir. 2008;145(1):16–9. https://doi.org/10.1016/s0021-7697(08)70283-7.
6. Chen J, Zhang B, Yan Z, Zhao H, Yang K, Yin Y, Jiang L. Exploratory laparoscopy combined with pathological examination in the diagnosis of obscure gastrointestinal bleeding in a child: a case report. BMC Pediatr. 2018;18(1):371. https://doi.org/10.1186/s12887-018-1339-9.
7. Mandrioli M, Inaba K, Piccinini A, Biscardi A, Sartelli M, Agresta F, et al. Advances in laparoscopy for acute care surgery and trauma. World J Gastroenterol. 2016;22(2):668–80.
8. Britannica, The Editors of Encyclopedia. "Laparoscopy". Encyclopedia Britannica. 2021. https://www.britannica.com/science/laparoscopy. Accessed 27 Apr 2021.
9. Sosa JL, Baker M, Puente I, et al. Negative laparotomy in abdominal gunshot wounds. Potential impact of laparoscopy. J Trauma. 1995;38:194–7.
10. Warren O, Kinross J, Paraskeva P, Darzi A. Emergency laparoscopy—current best practice. World J Emerg Surg. 2006;31(1):24. https://doi.org/10.1186/1749-7922-1-24.
11. Sauerland S, Agresta F, Bergamaschi R, Borzellino G, Budzynski A, Champault G, Fingerhut A, Isla A, Johansson M, Lundorff P, Navez B, Saad S, Neugebauer EA. Laparoscopy for abdominal emergencies: evidence-based guidelines of the European Association for Endoscopic Surgery. Surg Endosc. 2006;20(1):14–29. https://doi.org/10.1007/s00464-005-0564-0.
12. Neugebauer EAM, Sauerland S. Guidelines for emergency laparoscopy. World J Emerg Surg. 2006;1(1):31. https://doi.org/10.1186/1749-7922-1-31.
13. Agresta F, Ansaloni L, Baiocchi GL, Bergamini C, Campanile FC, Carlucci M, Cocorullo G, Corradi A, Franzato B, Lupo M, Mandalà V, Mirabella A, Pernazza G, Piccoli M, Staudacher C, Vettoretto N, Zago M, Lettieri E, Levati A, Pietrini D, Scaglione M, De Masi S, De Placido G, Francucci M, Rasi M, Fingerhut A, Uranüs S, Garattini S. Laparoscopic approach to acute abdomen from the consensus development conference of the Società Italiana di Chirurgia Endoscopica e nuove tecnologie (SICE), Associazione Chirurghi Ospedalieri Italiani (ACOI), Società Italiana di Chirurgia (SIC), Società Italiana di Chirurgia d'Urgenza e del trauma (SICUT), Società Italiana di Chirurgia nell'Ospedalità Privata (SICOP), and the European Association for Endoscopic Surgery (EAES). Surg Endosc. 2012;26(8):2134–64. https://doi.org/10.1007/s00464-012-2331-3.
14. Kazemier G, in't Hof KH, Saad S, Bonjer HJ, Sauerland S. Securing the appendiceal stump in laparoscopic appendectomy: evidence for routine stapling? Surg Endosc. 2006 Sep;20(9):1473–6. https://doi.org/10.1007/s00464-005-0525-7.
15. Soleimani M, Mehrabi A, Mood ZA, Fonouni H, Kashfi A, Büchler MW, Schmidt J. Partial cholecystectomy as a safe and viable option in the emergency treatment of complex acute cholecystitis: a case series and review of the literature. Am Surg. 2007;73(5):498–507.
16. Rogers SJ, Cello JP, Horn JK, Siperstein AE, Schecter WP, Campbell AR, Mackersie RC, Rodas A, Kreuwel HT, Harris HW. Prospective randomized trial of LC + LCBDE vs ERCP/S + LC for common bile duct stone disease. Arch Surg. 2010;145:28–33.
17. Adamson GD, Cuschieri A. Multimedia article. Laparoscopic infracolic necrosectomy for infected pancreatic necrosis. Surg Endosc. 2003;17(10):1675. https://doi.org/10.1007/s00464-003-0041-6.
18. Robertson GS, Wemyss-Holden SA, Maddern GJ. Laparoscopic repair of perforated duodenal ulcers. The role of laparoscopy in generalized peritonitis. Ann R Coll Surg Engl. 2000;82:6–10.
19. Sanabria AE, Morales CH, Villegas MI. Laparoscopic repair for perforated peptic ulcer disease. Cochrane Database Syst Rev. 2005;4:CD004778.
20. Yanar H, Taviloglu K, Ertekin C, Ozcinar B, Yanar F, Guloglu R, Kirtoglu M. Planned second-look laparoscopy in the management of acute mesenteric ischemia. World J Gastroenterol. 2007;13(24):3350–3.
21. Suter M, Zermatten P, Halkic N, Martinet O, Bettschart V. Laparoscopic management of mechanical small bowel obstruction: are there predictors of success or failure? Surg Endosc. 2000;14(5):478–83.
22. SAGES. Diagnostic laparoscopy guidelines. Surg Endosc. 2008;22:1353–83.
23. Dedemadi G, Sgourakis G, Radtke A, Dounavis A, Gockel I, Fouzas I, Karaliotas C, Anagnostou E. Laparoscopic versus open mesh repair for recurrent inguinal hernia: a meta-analysis of outcomes. Am J Surg. 2010;2:291–7.
24. Granberg S, Gjelland K, Ekerhovd E. The management of pelvic abscess. Best Pract Res Clin Obstet Gynaecol. 2009;23:667–78.
25. Dip F, Lo Menzo E, White KP, Rosenthal RJ. Does near-infrared fluorescent cholangiography with indocyanine green reduce bile duct injuries and conversions to open surgery during laparoscopic or robotic cholecystectomy? A meta-analysis. Surgery. 2021;169(4):859–67. https://doi.org/10.1016/j.surg.2020.12.008.
26. Wang C, Peng W, Yang J, et al. Application of near-infrared fluorescent cholangiography using Indocyanine green in laparoscopic cholecystectomy. J Int Med Res. 2020;48(12):300060520979224. https://doi.org/10.1177/0300060520979224.
27. Renz BM, Feliciano DV. Unnecessary laparotomies for trauma: a prospective study of morbidity. J Trauma. 1995;38:350–6.

28. Vega-Rivera F. Laparoscopia Exploradora Sistematizada para Trauma (LEST). In: de Vinatea J, editor. Ciencia y práctica en Cirugía Laparoscópica. 1st ed. Mexico City: Ed. Amolca; 2014. p. 103–20.
29. Loftus TJ, Croft CA, Rosenthal MD, Mohr AM, Efron PA, Moore FA, Upchurch GR Jr, Smith RS. Clinical impact of a dedicated trauma hybrid operating room. J Am Coll Surg. 2021;232(4):560–70. https://doi.org/10.1016/j.jamcollsurg.2020.11.008.
30. Choi S. A review of the ergonomic issues in the laparoscopic operating room. J Healthc Eng. 2012;3:587–604. https://doi.org/10.1260/2040-2295.3.4.587.
31. Ibrahim AM, Dimick JB, Joseph A. Building a better operating room: views from surgery and architecture. Ann Surg. 2017;265(1):34–6. https://doi.org/10.1097/SLA.0000000000001777.
32. Varela E, Brunt LM. SAGES laparoscopic surgery safety checklist. Boston: Springer; 2012. https://doi.org/10.1007/978-1-4419-7901-8_8.
33. Ahmad G, Baker J, Finnerty J, Phillips K, Watson A. Laparoscopic entry techniques. Cochrane Database Syst Rev. 2019;8:CD006583.
34. Tsybuliak GN. Diagnostic value of laparoscopy in closed trauma of the abdomen. VestnKhirIm I IGrek. 1966;96(5):75–7.
35. Kalnberz VK, Freĭdus BA. Laparoscopy in closed trauma to the stomach and organs of the abdominal cavity. VestnKhirIm I IGrek. 1968;101(10):33–8.
36. Heselson J. Peritoneoscopy in abdominal trauma. S Afr J Surg. 1970;8(3):53–61.
37. Cortesi N, Ferrari P, Romani M, Manenti A, Bruni GC. Preliminary studies of the diagnostic value of laparoscopy in polytraumatized persons. Minerva Chir. 1973;28(1):39–40.
38. Oliva V, Prete F, Neri V, Ianora A. Closed trauma and injuries of the liver and extrahepatic biliary ways. Diagnosis. Minerva Chir. 1974;29(10):626–44.
39. Gomel V. Laparoscopy. Can Med Assoc J. 1974;111(2):167–9.
40. Villavicencio RT, Aucar JA. Analysis of laparoscopy in trauma. J Am Coll Surg. 1999;189:11.
41. Carnevale N, Baron N, Delany HM. Peritoneoscopy as an aid in the diagnosis of abdominal trauma: a preliminary report. J Trauma. 1977;17:634.
42. Gazzaniga AB, Stanton WW, Bartlett RH. Laparoscopy in the diagnosis of blunt and penetrating injuries to the abdomen. Am J Surg. 1976;131:315.
43. Bickell WH, Wall MJ, Pepe PE, et al. Immediate versus delayed fluid resuscitation for hypotensive patients with penetrating torso injuries. NEJM. 1994;331(17):1105–9.
44. Kawahara NT, et al. Standard examination system for laparoscopy in penetrating abdominal trauma. J Trauma. 2009;67:589–95.
45. Sosa LJ, Arrillaga A, Puente I, et al. Laparoscopy in 121 consecutive patients with abdominal gunshot wounds. J Trauma. 1995;39:501.
46. Berci G, Sackier JM, Pas-Partlow M. Emergency laparoscopy. Am J Surg. 1991;161:332.
47. Di Saverio S, Birindelli A, Podda M, Segalini E, Piccinini A, Coniglio C, Frattini C, Tugnoli G. Trauma laparoscopy and the six w's: why, where, who, when, what, and how? J Trauma Acute Care Surg. 2019;86(2):344–67. https://doi.org/10.1097/TA.0000000000002130.
48. Johnson JJ, Garwe T, Raines AR, Thurman JB, Carter S, Bender JS, Albrecht RM. The use of laparoscopy in the diagnosis and treatment of blunt and penetrating abdominal injuries: 10-year experience at a level 1 trauma center. Am J Surg. 2013;205(3):317–21.
49. Dowson HM, Huang A, Soon Y, Gage H, Lovell DP, Rockall TA. Systematic review of the costs of laparoscopic colorectal surgery. Dis Colon Rectum. 2007;50(6):908–19.
50. Ballantyne GH. The pitfalls of laparoscopic surgery: challenges for robotics and telerobotic surgery. Surg Laparosc Endosc Percutan Tech. 2002;12(1):1–5.
51. Anteby SO, Schenker JG, Polishuk WZ. The value of laparoscopy in acute pelvic pain. Ann Surg. 1975;181:484–6.

# Esophageal Non-traumatic Emergencies

# 56

Luigi Bonavina, Emanuele Asti, and Tommaso Panici Tonucci

## 56.1 Introduction

**Learning Goals**
- To acquire knowledge about the clinical presentation of patients with non-traumatic esophageal emergencies (excluding blunt/penetrating traumatic injuries and caustic injuries).
- To acquire knowledge about the diagnostic pathways and the criteria guiding therapeutic decision-making.
- To acquire knowledge about non-operative and interventional management, including radiological, endoscopic, surgical, and hybrid techniques, to treat these emergencies.

L. Bonavina (✉)
Division of General and Foregut Surgery, Department of Biomedical Sciences for Health, University of Milan, IRCCS Policlinico San Donato, Milan, Italy

Department of Surgery, I.R.C.C.S. Policlinico San Donato, Milan, Italy
e-mail: luigi.bonavina@unimi.it

E. Asti · T. P. Tonucci
Division of General and Foregut Surgery, Department of Biomedical Sciences for Health, University of Milan, IRCCS Policlinico San Donato, Milan, Italy
e-mail: emanuele.asti@grupposandonato.it

### 56.1.1 Anatomy

The esophagus spans approximately 25 cm from the lower border of the cricoid to the esophago-gastric junction. There are three natural sites of anatomical narrowing along the esophagus: the first is at the level of the cricoid/upper esophageal sphincter (C6); the second is at the level of the aortic arch/left mainstem bronchus (T4–T5), and the third is at the level of the esophageal hiatus (T10). The esophageal wall includes four layers—mucosa, submucosa, muscularis propria, and adventitia—the latter being covered by visceral pleura. The lack of serosa allows spreading of infection laterally into the mediastinum, from the neck into the posterior mediastinum through the retropharyngeal space, and inferiorly into the upper abdomen. Knowledge of these anatomic compartments is essential to understand pathophysiology, properly interpret imaging, and plan appropriate management.

### 56.1.2 Background

The spectrum of esophageal non-traumatic emergencies is dominated by iatrogenic and barogenic perforations, obstruction from foreign bodies or incarcerated paraesophageal hernia, complications of esophageal surgery, descending necrotizing mediastinitis, and esophageal bleeding. Early and appropriate management of these conditions is crucial and represents the most important determinant of patient outcomes. Clinical manifestations in patients with esophageal emergencies include dysphagia, odynophagia, sialorrhea, food regurgitation, vomiting, hematemesis, chest pain, dyspnea, tachycardia, tachypnea, fever, and sepsis. On the other hand, some individuals may present with minimal or no symptoms and tolerance to sepsis. Prompt identification of esophageal perforation, conditions that may progress to perforation, cause, and site of esophageal obstruction, and source of bleeding are mandatory for selecting the most appropriate therapeutic strategy.

## 56.2 Clinical Presentation and Diagnosis

### 56.2.1 Esophageal Perforation

This is a trans-mural disruption of the esophageal wall and a highly heterogeneous clinical condition. Current reported mortality of esophageal perforation is up to 20% as a result of septic shock and cardiorespiratory failure. The common pathogenetic denominator is contamination of loose connective tissue surrounding the esophagus in the neck and mediastinum by digestive contents, with the potential for spread of infection to all contiguous anatomical spaces. This will initiate a systemic inflammatory response syndrome due to cytokine activation that may lead to sepsis with organ dysfunction [1, 2]. Typically, proximal perforations lead to formation of abscess in the retropharyngeal space and possible descent of infection into the posterior mediastinum through the fascial compartments of the neck. Esophageal perforation is caused by several mechanisms, which include direct piercing, shearing along the longitudinal axis, bursting from radial forces, or weakening of the esophageal wall due to necrosis [3–5].

*Iatrogenic perforations* represent the most frequent etiology and are related to either diagnostic or therapeutic procedures. Some perforations are due to direct injury from flexible or rigid upper gastrointestinal endoscopy at the Killian's triangle, often in the presence of an unknown Zenker's diverticulum. Other causes of perforation include endoscopic dilatation of caustic or peptic strictures, pneumatic dilation of the cardia for achalasia, stent placement, removal of impacted foreign bodies, removal of intragastric balloon for obesity, radiofrequency ablation for atrial fibrillation, endoscopic submucosal dissection, band ligation of esophageal varices, trans-esophageal cardiac ultrasound, and endotracheal intubation. Malignancy-related perforations are secondary to endoscopic dilation, stenting, and chemoradiation therapy or may occur spontaneously as a consequence of the natural history of esophageal cancer. Less frequent causes of iatrogenic perforations are injuries occurring as a result of surgical procedures, such as tracheostomy, cricopharyngeal myotomy for Zenker's diverticulum, cervical spine surgery, thyroidectomy, Heller myotomy for achalasia, resection of epiphrenic diverticula, gastric fundoplication, and lung resection.

*Barogenic perforation (Boerhaave's syndrome)* accounts for about 15% of esophageal full-thickness disruptions. Males in the sixth decade of life are predominantly affected, and association with alcohol ingestion is common. This type of perforation is induced by a sudden increase of intraluminal pressure secondary to forceful retching/vomiting, cough, or Valsalva maneuver, in the absence of upper esophageal sphincter relaxation. The rupture is typically longitudinal, of variable length, and located in the left posterolateral esophagus, near the left diaphragmatic crus. The mucosal tear is longer than the mucosal tear, may extend cranially, and rarely involves the intraperitoneal side. About 50% of Boerhaave's perforations occur in patients with hiatal hernia and gastroesophageal reflux disease as a consequence of the reduced abdomino-thoracic gradient [6, 7].

Time to treatment has long been considered the most significant predictor of survival in esophageal perforations, but time to diagnosis, site and size of injury, clinical severity at presentation according to Pittsburgh Severity Score (PSS), presence of underlying esophageal disorders, and modalities of initial treatment have an impact on postoperative morbidity, need for re-intervention, and length of hospital stay. The PSS stratifies patients into low-, intermediate-, and high-risk groups based on clinical variables at presentation, and increasing score is associated with increasing mortality [8, 9].

**Diagnosis** Iatrogenic perforations are often recognized or suspected during endoscopic or surgical procedures; therefore, an early diagnosis has a favorable impact on outcomes. Patients with proximal esophageal perforation present with neck pain, odynophagia, hoarseness, and subcutaneous air and crepitus at physical examination. A tracheoesophageal fistula should be suspected in critically ill patients subjected to prolonged mechanical ventilation or percutaneous tracheostomy who present with aspiration of gastric contents in the tracheobronchial tree or air leak around the cuffed tracheostomy tube and abdominal distension.

The classic presentation of Boerhaave's syndrome includes vomiting followed by chest pain and subcutaneous emphysema (Mackler's triad), but misdiagnosis with acute myocardial infarction, aortic dissection, perforated peptic ulcer, and acute pancreatitis is common. This may cause significant diagnostic delay and a late presentation with overt sepsis (Fig. 56.1). A history of vomiting should raise the suspicion of Boerhaave's syndrome, but errors in diagnosis are common and these patients may present late and be septic at the time of diagnosis [10]. A condition that may mimic a Boerhaave's syndrome is incarceration of a paraesophageal hernia with volvulus of the intrathoracic stomach leading to a closed-loop obstruction. This is associated with acute postprandial distress, chest pain resembling myocardial infarction, retching, and inability to vomit. Gastric gangrene and perforation can be developed as a consequence of acute gastric outflow obstruction, overdistension, and gastric wall ischemia [11, 12].

A timely diagnosis of esophageal perforation, possibly within 24 h, is critical to prevent sepsis secondary to mediastinal and pleural contamination and to decide the most appropriate therapeutic strategy. Tachycardia and tachypnea in the absence of fever can be a sole clinical manifestation of esophageal perforation. Routine blood testing can show initial signs of inflammation and sepsis, such as leukocytosis and high C-reactive protein levels. Anterior and lateral chest radiographs may show the typical Naclerio's sign, a V-shaped air transparency in the left lower mediastinal area indicating pneumomediastinum in the region of the distal esophagus [13]. Pneumothorax and pleural effusion are later signs of perforation. In stable patients, a gastrografin

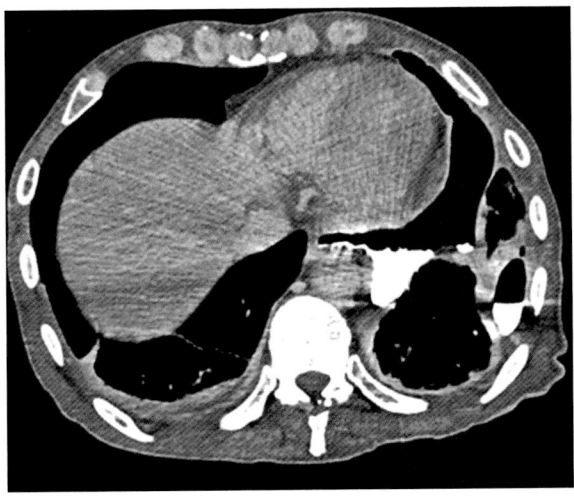 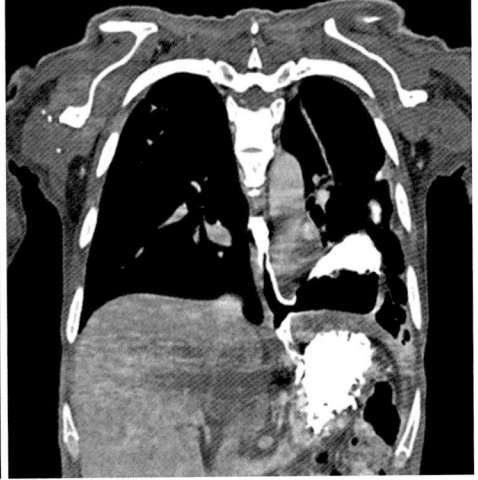

**Fig. 56.1** Axial and coronal CT scans showing inveterate Boerhaave's perforation with left esophagopleural fistula

swallow study can confirm the suspicion of esophageal leak. Computed tomography (CT) scan with oral and intravenous contrast should ideally be performed in all patients. A flexible upper gastrointestinal endoscopy can evaluate the location, the size, and the characteristics of the mucosal margins. Underlying esophageal conditions that may promptly be recognized by radiological/endoscopic imaging, and may influence the therapeutic strategy, include esophageal carcinoma, diverticula, achalasia, and hiatal hernia.

## 56.2.2 Foreign Body Ingestion

Ingestion of foreign bodies in adults may be accidental, intentional (prisoners and illicit drug dealers), or associated with cognitive impairment or psychiatric disorders. About 80% of ingested foreign bodies pass spontaneously through the gastrointestinal tract [14]. Esophageal foreign body impaction most commonly occurs at the level of hypopharynx/upper thoracic esophagus for anatomical (cricopharyngeus, aortic arch, and left main bronchus) and physiological (transition point between striated and smooth muscle fibers) reasons. The site of impaction also depends on the size and shape of the object. Sharp objects, such as meat/fish bones and dentures with clasps, have the potential to cause the most severe complications, including intramural perforation, penetration of contiguous structures, such as the aorta and the tracheobronchial tree, and periesophageal abscess. Food bolus impaction (steakhouse syndrome) typically occurs at the level of the distal esophagus and may be associated with underlying esophageal disorders, such as Schatzki ring, eosinophilic esophagitis, and esophageal cancer [15].

**Diagnosis** The clinical presentation is characterized by acute onset of dysphagia with inability to swallow saliva, which may be accompanied by sore throat, odynophagia, retrosternal pain, retching, drooling, and aspiration. Choking and dyspnea occur in patients with airway obstruction or aspiration. Initial assessment is based on patient's history, symptoms, and physical examination, including fever, neck tenderness, and subcutaneous emphysema. Plain neck, chest, and abdominal radiographs are useful to assess the presence, site of impaction, shape and size of the object, and indirect signs of perforation. Biplanar radiographs may reduce the false-negative rate and differentiate between airway and esophageal foreign body. Computed tomography should be performed when perforation is suspected, especially after ingestion of animal or fish bones. Contrast swallow studies are not recommended, especially in patients who are unable to swallow saliva because of the high risk of aspiration. Endoscopy has a diagnostic but also a therapeutic role in these patients. Patients with recurrent food bolus obstruction should be investigated for possible underlying esophageal disorders.

## 56.2.3 Complications of Esophageal Surgery

The anastomotic leak rate after esophagectomy and reconstruction with gastric, jejunal, or colonic conduit remains around 10%. Proper patient selection, choice of the operative strategy, pre-habilitation, and careful postoperative monitoring continue to play a crucial role, especially in the prevention of respiratory complications. Predictive factors of anastomotic leak are less defined, but the physiologic patient's status, comorbidity, neoadjuvant therapy, and anesthetic and intensive care approach may influence the risk of leak. Dehiscence of the anastomosis may occur as a result of faulty surgical technique, failure of the mechanical stapler, infection with perianastomotic abscess, or conduit ischemia [16].

Mechanical obstruction of the gastric conduit due to narrowing at the level of the crura, twisting of the stomach, paraconduit herniation [17], and chylothorax secondary to intraoperative damage of the thoracic duct are rare complications of esophagectomy [18]. Complications of surgery for benign esophageal conditions include recurrent hiatal herniation following repair of large paraesophageal hernia, stricture or erosion at the gastroesophageal junction from permanent prosthetic material used to buttress the cruroplasty, and leakage from stapled diverticulectomy or Heller's myotomy for achalasia.

**Diagnosis** Anastomotic leak can present with by tachycardia, tachypnea, and fever and be preceded by hypoxia, high levels of serum C-reactive protein [19], and/or high dosage of amylase in the pleural drain by postoperative day 3. New-onset atrial fibrillation is also an ominous clinical sign that should raise the suspicion of anastomotic leak. Neck pain and swelling, or the presence of saliva or pus in the drain, indicate a cervical anastomotic fistula. The diagnosis of anastomotic leak is confirmed by a gastrografin swallow study, CT scan with oral contrast, upper gastrointestinal endoscopy, and/or methylene blue test. The Clavien-Dindo and the Esophagectomy Complications Consensus Group (ECCG) are commonly used and validated tools to classify the severity of anastomotic disruption [20, 21].

Postoperative chest radiographs and CT scans can also identify mechanical obstruction of the gastric conduit requiring revisional surgery. On upper gastrointestinal endoscopy, curling and edema of the gastric folds should raise the suspicion of a twisted conduit. Chylothorax is easily diagnosed at bedside by the milky appearance of the pleural fluid and/or by dosage of triglycerides in the pleural fluid drain when the patient has resumed oral feeding. Occasionally, it may occur later during the postoperative course after the chest drain has been removed and present with dyspnea and pleural effusion. In such circumstances, a thoracentesis will be diagnostic.

Early recurrent herniation after hiatal hernia repair and fundoplication is promptly diagnosed by chest X-rays and CT scan. Stricture or erosion of the gastroesophageal junction from prosthetic material is a rather late postoperative event, which is usually diagnosed at a follow-up endoscopy.

### 56.2.4 Descending Necrotizing Mediastinitis

This is a severe form of deep infection with cellulitis, caused by mixed aerobic/anaerobic flora, due to retropharyngeal spread of odontogenic or peritonsillar abscesses along the deep fascial planes into the posterior mediastinum. The esophagus can be compressed by the abscess, or a late esophageal stricture can develop in survivors as a result of mediastinal fibrosis. The majority of patients have associated morbidities, such as diabetes, alcohol abuse, or immunodeficiency [22].

**Diagnosis** Patients are presented with odynophagia, neck pain and swelling, interscapular pain, dyspnea, fever, and sepsis. Contrast-enhanced CT scan is the main diagnostic tool and typically shows an abscess with gas bubbles above the tracheal bifurcation or extending below up to the diaphragm.

### 56.2.5 Esophageal Bleeding

Mallory–Weiss syndrome, intramural dissecting hematoma, acute esophageal necrosis (black esophagus), and severe reflux esophagitis with or without Barrett's esophagus are possible causes of esophageal bleeding [23–25]. Of these, the Mallory–Weiss syndrome is the most common and generally associated with vomiting and alcohol ingestion. Ischemia and/or coagulopathy play a major role in the pathogenesis of intramural hematoma and acute esophageal necrosis. Both Mallory–Weiss tears and intramural dissecting hematoma may be part of the spectrum of barogenic injuries. Aortoesophageal fistula can occur either in the setting of untreated thoracic aortic aneurysm, after surgical or endovascular repair, or after foreign body impaction. The Chiari's triad of chest pain, sentinel hematemesis, and final massive hemorrhage with exsanguination and death after a symptom-free interval is the typical presentation of an aortoesophageal fistula. The interval between the first episode of sentinel hemorrhage and the final diagnosis can range from 2 h to 6 months [26, 27].

Bleeding from esophageal varices is a catastrophic event in patients with liver cirrhosis and portal hypertension and is frequently associated with rebleeding, severe complications, and death. The mortality rate is 20% when variceal bleeding is the isolated complicating event of cirrhosis, rising to 80% if hepatic encephalopathy or ascites are present [28].

**Diagnosis** In patients presenting with esophageal bleeding, upper gastrointestinal endoscopy has the potential to identify the source of bleeding and to exclude the presence of impacted foreign bodies. Small mucosal erosions, oozing from a pin-hole erosion, ulcer with adherent clot over a pulsatile mass, or aortic graft exposure should suggest the presence of an aortoesophageal fistula. Attempts at endoscopic removal of the clot may cause exsanguination, therefore, urgent referral for angio-CT scan and possible endovascular treatment is recommended.

The diagnosis of variceal bleeding is suggested by the clinical history but should be confirmed by endoscopy after appropriate initial resuscitation to rule out other bleeding sources, such as erosive gastritis, gastric, and duodenal ulcer. An actively bleeding vessel and the presence of fibrin plug and red wale signs represent high-risk stigmata in patients with esophageal varices.

## 56.3 Treatment

### 56.3.1 Perforations

A variety of available management options have resulted in heterogeneous decision-making algorithms and large variations in reported outcomes. Initial management of esophageal perforation has traditionally relied upon open surgery consisting of primary suture repair with or without tissue reinforcement, esophageal diversion and exclusion, or esophageal resection. More recently, there has been a trend toward the adoption of minimally invasive surgical techniques and hybrid radiological, endoscopic, and/or thoracoscopic/laparoscopic procedures [29–32].

Unstable patients require airway stabilization, aggressive resuscitation, and possible damage control surgery, including surgical drainage or esophageal diversion, and feeding jejunostomy. Non-operative management (percutaneous drainage, antibiotics, and esophageal rest) can be considered only in stable patients with minimal symptoms, short interval between onset of symptoms and diagnosis, and contained esophageal leak, cavity well drained back into the esophagus, minimal evidence of clinical sepsis, and high degree of tolerance to mediastinal and pleural contamination [33, 34]. However, close clinical, laboratory, and imaging monitoring is mandatory (Table 56.1). Pre-existing esophageal or systemic morbidity and event-to-diagnosis interval have an impact on prognosis. The presence of sepsis, renal failure, and advanced age appears to be associated with higher mortality rates. A higher Pittsburgh Severity Score (PSS), old age, perforation located in the thoracic esophagus, and gross mediastinal/pleural contamination are predictive factors of treatment failure and leakage after primary suture repair [35, 36].

Cervical perforations are best treated by prompt surgical drainage and primary suture repair whenever possible through a left cervical incision along the anterior border of the sternocleidomastoid muscle. Post-intubation tracheoesophageal fistula is a distinct entity, which can be treated non-operatively if the patient is breathing spontaneously and respiratory parameters are stable. On the other hand, in patients requiring mechanical ventilation, placing the tip of the endotracheal tube distal to the fistula allows effective management of the airway. In case of extensive injury, surgical repair of the fistula on both the esophageal and tracheal side with interposition of a sternocleidomastoid flap is mandatory [37, 38].

**Table 56.1** Criteria for appropriate non-operative management in esophageal perforation

1. Contained mediastinal leak
2. Free flow of contrast back into esophagus
3. No or minimal symptoms
4. No evidence of sepsis
5. No or minimal mediastinal contamination
6. No gross pleural contamination
7. No pre-existing esophageal disease
8. Provision of enteral nutrition
9. Multidisciplinary care
10. Low threshold for aggressive intervention

Thoracic esophageal perforations require a multidisciplinary assessment and an individualized approach by considering patient's characteristics, comorbidities, etiology of perforation, site and size of perforation, degree of mediastinal/pleural contamination, evidence of sepsis, and PSS. The priority is to achieve a wide debridement of the mediastinum and pleural cavity in order to control infection and restore respiratory function and ensure an adequate nutritional support. Conservative treatment is feasible in highly selected patients with a small and contained leak and no evidence of sepsis. All other patients should undergo operative management, consisting of percutaneous or thoracoscopic drainage, primary endoscopic management, primary surgical repair, esophagectomy, or esophageal diversion [39, 40] (Flowchart 56.1).

Endoscopic management of esophageal perforation includes partially or totally covered stents, over the scope clips (Ovesco) [41], or endoluminal vacuum therapy [42]. Endoscopic treatment remains the first-choice approach for closing esophageal perforations that occur and are recognized during an endoscopic procedure. Initial endoscopic treatment with stents or clips is also

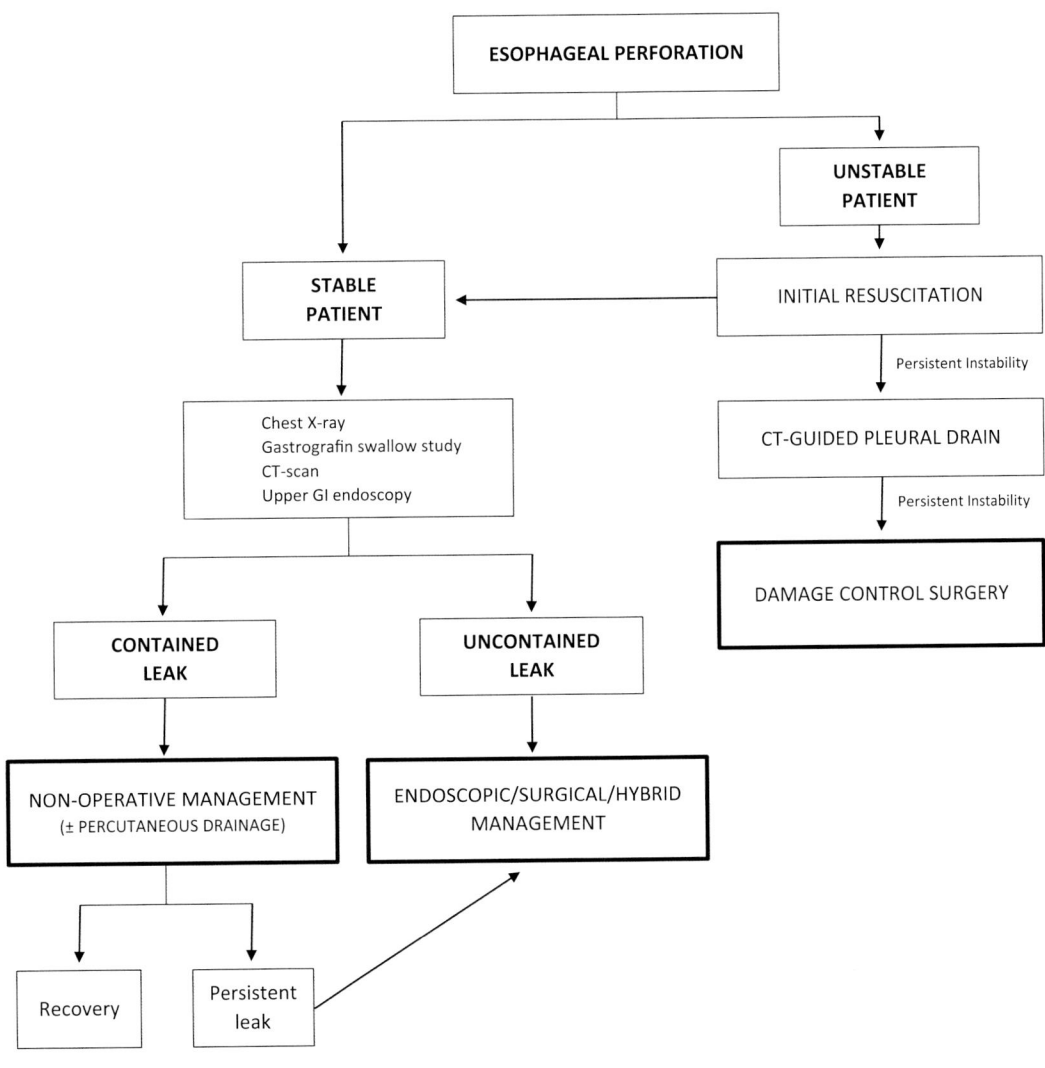

**Flowchart 56.1** Emergency management algorithm for esophageal perforation

reasonable in patients diagnosed early, with small leak and minimal periesophageal contamination, and in those who are unfit for surgery [43].

Primary surgical repair is traditionally accomplished via a right thoracotomy through the fifth intercostal space (middle third perforations) or a left thoracotomy in the seventh intercostal space (lower third perforations). Perforations of the esophagogastric junction can be accessed by either a left thoracotomy or an upper midline laparotomy. Primary repair should be preferred whenever possible in patients with Boerhaave's perforation. Intraoperative endoscopy can help for the assessment of mucosal viability and precise localization of the mucosal defect, which is usually longer than the muscular tear. The tear should be repaired with a double-layer suture (Fig. 56.2) that is buttressed with a gastric fundic patch, a pedicled intercostal muscle flap, or a pericardial/pleural/diaphragmatic flap. In patients diagnosed at an early stage, a minimally invasive thoracoscopic approach may be the preferred option, since it is better tolerated than open surgery and allows effective lavage/drainage and direct repair. When the distance of the perforation from the cardia is <5 cm, the leak is contained within the mediastinum, and there is no hemodynamic instability or signs of severe sepsis, a laparoscopic approach is also feasible (Fig. 56.3). Alternative options for primary suture repair in selected cases are esophagectomy, T-tube drainage to establish a controlled salivary fistula, esophageal exclusion and diversion, temporary exclusion without diversion [44], or a Thal repair [45]. Enteral nutrition through a nasogastric tube or jejunostomy should be provided to all these patients (Flowchart 56.2).

In individuals who present emergently with incarcerated hiatal hernia, decompression of the intrathoracic stomach by nasogastric tube or endoscopy should be a priority in stable patients. Often, it is impossible to blindly insert a nasogastric tube due to angulation of the distal esophagus. Endoscopy may be safely performed even in critically ill and frail patients when there are doubts about viability of the stomach [46]. In

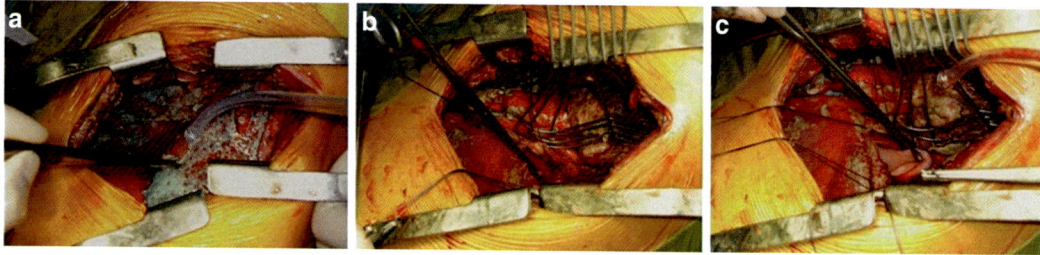

**Fig. 56.2** Trans-thoracic repair of Boerhaave's perforation: lung decortication (**a**), suture repair (**b**), and fundic patch (**c**)

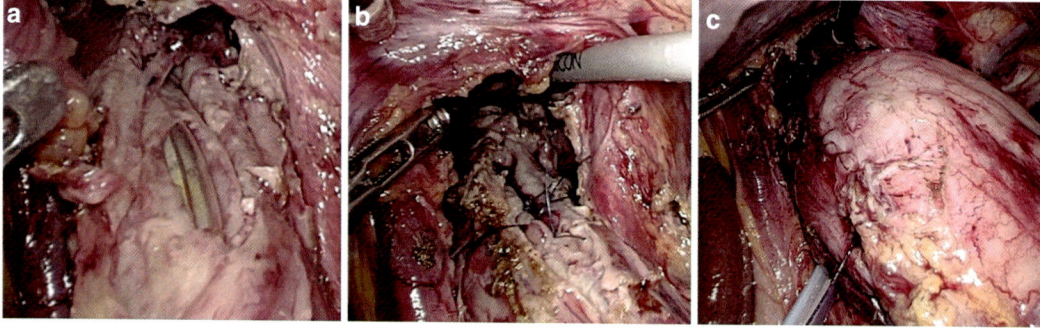

**Fig. 56.3** Laparoscopic approach for Boerhaave's perforation: nasogastric tube visible through the esophageal tear (**a**); double-layer suture repair of the esophagus (**b**); suture repair buttressed with a fundic patch (**c**)

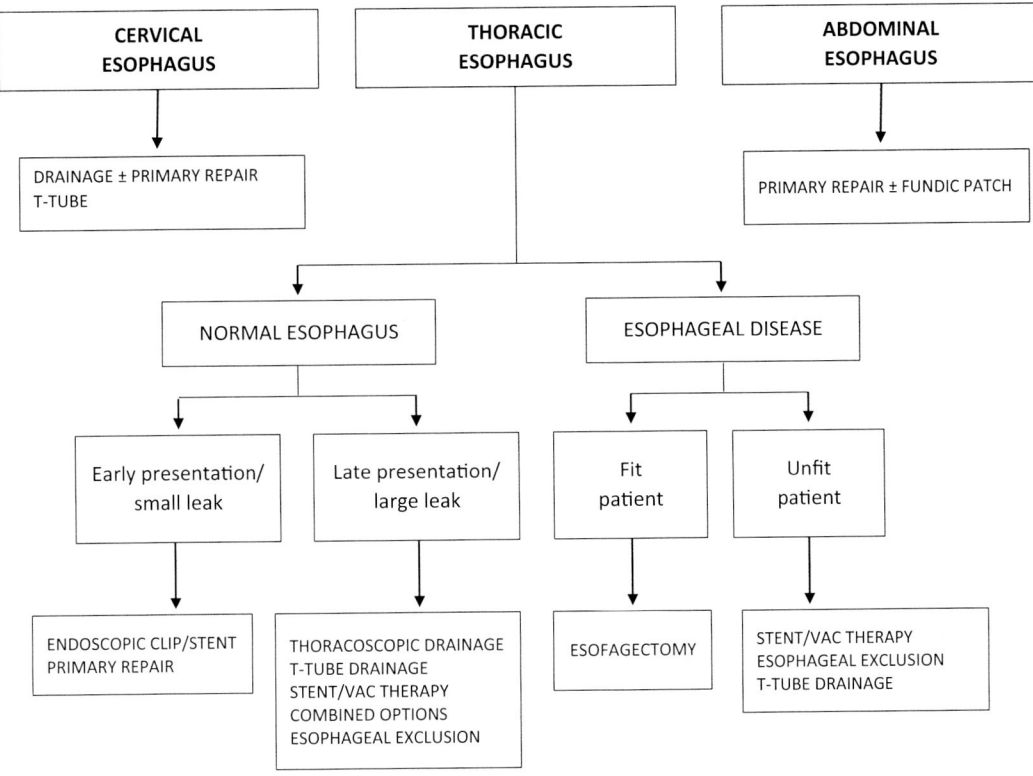

**Flowchart 56.2** Management algorithm for esophageal perforation according to site of injury

high-risk patients, endoscopic unfolding of the volvulus by a J or alpha loop maneuver and intra-abdominal repositioning of the stomach are occasionally feasible in the absence of gastric wall ischemia or perforation. However, this maneuver requires a skilled endoscopist and carries a risk of perforation, and recurrence is common [47]. An anterior gastropexy with or without percutaneous endoscopic gastrostomy should be considered in such circumstances to decrease the incidence of recurrent volvulus [48]. In stable patients, acute clinical presentations of paraesophageal hernia may be dealt with laparoscopy as an elective or semi-elective procedure, even in patients requiring wedge/sleeve gastric resections or segmental bowel resections. However, emergent situations in critically ill patients with sepsis and evidence of severe gastric ischemia or perforation do require an open approach. Damage control with total gastrectomy and exclusion diversion is necessary only in the occasional patient presenting with gastric gangrene [49].

### 56.3.2 Foreign Body Ingestion

Endoscopy is the recommended upfront treatment of impacted esophageal foreign bodies. Due to the risk of aspiration and/or perforation, flexible endoscopy should be performed within 2 h in patients with complete esophageal obstruction from food bolus and within 6 h in case of sharp objects, disc batteries, and magnets. Sharp or pointed objects that impacted on the upper esophagus can be difficult to remove and may require an overtube to reduce the trauma of repeated passages of the endoscope through the pharyngoesophageal junction. Manipulation is also necessary to grasp the blunt end of the foreign body first in order to avoid mucosal lacerations. In these patients, flexible and rigid endoscopy should be considered crossover techniques. Use of a bi-valved Weerda diverticuloscope under narcosis may be required and provides more working space and easier retrieval of large foreign bodies [50]. For other types of

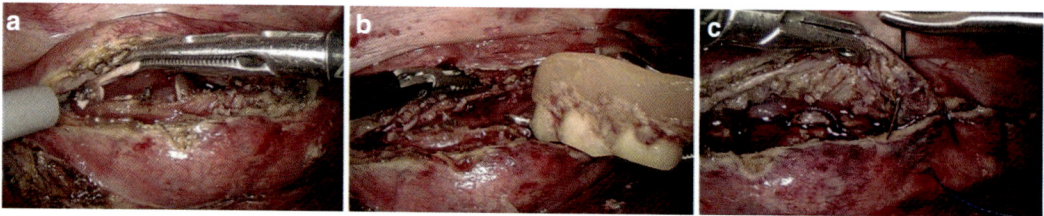

**Fig. 56.4** Thoracoscopic removal of foreign body (denture) impacted in the thoracic esophagus: removal after careful management of the clasps (**a**, **b**) and double-layer suture repair (**c**)

esophageal foreign bodies without complete obstruction, endoscopy should be performed within 24 h from ingestion. A concomitant assessment of underlying disease (hiatus hernia, peptic stricture, Schatzki ring, eosinophilic esophagitis, and tumors) possibly causing recurrent impaction is recommended. Food bolus obstruction can be successfully treated in most patients by air insufflation and gentle instrumental pushing after ensuring that there is no distal obstruction. In some circumstances, passage of a balloon catheter and a combination of other instruments (grasping forceps, snares, baskets, etc.) can help to disimpact the bolus, which can then be retrieved, especially if meat or fish bony components are present.

Surgical therapy is rarely required but remains mandatory for irretrievable foreign bodies, perforation, or foreign bodies in close proximity to the aorta or the airways. The surgical approach depends on the site of foreign body impaction and patient's comorbidities. Esophagotomy and foreign body extraction can be safely performed via left cervicotomy or via right thoracotomy or thoracoscopy [51] (Fig. 56.4).

### 56.3.3 Complications of Esophageal Surgery

Leakage of a cervical anastomosis has usually a benign course but should be promptly drained at bedside regardless of the presence of a frank neck abscess to allow open-wound treatment. Intrathoracic anastomotic leaks and gangrene of the gastric conduit are the most feared complications of esophagectomy. In case of early and large dehiscence, surgical exploration is indicated to repair or redo the anastomosis or to explant the gastric conduit if trans-mural ischemia is found. A more conservative approach using endoluminal vacuum therapy [52] or stenting combined with antibiotic therapy and nutritional support through nasojejunal tube or jejunostomy is reasonable in stable patients [53, 54] (Fig. 56.5). If necessary, ultrasound/CT scan-guided percutaneous drainage of mediastinal or pleural collections or videothoracoscopic lavage and drainage should be performed to minimize the risk of sepsis. Gangrene of the gastric conduit is a catastrophic complication requiring takedown of the stomach followed by cervical esophagostomy and feeding jejunostomy. The continuity of the alimentary tract can be restored at a later date by a colonic interposition.

Mechanical obstruction of the gastric conduit due to narrowing at the level of the crura or twisting of the stomach after intrathoracic pull-up requires a trans-abdominal and/or trans-thoracic approach to relieve the crura obstruction and/or to remodel the gastric conduit. Instead, patients with gastroparesis and pylorospasm may benefit from endoscopic pneumatic dilation.

Chylothorax may occur after trans-thoracic or trans-hiatal esophagectomy. After the diagnosis, the patient should receive total parenteral nutrition. Persistent and sustained (>500 mL/day) chyle leak requires trans-thoracic ligature of the thoracic duct via a right thoracoscopic approach. Administration of cream through a nasogastric tube 6 h before surgery is useful for easier identification of chyle leakage [55].

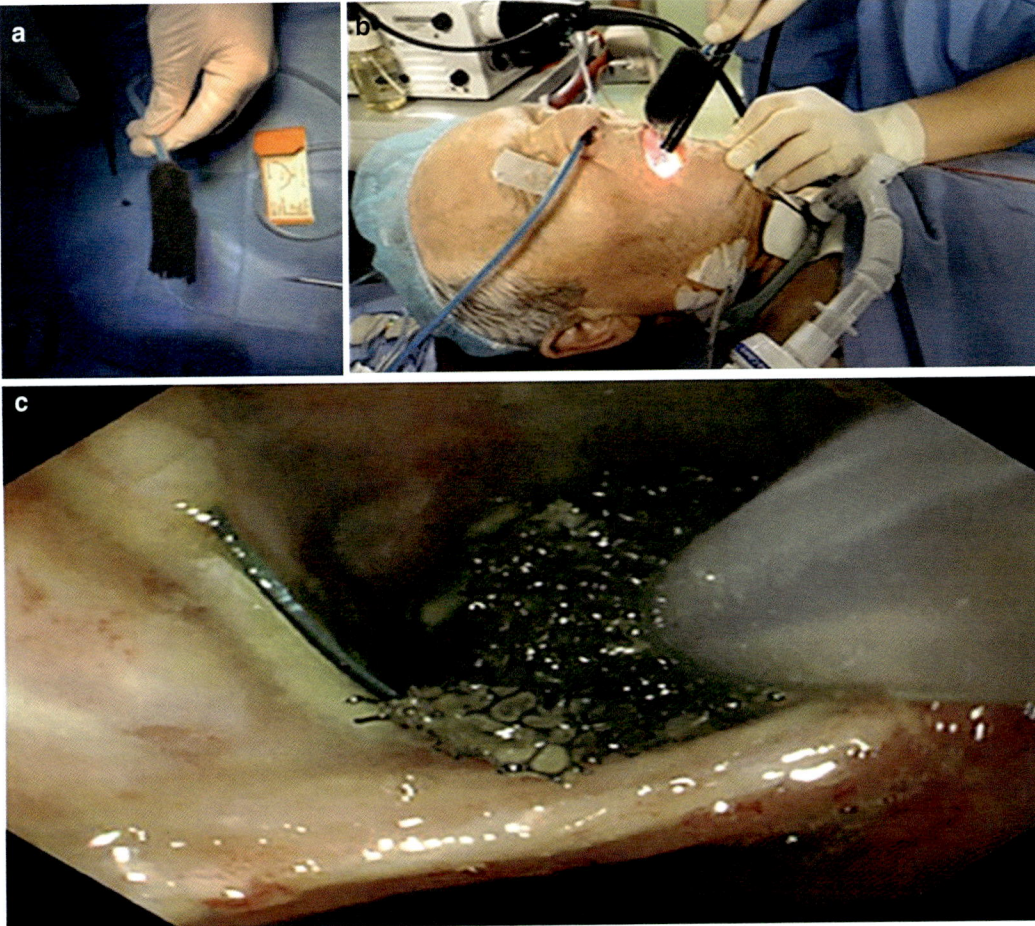

**Fig. 56.5** Endo-VAC therapy for esophagogastric anastomotic leakage: the polyurethane sponge is secured to a nasogastric tube (**a**); the sponge is advanced into the esophageal lumen under endoscopic guidance (**b**); and positioned across the anastomosis (**c**)

## 56.3.4 Descending Necrotizing Mediastinitis

Most cases of early diagnosed descending necrotizing mediastinitis that are limited to the upper mediastinal compartment can be adequately drained through a left cervical incision along the anterior border of the sternocleidomastoid muscle. In more advanced stages, a right-sided videothoracoscopy is the procedure of choice and can be performed either in the left-lateral or prone decubitus even in high-risk patients. Opening the mediastinal pleural reflection from above the arch of the azygos vein to the diaphragm allows extensive drainage of abscess loculations and debridement of necrotic tissue. Serial transcervical drainage and trans-thoracic debridement may be necessary for some patients with persistent/recurrent purulent discharge or sepsis.

## 56.3.5 Esophageal Bleeding

Most patients with esophageal bleeding can be treated non-operatively, except those presenting with tamponated aortoesophageal fistula during a free time interval before fetal exsanguination. In such circumstances and in fit patients, Thoracic

Endo-Vascular Repair (TEVAR) is the most common therapeutic option and a valid emergency alternative to direct open surgical aneurysm repair [56].

Management of variceal bleeding is aimed to control hemorrhage, prevent rebleeding, infection, and hepatorenal syndrome. Treatment of suspected acute variceal bleeding is based on appropriate volume resuscitation and a restrictive transfusion threshold of 7 g/dL, except for patients with massive hemorrhage or coronary heart disease. Endotracheal intubation and administration of vasoactive drugs (terlipressin and somatostatin), antibiotics, and proton-pump inhibitors represent the first-line approach. Once the patient is hemodynamically stable, upper gastrointestinal endoscopy should be performed within 12 h to confirm the source of bleeding. It is also useful to obtain an abdominal Doppler ultrasound to rule out portal vein thrombosis that may impact future treatment. Variceal band ligation combined with vasoactive drugs is the current standard of care. In patients with refractory hemorrhage, rescue treatment with balloon tamponade using a Sengstaken–Blakemore tube or a removable, self-expanding, and covered esophageal stent (SX-ELLA Danis) is recommended [57]. Balloon tamponade should be maintained for no longer than 24 h due to possible serious adverse events, such as esophageal ulceration, esophageal rupture, and aspiration pneumonia. The esophageal stent can remain in place for 1 week before removal. Further rescue treatments to be considered for refractory variceal bleeding are trans-jugular intrahepatic portosystemic shunt (TIPS) or a surgical portocaval anastomosis.

- Nil per os, parenteral/enteral nutrition, broad-spectrum antibiotics and fungal coverage (in immunocompromised patients) proton-pump inhibitors, nasogastric tube placement, and percutaneous drainage of chest air-fluid levels/periesophageal collections represent the mainstay of non-operative management in stable patients with contained esophageal perforation.
- Prompt neck drainage can prevent spread of infection to the posterior mediastinum in patients with cervical esophageal perforation.

**Don'ts**
- Whenever possible, avoid esophagectomy in patients with otherwise normal esophagus and in those with Boerhaave's perforation.
- Patients with intramural/dissecting esophageal hematoma or acute esophageal necrosis should be treated conservatively.
- Be aware of the risk of massive hematemesis from aortoesophageal fistula during endoscopic examination in patients with history of aortic stent or impacted sharp foreign bodies.

**Dos and Don'ts**
**Dos**
- Keep a high index of suspicion, especially after difficult or operative endoscopic procedures, and do not hesitate to order a gastrografin swallow study or computed tomography with intravenous and oral contrast. Early systemic signs of esophageal perforation include tachycardia and tachypnea, but fever may be delayed.

**Take-Home Messages**
- Management of esophageal emergencies should be multidisciplinary and involve a team of expert physicians.
- Early diagnosis and individualized management of perforations is crucial and may increase the chance of esophageal preservation.
- Non-operative management is a reasonable option in selected patients, but a low threshold of alert and an aggressive policy of percutaneous drainage are necessary to control sepsis.

- Minimally invasive and hybrid treatments can effectively replace open surgical approach in contained thoracic perforations.
- Prevention, early recognition, and a proactive attitude are the keys for successful treatment of esophageal emergencies. Changing the management algorithm with a more liberal use of radiological and endoscopic imaging and hybrid therapeutic approaches can lower the incidence of sepsis and improve overall outcomes.

## Multiple Choice Questions

1. **Which is the most common type of esophageal perforation?**
   A. External trauma
   B. Boerhaave's syndrome
   C. Instrumental
   D. Foreign body

2. **Perforation after balloon dilatation for achalasia usually requires:**
   A. Trans-hiatal esophagectomy
   B. Emergency Heller's myotomy and Dor fundoplication
   C. Trans-esophageal pigtail drainage
   D. None of the above

3. **Which is the approach of choice for a sharp foreign object (denture) impacted in the upper thoracic esophagus for longer than 24 h?**
   A. Flexible endoscopic removal under mild sedation
   B. Esophagotomy and removal through left thoracotomy
   C. Esophagotomy and removal through left cervicotomy
   D. Esophagotomy and removal through right thoracoscopy

## References

1. Singer M, Deutschman CS, Seymour CW. The third international consensus definitions for sepsis and septic shock (sepsis-3). JAMA. 2016;315(8):801–10.
2. van der Steen M, Verhage R, Singer M, Pickkers P. Overview of the third international consensus definitions for sepsis and shock (sepsis-3). Neth J Crit Care. 2016;24:6–9.
3. Wahed S, Dent B, Jones R, Griffrin SM. Spectrum of oesophageal perforations and their influence on management. Br J Surg. 2014;101:e156–62.
4. Axtell AL, Gaissert HA, Morse CR, et al. Management and outcomes of esophageal perforation. Dis Esophagus. 2021;35(1):doab039. https://doi.org/10.1093/dote/doab039.
5. Wu JT, Mattox KL, Wall MJ. Esophageal perforations: new perspectives and treatment paradigms. J Trauma. 2007;63:1173–84.
6. Korn O, Onate JC, Lopez R. Anatomy of the Boerhave syndrome. Surgery. 2007;141:222–8.
7. Griffin SM, Lamb PJ, Shenfine J, et al. Spontaneous rupture of the oesophagus. Br J Surg. 2008;95:115–20.
8. Schweigert M, Sousa HS, Solymosi N, et al. Spotlight on esophageal perforation: a multinational study using the Pittsburgh esophageal perforation severity scoring system. J Thorac Cardiovasc Surg. 2016;151(4):1002–9.
9. Wigley C, Athanasiou A, Bhatti A, et al. Does the Pittsburgh Severity Score predict outcome in esophageal perforation? Dis Esophagus. 2019;32(2):doy109. https://doi.org/10.1093/dote/doy109.
10. Chirica M, Kelly MD, Siboni S, et al. Esophageal emergencies: WSES guidelines. World J Emerg Surg. 2019;14(1):20. https://doi.org/10.1186/s13017-019-0245-2.20.
11. Hill LD. Incarcerated paraesophageal hernia. A surgical emergency. Am J Surg. 1973;126:286–91.
12. Bonavina L, Inaba K. Incarcerated hiatal hernia. In: Galante J, Coimbra R, editors. Thoracic surgery for the acute surgeon, hot topics in acute care surgery and trauma. Cham: Springer Nature; 2021. p. 43–51.
13. Sinha R. Naclerio's V sign. Radiology. 2007;245:296–7.
14. Aiolfi A, Ferrari D, Riva CG, Toti F, Bonitta GL, Bonavina L. Esophageal foreign bodies in adults: systematic review of the literature. Scand J Gastroenterol. 2018;53(10–11):1171–8. https://doi.org/10.1080/00365521.2018.1526317.
15. Ferrari D, Siboni S, Riva CG, et al. Esophageal foreign bodies: observational cohort study and factors associated with recurrent impaction. Eur J Gastroenterol Hepatol. 2020;32(7):827–31.
16. Verstegen MHP, Bouwense SAW, van Workum F, et al. Management of intrathoracic and cervical anastomotic leakage after esophagectomy for esophageal cancer: a

systematic review. World J Emerg Surg. 2019;14:17. https://doi.org/10.1186/s13017-019-0235-4.
17. Brenkman HJF, Parry K, Noble F, et al. Hiatal hernia after esophagectomy for cancer. Ann Thorac Surg. 2017;103:1055–62.
18. Lagarde SM, Omloo JMT, de Jong K, et al. Incidence and management of chyle leakage after esophagectomy. Ann Thorac Surg. 2005;80:449–54.
19. Asti E, Bonitta G, Melloni M, et al. Utility of C-reactive protein as predictive biomarker of anastomotic leak after minimally invasive esophagectomy. Langenbecks Arch Surg. 2018;403:235–44. https://doi.org/10.1007/s00423-018-1663-4.
20. Dindo D, Demartines N, Clavien PA. Classification of surgical complications. A new proposal with evaluation in a cohort of 6336 patients and results of a survey. Ann Surg. 2004;240(2):205–13.
21. Low DE, Alderson D, Cecconello I, et al. International consensus on standardization of data collection for complications associated with esophagectomy: esophagectomy complications consensus group (ECCG). Ann Surg. 2015;262:286–94.
22. Ridder GJ, Maier W, Kinzer S, et al. Descending necrotizing mediastinitis. Contemporary trends in etiology, diagnosis, management, and outcome. Ann Surg. 2010;251(3):528–34.
23. Wangrattanapranee P, Khrucharoen U, Jensen DM, et al. Severe upper gastrointestinal hemorrhage caused by reflux esophagitis. Dig Dis Sci. 2022;67:159–69.
24. Byrne JJ, Moran JM. The Mallory–Weiss syndrome. N Engl J Med. 1965;272:398–400.
25. Gurvits GE, Cherian K, Shami MF, et al. Black esophagus: new insights and multicenter international experience in 2014. Dig Dis Sci. 2015;60:444–53.
26. Hollander JE, Quick J. Aortoesophageal fistula: a comprehensive review of the literature. Am J Med. 1991;91:279–87.
27. Grimaldi S, Milito P, Lovece A, et al. Dysphagia aortica. Eur Surg. 2021;54:228–39. https://doi.org/10.1007/s10353-021-00741-9.
28. Karstensen JG, Ebigbo A, Bhat P, et al. Endoscopic treatment of variceal upper gastrointestinal bleeding: European Society of Gastrointestinal Endoscopy (ESGE) Cascade guideline. Endosc Intern Open. 2020;8:E990–7.
29. Kuppusamy M, Hubka M, Felisky CD, et al. Evolving management strategies in esophageal perforation: surgeons using nonoperative techniques to improve outcomes. J Am Coll Surg. 2011;213:164–72.
30. Biancari F, Saarnio J, Mennander A, et al. Outcome of patients with esophageal perforations: a multicenter study. World J Surg. 2014;38(4):902–9.
31. Biancari F, Gudbjartsson T, Mennander A, et al. Treatment of esophageal perforation in octogenarians: a multicenter study. Dis Esophagus. 2014;27(8):715–8.
32. Ali JT, Rice RD, David EA, et al. Perforated esophageal intervention focus (PERF) study: a multicenter examination of contemporary treatment. Dis Esophagus. 2017;30:1–8.
33. Altorjay A, Kiss J, Voros A, et al. Nonoperative management of esophageal perforations. Is it justified? Ann Surg. 1997;225(4):415–21.
34. Sudarshan M, Elharram M, Spicer J, et al. Management of esophageal perforation in the endoscopic era: is operative repair still relevant? Surgery. 2016;160(4):1104–10.
35. Abbas G, Schuchert MJ, Pettiford BL, et al. Contemporaneous management of esophageal perforation. Surgery. 2009;146(4):749–55.
36. Ferguson MK, Reeder LB, Olak J. Outcome after failed initial therapy for rupture of the esophagus or intrathoracic stomach. J Gastrointest Surg. 1997;1:34–9.
37. Conti M, Pougeoise M, Wurtz A, et al. Management of postintubation tracheobronchial ruptures. Chest. 2006;130:412–8.
38. Foroulis CN, Nana C, Kleontas A, et al. Repair of post-intubation tracheoesophageal fistulas through the left pre-sternocleidomastoid approach: a recent case-series of 13 patients. J Thorac Dis. 2015;7(S1):S20–6.
39. Sdralis EIK, Petousis S, Rashid F, et al. Epidemiology, diagnosis and management of esophageal perforations: systematic review. Dis Esophagus. 2017;30(8):1–6.
40. Tang A, Ahmad U, Raja S, et al. Repair, reconstruct, or divert. The fate of the perforated esophagus. Ann Surg. 2021;274:e417–24.
41. Bona D, Aiolfi A, Rausa E, Bonavina L. Management of Boerhaave's syndrome with an over-the-scope-clip. Eur J Cardio Thorac Surg. 2013;45:752–4.
42. Moore CB, Almoghrabi O, Hofstetter W, Veeramachanen N. Endoluminal wound vac: an evolving role in treatment of esophageal perforation. J Vis Surg. 2020;6:43.
43. Vermeulen BD, Van der Leeden B, Ali JT, et al. Early diagnosis is associated with improved clinical outcomes in benign esophageal perforation: an individual patient data meta-analysis. Surg Endosc. 2020;35:3492–505. https://doi.org/10.1007/s00464-020-07806-y.
44. Bardini R, Bonavina L, Pavanello M, Asolati M, Peracchia A. Temporary double exclusion of the perforated esophagus using absorbable staples. Ann Thorac Surg. 1992;54:1165–7.
45. Thal AP, Hatafuku T. Improved operation for esophageal rupture. JAMA. 1964;188:126–8.
46. Bawahab M, Mitchell P, Church N, Debru E. Management of acute paraesophageal hernia. Surg Endosc. 2009;23:255–9.
47. Tsang TK, Walker R, Yu DJ. Endoscopic reduction of gastric volvulus: the alpha-loop maneuver. Gastrointest Endosc. 1995;42:244–8.
48. Kercher KW, Matthews BD, Ponsky JL, et al. Minimally invasive management of paraesophageal herniation in the high-risk surgical patient. Am J Surg. 2001;182:510–4.
49. Light D, Links D, Griffin M. The threatened stomach: management of the acute gastric volvulus. Surg Endosc. 2016;30:1847–52.

50. Ferrari D, Aiolfi A, Bonitta G, et al. Flexible versus rigid endoscopy in the management of esophageal foreign body impaction: systematic review and meta-analysis. World J Emerg Surg. 2018;13:42.
51. Bonavina L, Aiolfi A, Siboni S, Rausa E. Thoracoscopic removal of dental prosthesis impacted in the upper thoracic esophagus. World J Emerg Surg. 2014;9:5.
52. Rausa E, Asti E, Aiolfi A, Bianco F, Bonitta G, Bonavina L. Comparison of endoscopic vacuum therapy versus endoscopic stenting for esophageal leaks: systematic review and meta-analysis. Dis Esophagus. 2018;31(11):doy060. https://doi.org/10.1093/dote/doy060.
53. Van Boeckel PGA, Sijbring A, Vleggaar FP, Siersema PD. Systematic review: temporary stent placement for benign rupture or anastomotic leak of the oesophagus. Aliment Pharmacol Ther. 2011;33(12):1292–301.
54. Dent B, Griffin SM, Jones R, Wahed S, Immanuel A, Hayes N. Management and outcomes of anastomotic leaks after oesophagectomy. Br J Surg. 2016;103:1033–8.
55. Bonavina L, Saino G, Bona D, et al. Thoracoscopic management of chylothorax complicating esophagectomy. J Laparoendosc Surg Adv Surg Tech. 2001;11(6):367–9.
56. Chiesa R, Melissano G, Marone EM, et al. Endovascular treatment of aortoesophageal and aortobronchial fistulae. J Vasc Surg. 2010;51:1195–202.
57. Escorsell A, Pavel O, Cardenas A, et al. Esophageal balloon tamponade versus esophageal stent in controlling acute refractory variceal bleeding: a multicenter randomized controlled trial. Hepatology. 2016;63:1957–67.

## Further Reading

Cameron JL, Kieffer RF, Hendrix TR, et al. Selective non operative management of contained intrathoracic esophageal disruptions. Ann Thorac Surg. 1979;27:404–8.

Chirica M, Kelly MD, Siboni S, et al. Esophageal emergencies: WSES guidelines. World J Emerg Surg. 2019;14:26. https://doi.org/10.1186/s13017-019-0245-2.20.

Griffin SM, Lamb PJ, Shenfine J, et al. Spontaneous rupture of the oesophagus. Br J Surg. 2008;95:115–20.

Kuppusamy M, Hubka M, Felisky CD, et al. Evolving management strategies in esophageal perforation: surgeons using nonoperative techniques to improve outcomes. J Am Coll Surg. 2011;213:164–72.

# Esophageal Trauma

**57**

Michael D. Kelly and Mircea Chirica

## 57.1 Introduction

> **Learning Goals**
> - Improve the practitioner's ability to diagnose and manage patients in the initial phase of esophageal trauma.
> - To maintain a high degree of suspicion for rare esophageal injury in blunt trauma.

Injury to the esophagus by external trauma is a rare but potentially life-threatening condition. The esophagus traverses three body compartments the neck, chest, and abdomen and is surrounded by vital structures. Therefore, injuries may present with wide ranging symptomatology and management may be complex. Despite the relative rarity, clinicians from multiple specialties including emergency medicine, general, and trauma surgery may be called upon to diagnosis and management this condition. Because of the low incidence of esophageal injuries, high-quality evidence is lacking and the majority of publications in the literature are case reports, case series, or literature reviews.

Traumatic injury of the esophagus (TIE) accounts for less than 15% of all esophageal injuries [1, 2] and was recorded in less than 1% of patients managed in 20 Level I trauma centers across a 6-year period [3]. They are classified according to the anatomic location being cervical, thoracic, or abdominal and according to the mechanism of injury being penetrating or blunt trauma. Due to the anatomical location of the esophagus, they are usually associated with injuries to airway, lungs, major vascular structures and heart, spinal cord airway, and abdominal viscera and this worsens the prognosis [4]. TIE occurs mostly in young males and the most frequently encountered presentation is that of a penetrating injury to the cervical esophagus. Mortality of TIE is high with most deaths occurring within 24 h because of severe associated injuries [2]. Trauma to the thoracic esophagus is especially associated with high mortality rates [5]. Early diagnosis of TIE is mandatory to improve outcomes and requires a high level of suspicion.

M. D. Kelly
Medalliance, Albury, NSW, Australia
e-mail: mk@mdkelly.com

M. Chirica (✉)
Service de Chirurgie Digestive, Centre Hospitalier Universitaire Grenoble Alpes, La Tronche, France

## 57.1.1 Epidemiology and Etiology

External TIE is a rare condition. The literature overall confirms that penetrating injuries are more common than blunt injuries [6]. However, the heterogeneity of the condition will vary this ratio between different societies and trauma systems. In the United States of America about 90% are penetrating injuries and the most common penetrating etiology is gunshot wound (75%), followed by stab wounds [4, 6]. In a large prospective trauma study of esophageal perforations from Scotland, blunt trauma (57%) was slightly more common than penetrating injuries [7].

The mechanism whereby blunt chest or upper abdominal trauma leads to esophageal rupture is conjectural. Some authors postulate pressurization of air within the esophagus with closed sphincters. An unusual cause of blunt TIE is barotrauma by external air-blast injuries [8].

## 57.1.2 Classification

Injuries may be easily and usefully classified as either blunt or penetrating and involving the cervical, thoracic, or abdominal segment of the esophagus. The American Association for the Surgery of Trauma injury scale is shown in Table 57.1 [9].

**Table 57.1** Esophagus injury scale

| Grade[a] | Description of injury | ICD-9 | AIS-90 |
|---|---|---|---|
| I | Contusion/hematoma | 862.22/0.32 | 2 |
|   | Partial thickness laceration | 862.22/0.32 | 3 |
| II | Laceration <50% circumference | 862.22/0.32 | 4 |
| III | Laceration >50% circumference | 862.22/0.32 | 4 |
| IV | Segmental loss or devascularization <2 cm | 862.22/0.32 | 5 |
| V | Segmental loss or devascularization >2 cm | 862.22/0.32 | 5 |

[a]Advance one grade for multiple lesions up to grade III

## 57.2 Diagnosis

### 57.2.1 Clinical Presentation and Investigations

There are no specific symptoms or pathognomonic signs of TIE. Physical examination is not reliable for early diagnosis of TIE. The presentation will depend the mechanism of injury, whether blunt or penetrating and the site of injury being neck or chest. Symptoms such as chest pain, dyspnea, subcutaneous emphysema, and dysphagia may be present. Symptoms related to damage of neighboring vital structures (large vessels, heart, lungs) usually hide more discreet manifestations due to esophageal involvement.

Laboratory studies are not useful for early diagnosis of TIE; however, imaging studies are critically important. Chest X-ray may show pneumomediastinum or soft tissue air in the neck but is not specific for TIE. Contrast-enhanced computed tomography (CT) and CT esophagography should be performed in hemodynamically stable patients with suspicion of TIE [10]. Contrast-enhanced CT is useful to identify associated injuries and can provide important information regarding the trajectory of the penetrating agent (bullet, stab wound). CT may also show indirect signs of esophageal perforation (paraesophageal collections, free air, pleural effusions).

Formal contrast swallow esophagogram requires a stable and cooperative patient and is not suitable in many trauma scenarios. Usually, a water-soluble agent such as gastrografin is used and barium is avoided. CT esophagram has largely replaced contrast swallows but can miss up to 30% of small esophageal perforations [10]. One major drawback of esophageal opacification techniques is the fact that swallowing is only possible in patients who are well and nasogastric tube-administered contrast may miss esophageal perforations.

Flexible endoscopy should be performed as an adjunct to CT in patients with suspected TIE. Endoscopy provides direct visualization of the injury site and may be useful in patients with equivocal CT findings. Other advantages include easy availability in most trauma centers and the possibility of use in intubated and unstable patients. In combination with contrast-enhanced CT, flexible endoscopy allows the accurate diagnosis of TIE in more than 90% of cases [10]. The use of endoscopy has been shown to alter surgical management in 69% of patients [10]. In unstable patients rushed to the operative room, intraoperative endoscopy can be employed to rule out esophageal perforation. Under such circumstances triple endoscopy (esophagoscopy, laryngoscopy, and bronchoscopy) is indicated as injury of one of these structures should raise the suspicion of damage to the adjacent organs. There is the theoretical risk of insufflation during the procedure promoting mediastinal contamination or increasing the size of the perforation and "air embolism"; for this reason low-flow insufflation and use of $CO_2$ rather than air are recommended [10].

An esophagogram should be considered for patients suffering from external air-blast injury who presented symptoms of chest pain, dyspnea, or subcutaneous emphysema.

It is mandatory to diagnose, define the location and the extent of esophageal damage; any delay in the management of overlooked esophageal perforations can impair patient outcomes. It is also essential to detect injury to adjacent structures, such as the trachea, and a delay in diagnosis of 24 h are associated with a poor outcome, associated injuries that may affect management and survival [10].

## 57.3 Medical Treatment

Patients with TIE undergo non-operative management (NOM) if they have no esophageal perforation. Patients with esophageal perforation can be offered NOM in certain circumstances. Again, the location and mechanism of injury is so variable that definitive recommendations cannot be made. As a general rule penetrating injuries by their nature will require exploration.

NOM for TIE should be offered only if intense monitoring in an intensive care unit setting, surgical expertise and interventional radiology skills are available. NOM requires keeping patients nil by mouth, use of broad spectrum antibiotic coverage, proton pump inhibitor, placement of a nasogastric tube, and early introduction of nutritional support via the use of either enteral feeding or total parenteral nutrition. Additional measures such as percutaneous radiological drainage of peri-esophageal or pleural collections may be needed in select cases.

The use of an endoscopically placed self-expanding metal stent (SEMS) (fully covered, removable) to cover a perforation due to external TIE is an attractive option. Stent migration is a real issue when these stents are used for non-malignant conditions but they certainly have a role in TIE where primary repair has failed [11].

## 57.4 Surgical Treatment

Surgical exploration is performed in most TIE patients and is dictated by damage to adjacent structures. Management is conditioned by location of the perforation, the tissue injury itself and any concomitant injuries. The majority of cases are amenable to primary repair with flap re-enforcement. Other principles include adequate external drainage of the area and around the repair, decompression of the esophagus and stomach (via nasogastric tube or gastrostomy tube), and distal enteral nutrition (feeding jejunostomy) [6, 10].

Other surgical procedures include simple drainage, esophageal exclusion with esophagostomy, gastrostomy or jejunostomy, and esophagectomy followed by esophageal reconstruction.

Patients with TIE should undergo immediate surgical treatment if they have hemodynamic instability, obvious non-contained extravasation of contrast material, or systemic signs of sepsis. In these patients, surgery should be undertaken as soon as possible; a large body of literature shows that delayed (>24 h) surgical management of esophageal perforation results in increased morbidity and mortality rates. Recent studies suggest that while delayed surgical treatment does not affect mortality rates, it did nevertheless reduce the odds of successful primary esophageal repair. If emergency surgery was prompted by associated injuries an esophageal perforation should be sought intraoperatively by direct inspection, intraluminal instillation of dye (methylene blue), or endoscopy [10].

Delayed surgical treatment is indicated in patients with TIE-related esophageal perforation in whom primary repair of the esophagus was not feasible or had failed. TIE patients with esophageal perforation who are ineligible for primary repair undergo either esophageal resection or exclusion–diversion procedures. If they survive, patients require a second procedure to restore continuity of the gastrointestinal tract. Esophageal reconstruction by colon or gastric interposition is usually scheduled 6–12 months after TIE [6, 10].

For TIE located in the neck, direct repair of the esophageal perforation should be attempted whenever feasible. If direct repair is not feasible, esophagostomy and cervical drainage are recommended [10, 12]. Appropriate treatment of associated injuries (tracheal, carotid) is essential under these circumstances as these can pose specific problems (tracheo-esophageal fistula, postoperative carotid disruption). Avoiding formation of a tracheotomy, buttressing repairs with viable tissue, and drainage through the contralateral neck have all been recommended to prevent such complications [10].

Operative repair is the treatment of choice for TIE with free perforation of the thoracic esophagus. If primary repair is not feasible, diversion, exclusion, or resection of the thoracic esophagus should be performed. Usually a right posterolateral thoracotomy will be used although distal lesions may be approached from the abdomen or the left chest. Damage to the spine, the great vessels, the heart, and the lungs may be associated and will determine survival in the short term; their treatment takes priority over esophageal injuries and may require a damage control approach [10].

Operative repair is the treatment of choice for TIE with free perforation of the abdominal esophagus [10]. In some cases, it may be possible to cover with a Nissen fundoplication. This injury may be associated with bleeding from coexistent liver, spleen, or great vessel injuries and will take priority.

Principles of damage control surgery and of damage control reanimation should be applied to hemodynamically unstable patients with TIE. In one study, mortality of TIE was 44% with 92% of the deaths occurring within 24 h of presentation; mortality was related to the injury severity score (ISS) and not to the esophageal injuries [10]. Thus, abbreviated source control surgery followed by transfer to the intensive care unit for physiological resuscitation is paramount in hemodynamically unstable TIE patients; a second look procedure in the operating room is then required for definitive surgical management of esophageal and other associated injuries. External drainage, esophageal exclusion, or expeditious resection should be undertaken in parallel with bleeding control measures; specific esophageal reconstruction would be undertaken in survivors as previously described [10].

### Dos and Don'ts

**Dos**

- Protect the airway by intubating the patient early and follow trauma guidelines as injuries to concomitant structures will be more lethal in the short term.
- Perform emergency CT evaluation, ideally with enteral water-soluble contrast.
- Perform surgical exploration early as most significant injuries will have septic contamination of the surrounding tissue spaces.
- Transfer hemodynamically stable patients to high volume trauma centers.
- Consider damage control surgery in patients with TIE and severe damage of vital organs.

### Don'ts

- Don't forget the esophagus in gunshot, knife, or blunt injuries to the chest, neck, and abdomen.
- Don't miss esophageal injuries in blunt thoracic traumas.
- Don't attempt complex esophageal reconstruction in unstable patients.

### Take-Home Messages

- Physical examination and laboratory studies are not useful for early diagnosis of esophageal trauma.
- Contrast-enhanced CT and CT esophagography should be performed in hemodynamically stable patients suspected of esophageal injury.
- Intraoperative flexible endoscopy is useful for unstable patients with minimal preoperative workup. The role of stenting is unknown at this time.
- Patients with esophageal injury can be offered non-operative management if they do not have perforation and meet NOM criteria.
- Patients with esophageal injury should undergo immediate surgical exploration if they have hemodynamic instability, obvious non-contained extravasation of contrast material on CT or systemic signs of severe sepsis.
- The type of operative repair will depend on the site and degree of injury and any associated injuries to concomitant structures.
- Associated injuries are common and their appropriate management conditions immediate patient survival.

### Questions

1. **External trauma causing esophageal injury**
   A. Does not need operation in most cases
   B. **Is rare**
   C. Has an easily definable clinical course
   D. Is easily diagnosed
2. **Penetrating esophageal injury**
   A. Is usually treated non-operatively
   B. Endoscopy is mandatory
   C. **Usually diagnosed by CT**
   D. Usually an isolated injury
3. **Blunt chest trauma**
   A. **May cause isolated esophageal injury**
   B. Never causes esophageal rupture
   C. Barotrauma does not affect the esophagus
   D. Is a commoner cause of injury to the esophagus than penetrating
4. **Pneumomediastinum**
   A. Is always due to esophageal rupture
   B. Always requires contrast studies
   C. **May be unrelated to rupture of esophagus**
   D. May have minimal symptoms

## References

1. Petrone P, Kassimi K, Jimenez-Gomez M, et al. Management of esophageal injuries secondary to trauma. Injury. 2017;48(8):1735–42.
2. Patel MS, Malinoski DJ, Zhou L, et al. Penetrating oesophageal injury: a contemporary analysis of the National Trauma Data Bank. Injury. 2013;44(1):48–55.
3. Makhani M, Midani D, Goldberg A, et al. Pathogenesis and outcomes of traumatic injuries of the esophagus. Dis Esophagus. 2014;27(7):630–6.
4. Asensio JA, Chahwan S, Forno W, et al. Penetrating esophageal injuries: multicenter study of the

American Association for the Surgery of Trauma. J Trauma. 2001;50(2):289–96.
5. Aiolfi A, Inaba K, Recinos G, et al. Non-iatrogenic esophageal injury: a retrospective analysis from the National Trauma Data Bank. World J Emerg Surg. 2017;12:19–106.
6. Biffl WL, Moore EE, Feliciano DV, et al. Western trauma association critical decisions in trauma: diagnosis and management of esophageal injuries. J Trauma Acute Care Surg. 2015;79:1089.
7. Skipworth RJ, McBride OM, Kerssens JJ, Paterson-Brown S. Esophagogastric trauma in Scotland. World J Surg. 2012;36:1779.
8. Roan JN, Wu MH. Esophageal perforation caused by external air-blast injury. J Cardiothorac Surg. 2010;5:130.
9. Moore EE, Jurkovich GJ, Knudson MM, Cogbill TH, Malangoni MA, Champion HR, et al. Organ injury scaling VI: extrahepatic biliary, esophagus, stomach, vulva, vagina, uterus (nonpregnant), uterus (pregnant), fallopian tube, and ovary. J Trauma Acute Care Surg. 1995;39(6):1069–70.
10. Chirica M, Kelly MD, Siboni S, Aiolfi A, Riva CG, Emanuele A, et al. Esophageal emergencies: WSES guidelines. World J Emerg Surg. 2019;14:26.
11. Muneer M, Abdelrahman H, El-Menyar A, Afifi I, Al-Hassani A, AlMadani A. External air compression: a rare cause of blunt esophageal injury, managed by a stent. Int J Surg Case Rep. 2014;5(9):620–3.
12. Ivatury RR, Moore FA, Biffl W, Leppeniemi A, Ansaloni L, Catena F, et al. Oesophageal injuries: position paper, WSES, 2013. World J Emerg Surg. 2014;9:9.

# Caustic Ingestion

## 58

Mircea Chirica, Helene Corte, and Pierre Cattan

**Learning Goals**
- Improve the practitioner's ability to manage patients in the initial phase of caustic ingestion.
- Enable appropriate emergency decision-making based on computed tomography evaluation of the severity of digestive injuries.
- Become familiar with outcomes of caustic ingestions and be able provide reliable step-by step information to patients and relatives.

## 58.1　Introduction

Ingestion of caustic substances agents accidentally or with suicidal intent is a rare event with potential devastating consequences [1, 2]. Most patients present with mild digestive injuries tract that don't necessitate specific intervention and resolve without sequels. A small number of patients need emergency lifesaving surgery for the treatment of transmural necrosis of the upper digestive tract [3]. Complex reconstructive surgery may be required following emergency esophageal resection and for the treatment refractory esophageal strictures [4]. Coordinate intervention and close collaboration of several specialists (emergency care physicians, radiologists, anesthesiologists surgeons, otorhinolaryngologists, gastroenterologists, and psychiatrists) are necessary during the emergency management of caustic injuries [1, 2]. During the last decade, the progressive replacement of endoscopy by computed tomography for the evaluation of gastrointestinal necrosis represents a major paradigm shift in the emergency management of caustic injuries [5–8].

## 58.2　Epidemiology

Worldwide caustic ingestion is underreported, and for this reason, reliable epidemiologic data are lacking in the literature [2, 9]. A recent report from France showed that caustic injuries represented 0.016% of all adult emergency department admissions during the last decade. Caustic ingestion was intentional in 89% of patients and 72% of them had a previous history of psychiatric disease (Challine et al. in press). In contrast, accidents are more frequent in children [2, 9–11] with some 1000 children admitted to hospital

M. Chirica (✉)
Service de Chirurgie Digestive, Centre Hospitalier Universitaire Grenoble Alpes, La Tronche, France

H. Corte · P. Cattan
Service de Chirurgie Générale, Digestive et Endocrinienne, Hôpital Saint-Louis, Paris, France
e-mail: helene.corte@aphp.fr; pierre.cattan@aphp.fr

every year in the US [12]. Worldwide the incidence in this population is increasing steadily, especially in developing countries which lack effective regulatory measures and structured prevention programs [2, 13, 14].

## 58.3 Corrosive Agents

Acids, alkalis, and oxidative agents (i.e., bleach) are the most frequently involved agents. Strong acids are thought to produce coagulation necrosis which lessens tissue penetration sparing the esophagus and inducing severe gastric damage [11] while alkalis are responsible of liquefaction necrosis and induce immediate severe injuries at all levels of the gastrointestinal tract [2, 9–11]. Nevertheless, in case of massive ingestion, transmural necrosis occurs at all levels of the gastrointestinal irrespective of the nature of the causal agent [15]. The pattern of ingestion is different across the world depending on local customs and population access to corrosives agents; bleach and alkalis are often employed in Europe and North America while acids are most frequently ingested in Asia [1, 12].

Severe systemic effects have been described with some agents such as hypocalcemia (phosphoric, hydrofluoric acids), hyponatremia (strong acids/alkalis), hypokalemia, and hypomagnesaemia (hydrofluoric acids) [1, 12]. The extent of digestive involvement is directly related to the quantity ingested but this information is seldom available [2, 9].

## 58.4 Emergency Management

During the initial approach, the main goals include avoid aggravating the degree of caustic lesions, obtain the control of organ failures, address potential systemic effects, and evaluate the transmural character of caustic damage.

### 58.4.1 Prehospital Management

During the initial phase, it is paramount to establish the diagnosis of caustic agent ingestion and determine the quantity, the nature, and the physical form (solid, liquid, gel, vapors-concomitant aspiration) of the ingested agent [16]. Evaluation of the accidental–intentional character of the ingestion and detection of co-ingestion of alcohol and/or drugs is important. The presence of additional risk factors such as extreme ages (young children, elderly), pregnancy, and underlying diseases (cancer, cirrhosis) would condition management and outcomes [17]. Patients should be transported rapidly to the hospital, and any maneuver likely to induce a second esophageal passage of the corrosive agent (strict supine position, provoked vomiting, gastric lavage, ingestion of diluents) should be prohibited. Attempts at pH neutralization by ingestion of weak acids or alkalis would only produce further damage by exothermic reactions and should be avoided [12, 17].

### 58.4.2 In Hospital Management

Symptomatic treatment should be pursued after hospital admission in parallel with the assessment of the severity of gastrointestinal damage. Respiratory distress due to severe pharyngeal involvement requires airway securing by tracheal intubation; fiberoptic laryngoscopy is preferable to blind intubation under such circumstances [17]. Contact of Poison Control Centers is recommended if uncertainty persists regarding systemic toxicity. Insertion of nasogastric tubes during early management should be avoided as there is no proven benefit but increased risks of caustic pneumonia and digestive perforation [17]. Systematic use of proton-pump inhibitors, H2 blockers, corticosteroids, and broad-spectrum antibiotics outside controlled trials is not recommended in the absence of valid proof regarding their efficacy [1, 9, 10].

## 58.4.3 Evaluation of Digestive Caustic Injuries

### 58.4.3.1 Symptoms

The clinical presentation is directly related to the nature, the quantity, and physical form of the ingested corrosives. Solid agents induce maximum damage to the mouth and pharynx while liquids transit rapidly and involve the esophagus and the stomach; in some situations, the aspiration of caustic vapors may induce caustic pneumonia. Digestive perforation and clinical signs of peritonitis (abdominal tenderness/rebound, subcutaneous emphysema, hemodynamic instability) should prompt immediate surgery. Such signs are infrequent on presentation, and their absence should not delay management [3, 18]. Hoarseness, stridor, and dyspnea are suggestive of laryngeal/epiglottis involvement. Dysphagia, drooling, and odynophagia usually reflect pharyngeal and esophageal damage while epigastric pain and hematemesis suggest gastric injuries. Nevertheless, it is commonly agreed that symptom intensity correlates poorly with the extent of gastrointestinal damage, and transmural digestive necrosis may be accompanied by discrete symptoms in the initial phase [2, 9, 10].

### 58.4.3.2 Laboratory Studies

A wide range of laboratory tests is performed in the emergency setting including liver function tests, $Na^+$, $K^+$, $Cl^-$, urea, creatinine, $Ca^{2+}$, $Mg^+$, leucocytes, hemoglobin, platelets, TP, and serum lactates. In young women of childbearing age, β-HCG levels should be measured, and serum alcohol levels should be checked in all patients [17]. Laboratory parameters may predict the severity of caustic injuries: leukocytosis, thrombocytopenia, elevated serum C-reactive protein levels, acidosis, renal failure, and the perturbation of liver function tests have been shown to correlate with transmural necrosis and poor outcomes [2, 9, 10]. The dynamic evolution of laboratory parameters is useful in monitoring patients during non-operative management [19].

### 58.4.3.3 Computed Tomography

Computed tomography (CT) has replaced endoscopy in the emergency setting for the assessment of upper digestive injuries and is currently the mainstay of damage extent evaluation after caustic ingestion [8]. CT of the neck, the thorax, and the abdomen should be performed 3–12 h after ingestion; intravenous injection of a nonionic contrast agent (2 mL/kg) with an 18–25-s acquisition time and a 90-s scan delay is mandatory. Oral contrast is not recommended as it may induce difficulties in slide interpretation without providing significant benefit. Several recent reports have shown that CT outperformed endoscopy in selecting patients for surgery [6, 7, 20] and in predicting risks of esophageal stricture [5]. A simple and highly reproducible CT classification [1, 8] of caustic injuries has been recently proposed. Esophageal injuries were classified as Grade I: normal wall enhancement, no edema, no peri-esophageal fat stranding; Grade IIa "target-like" wall enhancement, wall edema, peri-esophageal fat stranding; Grade IIb rim enhancement of the outer wall, edema, peri-esophageal fat stranding; Grade IV absence of post-contrast wall enhancement, peri-esophageal fat blurring. Gastric injuries were classified as Grade I: normal wall enhancement, no edema; Grade II continuous wall enhancement, edema; Grade III absence of post-contrast wall enhancement (Table 58.1). CT features of esophageal and gastric caustic injuries are shown in Fig. 58.1. As a general rule, patients with Grade III injuries should be considered for emergency surgical exploration while patients with less severe involvement can be offered non-operative management (Fig. 58.2). Between 2015 and 2020, 294 patients were managed using a CT-only management algorithm without endoscopy at the Saint Louis Hospital in Paris. Their early outcomes, nutritional results, and long-term survival were similar to those of 120 patients managed by a combined CT-endoscopy algorithm between 2012 and 2015 (unpublished data).

**Table 58.1** CT classification of caustic injuries

| Severity of caustic injuries | | | |
|---|---|---|---|
| Esophagus | | | |
| Grade I | • Normal aspect<br>• Esophageal wall enhancement<br>• No edema<br>• No stranding | | • No significant esophageal damage<br>• Immediate feeding<br>• Quick discharge |
| Grade Ia | • Esophageal mucosa enhancement<br>• Thickened esophageal wall<br>• Enhancement of outer esophageal wall confers "target aspect" | | • Mild injuries<br>• Oral nutrition usually well tolerated<br>• Stricture risks <20% |
| Grade IIb | • Rim enhancement of outer esophageal wall<br>• No enhancement of necrosed mucosa which fills the esophageal lumen | | • Severe injuries<br>• Oral nutrition difficult<br>• Enteral or parenteral nutritional support may be required<br>• Stricture risks >80% |
| Grade III | • No enhancement of the esophageal wall<br>• Peri-esophageal fat blurring | | • Transmural necrosis<br>• Indication for emergency esophagectomy |
| Stomach | | | |
| Grade I | • Normal wall enhancement<br>• No edema | | • No significant esophageal damage<br>• Immediate feeding<br>• Quick discharge |
| Grade II | • Continuous enhancement of the gastric wall<br>• Edema | | • Mild injuries<br>• Oral nutrition usually well tolerated |
| Grade III | • No enhancement of the gastric wall | | • Transmural necrosis<br>• Indication for emergency laparotomy |

**Fig. 58.1** Computed tomographic classification of caustic injuries of the esophagus and the stomach

**ESOPHAGUS**

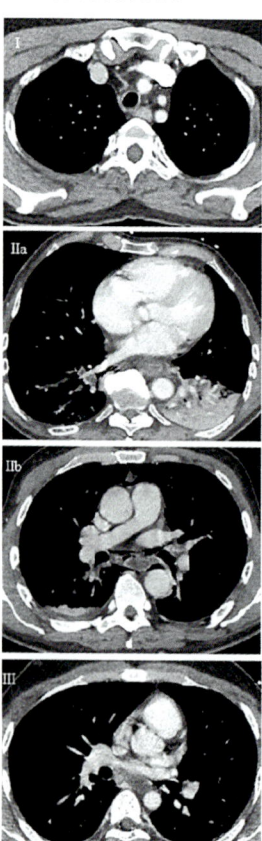

**STOMACH**

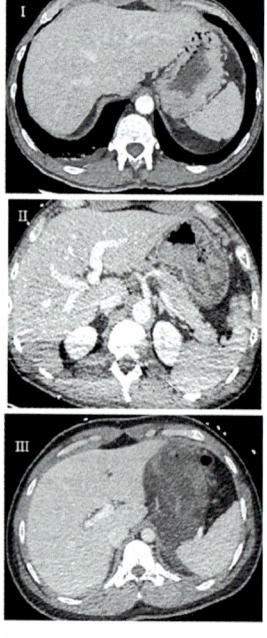

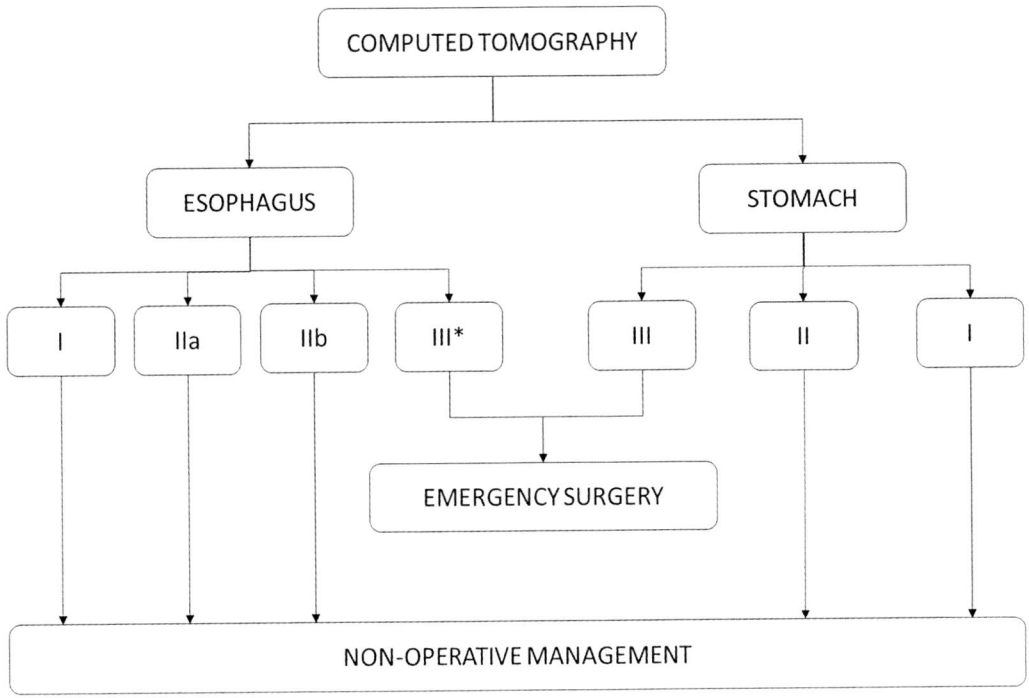

\* Non-operative management if gastric injuries Grade I-II

**Fig. 58.2** Computed tomography-based algorithm for the management of caustic ingestion

### 58.4.3.4 Endoscopy

Esophagogastroduodenoscopy which used to be the cornerstone of caustic ingestion management algorithms worldwide [2, 9, 11] can be safely abandoned during the emergency work-up of caustic ingestion. However, upfront endoscopy is still recommended in children [12] and in patients contraindicated to CT (i.e., severe iodine allergy, renal failure) [1]. Endoscopy should also be used in low-resource settings when CT is unavailable. The Zargar classification should be employed for the grading of caustic injuries (Fig. 58.3); patients with Grade IIIb injuries should be considered for emergency resection. If esophageal resection is considered based on endoscopy findings, CT confirmation of transmural necrosis is necessary prior to surgery. Endoscopy is still the mainstay for the diagnosis and the upfront treatment of caustic strictures [5].

**Fig. 58.3** Endoscopic classification of corrosive injuries Grade I: edema and hyperemia of the mucosa; Grade IIa: superficial localized ulcerations, friability, and blisters; Grade IIb: circumferential and deep ulcerations; Grade IIIa: small scattered areas of necrosis; Grade IIIb: extensive necrosis

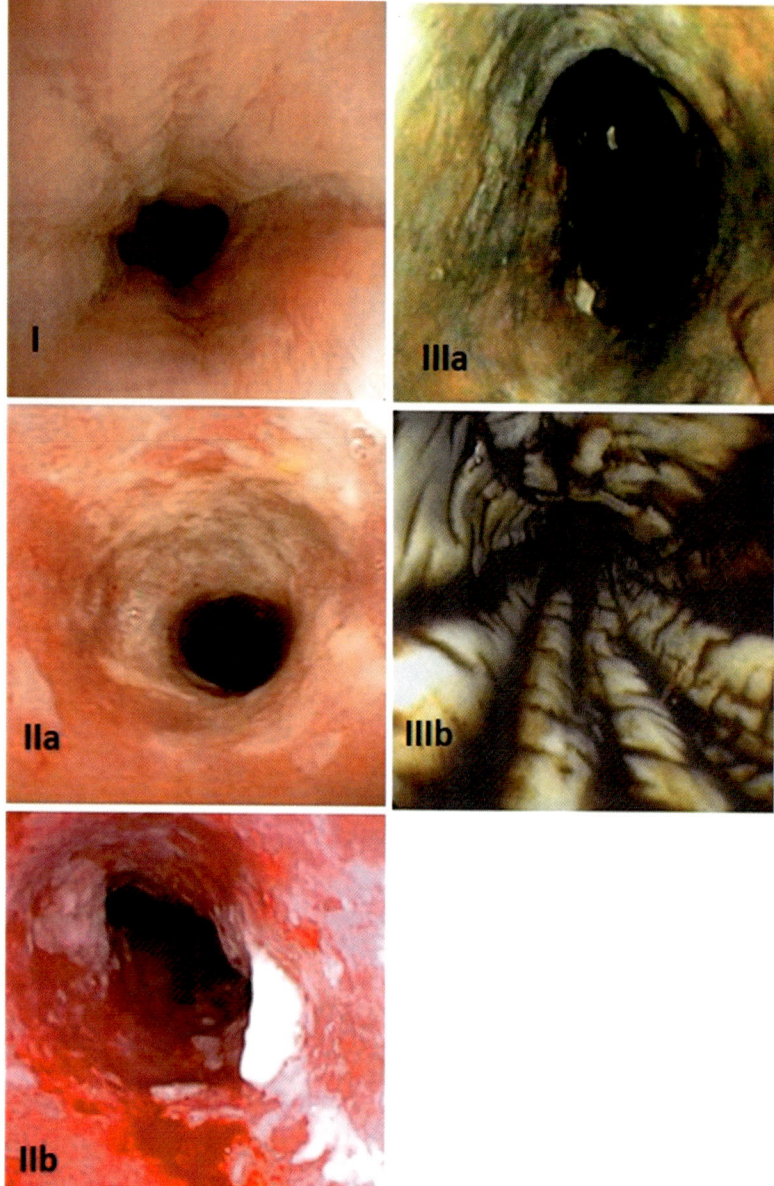

## 58.4.4 Injury Directed Management

#### Dos and Don'ts

#### Dos
- Quickly assess the ingestion circumstances and the patient's condition during the initial phase.
- Protect the airway by intubating the patient if necessary.
- Involve several different specialists from the start of the treatment.
- Perform emergency CT evaluation of the severity of caustic injuries.
- Perform surgical exploration if suspected transmural necrosis.
- Perform systematic airway evaluation prior to surgery.

#### Don'ts
- Don't try chemical or mechanical reversal of the effects of corrosive agents.
- Don't perform decision-making based on endoscopy findings alone.
- Don't resect the esophagus in the absence of transmural gastric necrosis.
- Never undertake esophageal reconstruction at the time of the emergency operation.
- Transfer patients to higher volume centers if appropriate local expertise is lacking.

A CT based management algorithm is shown in (Fig. 58.2).

### 58.4.4.1 Non-operative Treatment
A non-operative approach can be offered to 70–80% of patients after caustic ingestion [1]. Patients eligible for non-operative treatment may resume oral alimentation as soon they can swallow. After psychiatric consultation, these patients can be discharged as soon as they eat normally [8]. Patients with severe esophageal injuries (CT grade II) may develop early dysphagia within 10–21 days of ingestion; endoscopic evaluation should be performed as soon as symptoms appear but endoscopic dilation should be withhold during the first 3–6 weeks because local inflammation may increase perforation risks [1, 2]. Under such circumstances, jejunostomy construction should be considered before hospital discharge in order to allow enteral feeding. Patients with severe injuries require close monitoring; deterioration of clinical and/or laboratory tests (abdominal pain, rebound tenderness, shock, need for ventilatory support, renal failure, peripheral-blood leukocytosis, and/or acidosis) should prompt repeat CT evaluation [6]. Although ongoing digestive necrosis requiring surgical resection is anecdotal after initial CT guided non-operative management (only one of more than 500 patients in our recent experience), severe complications have been reported in 10–20% of patients and mortality in 2–6% (Challine et al. in press).

An outpatient visit should be scheduled 4 months after ingestion; if patients eat normally, long-term follow-up is not required as beyond this delay stricture formation is unusual [5]. In patients who develop caustic strictures, management options range from endoscopic dilation to complex reconstructive surgery [1].

### 58.4.4.2 Emergency Surgery
Emergency surgery should be offered to those patients in whom CT shows transmural necrosis of digestive organs. Prompt operation in such patients aims to prevent perforation and spillage of digestive content in the mediastinum and the peritoneum which lead invariably to death [3]. In one report, emergency surgery was performed in 24 (20%) of 120 consecutive caustic ingestion patients [7]. However in our more recent experience as well as in a recent nationwide French study [21], the rates of emergency surgery have decreased to 10%; subtle changes in ingestion patterns may explain this trend. Fiberoptic bronchoscopy to rule out airway involvement is mandatory before surgery even if the surgeon feels that resection might not be necessary. Emergency surgery for caustic injuries is usually performed through a midline laparotomy but successful laparoscopic exploration

has been reported [22]. Surgical management of transmural caustic necrosis requires resection of the involved organs, mainly the stomach and the esophagus; in rare occasions resection of other abdominal organs such as the duodenum, the pancreas, the colon, and the bowel may be lifesaving [23].

## Oesophagogastrectomy (OGT)

OGT through a combined abdominal and cervical approach is the most frequently employed resection procedure [3]. In the absence of tracheobronchial necrosis, esophageal stripping is usually employed to remove the esophagus. OGT is indicated when CT suggests transmural esophageal necrosis and laparotomy confirms transmural gastric necrosis. Feeding jejunostomy allows enteral nutrition [3] while waiting for reconstruction which should be delayed for at least 6 months [24]. The existence of isolated esophageal necrosis has been recently challenged [7, 19]; of 37 resections performed by our team during the last 8 years, the only isolated esophagectomy was due to the misinterpretation of CT slides. For this reason, if CT and /or laparotomy definitely rule out gastric necrosis we do not recommend esophageal resection even if CT is suggestive of transmural esophageal necrosis (Fig. 58.2). Esophageal reconstruction should never be attempted during the emergency operation because delayed formation of pharyngeal strictures might compromise nutritional outcomes [4] and necessitate secondary complex reconstructive procedures [25].

## Gastrectomy

In the absence of relevant data regarding outcomes of partial gastrectomy for caustic necrosis, most authors agree that the stomach should be completely removed in such cases [26]. Total gastrectomy with esophagojejunostomy (EJ) is increasingly undertaken in stable patients; intraoperative exploration usually reveals that the esophageal mucosa is burned but the presence of thickened walls of the abdominal esophagus allows safe immediate reconstruction. Actually, leakage of the EJ in this setting is rare [26]. However if the viability of the abdominal esophagus is doubtful or the surgeon is not at ease with EJ, esophagectomy or a damage control procedure (esophageal exclusion, external drainage) should be favored [1]. In our experience, all but 1 of 40 patients developed refractory esophageal strictures which required esophagocoloplasty reconstruction after total gastrectomy and EJ; for this reason, construction of a feeding jejunostomy is mandatory at the end of the procedure. The main argument supporting total gastrectomy and EJ rather than OGT in patients with isolated gastric necrosis is the high mortality associated with esophagectomy "per se" [3].

## Extended Resections

After massive ingestion of strong caustic agents, all transmural necrosis injuries should be resected during the initial procedure; second-look procedures should only be performed if clinical and biological data suggest ongoing necrosis [23]. After completion of the OGT procedure, pancreatoduodenectomy (PD), resection of the colon, the spleen, and bowel may be required in up to 20% of patients [3]. Following PD, immediate reconstruction of the bile duct and the pancreas is recommended as it may decrease the rate of specific pancreatobiliary complications [27]; external drainage is a valid option in unstable patients and/or if surgical expertise is not available. Abortion of the procedure should be considered in the presence of extensive bowel necrosis which is associated with prohibitive mortality and compromised nutritional outcomes. With this exception, the decision to abort potentially lifesaving emergency resection should not be guided by quality of life related issues [28, 29]. Perceived inability to perform future esophageal reconstruction by the emergency surgeon should not influence emergency surgical strategies. Actually, highly specialized centers may offer technical solutions to complex reconstructive challenges [25], and even in case of functional failure, patients may lead quite normal lives on definitive enteral nutrition [28, 29].

### Tracheobronchial Necrosis (TBN)

On rare occasions, direct extension of esophageal necrosis to the tracheobronchial tree may induce caustic necrosis of the trachea, the carina, and/or the left bronchus. Under such circumstances, blind stripping of the thoracic esophagus may result in concomitant stripping of the airway with high risks of intraoperative death. Thus if TBN is certified by preoperative bronchoscopy, esophageal resection should be performed by a right thoracic approach to allow visual control and airway repair [30].

### Results of Emergency Surgery

The extent of resection is the major determinant of early outcomes. In a recent report mortality after gastrectomy, OGT, PD, and TBN for caustic injuries reached 11%, 14%, 39%, and 45% and morbidity rates were 63%, 65%, 94%, and 100%, respectively [3]. The standardized mortality ratio (SMR) after emergency surgery for caustic injuries was 21.5 when compared with the general French population [3]. Factors that have negative impact on long-term survival and functional outcomes include advanced age and the extent of caustic necrosis [3].

## 58.5 Conclusion

Caustic ingestion has a terrible influence on survival, nutritional results, and patient's quality of life. Efforts directed at improving patient selection for surgery by using CT evaluation have been shown to improve outcomes and are progressively endorsed by surgical societies worldwide. The implementation of national health programs directed at public education and the introduction of effective measures limiting access to strong corrosive substances are probably the only way which may help eradicate this condition.

> **Take-Home Messages**
> - Computed tomography has replaced endoscopy and is currently the mainstay for the evaluation of caustic injuries severity
> - Aggressive resection of all transmural necrosis areas may be lifesaving after massive caustic ingestion
> - Patients on lifelong enteral nutrition may lead normal lives; quality of life issues should not be used to decide the abortion of a potentially lifesaving procedure

> **Questions**
> 1. **Caustic ingestion in adults**
>    A. Is a frequent condition
>    B. **Is most often intentional**
>    C. The incidence is increasing steadily worldwide
>    D. Occurs in the absence of psychiatric disease
> 2. **With regard to the nature of the ingested agent**
>    A. Acids produce liquefaction necrosis
>    B. Alkalis spare the esophagus
>    C. **Massive ingestion of strong acid may result in transmural necrosis of the esophagus**
>    D. Bleach induced injuries are always mild
> 3. **During the prehospital management phase**
>    A. **Alcohol co-ingestion should be sought**
>    B. The quantity ingested is easy to determine
>    C. Gastric lavage is indicated in children
>    D. Milk should be administered after acid ingestion

4. **Following hospital admission**
   A. Nasogastric tube insertion is recommended
   B. Broad spectrum antibiotics may decrease the rate of pulmonary complications
   C. **Intubation may be necessary to secure the airway**
   D. Corticoids decrease risks of esophageal stricture formation
5. **Regarding the clinical presentation after caustic ingestion:**
   A. Severe abdominal pain is closely correlated with the extent of gastric necrosis
   B. Esophageal perforation is frequently encountered
   C. Solid agents spare the pharynx
   D. **Aspiration of caustic vapors induces severe pneumonia**
6. **Laboratory tests in patients who ingested corrosive agents: in all**
   A. Are not required in the emergency setting
   B. β-HCG levels should be measured in all patients
   C. Leukocytosis is a sign of pharyngeal necrosis
   D. **Dynamic evolution is useful in monitoring patients after non-operative management**
7. **Computed tomography after caustic ingestion**
   A. Should always be performed after endoscopy
   B. Requires oral contrast administration
   C. **Outperforms endoscopy in detecting transmural caustic necrosis**
   D. Should be used as first line exam in children
8. **The CT classification of caustic injuries**
   A. **Is useful in establishing management algorithms**
   B. Grade III gastric injuries require close surveillance
   C. Grade I esophageal injuries have a high risk of stricture formation
   D. Grade IIb esophageal injuries require emergency esophagectomy
9. **Regarding non-operative management of caustic injuries**
   A. About half of patients can be offered non-operative management
   B. **Patients can resume oral alimentation when able to swallow**
   C. Psychiatric evaluation is not necessary in patients with mild injuries
   D. Mortality is nil in this population
10. **Emergency surgery for caustic injuries**
    A. Should be aborted in case of transmural necrosis of the duodenum
    B. **May be lifesaving even in the presence of pancreatic necrosis**
    C. Esophagocoloplasty may be attempted immediately after esophagogastrectomy
    D. The colon should never be resected as it may compromise reconstruction

## References

1. Chirica M, Bonavina L, Kelly MD, Sarfati E, Cattan P. Caustic ingestion. Lancet. 2017;389(10083):2041–52.
2. Contini S, Scarpignato C. Caustic injury of the upper gastrointestinal tract: a comprehensive review. World J Gastroenterol. 2013;19(25):3918–30.
3. Chirica M, Resche-Rigon M, Bongrand NM, Zohar S, Halimi B, Gornet JM, et al. Surgery for caustic injuries of the upper gastrointestinal tract. Ann Surg. 2012;256(6):994–1001.
4. Chirica M, Brette MD, Faron M, Munoz Bongrand N, Halimi B, Laborde C, et al. Upper digestive tract reconstruction for caustic injuries. Ann Surg. 2015;261(5):894–901.
5. Bruzzi M, Chirica M, Resche-Rigon M, Corte H, Voron T, Sarfati E, et al. Emergency computed tomography predicts caustic esophageal stricture formation. Ann Surg. 2018;270(1):109–14.
6. Chirica M, Resche-Rigon M, Pariente B, Fieux F, Sabatier F, Loiseaux F, et al. Computed tomography evaluation of high-grade esophageal necrosis after corrosive ingestion to avoid unnecessary esophagectomy. Surg Endosc. 2015;29(6):1452–61.

7. Chirica M, Resche-Rigon M, Zagdanski AM, Bruzzi M, Bouda D, Roland E, et al. Computed tomography evaluation of esophagogastric necrosis after caustic ingestion. Ann Surg. 2016;264(1):107–13.
8. Chirica M, Bonavina L, Cattan P. Ingestion of caustic substances. N Engl J Med. 2020;383(6):600.
9. Hugh TB, Kelly MD. Corrosive ingestion and the surgeon. J Am Coll Surg. 1999;189(5):508–22.
10. Keh SM, Onyekwelu N, McManus K, McGuigan J. Corrosive injury to upper gastrointestinal tract: still a major surgical dilemma. World J Gastroenterol. 2006;12(32):5223–8.
11. Ramasamy K, Gumaste VV. Corrosive ingestion in adults. J Clin Gastroenterol. 2003;37(2):119–24.
12. Hoffman RS, Burns MM, Gosselin S. Ingestion of caustic substances. N Engl J Med. 2020;382(18):1739–48.
13. Contini S, Garatti M, Swarray-Deen A, Depetris N, Cecchini S, Scarpignato C. Corrosive oesophageal strictures in children: outcomes after timely or delayed dilatation. Dig Liver Dis. 2009;41(4):263–8.
14. Contini S, Swarray-Deen A, Scarpignato C. Oesophageal corrosive injuries in children: a forgotten social and health challenge in developing countries. Bull World Health Organ. 2009;87(12):950–4.
15. Ducoudray R, Mariani A, Corte H, Kraemer A, Munoz-Bongrand N, Sarfati E, et al. The damage pattern to the gastrointestinal tract depends on the nature of the ingested caustic agent. World J Surg. 2016;40(7):1638–44.
16. Chirica M, Kelly MD, Siboni S, Aiolfi A, Riva CG, Asti E, et al. Esophageal emergencies: WSES guidelines. World J Emerg Surg. 2019;14:26.
17. Bonavina L, Chirica M, Skrobic O, Kluger Y, Andreollo NA, Contini S, et al. Foregut caustic injuries: results of the world society of emergency surgery consensus conference. World J Emerg Surg. 2015;10:44.
18. Tohda G, Sugawa C, Gayer C, Chino A, McGuire TW, Lucas CE. Clinical evaluation and management of caustic injury in the upper gastrointestinal tract in 95 adult patients in an urban medical center. Surg Endosc. 2008;22(4):1119–25.
19. Zerbib P, Voisin B, Truant S, Saulnier F, Vinet A, Chambon JP, et al. The conservative management of severe caustic gastric injuries. Ann Surg. 2011;253(4):684–8.
20. Mensier A, Onimus T, Ernst O, Leroy C, Zerbib P. Evaluation of severe caustic gastritis by computed tomography and its impact on management. J Visc Surg. 2020;157(6):469–74.
21. Observational Study JAMA Surg. 2022;157(2):112–119. https://doi.org/10.1001/jamasurg.2021.6368. Outcomes Associated With Caustic Ingestion Among Adults in a National Prospective Database in France Alexandre Challine 1 2, Léon Maggiori 1, Sandrine Katsahian 2 3, Hélène Corté 1, Diane Goere 1, Andrea Lazzati 4 5, Pierre Cattan 1, Mircea Chirica 6 Affiliations expand PMID: 34878529; PMCID: PMC8655661. https://doi.org/10.1001/jamasurg.2021.6368
22. Di Saverio S, Biscardi A, Piccinini A, Mandrioli M, Tugnoli G. Different possible surgical managements of caustic ingestion: diagnostic laparoscopy for Zargar's grade 3a lesions and a new technique of "duodenal damage control" with "4-tubes ostomy" and duodenal wash-out as an option for extensive 3b lesions in unstable patients. Update Surg. 2015;67(3):313–20.
23. Cattan P, Munoz-Bongrand N, Berney T, Halimi B, Sarfati E, Celerier M. Extensive abdominal surgery after caustic ingestion. Ann Surg. 2000;231(4):519–23.
24. Chirica M, Veyrie N, Munoz-Bongrand N, Zohar S, Halimi B, Celerier M, et al. Late morbidity after colon interposition for corrosive esophageal injury: risk factors, management, and outcome. A 20-year experience. Ann Surg. 2010;252(2):271–80.
25. Chirica M, Vuarnesson H, Zohar S, Faron M, Halimi B, Munoz Bongrand N, et al. Similar outcomes after primary and secondary esophagocoloplasty for caustic injuries. Ann Thorac Surg. 2012;93(3):905–12.
26. Chirica M, Kraemer A, Petrascu E, Vuarnesson H, Pariente B, Halimi B, et al. Esophagojejunostomy after total gastrectomy for caustic injuries. Dis Esophagus. 2013;27(2):122–7.
27. Lefrancois M, Gaujoux S, Resche-Rigon M, Chirica M, Munoz-Bongrand N, Sarfati E, et al. Oesophagogastrectomy and pancreatoduodenectomy for caustic injury. Br J Surg. 2011;98(7):983–90.
28. Faron M, Corte H, Poghosyan T, Bruzzi M, Voron T, Sarfati E, et al. Quality of life after caustic ingestion. Ann Surg. 2020;274(6):e529–34.
29. Raynaud K, Seguy D, Rogosnitzky M, Saulnier F, Pruvot FR, Zerbib P. Conservative management of severe caustic injuries during acute phase leads to superior long-term nutritional and quality of life (QoL) outcome. Langenbecks Arch Surg. 2015;401(1):81–7.
30. Benjamin B, Agueb R, Vuarnesson H, Tranchart H, Bongrand NM, Sarfati E, et al. Tracheobronchial necrosis after caustic ingestion. Ann Surg. 2015;263(4):808–13.

# 59. Surgical Jaundice and Cholangitis

Aleksandar R. Karamarkovic, Jovan T. Juloski, and Vladica V. Cuk

## 59.1 Introduction

Jaundice is yellowish discoloration of the skin and sclera. It is a result of elevated bilirubin levels in blood. Various conditions can lead to elevated blood bilirubin and these are discussed further in this chapter, but obstruction of the biliary tree, which can be managed surgically, is the main focus of surgeons. Cholangitis is an infection of the biliary system, and is generally associated with the presence of biliary obstruction. Cholangitis occurs when partial or complete obstruction of the bile duct exists, resulting in increased intraluminal pressure and infection of the retained bile proximal to the obstruction. All this can lead to a life-threatening condition, such as sepsis and multiorgan failure and finally death.

> **Learning Goals**
> - Jaundiced patients are at increased risk for renal dysfunction, hepatic failure, cardiovascular impairments, nutritional deficiencies, bleeding entanglements, infections, and wound complications, and their perioperative mortality and morbidity are increased.
> - Cholangitis is not just one entity with a clear-cut clinical presentation but more as a scope of disease that presents diversely with a wide range of severity.
> - The management of cholangitis should follow three steps: resuscitation, broad spectrum parenteral antibiotics, and biliary decompression. Sepsis caused by untreated cholangitis is almost always fatal, and the potential for the progression from mild to severe cholangitis can be swift and beyond recall.

### 59.1.1 Epidemiology

The incidence of biliary obstruction in the United States is approximately 5 cases per 1000 people [1]. Gallstones are one of the most common diseases of digestive system and most common cause of biliary obstruction [2]. Persons of Hispanic origin and Northern Europeans have a higher risk of gallstones compared to people from Asia and Africa [1]. Women are much more likely to develop gallstones than men [1]. By the sixth decade, almost 25% of American women develop gallstones, with as many as 50% of women aged

A. R. Karamarkovic (✉) · J. T. Juloski · V. V. Cuk
Faculty of Medicine, University of Belgrade, Belgrade, Serbia

Surgical Clinic "Nikola Spasic", Zvezdara University Medical Center, Belgrade, Serbia
e-mail: alekara@sbb.rs

75 years developing gallstones [1]. This increased risk is likely caused by the effect of estrogen on the liver, causing it to remove more cholesterol from the blood and diverting it into the bile [1]. Gallbladder cancer is also more common in females than in males [3]. Approximately 20% of men aged 75 years have gallstones, with more complicated disease courses occurring in those who have had cholecystectomies [1].

Cholangitis is a result of biliary obstruction and bacterial superinfection, and the most common cause of obstruction is choledocholithiasis [4]. The condition is reported in both sexes and throughout all continents with similar frequencies, except from oriental cholangio-hepatitis or recurrent pyogenic cholangitis which is more frequent in Southeast Asia [5]. The median age of presentation is between 50 and 60 years of age, with, as said earlier, biliary stones as the main cause [6]. In neonate's extrahepatic biliary atresia can cause cholangitis, as can choledochal cysts in young adults [6].

## 59.1.2 Etiology

Various reasons can cause elevated bilirubin levels. Increased bilirubin production, flawed bilirubin uptake into the hepatocytes, reduces bilirubin conjugation, impaired excretion of bilirubin into the bile ducts and finally, obstruction of the biliary tree at any level [7]. Duct obstructions, the main surgical interest, are caused most frequently by choledocholithiasis and benign or malignant strictures/obstructions [7].

The two most common causes of cholangitis are common bile duct stones and biliary tract manipulations, including cholangitis after biliary-enteric anastomosis [6, 8, 9]. Other possible causes of biliary tract obstruction that may lead to infection include strictures, tumors, choledochal/biliary cysts, or sump syndrome. Hepatolithiasis is also a possible cause of cholangitis and is observed more frequently in East Asia [10]. Being the result of biliary stasis and bacterial superinfection, cholangitis can be a result of other, not so frequent causes such as AIDS cholangiopathy and *Ascaris lumbricoides* infection [6, 9].

## 59.1.3 Classification

Increase in bilirubin production, impaired hepatocyte uptake of bilirubin, reduction of bilirubin conjugation, altered transport or excretion of bilirubin into the bile ducts, or obstruction of the intrahepatic or extrahepatic biliary tree can all cause jaundice (Table 59.1) [7]. Increase in production, impaired uptake, and reduced conjugation of bilirubin all lead to a predominantly unconjugated hyperbilirubinemia. Altered transport and excretion and biliary ductal obstruction result in predominantly conjugated hyperbilirubinemia. This classification merely represents all

**Table 59.1** Classification of jaundice

| Classification of jaundice | | |
|---|---|---|
| Defect in bilirubin metabolism | Predominant hyperbilirubinemia | Examples |
| Increased production | Unconjugated | Congenital hemoglobinopathies, hemolysis, multiple transfusions, sepsis, burns |
| Impaired hepatocyte uptake | Unconjugated | Gilbert's disease, drug induced |
| Reduced conjugation | Unconjugated | Neonatal jaundice, Crigler–Najjar syndrome |
| Altered transport and excretion | Conjugated | Hepatitis, cirrhosis, Dubin–Johnson syndrome, Rotor's syndrome |
| Biliary obstruction | Conjugated | Choledocholithiasis, benign strictures, chronic pancreatitis, sclerosing cholangitis, periampullary cancer, biliary malignancies |

This table was published in BLUMGART'S Surgery of the Liver, Biliary Tract, and Pancreas. 6th edition. Reproduced with the permission from Elsevier levels of bilirubin metabolism that can be disturbed. Great deal of cases can have more than one of these disturbances, so patients can have more complex illnesses [7]. Obstruction of biliary ducts can be divided into: complete obstruction, intermittent obstruction, chronic incomplete obstruction, or segmental duct obstruction (Table 59.2) [7]. Clinically visible jaundice is present in those cases with complete obstruction, while intermittent obstruction can lead to biochemical changes and symptoms such as fever, pain or pruritus, but not necessarily jaundice.

According to latest Tokyo guidelines from 2018, acute cholangitis is classified into three grades: mild (grade I), moderate (grade II), severe (grade III) [11]. This classification is based on the severity of patient's status, taking into consideration age, white blood count (WBC), bilirubin, albumin levels, presence of fever, platelet count, international normalized ratio (INR) values, blood urea nitrogen (BUN), etc.

### 59.1.4 Pathophysiology

Acute cholangitis is an ascending bacterial infection in association with partial or complete obstruction of the bile ducts [9]. Hepatic bile is sterile and the bile in the bile ducts is kept sterile by continuous flow and by the presence of antibacterial material such as immunoglobulins. Bacterial contamination of the bile itself doesn't lead to clinical cholangitis, only in combination with stasis of the bile it can cause cholangitis [9, 12]. The most common strains cultured form bile in patient with cholangitis are *Klebsiella pneumoniae*, *Escherichia coli*, *Streptococcus faecalis*, *Enterobacter*, and *Bacteroides fragilis* [9, 12, 13]. Biliary obstruction has local effects on the bile ducts, which further lead to impaired function of hepatocytes and, ultimately, to widespread systemic effects due cholangiolymphatic and cholangiovenous reflux. Jaundiced patients are at increased risk for hepatic and renal failure, cardiovascular disturbances, nutritional deficiencies, coagulopathy, immunodeficiencies, healing impairments and their perioperative mortality and morbidity are increased [7]. Besides these effects, when infection of the bile is present, pathogens eventually overcome the blood barrier and enter the blood stream. This eventually leads to septicemia, sepsis, multiorgan failure, and finally septic shock [9, 11, 12].

**Table 59.2** Lesions commonly associated with biliary tract obstruction

| Lesions commonly associated with biliary tract obstruction |
|---|
| **Type I: Complete obstruction** |
| Tumors of the head of the pancreas |
| Common bile duct ligation |
| Cholangiocarcinoma |
| Gallbladder cancer |
| Parenchymal liver tumors (primary or secondary) |
| **Type II: Intermittent obstruction** |
| Choledocholithiasis |
| Periampullary tumors |
| Duodenal diverticula |
| Choledochal cyst |
| Polycystic liver disease |
| Biliary parasites |
| Hemobilia |
| **Type III: Chronic incomplete obstruction** |
| Strictures of the common bile duct |
| Congenital biliary atresia |
| Traumatic (iatrogenic) |
| Sclerosing cholangitis |
| Post radiotherapy |
| Stenosis of biliary-enteric anastamosis |
| Chronic pancreatitis |
| Cystic fibrosis |
| Sphincter of Oddi stenosis |
| **Type IV: Segmental obstruction** |
| Traumatic |
| Intrahepatic stones |
| Sclerosing cholangitis |
| Cholangiocarcinoma |

This table was published in BLUMGART'S Surgery of the Liver, Biliary Tract, and Pancreas. 6th edition. Reproduced with the permission from Elsevier

## 59.2 Diagnosis

### 59.2.1 Clinical Presentation

As said earlier in this chapter, cholangitis is not a single, with well-defined clinical presentation, disease, but can present as anything from mild and self-limited illness to a fulminant, life-threatening septicemia [9, 11]. Classic symptoms, fever, epigastric or right upper quadrant pain, and jaundice, first described by Charcot in 1877 [9], are present in only about two thirds of patients [12]. Further progression leads to septicemia and mental deterioration, also known as Reynold's pentad, originally described by Reynold and Dargan in 1959 [9]. Atypical presentation is also possible, especially in the elderly, who may have little, if any symptoms, until they collapse with septicemia [12]. Patients with stents usually do not develop jaundice, and on physical examination precise diagnosis can be challenging [12].

### 59.2.2 Tests

In order to diagnose and adequately grade the severity of cholangitis, according to Tokyo guidelines, following laboratory test should be done: blood tests, especially white blood cell count and platelet count, C-reactive protein (CRP), blood gas analysis, albumin, alkaline phosphatase (ALP), gamma-glutamyl transferase (GGT), aspartate aminotransferase (AST), alanine aminotransferase (ALT), bilirubin, blood urea nitrogen (BUN), creatinine, prothrombin time (PT), and PT-international normalized ratio (INR) [11]. Blood culture should be performed if high fever is present [11].

Imaging tools that are being used are: transabdominal ultrasound (US), endoscopic ultrasound (EUS), intraductal sonography (IDUS), endoscopic retrograde cholangiography (ERCP), percutaneous cholangiography (PTC), computed tomography (CT), and nuclear magnetic resonance/magnetic resonance cholangiopancreatography (NMR/MRCP). Abdominal ultrasound is simple, cheap, widely used, minimally invasive, and should be firstly performed in patients with suspected biliary infection [9]. It will document the presence of gallbladder stones, demonstrate dilated ducts, and possibly pinpoint the site of obstruction. One should not forget its disadvantages such as the fact that the results are easily affected by the operator's skill and the patient's condition [9, 11]. EUS is superior to transabdominal US and CT, and equivalent to ERCP or MRCP. EUS can be combined with fine needle aspiration to provide tissue diagnosis, important in the case of biliary malignancy [9]. IDUS is a relatively new technology, and has shown to be a very useful adjunct to ERCP when imaging the proximal bile ducts and also provides more accurate characteristics of bile duct lesions [9].

The definitive diagnostic tests are ERCP and PTC, beside that they will show the level and the reason for the obstruction, they also allow sampling of the bile for microbiology, removal of stones if present, and allow drainage of the bile ducts with drainage catheters or stents [12]. CT and NMR will show pancreatic and periampullary masses, if present, in addition to the ductal dilatation [12].

> **Differential Diagnosis**
>
> As said earlier, cholangitis is not a single entity, yet a variety of clinical appearances [9]. Since pregnant women are prone to symptomatic gallstones, consider cholangitis in pregnant, febrile, or jaundiced patients. Here one must be careful and differentiate cholangitis from HELLP syndrome in preeclampsia (hemolysis, elevated liver enzymes, low platelet count), since it also causes abdominal pain and elevated liver enzymes, but patients here are hypertensive, and arterial tension may be lowered in cholangitis [14]. Cholelithiasis and cholangitis are uncommon in children, except in those with underlying hemolytic disorders or biliary anomalies. The incidence of cholangitis is higher in elderly persons, most likely due to the increased prevalence of common bile duct stones with age. As in other infections and abdominal processes, elderly patients frequently do not manifest pathology in a classic pattern. Consider cholangitis in febrile or hypotensive elderly patients [12]. Other conditions to consider in patients with suspected acute cholangitis include the following: cirrhosis, liver failure, liver abscess, acute appendicitis, perforated peptic ulcer, pyelonephritis, right colon diverticulitis, acute pancreatitis, mesenteric ischemia, septic shock, viral hepatitis.

## 59.3 Treatment

### 59.3.1 Medical Treatment

Historically speaking, operative management was the only option for treatment of obstructive jaundice; however, nowadays there are other treatment options, like endoscopic biliary drainage (EBD), percutaneous transhepatic biliary drainage (PTBD), balloon dilatation, and endoscopic sphincterotomy. Patients with jaundice have increased risk of developing kidney failure, gastrointestinal bleeding, cardiopulmonary complications, and infections.

#### 59.3.1.1 Cardiopulmonary

In assessing cardiopulmonary status, age of patient, recent myocardial infarction (heart attack), presence of congestive heart failure, significant valvular heart disease, and heart rhythm disorder are all connected with increased operative risk. In addition, patients with severe lung disease are not candidates for major abdominal surgery (extensive abdominal interventions) [15].

#### 59.3.1.2 Renal

Patients with jaundice, especially those with liver cirrhosis and cholangitis, have increased risk of renal failure. Maintaining appropriate blood volume and treatment of dehydration are extremely important for preventing renal failure. In this regard, patients can benefit of invasive hemodynamic monitoring using a central venous catheter or pulmonary artery catheter to evaluate intravascular volume. Per os application of 500 mg of sodium deoxycholate three times a day, 48 h before surgery has protective effect on the development of systemic endotoxemia. Certain oral bile salts have been shown to be efficacious in preventing the development of postoperative kidney injury. In a study by Cahill (1983) 54% of 24 patients with jaundice not given oral bile salts before surgery were found to have systemic endotoxemia, which was associated with renal impairment in two-thirds of the cases [16].

#### 59.3.1.3 Nutrition

Malnutrition is significant risk factor for surgery in case of obstructive jaundice. Patients with malignant obstructive jaundice have varying degrees of malnutrition so they need adequate nutritional support. Operative morbidity and mortality rates are significantly reduced in patients undergoing nutritional hyperalimentation 20 days before percutaneous biliary drainage [17].

#### 59.3.1.4 Coagulation

Patients with obstructive jaundice, cholangitis, or cirrhosis are prone to excessive intraoperative bleeding. The most common coagulopathy in these patients is reflected in prolongation in prothrombin time (PT), which is reversible by giving vitamin K parenterally. Patients with severe jaundice and/or cholangitis can also develop disseminated intravascular coagulopathy (DIC), which may require infusion of platelets, fresh frozen plasma, and humane recombinant soluble thrombomodulin (rTM) [18, 19]. Treatment of DIC also requires source control for biliary sepsis, which, in addition to the use of systemic antibiotics, also includes urgent biliary decompression. In patients with cirrhosis, coagulopathies are often multifactorial and include secondary thrombocytopenia, prolongation of PT, and partial thromboplastin time (PTT) and fibrinolysis. Vitamin K should be given if PT is prolonged. If no effect is seen and/or PTT is also prolonged, fresh frozen plasma should be given. Thrombocytopenia can be corrected by platelet transfusion. If patient has a shortened coagulation lysis time and hypofibrinogenemia ε-aminocaproic acid can be given.

Endoscopic treatment is considered the first line of treatment for benign strictures, because of its safety, efficiency, and less invasive nature compared to surgery or percutaneous techniques. Alternative techniques of EBD are EUS-assisted biliary drainage (EUS-BD), which is PTBD. In patients with unresectable tumor of distal half of main biliary duct, endoscopic biliary stenting is performed for the purpose of palliation. In hilar lesions preference is given to PTBD. Also, in inoperable tumors of distal choledochus, endobiliary photodynamic therapy (PTD), radio frequency ablation (RFA), and drug-eluting stent (DES) are used; first two techniques are yielding promising results for now [20].

Initial treatment of acute cholangitis implies infusion of sufficient amounts of fluids, application of antibiotics and analgesics with careful monitoring of blood pressure, heart rate, and diuresis. Based on Tokyo guideline for treatment of acute cholangitis (TG18) [11], the treatment depends on severity of symptoms (Fig. 59.1) [21].

### 59.3.1.5 Grade I (Mild Acute Cholangitis)

In most cases, an initial treatment that includes antibiotics is sufficient, and most patients don't need biliary drainage. However, biliary drainage should be considered if the patient does not respond to initial treatment. Endoscopic sphincterotomy (EST) and following choledocholithotomy can be performed simultaneously with biliary drainage [21].

### 59.3.1.6 Grade II (Moderate Acute Cholangitis)

Moderate acute cholangitis is a cholangitis that is not severe but requires early biliary drainage. Early endoscopic or percutaneous transhepatic biliary drainage is indicated. Depending on etiology, if surgical treatment is required, it should be performed after improvement of the general condition, while EST and subsequent choledocholithotomy may be performed during biliary drainage, depending on the cause of cholangitis [21].

### 59.3.1.7 Grade III (Severe Acute Cholangitis)

Severe acute cholangitis is cholangitis with organ damage caused by sepsis. How the patient's condition can quickly deteriorate, a rapid response is needed, including appropriate organ support (endotracheal intubation and artificial ventilation and use of inotropic and vasopressor drugs). Endoscopic or percutaneous biliary drainage should be performed as soon as possible after the patient's condition has improved with initial treatment and cardiovascular and respiratory support. If treatment of basic etiology is necessary, it should be provided after the improvement of the general condition of the patient [21].

If the health facility isn't equipped for biliary drainage or appropriate intensive care, it is desirable to transport patients with severe or moderate form of cholangitis to an institution that is capable of providing these interventions, whether or

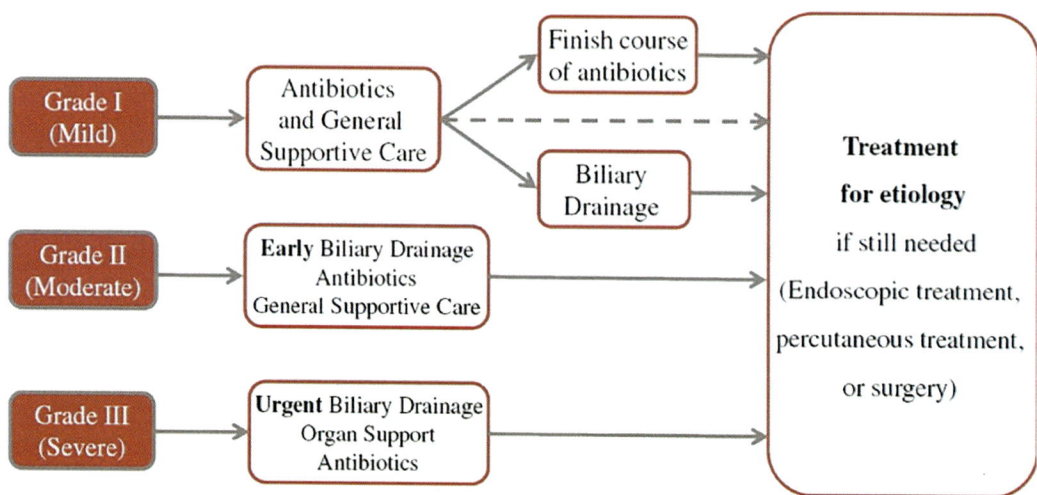

**Fig. 59.1** TG18 flowchart for the management of acute cholangitis. Cited and modified from Miura et al. [21] *Blood culture should be taken into consideration before antibiotics are started. Bile samples should be taken during biliary drainage and cultured. †Principles of treatment for acute cholangitis consist of antimicrobial administration, biliary drainage, and treatment of the etiology. For patients with mild or moderate choledocholithiasis, if possible the etiology should be treated at the same time as biliary drainage is performed

not they are really needed at a given time (Table 59.3) [22].

When choosing antimicrobial therapy, microbiological agent, pharmacokinetics and pharmacodynamics, local antibiogram, history of antimicrobial drug use, allergies and adverse events, kidney and liver function should all be considered. An anaerobic therapy is required in bilio-digestive anastomosis [13].

Patients with septic shock should receive appropriate antimicrobial therapy within 1 h [23].

In other patients with milder form of the disease, therapy should be administered within 6 h of diagnosis [24].

In light of the growing incidence of cephalosporin-, penicillin derivatives-, and fluoroquinolone-resistant strains of *E. coli* and *Klebsiella*, in empirical treatment should be used carbapenems, piperacillin/tazobactam, tigecycline, amikacin, as well as newer generation drugs such as ceftazidime/avibactam and ceftolozane/tazobactam, until sensitivity to narrow-spectrum of antibiotics is demonstrated.

For acute cholangitis of III degree, as initial (empirical) therapy, the use of vancomycin and antibiotics with antipseudomonal effect is recommended until the causes are identified and antibiogram is determined, given that *Enterococcus* spp., and in particular *Pseudomonas aeruginosa*, are virulent pathogens and increase mortality. In case of resistance of *Enterococcus* spp., linezolid or daptomycin is used instead of vancomycin. For grade I and II cholangitis, due to *Bacteroides* spp. resistance, the use of cefmetazole, flomoxef, and cefoperazone/sulbactam is recommended [24]. Once control of the source of infection has been established in patients with acute cholangitis, antimicrobial therapy for 4–7 days is recommended. If bacteremia is caused by gram-positive cocci, such as *Enterococcus* spp., *Streptococcus* spp., it is recommended to use antibiotics for at least 2 weeks [13]. Randomized clinical studies showed that early and proactive use of analgesics in acute cholangitis does not lead to late and misdiagnosis. The use of morphine-hydrochloride and similar opioids should be avoided due to spasm of Ody's sphincter and a consequent, additional increase in pressure in the biliary tree [25, 26].

In acute cholangitis, patients who do not respond to initial drug treatment within 12–48 h should receive emergency decompression of the biliary tree, which is essential and occupies, along with antibiotic therapy, a central place in treatment. Biliary tract decompression can be endoscopic (EBD), percutaneous biliary drainage (PTBD), or surgical. EBD includes external nasobiliar drainage (ENBD) and endoscopical retrograde biliary drainage (ERBD, ERCP). Initial non-surgical biliary drainage is recommended [21].

### 59.3.2 Surgical Treatment

Surgical treatment of jaundice depends on its cause (Table 59.4) [27]. In acute cholangitis caused by choledocholithiasis, open drainage should only be used on patients for whom endoscopic or percutaneous transhepatic drainage is contraindicated or in those in which it has been unsuccessfully performed. In such difficult conditions, the primary goal is efficient decompression of the bile duct. In this case, the recommendation is to complete operation quickly by placing a T-drain, and without spending additional time on extraction of calculus [28]. After remediation of acute cholangitis due to choledocholithiasis, prophylactic laparoscopic cholecystectomy has clinical value [29].

**Table 59.3** Transfer criteria for acute cholangitis [22]

**Severe acute cholangitis (grade III)**
Patients who require emergency biliary drainage as well as critical care should be transferred immediately to a hospital where this can be provided

**Moderate acute cholangitis (grade II)**
Patients should be treated in a hospital where biliary drainage and systemic management can be performed. If a hospital is not equipped to perform biliary drainage, they should be transferred to a hospital where this can be provided

**Mild acute cholangitis (grade I)**
If a calculus is present in the common bile duct or there is no response to initial treatment (within 24 h), a similar response to that for moderate acute cholangitis should be considered

**Table 59.4** Surgical options specific to pathology [27]

| Pathology | Surgical options | Alternatives |
|---|---|---|
| Acute choledocholithiasis | Cholecystectomy with bile duct exploration and T-tube drainage | Cholecystectomy with ERCP |
| Stone impaction at ampulla | Cholecystectomy with bile duct exploration and T-tube drainage | Cholecystectomy with ERCP |
| Mirizzi's syndrome | Cholecystectomy with bile duct exploration and T-tube drainage | Roux-en-Y hepaticojejunostomy |
| Stenosis of sphincter of Oddi | Transduodenal sphincteroplasty | Choledochoduodenostomy or Roux-en-Y hepaticojejunostomy |
| Gallstone pancreatitis (primary stones and common channel) | Transduodenal sphincteroplasty | Roux-en-Y hepaticojejunostomy |
| Chronic pancreatitis with obstructed jaundice (benign) | Choledochoduodenostomy | Roux-en-Y hepaticojejunostomy |
| Ischemic biliary strictures | Roux-en-Y hepaticojejunostomy | |
| Primary sclerosing cholangitis | Roux-en-Y hepaticojejunostomy | |
| Choledochal cysts | Roux-en-Y hepaticojejunostomy | |
| Cholangiocarcinoma | Radical resection with Roux-en-Y hepaticojejunostomy | Palliative Roux-en-Y hepaticojejunostomy |
| Gallbladder carcinoma | Radical resection with roux-en-Y hepaticojejunostomy | Palliative Roux-en-Y hepaticojejunostomy |
| Pancreatic carcinoma | Radical resection with Roux-en-Y hepaticojejunostomy | Palliative Roux-en-Y hepaticojejunostomy |

### 59.3.3 Prognosis

The prognosis for the treatment of surgical jaundice certainly depends on its cause. The goal of biliary drainage in unresectable cancers is to improve the quality of life and the use of palliative chemotherapy in those patients whose general condition allows it [30, 31]. Thirty-day mortality was similar in PTBD and EBD in the treatment of malignant jaundice by 23.1% [32, 33]. In these patients, surgical drainage is associated with higher mortality, morbidity, and longer hospitalizations compared with non-surgical interventions [34]. Routine use of preoperative biliary drainage in resectable tumors of the pancreas and the biliary tract leads to higher incidence of postoperative complications and mortality [35, 36].

The most significant complications related to biliary stent include recurrent obstruction (RBO) which was defined by recurrent jaundice and/or cholangitis after stent placement based on the Tokyo Criterion 2014. Other complications include pancreatitis, cholecystitis, non-occlusive cholangitis, bleeding, ulceration, penetration. Cholangitis in patients with persistent biliary stent suggests the development of RBO and requires early endoscopic reintervention [37].

Treating cholangitis only conservatively leads to mortality rate of 87–100% [38, 39]. Emergency surgical treatment is associated with significant morbidity and mortality rate; therefore, both EBD and PTBD have been proposed as effective therapy for 5–10% of patients with acute cholangitis who do not respond to conservative therapy [40]. Mortality after endoscopic biliary decompression is 10% while in open procedure is 32%. The percentage of complications of endoscopic drainage is 34% and in open procedure 66% [41]. Endoscopic sphincterotomy (EST) is contraindicated in coagulopathy, systemic sepsis, and hemodynamic instability, except in patients who have clinically worsened after initial aggressive drug therapy. Emergency EST in bile duct decompression should be avoided especially in elderly patients due to high mortality rates (18.8%). In elderly patients it was observed that only endoscopic drainage results in lower morbidity (16.7%) and mortality rates (5.6%) compared to morbidity and mortality rates in surgical (87.5% and 25% respectively) and percutaneous drainage (36.4%; 9.1%) [42].

### Dos and Don'ts

- In unresectable cancers, jaundice should be treated by non-surgical procedures.
- Patients with septic shock should receive appropriate antimicrobial therapy within 1 h. In other patients with milder form of the disease, therapy should be administered within 6 h of diagnosis.
- In acute cholangitis, patients who do not respond to initial drug treatment within 12–48 h, non-surgical biliary drainage is recommended.
- Routine use of preoperative biliary drainage in resectable tumors of the pancreas and the biliary tract is not recommended.
- Endoscopic sphincterotomy (EST) is contraindicated in coagulopathy, systemic sepsis, and hemodynamic instability. Emergency EST in bile duct decompression should be avoided especially in elderly patients.

### Take-Home Messages

- Treatment of surgical jaundice is complex and multidisciplinary and is not focused only on the hepatobiliary system but also on maintaining the homeostasis of all organ systems;
- Rehydration therapy, administration of broad-spectrum antibiotics, and emergency decompression of the biliary tree are key to treating acute cholangitis;
- Initial biliary decompression requires endoscopic or percutaneous biliary drainage;
- Surgical treatment should be undertaken in case of unsuccessful endoscopic or percutaneous treatment.

### Multiple Choice Questions

1. The incidence of biliary obstruction in the United States is approximately:
   A. **5 cases per 1000 people;**
   B. 10 cases per 1000 people;
   C. 15 cases per 1000 people;
   D. 23 cases per 1000 people.
2. Biliary duct obstructions are caused most frequently by:
   A. Choledocholithiasis;
   B. Benign strictures/obstructions;
   C. Malignant strictures/obstructions;
   D. **All of the above.**
3. According to Tokyo guidelines from 2018, acute cholangitis is classified into:
   A. Two grades;
   B. **Tree grades;**
   C. Four grades;
   D. Six grades.
4. Biliary ductal obstruction results in predominantly:
   A. **Conjugated hyperbilirubinemia;**
   B. Unconjugated hyperbilirubinemia;
   C. Conjugated and unconjugated hyperbilirubinemia;
   D. Hypercholesterolemia.
5. Charcot triad consists of:
   A. Septicemia, right upper quadrant pain, and jaundice;
   B. **Fever, epigastric or right upper quadrant pain and jaundice;**
   C. Septicemia, mental deterioration, and epigastric or right upper quadrant pain;
   D. Septicemia, mental deterioration, and jaundice.
6. Patients with severe jaundice and/or cholangitis can also develop disseminated intravascular coagulopathy (DIC), which may require medical treatment consist of:
   A. Infusion of platelets;
   B. Fresh frozen plasma;
   C. Humane recombinant soluble thrombomodulin (rTM).
   D. **All of the above.**

7. Patients with acute cholangitis and septic shock should receive appropriate antimicrobial therapy within:
   A. 6 hours;
   B. 12 hours;
   C. **1 hour;**
   D. 24–48 hours.
8. For acute cholangitis of III degree, as initial (empirical) antimicrobial therapy is the use of:
   A. Cephalosporin-derivatives;
   B. Tigecycline;
   C. Amikacin;
   D. **Vancomycin and antibiotics with antipseudomonal effect.**
9. In case of failure of medical treatment of acute cholangitis, the procedure of choice for emergency biliary decompression is:
   A. Surgical procedure;
   B. Endoscopic biliary drainage;
   C. Percutaneous biliary drainage;
   D. **B and C.**
10. Choose the correct statement:
    A. In acute cholangitis, mortality after endoscopic biliary decompression is 32%;
    B. **Emergency surgical treatment is associated with significant morbidity and mortality rate;**
    C. Emergency EST in bile duct decompression should be performed especially in elderly patients;
    D. Routine use of preoperative biliary drainage in resectable tumors of the pancreas and the biliary tract leads to lower incidence of postoperative complications and mortality.

# References

1. Bonheur JL. Biliary obstruction. Mescape. 2019. https://emedicine.medscape.com/article/187001-overview#a6.
2. Cai JS, Qiang S, Bao-Bing Y. Advances of recurrent risk factors and management of choledocholithiasis. Scand J Gastroenterol. 2017;52(1):34–43. https://doi.org/10.1080/00365521.2016.1224382.
3. Zhu AX, Hong TS, Hezel AF, Kooby DA. Current management of gallbladder carcinoma. Oncologist. 2010;15(2):168–81. https://doi.org/10.1634/theoncologist.2009-0302.
4. Lan Cheong Wah D, Christophi C, Muralidharan V. Acute cholangitis: current concepts. ANZ J Surg. 2017;87(7–8):554–9. https://doi.org/10.1111/ans.13981.
5. Lee KF, Chong CN, Ng D, Cheung YS, Ng W, Wong J, et al. Outcome of surgical treatment for recurrent pyogenic cholangitis: a single-centre study. HPB (Oxford). 2009;11(1):75–80. https://doi.org/10.1111/j.1477-2574.2008.00018.x.
6. Shojamanesh H. Cholangitis. Medscape. 2020. https://emedicine.medscape.com/article/184043-overview#a6. Accessed 11 Mar 2020.
7. Pitt HA. Bile secretion and pathophysiology of biliary tract obstruction. In: Jarnagin WR, editor. BLUMGART'S surgery of the liver, biliary tract, and pancreas. 6th ed. Philadelphia: Elsevier; 2017. p. 123–32.
8. Shojaiefard A, Esmaeilzadeh M, Ghafouri A, Mehrabi A. Various techniques for the surgical treatment of common bile duct stones: a meta review. Gastroenterol Res Pract. 2009;2009:840208. https://doi.org/10.1155/2009/840208.
9. Calvino AS, Espat NJ. Cholangitis. In: Jarnagin WR, editor. BLUMGART'S surgery of the liver, biliary tract and pancreas. 6th ed. Philadelphia: Elsevier; 2017. p. 714–24.
10. Li FY, Cheng NS, Mao H, Jiang LS, Cheng JQ, Li QS, et al. Significance of controlling chronic proliferative cholangitis in the treatment of hepatolithiasis. World J Surg. 2009;33(10):2155–60. https://doi.org/10.1007/s00268-009-0154-8.
11. Miura F, Okamoto K, Takada T, Strasberg SM, Asbun HJ, Pitt HA, et al. Tokyo guidelines 2018: initial management of acute biliary infection and flowchart for acute cholangitis. J Hepatobiliary Pancreat Sci. 2018;25(1):31–40. https://doi.org/10.1002/jhbp.509.
12. Pham TH, Hunter JG. Gallbladder and the extrahepatic biliary system. In: Brunicardi FC, editor. Schwartz's principles of surgery. New York: McGraw Hill; 2015. p. 1311–40.
13. Gomi H, Solomkin JS, Schlossberg D, Okamoto K, Takada T, Strasberg SM, et al. Tokyo guidelines 2018: antimicrobial therapy for acute cholangitis and cholecystitis. J Hepatobiliary Pancreat Sci. 2018;25(1):3–16. https://doi.org/10.1002/jhbp.518.
14. Wallace K, Harris S, Addison A, Bean C. HELLP syndrome: pathophysiology and current therapies. Curr Pharm Biotechnol. 2018;19(10):816–26. https://doi.org/10.2174/1389201019666180712115215.
15. Goldman L, et al. Multifactorial index of cardiac risk in noncardiac surgical procedures. N Engl J Med. 1977;297:845–50.

16. Cahill CJ. Prevention of postoperative renal failure in patients with obstructive jaundice: the role of bile salts. Br J Surg. 1983;70:590–5.
17. Foschi D, et al. Hyperalimentation of jaundiced patients on percutaneous transhepatic biliary drainage. Br J Surg. 1986;73:716–9.
18. Suetani K, Okuse C, Nakahara K, Michikawa Y, Noguchi Y, Suzuki M, et al. Thrombomodulin in the management of acute cholangitis-induced disseminated intravascular coagulation. World J Gastroenterol. 2015;21:533–40.
19. Nakahara K, Okuse C, Adachi S, Suetani K, Kitagawa S, Okano M, et al. Use of antithrombin and thrombomodulin in the management of disseminated intravascular coagulation in patients with acute cholangitis. Gut Liver. 2013;7:363–70.
20. Nakai Y, Isayama H, Wang HP, et al. International consensus statements for endoscopic management of distal biliary stricture. J Gastroenterol Hepatol. 2020;35(6):967–79. https://doi.org/10.1111/jgh.14955.
21. Miura F, Takada T, Strasberg SM, Solomkin JS, Pitt HA, Gouma DJ, et al. TG13 flowchart for the management of acute cholangitis and cholecystitis. J Hepatobiliary Pancreat Sci. 2013;20:47–54.
22. Tokyo Guidelines. The revision committee for the guidelines of acute cholangitis and cholecystitis. Guidelines of acute cholangitis and cholecystitis 2013. Tokyo: Igakutosho-shuppan Ltd.; 2013.
23. Rhodes A, Evans LE, Alhazzani W, Levy MM, Antonelli M, Ferrer R, et al. Surviving sepsis campaign: international guidelines for management of sepsis and septic shock: 2016. Intensive Care Med. 2017;43:304–77.
24. Solomkin JS, Mazuski JE, Bradley JS, Rodvold KA, Goldstein EJC, Baron EJ, et al. Diagnosis and management of complicated intra-abdominal infection in adults and children: guidelines by the surgical infection society and the Infectious Diseases Society of America. Clin Infect Dis. 2010;50:133–6.
25. Thomas SH, Silen W, Cheema F, Reisner A, Aman S, Goldstein JN, et al. Effects of morphine analgesia on diagnostic accuracy in emergency department patients with abdominal pain: a prospective, randomized trial. J Am Coll Surg. 2003;196:18–31.
26. Gallagher EJ, Esses D, Lee C, Lahn M, Bijur PE. Randomized clinical trial of morphine in acute abdominal pain. Ann Emerg Med. 2006;48(2):150–60.
27. Kukar M, Wilkinson N. Surgical management of bile duct strictures. Indian J Surg. 2015;77:125–32.
28. Saltzstein EC, Peacock JB, Mercer LC. Early operation for acute biliary tract stone disease. Surgery. 1983;94:704–8.
29. Boerma D, Rauws EA, Keulemans YC, Janssen YC, Bolwerk CJ, Timmer R, et al. Wait-and-see policy or laparoscopic cholecystectomy after endoscopic sphincterotomy for bile duct stones: a randomized trial. Lancet. 2002;360:739–40.
30. Saluja SS, Gulati M, Garg PK, et al. Endoscopic or percutaneous biliary drainage for gallbladder cancer: a randomized trial and quality of life assessment. Clin Gastroenterol Hepatol. 2008;6:944–50.
31. Barkay O, Mosler P, Schmitt CM, et al. Effect of endoscopic stenting of malignant bile duct obstruction on quality of life. J Clin Gastroenterol. 2013;47:526–31.
32. Zhao XQ, Dong JH, Jiang K, et al. Comparison of percutaneous transhepatic biliary drainage and endoscopic biliary drainage in the management of malignant biliary tract obstruction: a meta-analysis. Dig Endosc. 2015;27:137–45.
33. van Delden OM, Laméris JS. Percutaneous drainage and stenting for palliation of malignant bile duct obstruction. Eur Radiol. 2008;18:448–56. https://doi.org/10.1007/s00330-007-0796-6.
34. Smith AC, Dowsett JF, Russell RC, et al. Randomised trial of endoscopic stenting versus surgical bypass in malignant low bileduct obstruction. Lancet. 1994;344:1655–60. https://doi.org/10.1016/S0140-6736(94)90455-3.
35. Sewnath ME, et al. Meta-analysis on the efficacy of preoperative biliary drainage for tumors causing obstructive jaundice. Ann Surg. 2002;236:17–27.
36. Sohn TA, et al. Do preoperative biliary stents increase post pancreaticoduodenectomy complications? J Gastrointest Surg. 2000;4:258–68.
37. Isayama H, Hamada T, Yasuda I, et al. TOKYO criteria 2014 for transpapillary biliary stenting. Dig Endosc. 2015;27:259–64.
38. O'Connor MJ, Schwartz ML, McQuarrie DG, Sumer HW. Acute bacterial cholangitis: an analysis of clinical manifestation. Arch Surg. 1982;117:437–41.
39. Welch JP, Donaldson GA. The urgency of diagnosis and surgical treatment of acute suppurative cholangitis. Am J Surg. 1976;131:527–32.
40. Gigot JF, et al. Acute cholangitis: multivariate analysis of risk factors. Ann Surg. 1989;209:435–8.
41. Lai EC, Mok FP, Tan ES, Lo CM, Fan ST, You KT, et al. Endoscopic biliary drainage for severe acute cholangitis. N Engl J Med. 1992;24:1582–6.
42. Boender J, Nix GA, de Ridder MA, Dees J, Schutte HE, van Buuren HF, et al. Endoscopic sphincterotomy and biliary drainage in patients with cholangitis due to common bile duct stones. Am J Gastroenterol. 1995;90:233–8.

## Further Reading

Calvino AS, Espat NJ. Cholangitis. In: Jarnagin WR, editor. BLUMGART'S surgery of the liver, biliary tract and pancreas. 6th ed. Philadelphia: Elsevier; 2017. p. 714–24.

Miura F, Okamoto K, Gomi H, Solomkin JS, Schlossberg D, Okamoto K, Takada T, Strasberg SM, et al. Tokyo guidelines 2018: antimicrobial therapy for acute cholangitis and cholecystitis. J Hepatobiliary Pancreat Sci. 2018;25(1):3–16. https://doi.org/10.1002/jhbp.518.

Pitt HA. Bile secretion and pathophysiology of biliary tract obstruction. In: Jarnagin WR, editor. BLUMGART'S surgery of the liver, biliary tract, and pancreas. 6th ed. Philadelphia: Elsevier; 2017. p. 123–32.

Takada T, Strasberg SM, Asbun HJ, Pitt HA, et al. Tokyo guidelines 2018: initial management of acute biliary infection and flowchart for acute cholangitis. J Hepatobiliary Pancreat Sci. 2018;25(1):31–40. https://doi.org/10.1002/jhbp.509.

# Biliary Colic and Acute Cholecystitis

## 60

Paola Fugazzola, Mario Improta, and Luca Ansaloni

## 60.1 Introduction

**Learning Goals**

- Be able to make differential diagnosis between biliary colic and acute cholecystitis.
- Understand the pathogenesis that leads to the development of inflammation of the gallbladder and therefore to cholecystitis, and understanding of its severity classification.
- Understand the management options and timing of intervention, ranging from pure pain management to laparoscopic early cholecystectomy.

### 60.1.1 Epidemiology

In the United States, up to 20 million people among men and women, with a rate of 1:5, suffer from gallbladder disease. The prevalence of gallstones in the general population is 10–15% and 40% of those will develop gallstone-related complication [1–3]. The typical patient is a female in its 40 s or 50 s (the 4F: female, fat, fertile, forty).

### 60.1.2 Etiology

Gallstones cause all episodes of biliary colic and the most of episodes of cholecystitis. High levels of serum lipids, high cholesterol, or rapid weight loss (liver metabolize fats and more cholesterol are secreted into the gallbladder) can facilitate the formation of gallstones [4].

Up to 80% of gallstones are made of cholesterol, while 20% are formed by bilirubin conjugated with cholesterol itself in mixed form or with calcium [5].

### 60.1.3 Classification

Biliary colic consists of pain in the right upper quadrant associated with the presence of gallstones, usually rises after a fat-rich meal. Acute cholecystitis is the presence of inflammation of the gallbladder with or without the presence of gallstones.

Once the diagnosis of acute calculous cholecystitis (ACC) is made (see diagnostic criteria in the next section), the severity of the cholecystitis must be assessed to ensure the best treatment.

---

P. Fugazzola (✉) · M. Improta · L. Ansaloni
General and Emergency Surgery Unit, General Surgery 1 Department, IRCCS San Matteo Hospital, University of Pavia, Pavia, Italy

Classification of severity for acute cholecystic has been proposed by the Tokyo guidelines (TG) group [4].

1. Grade I, *Mild ACC*: does not meet the criteria of "Grade III" or "Grade II" ACC: grade I can also be defined as ACC in a healthy patient with no organ dysfunction and mild inflammatory changes in the gallbladder, making cholecystectomy a safe and low-risk operative procedure.
2. Grade II, *Moderate ACC*, associated with any one of the following conditions:
   (a) Elevated white blood cell count (>18,000/mm$^3$);
   (b) Palpable tender mass in the right upper abdominal quadrant;
   (c) Duration of complaints >72 h;
   (d) Marked local inflammation (gangrenous cholecystitis, pericholecystic abscess, hepatic abscess, biliary peritonitis, emphysematous cholecystitis).
3. Grade III, *Severe ACC*: an ACC associated with organ dysfunction.
   (a) Cardiovascular dysfunction: hypotension with dopamine >5 μg/kg/min, or norepinephrine, any dose;
   (b) Neurological dysfunction: decreased level of consciousness;
   (c) Respiratory dysfunction: PaO$_2$/FiO$_2$ ratio <300;
   (d) Renal dysfunction: oliguria, creatinine >2.0 mg/dL;
   (e) Hepatic dysfunction: PT-INR >1.5;
   (f) Hematological dysfunction: platelet count <100,000/mm$^3$.

## 60.1.4 Pathophysiology

Except for some cases of acalculous cholecystitis [mostly due to trauma, burns, parenteral nutrition, chronic liver disease, multiorgan failures (MOFs)], most cholecystitis are associated with the presence of gallstone. The natural history of biliary colic and cholecystitis is different. In the biliary colic, a gallstone impacts the cystic duct usually after a fat meal that causes the gallbladder to shrink. The gallbladder will then contract in an attempt to remove the gallstone and to have it pass through the cystic duct, this itself produces the pain [7]; in the biliary colic, the gallstone eventually will pass through the cystic duct if small enough, or if too big to pass will move away from the efflux tract with the resolution of symptoms. Sometimes, if it can pass in the main biliary duct (NBD), obstructive jaundice can be caused. In contrast, when the gallstone fails to move away from the cystic duct, the bile starts to accumulate causing gallbladder distention, thus inability to lymphatic drainage and later bacterial overgrowth and infection (Fig. 60.1).

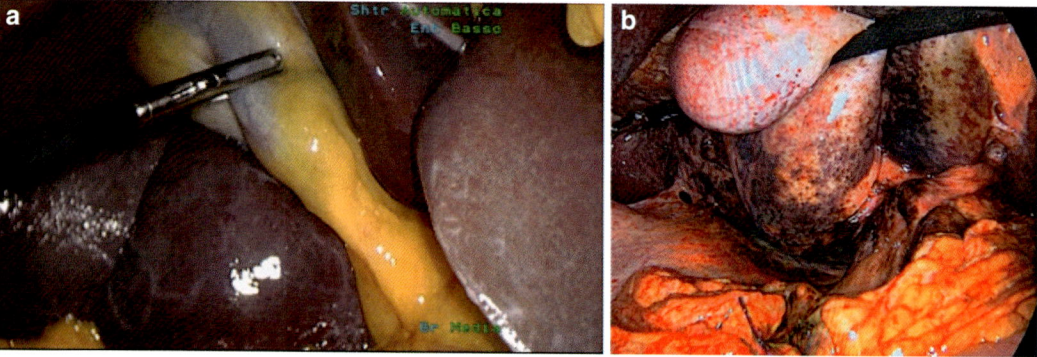

**Fig. 60.1** (a) Intraoperative image of a patient undergoing laparoscopic cholecystectomy for biliary colics. (b) Intraoperative image of a patient with acute cholecystitis

## 60.2 Diagnosis

### 60.2.1 Clinical Presentation

The typical presentation is pain in the right upper quadrant (associated with fever in acute cholecystitis) that can be irradiated to the right shoulder or scapula. Fever and vomiting are frequent in acute cholecystitis while these are absent in biliary colic, as a marker of systemic inflammation. The pain is continuous and makes the name "colic" misleading since it derives from the stretching of the walls of the gallbladder; usually, it starts after a fat-rich meal. Acute abdomen is rare except in the event of a perforation of the gallbladder; if perforation occurs on the liver side, in contrast, there will be no peritonitis but the development of a peri-liver abscess.

The "Murphy" sign is the pain and momentary arrest of breathing at the palpation of the costal margin in the right upper quadrant, while the patient is asked to take a big breath. Breathing lowers the diaphragm that pushes the liver and the gallbladder more anteriorly and inferior to the costal margin, so when the operator push with his hand under the costal margin the breathing is stopped due to intense pain.

### 60.2.2 Tests

Alteration of laboratory markers is unusual in biliary colic, except if the gallstone passes in the main biliary duct, while it is common in acute cholecystitis. Leukocytosis and elevation of C reactive protein (CRP) are suggestive of local inflammation; alteration of serum bilirubin, liver function tests (LFTs), and cholestasis markers such as alkaline phosphatase and gamma-glutamyl transferase (GGT) are uncommon and suggestive of potential involvement of the common bile duct and therefore should prompt further investigation.

Ultrasound investigation alone is enough to confirm the diagnosis of biliary colic. Gallstones appear as hyperechoic comma with posterior shadowing, those are mobile and can be multiple. In the case of a gallstone impacted in the cystic duct, the infundibulum of the gallbladder will not be visible and will be masked by the gallstones that are firm.

**In the event of acute cholecystitis besides the presence of gallstones, ultrasound signs are**
1. thickening of the gallbladder wall (some author uses 3 mm as cutoff while others use 5 mm) (Fig. 60.2),
2. presence of pericholecystic fluid,
3. ultrasound-murphy sign.

### 60.2.3 Diagnostic Criteria

In 2018, the TG group proposed three criteria to take into account for the diagnosis of ACC [4] (Table 60.1)
1. the presence of local inflammation, such as right upper quadrant pain and/or Murphy's sign;
2. the presence of systemic inflammation, identified by the presence of fever or alteration of laboratory findings (leukocytosis, elevation of CRP);
3. imaging findings characteristic of ACC.

To confirm a diagnosis of acute cholecystitis, each item of the three criteria must be present.

Accuracy of the diagnostic criteria of the TG 2018 is up to 95% but other studies showed poor sensitivity.

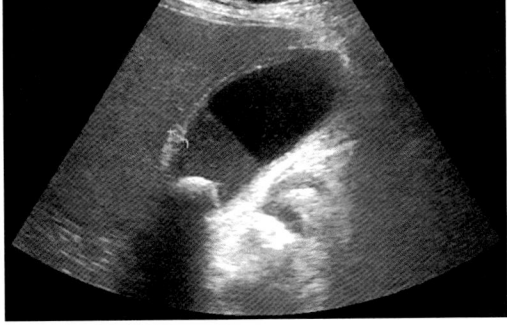

**Fig. 60.2** Acute cholecystitis with gallstone impacted in the infundibulum. Note the cholecystic wall thickening, the acoustic shadowing of the gallstone, and the isoechoic sludge inside the gallbladder

**Table 60.1** Diagnostic criteria for suspected and definitive diagnosis of acute cholecystitis

| |
|---|
| **1. Local inflammation** |
| – Murphy sign's |
| – RUQ palpable mass |
| – RUQ tenderness |
| **2. Systemic inflammation** |
| – Fever |
| – Leukocytosis |
| – Elevated CRP |
| **3. Suggestive imaging** |
| – Impacted gallstone |
| – Wall thickening |
| – Pericholecystic fluid |
| **Suspected diagnosis** |
| One item in A + one item in B |
| **Definitive diagnosis** |
| One item in A + one item in B + one item in C |

A study found that, among fever, inflammatory markers, and ultrasound (US) findings, the only neutrophil count was statistically associated with the diagnosis of cholecystitis [1]. The study showed that the overall accuracy of TG 2013 criteria was 60.3% and TG 2013 over-diagnosed ACC in 62.5% of normal gallbladders. Then, according to 2016 and 2020 WSES guidelines (GL) there is no single clinical or laboratory finding with sufficient diagnostic accuracy to establish or exclude ACC. Only a combination of detailed history, complete clinical examination, laboratory tests and imaging investigations may strongly support the diagnosis of ACC, although the best combination is not yet known [6, 7].

## 60.3 Treatment

### 60.3.1 Biliary Colic

Pain management is the only urgent intervention that is needed in case of biliary colic without the occurrence of acute cholecystitis. Biliary colic should be treated with non-steroidal anti-inflammatory drugs and spasmolytics. Definitive treatment for biliary colic is the laparoscopic cholecystectomy which can be postponed and performed not in an emergency setting. Routine treatment is not recommended for patients with asymptomatic gallbladder stones [8].

### 60.3.2 Acute Cholecystitis

The definitive treatment of ACC is laparoscopic cholecystectomy (LP), but the decision to operate should take into account a lot of factors such as time from the onset of symptoms to intervention, performance status of the patient, and according to TG 2018, the severity of the acute cholecystitis [4, 9]. During these years a lot reports, case series and randomized controlled trials have been published discussing the better timing for laparoscopic cholecystectomy in ACC, early (EC) or delayed (DC).

EC is defined as an intervention performed *as soon as possible* (usually within 24–72 h from hospital access) but at max within 7 days from hospital admission and within 10 days from the onset of symptoms. DC is defined as cholecystectomy performed at least 6 weeks after the resolution of acute cholecystitis. Intermediate Laparoscopic Cholecystectomy (ILC) is defined as cholecystectomy performed from 10 days to 6 weeks from the acute episode [10].

**TG suggest a treatment flowchart based on the clinical classification of ACC (see Sect. 60.1.3, Classification) as follows**

- Mild Cholecystitis—if patient performance status (PS) allows intervention, EC should be performed. If the patient is unfit for surgery (e.g., Charlson index >6 or ASA-PS >3) "conservative management" with antibiotics is advocated, followed by DC.
  - Moderate Cholecystitis—EC in an advanced surgical center is recommended if the CCI and ASA-PS scores suggest the patient can withstand surgery (CCI <6 and ASA-PS <3). In case of difficult cholecystectomy, switch to open or subtotal cholecystectomy could be considered. If patient cannot withstand surgery, TG suggested conservative management and, if patient does not respond to initial medical treatment, biliary drainage (BD) (consider DC).
  - Severe Cholecystitis—attempts should be made to normalize organ function through organ support, alongside administration of antimicrobials. EC in an advanced surgical

center is recommended if the patient is judged to be able to withstand surgery (no neurological and respiratory dysfunction, total bilirubin <2 mg/dL, CCI <4 and ASA-PS <3). In case of difficult cholecystectomy, switch to open or subtotal cholecystectomy could be considered. If patient cannot withstand surgery, TG suggested conservative management and, if patient does not respond to initial medical treatment, biliary drainage (BD) (consider DC).

WSES GL recommended EC as the first-line therapy for ACC, after a risk stratification for common bile duct stones (CBDS). The only contraindications to EC are septic shock or absolute anesthesiology contraindications. WSES 2020 GL recommended laparoscopic or open subtotal cholecystectomy in situations in which anatomic identification is difficult and in which the risk of iatrogenic injuries is high [6].

Focusing on timing of cholecystectomy, WSES recommendation is EC, given that ILC and DC showed higher complication rates and costs. If EC is not feasible, DC should be proposed. ILC has shown to be a higher risk and therefore should be discouraged [10] (Fig. 60.3).

Alternative or complementary to surgical therapy, antibiotic therapy in patients with ACC can be used on three occasions: (1) when the patient is unfit for surgery and conservative management is chosen; (2) when the patient refuses surgery even in the setting of a timely intervention; (3) as bridge therapy for patients with septic shock that

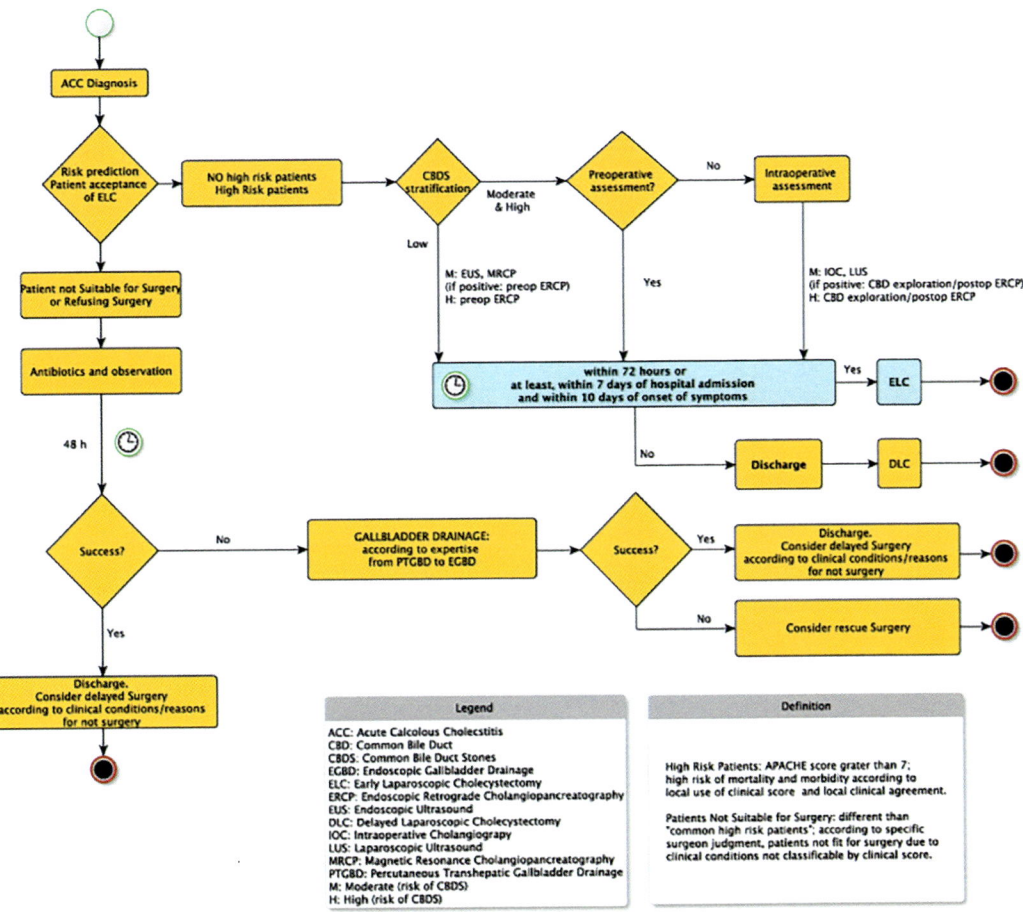

**Fig. 60.3** Algorithm for the management of acute cholecystitis after CBDS assessment adapted from WSES guidelines [6] with permission

later will undergo intervention or patients with CBDS (common bile duct stone) as a bridge while endoscopic intervention for stone removal is performed.

If cholecystectomy is performed, discontinuation of antibiotic therapy after an intervention is recommended by WSES GL, taken into account randomized studies that showed no difference in the incidence of postoperative infections between patients who undergone a 5 day-trial of postoperative antibiotic versus patients who discontinued therapy [6]. TG suggested postoperative antibiotic therapy for a duration of 4–7 days only in case of grade III or complicated ACC.

If surgical therapy is not feasible and antibiotic therapy alone fails to improve patient symptoms (e.g., worsening of pain and/or laboratory markers of infection, and new-onset organ damage), BD should be considered. BD removes the infected bile from gallbladder and therefore helps the resolution of inflammation. It could be performed percutaneously (US-guided, Fig. 60.4) or endoscopically.

The CHOCOLATE study, a randomized controlled trial [11] comparing EC and percutaneous biliary drainage in high-risk patients (APACHE II score ≥7) with ACC, showed a higher major complication rate, a higher reintervention rate and a higher rate of recurrent biliary disease in the BD arm. Another recent trial, the DRAC 1 trial [12], compared endoscopic ultrasound (EUS)-guided with percutaneous biliary drainage in high-risk patients (age ≥80, ASA-PS score ≥3, age-adjusted CCI >5 or Karnofsky score <50) with ACC, finding improved outcomes in EUS-guided arm in terms of adverse events, reintervention rate, readmissions, and recurrent cholecystitis. Furthermore, the introduction of EUS-guided biliary drainage with lumen-apposing self-expandable metal stents (LAMSs) seems to have promising results in this patient population [6].

### 60.3.3 Common Bile Duct Stones Associated with Acute Cholecystitis

Since acute cholecystitis and biliary colic are mostly caused by gallstones, the risk that some of those gallstones pass the cystic duct and obstruct the common bile duct exists. Liver laboratory tests should be performed to evaluate the presence of CBDS which can occur up to 25% in combination with acute cholecystitis [3]. The most reliable tests are GGT (gamma-glutamyl transferase, sensitivity of 80.6%, specificity of 75.3%, using a cut-off of 224 U/L) and serum bilirubin level (specificity 60% with a cut-off level of 1.7 mg/dL and 75% with a cut-off level of 4 mg/dL) but WSES GL recommend against the use of laboratory markers alone to make the diagnosis of CBDS [13].

Some scores were developed and validated to assess the risk of CBDS. The score proposed by the American Society of Gastrointestinal Endoscopy (ASGE) and the Society of American Gastrointestinal Endoscopic Surgeon (SAGES) and modified by WSES [6, 14], considers the evidence of CBDS at abdominal ultrasound, the presence of cholangitis, the common bile duct diameter, the total serum bilirubin, the finding of abnormal liver test, the age, and the presence of pancreatitis. With these parameters patients are stratified in three risk classes. Only patients with

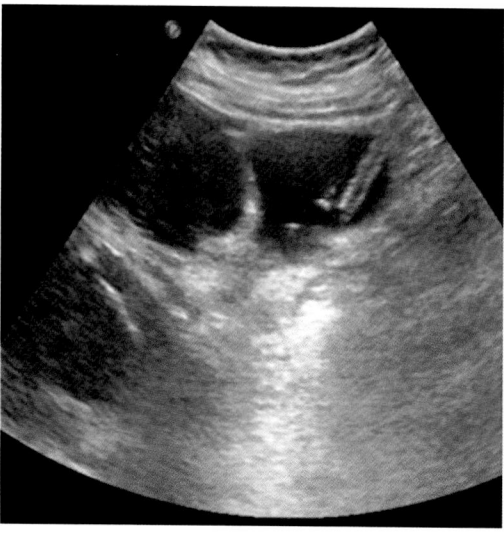

**Fig. 60.4** Percutaneous ultrasound-guided biliary drainage. Note the arrow that points to the hyperechoic drainage

evidence of CBDS at abdominal US should be considered at high risk and should directly undergo Endoscopic Retrograde Cholangio-Pancreatography (ERCP). Patients at intermediate risk should undergo second level investigations such as Endoscopic Ultrasound (EUS) or Magnetic Resonance Cholangio-Pancreatography (MRCP), Laparoscopic Ultrasound (LUS) or Intraoperative Cholangiography (IOC), depending on local expertise and availability. Low-risk patients could directly receive EC (Table 60.2).

A recently validated score, the Israelian Score (IS) ideated on patients with ACC, included common bile duct diameter, age, and total serum bilirubin. It stratifies patients in three risk class: in case of IS equals to 2, the patient should undergo preferentially a preoperative EUS or a MRCP to investigate CBDS. In case of confirmation of CBDS or in case of IS equals to 3, an ERCP prior to EC should be performed. In case of score equals to 0 or 1, the patient could be directly subjected to EC [15] (Table 60.3).

**Table 60.2** Risk factors and classification of risk of CBDS according to WSES GL 2020

| Predictive factor for choledocholithiasis | |
|---|---|
| Very strong | Evidence of CBD stone at abdominal ultrasound |
| | Ascending cholangitis |
| Strong | Common bile duct diameter >6 mm (with gallbladder in situ) |
| | Total serum bilirubin >1.8 mg/dL |
| Moderate | Abnormal liver biochemical test other than bilirubin |
| | Age older than 55 years |
| | Clinical gallstone pancreatitis |

| Risk class for choledocholithiasis | |
|---|---|
| High | Presence of any very strong |
| Low | No predictors present |
| Intermediate | All other patients |

**Table 60.3** Israelian Score for CBDS

| Predictive factor for choledocholithiasis | |
|---|---|
| Parameters | Score |
| CBD width by US ≥7 mm | 1 |
| Age (years) ≥70 | 1 |
| Total bilirubin ≥1.8 | 1 |

### Dos and Don'ts

**Dos**
- Perform ultrasound, inflammatory marker, and liver blood exams in the suspect of biliary colic or cholecystitis
- Obtain history to assess the timing of the onset of symptoms
- Stratify the risk of main biliary duct stones
- In case of ACC, perform cholecystectomy as soon as possible, however, within 10 days from the onset of symptoms

**Don'ts**
- Misdiagnose biliary colic for acute cholecystitis (remember the presence of signs of inflammation: fever, labs)
- Perform CT as the first-choice exam in suspect of gallbladder pathology (unless other causes of the acute abdomen are suspected, e.g., perforation)
- Perform cholecystectomy without ruling out main biliary duct stones

### Take-Home Messages

- Biliary colic and cholecystitis are differentiated by the presence of local and systemic inflammation and/or infection.
- The combination of detailed history, complete clinical examination, laboratory tests, and imaging investigation may strongly support the diagnosis of ACC.
- Early laparoscopic cholecystectomy (performed as soon as possible, however, within 10 days from onset of symptoms) is the treatment of choice for ACC.
- Common bile duct stones must be indagated in all patients with biliary colic or cholecystitis.

**Multiple Choice Questions (An Always Right Answer)**

1. What is the difference between biliary colic and acute cholecystitis?
   A. The presence of local and/or systemic inflammation
   B. The presence of impacted common bile duct stone
   C. The absence of pain in the right upper quadrant
   D. A and C both right
2. What is the most common cause of biliary colic and cholecystitis?
   A. The presence of gallstones
   B. Infection of the fourth segment of the liver
   C. Antibiotics and pain management assumption
   D. All answers are wrong
3. What are the manifestation of acute cholecystitis?
   A. All answers are right
   B. Pain at the right upper quadrant with or without vomiting
   C. Fever and chills
   D. Positivity of the murphy sign
4. Which of these criteria confirm a diagnosis of acute cholecystitis?
   A. All answers are wrong
   B. The presence of pain in the right upper quadrant only
   C. The presence of pain in the right upper quadrant associated with elevated serum bilirubin
   D. The presence of pain in the right upper quadrant associated with free peritoneal fluid seen at the ultrasound
5. Which of the following is true?
   A. Severe cholecystitis is identified from the presence of organ damage
   B. Mild cholecystitis should be treated as out department patients and without surgery
   C. The absence of pain in the right upper quadrant excludes the diagnosis of cholecystitis
   D. A and C both true
6. Which of the following is false?
   A. All answers are false
   B. In the presence of fever, antibiotic therapy should always be started
   C. If cholecystectomy can't be performed within 72 h it should be delayed
   D. Open cholecystectomy should never be performed
7. Which one is the best diagnostic test for acute cholecystitis?
   A. Ultrasound
   B. CT without contrast
   C. Contrast-enhanced CT
   D. Abdominal X-ray
8. Which is the definition of early cholecystectomy?
   A. Cholecystectomy performed as soon as possible, within 72 h and no longer than 10 days from the onset of symptoms
   B. Cholecystectomy performed as soon as possible, within 72 h and no longer than 7 days from the onset of symptoms
   C. Cholecystectomy performed as soon as possible, within 72 h
   D. Cholecystectomy performed within 6 weeks from the onset of symptoms
9. Which is the most reliable sign of CBDS?
   A. A combination of ultrasound, laboratory exam, and age
   B. Serum bilirubin

C. CT scan with stones in the gallbladder
D. Ultrasound examination

10. Which is the indication to perform biliary drainage?
    A. Moderate or severe cholecystitis in patients unfit for surgery that fails to respond to antibiotic treatment
    B. Severe cholecystitis that responds to antibiotic treatment
    C. All severe cholecystitis
    D. Severe cholecystitis that fails to respond to antibiotic treatment in patients fit for surgery

## References

1. Naidu K, Beenen E, Gananadha S, Mosse C. The yield of fever, inflammatory markers and ultrasound in the diagnosis of acute cholecystitis: a validation of the 2013 Tokyo guidelines. World J Surg. 2016;40:2892–7. https://doi.org/10.1007/s00268-016-3660-5.
2. Regimbeau JM, Fuks D, Pautrat K, et al. Effect of postoperative antibiotic administration on postoperative infection following cholecystectomy for acute calculous cholecystitis: a randomized clinical trial. JAMA. 2014;312:145–54. https://doi.org/10.1001/jama.2014.7586.
3. Shaffer EA. Epidemiology and risk factors for gallstone disease: has the paradigm changed in the 21st century? Curr Gastroenterol Rep. 2005;7:132–40. https://doi.org/10.1007/s11894-005-0051-8.
4. Yokoe M, Hata J, Takada T, et al. Tokyo guidelines 2018: diagnostic criteria and severity grading of acute cholecystitis (with videos). J Hepatobiliary Pancreat Sci. 2018;25:41–54. https://doi.org/10.1002/jhbp.515.
5. Jarrar BM, Al-Rowaili MA. Chemical composition of gallstones from Al-Jouf Province of Saudi Arabia. Malays J Med Sci. 2011;18:47–52.
6. Pisano M, Allievi N, Gurusamy K, et al. 2020 World Society of Emergency Surgery updated guidelines for the diagnosis and treatment of acute calculus cholecystitis. World J Emerg Surg. 2020;15:61. https://doi.org/10.1186/s13017-020-00336-x.
7. Byrne JJ, Berger RL. The pathogenesis of acute cholecystitis. Arch Surg. 1960;81:812–6. https://doi.org/10.1001/archsurg.1960.01300050134024.
8. EASL Clinical Practice Guidelines on the prevention. Diagnosis and treatment of gallstones. J Hepatol. 2016;2016:005. https://doi.org/10.1016/j.jhep.2016.03.005.
9. Mayumi T, Okamoto K, Takada T, et al. Tokyo guidelines 2018: management bundles for acute cholangitis and cholecystitis. J Hepatobiliary Pancreat Sci. 2018;25:96–100. https://doi.org/10.1002/jhbp.519.
10. Gutt CN, Encke J, Köninger J, et al. Acute cholecystitis: early versus delayed cholecystectomy, a multicenter randomized trial (ACDC study, NCT00447304). Ann Surg. 2013;258:385–93. https://doi.org/10.1097/sla.0b013e3182a1599b.
11. Loozen CS, Van Santvoort HC, Van Duijvendijk P, Besselink MG, Gouma DJ, Nieuwenhuijzen GA, et al. Laparoscopic cholecystectomy versus percutaneous catheter drainage for acute cholecystitis in high risk patients (CHOCOLATE): multicentre randomised clinical trial. BMJ. 2018;363:k3965.
12. Teoh AYB, Kitano M, Itoi T, Pérez-Miranda M, Ogura T, Chan SM, et al. Endosonography-guided gallbladder drainage versus percutaneous cholecystostomy in very high-risk surgical patients with acute cholecystitis: an international randomised multicentre controlled superiority trial (DRAC 1). Gut. 2020;69(6):1085–91.
13. Maple JT, Ben-Menachem T, Anderson MA, Appalaneni V, Banerjee S, Cash BD, et al. The role of endoscopy in the evaluation of suspected choledocholithiasis. Gastrointest Endosc. 2010;71(1):1–9.
14. Williams EJ, Green J, Beckingham I, et al. Guidelines on the management of common bile duct stones (CBDS). Gut. 2008;57:1004–21. https://doi.org/10.1136/gut.2007.121657.
15. Khoury T, Kadah A, Mari A, et al. A validated score predicting common bile duct stone in patients hospitalized with acute calculus cholecystitis: a multi-center retrospective study. Surg Endosc. 2021;35:3709–15. https://doi.org/10.1007/s00464-020-07853-5.

## Further Reading

Mayumi T, Okamoto K, Takada T, et al. Tokyo guidelines 2018: management bundles for acute cholangitis and cholecystitis. J Hepatobiliary Pancreat Sci. 2018;25:96–100. https://doi.org/10.1002/jhbp.519.

Pisano M, Allievi N, Gurusamy K, et al. 2020 World Society of Emergency Surgery updated guidelines for the diagnosis and treatment of acute calculus cholecystitis. World J Emerg Surg. 2020;15:61. https://doi.org/10.1186/s13017-020-00336-x.

Yokoe M, Hata J, Takada T, et al. Tokyo guidelines 2018: diagnostic criteria and severity grading of acute cholecystitis (with videos). J Hepatobiliary Pancreat Sci. 2018;25:41–54. https://doi.org/10.1002/jhbp.515.

# Hepatic Abscesses

Kyra N. Folkert, Sarah Khalil, and Robert Sawyer

## 61.1 Introduction

Hepatic abscesses although rare carry a significant mortality rate. They may develop as a result of both intra- and extra-abdominal infection. They are typically broken down into pyogenic or amebic, although they may also be caused by fungal and mixed infections. Successful treatment relies on prompt diagnosis and appropriate management. Different imaging modalities have distinct radiological findings, which may help one identify a liver abscess. Treatment has evolved in recent years and can range from antibiotics, percutaneous intervention, and even surgical intervention depending on the disease severity and response to minimally invasive treatments.

> **Learning Goals**
>
> - Understand the etiology, epidemiology, and common clinical presentation of hepatic abscesses
> - Be able to detect and interpret common laboratory and radiologic findings to assist with diagnosis
> - Identify and apply optimal treatment of hepatic abscesses in clinical practice

### 61.1.1 Epidemiology

Hepatic abscesses are a relatively uncommon disease process estimated only to account for 2.3 per 100,000 population in North America [1, 2]. Studies in Taiwan have noted considerably higher rates of disease up to 17.6 cases per 100,000 people [3]. Liver abscesses can be broken down further into pyogenic, amebic, fungal, and mixed. Hydatid disease should also be included in the spectrum of liver abscesses. Men have been noted to have a greater risk of acquiring a pyogenic liver abscess compared to women at a rate of 3.3 vs. 1.3 per 100,000 [2]. Mortality rate for hepatic abscesses varies widely across most studies and can range between 10 and 40% [1]. Incidence of pyogenic liver abscesses appears to increase with increasing age. Risk factors for the development of pyogenic liver abscesses include diabetes,

K. N. Folkert · S. Khalil · R. Sawyer (✉)
Western Michigan University Homer Stryker MD School of Medicine, Kalamazoo, MI, USA
e-mail: kyra.folkert@med.wmich.edu;
sarah.khalil@med.wmich.edu;
robert.sawyer@med.wmich.edu

© The Author(s), under exclusive license to Springer Nature Switzerland AG 2023
F. Coccolini, F. Catena (eds.), *Textbook of Emergency General Surgery*,
https://doi.org/10.1007/978-3-031-22599-4_61

liver transplant, cancer, and chronic proton pump inhibitor use [2, 4–8]. Patients with amebic liver abscesses are typically younger, with most cases occurring before the fifth decade of life [9]. Notably, 80% of the reported pyogenic liver abscess cases reported in the literature have occurred in East Asian countries [5].

An estimated 10% of the world's population is infected with *Entamoeba histolytica*, with the highest incidence in tropical countries. Amebiasis is one of the top three leading causes of parasite death in the world [10, 11] Those at greatest risk of infection are individuals with lower socioeconomic status living in overcrowded areas or areas with poor sanitation [11]. Most individuals will remain asymptomatic but around 5% may develop hepatic abscesses [12]. It should be noted that of those affected men are more commonly affected than women at a rate of 10:1, and those with chronic corticosteroid use are at higher risk of hepatic abscess development [12]. It is estimated that between 40,000 and 110,000 individuals per year die due to amoebic liver abscess [13].

Hydatid disease, caused by the tapeworm *Echinococcus granulosus*, is endemic in South America, Eastern Europe, and the Middle East according to the WHO. Its intermediate hosts are farm animals, such as sheep, goats, pigs, horses, and cattle. Prevalence can vary from 20 to 95%, particularly in areas near slaughterhouses, and the incidence of infected humans is thought to be far greater than the incidence of surgical cases [14].

Fungal abscesses are the least common cause of hepatic abscesses but typically occur in patients with a history of hematologic malignancy who have undergone chemotherapy treatment with a resultant neutropenia [15]. Fungal abscesses are also rarely associated with liver transplant and transarterial chemoembolization of liver tumors [1].

## 61.1.2 Etiology

Historically appendicitis was the leading cause of pyogenic liver abscess. Many studies are now showing that appendicitis causes pyogenic liver abscess <10% of the time [10, 16]. Most liver abscesses are now known to be associated with varying forms of biliary tract disease and biliary instrumentation [8]. Certain organisms are known to be associated with causes of liver abscesses (Table 61.1). *Escherichia coli* is the most common bacteria associated with liver abscesses [17, 18]. *Klebsiella pneumoniae* liver abscess is much more common in Asian countries [8]. It is also the most common organism associated with colorectal cancer in patients diagnosed with pyogenic liver abscess and some believe those with *K. pneumoniae* pyogenic liver abscess should undergo colonoscopy to screen for occult malignancy [19]. *K. pneumoniae* has also been known to be associated with cryptogenic liver abscesses. Many cases of hepatic abscess are cryptogenic in origin and up to 50% of liver abscesses are reported to be cryptogenic [8]. Less commonly, patients may develop pyogenic liver abscesses due to ingestion and migration of foreign bodies, such as toothpicks and fishbones [20]. Pyogenic liver abscess caused by staphylococcus and streptococcus species is typically associated with underlying endocarditis [16]. Anaerobic abscess can also develop and is more common in patients with blunt traumatic liver injury [21].

Amebic liver abscess develops as a result of *Entamoeba histolytica* infection, which is spread via fecal-oral transmission [6, 12]. Poor sanitation is the greatest risk factor for *E. histolytica*, as ingestion of contaminated food or water is the most common source of infection in humans; however, it can also be transmitted by oral and anal sex [6].

**Table 61.1** Classification of hepatic abscess by type and the most common organisms

| Abscess source | Most common organisms |
|---|---|
| Biliary | *Escherichia coli, Klebsiella pneumoniae,* enterococcus |
| Hematogenous | *Staphylococcus* and *Streptococcus* species |
| Diverticulitis, appendicitis | *Bacteroides fragilis,* anaerobic bacteria, mixed species |
| Immunocompromised | *Candida species, aspergillus, cryptococcus* |
| Cryptogenic | *Klebsiella pneumoniae* (especially in Asia), anaerobes |
| Amebic | *Entamoeba histolytica* |
| Hydatid | *Echinococcal* species |

*Echinococcus granulosus* is a small tapeworm that is commonly found in farming communities and the Mediterranean. Its definitive hosts are dogs and wolves, who become infected after ingesting infected meat. It lives as an adult tapeworm inside the intestine of its definitive hosts and releases proglottids carrying eggs into the intestinal lumen [22]. It infects intermediate hosts, such as sheep and pigs, after ingestion of water contaminated by infected feces. When ingested it remains attached to the intestinal mucosa and sheds proglottids carrying hundreds of eggs. When it enters intermediate hosts, it matures into cysts and daughter cysts. Humans are accidental intermediate hosts, becoming infected after direct contact with a dog contaminated with egg-bearing feces or by ingesting contaminated food or water [14, 22].

## 61.1.3 Classification

There are four main types of hepatic abscesses. These include:

1. Pyogenic
   (a) Can be polymicrobial
   (b) Arise from a number of different sources
2. Amebic
   (a) Infection with *Entamoeba histolytica*
3. Hydatid
   (a) Infection with *Echinococcus granulosus* or other Echinococcal species
4. Fungal
   (a) Typically caused by *Candida species*

As there are considerable differences between the types of abscess and their management, each chapter subsegment will further be divided into sections specific to each type of abscess.

## 61.1.4 Pathophysiology

The dual blood supply of liver from portal and systemic circulation makes the liver particularly susceptible to pyogenic abscess from hematogenous spread [6, 23]. This is particularly true in endocarditis, where septic microemboli travel through the bloodstream and seed the liver, causing multiple small abscesses that can coalesce to form a large abscess [8]. Central-line associated infection, periodontal disease, and bacteremia from any cause of sepsis can also result in abscess formation in this manner [6]. Seeding of the portal vein from intra-abdominal infection, such as appendicitis or diverticulitis, was historically the most common route for abscess development [6]. This has changed in recent years with faster time to detection and treatment of intraabdominal infection [6].

Pyogenic liver abscesses of biliary origin are thought to develop after inoculation of the biliary tree with enteric flora. The biliary tree is sterile in most patients as the sphincter of Oddi prevents bacteria from entering the bile duct. In patients with choledocholithiasis, biliary stents, or biliary-intestinal anastomoses, enteric flora are able to enter the biliary tree and can result in the development of cholangitis if the bile duct is occluded by stricture or stone [24]. In some cases, biliary-intestinal anastomosis or stenting can result in chronic infection of the bile duct and repeated episodes of cholangitis, which can eventually result in formation of liver abscess [24]. Pyogenic abscess can also develop as direct extension from cholecystitis, perinephric abscess, and subphrenic abscess [6].

Liver trauma can also result in abscess formation, including any surgical intervention or chemoembolization [6, 23]. Abscess development can be secondary to direct inoculation of the liver via a penetrating mechanism, but the predominant risk factor for abscess development is thought to be necrosis after liver trauma [6].

Amebic liver abscess is the most common extraintestinal manifestation of amebiasis and is believed to be caused by ascending infection through the portal system [25]. *E. histolytica* has two stages in its life cycle, the cyst and the trophozoite [6]. *E. histolytica* ingested in the cyst stage travels through the small intestine, where it develops into trophozoites and invades the intestinal mucosa [6]. Most cases of amebiasis are confined to the intestine and result in diarrhea; however, extraintestinal manifestations of disease are seen when *E. histolytica* invades the intestine and enters the bloodstream [11]. From there it can travel to the liver, where trophozoites are thought to both lyse neutrophils, directly injure hepatocytes and cause hepatic venule obstruction [8, 12, 25]. The abscess then typically consists of infarcted hepatic parenchyma and liquefied hepatic cells which are encapsulated with a rib of connective tissue causing the characteristic rib enhancement on computed tomography scan [12, 25]. This liquified material is what is typically referred to as the characteristic finding of "anchovy paste" on aspiration. The cyst itself can vary greatly in size and has been noted to range on average from 5 to 15 cm, with the majority occurring in the right lobe of the liver due to the nature of portal blood flow [11, 12].

When Echinococcus is ingested by humans, it first enters an asymptomatic incubation period within the intestine, in which oncospheres are released by eggs that can penetrate the intestinal wall. These oncospheres travel through the portal venous system and can travel to organs such as the liver and lungs [12]. In the liver, oncospheres begin cyst development. These cysts are usually unilocular and grow 1–3 cm per year [12]. They remain asymptomatic for many years until they begin to impinge on nearby structures, causing venous obstruction, portal hypertension, and biliary obstruction. Fistulous communication with the biliary tract can occur and cholangitis can develop [14]. When cysts rupture into the peritoneal cavity they can cause anaphylaxis via an IgE-mediated response, as well as a secondary infection of the peritoneal cavity with hydatid disease [14]. They can also perforate the diaphragm and cause empyema or biliary-bronchial fistula [12].

## 61.2 Diagnosis

### 61.2.1 Clinical Presentation

Fever is the most common symptom reported in patients with hepatic abscesses, and up to 90% of patients with a hepatic abscess will present with fever [26]. Patients with pyogenic abscesses tend to have a more indolent course of symptoms and they often report more nonspecific pain compared to those with amebic liver abscesses [9]. Patients with pyogenic liver abscesses typically do not have fevers or localized right upper quadrant pain until late in the disease process [8]. Less common symptoms include anorexia, jaundice, and malaise. Patients with pyogenic abscess of biliary origin will present with nonspecific findings but will have a history of cholangitis or biliary-enteric anastomosis [24]. Ruptured abscess can present with peritonitis and sepsis [6].

In patients with amebic or echinococcal abscess, history will also include travel to endemic areas [27]. Amebic liver abscesses can develop years after *E. histolytica* infection, and so it is important to take a thorough history, particularly if the patient is not currently living in an endemic area [6]. Despite a large number of individuals infected with *E. histolytica*, many individuals are carriers and do not exhibit clinical signs of disease. It is unknown what factors predispose someone to develop invasive disease after infection [6]. Up to 80% of patients with amebic liver abscess experience fevers and right upper quadrant pain. Time to symptom onset can vary greatly but typically occurs 8–20 weeks from the time of exposure [12, 27]. These lesions can vary greatly in size and have been noted to range on average from 5 to 15 cm, with the majority occurring in the right lobe of the liver [11, 12].

Patients with hydatid disease will often present with abdominal pain, obstructive jaundice, and pruritus secondary to bile duct obstruction [14, 22]. Depending on the location of the cyst, nausea and vomiting can also be a presenting symptom if the cyst compresses the stomach or intestine [22]. A mass can sometimes be appreciated with palpation of the liver. In the case of cyst-biliary fistula, patients can present with cholangitis [12]. Cyst rupture can occur spontaneously or as a result of trauma. As previously stated above, in the event of cyst rupture, these patients often present with anaphylaxis [14]. More rarely, diaphragmatic perforation occurs and a patient will present with symptoms of pneumonia or empyema [12, 14].

Unfortunately, patients with fungal liver abscesses typically have delayed diagnosis for a multitude of reasons. Many of these patients are those with hematologic malignancy who are immunosuppressed. These patients typically present with fever, jaundice, and vague abdominal pain. They are often less likely to display the symptoms of malaise and anorexia seen in those with pyogenic liver abscesses [15]. One needs to maintain a high index of suspicion for fungal abscess in an immunocompromised individual, transplant recipients or those with a history of ablative procedures who present with fevers which do not improve with conventional antibiotic treatment [26].

## 61.2.2 Tests

Imaging workup is necessary to aid in the diagnosis of hepatic abscess as most patients present with nonspecific symptoms. Laboratory evaluation can reveal signs of sepsis, obstructive jaundice, or cholangitis but imaging will further differentiate between hepatic abscess and other hepatic pathology. Most patients will have no findings on chest X-ray, although rarely patients may have evidence of pleural effusions or an elevated right hemidiaphragm [26]. Initial imaging is typically with ultrasound which ranges from 75 to 95% sensitive in detection of hepatic abscesses. Based on the progress and stage of disease, the lesion may appear as hypo- or hyperechoic [8]. Computed tomography with IV contrast can be 95% sensitive in the detection of hepatic abscesses [8]. Some studies report no missed cases by ultrasound which were later found on CT, suggesting that an adequate liver ultrasound may be sufficient imaging for abscess detection [9]. Imaging typically shows a well-defined mass with a peripherally enhancing rim, although this can vary based on the life cycle of the abscess [26]. *Klebsiella pneumoniae* abscesses may also have air-fluid levels on CT and ultrasound imaging [26]. In cases of pyogenic disease, blood cultures may be positive in up to 50% of cases and aspiration almost always has bacteria evident on gram stain and culture [9]. Notably, CT scan cannot differentiate between pyogenic and amebic abscess and in the presence of positive history findings, amebic serologies should be obtained to definitively make the diagnosis [27].

Diagnosis of amebic liver abscess relies on characteristic symptoms, imaging findings, and serum antibody testing. These patients do not require aspiration in order to make the diagnosis of amebic liver abscess [9]. Antibody testing is >94% sensitive and >95% specific for amebic liver abscess [25]. Reports of false negative testing are typically due to testing too early. Most patients are not serum antibody positive until 7–10 days after infection [11, 12, 25]. Some studies have noted that alkaline phosphatase and erythrocyte sedimentation rate are typically elevated in these patients [8, 10, 11, 25]. Stool microscopy has been used in the past but is less useful due to its low sensitivity rates. Stool microscopy is also unable to distinguish between *E. histolytica,* and *Entamoeba dispar* and *Entamoeba moshkovskii moshkovskii,* unless the *E. histolytica* trophozoites have ingested red blood cells [28, 29]. The latter two organisms frequently colonize the lower gastrointestinal tract but are nonpathogenic [25, 29]. On contrast-enhanced CT, amebic liver abscesses present as round with an enhancing wall, with or without surrounding edema [26].

Diagnosis of hydatid disease can be difficult from serum studies, as there is often very little immune response, which depends on the cyst location, size, and intactness of the cyst wall [30]. Serum tests rely on the antibody response to Echinococcal infection, specifically for IgG, IgM, and IgE antibodies. These include immunoblot assay, ELISA, and immunoelectrophoresis [14]. They are generally thought to have low sensitivity due to undetectable immune response [14, 22]. To avoid the high false-positive rates, confirmatory electrophoresis may be used as an adjunct to increase accuracy [12]. Liver enzyme tests are abnormal in only 40% of infected patients [22]. Eosinophilia can also be present in up to 40% of patients [22]. Ultrasound is the gold standard for diagnostic imaging and has the highest sensitivity for the detection of membranes, septa, and hydatid sand [22]. The characteristic finding on ultrasound is a cyst with a calcified rim and a "water lily sign," which occurs after the detachment of the pericyst from the endocyst membrane and resembles a water lily floating in a pond [30]. CT scan can be useful in the diagnosis of hydatid cyst, as it can aid in determining cyst size, proximity to bile ducts, number of septations, membrane integrity, and the condition of the surrounding liver parenchyma. MRI can also provide detailed information about the membrane as well as the presence of daughter cysts and scoleces, known as hydatid sand. Cyst rupture can also be evident on imaging, as the cyst will decrease in size if it has fistulized to the nearby biliary tree or ruptured into the peritoneal or pleural space [22].

Due to its association with immunosuppression, fungal liver abscesses may be harder to detect with labs alone. These patients often do not show the typical leukocytosis or hyperbilirubinemia seen in those with pyogenic liver abscesses. Diagnosis of fungal abscesses relies on high clinical suspicion and imaging findings. Imaging may vary greatly in those with fungal liver abscesses. Ultrasound often shows hypoechoic lesions with a "bull's-eye" appearance due to a central hyperechoic nodule caused by fibrosis [26]. Contrast-enhanced CT will show hypoattenuating lesions on the arterial phase and this can occur with or without contrast enhancement [26]. Patients with disseminated candidiasis may also frequently have splenic manifestations on imaging. Patients with the disseminated fungal infection do not frequently have positive blood cultures and diagnosis relies on culturing of the organism or identification with β-$d$-glucan testing, which unfortunately can have low sensitivity [26, 31].

**Differential Diagnosis**
As hepatic abscess generally has an indolent course and vague symptomatology, the differential diagnosis is fairly broad. It includes hepatitis, malignancy, cholangitis, cholecystitis, primary and secondary liver tumors, and right lower lobar pneumonia. Laboratory evaluation can help to narrow a hepatic source of symptoms but cannot differentiate between different intrahepatic pathology. In those with solid hepatic tumors with necrosis, it can be difficult to differentiate this from a liver abscess. However, necrotic tumors may have other features on imaging including focal calcifications and transient areas of segmental enhancement on CT imaging [26]. More rarely disseminated tuberculosis and bartonellosis can present with multiple hypoattenuating lesions in the liver on contrast-enhanced CT [26]. Differentiating factors between abscess and other possible diagnoses include specific history findings as well as imaging studies as detailed above.

## 61.3 Treatment

### 61.3.1 Medical Treatment

Pyogenic liver abscess treatment typically consists of 14 days of parenteral antibiotics followed by oral antibiotics for a total duration of 6 weeks of antibiotics. Coverage will vary based on the suspected source of pyogenic liver abscess but in general should cover for gram-negative aerobe, gram-positive cocci, and anaerobic bacteria [1, 16]. Typical medical treatment includes a penicillin, a third-generation cephalosporin, and metronidazole [1, 9]. Uniloculated cysts <5 cm in size are often managed with antibiotics and cyst aspiration, whereas cysts >5 cm are better managed with image-guided drain placement after aspiration (Fig. 61.1) [16, 26, 32]. Percutaneous aspiration of the abscess is important in order to de-escalate antibiotics and narrow coverage as indicated [9]. Patients with pyogenic liver abscess may have fevers that persist for up to 2 weeks despite appropriate antimicrobial coverage. Percutaneous drainage, as well as surgical drainage, typically does not need to be considered unless the fevers persist

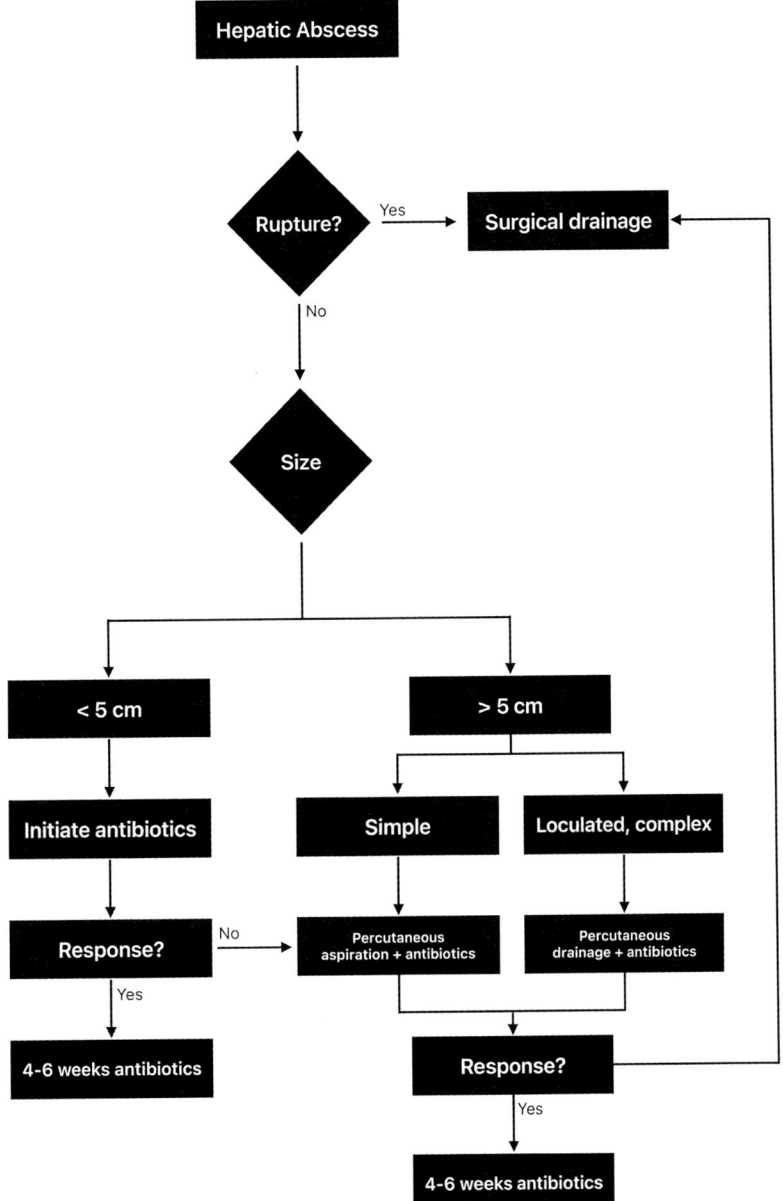

**Fig. 61.1** Hepatic abscess treatment algorithm

beyond 2 weeks or the patient clinically deteriorates [9]. However, in patients with large or multi-loculated liver abscesses, first-line treatment involves placement of a percutaneous drainage catheter typically ranging in size from 8 to 14 Fr. These catheters are often left to gravity until the abscess is thought to be fully drained, or they can be upsized if there is a concern for inadequate drainage [1, 9]. Success rates vary by study but percutaneous drainage with appropriate antibiotics has been noted to be up to 90% successful [1, 16].

In order to truly eradicate hepatic amebiasis both the liver manifestations of the disease and the intraluminal *E. histolytica* must be treated [12]. It is especially important to consider *E. histolytica* in the differential diagnosis of patients with hepatic abscesses, especially those who have traveled to endemic countries. Literature suggests treating individuals with high enough suspicion for the disease even with negative serology given the lag time between infection and positive serology results [13]. The current treatment of choice for amebic liver abscesses is metronidazole 500 mg every 8 h for 7–14 days [11, 12]. Patients can typically be monitored clinically without the need for repeat ultrasounds, with most patients typically experiencing an improvement in symptoms within the first 3 days of treatment, especially reduction in fevers [9, 10]. After completion of metronidazole therapy for the hepatic disease, treatment for intestinal disease should be initiated with paromomycin 25–30 mg/kg/day every 8 h for 7 days. An alternative regimen using diloxanide furoate 500 mg every 8 h for 7 days is also effective at the elimination of the intraluminal cysts, although this drug is not readily available in the United States [10, 12, 25]. The majority of patients with amebic liver abscess will resolve with oral medications alone. A prospective randomized trial comparing percutaneous aspiration + oral antibiotics vs. antibiotics alone showed no statistically significant benefit in patients undergoing aspiration when evaluation length of time to becoming afebrile and hospital length of stay [33]. Patients with large abscesses (>10 cm) are at risk of treatment failure or abscess rupture and may eventually require percutaneous aspiration, although this is typically rare [10, 11, 34]. Patients with large left lobe abscesses should be considered for percutaneous aspiration due to the risk of rupture into the pericardium [9].

Management of hydatid disease depends on the extent of organ involvement, degree of dissemination of disease, and presence of cyst–biliary communication, with the ultimate goal of treatment to eliminate the germinal layer of the cyst. Medical therapy should be considered in patients with inoperable disease or to reduce risk of secondary seeding prior to further intervention. Contraindications to medical therapy include large cysts with impending rupture, cysts with heavily calcified rim, pregnancy, and chronic liver disease [14]. The mainstay of medical therapy is albendazole and mebendazole, with albendazole found to be superior to mebendazole [14]. The treatment algorithm for a 70 kg male is 400 mg BID for 28 days [14]. A second agent, praziquantel, may be used in conjunction with albendazole therapy but is not sufficient as a single agent [30]. Smaller cysts were found to have the best response to medical therapy. Aspiration can be an option in select cases; however, the definitive treatment for hydatid cyst is surgical resection, to be discussed below.

Patients with fungal liver abscesses typically have a high mortality rate, especially in the setting of fungemia [15]. Current literature suggests that if fungal infection is suspected and the patient has known risk factors for the development of a fungal liver abscess, such as immunosuppression or hematologic malignancy, early initiation of antifungal medications is key to reduce mortality risk [15, 16]. The goal standard of treatment for patients with fungal liver abscesses is percutaneous aspiration and drainage with antimycotic therapy. Initial treatment is typically with amphotericin B which must be initiated early and is associated with decreased mortality if initiated prior to the onset of fungemia [15]. Newer literature also supports the use of micafungin and caspofungin for long-term antimycotic therapy and cautions against fluconazole treatment due to increasing *Candida* species resistance [16].

## 61.3.2 Surgical Treatment

Until the late 1970s surgical drainage was considered the standard of care treatment for hepatic abscesses [9]. With advances in interventional radiology, image-guided percutaneous approaches for management have been proven to be safe and efficacious methods for treatment and are now the preferred approach in most patients with pyogenic abscess [6].

There is still a role in surgical management of pyogenic abscesses, particularly in patients with ascites, large, loculated abscesses, or thick material that cannot be aspirated. Surgical intervention is also indicated in the case of a ruptured abscess with peritonitis [1]. Surgical approach for pyogenic abscess can be laparoscopic or open. Techniques for management include fenestration and drainage for superficial abscesses, but for complex or deep cysts partial hepatectomy may be necessary [6, 16, 35]. Intraoperative ultrasound can also be used for deep abscesses that are not easily visualized.

Surgical resection of hydatid disease is considered the standard of therapy, as cyst rupture or intraperitoneal spillage of cyst contents can result in anaphylaxis; however, for simple cysts, there is a role for percutaneous management. The Percutaneous Aspiration Injection and Re-aspiration (PAIR) procedure rely on CT guidance to identify and aspirate cyst contents, instill a scolicidal agent, and aspirate the cyst contents. The typical scolicidal agents of choice are 20% sterile saline or ethyl alcohol [12]. Aspiration is contraindicated in cysts that are not amenable to percutaneous access, cysts communicating with biliary structures, superficial cysts at risk of spillage, and complex, multiseptated cysts. Cysts that communicate with the biliary tree are at risk of causing sclerosing cholangitis if ethyl alcohol is injected into the cyst cavity [11]. If there is concern for cysto-biliary communication, a cholangiogram may be performed prior to injection of scolicidal agents. In the event of intraperitoneal spillage, irrigation with hypertonic saline and use of a scolicidal agent must be used immediately; however, the patient must be closely monitored for fatal hypernatremia [36].

The goal of surgical therapy in hydatid disease is twofold: cyst removal and obliteration of the cyst cavity. This may be achieved by simple cyst resection or partial hepatectomy. An open pericystectomy consists of cyst drainage, injection of a scolicidal agent, and removal of the pericyst and its contents, whereas a closed pericystectomy consists of cyst resection without drainage. Concurrent medical treatment with albendazole should begin at least 7 days prior to any intervention and should continue for at least 4 weeks after treatment [14]. In patients with complicated cases, this treatment may be extended up to 6 months.

### 61.3.3 Prognosis

After drainage of hepatic abscess, antimicrobial therapy should be tailored to the specific infectious agent. Further imaging is not needed unless there is less drainage than expected or persistence of symptoms. Predictors of treatment failure or disease recurrence include multiple abscesses, mixed bacterial and fungal abscesses, respiratory symptoms, associated malignancy, and size >5 cm. Mortality after percutaneous drainage can range from 2 to 12% and is higher in patients who require open drainage, have associated malignancy, or have anaerobic or fungal abscess [26].

Over 90% of patients with amebic liver abscesses will respond to medical treatment alone and not require further intervention [34]. Mortality rates are notably higher for patients with pyogenic liver abscesses versus those with amebic liver abscesses. There are multiple speculated reasons for this phenomenon including delayed time to diagnosis due to nonspecific symptoms and a typically older patient population [9]. Pyogenic liver abscess patients are also typically in the hospital for a longer length of time than those with amebic liver abscess which also increases the risk of hospital acquired infections [9].

Unfortunately, patients diagnosed with fungal abscesses have overall mortality rates of around 50% [15, 16]. Those with fungemia prior to initiation of treatment are at higher risk of mortality than those diagnosed prior to the onset of fungemia. Even with early identification, appropriate drainage, either aspiration or catheter placement, and prompt initiation of antifungal treatment these patients may still have mortality rates of up to 20% [16].

---

**Dos and Don'ts**

**Treatment Dos**
- Consider the underlying pathology leading to the abscess
- Correct any underlying pathology leading to the abscess
- Use the least invasive method with a good chance of success to drain the abscess
- Send cultures and other appropriate diagnostic studies
- Tailor antimicrobials base on cultures

- Limit the duration of antimicrobials to 4–5 days if source control has been achieved
- Be willing to administer long-term antimicrobials for multiple abscesses that cannot be drained

**Treatment Don'ts**
- Fail to perform a full diagnostic evaluation to determine the source of the abscess
- Consider multiple abscesses that cannot be drained "untreatable"
- Become discouraged if multiple interventions are required over time

**Take-Home Messages**

- Although rare, hepatic abscesses have a high mortality rate and can have devastating extrahepatic complications and prompt recognition can significantly improve patient outcomes
- The majority of pyogenic abscesses are secondary to other pathology (biliary tract disease, gastrointestinal infections, bloodstream infections, vascular insufficiency to the biliary treat, etc.) and the primary pathology must be identified and corrected
- High clinical suspicion is imperative to early diagnosis and treatment of fungal hepatic abscesses, especially in those with history of hematologic malignancy or immunosuppression
- The least invasive intervention with a reasonable likelihood of success should be tried first, for example, percutaneous rather than open drainage, and will result in the lowest morbidity
- Abscesses that cannot be drained due to location or number can still be successfully treated with long-term antimicrobials

**Questions**

1. Factors associated with pyogenic hepatic abscesses include:
   A. Hypertension
   B. Lower age
   C. **Malignancy**
   D. Mediterranean diet
2. The risk factor most commonly associated with hepatic abscess following trauma is:
   A. Direct seeding from bullets
   B. **Necrosis of liver tissue**
   C. Previously undiagnosed choledocholithiasis
   D. Spillage from bowel repair
3. Gold standard of therapy for treatment of hydatid disease is:
   A. Albendazole therapy alone
   B. Metronidazole therapy alone
   C. Percutaneous aspiration
   D. **Surgical resection**
4. If there is concern for *Candida* species resistance when treating fungal liver abscesses, the medication of choice is:
   A. **Caspofungin**
   B. Fluconazole
   C. Metronidazole
   D. Praziquantel
5. Fungal liver abscesses may present with what finding on ultrasound imaging:
   A. **"Bull's eye" appearance**
   B. Peripherally enhancing rim
   C. Air fluid levels
   D. "Water lily" sign
6. The most common symptom reported in patients with hepatic abscesses is:
   A. Anorexia
   B. **Fever**
   C. Peritonitis
   D. Right upper quadrant pain
7. A patient presents with a 5.5 cm simple hepatic abscess, the best management for this patient is:
   A. Antibiotics alone
   B. Aspiration alone

C. **Aspiration and antibiotics**
D. Laparoscopic drainage

8. A patient with a 3 cm amebic hepatic abscess undergoes treatment with antibiotics, how quickly do typically you expect to see resolution of fevers?
   A. **1–3 days**
   B. 1–2 weeks
   C. 1–2 months
   D. 1 year

9. What organism is most commonly associated with colorectal cancer patients diagnosed with liver abscesses?
   A. *Echinococcus granulosus*
   B. *Entamoeba histolytica*
   C. *Escherichia coli*
   D. ***Klebsiella pneumoniae***

10. Most common organism associated with hematogenous causes of liver abscesses:
    A. *Bacteroides fragilis*
    B. *Enterococcus* species
    C. *Escherichia coli*
    D. ***Staphylococcus* species**

# References

1. Mavilia MG, Molina M, Wu GY. The evolving nature of hepatic abscess: a review. J Clin Transl Hepatol. 2016;4(2):158–68.
2. Kaplan GG, Gregson DB, Laupland KB. Population-based study of the epidemiology of and the risk factors for pyogenic liver abscess. Clin Gastroenterol Hepatol. 2004;2(11):1032–8.
3. Tsai FC, Huang YT, Chang LY, Wang JT. Pyogenic liver abscess as endemic disease. Taiwan Emerg Infect Dis. 2008;14(10):1592–600.
4. Lardière-Deguelte S, Ragot E, Amroun K, Piardi T, Dokmak S, Bruno O, et al. Hepatic abscess: diagnosis and management. J Visc Surg. 2015;152(4):231–43.
5. Qu K, Liu C, Wang ZX, Tian F, Wei JC, Tai MH, et al. Pyogenic liver abscesses associated with nonmetastatic colorectal cancers: an increasing problem in Eastern Asia. World J Gastroenterol. 2012;18(23):2948–55.
6. Roediger R, Lisker-Melman M. Pyogenic and amebic infections of the liver. Gastroenterol Clin N Am. 2020;49(2):361–77.
7. Lin HF, Liao KF, Chang CM, Lin CL, Lai SW. Correlation between proton pump inhibitors and risk of pyogenic liver abscess. Eur J Clin Pharmacol. 2017;73(8):1019–25.
8. Reid-Lombardo KM, Khan S, Sclabas G. Hepatic cysts and liver abscess. Surg Clin N Am. 2010;90(4):679–97.
9. Barnes PF, De Cock KM, Reynolds TN, Ralls PW. A comparison of amebic and pyogenic abscess of the liver. Medicine (Baltimore). 1987;66(6):472–83.
10. Krige JEJ, Beckingham J. Liver abscesses and hydatid disease. Bmj. 2001;322:537–40.
11. Torre A, Kershenobich D. Amebic liver abscess. Ann Hepatol. 2002;1(1):45–7.
12. Mulholland MW, Lillemoe KD, Doherty GM, Upchurch GR Jr, Alam HB, Pawlik TM. Greenfield's surgery. 6th ed. Baltimore: Wolters Kluwer; 2017. p. 930–41.
13. Marn H, Ignatius R, Tannich E, Harms G, Schürmann M, Dieckmann S. Amoebic liver abscess with negative serologic markers for *Entamoeba histolytica*: mind the gap! Infection. 2012;40(1):87–91.
14. Pakala T, Molina M, Wu GY. Hepatic echinococcal cysts: a review. J Clin Transl Hepatol. 2016;4(1):39–46. https://doi.org/10.14218/JCTH.2015.00036.
15. Lipsett PA, Huang CJ, Lillemoe KD, Cameron JL, Pitt HA. Fungal hepatic abscesses: characterization and management. J Gastrointest Surg. 1997;1(1):78–84.
16. Cameron JL, Cameron AM. Current surgical therapy. 13th ed. Amsterdam: Elsevier; 2020. p. 388–93.
17. Johannsen EC, Sifri CD, Madoff LC. Pyogenic liver abscesses. Infect Dis Clin N Am. 2000;14(3):547–63.
18. Serraino C, Elia C, Bracco C, et al. Characteristics and management of pyogenic liver abscess: a European experience. Medicine (Baltimore). 2018;97(19):e0628.
19. Huang W-K, Chang JW-C, See L-C, Tu H-T, Chen J-S, Liaw C-C, et al. Higher rate of colorectal cancer among patients with pyogenic liver abscess with *Klebsiella pneumoniae* than those without: an 11-year follow-up study. Color Dis. 2012;14(12):e794–801.
20. Leggieri N, Marques-Vidal P, Cerwenka H, Denys A, Dorta G, Moutardier V, et al. Migrated foreign body liver abscess illustrative case report, systematic review, and proposed diagnostic algorithm. Medicine (Baltimore). 2010;89(2):85–95.
21. Nachman S, Kaul A, Li KI, Slim MS, Filippo JAS, Van Horn K. Liver abscess caused by *Clostridium bifermentans* following blunt abdominal trauma. J Clin Microbiol. 1989;27(5):1137–8.
22. Bhutani N, Kajal P. Hepatic echinococcosis: a review. Ann Med Surg (Lond). 2018;36:99–105. https://doi.org/10.1016/j.amsu.2018.10.032.
23. Webb GJ, Chapman TP, Cadman PJ, Gorard DA. Pyogenic liver abscess. Frontline Gastroenterol. 2014;5(1):60–7.
24. Shi SH, Zhai ZL, Zheng SS. Pyogenic liver abscess of biliary origin: the existing problems and their strategies. Semin Liver Dis. 2018;38(3):270–83. https://doi.org/10.1055/s-0038-1661363.

25. Stanley SL Jr. Amoebiasis. Lancet. 2003;361:1025–35.
26. Bächler P, Baladron MJ, Menias C, Beddings I, Loch R, Zalaquett E, et al. Multimodality imaging of liver infections: differential diagnosis and potential pitfalls. Radiographics. 2016;36(4):1001–23.
27. Conter RL, Pitt HA, Tompkins RK, Longmire WP Jr. Differentiation of pyogenic from amebic hepatic abscesses. Surg Gynecol Obstet. 1986;162(2):114–20.
28. Ngui R, Angal L, Fakhrurrazi SA, Lian YLA, Ling LY, Ibrahim J, et al. Differentiating *Entamoeba histolytica*, *Entamoeba dispar* and *Entamoeba moshkovskii* using nested polymerase chain reaction (PCR) in rural communities in Malaysia. Parasites Vectors. 2012;5(1):1.
29. Skappak C, Akierman S, Belga S, Novak K, Chadee K, Urbanski SJ, et al. Invasive amoebiasis: a review of Entamoeba infections highlighted with case reports. Can J Gastroenterol Hepatol. 2014;28(7):355–9.
30. Macpherson CN, Bartholomot B, Frider B. Application of ultrasound in diagnosis, treatment, epidemiology, public health and control of *Echinococcus granulosus* and *E. multilocularis*. Parasitology. 2003;127(Suppl):S21–35. https://doi.org/10.1017/s0031182003003676.
31. Theel ES, Doern CD. β-D-Glucan testing is important for diagnosis of invasive fungal infections. J Clin Microbiol. 2013;51(11):3478–83.
32. Cai YL, Xiong XZ, Lu J, et al. Percutaneous needle aspiration versus catheter drainage in the management of liver abscess: a systematic review and meta-analysis. HPB (Oxford). 2015;17(3):195–201. https://doi.org/10.1111/hpb.12332.
33. Van Allan RJ, Katz MD, Johnson MB, Laine LA, Liu Y, Ralls PW. Uncomplicated amoebic liver abscess: prospective evaluation of percutaneous aspiration. Radiology. 1992;183:827–30.
34. Weinke T, Grobusch MP, Güthoff W. Amebic liver abscess—rare need for percutaneous treatment modalities. Eur J Med Res. 2002;7(1):25–9.
35. Heneghan HM, Healy NA, Martin ST, et al. Modern management of pyogenic hepatic abscess: a case series and review of the literature. BMC Res Notes. 2011;4:80.
36. Zeng R, Wu R, Lv Q, Tong N, Zhang Y. The association of hypernatremia and hypertonic saline irrigation in hepatic hydatid cysts. Medicine (Baltimore). 2017;96(37):e7889.

## Further Reading

Bächler P, Baladron MJ, Menias C, Beddings I, Loch R, Zalaquett E, et al. Multimodality imaging of liver infections: differential diagnosis and potential pitfalls. Radiographics. 2016;36(4):1001–23.

Barnes PF, De Cock KM, Reynolds TN, Ralls PW. A comparison of amebic and pyogenic abscess of the liver. Medicine (Baltimore). 1987;66(6):472–83.

Lipsett PA, Huang CJ, Lillemoe KD, Cameron JL, Pitt HA. Fungal hepatic abscesses: characterization and management. J Gastrointest Surg. 1997;1(1):78–84.

Mavilia MG, Molina M, Wu GY. The evolving nature of hepatic abscess: a review. J Clin Transl Hepatol. 2016;4(2):158–68.

Reid-Lombardo KM, Khan S, Sclabas G. Hepatic cysts and liver abscess. Surg Clin N Am. 2010;90(4):679–97.

# Spleen Non-traumatic Acute Surgical Conditions

## 62

Marco Ceresoli and Luca Degrate

---

**Learning Goals**

- To know etiology and pathophysiology, diagnosis and management of splenic abscess
- To know etiology and pathophysiology, diagnosis and management of nontraumatic splenic rupture
- To know how the management after splenectomy

---

## 62.1 Splenic Abscess

### 62.1.1 Epidemiology

Splenic abscess is a very rare clinical condition, with an estimated incidence between 0.2 and 0.7% at autopsy reports. However, the associated mortality is high, ranging from 15 to 20% among immunocompetent patients to 80% among patients with immunodeficiency [1]. Due to the increased incidence of acquired immunodeficiency syndrome (AIDS) and other immunocompromised states associated with chronic corticosteroid use and chemotherapy, the incidence of splenic abscesses is increasing, showing a bimodal age distribution with peaks in the third and sixth decade of life [2].

### 62.1.2 Etiology

Microorganisms related to the formation of splenic abscesses are either bacterial or fungal. The most common bacteria found in the cultures from splenic abscesses are Gram-positive aerobic bacteria, such as Staphylococcus (16–20%), Streptococcus (6–22%) or Gram-negative as Salmonella (11–16%). Fungal organisms such as Candida, Aspergillus, and mycobacteria represent nearly 8% of all cases and are especially found in immunodeficient patients. Polymicrobial flora may be found in almost 50% of the cases, while rare organisms associated with splenic abscesses are *Burkholderia pseudomallei*, *Actinomycetes*, *Brucella melitensis*, and *Klebsiella pneumoniae* [3].

### 62.1.3 Classification

Splenic abscesses can be classified according to the type of associated microorganisms and to the involvement of the spleen. Abscesses can be sol-

---

M. Ceresoli (✉)
School of Medicine and Surgery, University of Milano-Bicocca, Monza, Italy

General and Emergency Surgery, Fondazione IRCCS San Gerardo dei Tintori, Monza, Italy

L. Degrate
General and Emergency Surgery, ASST Monza, San Gerardo Hospital, Monza, Italy

© The Author(s), under exclusive license to Springer Nature Switzerland AG 2023
F. Coccolini, F. Catena (eds.), *Textbook of Emergency General Surgery*,
https://doi.org/10.1007/978-3-031-22599-4_62

itary or multifocal within the spleen parenchyma. Moreover, the absence or presence of septa may render the abscess unilocular or multilocular. Approximately two-thirds of splenic abscesses in adults are solitary, while one-third splenic abscesses are multiple. Multifocal abscesses are frequently seen in immunocompromised patients.

## 62.1.4 Pathophysiology

The majority (up to 70% of cases) of splenic abscesses are related to the hematogenous spread of microorganisms from a primary site of infection, as in the case of endocarditis or osteomyelitis. In some cases, the splenic abscess occurs from the spread of a contiguous focus of infection that has involved organs like the left kidney, pancreatic tail, left colon, or stomach (in this case, notably following bariatric surgery). In other cases, splenic abscesses are caused by superinfection of infarctual area of the spleen, which may be the result of cardiac embolism or the effect of interventional radiology embolization, as in the case of treatment of splenic artery aneurysms or splenic traumatic injuries. Abscesses have also been found to be associated with parasitic infection of the spleen.

Hemoglobinopathies, immunodeficiencies (HIV, chemotherapy, corticosteroid use), diabetes mellitus, intravenous drug abuse, cancer and trauma are common associated risk factors for splenic abscess development [4].

## 62.1.5 Diagnosis

### 62.1.5.1 Clinical Presentation

Clinical manifestations of a splenic abscess are often unspecific and the diagnosis may be a clinical challenge. Patients usually show general signs and symptoms of infection such as fever and chills and complain of pain in the left hypochondrium or lower left chest. The clinical triad of fever, abdominal pain, and leukocytosis is present in most of the patients. However, other unspecific symptoms may be present, such as vomiting, nausea, and left shoulder pain.

Physical examination may reveal splenomegaly, tenderness in the left hypochondrium, left basilar rales, and dullness at the left lung base.

### 62.1.5.2 Tests

Laboratory tests will reveal leukocytosis and increased inflammatory markers (C-reactive protein, procalcitonin), while blood cultures may be positive.

Plain chest radiographs can show elevation of the left hemidiaphragm and the left-sided pleural effusion with or without left basal atelectasis. However, the imaging diagnostic procedures of choice are abdominal ultrasound and computed tomography (CT). Ultrasound can demonstrate a poorly defined hypo- or anechoic lesion with irregular walls and splenomegaly. Sometimes hyperechoic appearance with distal shadowing due to the presence of gas may be observed.

Multidetector contrast-enhanced computed tomography (CT) is the gold standard for diagnosis and it helps to plan the treatment by delineating the details of the abscess and the topography of the surrounding structures. The typical CT appearance of a splenic abscess is that of a focal well-demarcated hypodense lesion, sometimes loculated with septations. The size might vary from sub centimeters to several centimeters. The presence of gas, although uncommon, is considered diagnostic, while multiple small hypodense lesions may be seen in immunocompromised patients and/or with fungal infections, abdominal tuberculosis, and atypical mycobacterial infections (Fig. 62.1).

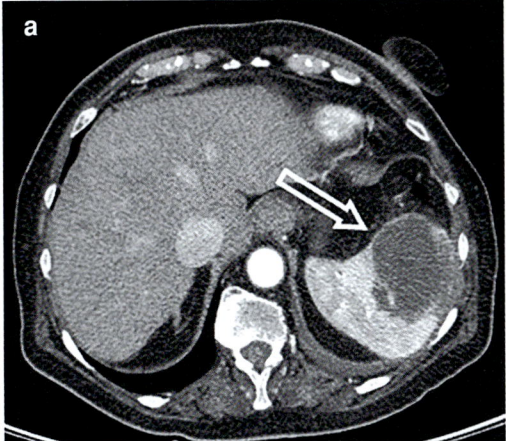
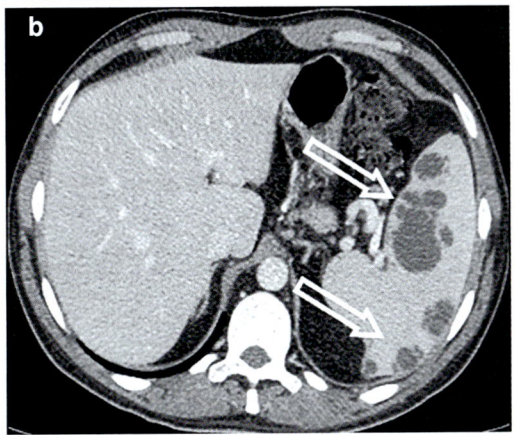
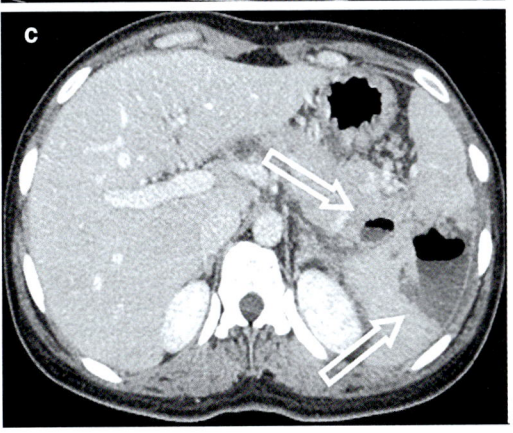

**Fig. 62.1** Multidetector computed tomography of different splenic abscesses. (**a**) Unilocular splenic abscess of the superior pole of the spleen, due to *Enterococcus faecalis* endocarditis. (**b**) Multifocal splenic abscesses and splenomegaly. (**c**) Intraparenchymal and perihilar splenic abscesses with gas-fluid levels (arrowheads) due to *Mycobacterium tuberculosis* complex with superinfection by candida and Gram + anaerobes

Magnetic resonance imaging can be useful to differentiate splenic abscesses from other cystic splenic lesions. The abscesses display variable, fluid-like low T1 and high T2 signal intensity, with some peripheral enhancement [5, 6].

> **Differential Diagnosis**
>
> Splenic abscesses should be differentiated from other pathologies such as splenic infarction, cysts, primary and secondary neoplasms and from localized purulent collections inside the peritoneal cavity in the left hypochondrium, following bariatric surgery or left colonic flexure perforation.
>
> Percutaneous aspiration, under ultrasound or CT guidance, can help to confirm the diagnosis and it is considered a safe and effective modality to determine whether there is a bacterial or fungal etiology, in order to direct antimicrobial therapy.

## 62.1.6 Treatment

### 62.1.6.1 Medical Treatment

A patient with a splenic abscess should be immediately treated with parenteral high-dose broad-spectrum antibiotics. Antibiotic therapy is of paramount importance while further therapeutic arrangements are made and the choice of antibiotics should be guided by the culture results. Medical treatment alone is not recommended because of high mortality rates up to 50% in those patients only managed with antibiotics.

The gold standard of treatment of splenic abscesses is splenectomy; however, percutaneous aspiration of the abscess can be considered as a less invasive option in selected high risk for surgery patients or as a bridge to surgery in case of life-threatening septic conditions requiring stabilization prior to surgical intervention. Percutaneous drainage may be performed under ultrasound or CT guidance and it is more appropriate and effective in case of a solitary, unilocular, liquefied-content abscess. Conversely, it is less likely to be successful in patients presenting multiple or multilocular abscesses or in presence of septations and necrotic debris inside the abscess, or in absence of a well-defined wall. Contraindications to percutaneous drainage are coagulopathy, presence of multiple small abscesses, cavities filled with necrotic debris, diffuse ascites, or difficult percutaneous access.

In case of no response to medical therapy, appropriate treatment for fungi, actinomycetes, or Mycobacterium should be taken into consideration. Antifungal therapy alone may be used with success in fungal splenic abscesses because the presence of abscess within the spleen is often a manifestation of a disseminated fungal infection. As this approach appears to be effective for fungal abscesses, splenectomy should yet be considered as a definitive treatment for those patients with bacterial splenic abscesses with no response to medical therapy and percutaneous drainage [7].

### 62.1.6.2 Surgical Treatment

Splenectomy is the last choice treatment option for splenic abscess and it has been found to be the most effective and definitive procedure for the majority of patients compared to drainage or medical therapy alone [8].

Splenectomy is indicated in case of multiple or multilocular abscesses, in case of contraindications to percutaneous drainage or in case of patients with no response to medical therapy. It may be performed either laparoscopically or through laparotomy, and a drainage of the splenic bed is recommended at the end of operation. The reported morbidity after open splenectomy for abscess ranges from 28 to 43%. Postoperative mortality rates are high up to 16.9%; however, the mortality rate of splenectomy for failed percutaneous drainage is similar to that of splenectomy alone as first-line therapy. Laparoscopic splenectomy is an alternative to the open method and it is associated with faster postoperative recovery and reduced hospital stay [9]. A preoperative detailed study of the CT scans helps to determine the possibility to perform splenectomy laparoscopically, because the large size of the spleen, close location of the pancreatic tail and diffuse surrounding inflammation may render challenging this approach. During surgery, a careful manipulation of the spleen is necessary in order to avoid capsular injury and spillage of abscess contents into the peritoneal cavity (Fig. 62.2).

### 62.1.6.3 Prognosis

An appropriate and immediate management of splenic abscess is essential because it is associated with high mortality rates without a prompt treatment. Mortality mostly depends on the immune status of the patient and the typology of the abscess. It ranges from 15 to 20% in immunocompetent patients with unilocular abscesses to 80% in immunocompromised patients with multilocular abscesses.

With no treatment, splenic abscesses may propagate to the diaphragm, abdominal wall, and near organs, leading to the formation of fistula that should be managed by surgery. Pneumoperitoneum may represent the complication of gas-containing splenic abscesses, while pneumonia, atelectasis, or left-sided pleural effusions are common respiratory complications associated with the presence of a splenic abscess.

> **Dos and Don'ts**
> - Administer broad-spectrum parenteral antibiotics
> - Obtain a specimen for cultural examination in order to administer the proper therapy
> - Evaluate the best treatment from percutaneous drainage, laparotomic or laparoscopic splenectomy

## 62.2 Atraumatic/Pathologic Splenic Rupture

### 62.2.1 Epidemiology

Atraumatic and spontaneous splenic rupture is a rare but potentially lethal condition. No exact data about epidemiology and etiology are available in the literature and evidences derive from case reports and small case series. A 2008 systematic review of the existing literature about atraumatic splenic rupture reported a total 845 cases published in 632 articles (from 1980 to 2008) [10].

Atraumatic splenic rupture was more common in men (66.7%) and mean age was 45 years (range: 18–86). No definitive data about the real incidence exist.

### 62.2.2 Etiology and Pathophysiology

Atraumatic splenic rupture is caused by several conditions; its exact pathophysiology is not known and several mechanisms could be hypothesized, such as the presence of pathologic tissue (neoplastic or inflammatory), the presence of ischemic area, the effect of local inflammation as in acute and chronic pancreatitis and the enlargement of the spleen. Table 62.1 reports the commonest causes of splenomegaly. Spontaneous rupture can be observed even in nonpathological spleens but it is more common in enlarged spleens or pathological conditions. Among the described cases the most common etiologies are represented by hematological malignancies and viral infections as EBV or CMV [10–12].

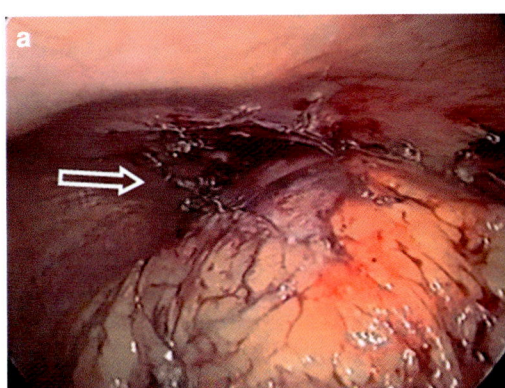
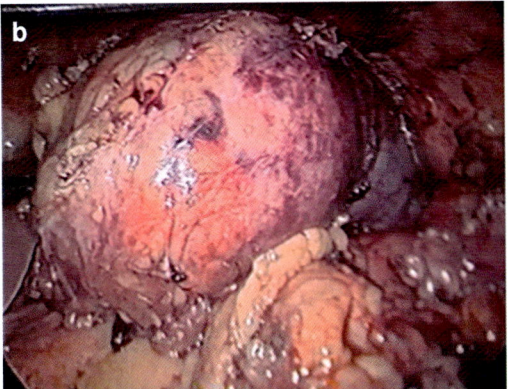
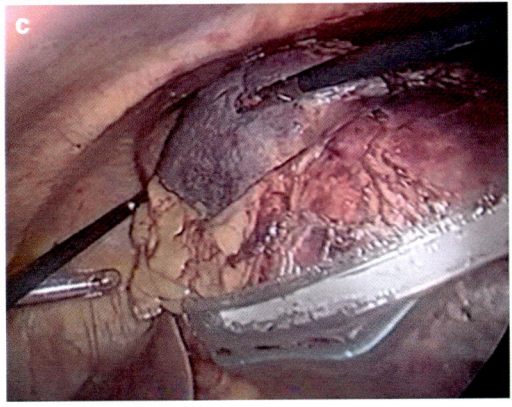

**Fig. 62.2** Intraoperative view of inferior pole splenic abscess, during laparoscopic splenectomy. (**a**) Adhesions between the splenic abscess and the diaphragmatic peritoneum (arrowhead). (**b**) Complete isolation of the inferior pole of the spleen. (**c**) Extraction of the spleen by endobag

**Table 62.1** Principal causes of splenomegaly

| Hematologic malignancies and diseases | |
|---|---|
| | Congestive |
| Lymphoma | Liver cirrhosis |
| Leukemias | Heart failure |
| Polycythemia vera | Thrombosis of portal, hepatic, or splenic veins |
| Essential thrombocythemia | |
| Primary myelofibrosis | **Other** |
| Chronic hemolytic anemias | Sarcoidosis |
| Sickle cell disease | Amyloidosis |
| | Lysosomal storage diseases |
| **Infections** | Postgranulocyte colony-stimulating factor (GCS-F) |
| EBV infection, mononucleosis | |
| Schistosomiasis | |
| Malaria | |

**Table 62.2** Splenic injuries classifications

| Grade | Injury |
|---|---|
| AAST | |
| I | Subcapsular hematoma <10% surface area; laceration <1 cm |
| II | Subcapsular hematoma 10–50% surface area; intraparenchymal hematoma <5 cm; laceration 1–3 cm |
| III | Subcapsular hematoma >50% surface area or expanding, Intraparenchymal hematoma >5 cm; laceration >3 cm |
| IV | Laceration of segmental or hilar vessels producing major devascularization (>25% of spleen) |
| V | Completely shatters spleen; hilar injury with devascularization |
| WSES | |
| I | AAST grade I–II with stable hemodynamic |
| II | AAST grade III with stable hemodynamic |
| III | AAST grade IV–V with stable hemodynamic |

## 62.2.3 Classification

Nontraumatic splenic ruptures are very uncommon and no specific classification exists. They can be classified using the grading of traumatic splenic injuries proposed by the American Association of the Surgery of Trauma [13] or with the classification by the WSES (Table 62.2) [14]. Splenic ruptures can be also classified accordingly to the underlying disease.

## 62.2.4 Diagnosis

### 62.2.4.1 Clinical Presentation

The clinical presentation of nontraumatic spleen rupture could be very variable, depending on the extent of the rupture and the diagnosis may be very insidious. Patients could complain a vague abdominal pain, localized in the left upper quadrant in case of limited subcapsular hematoma, or diffuse abdominal pain if hemoperitoneum is present (Fig. 62.3a, b). A possible clinical presentation could be syncope or lipothymia, while in some cases patients may present a hemorrhagic shock that requires prompt diagnosis and treatment.

In absence of trauma events, an accurate anamnesis is crucial in order to suspect the presence of pathological conditions and a possible spontaneous splenic rupture. The diagnostic work-up should be always evaluated according to the hemodynamic status of the patient [15].

### 62.2.4.2 Tests

Laboratory tests are useful to identify a possible etiology if unknown; the finding of anemia is inconstant, depending on the extent of the rupture; similarly to trauma patients, it is crucial to evaluate the serum lactate level and base excess in order to identify hemorrhagic shock.

First-level imaging should be US examination: principal findings are an enlarged spleen and, significantly, the presence of free fluid in the peritoneal cavity. In the case of the patient's hemodynamic stability, a contrast-enhanced abdominal CT scan is mandatory to confirm or identify the splenic rupture and to describe the possible presence of arterial of venous contrast extravasation (blushing). Other imaging techniques are not useful nor indicated in case of suspected nontraumatic splenic rupture.

> **Differential Diagnosis**
> Atraumatic splenic rupture should be differentiated by the rupture of splenic artery aneurysm.

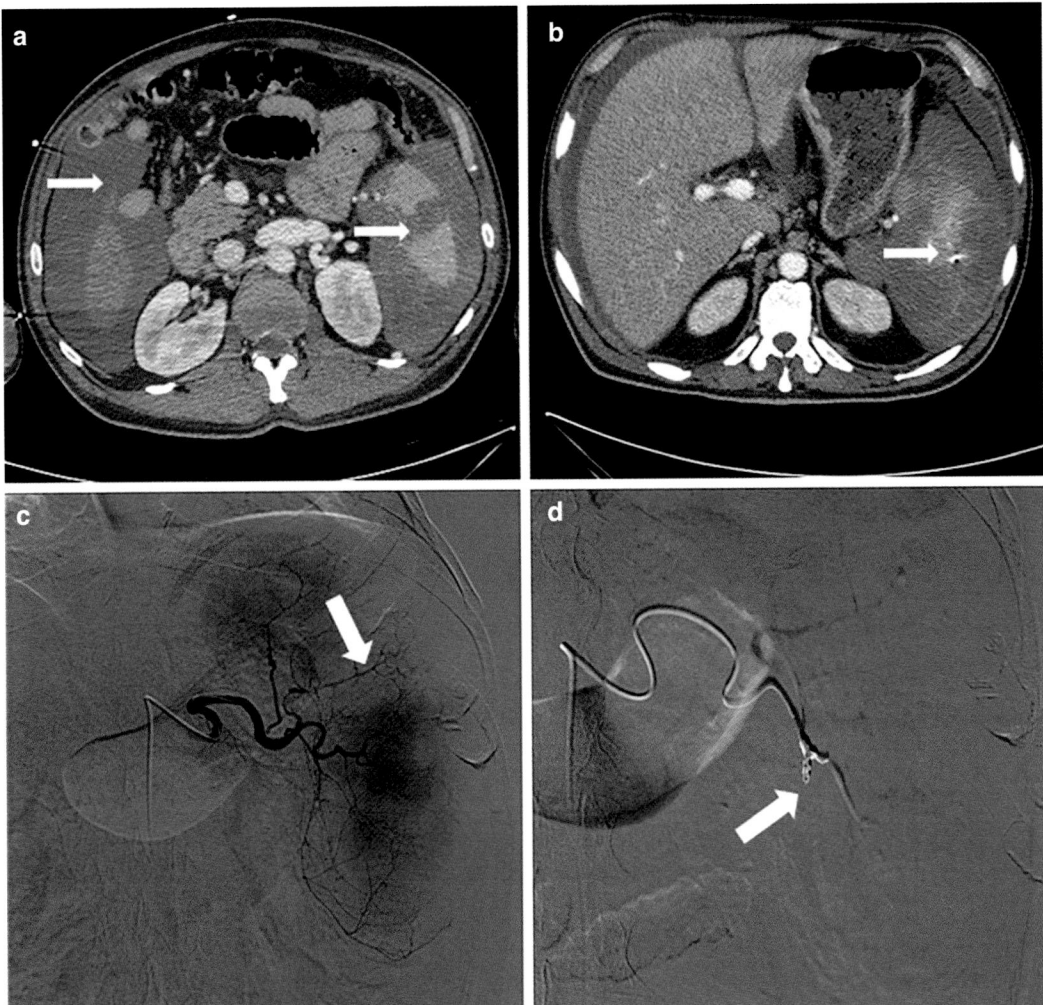

**Fig. 62.3** (a) Splenic rupture (arrow) with massive hemoperitoneum (arrow). (b) Splenic rupture with intraparenchymal hematoma and arterial blushing (arrow). (c) Angiography with arterial blushing (arrow). (d) Distal angioembolization with metallic coils (arrow)

## 62.2.5 Treatment

### 62.2.5.1 Medical Treatment

Similarly to traumatic splenic injuries the treatment should be evaluated according to the extent of the injury, the patient's hemodynamic status, and the available facilities and skills. In case of hemodynamic instability, nonoperative management is not indicated, and open splenectomy is mandatory.

In case of low-grade injuries (WSES grade I and II) and with hemodynamic stability, a conservative treatment should be always attempted. Patient should be observed with serial evaluations of the hemodynamic status and eventual bleeding, with laboratory tests. High-grade injuries with hemodynamic stability (WSES grade III) could be treated with an attempt of conservative treatment in selected patients when facilities are available: patients should be admitted to ICU with continuous monitoring of hemodynamic status.

In case of hemodynamic stability and with the presence of arterial blushing at CT scan, angiography with angioembolization is indicated, if available (Fig. 62.3b–d); if this service is not available, a conservative treatment should not be attempted. The pooled success of nonoperative treatment is nearly 80% [10].

### 62.2.5.2 Surgical Treatment

In case of hemodynamic instability (WSES grade IV), failure of nonoperative treatment or conservative treatment not feasible, splenectomy is indicated [16, 17]. As in trauma patients, a median laparotomy is suggested as a surgical approach that allows a better exposition of the surgical field and exploration of all the peritoneal cavities. Organ preserving surgery, such as splenic repair or splenorrhaphy, is not suggested due to a high failure rate associated with the presence of pathologic tissue. In very selected cases, when skills are available and in the presence of stable hemodynamic and no massive hemoperitoneum, laparoscopic splenectomy could be attempted. At the end of the operation, the positioning of a drainage is suggested, allowing to early identification of postoperative bleeding, prevention of fluid collections, and management of a possible postoperative pancreatic fistula.

> **Dos and Don'ts**
>
> - Evaluate the hemodynamic status of the patient and plan the treatment according to it
> - Evaluate the extent of the splenic injury and plan the treatment accordingly
> - Do not plan nonoperative management in an unstable patient
> - Do not plan nonoperative management in high-grade injury with hemodynamic stability if there are no facilities to serial and continuous monitoring of the patient

### 62.2.5.3 Prognosis

The prognosis of the patient is mostly related to the underlying disease and the cause of splenic rupture. The reported pooled mortality of nontraumatic splenic rupture is 12% [10]. Factors that affect mortality are splenomegaly, age above 40 years, and the presence of malignant disease. Possible complications after splenectomy are hemorrhage and hematoma, infected fluid collection, pancreatitis, and pancreatic fistula. Long-term complications after splenectomy are the overwhelming post-splenectomy infections (OPSI).

## 62.3 Splenic Artery Aneurism

See Chap. 104—**visceral aneurism**.

## 62.4 Postsplenectomy Management

Asplenic or hyposplenic patients, as those who underwent splenectomy, are susceptible to a variety of different infections, more likely to be caused by encapsulated organisms as they are more resilient to phagocytosis. The most dreadful complication of splenectomy is overwhelming postsplenectomy infection (OPSI), which is associated with significant morbidity and mortality rates especially in young people [18]. This highlights the importance of preventive strategies in the management of splenectomized individuals. First of all, patients and their family members should be educated regarding their asplenic status and be aware of their increased susceptibility to infectious diseases and the need to take relevant health precautions. Splenectomized patients should seek immediate medical attention in case of fever, chills, myalgia, headache, vomiting, and abdominal pain or in case of animal bites; they should always carry antibiotic supplies with them and ask for medical advice prior to traveling, especially before visiting a malaria-endemic area.

Second, in order to reduce the risk of OPSI, patients should be vaccinated against *Streptococcus pneumoniae*, *Neisseria meningitidis*, *Haemophilus influenzae* type b, and annual influenza virus [19]. Vaccines should be administered at least 2 weeks before surgery in elective cases or at least 2 weeks after the surgical intervention in emergency cases.

Third, postsplenectomy patients should early start empirical antimicrobial therapy with amoxicillin–clavulanic acid, trimethoprim/sulfamethoxazole, or cefuroxime in case of febrile episodes.

Moreover, malaria prophylaxis, mosquito repellents, and other barrier precautions are recommended for travelers in malaria-endemic areas.

**Take-Home Messages**

- Splenic abscesses are very uncommon and affect typically immunocompromised patients
- Mortality is high and treatment of splenic abscess should be tailored to patient's condition and abscess extent, comprehending antibiotic therapy and percutaneous or surgical drainage
- Nontraumatic splenic rupture is very uncommon and affects patients with splenomegaly and or the presence of pathologic splenic tissue
- The evaluation of hemodynamic is fundamental in the definition of the treatment
- Always perform emergency splenectomy in case of hemodynamic instability; consider nonoperative management in case of low-grade injuries and hemodynamic stability
- Perform vaccination against capsulated bacteria after splenectomy and recommend early antibiotic treatment in case of fever

**Multiple Choice Questions**

1. Splenic abscesses are most common in:
   A. Trauma patients
   B. **Immunocompromised patients**
   C. Elderly
   D. Children
2. The most common microorganisms in splenic abscesses are:
   A. Gram-negative bacteria
   B. **Gram-positive bacteria**
   C. Fungi
   D. Intracellular bacteria
3. Which is the first choice treatment of splenic abscesses?
   A. Open surgery
   B. **Antibiotic therapy**
   C. Percutaneous drainage
   D. Minimally invasive surgery
4. Which of the following has the higher diagnostic accuracy for splenic abscesses?
   A. **Contrast-enhanced CT scan**
   B. MRI
   C. Abdominal ultrasound
   D. Plain abdominal X-rays
5. Which of the following is the commonest cause of splenomegaly?
   A. **Hematologic malignancy**
   B. Malaria
   C. Hearth failure
   D. Lysosomal storage disease
6. Spontaneous splenic rupture is more common in:
   A. Young men in normal health
   B. Young men with malaria
   C. **Old men with disseminated lymphoma**
   D. Young pregnant women
7. Splenectomy:
   A. Is always recommended in all cases of splenic rupture
   B. Is recommended only in low-grade splenic lesions (AAST I–II)

C. Is contraindicated in patients with low-grade lesions
   D. **Is mandatory in case of hemodynamic instability**
8. Conservative treatment in case of spontaneous splenic rupture:
   A. Is always contraindicated
   B. **It requires the presence of a proper patients monitoring**
   C. Is the first therapeutic choice in all cases of spontaneous splenic rupture
   D. In case of spontaneous splenic rupture, angioembolization is always ineffective
9. The acronym OPSI stays for:
   A. Obnubilating psychiatric surgical infection
   B. Overwhelming prophylactic serum injection
   C. **Overwhelming postsplenectomy infections**
   D. Ostile pseudomonas streptococcus infection
10. For which of the following bacteria a patient who underwent splenectomy should be vaccinated?
    A. *Streptococcus anginosus*
    B. *Streptococcus bovis*
    C. *Neisseria meningitidis*
    D. ***Haemophilus influenzae***

## References

1. Lee WS, Choi ST, Kim KK. Splenic abscess: a single institution study and review of the literature. Yonsei Med J. 2011;52(2):288–92.
2. Lee MC, Lee CM. Splenic abscess: an uncommon entity with potentially life-threatening evolution. Can J Infect Dis Med Microbiol. 2018;2018:8610657. https://doi.org/10.1155/2018/8610657.
3. Yilmaz M, Arslan F, Başkan Ö, Mert A. Splenic abscess due to brucellosis: a case report and a review of the literature. Int J Infect Dis. 2014;20:68–70. https://doi.org/10.1016/j.ijid.2013.11.010.
4. Liu YH, Liu CP, Lee CM. Splenic abscesses at a tertiary medical center in northern Taiwan. J Microbiol Immunol Infect. 2014;47(2):104–8. https://doi.org/10.1016/j.jmii.2012.08.027.
5. Tonolini M, Bianco R. Nontraumatic splenic emergencies: cross-sectional imaging findings and triage. Emerg Radiol. 2013;20(4):323–32.
6. Nieciecki M, Kożuch M, Czarniecki M, et al. How to diagnose splenic abscesses? Acta Gastroenterol Belg. 2019;82:421–6.
7. Divyashree S, Gupta N. Splenic abscess in immunocompetent patients managed primarily without splenectomy: a series of 7 cases. Perm J. 2017;21:16–139. https://doi.org/10.7812/TPP/16-139.
8. Carbonell AM, Kercher KW, Matthews BD, et al. Laparoscopic splenectomy for splenic abscess. Surg Laparosc Endosc Percutaneous Tech. 2004;14(5):289–91. https://doi.org/10.1097/00129689-200410000-00013.
9. Gelmini R, Romano F, Quaranta N, et al. Sutureless and stapleless laparoscopic splenectomy using radiofrequency: LigaSure device. Surg Endosc Other Interv Tech. 2006;20(6):991–4. https://doi.org/10.1007/s00464-005-0470-5.
10. Renzulli P, Hostettler A, Schoepfer AM, et al. Systematic review of atraumatic splenic rupture. Br J Surg. 2009;96:1114–21. https://doi.org/10.1002/bjs.6737.
11. Odalović B, Jovanović MD, Stolić R, et al. Spontaneous splenic rupture in infectious mononucleosis. Srp Arh Celok Lek. 2018;146:320–2. https://doi.org/10.2298/SARH160629207O.
12. Imbert P, Rapp C, Buffet PA. Pathological rupture of the spleen in malaria: analysis of 55 cases (1958–2008). Travel Med Infect Dis. 2009;7:147–59. https://doi.org/10.1016/j.tmaid.2009.01.002.
13. Moore EE, Cogbill TH, Jurkovich GJ, et al. Organ injury scaling: spleen and liver (1994 revision). J Trauma. 1995;38(3):323–4.
14. Coccolini F, Fugazzola P, Morganti L, et al. The World Society of Emergency Surgery (WSES) spleen trauma classification: a useful tool in the management of splenic trauma. World J Emerg Surg. 2019;14:30. https://doi.org/10.1186/s13017-019-0246-1.
15. Coccolini F, Montori G, Catena F, et al. Splenic trauma: WSES classification and guidelines for adult and pediatric patients. World J Emerg Surg. 2017;12:40. https://doi.org/10.1186/s13017-017-0151-4.
16. Renzulli P, Gross T, Schnüriger B, et al. Management of blunt injuries to the spleen. Br J Surg. 2010;97:1696–703. https://doi.org/10.1002/bjs.7203.
17. Coco D, Leanza S. Indications for surgery in non-traumatic spleen disease. Open Access Maced J Med Sci. 2019;7:2958–60. https://doi.org/10.3889/oamjms.2019.568.
18. Tahir F, Ahmed J, Malik F. Post-splenectomy sepsis: a review of the literature. Cureus. 2020;12:e6898. https://doi.org/10.7759/cureus.6898.
19. Bonanni P, Grazzini M, Niccolai G, et al. Recommended vaccinations for asplenic and hyposplenic adult patients. Hum Vaccin Immunother. 2017;13(2):359–68.

## Further Reading

Carbonell AM, Kercher KW, Matthews BD, Joels CS, Sing RF, Heniford BT. Laparoscopic splenectomy for splenic abscess. Surg Laparosc Endosc Percutan Tech. 2004;14(5):289–91. https://doi.org/10.1097/00129689-200410000-00013.

Coccolini F, Fugazzola P, Morganti L, et al. The World Society of Emergency Surgery (WSES) spleen trauma classification: a useful tool in the management of splenic trauma. World J Emerg Surg. 2019;14:30. https://doi.org/10.1186/s13017-019-0246-1.

Lee WS, Choi ST, Kim KK. Splenic abscess: a single institution study and review of the literature. Yonsei Med J. 2011;52(2):288–92. https://doi.org/10.3349/ymj.2011.52.2.288.

Renzulli P, Hostettler A, Schoepfer AM, Gloor B, Candinas D. Systematic review of atraumatic splenic rupture. Br J Surg. 2009;96(10):1114–21. https://doi.org/10.1002/bjs.6737.

Tahir F, Ahmed J, Malik F. Post-splenectomy sepsis: a review of the literature. Cureus. 2020;12(2):e6898. https://doi.org/10.7759/cureus.6898.

# Acute Adrenal Conditions: Pheochromocytoma Emergencies

## 63

Gabriele Materazzi, Leonardo Rossi, and Piermarco Papini

Pheochromocytoma and paragangliomas (PPGL) are rare chromaffin cell tumors characterized by the production of catecholamines and their metabolites and that can be fatal if left undiagnosed. The diagnosis and management of these neoplasms may result in very challenging due to the organ-specific effects of high production of catecholamines and their related consequences [1, 2].

Unfortunately, since these neuroendocrine tumors are often not recognized or misdiagnosed and consequently not well treated, they may present in several possible situations that could evolve suddenly or slowly to true emergency conditions [1].

## 63.1 Introduction

> **Learning Goals**
> - Although rarely, pheochromocytomas and paragangliomas may request an emergency treatment.
> - The effect of catecholamines may result in several acute presentation, mostly related the cardiovascular system.
> - A prompt diagnosis is crucial to perform the correct treatment.

G. Materazzi (✉) · L. Rossi · P. Papini
Endocrine Surgery Unit, Department of Surgery, Pisa University Hospital, Pisa, Italy
e-mail: gabriele.materazzi@unipi.it

### 63.1.1 Epidemiology

Pheochromocytomas and paragangliomas are relatively rare catecholamine-producing tumors with an estimated annual incidence of 2–8 per million population. They occur mostly between the third and the fifth decades of life, although 20% of cases occur in pediatric age. Both genders are affected equally. Moreover, the prevalence among hypertensive patients ranges between 0.1% and 0.6% in adults and between 2% and 4.5% in the pediatric population [3].

PPGL are diagnosed incidentally during imaging scans in 10–49% of cases and 4–8% of adrenal incidentalomas are pheochromocytomas.

Overall, among these catecholamine-producing tumors, 80–85% are pheochromocytomas and 15–20% are paragangliomas [3].

### 63.1.2 Etiology

Pheochromocytomas and paragangliomas occur as sporadic tumors or in a familial context. It is reported that around 24–27% of cases carry a germline mutation [4, 5]. Nowadays, genetic screening plays a key role in diagnosis [6].

The main syndromes associated with pheochromocytoma are multiple endocrine neoplasia type IIA (MEN-IIA), von Hippel-Lindau (VHL) disease, or neurofibromatosis type I (NF-1). Multiple endocrine neoplasia type IIA consists in

© The Author(s), under exclusive license to Springer Nature Switzerland AG 2023
F. Coccolini, F. Catena (eds.), *Textbook of Emergency General Surgery*,
https://doi.org/10.1007/978-3-031-22599-4_63

the familial association of medullary thyroid cancer, pheochromocytoma, and parathyroid hyperplasia. Patients affected by von Hippel-Lindau disease are characterized by the association of the following conditions with early onset: bilateral kidney tumors and cysts, pheochromocytomas, pancreatic tumors, cerebellar and spinal hemangioblastomas and retinal angiomas [7]. Hallmark of neurofibromatosis 1 includes cafè-au-lait spots, neoplasms of the peripheral and central nervous systems and cutaneous neurofibromas. Moreover, pheochromocytomas are reported to be associated with NF-1: their incidence is approximately 0.1–5.7% and it increases to 20–50% in patients with hypertensive status [8].

Overall, hereditary pheochromocytomas are typically intra-abdominal and bilateral and present an earlier onset compared to those with sporadic disease [7].

## 63.1.3 Classification

According to the updated 2017 World Health Organization (WHO) Classification of Tumors of Endocrine Organs, the term pheochromocytoma is referred to intra-adrenal tumor, whereas similar tumors arising outside the adrenal gland are defined as extra-adrenal paragangliomas and further named on the basis of their anatomic origin. Moreover, the well-known 10% rule (10% familial, 10% malignant, and 10% extra-adrenal) for sympathetic paragangliomas is no longer considered applicable since the rate of heritable lesions is reported to be up to 30% [9].

Notably, it is worth to be taken into account that around 10% of pheochromocytomas and 30–40% of paragangliomas are malignant [10]. Although scoring systems for histological evaluation of PPGL are reported, it is not possible to differentiate benign from malignant lesions by histopathology. The evidence of malignancy in these tumors can be defined for the presence of invasion of adjacent tissues or metastasis at presentation or during the follow-up [3, 10].

## 63.1.4 Pathophysiology

PPGL are tumors that release in the bloodstream an excess of catecholamines and therefore enhances the sympathetic nervous system leading to symptoms such as hypertension and palpitations, headaches, and sweating. Catecholamine production takes place in both the adrenal gland, as well as sympathetic paraganglia [11].

The secretory pattern of PPGL varies considerably on the basis of the type of tumors and depends on the pathway of the intracellular enzymes dedicated to product catecholamines. It is suggested that pheochromocytomas typically produce epinephrine, whereas paragangliomas have predominant or exclusive secretion of norepinephrine [12, 13]. Moreover, certain PPGL can secrete dopamine, sometimes in isolation, due to the lack of dopamine-β-hydroxylase [14].

Moreover, it is reported that among hereditary PPGL, the pattern of catecholamine production can depend on the underlying mutation. In particular, patients affected by von Hippel–Lindau syndrome are characterized by typical norepinephrine production, whereas patients affected by MEN type 2 are characterized by a production of a mixture of epinephrine and norepinephrine. Noradrenergic tumors and adrenergic tumors have distinct patterns of gene expression that are retained even when there is no clear hereditary basis [12].

On a biochemical point of view, norepinephrine typically acts on alpha-1, alpha-2, and beta-1 receptors, leading to the clinical presentation characterized by sustained hypertension. On the other hand, epinephrine mainly stimulates beta-1 and beta-2 receptors and patients with predominantly epinephrine-secreting tumors exhibited paroxysmal hypertension attributed to episodic catecholamine release and beta-2 receptor-mediated vasodilatation in skeletal muscles. Finally, the hemodynamic effects of dopamine are mainly related to the dose of the hormone in the bloodstream. Indeed, when the serum levels of dopamine are within the normal ranges, this catecholamine acts mainly on dopamine receptors, resulting in renal artery dilatation and negative cardiac inotropic action [15, 16]. On the contrast, as the dopamine serum concentration rises, dopamine can stimulate alpha- and beta-adrenergic receptors, resulting in variable degrees of hypertension and tachycardia. As a result, patients with dopamine-secreting tumors may exhibit labile blood pressure, varying from normotension to postural hypotension or hypertension [17].

## 63.2 Diagnosis

Although PPGL are diagnosed and treated rarely in the Emergency Unit, they represent an important entity to be considered in the setting of differential diagnosis of several clinical presentations. PPGL may present with a wide spectrum of clinical presentations, ranging from a multisystemic or hypertensive crisis to more subtle symptoms masquerading as anxiety attacks [7]. It is crucial to not overlook the possibility of PPGL in case of an emergency situation where the conventional therapy fails to achieve control. Physicians must keep in mind this rare entity and try to obtain a prompt diagnosis in order to undertake an adequate therapy.

Diagnosis of PPGL is obtained via biochemical confirmation of catecholamines excess, followed by anatomical localization of the tumor(s).

### 63.2.1 Clinical Presentation

Excess release and high levels of circulating catecholamines are responsible for the typical symptoms. Characteristically, patients present with hypertension (sustained or, most often, paroxysmal), usually associated with the classic triad of headache, palpitations, and sweating [7]. Furthermore, patients with elevated levels of circulating catecholamines may suffer of an anxiety status and a sense of impending doom.

This wide spectrum of signs and symptoms has led to the label pheochromocytoma as *"the great masquerader"* since the clinical presentation is often nonspecific and raises up the suspicious of more common conditions, such as hypertension, arrhythmias, and anxiety and thus leading to acute or chronic complications without obtaining a correct diagnosis [1]. Moreover, it is reported that patients with mild hypercatecholaminemia can be relatively asymptomatic or mildly symptomatic and the disease may remain undiagnosed [1].

Nevertheless, severe hypercatecholaminemia is markedly symptomatic and may require emergency interventions due to the high risk of morbidity and mortality. In this situation, the clinical suspicion is an absolute cornerstone of the management and an eventual delay in diagnosis is adversely proportional to the overall outcome. Hereby we reported the acute conditions associated with PPGL which require an emergency management. Main clinical presentations are summarized in Table 63.1.

#### 63.2.1.1 Multisystemic Failure

Even though multisystem failure (MSF) is a rare presentation of pheochromocytoma, it represents the most deadly complication due to its high morbidity and mortality and its rapid and unpredictable evolution and requires a prompt detection. This feared condition is defined as multi-organs failure usually associated with a temperature greater than 40 °C, hypertension or hypotension and encephalopathy [18]. Notably, multisystemic failure is not synonymous with malignant hypertension: indeed, several cases are reported in which this condition is associated with a normotensive or hypotensive status [19, 20]. Moreover, although MSF is usually preceded by hypertensive crisis, it may occur with mild and unspecific symptoms, especially in fragile patients. Besides,

**Table 63.1** Main clinical presentations of PPGL

| Emergency presentations | Elective presentations |
|---|---|
| Multisystemic crisis | Asymptomatic |
| Hypertensive crisis | Paroxysmal hypertension |
| Severe hypotension/cardiogenic shock | Sustained hypertension |
| Ventricular tachyarrhythmias/fibrillation | Headaches, palpitation, sweating |
| Pulmonary edema | Supraventricular arrhythmias |
| Acute coronary syndrome | Anxiety status, sense of impending doom |

MSF may be associated even with less common signs and symptoms, such as abdominal pain, nausea, back pain, anemia, dyspnea, and renal failure [20].

Pheochromocytoma multisystemic crisis can occur spontaneously or may arise from the manipulation of the tumor, from an abdominal trauma or surgery, or the use of some medications [21–23].

Overall, pheochromocytoma multisystemic crisis is associated with a high mortality rate and clinical outcomes mostly depend on delays in diagnosis and the time of initiation of an appropriate therapy [24].

### 63.2.1.2 Hypertensive Crisis

Pheochromocytoma hypertensive crisis is a life-threatening condition secondary to a massive catecholamines secretion into the bloodstream and may result in severe complications, such as cardiovascular collapse, pulmonary edema, and sometimes acute respiratory failure with deadly outcomes [25]. The crisis is usually sprung from severe stress or pain, trauma, postural changes, local manipulation, all conditions which increase the intra-abdominal pressure or administration of some medications. Anyway, the spontaneous hypertensive crisis has been reported without any exogenous stress [26, 27]. As previously reported, this condition is most often related to norepinephrine-secreting tumors, which leads to alpha 1-adrenoceptors mediated peripheral vasoconstriction [26].

### 63.2.1.3 Hypotension and Cardiogenic Shock

It is of paramount importance to keep in mind that, occasionally, pheochromocytoma may present with severe hypotension: this clinical presentation occurred in the case of tumors that secrete mainly epinephrine. Indeed, epinephrine acts mainly on beta2-adrenoceptors, which leads to peripheral vasodilatation [25]. Besides, hypotension may also be secondary to the sudden cessation of catecholamines secretion after pheochromocytoma removal in a patient with very low circulatory volume secondary to vasoconstriction and desensitized beta-adrenoceptors [28]. It is reported in the literature that around 20% of patients affected by pheochromocytoma may have hypotension; further, up to 2% of patients may present with cardiogenic shock [29].

Cardiogenic shock is typically caused by pump failure due to severe left ventricular dysfunction. However, it should be remembered that severe hypotension may be due to severe left ventricular outlet tract obstruction as a complication of mid-apical Tako-Tsubo triggered by PPGL: it is crucial to not overlook this complication since its treatment differs completely from the one of cardiogenic shock caused by cardiac pump failure [25].

### 63.2.1.4 Arrhythmias

It is well known that PPGL have been reported associated with several forms of tachyarrhythmias, usually perceived by the patients as palpitations [30]. Lenders et al. reported that around 50–70% of patients affected by pheochromocytoma experienced palpitations [31].

Arrhythmias are related to the action of catecholamines on beta-adrenergic receptors. Although usually supraventricular, including atrial fibrillation and flutter, pheochromocytoma may be rarely associated with serious and potentially fatal ventricular arrhythmias, such as ventricular tachyarrhythmias, ventricular fibrillation, and torsade de pointes [25].

### 63.2.1.5 Acute Coronary Syndrome

Patients affected by PPGL may also be presented with symptoms, laboratory and ECG finding suggestive of the acute coronary syndrome. This worrisome complication is due to the action of catecholamines which leads to vasoconstriction of the coronary arteries along with an increasing oxygen request from the myocardial tissue sustained by the stimulation of the heart rate and contractility [2].

Distinguishing patients with acute coronary syndrome sustained by pheochromocytoma or heart disease may be very challenging. Retrosternal pain radiating to both upper limbs, palpitations, and anxiousness are commonly shared, as well as ECG findings [32].

On the other hand, severe hypertension accompanied by headache and profuse sweating, and history of paroxysmal attack may be suggestive of pheochromocytoma. Furthermore, if coronary arteries appear normal at angiography a pheochromocytoma should be suspected [2].

### 63.2.1.6 Myocarditis and Cardiomyopathy

Pheochromocytoma may present even as myocarditis or cardiomyopathy. These conditions may be related to direct myocardial toxicity of prolonged high levels of catecholamines, as well as prolonged hypertension or a coronary event. Three types of cardiomyopathies are reported: dilated, hypertrophic, and Tako-Tsubo like [32].

Clinically, patients may present a congestive heart failure, hypotension, pulmonary edema, or cardiogenic shock associated with diffuse left ventricular dysfunction [33, 34].

The myocardial changes documented in the case of cardiomyopathy sustained by pheochromocytoma usually improve after the administration of appropriate pharmacologic medications and resection of the tumor [32].

### 63.2.1.7 Pulmonary Edema

Rarely pheochromocytoma may manifest as pulmonary edema (PE). In this cohort of patient, pulmonary edema has usually a cardiogenic origin; nonetheless, noncardiogenic PE is reported and is believed that this condition is the result of a catecholamine-induced increasing of pulmonary capillary pressure and permeability as well as neutrophil accumulation and increased hydrostatic pressure due to overfilling or constriction of the pulmonary veins [35, 36].

### 63.2.1.8 Gastrointestinal, Nephrological, and Neurological Emergencies

Rarely, pheochromocytoma may present as gastrointestinal, nephrological, or neurological emergencies. In the former case, the cause may be an hemorrhage of the tumor with huge secretion of catecholamines leading to a hypertensive crisis associated with severe abdominal pain and vomiting. Alternatively, a prolonged exposure to high level of catecholamines may determine vasoconstriction of mesenterial arteries, which results in bowel ischemia requiring emergency surgery [2, 37].

Moreover, acute renal failure may be the result of rhabdomyolysis followed by myoglobinuric renal failure caused by extreme vasoconstriction related to an elevated levels of catecholamines [38].

Finally, most of the neurological symptoms caused by pheochromocytoma are the result of cerebral hemorrhage due to paroxysmal attacks of hypertension [2, 39].

## 63.2.2 Tests

### 63.2.2.1 Biochemical Tests

The diagnosis of pheochromocytoma depends crucially on the demonstration of excessive production of catecholamines. Currently, the diagnosis is established by elevated plasma metanephrines or elevated 24-h urinary metanephrines. Exception to this are tumors smaller than 1 cm which do not release catecholamines and the exceptional cases of tumors that purely produce dopamine [40, 41].

Notably, it is well known that, on the contrast of catecholamine which is secreted episodically and has a relatively short half-life, their O-methylated metabolites are produced continuously within tumor cells and have relatively longer plasma half-lives, making metanephrines more reliable for the diagnosis of pheochromocytoma [42, 43].

Important to keep in mind that when measuring the 24 h urinary excretion of metanephrines, urinary creatinine should be measured to verify the completeness of the urine collection. Regarding the assay of plasma metanephrines, it should be performed with the patient recumbent for at least 30–40 min and this test helps to differentiate neurogenic from hypertension caused by pheochromocytoma.. A value of plasma metanephrines of more than fourfold above the upper reference limit is reported to be associated with close to 100% probability of the tumor [44]. On the other hand, in patients with plasma metanephrine values above the upper reference limit and less than fourfold above that limit, the clonidine suppression test combined may be useful [44]. In particular, a clonidine suppression test that does not suppress the elevated plasma normetanephrine levels to <40% after 3 h of administration has a very high sensitivity and specificity (100% and 96%, respectively) for diagnosing pheochromocytoma [40, 45].

Moreover, when a biochemical test is going to be performed, caffeinated beverages, strenuous physical activity, and smoking must be avoided at least about 8–12 h before the testing [46]. Likewise, some medications, such as isoproterenol, methyldopa, levodopa, tricyclic antidepressants, sympathomimetics, phenoxybenzamine, labetalol, acetaminophen, monoamine-oxidase inhibitors, beta-adrenergic blocking agents, calcium channel blockers, which are reported to interfere with assays of plasma and urinary metanephrines, should be discontinued at least 1 week before tests [40, 41].

Anyway, one clinical dilemma is whether to measure catecholamines metabolites in the blood or in a 24 h urine collection. Lenders et al. performed a multicenter study in 2002 and concluded that plasma-free metanephrines constitute the best test for excluding or confirming pheochromocytoma and should be the test of first choice for diagnosis of the tumor. They reported that a negative test result virtually excludes pheochromocytoma [42]. Moreover, the high diagnostic accuracy of measurements of plasma-free metanephrines has been confirmed by several independent studies [47–49]. On the other hand, Perry et al. reported that measurements of urine fractionated metanephrines by mass spectrometry provide excellent sensitivity (97%) and specificity (91%) for the diagnosis of PPGL [50].

All in all, the Clinical Practical Guidelines of Pheochromocytoma and Paraganglioma does not recommend that one test is superior to the other and concluded only that the initial biochemical testing for PPGL should include measurements of plasma-free metanephrines or urinary fractionated metanephrines [51].

### 63.2.2.2 Imaging Studies

Anatomic localization of a catecholamine-secreting tumor should be performed only after a biochemical diagnosis has been confirmed. Computer tomography (CT) is considered the gold standard imaging modality due to its excellent spatial resolution for thorax, abdomen, and pelvis [51]. CT is characterized by high sensitivity (88–100%) for the diagnosis of pheochromocytoma, although it decreases to approximately 90% in the case of paraganglioma [51, 52]. Anyway, CT lacks specificity, since pheochromocytoma may be either homogeneous and heterogeneous, solid, cystic, and necrotic with calcifications [51].

MRI, on the other hand, provides superior contrasting effects in soft tissues and therefore may be better for differentiating pheochromocytomas from adrenal adenomas. Moreover, it provides a better evaluation of the relationship between the tumor and the surrounding tissues, resulting in great support to exclude or confirm vessel invasion. Furthermore, iodide contrast agent is not necessary and the method does not use radiation: this makes MRI preferred in case of pregnant women and children [53]. Clinical Guidelines recommend MRI in patients with metastatic PPGLs, for detection of the skull base and neck paragangliomas, in patients with an allergy to CT contrast, and when radiation exposure should be limited [51].

Complementary to a CT scan or MRI, 123I-MIBG scintigraphy is a highly specific method. 123I-MIBG is administered intravenously and body scans are performed after 4 and 24 h. The main purpose of 123I-MIBG scintigraphy is to functionally confirm tumor tissue that has been localized via CT scan or MRI. It resulted also helpful to diagnose extra-adrenal pheochromocytomas and remaining tumor tissue after surgery. The specificity of this method is very high (95–100%); however, its sensitivity is significantly lower (77–90%) [6, 53].

### Differential Diagnosis

As stated above, pheochromocytoma has been labeled *"the great masquerader"* for the wide spectrum of possible presentations which may mimic other more common clinical conditions.

Pheochromocytoma should be taken into consideration in cases of unexplained shock, especially when abdominal pain and pulmonary edema are associated. Likewise, pheochromocytoma should be considered in case of multiple organ failure, high fever, encephalopathy, and severe hypertension or hypotension. Moreover, consumption of certain illegal substances, such as amphetamine, cocaine, and lysergic acid, as well as some cardiological (arrhythmias such as paroxysmal supraventricular tachycardia, essential or renovascular hypertension) or psychological (anxiety disorders) conditions may cause manifestations mimicking pheochromocytoma [10].

Besides, worthy to be underlined that many types of stress can also significantly elevate concentrations of plasma and urinary catecholamines and their metabolites, but rarely they reach the levels typical of pheochromocytoma [10].

Physicians must forever recall that pheochromocytoma wears many disguises. The first step to obtain a correct diagnosis of pheochromocytoma is *think to pheochromocytoma*!

## 63.3 Treatment

### 63.3.1 Preoperative Management

Management of PPGL emergencies results directly correlated to symptoms and clinical presentation of the patient. Nevertheless, either it matters of an elective or emergency situation, administration of preoperative nonselective alpha-adrenoreceptor blockers (phenoxybenzamine) or alpha-1-selective adrenoreceptors blockers (doxazosin, prazosin, and terazosin) is recommended for all patients affected by hormonally functional PPGLs to prevent perioperative cardiovascular complications [51]. Anyhow, although performed by most of Institutions, to date, randomized controlled trials to support the use of pre-operative alpha-blockade are lacking and successful removal of PPGL has been reported without preparation of the patient with alpha-adrenergic blockade [54–56]. As second-line therapy, if the patient's blood pressure cannot be controlled with the alpha-adrenoreceptors blockade alone, additional calcium channel blocker can be administered. Besides, calcium channel blocker can be used in monotherapy in patients with normotensive or mild hypertension [57].

Moreover, if the heart rate is above 100 bpm 3–4 days after alpha-blockade is introduced, beta-adrenoreceptor blockers (such as propranolol or atenolol) should be administered to control tachycardia. It is crucial to keep in mind that the use of beta-adrenoreceptor blockers without therapy with alpha-adrenoreceptor blockers is contraindicated due to the risk of hypertensive crises caused by the unopposed stimulation of alpha-adrenergic receptors [51, 58]. Practical guidelines recommend preoperative medical treatment for 7–14 days to allow adequate time to normalize blood pressure and heart rate [51].

Further, the alpha-adrenergic blockade should be accompanied by a high-dose sodium diet (5000 mg/day) and adequate daily fluid intake (2.5 L/day) to prevent severe hypotension after tumor removal. Alternatively, patients should receive 1–2 L of intravenous saline (0.9% NaCl) solution one day before the surgery [51, 58]. Expanding the blood volume helps to mitigate or even avoid hypotension once the adrenergic stimulus has been removed in the postoperative period, although only retrospective data exist to support the practice [59].

The aim of the preoperative medical preparation in patients who request adrenalectomy for a PPGL should be to keep the blood pressure below 130/80 mmHg while sitting and not lower than 80/45 mmHg while standing. The target in the heart rate is 60–70 bpm while sitting and 70–80 bpm while standing [59].

Metyrosine is a catecholamine synthesis inhibitor, which may be reserved in combination with alpha-adrenergic receptor blockers in case of refractory hypertension [57]. Anyway, many experts do not recommend Metyrosine due to its potential negative effects on cardiac function. Moreover, it is associated with several side effects, such as sedation, depression, and extrapyramidal manifestations [11].

Patients who present with PPGL crisis should be admitted to hospital for aggressive medical management of symptoms before surgical treatment [57]. In these cases, immediate surgical intervention without stabilization of vital parameters is associated with high morbidity and mortality. Although many of these patients can be stabilized by means of alpha-adrenoreceptors blockers, a multidisciplinary approach is required. Occasionally, intra-aortic balloon pump (IABP) or extracorporeal membrane oxygenation (ECMO) may be required to manage severe cardiogenic shock [23, 60].

Overall, adrenalectomy can be performed within 1–2 weeks in patients who generally recover with medical and intensive care support. However, emergency surgery may be necessary in rare case of tumor rupture or uncontrolled bleeding [58].

The recommended pre-operative protocol is summarized in Flowchart 63.1.

### 63.3.2 Intra-Operative Management

It is crucial to achieve a successful treatment that the surgical and anesthesiologic team collaborate during the operation. The manipulation of the tumor may lead to an increase of the blood pressure or heart rate and surgeons may be asked to stop the surgical action to restore the vital parameters within the limits. Esmolol is usually administered in case of intra-operative hypertension;

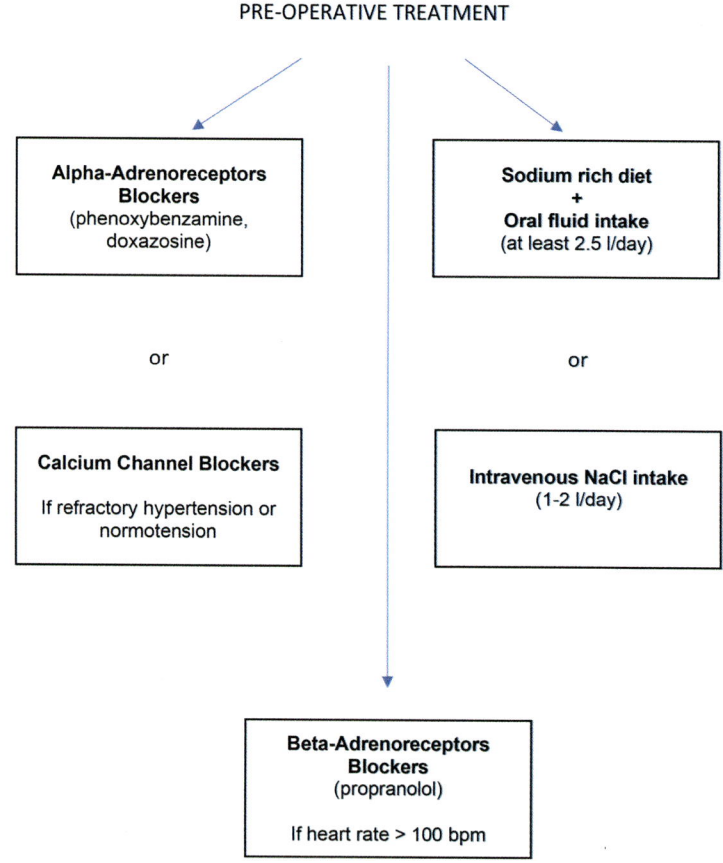

**Flowchart 63.1** Preoperative management

moreover, intravenous magnesium sulfate can be used to manage refractory hypertension [58].

Once the tumor has been removed, hypotension may occur: administration of intravenous isotonic fluid (0.9% NaCl) may help to face this situation. Besides, bolus or infusion of ephedrine or phenylephrine can be administered if needed [58].

### 63.3.3 Medical Treatment

Rupture of an adrenal pheochromocytoma is extremely rare and can be fatal due to sudden cardiovascular consequences with high mortality rate [61]. The exact mechanism of pheochromocytoma rupture is debated, but high blood pressure attributable to a massive release of catecholamines into the bloodstream is likely associated with vasoconstriction within the tumor and subsequent hemorrhage and necrosis. Furthermore, rapid tumor growth may play a role to determine high intracapsular pressure, which may lead to capsular tear and retroperitoneal bleeding [62].

In case of failure of medical conservative management and hemodynamic instability, transarterial embolization has been reported to be a viable option in case of pheochromocytoma rupture. Although emergency adrenalectomy for ruptured pheochromocytoma has been associated with a high mortality rate, endearing outcomes have been reported for cases in which transarterial embolization was used for hemostasis and patient stabilization until elective surgery can be performed [63–66].

### 63.3.4 Surgical Treatment

As stated above, emergency surgery in case of acute adrenal conditions is not recommended except for very selective cases. First of all, an extraordinary effort should be performed to stabilize the patient by means of medical management; surgery can be safely performed within 1–2 weeks after the patient's recovery [24].

Laparoscopic removal of pheochromocytomas and paragangliomas is worldwide considered the "gold standard technique" due to its high reproducibility associated with low postoperative morbidity, short hospital stay and operative time, fast postsurgical recovery, and high patient satisfaction [51].

Since the era of open adrenalectomy, the dogma has always been to ligate the adrenal vein as early as possible to prevent catecholamine surges related to gland manipulation (Fig. 63.1). Notwithstanding the rule "*the vein first*" is still followed in several institutions, recent studies reported that delayed adrenal vein ligation is safe and effective [67].

Although the trans-peritoneal approach is the most commonly used technique to remove pheochromocytoma, the retroperitoneoscopic route, popularized by MK Walz and his team, is progressively gaining more and more consensus [68]. Besides, a cortical-sparing surgery is considered suitable in the case of hereditary or bilateral pheochromocytoma to prevent postsurgical adrenal failure [51].

Finally, practical guidelines recommend open resection for large (more than 6 cm in diameter) or invasive lesions, as well as for pheochromocytoma with suspicion of malignancy [51].

### 63.3.5 Prognosis

Patients presenting with pheochromocytoma crisis suffer from a mortality rate approximately of 15% [69]. About 25% of patients remain hyper-

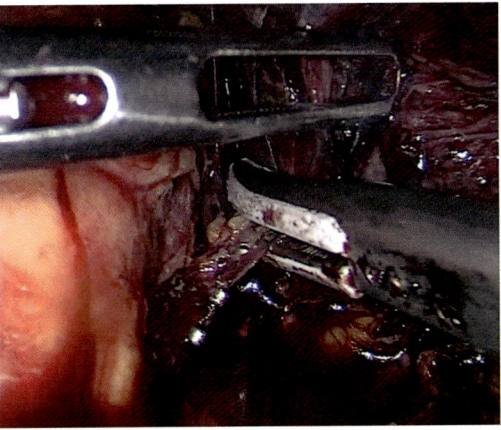

**Fig. 63.1** The middle adrenal vein is ligated as early as possible

tensive following adrenalectomy: this may be due to coexisting essential hypertension or rarely to tumor relapse. Five-year survival for patients with benign pheochromocytoma is 95%, but varies from 36% to 50% in the case of malignant tumors [10].

> **Dos and Don'ts**
>
> - Emergency surgery in case of pheochromocytoma crisis is not recommended.
> - Administration of alpha-adrenoreceptor blockers (eventually associated with beta-adrenoreceptor blockers) is recommended for all hormonally functional pheochromocytoma.
> - The use of beta-adrenoreceptor blocker without alpha-adrenoreceptor blockers is not indicated and may lead to a hypertensive crisis.

> **Take-Home Messages**
>
> - Pheochromocytoma emergencies are rare but harbor high morbidity and mortality.
> - A multidisciplinary evaluation is crucial for the management of adrenal emergencies related to pheochromocytoma.
> - It is of paramount importance effort to obtain hemodynamic stability.
> - The use of alpha-adrenoreceptor blockers is recommended before surgery.
> - Adrenalectomy can be performed within 1–2 weeks in patients who generally recover with medical and intensive care support.

**Multiple Choice Questions**

1. Which is the main difference between pheochromocytoma and paraganglioma?
    A. The former is located inside the adrenal gland, the latter outside the adrenal gland (X)
    B. The former is located outside the adrenal gland, the latter inside the adrenal gland
    C. The former produces catecholamines, the latter glucocorticoids
    D. The former produces catecholamines, the latter sexual hormones
2. Pheochromocytoma may occur in a familial context. Which are the main associated syndromes?
    A. MEN I, MEN 2B, VHL syndrome
    B. MEN IIA, VHL syndrome, NF I (X)
    C. Conn Disease, MEN II B, NF II
    D. Cushing disease, MEN IIA, VHL syndrome
3. Which is the most common clinical presentation of PPGL?
    A. Headache, sweating, palpitations (X)
    B. Hypertensive crisis
    C. Multisystemic failure
    D. Acute abdomen
4. Which of the following actions may spring a pheochromocytoma crisis?
    A. Manipulation during surgery
    B. Trauma
    C. Administration of some medications (such as tricyclic antidepressants, levodopa, labetalol)
    D. All the above-mentioned answers (X)

5. What is the main cause of the complications of PPGL?
   A. Mass-effect
   B. Rupture
   C. Tumor necrosis
   D. High levels of circulating catecholamines (X)
6. Which is the first level test for a proper diagnosis of pheochromocytoma?
   A. CT scan
   B. US scan
   C. MRI scan
   D. Biochemical test (serum or 24-h urinary metanephrines level) (X)
7. Which is the best imaging study to localize pheochromocytoma?
   A. US scan
   B. CT scan (X)
   C. MRI scan
   D. 123I-MIBG scintigraphy
8. Which is the optimal pre-operative treatment of PPGL?
   A. Alpha-adrenoreceptor blockers + intense hydration ± beta-adrenoreceptor blockers (X)
   B. Beta-adrenoreceptor blockers + intense hydration
   C. Alpha-adrenoreceptor blockers
   D. Calcium channel blockers + intense hydration ± beta-adrenoreceptor blockers
9. In case of emergency presentation of pheochromocytoma, which is the best management?
   A. Emergency surgery
   B. Medical therapy associated with intensive care to stabilize the patient (X)
   C. Trans-arterial embolization
   D. None of the above mentioned answers
10. Which is the gold standard technique for the adrenal removal?
    A. Laparoscopic adrenalectomy (transperitoneal or retroperitoneal) (X)
    B. Robotic adrenalectomy
    C. Open adrenalectomy
    D. Depends on the experience of the surgeon

## References

1. Kantorovich V, Pacak K. Emergencies related to pheochromocytoma/paraganglioma syndrome. 2019. In: Feingold KR, Anawalt B, Boyce A, Chrousos G, de Herder WW, Dhatariya K, Dungan K, Grossman A, Hershman JM, Hofland J, Kalra S, Kaltsas G, Koch C, Kopp P, Korbonits M, Kovacs CS, Kuohung W, Laferrère B, EA MG, McLachlan R, Morley JE, New M, Purnell J, Sahay R, Singer F, Stratakis CA, Trence DL, Wilson DP, editors. Endotext. South Dartmouth, MA: MDText.com, Inc.; 2000.
2. Brouwers FM, Lenders JW, Eisenhofer G, Pacak K. Pheochromocytoma as an endocrine emergency. Rev Endocr Metab Disord. 2003;4(2):121–8. https://doi.org/10.1023/a:1022981801344.
3. Aygun N, Uludag M. Pheochromocytoma and paraganglioma: from epidemiology to clinical findings. Sisli Etfal Hastan Tip Bul. 2020;54(2):159–68. https://doi.org/10.14744/SEMB.2020.18794.
4. Neumann HP, Bausch B, SR MW, Bender BU, Gimm O, Franke G, Schipper J, Klisch J, Altehoefer C, Zerres K, Januszewicz A, Eng C, Smith WM, Munk R, Manz T, Glaesker S, Apel TW, Treier M, Reineke M, Walz MK, Hoang-Vu C, Brauckhoff M, Klein-Franke A, Klose P, Schmidt H, Maier-Woelfle M, Pęczkowska M, Szmigielski C, Eng C, Freiburg-Warsaw-Columbus Pheochromocytoma Study Group. Germ-line mutations in nonsyndromic pheochromocytoma. N Engl J Med. 2002;346(19):1459–66. https://doi.org/10.1056/NEJMoa020152.
5. Amar L, Bertherat J, Baudin E, Ajzenberg C, Bressac-de Paillerets B, Chabre O, Chamontin B, Delemer B, Giraud S, Murat A, Niccoli-Sire P, Richard S, Rohmer V, Sadoul JL, Strompf L, Schlumberger M, Bertagna X, Plouin PF, Jeunemaitre X, Gimenez-Roqueplo AP. Genetic testing in pheo-

chromocytoma or functional paraganglioma. J Clin Oncol. 2005;23(34):8812–8. https://doi.org/10.1200/JCO.2005.03.1484.
6. Reisch N, Peczkowska M, Januszewicz A, Neumann HP. Pheochromocytoma: presentation, diagnosis and treatment. J Hypertens. 2006;24(12):2331–9. https://doi.org/10.1097/01.hjh.0000251887.01885.54.
7. Torrey SP. Recognition and management of adrenal emergencies. Emerg Med Clin North Am. 2005;23(3):687–702, viii. https://doi.org/10.1016/j.emc.2005.03.003.
8. Walther MM, Herring J, Enquist E, Keiser HR, Linehan WM. von Recklinghausen's disease and pheochromocytomas. J Urol. 1999;162(5):1582–6.
9. Guilmette J, Sadow PM. A guide to pheochromocytomas and paragangliomas. Surg Pathol Clin. 2019;12(4):951–65. https://doi.org/10.1016/j.path.2019.08.009. Epub 2019 Sep 28.
10. Manger WM, Gifford RW. Pheochromocytoma. J Clin Hypertens (Greenwich). 2002;4(1):62–72. https://doi.org/10.1111/j.1524-6175.2002.01452.x.
11. Wang H, Jepegnanam C. Recognition and management of phaeochromocytoma and paraganglioma. Anaesth Intensive Care Med. 2017; https://doi.org/10.1016/j.mpaic.2017.06.022.
12. Eisenhofer G, Lenders JW, Goldstein DS, Mannelli M, Csako G, Walther MM, Brouwers FM, Pacak K. Pheochromocytoma catecholamine phenotypes and prediction of tumor size and location by use of plasma free metanephrines. Clin Chem. 2005;51(4):735–44. https://doi.org/10.1373/clinchem.2004.045484. Epub 2005 Feb 17.
13. van der Harst E, de Herder WW, de Krijger RR, Bruining HA, Bonjer HJ, Lamberts SW, van den Meiracker AH, Stijnen TH, Boomsma F. The value of plasma markers for the clinical behaviour of phaeochromocytomas. Eur J Endocrinol. 2002;147(1):85–94. https://doi.org/10.1530/eje.0.1470085.
14. Eisenhofer G, Goldstein DS, Sullivan P, Csako G, Brouwers FM, Lai EW, Adams KT, Pacak K. Biochemical and clinical manifestations of dopamine-producing paragangliomas: utility of plasma methoxytyramine. J Clin Endocrinol Metab. 2005;90(4):2068–75. https://doi.org/10.1210/jc.2004-2025. Epub 2005 Jan 11.
15. Zuber SM, Kantorovich V, Pacak K. Hypertension in pheochromocytoma: characteristics and treatment. Endocrinol Metab Clin N Am. 2011;40(2):295–311, vii. https://doi.org/10.1016/j.ecl.2011.02.002.
16. Isaacs M, Lee P. Preoperative alpha-blockade in phaeochromocytoma and paraganglioma: is it always necessary? Clin Endocrinol (Oxf). 2017;86(3):309–14. https://doi.org/10.1111/cen.13284. Epub 2016 Dec 15.
17. Foo SH, Chan SP, Ananda V, Rajasingam V. Dopamine-secreting phaeochromocytomas and paragangliomas: clinical features and management. Singap Med J. 2010;51(5):e89–93.
18. Newell KA, Prinz RA, Pickleman J, Braithwaite S, Brooks M, Karson TH, Glisson S. Pheochromocytoma multisystem crisis. A surgical emergency. Arch Surg. 1988;123(8):956–9. https://doi.org/10.1001/archsurg.1988.01400320042007.
19. Herbland A, Bui N, Rullier A, Vargas F, Gruson D, Hilbert G. Multiple organ failure as initial presentation of pheochromytoma. Am J Emerg Med. 2005;23(4):565–6. https://doi.org/10.1016/j.ajem.2004.12.001.
20. Kakoki K, Miyata Y, Shida Y, Hakariya T, Takehara K, Izumida S, Sekino M, Kinoshita N, Igawa T, Fukuoka J, Sakai H. Pheochromocytoma multisystem crisis treated with emergency surgery: a case report and literature review. BMC Res Notes. 2015;8:758. https://doi.org/10.1186/s13104-015-1738-z.
21. Eisenhofer G, Rivers G, Rosas AL, Quezado Z, Manger WM, Pacak K. Adverse drug reactions in patients with phaeochromocytoma: incidence, prevention and management. Drug Saf. 2007;30(11):1031–62. https://doi.org/10.2165/00002018-200730110-00004.
22. Greaves DJ, Barrow PM. Emergency resection of phaeochromocytoma presenting with hyperamylasaemia and pulmonary oedema after abdominal trauma. Anaesthesia. 1989;44(10):841–2. https://doi.org/10.1111/j.1365-2044.1989.tb09105.x.
23. Takagi S, Miyazaki S, Fujii T, Daikoku S, Sutani Y, Morii I, Yasuda S, Goto Y, Nonogi H. Dexamethasone-induced cardiogenic shock rescued by percutaneous cardiopulmonary support (PCPS) in a patient with pheochromocytoma. Jpn Circ J. 2000;64(10):785–8. https://doi.org/10.1253/jcj.64.785.
24. Scholten A, Cisco RM, Vriens MR, Cohen JK, Mitmaker EJ, Liu C, Tyrrell JB, Shen WT, Duh QY. Pheochromocytoma crisis is not a surgical emergency. J Clin Endocrinol Metab. 2013;98(2):581–91. https://doi.org/10.1210/jc.2012-3020. Epub 2013 Jan 2.
25. Y-Hassan S, Falhammar H. Cardiovascular manifestations and complications of pheochromocytomas and paragangliomas. J Clin Med. 2020;9(8):2435. https://doi.org/10.3390/jcm9082435.
26. Pappachan JM, Tun NN, Arunagirinathan G, Sodi R, Hanna FWF. Pheochromocytomas and hypertension. Curr Hypertens Rep. 2018;20(1):3. https://doi.org/10.1007/s11906-018-0804-z.
27. Falhammar H, Kjellman M, Calissendorff J. Initial clinical presentation and spectrum of pheochromocytoma: a study of 94 cases from a single center. Endocr Connect. 2018;7(1):186–92. https://doi.org/10.1530/EC-17-0321. Epub 2017 Dec 7.
28. Olson SW, Deal LE, Piesman M. Epinephrine-secreting pheochromocytoma presenting with cardiogenic shock and profound hypocalcemia. Ann Intern Med. 2004;140(10):849–51. https://doi.org/10.7326/0003-4819-140-10-200405180-00033.
29. Bergland BE. Pheochromocytoma presenting as shock. Am J Emerg Med. 1989;7(1):44–8. https://doi.org/10.1016/0735-6757(89)90084-3.
30. Zelinka T, Petrák O, Turková H, Holaj R, Strauch B, Kršek M, Vránková AB, Musil Z, Dušková J, Kubinyi J, Michalský D, Novák K, Widimský J. High inci-

dence of cardiovascular complications in pheochromocytoma. Horm Metab Res. 2012;44(5):379–84. https://doi.org/10.1055/s-0032-1306294. Epub 2012 Apr 19.
31. Lenders JW, Eisenhofer G, Mannelli M, Pacak K. Phaeochromocytoma. Lancet. 2005;366(9486):665–75. https://doi.org/10.1016/S0140-6736(05)67139-5.
32. Santos JRU, Brofferio A, Viana B, Pacak K. Catecholamine-induced cardiomyopathy in pheochromocytoma: how to manage a rare complication in a rare disease? Horm Metab Res. 2019;51(7):458–69. https://doi.org/10.1055/a-0669-9556. Epub 2018 Sep 18.
33. Baker G, Zeller NH, Weitzner S, Leach JK. Pheochromocytoma without hypertension presenting as cardiomyopathy. Am Heart J. 1972;83(5):688–93. https://doi.org/10.1016/0002-8703(72)90410-3.
34. Garcia R, Jennings JM. Pheochromocytoma masquerading as a cardiomyopathy. Am J Cardiol. 1972;29(4):568–71. https://doi.org/10.1016/0002-9149(72)90452-3.
35. Takeshita T, Shima H, Oishi S, Machida N, Uchiyama K. Noncardiogenic pulmonary edema as the first manifestation of pheochromocytoma: a case report. Radiat Med. 2005;23(2):133–8.
36. Nepal S, Giri S, Bhusal M, Siwakoti K, Pathak R. An uncommon cause of acute pulmonary edema. JAAPA. 2016;29(9):1–4. https://doi.org/10.1097/01.JAA.0000490945.35987.83.
37. Hendrickson RJ, Katzman PJ, Queiroz R, Sitzmann JV, Koniaris LG. Management of massive retroperitoneal hemorrhage from an adrenal tumor. Endocr J. 2001;48(6):691–6. https://doi.org/10.1507/endocrj.48.691.
38. Shemin D, Cohn PS, Zipin SB. Pheochromocytoma presenting as rhabdomyolysis and acute myoglobinuric renal failure. Arch Intern Med. 1990;150(11):2384–5.
39. Fox JM, Manninen PH. The anaesthetic management of a patient with a phaeochromocytoma and acute stroke. Can J Anaesth. 1991;38(6):775–9. https://doi.org/10.1007/BF03008459.
40. van Berkel A, Lenders JW, Timmers HJ. Diagnosis of endocrine disease: Biochemical diagnosis of phaeochromocytoma and paraganglioma. Eur J Endocrinol. 2014;170(3):R109–19. https://doi.org/10.1530/EJE-13-0882.
41. Farrugia FA, Martikos G, Tzanetis P, Charalampopoulos A, Misiakos E, Zavras N, Sotiropoulos D. Pheochromocytoma, diagnosis and treatment: Review of the literature. Endocr Regul. 2017;51(3):168–81. https://doi.org/10.1515/enr-2017-0018.
42. Lenders JW, Pacak K, Walther MM, Linehan WM, Mannelli M, Friberg P, Keiser HR, Goldstein DS, Eisenhofer G. Biochemical diagnosis of pheochromocytoma: which test is best? JAMA. 2002;287(11):1427–34. https://doi.org/10.1001/jama.287.11.1427.
43. Eisenhofer G, Huynh TT, Hiroi M, Pacak K. Understanding catecholamine metabolism as a guide to the biochemical diagnosis of pheochromocytoma. Rev Endocr Metab Disord. 2001;2(3):297–311. https://doi.org/10.1023/a:1011572617314.
44. Eisenhofer G, Goldstein DS, Walther MM, Friberg P, Lenders JW, Keiser HR, Pacak K. Biochemical diagnosis of pheochromocytoma: how to distinguish true- from false-positive test results. J Clin Endocrinol Metab. 2003;88(6):2656–66. https://doi.org/10.1210/jc.2002-030005.
45. Maurea S, Cuocolo A, Reynolds JC, Neumann RD, Salvatore M. Diagnostic imaging in patients with paragangliomas. Computed tomography, magnetic resonance and MIBG scintigraphy comparison. Q J Nucl Med. 1996;40(4):365–71.
46. Francis IR, Korobkin M. Pheochromocytoma. Radiol Clin N Am. 1996;34(6):1101–12.
47. Raber W, Raffesberg W, Bischof M, Scheuba C, Niederle B, Gasic S, Waldhäusl W, Roden M. Diagnostic efficacy of unconjugated plasma metanephrines for the detection of pheochromocytoma. Arch Intern Med. 2000;160(19):2957–63. https://doi.org/10.1001/archinte.160.19.2957.
48. Sawka AM, Jaeschke R, Singh RJ, Young WF Jr. A comparison of biochemical tests for pheochromocytoma: measurement of fractionated plasma metanephrines compared with the combination of 24-hour urinary metanephrines and catecholamines. J Clin Endocrinol Metab. 2003;88(2):553–8. https://doi.org/10.1210/jc.2002-021251.
49. Unger N, Pitt C, Schmidt IL, Walz MK, Schmid KW, Philipp T, Mann K, Petersenn S. Diagnostic value of various biochemical parameters for the diagnosis of pheochromocytoma in patients with adrenal mass. Eur J Endocrinol. 2006;154(3):409–17. https://doi.org/10.1530/eje.1.02097.
50. Perry CG, Sawka AM, Singh R, Thabane L, Bajnarek J, Young WF Jr. The diagnostic efficacy of urinary fractionated metanephrines measured by tandem mass spectrometry in detection of pheochromocytoma. Clin Endocrinol (Oxf). 2007;66(5):703–8. https://doi.org/10.1111/j.1365-2265.2007.02805.x. Epub 2007 Mar 27.
51. Lenders JW, Duh QY, Eisenhofer G, Gimenez-Roqueplo AP, Grebe SK, Murad MH, Naruse M, Pacak K, Young WF Jr, Endocrine Society. Pheochromocytoma and paraganglioma: an endocrine society clinical practice guideline. J Clin Endocrinol Metab. 2014;99(6):1915–42. https://doi.org/10.1210/jc.2014-1498.
52. Mannelli M, Ianni L, Cilotti A, Conti A. Pheochromocytoma in Italy: a multicentric retrospective study. Eur J Endocrinol. 1999;141(6):619–24. https://doi.org/10.1530/eje.0.1410619.
53. Ilias I, Pacak K. Current approaches and recommended algorithm for the diagnostic localization of pheochromocytoma. J Clin Endocrinol

Metab. 2004;89(2):479–91. https://doi.org/10.1210/jc.2003-031091.
54. Shao Y, Chen R, Shen ZJ, Teng Y, Huang P, Rui WB, Xie X, Zhou WL. Preoperative alpha blockade for normotensive pheochromocytoma: is it necessary? J Hypertens. 2011;29(12):2429–32. https://doi.org/10.1097/HJH.0b013e32834d24d9.
55. Ulchaker JC, Goldfarb DA, Bravo EL, Novick AC. Successful outcomes in pheochromocytoma surgery in the modern era. J Urol. 1999;161(3):764–7.
56. Groeben H, Nottebaum BJ, Alesina PF, Traut A, Neumann HP, Walz MK. Perioperative α-receptor blockade in phaeochromocytoma surgery: an observational case series. Br J Anaesth. 2017;118(2):182–9. https://doi.org/10.1093/bja/aew392.
57. Wiseman D, Lakis ME, Nilubol N. Precision surgery for pheochromocytomas and paragangliomas. Horm Metab Res. 2019;51(7):470–82. https://doi.org/10.1055/a-0926-3618. Epub 2019 Jul 15.
58. Aygun N, Uludag M. Pheochromocytoma and paraganglioma: from treatment to follow-up. Sisli Etfal Hastan Tip Bul. 2020;54(4):391–8. https://doi.org/10.14744/SEMB.2020.58998.
59. Pacak K. Preoperative management of the pheochromocytoma patient. J Clin Endocrinol Metab. 2007;92(11):4069–79. https://doi.org/10.1210/jc.2007-1720.
60. Suh IW, Lee CW, Kim YH, Hong MK, Lee JW, Kim JJ, Park SW, Park SJ. Catastrophic catecholamine-induced cardiomyopathy mimicking acute myocardial infarction, rescued by extracorporeal membrane oxygenation (ECMO) in pheochromocytoma. J Korean Med Sci. 2008;23(2):350–4. https://doi.org/10.3346/jkms.2008.23.2.350.
61. Kobayashi T, Iwai A, Takahashi R, Ide Y, Nishizawa K, Mitsumori K. Spontaneous rupture of adrenal pheochromocytoma: review and analysis of prognostic factors. J Surg Oncol. 2005;90(1):31–5. https://doi.org/10.1002/jso.20234.
62. Maruyama M, Sato H, Yagame M, Shoji S, Terachi T, Osamura RY. Spontaneous rupture of pheochromocytoma and its clinical features: a case report. Tokai J Exp Clin Med. 2008;33(3):110–5.
63. Edo N, Yamamoto T, Takahashi S, Mashimo Y, Morita K, Saito K, Kondo H, Sasajima Y, Kondo F, Okinaga H, Tsukamoto K, Ishikawa T. Optimizing hemodynamics with transcatheter arterial embolization in adrenal pheochromocytoma rupture. Intern Med. 2018;57(13):1873–8. https://doi.org/10.2169/internalmedicine.9907-17. Epub 2018 Feb 28.
64. Habib M, Tarazi I, Batta M. Arterial embolization for ruptured adrenal pheochromocytoma. Curr Oncol. 2010;17(6):65–70. https://doi.org/10.3747/co.v17i6.597.
65. Park JH, Kang KP, Lee SJ, Kim CH, Park TS, Baek HS. A case of a ruptured pheochromocytoma with an intratumoral aneurysm managed by coil embolization. Endocr J. 2003;50(6):653–6. https://doi.org/10.1507/endocrj.50.653.
66. Pua U, Wong DE. Transarterial embolisation of spontaneous adrenal pheochromocytoma rupture using polyvinyl alcohol particles. Singap Med J. 2008;49(5):e126–30.
67. Vassiliou MC, Laycock WS. Laparoscopic adrenalectomy for pheochromocytoma: take the vein last? Surg Endosc. 2009;23(5):965–8. https://doi.org/10.1007/s00464-008-0264-7. Epub 2008 Dec 31.
68. Walz MK, Alesina PF, Wenger FA, Koch JA, Neumann HP, Petersenn S, Schmid KW, Mann K. Laparoscopic and retroperitoneoscopic treatment of pheochromocytomas and retroperitoneal paragangliomas: results of 161 tumors in 126 patients. World J Surg. 2006;30(5):899–908. https://doi.org/10.1007/s00268-005-0373-6.
69. Meijs AC, Snel M, Corssmit EPM. Pheochromocytoma/paraganglioma crisis: case series from a tertiary referral center for pheochromocytomas and paragangliomas. Hormones (Athens). 2021; https://doi.org/10.1007/s42000-021-00274-6. Epub ahead of print.

# Nontraumatic Liver Hemorrhage

## 64

Amudan J. Srinivasan and Andrew B. Peitzman

## 64.1 Introduction

**Learning Objectives**

- Define the common and uncommon etiologies of nontraumatic hepatic hemorrhagic disease.
- Identify priorities in the diagnosis and initial management of a patient with suspected nontraumatic liver hemorrhage.
- Understand operative and nonoperative approaches to management of nontraumatic liver hemorrhage.

### 64.1.1 Epidemiology

Overall, nontraumatic liver hemorrhage (NLH) is a rare clinical entity. For patients presenting with spontaneous hemoperitoneum, the liver is the most common source of hemorrhage, followed by the spleen [1]. It is estimated that there were fewer than 100 cases of NLH reported in the medical literature prior to 1980, though it is now estimated that NLH is the admitting diagnosis for approximately 1% of admissions to hepatic specialty units [2, 3]. Within areas of high prevalence of hepatocellular carcinoma (HCC), tumor rupture with intraperitoneal hemorrhage can be the initial presentation for between 3% and 20% of cases, though efforts to improve early detection of HCC have decreased the frequency of initial hemorrhagic presentation in certain regions [4]. HCC represents the most common etiology of NLH in regions where it remains prevalent; in areas where HCC is comparatively rarer, the most common cause of NLH is a ruptured hepatic adenoma.

### 64.1.2 Etiology and Classification

Multiple etiologies exist for NLH, as the hemorrhagic focus is usually a structural lesion of some type. These etiologies can be broadly classified into benign hepatic lesions, malignant hepatic lesions, vascular/autoimmune diseases, and obstetric hepatic pathology. Table 64.1 further expands the entities within each of these classifications. Following a discussion regarding the presentation and initial workup of patients with suspected NLH, the bulk of this chapter is devoted to a more in-depth analysis of the pathophysiology of these numerous etiologies and provides specific guidance for each.

A. J. Srinivasan · A. B. Peitzman (✉)
Department of Surgery, University of Pittsburgh, Pittsburgh, PA, USA
e-mail: srinivasanaj@upmc.edu;
peitzmanab@upmc.edu

**Table 64.1** Etiologies of nontraumatic liver hemorrhage

| | |
|---|---|
| Benign hepatic lesions | Hepatic adenoma |
| | Cyst |
| | Focal nodular Hyperplasia |
| | Hemangioma |
| | Nodular regenerative hyperplasia |
| | Biliary cystadenoma |
| | Angiomyolipoma |
| Malignant hepatic lesions | Hepatocellular carcinoma |
| | Angiosarcoma |
| | Epithelioid Hemangioendothelioma |
| | Hepatoblastoma |
| | Rhabdoid sarcoma |
| | Metastatic disease to liver |
| Vascular/ autoimmune/ connective tissue | Peliosis hepatis |
| | Amyloidosis |
| | Systemic lupus erythematosus |
| | Polyarteritis nodosa/vasculitides |
| Obstetric hepatic disease | HELLP syndrome |
| | Acute fatty liver of pregnancy |

## 64.2 Common Principles in Diagnosis and Management

### 64.2.1 Clinical Presentation

Regardless of underlying etiology, patients with NLH can have a wide variety of clinical presentations depending upon the severity of their bleed, ranging from the asymptomatic patient with a hemorrhagic lesion discovered on imaging obtained for another indication, to patients presenting *in extremis* due to catastrophic intra-abdominal hemorrhage. Most commonly, however, these patients will present with acute-onset abdominal pain, which may be associated with nausea, emesis, and abdominal distension. Pain may be confined to the right upper abdominal quadrant, though with enough intraperitoneal hemorrhage the pain may become diffuse, and may be associated with peritoneal signs on physical exam. On physical examination, identify the patients at risk for clinical decompensation; tachycardia, pallor, and alterations of mental status should be concerning findings as they precede overt hypotension. Patients who are hypotensive on initial presentation will require more aggressive management and may require emergent operative management prior to imaging if the patient cannot be stabilized for the trip to radiology. Physical examination may also reveal stigmata of chronic liver disease, such as icterus, gynecomastia, telangiectasia, and caput medusae/superficial varices, all of which should alert the astute examiner to the possibility of hepatic pathology contributing to the patient's acute presentation, as well as the possible presence of underlying cirrhotic coagulopathy.

### 64.2.2 Laboratory Testing

Laboratory testing and imaging can help clarify etiology of NLH, though it should be emphasized that formal diagnostic testing should only be performed in patients who are hemodynamically stable. Patients presenting with acute-onset severe abdominal pain should receive a baseline set of bloodwork to include a complete blood count, basic metabolic panel, hepatic function panel, and coagulation studies. While a low hemoglobin may imply abdominal hemorrhage, patients with NLH can be similar to trauma patients in that a significant amount of hemorrhage can occur before the blood loss is reflected in the hemoglobin measurement. An elevated bilirubin and international normalized ratio (INR) along with hyponatremia suggest cirrhosis or otherwise significant hepatic synthetic dysfunction. The creatinine and blood urea nitrogen (BUN) can provide evidence of current renal function, which may be impaired in the setting of acute hemorrhagic prerenal insult; the renal function is particularly important to take into consideration when planning interventional studies involving the use of contrast dye. Certain laboratory tests may contribute diagnostic or prognostic value regarding the underlying etiology, such as the alpha-fetoprotein (AFP) level in HCC—these specific diagnostics are detailed later along with their relevant etiologies.

### 64.2.3 Imaging

In the context of emergency imaging, the major modalities that play a role in diagnosis and workup of NLH are computed tomography (CT) and ultrasonography (US). While magnetic resonance imaging (MRI) has a well-defined role in the diagnosis of liver lesions, its time constraints and accessibility issues render its utility limited in the emergent setting. Accordingly, the discussion of this chapter will focus on the use of CT and US in the initial workup of NLH.

Ultrasound is an excellent imaging modality in the diagnosis of NLH, but has several important limitations. Foremost among those limitations is its reliance on operator expertise, though the modern omnipresence of the ultrasound machine within the emergency department and intensive care setting has allowed many physicians and surgeons to become proficient in its use. US is a relatively inexpensive and rapid imaging test and can be performed at the patient's bedside, thereby obviating the need for patients to be transported. In addition, ultrasound can easily be repeated. The role of the focused assessment with sonography in trauma (FAST) as an adjunct tool in the workup of trauma patients has been well-established and in the hands of trained operators can achieve reasonable sensitivity, usually in the range of 80–90%, with specificity usually above 90–95% based on case series [5]. While the NLH population is distinct from the trauma population, the use of a FAST-type exam can offer utility in these patients, particularly in those with clinical instability. Free intraperitoneal fluid is noted as a hypo- or anechoic region, usually visualized at the interface between intraperitoneal and retroperitoneal structures (e.g., Morrison's pouch: between the liver and kidney). Of note, however, the FAST is limited in its ability to distinguish between types of intraperitoneal fluid, and patients with a moderate to large ascites burden, possibly from chronic liver disease, may be difficult to distinguish from patients who have acutely bled from a hepatic lesion. Layering within the fluid, areas of echogenicity, or a heterogeneous appearance of the intraperitoneal fluid point toward hemoperitoneum instead of ascites or simple fluid. A further limitation of US is the inability to determine active extravasation, for which angiographic or cross-sectional imaging would be required [6].

Due to its speed of performance and diagnostic accuracy, CT imaging is recommended for all patients with a sufficient level of hemodynamic stability. Furthermore, it is recommended that patients suspected to have NLH undergo a multiphase CT when possible. The use of arterial phase and portal venous phase imaging helps better discern certain culprit hepatic lesions as discussed in more detail below. Many trauma protocol CTs at trauma centers are designed to allow for arterial phase imaging of the upper abdomen including the liver and spleen prior to a complete portal venous phase abdomen/pelvis CT, and similar imaging may have value in the patient suspected to have NLH. Contrast-enhanced imaging has the additional benefit of identifying active extravasation on both arterial and venous phase imaging, which allows for a more targeted approach to angiographic interventions. In the CT with evidence of intraperitoneal hemorrhage, the appearance of the blood may vary based on the acuity of the hemorrhage. Acute bleeding can be identified as intraperitoneal fluid with density in the 30–45 Hounsfield Unit (HU) range. After several hours, the blood can assume a more hyperattenuating appearance, with 40–70 HU density, due to coagulation and increased physical density of the blood products. Hemoperitoneum can also be distinguished from concomitant ascites as the two fluids will have a demarcating line at their interface [7–9].

### 64.2.4 Management

The initial management of a patient with NLH is similar to the initial management of the trauma patient. Attention should initially be directed to stabilizing the patient's cardiopulmonary state, which may require endotracheal intubation and mechanical ventilation if the patient is *in extremis*. Rapid venous access should be obtained—ideally, multiple large-bore peripheral intravenous lines are preferable to central access, though a short, large-bore central line such as a sheath/introducer can provide adequate access for resuscitation as well. In patients with evidence of hemodynamic instability, early blood product transfusion is recommended as part of resuscitation and blood products should be used preferentially in these patients over crystalloid or colloid. Though no trials have directly compared transfusion strategies for patients with NLH, in the absence of this evidence it is likely reasonable to pursue a component transfusion strategy similar to the 1:1:1 ratio of packed red blood cell units to fresh frozen plasma to platelets that was developed by the PROPPR trial [10]. In patients who are hemodynamically stable packed red blood cell transfusion should be initiated at a hemoglobin <7 g/dL unless patient-specific cardiopulmonary comorbidities would indicate transfusion at 8 g/dL. Any existing coagulopathy, which may be inherent to the patient due to comorbid conditions, or may arise in the setting of massive hemorrhage itself, should be aggressively corrected. Thromboelastography can guide correction of coagulopathy, though it may not be available at all institutions. At institutions where coagulopathy correction is guided by laboratory coagulation parameters, physicians should attempt to correct INR to <1.5 and transfuse platelet products to maintain concentrations >50,000/μL.

If the patient remains hemodynamically unstable following the volume challenge of initial resuscitation, proceed promptly to the operating room for direct control of hemorrhage. The patient should be positioned supine with arms abducted, a urinary catheter should be placed, and the skin should be prepped with an appropriate antiseptic solution. The initial conduct of the operation is similar to a trauma laparotomy, as the hemodynamically unstable patient may not have undergone imaging to establish their NLH diagnosis. Accordingly, a midline laparotomy is the recommended initial incision. Upon entry into the abdomen, laparotomy pads should be used to pack all quadrants to obtain temporary hemostasis and allow the anesthesia team to catch up on resuscitation. As the quadrants are serially inspected and packs removed, the hemorrhagic lesion may become apparent on inspection or palpation of the liver. The operation at this point should be tailored to the patient's physiology, and patients who have non-reassuring hemodynamics or persistent acidosis should be considered for a damage-control procedure with temporary abdominal closure and plan for return to the operating room within 24–48 h following resuscitation and correction of physiologic aberrancy. If a mass lesion is the suspected source of the hemorrhage, obtain biopsies prior to abdominal closure, as the pathology report will facilitate further management.

In the setting of a damage control procedure, packing can provide adequate hemostasis, and a common strategy using packs around the liver to manually restore the normal anatomic configuration (particularly if there is a large lesion or laceration associated with the lesion). Surgical energy devices, such as argon-beam coagulation or bipolar devices such as the Aquamantys™ (Medtronic, Minneapolis, MN), contribute to hemostasis of raw liver surface. Large sutures of chromic gut or similar absorbable material can be used to reapproximate areas of capsular violation and tamponade bleeding from the exposed surface as well. Altogether, packing and local control of hemorrhage can bring about hemostasis in approximately one-third of cases. For bleeding refractory to these means of local control, inflow occlusion with Pringle's maneuver at the porta hepatis can help dry the field enough. Many of the causative lesions, such as HCC, draw their primary vascular supply from the hepatic arterial distribution, and angioembolization can be lifesaving in these patients. Ideally, the patient bleeding from an HCC can be managed in a hybrid operating room. Failure of these techniques would constitute an indication for upfront resection of the hemorrhagic lesion. Of note, a nonanatomic resection is a reasonable technique in the setting of acute hemorrhage and can be followed by subsequent anatomic resection if indicated in the stabilized patient. Nonanatomic resection can be performed by first mobilizing the liver (i.e., taking down the triangular ligaments), marking the border of resection using electrocautery on Glisson's capsule, and dividing the parenchyma using one or more of several accepted techniques (crush/clamp, tissue-sealing bipolar energy, ultrasonic dissectors, or vascular-load staplers). Care should be taken to oversew any large exposed vascular structures within the parenchymal transection line to minimize risks of delayed hemorrhage or bile leak [2, 11] (Fig. 64.1).

The hemodynamically stable patient, or patient who responds well to initial resuscitation, may be considered for initial nonoperative management with or without adjunctive use of embolization. In almost half of all cases, nonoperative management alone with close monitoring, serial hemoglobin measurements, and transfusion as needed can be adequate as initial management. For those patients who fail nonoperative management due to ongoing transfusion requirement in the setting of stable hemodynamic parameters, angioembolization is a vital adjunct that can lead to hemostasis in approximately 80%. When the exact etiology of the bleeding lesion is not known, coil embolization should be avoided initially as the use of Gelfoam allows for subsequent chemoembolization as a treatment modality if indicated. It is important to realize that up to 20% of patients who undergo embolization may have repeat bleeding episodes which may require re-embolization or operative exploration [2].

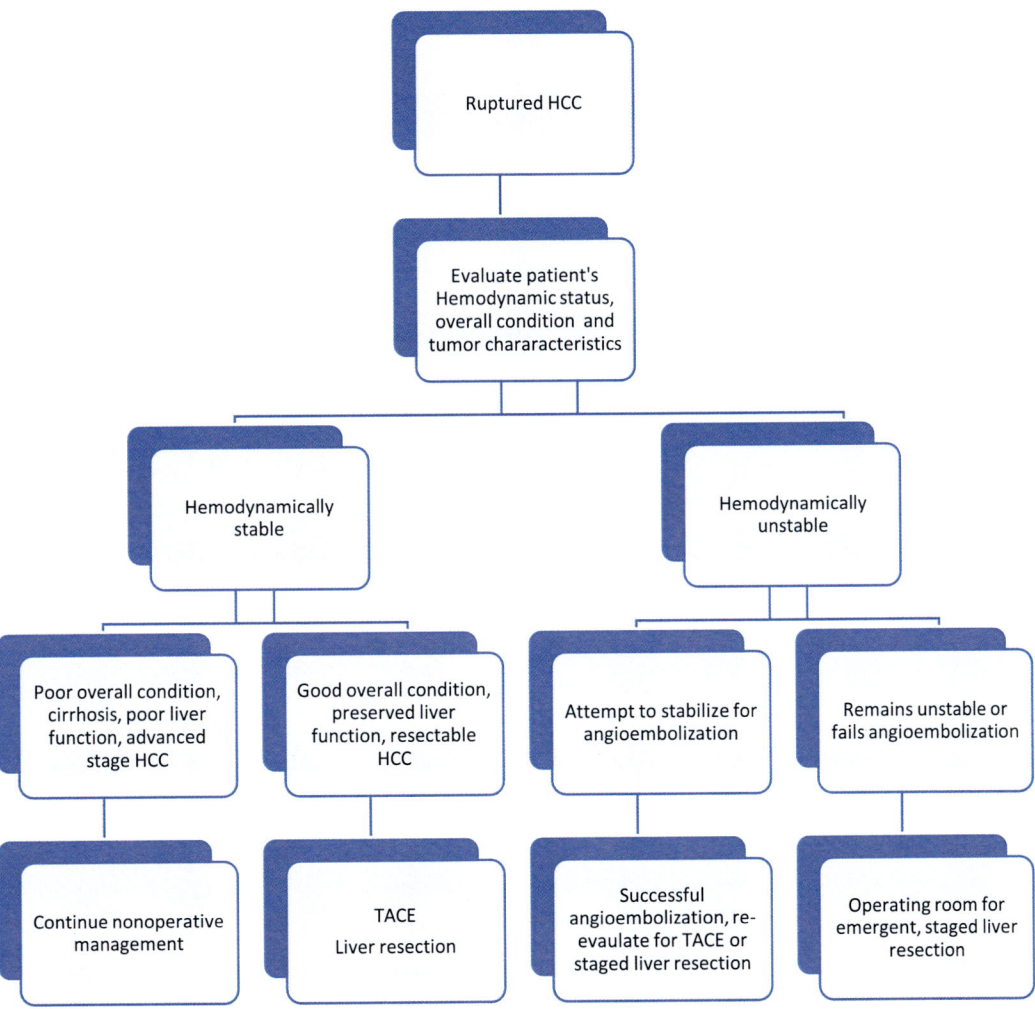

**Fig. 64.1** Algorithm for the management of ruptured hepatocellular cancer (HCC). *TACE* transarterial chemoembolization

## 64.3 Etiologies of NLH

### 64.3.1 Benign Hepatic Lesions

#### 64.3.1.1 Hepatic Adenoma

Adenomas represent a benign neoplastic proliferation of hepatocytes and the most common cause for NLH in regions where HCC is not highly prevalent. Hepatic adenomas are relatively rare, with an overall incidence around 3–4 per 100,000, and classically affect women in their third and fourth decades of life who have had exposure to hormonal therapy, usually in the form of oral contraceptive pills (OCPs). Other populations at risk include persons with thalassemia, hemochromatosis, glycogen storage disorders, and persons who use anabolic steroids. In most cases, adenomas are solitary lesions, though up to 20% of patients can have multiple lesions at presentation [12, 13].

Hepatic adenomas have historically been managed on the basis of size alone as a proxy for risk of hemorrhage and malignant transformation, though newer understanding of the molecular pathophysiology of these lesions has influenced management significantly. Modern classification schemes identify five subtypes of hepatic adenoma. The first, hepatocyte nuclear factor 1α (HNF-1α)-inactivated, is relatively indolent, accounts for 30–40% of all adenomas, and is associated with a lower risk for both malignant transformation and hemorrhage. By comparison, the β catenin-activated adenoma subtype (~10% of all adenomas) can be associated with significant cellular atypia at pathology and can have a rate of malignant transformation of 46% in series evaluating specific activating mutations. Inflammatory adenomas comprise approximately 40% of all hepatic adenomas, are due to aberrant regulation of the Janus kinase, and are more common in obese patients. They have a risk of malignant transformation but this risk is much lower than in the β catenin-activated subtype. Sonic hedgehog adenomas account for fewer than 5% of cases, but are associated with higher rates of spontaneous hemorrhage without elevated risks of malignancy. Finally, unclassified adenomas comprise the remainder of these lesions and do not have unifying histologic or molecular features. Further cohort studies have noted a markedly higher risk of malignant transformation in male patients compared to female patients. In accordance with the above, Krause and Tanabe proposed a modernized algorithm for the management of hepatic adenomas in the elective setting which can be seen in Fig. 64.2 [14–16].

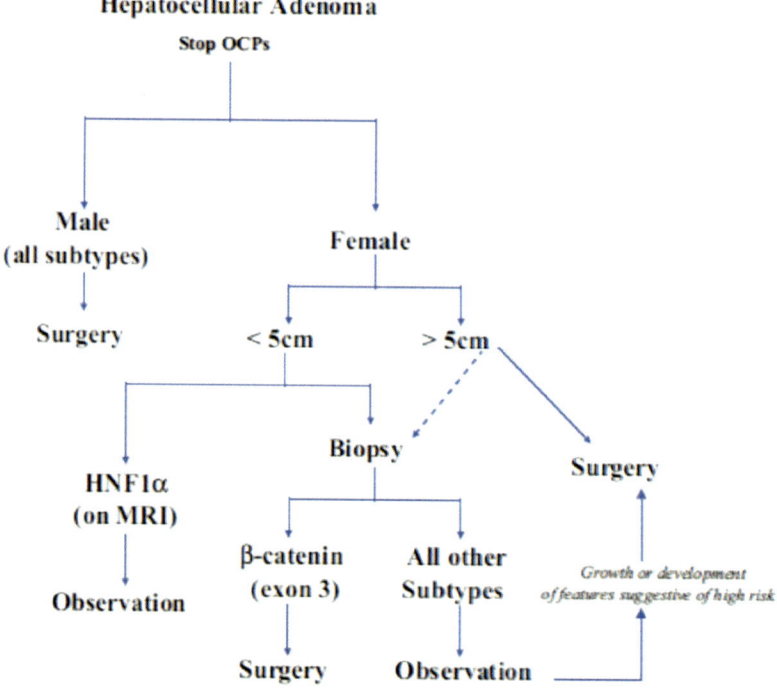

Fig. 64.2 Management of hepatic adenoma in the elective setting. (With permission from Krause and Tanabe, A shifting paradigm in diagnosis and management of hepatic adenoma. Ann Surg Oncol, 2020: 27, page 3336) [16]

While larger lesions have a greater propensity for hemorrhage, it is important to realize that any size lesion can cause spontaneous hemorrhage [17, 18]. On CT, a bleeding adenoma will appear as a hyperattenuating mass lesion within the liver, with associated subcapsular hematoma or intraperitoneal blood. On US/FAST, the lesion is usually hypoechoic, possibly with internal hyperechoic areas, and can have large vessels at the periphery [9].

Embolization should be strongly considered for bleeding adenomas, as bland embolization cannot only bring about appropriate hemostasis, it can also decrease the size of the offending lesion, which can facilitate staged resection following resolution of the hemorrhagic episode. Resection is recommended for lesions greater than the 4–5 cm threshold but also for culprit lesions following an episode of NLH. Given its benign nature, a nonanatomic resection is sufficient unless malignancy is found on the final pathology [19, 20] (Fig. 64.3).

### 64.3.1.2 Hepatic Cyst

Benign hepatic cysts are relatively common lesions that are very infrequent causes of NLH. Cysts generally arise from the biliary epithelium, and it is estimated that between 2% and 5% of the population has at least one. Patients are generally asymptomatic from benign cysts but can develop symptoms if the cysts grow large to the point of exerting a mass effect on surrounding structures. Cyst rupture with hemorrhage is exceedingly rare, and there are a sparse few case reports detailing intraperitoneal hemorrhage due to benign cyst rupture [22, 23]. More commonly, asymptomatic intracystic hemorrhage occurs but does not extend beyond the cyst wall. Larger lesions, and patients with polycystic liver disease, are more likely to undergo cyst rupture, which may or may not be associated with hemorrhage [24]. Ultrasound of these lesions may demonstrate anechoic or hypoechoic, well-demarcated structures without internal flow. CT similarly demonstrates well-demarcated structures with hypoattenuating homogeneous internal component. Hydatid cysts are infectious in nature and arise due to *Echinococcus* species. On imaging, they can appear to have smaller cystic substructures within a larger cyst. Classically, these lesions are more prone to perforation, which can precipitate anaphylaxis due to the cyst contents. However, it is possible for these lesions to cause intraperitoneal hemorrhage, though due to the rarity of these occurrences it is not known what lesion and patient factors predispose to this outcome [25].

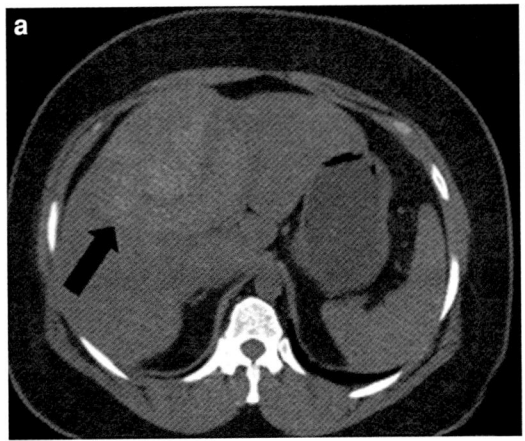
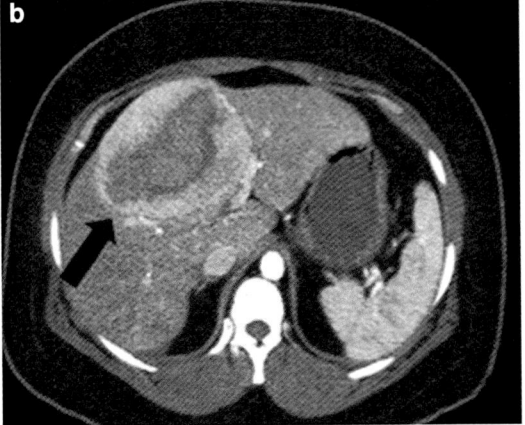

**Fig. 64.3** A 27-year-old woman who presented with RUQ pain. (**a**) Axial unenhanced CT image and (**b**) arterial phase contrast-enhanced CT image show an 11 cm subcapsular adenoma that exhibits high-density hemorrhage (arrow in **a**) and heterogenous arterial enhancement (arrow in **b**). Pathology confirmed this was a ruptured inflammatory hepatocellular adenoma. (With permission from Dharmana et al., Hepatocellular adenoma: imaging review of the various molecular subtypes. Clin Radiol 2017; 72: page 278) [21]

### 64.3.1.3 Focal Nodular Hyperplasia (FNH)

FNH represents the second most common benign liver lesion after hemangioma and is also classically seen in women in their third and fourth decades of life, similar to adenoma. Oral contraceptives may accelerate their growth but the relationship is not as well established as it is for adenoma. On histology, FNH consists of aggregates of hyperplastic hepatocytes separated by fibrous septa, and large feeding vessels can be present at the periphery and in the classic central fibrous scar seen in these lesions. FNH is usually asymptomatic but can cause abdominal discomfort or compressive symptoms due to mass effect in larger lesions. Intraperitoneal hemorrhage is rare, though it is conjectured that lesions which are larger and more peripheral may be at higher risk. Pregnancy is also thought to be a risk for NLH from these lesions [26–28]. On CT, FNH is suspected with arterially enhancing lesions, which are isoattenuating in the venous phase, with a prominent and hypoattenuating central scar [9]. While asymptomatic FNH is usually managed expectantly, FNH lesions associated with spontaneous hemorrhage should undergo resection following the acute episode.

### 64.3.1.4 Hemangioma

Hemangioma is the most common benign liver lesion, with an estimated prevalence of 5–10%. They are more common in women, and can be classified on the basis of size, with lesions >4 cm in size being termed "giant hemangiomas." Lesion rupture is a rare entity—there are fewer than 100 cases reported in the literature, and half of these cases had some form of antecedent trauma. Risk factors for nontraumatic hemorrhage include active pregnancy, lesions >11 cm in diameter, and peripheral lesion location with exophytic/extrahepatic component [29]. The overall mortality described in the literature for hemangioma rupture approaches 35%, though the majority of that mortality was documented prior to 1990 and contemporary advances may render this figure a gross overestimate [30, 31]. On ultrasound, hemangiomas tend to be well-demarcated hyperechoic lesions, and on CT these lesions are usually hypoechoic on noncontrast imaging with peripheral nodular arterial enhancement [9]. As with other benign lesions, staged resection should be performed for hemorrhagic hemangiomas, though the large size of some lesions may require considerable hepatic resection.

### 64.3.1.5 Nodular Regenerative Hyperplasia (NRH)

Nodular regenerative hyperplasia is a rare parenchymal transformative process whereby the hepatic tissue undergoes morphological transformation at the histologic level into a nonfibrotic regenerative nodular architecture. It is a documented cause of portal hypertension due to changes within the resistance profile of the hepatic parenchyma, though this occurs in the setting of normal hepatic synthetic function and no significant cirrhosis. There are associations between NRH and certain autoimmune disorders (such as lupus, rheumatoid arthritis, and vasculitides), hematologic disorders (immune thrombocytopenia, leukemias, and lymphomas), and medications (azathioprine). The diagnosis of NRH is typically made on biopsy, though CT imaging can sometimes show a miliary appearance to the hepatic parenchyma, as well as intra-abdominal sequela of portal hypertension, such as splenomegaly and variceal disease [32]. There is a single case report of spontaneous intraperitoneal hemorrhage due to NRH, making it an extremely rare cause. However, an important point to note is the "field defect" nature of NRH which may render certain operative techniques ineffective for lasting hemostasis depending on the parenchymal texture and its response to these interventions. In the single case report, the patient in question failed nonoperative management with embolization and required an anatomic right hepatectomy [3].

### 64.3.1.6 Biliary Cystadenoma

Biliary cystadenomas are rare multilocular cysts arising from biliary epithelium, and only comprise 1% of hepatic cystic lesions. They are much better known for their ability to undergo malignant transformation to biliary cystadenocarcinoma, which can happen in almost 20% of cases [33]. On CT imaging, these lesions appear multilobular with hypoattenuating cyst contents and septations/loculations within the cyst cavity [34]. Bleeding has been reported rarely as a result of proven biliary cystadenoma. While nonoperative management and embolization may suffice for the initial management of these lesions, biliary cystadenomas should be formally resected following the acute phase for their risk of malignant transformation [35].

### 64.3.1.7 Angiomyolipoma (AMLs)

Angiomyolipomas are benign tumors composed of vascular, muscle, and fat elements. More commonly occurring in the kidneys, they can also occur in the liver, where it can be difficult to differentiate their imaging characteristics from HCC or hepatic adenoma unless there is a significant proportion of fat in their composition [36]. Renal AMLs have been known to have hemorrhagic complications, and current guidelines recommend resection or embolization when greater than 4 cm in diameter or with identified intralesional aneurysms. AMLs in general can be associated with tuberous sclerosis and its variants [37]. There have only been a handful of cases of NLH resulting from hepatic AMLs, though their vascularity and propensity for aneurysmal degeneration can in theory predispose these lesions to hemorrhage [38]. Following initial control of hemorrhage by nonoperative or operative means, these lesions should be resected if hemorrhagic to prevent recurrent hemorrhage.

## 64.3.2 Malignant Hepatic Lesions

### 64.3.2.1 Hepatocellular Carcinoma (HCC)

HCC is the most common primary malignancy of the liver, occurring over 80% of the time in the context of underlying cirrhosis which may be due to chronic hepatitis B/C infection, alcoholic liver disease, or nonalcoholic fatty liver disease, among other etiologies. It is estimated that between 3% and 20% of HCC can present with NLH as the initial symptom, depending on cohort [39]. In areas where HCC is prevalent, it accounts for the most common underlying etiology in cases of NLH. Several factors inherent to the tumor are hypothesized to enable hemorrhagic tumor rupture: rapid growth in the setting of fibrotic/cirrhotic surrounding liver parenchyma, loss of vascular integrity, and arterial remodeling (the latter two of which occur in the context of tumor neovascularization) all potentially contribute to fragile tumors and friable vessels which are prone to hemorrhage [40].

Overall mortality from NLH with a culprit HCC lesion is difficult to definitively measure due to regional differences in disease prevalence and interventional capabilities but ranges from 15% to 70% based on cohort. At least some part of this mortality figure is spurred on by the estimated 10–40% risk of acute hepatic decompensation which can follow hemorrhagic tumor rupture due to hemodynamic effects and dysfunction of other organ systems [4, 41]. Risk factors for intraperitoneal HCC rupture include larger tumor size, peripheral tumor location within the liver, exophytic tumor morphology, and degree of underlying cirrhosis/elevated model for end-stage liver disease (MELD) score [42].

If a liver-protocol CT can be obtained, HCC lesions classically enhance on arterial phase with evidence of washout on venous phase imaging and are sometimes observed to have a lesion capsule or pseudocapsule. Contrast-enhanced imaging may show contrast blush if there is active extravasation. On ultrasound, hemorrhagic HCC lesions will appear as hyperechoic liver masses with surrounding hemoperitoneum [9].

Bland embolization for the ruptured HCC is a good initial strategy and has been associated with decreased hospital mortality and length of stay for patients presenting with NLH secondary to HCC lesions. However, up to 20% of patients managed with nonresectional means can experience rebleeding episodes. While the initial management of these episodes can include repeat embolization, the overall mortality for patients who re-bleed approaches 50% [43]. The use of Gelfoam during initial embolization allows the subsequent use of chemo-embolization as a means of oncologic therapy following the acute phase. At certain capable centers, patients presenting with hemorrhagic HCC lesions have undergone direct transcatheter arterial chemoembolization (TACE) at their index presentation; a review of this practice has found decreased early complications but similar long-term survival to patients who undergo upfront resection [44].

Operative resection at the time of initial NLH presentation is a morbid, but viable means of controlling hemorrhage and the culprit lesion. However, it is associated with high in-hospital mortality, approaching 25–40%, and 1-year survival around 50%. A considerably less morbid strategy is to obtain hemostasis during the index episode and attempt to get the patient to a staged, elective resection. Staged resection in the elective setting for hemorrhagic HCC lesions carries a much lower 0–10% risk of in-hospital mortality and a corresponding 1-year survival of 60–100% [41] (Fig. 64.4).

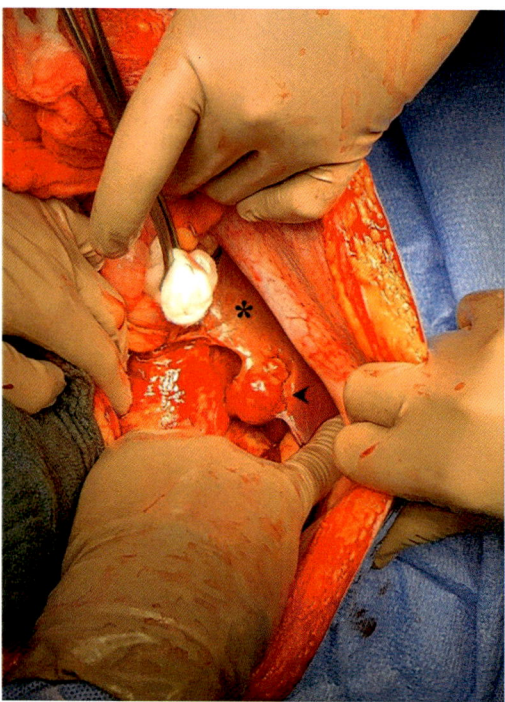

**Fig. 64.4** Intraoperative photograph of a hemorrhagic HCC (arrow) in a 31-year-old female primigravida who was 40 weeks pregnant and developed severe abdominal pain associated with significant free blood-density fluid on abdominal ultrasound. (From Scioscia et al., Spontaneous bleeding of hepatocellular carcinoma during pregnancy, Archives of Gynecology and Obstetrics, 2021; 303: 279, open access) [45]

### 64.3.2.2 Angiosarcoma

Accounting for fewer than 2% of all primary hepatic malignancies, angiosarcoma is a mesenchymal tumor that is classically associated with exposure to vinyl chloride, thorium dioxide/thorotrast, or anabolic steroids, though the majority of these lesions occur in patients who have no significant exposure history. They are vascular by nature, arising from endothelium, and this in combination with their aggressive growth predisposes these lesions to intraperitoneal hemorrhage—it is estimated that 15–25% of cases will have NLH at the time of initial presentation [46]. The tumor is frequently advanced or metastatic at the time of diagnosis, and this confers an overall poor prognosis, with median survival around 1 year from diagnosis. Their appearance on CT can be variable, but they are generally hypoattenuating masses with peripheral nodular arterial enhancement. Some may show evidence of heterogeneity within the mass, with regions of hyperattenuation. Following stabilization, there is a reasonable argument to be made for the resection of a hemorrhagic primary lesion in the elective setting, though the oncologic benefit of such an operation may be unclear if there are metastatic lesions [47, 48].

### 64.3.2.3 Epithelioid Hemangioendothelioma (EHE)

Another vascular sarcoma arising from the endothelium, epithelioid hemangioendothelioma is rarer still compared to hepatic angiosarcoma with an estimated incidence of fewer than 1 per million. Much more indolent and low grade compared to angiosarcoma, patients are commonly asymptomatic or have nonspecific abdominal complaints at the time of tumor diagnosis. Due to its vascular origin, it can also present with intraperitoneal hemorrhage, though the exact proportion of lesions that do so is difficult to ascertain due to disease rarity. On CT, these lesions can be hypoattenuating and may or may not exhibit calcifications. They enhance peripherally on the arterial phase in a ring-like configuration and show stronger contrast enhancement on the venous phase. They are reasonable targets for embolization in the acute phase, though patients should be considered for either anatomic resection (if feasible given tumor burden) or liver transplantation following recovery from the acute NLH episode [49, 50].

### 64.3.2.4 Hepatoblastoma

Hepatoblastoma is a major cause of NLH in the pediatric population, as it represents the most common primary hepatic malignancy in children. Most commonly diagnosed before the age of 2, it is extremely rare in the adult population. Intraperitoneal rupture and hemorrhage occur in up to 30% of cases. Since the disease can be present congenitally, there is even a report of intraperitoneal hemorrhagic rupture occurring in the course of uncomplicated vaginal delivery [51]. Imaging with plain films may sometimes reveal a nonspecific mass in the right upper quadrant with calcifications, and ultrasound will show an echogenic soft tissue-density mass, possibly with calcifications. CT is obtained less frequently in the pediatric population in the interest of sparing ionizing radiation, though can be beneficial for operative planning in the setting of suspected NLH. On CT, hepatoblastoma will usually be a well-defined heterogeneous but overall hypoattenuating mass that may have areas of necrosis or calcification. Initial management of NLH in the pediatric population is similar to that in the adult, and embolization can be undertaken in these patients using the classical vascular access points or even the umbilical artery in the neonatal patient [52, 53]. Since hepatoblastoma is commonly managed with neoadjuvant platinum-based chemotherapy prior to resection in the nonruptured setting, multidisciplinary consultation is recommended to determine the appropriate sequence of therapy and resection in a patient who has recovered from acute NLH [54].

### 64.3.2.5 Rhabdoid Sarcoma

Another malignant cause of NLH in the pediatric population is rhabdoid sarcoma, a rare, aggressive tumor of mesenchymal origin that usually is diagnosed in early childhood. Patients may have a palpable mass of the right upper quadrant at diagnosis, though the disease is frequently metastatic when diagnosed leading to a rather dismal median survival of 2 months. Spontaneous rupture with intraperitoneal hemorrhage has been documented multiple times in the literature, though the rarity of the primary tumor makes further granular data difficult to obtain [55, 56]. Ultrasound will frequently show a complex cystic mass with heterogeneous stroma, and CT shows a heterogeneous mass lesion, which is usually isodense to hypodense, possibly with cystic septate components of the larger mass [57]. Management is similar to hepatoblastoma in that consideration should be given to chemotherapy prior to a definitive staged resection following recovery from the acute bleed.

### 64.3.2.6 Metastatic Disease to the Liver

The liver is a common site for metastatic disease due in large part to its dual blood supply as well as its exposure to the near-complete venous drainage of the gastrointestinal tract. Overall, metastatic liver lesions are much more common than primary liver tumors, though they represent a relatively small fraction of hepatic lesions associated with intraperitoneal hemorrhage. Nonetheless, there are case reports within the literature that discuss hemorrhage from a variety of primary tumor types, including nasopharyngeal, breast, lung, pancreas, colon, lymphoma, and melanoma [58–60]. While not formally studied, it has been theorized that peripheral and subcapsular lesions are more likely to produce NLH due to the propensity for a capsular tear from the mass effect of tumor growth. On imaging, metastatic lesions are usually multiple well-defined rounded tumors that can have variable imaging characteristics based on the specific primary but are usually hypoechoic on ultrasound and hypoattenuating and hypoenhancing on CT [9]. As metastatic lesions usually derive blood supply from the hepatic arterial distribution, they are reasonable candidates for embolization, though the patient's overall prognosis is usually poor in the setting of metastatic disease.

## 64.3.3 Vascular/Autoimmune/ Connective Tissue

### 64.3.3.1 Peliosis Hepatis

Peliosis hepatis is a rare, idiopathic disorder that causes dilation of the hepatic sinusoids leading to the formation of blood-filled cavities within the liver. It is frequently asymptomatic in the affected individuals, and historically the disease was noted only as an incidental finding at autopsy. The liver generally maintains normal synthetic function and does not have any notable biochemical aberrations, and currently, the diagnosis is sometimes made incidentally on imaging. The disease has associations with *Bartonella* infection, HIV infection/AIDS, end-stage renal disease, hematologic malignancies, and certain drugs such as steroids and azathioprine. Intraperitoneal hemorrhage is rare, but there are multiple cases reported in the literature [61–63]. On ultrasound, the peliosis lesions can appear as irregular, hypoechoic masses, sometimes with cystic components. Contrast-enhanced CT will demonstrate hypoattenuating lesions, which exhibit centrifugal arterial enhancement (starting from the center of the lesion and extending radially) with persistent enhancement and no evidence of washout on the venous phase. It is particularly important to note that these lesions may or may not be amenable to embolization, as they are known to have aberrant vascular anatomy at the lesion periphery [64].

### 64.3.3.2 Amyloidosis

A condition usually affecting multiple organ systems, amyloidosis occurs due to the widespread deposition of misfolded light chain protein within various tissues of the body, causing organ dysfunction as a result of these protein aggregates. Hepatomegaly is common in light-chain amyloidosis though the hepatic synthetic function is usually preserved. More relevant to NLH, amyloidosis can change the tissue texture of the hepatic parenchyma, resulting in a more fragile organ overall that can be prone to spontaneous hemorrhage. While NLH due to amyloidosis is uncommon, there have been multiple case reports within the literature describing instances [65]. Imaging usually only shows the nonspecific changes of hepatomegaly and changes in the parenchymal echotexture or attenuation, though in the setting of hemoperitoneum this may alert the interpreting physician to the possibility of amyloid.

Management can be more nuanced due to the propensity for lacerations to expand in the setting of the abnormal parenchymal texture, hemorrhage may not be due mainly to arterial branches and may have elements of portal or hepatic venous hemorrhage as well, which may not readily be amenable to angiographic control [66]. Further, the altered hepatic texture may not respond predictably to techniques of local control, including deep liver sutures or other means of hepatic plication. In these settings, anatomic resection may be indicated if other less radical means have failed to produce hemostasis [67]. Of note, there are reports of successful emergent liver transplantations for spontaneously hemorrhaging amyloid liver—however, the immediate benefit of this major intervention should be balanced with the fact that the allograft will inevitably develop amyloid-related changes due to the unchanged systemic disease [68].

### 64.3.3.3 Systemic Lupus Erythematosus (SLE)

A rheumatologic disease with multiple systemic manifestations across several organ systems, SLE can also cause NLH though it is extremely rare. Approximately one-third of patients can develop a degree of hepatomegaly, though the etiology of this development is not known and may not be due to a singular unifying etiology. Due to the fact that many of these patients remain on long-term corticosteroids, it has been conjectured that NLH may be precipitated by tissue fragility spurred by this steroid use [69]. Emergency imaging is unlikely to be revealed in the setting of SLE-induced NLH and may just show hemoperitoneum and hepatomegaly. Management is generally similar to that of amyloid-induced NLH [70, 71].

### 64.3.3.4 Polyarteritis Nodosa and Other Vasculitides

Polyarteritis nodosa is a relatively rare medium-vessel vasculitis with an estimated incidence of 2–9 per million population. The transmural vascular inflammation gives rise to multiple aneurysmal dilatations within the affected vessels and can produce an angiographic "rosary sign" (small aneurysms strung like the beads of a rosary) that may suggest the diagnosis. Hepatic artery aneurysmal disease is not common but possible as a result of polyarteritis nodosa and other vasculitides. While there are more reports of spontaneous retroperitoneal hemorrhage than intraperitoneal hemorrhage resulting from vasculitis, the latter is possible and has been reported, though remains an overall rare entity [72]. On imaging, ultrasound or arterial-phase CT may show microaneurysmal disease within the hepatic arterial distribution, which suggests the presence of vasculitis, and the arterial-phase CT may also demonstrate active extravasation from a ruptured aneurysm [73]. Due to the vascular nature of these lesions, they are readily amenable to embolization.

### 64.3.4 Obstetric Hepatic Disease

#### 64.3.4.1 Hemolysis, Elevated Liver Enzymes, and Low Platelets (HELLP) Syndrome

The HELLP syndrome is an idiopathic clinical entity that is thought to share a pathologic etiology with preeclampsia/eclampsia, characterized by microangiopathic hemolytic anemia, elevations in transaminases, and thrombocytopenia. Approximately 4–12% of cases of severe preeclampsia have an associated component of HELLP syndrome. Though the suspected root cause of preeclampsia is abnormal placental development, perhaps at the vascular interfaces of maternal/fetal circulation, it is believed that some component of endothelial damage is associated with the development of HELLP. This endotheliopathy and corresponding microangiopathy can create perturbations in hepatic sinusoidal flow, causing congestion and hepatocyte necrosis [74]. In this setting, spontaneous hepatic hemorrhage can occur and can breach the liver capsule causing NLH. This can be extremely morbid, with mortality ranging from 18% to 86% depending on cohort, though it is rare even in the context of HELLP syndrome—less than 1–2% of all HELLP cases. Most commonly occurring in the right hepatic lobe (75%), most likely due to the greater tissue mass in that lobe, it presents most commonly between 28 and 36 weeks of gestation [75]. HELLP-associated NLH should be strongly suspected in any pregnant patient presenting with acute hemodynamic instability and an acute abdomen.

Ultrasound will show evidence of hemoperitoneum but may not show additional significant findings. CT or CT angiography can be obtained in the hemodynamically stable patient and should be strongly considered in this population despite the concerns regarding fetal ionizing radiation exposure as the condition poses a direct threat to the life of both the mother and the fetus. CT angiography can guide interventional management, but these patients will frequently proceed straight to the operating room as the definitive management of HELLP/severe preeclampsia is prompt delivery of the fetus and placenta. At the time of the caesarian section, a midline laparotomy should be used to allow extensile exposure of the upper abdomen and direct control of hemorrhage. While preoperative angiographic management may be considered for hemorrhage with active extravasation, it should not delay operative management if there is evidence of fetal or maternal distress [76, 77] (Fig. 64.5).

#### 64.3.4.2 Acute Fatty Liver of Pregnancy

Rarer than the HELLP syndrome, acute fatty liver of pregnancy is another idiopathic syndrome of acute, a fulminant hepatic failure that primarily occurs in third-trimester patients. While it also is associated with preeclampsia, the cause of the rapid hepatic decompensation is even less well understood, with speculation that the disorder may relate to acute mitochondrial dysfunction or acute acquired impairments of fatty acid metabolism [79]. These patients may present

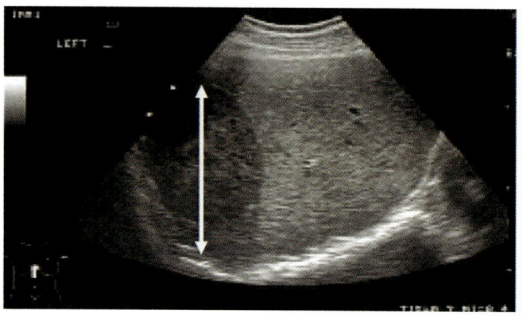 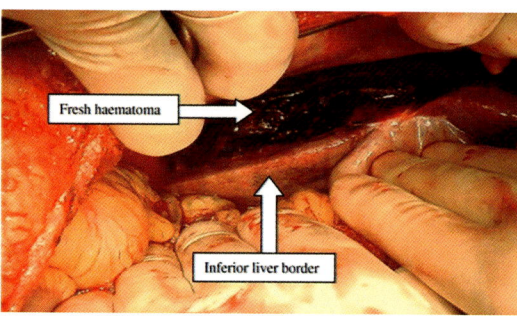

**Fig. 64.5** NLH secondary to HELLP syndrome in a 35-year-old female. The image at left demonstrates a large subcapsular hematoma, and the image at right demonstrates the intraoperative appearance of this lesion. (From Kelly et al., Second-trimester hepatic rupture in a 35-year-old nulliparous woman with HELLP syndrome: a case report, World Journal of Emergency Surgery, 2009; 4:23: page 2, open access) [78]

with jaundice, abdominal pain, gastrointestinal bleeding, and coagulopathy (classically disseminated intravascular coagulopathy). Laboratory evaluations may demonstrate hepatic synthetic failure. While spontaneous rupture is a rare event in an already rare disease state, it is documented in the literature. Both CT and US will show signs of hepatic steatosis and likely hepatomegaly with evidence of hemoperitoneum [80].

The acute management of NLH in the setting of acute fatty liver of pregnancy is similar to that of HELLP syndrome: prompt fetal delivery via laparotomy and caesarian section, with operative control of hepatic hemorrhage. Angiography can be a useful adjunct but again should not delay the definitive management: fetal delivery is necessary for any chance at the recovery of hepatic function [81]. Of note, liver transplantation is a viable means of managing the fulminant hepatic failure, with eight transplants occurring between 1987 and 2003 for this indication [79].

### Dos and Don'ts

- <u>Do</u> perform a rapid, systematic workup in any patient with suspected NLH and prioritize determination and management of hemodynamic status.
- <u>Do</u> ensure appropriate venous access in the actively hemorrhaging patient and begin early balanced blood product resuscitation.
- <u>Do</u> expedite hemodynamically unstable vpatients to the operating room for laparotomy.
- <u>Do</u> obtain biopsies of hemorrhagic mass lesions intraoperatively to determine the need for additional staged procedures.
- <u>Do</u> consider a liver-protocol CT in patients with the hemodynamic status to tolerate it, or a FAST exam/point of care ultrasound in patients with more tenuous hemodynamics.
- <u>Don't</u> feel compelled to perform resection of a mass lesion at the time of exploration for acute NLH; damage control is a viable option and outcomes are better with staged resection.
- <u>Don't</u> pursue angioembolization in the hemodynamically unstable patient, though it can be a very useful adjunct for hemorrhage control.

### Take-Home Messages

- Nontraumatic liver hemorrhage is a rare disease that can be caused by a variety of benign and malignant hepatic lesions, autoimmune/vascular disorders, or

causes unique to the obstetric population.
- Priorities in workup and management include the establishment of appropriate venous access, initiation of early blood product resuscitation, and early hemorrhage control.
- Unstable patients should be operatively explored. Damage control is a viable strategy, though numerous methods exist to aid in local control (suture plication, energy-based coagulation). Perform resection at the time of initial exploration only if the hemorrhage is refractory to other means of control.
- Imaging in the emergent setting can include ultrasound/FAST exam, or CT scan if stable. CT should be obtained using a liver protocol if possible.
- Angioembolization is a useful adjunct method of hemostasis. Gelfoam should be used when able to facilitate later angiographic interventions.

**Chapter Questions**

1. A 43-year-old female presents to your emergency department with acute-onset severe abdominal pain. Her medical history is significant for menometrorrhagia for which she takes a daily combined oral contraceptive pill. On evaluation, her vital signs are significant for a pulse of 134, blood pressure of 88/54, and she is pale and lethargic. A FAST exam identifies free fluid in the right upper quadrant with a hypoechoic liver lesion. What is the most appropriate next step in management?
   A. Triphasic CT scan of the abdomen and pelvis
   B. Diagnostic peritoneal lavage
   C. **Initiation of large bore intravenous access and blood product resuscitation**
   D. IR angioembolization
2. What is the most likely etiology for the patient referenced in question 1?
   A. Hepatocellular carcinoma
   B. **Hepatic adenoma**
   C. HELLP
   D. Vasculitis or autoimmune disorders
3. Which of the following is true regarding angioembolization of hemorrhagic hepatic lesions?
   A. Coils should be used for embolization when possible
   B. Embolization is an option for patients who remain hypotensive after initial blood product resuscitation
   C. Chemoembolization/TACE should be performed preferentially for hemorrhagic liver lesions
   D. **Up to 20% of patients undergoing angioembolization for a hemorrhagic hepatic lesion may require repeat embolization or operative control of ongoing hemorrhage**
4. You have brought a 67-year-old male to the OR for hemoperitoneum with hemodynamic instability. After performing a midline laparotomy and packing the abdominal quadrants, you begin to remove packs and have identified a fungating, exophytic mass in the right lobe of the liver as the source of the hemorrhage. Your packs provide adequate hemostasis. You are alerted by your anesthesiologist that the patient is acidotic and has a core temperature of 34 °C. The most prudent course of action is:
   A. **Apply a temporary abdominal closure after hemostasis is achieved and resuscitate the patient in the ICU before second-look laparotomy**
   B. Perform an oncologic/anatomic resection of the right lobe lesion
   C. Transport the patient to IR for urgent angioembolization

D. Perform a nonanatomic resection of the right lobe lesion for control of hemorrhage

5. The most common hemorrhagic abdominal malignancy in the pediatric population is:
   A. Rhabdoid sarcoma
   B. Hepatocellular carcinoma
   C. Hemangiosarcoma
   D. **Hepatoblastoma**

6. Which of the following descriptions of CT findings most accurately describes a hepatocellular carcinoma?
   A. Peripheral nodular enhancement with persistence of contrast on venous phase
   B. Stellate central scar
   C. **Brisk arterial enhancement with venous phase washout and pseudocapsule**
   D. Hypoattenuating and nonenhancing

7. A 68-year-old male is found to have nontraumatic liver hemorrhage. His medical history is significant for restrictive cardiomyopathy and progressive chronic kidney disease. Imaging demonstrates an enlarged liver with heterogeneous parenchymal attenuation and surrounding hemoperitoneum. The most likely underlying etiology for this patient's hemorrhage is:
   A. **Amyloidosis**
   B. Nodular regenerative hyperplasia
   C. Peliosis hepatis
   D. Polyarteritis nodosa

8. Which of the following hepatic adenomas may undergo surveillance instead of elective operative resection?
   A. 4.2 cm hepatic adenoma in the left lateral segment of a 34-year-old male
   B. **2.1 cm inflammatory-subtype adenoma in the left lateral segment of a 28-year-old female**
   C. 5.6 cm HNF-1α inactivated lesion in segment 4 in a 43-year-old female
   D. 3.2 cm segment 6 lesion in a 28-year-old female, found to be a β-catenin activated lesion on biopsy

9. The most appropriate fluid for resuscitation of the hypotensive patient with non-traumatic liver hemorrhage is:
   A. Normal saline
   B. Albumin
   C. **Blood products**
   D. Lactated ringers

10. A 37-year-old female, gravida 2 para 1, at 34 weeks' gestation, presents to the emergency department with severe abdominal pain. Her pregnancy has been complicated by hypertension and proteinuria. She is found to have hemoperitoneum and her biochemical workup demonstrates an elevated lactate dehydrogenase and thrombocytopenia. She is tachycardic with a heart rate of 120 but is normotensive. Fetal monitoring reveals late decelerations. Large bore IV access has been established. What is the next best step in management of this patient?
    A. IR angioembolization of the hemorrhagic foci
    B. Labor induction with oxytocin drip
    C. Immediate OR for low transverse c-section
    D. **Immediate OR for midline laparotomy and c-section**

## References

1. Kasotakis G. Spontaneous hemoperitoneum. Surg Clin N Am. 2014;94:65–9 [cited 2021 Feb 5]. Available from: https://pubmed.ncbi.nlm.nih.gov/24267498/.
2. Srinivasa S, Lee WG, Aldameh A, Koea JB. Spontaneous hepatic haemorrhage: a review of pathogenesis, aetiology and treatment. HPB. 2015;17:872–80 [cited 2021 Feb 5]. Available from: https://www.ncbi.nlm.nih.gov/pmc/articles/PMC4571754/?report=abstract.
3. Battula N, Tsapralis D, Takhar A, Coldham C, Mayer D, Isaac J, et al. Aetio-pathogenesis and the management of spontaneous liver bleeding in the West: a 16-year

single-centre experience. HPB. 2012;14(6):382–9 [cited 2021 Feb 20]. Available from: http://www.ncbi.nlm.nih.gov/pubmed/22568414.
4. Lai ECH, Lau WY. Spontaneous rupture of hepatocellular carcinoma: a systematic review. Arch Surg. 2006;141:191–8 [cited 2021 Feb 5]. Available from: https://pubmed.ncbi.nlm.nih.gov/16490898/.
5. Schwed AC, Wagenaar A, Reppert AE, Gore AV, Pieracci FM, Platnick KB, et al. Trust the FAST: confirmation that the FAST examination is highly specific for intra-abdominal hemorrhage in over 1,200 patients with pelvic fractures. J Trauma Acute Care Surg. 2021;90(1):137–42 [cited 2021 Mar 10]. Available from: https://pubmed.ncbi.nlm.nih.gov/32976327/.
6. Lucey BC, Varghese JC, Soto JA. Spontaneous hemoperitoneum: causes and significance. Curr Probl Diagn Radiol. 2005;34:182–95 [cited 2021 Feb 5]. Available from: https://pubmed.ncbi.nlm.nih.gov/16129236/.
7. Lucey BC, Varghese JC, Anderson SW, Soto JA. Spontaneous hemoperitoneum: a bloody mess. Emerg Radiol. 2007;14:65–75.
8. Furlan A, Fakhran S, Federle MP. Spontaneous abdominal hemorrhage: causes, CT findings, and clinical implications. Am J Roentgenol. 2009;193(4):1077–87 [cited 2021 Feb 5]. Available from: https://pubmed.ncbi.nlm.nih.gov/19770332/.
9. Casillas VJ, Amendola MA, Gascue A, Pinnar N, Levi JU, Perez JM. Imaging of nontraumatic hemorrhagic hepatic lesions. Radiographics. 2000;20(2):367–78 [cited 2021 Feb 5]. Available from: https://pubmed.ncbi.nlm.nih.gov/10715337/.
10. Holcomb JB, Tilley BC, Baraniuk S, Fox EE, Wade CE, Podbielski JM, et al. Transfusion of plasma, platelets, and red blood cells in a 1:1:1 vs a 1:1:2 ratio and mortality in patients with severe trauma: the PROPPR randomized clinical trial. JAMA. 2015;313(5):471–82 [cited 2021 Mar 11]. Available from: https://pubmed.ncbi.nlm.nih.gov/25647203/.
11. Liu CL, Fan ST, Lo CM, Tso WK, Tung-Ping Poon R, Lam CM, et al. Management of spontaneous rupture of hepatocellular carcinoma: Single-center experience. J Clin Oncol. 2001;19(17):3725–32 [cited 2021 Mar 11]. Available from: http://ascopubs.org/doi/10.1200/JCO.2001.19.17.3725.
12. Thomeer MG, Broker M, Verheij J, Doukas M, Terkivatan T, Bijdevaate D, et al. Hepatocellular adenoma: when and how to treat? Update of current evidence. Therap Adv Gastroenterol. 2016;9:898–912 [cited 2021 Feb 19]. Available from: https://www.ncbi.nlm.nih.gov/pmc/articles/PMC5076773/.
13. Myers L, Ahn J. Focal nodular hyperplasia and hepatic adenoma: evaluation and management. Clin Liver Dis. 2020;24:389–403 [cited 2021 Feb 19]. Available from: https://pubmed.ncbi.nlm.nih.gov/32620279/.
14. Tsilimigras DI, Rahnemai-Azar AA, Ntanasis-Stathopoulos I, Gavriatopoulou M, Moris D, Spartalis E, et al. Current approaches in the management of hepatic adenomas. J Gastrointest Surg. 2019;23(1):199.
15. Rodrigues BT, Mei SLCY, Fox A, Lubel JS, Nicoll AJ. A systematic review on the complications and management of hepatic adenomas: a call for a new approach. Eur J Gastroenterol Hepatol. 2020;32(8):923.
16. Krause K, Tanabe KK. A shifting paradigm in diagnosis and management of hepatic adenoma. Ann Surg Oncol. 2020;27(9):3330.
17. Deneve JL, Pawlik TM, Cunningham S, Clary B, Reddy S, Scoggins CR, et al. Liver cell adenoma: a multicenter analysis of risk factors for rupture and malignancy. Ann Surg Oncol. 2009;16(3):640–8 [cited 2021 Feb 19]. Available from: https://pubmed.ncbi.nlm.nih.gov/19130136/.
18. Cho SW, Marsh JW, Steel J, Holloway SE, Heckman JT, Ochoa ER, et al. Surgical management of hepatocellular adenoma: take it or leave it? Ann Surg Oncol. 2008;15(10):2795–803 [cited 2021 Feb 19]. Available from: https://pubmed.ncbi.nlm.nih.gov/18696154/.
19. Stoot JHMB, van der Linden E, Terpstra OT, Schaapherder AFM. Life-saving therapy for haemorrhaging liver adenomas using selective arterial embolization. Br J Surg. 2007;94(10):1249–53 [cited 2021 Feb 19]. Available from: https://pubmed.ncbi.nlm.nih.gov/17696216/.
20. Erdogan D, van Delden OM, Busch ORC, Gouma DJ, van Gulik TM. Selective transcatheter arterial embolization for treatment of bleeding complications or reduction of tumor mass of hepatocellular adenomas. Cardiovasc Intervent Radiol. 2007;30(6):1252–8 [cited 2021 Feb 19]. Available from: https://pubmed.ncbi.nlm.nih.gov/17605070/.
21. Dharmana H, Saravana-Bawan S, Girgis S, Low G. Hepatocellular adenoma: imaging review of the various molecular subtypes. Clin Radiol. 2017;72(4):276.
22. Marion Y, Brevart C, Plard L, Chiche L. Hemorrhagic liver cyst rupture: an unusual life-threatening complication of hepatic cyst and literature review. Ann Hepatol. 2013;12(2):336–9.
23. Agrawal S, Khurana J, Sahu M. Hemorrhagic liver cyst. J Gastrointest Surg. 2012;16(8):1629–31 [cited 2021 Feb 19]. Available from: https://pubmed.ncbi.nlm.nih.gov/22350722/.
24. Fong ZV, Wolf AM, Doria C, Berger AC, Rosato EL, Palazzo F. Hemorrhagic hepatic cyst: report of a case and review of the literature with emphasis on clinical approach and management. J Gastrointest Surg. 2012;16(9):1782–9 [cited 2021 Feb 19]. Available from: https://pubmed.ncbi.nlm.nih.gov/22688416/.
25. Amaral MJ, Serôdio M, Koch MJ, Almeida R, Campos JC, Tralhão JG. Ruptured hemorrhagic hepatic cyst: an unusual case report. GE Port J Gastroenterol. 2020;27:124–7 [cited 2021 Feb 19]. Available from: https://www.ncbi.nlm.nih.gov/pmc/articles/PMC7113593/.
26. Li T, Qin LX, Ji Y, Sun HC, Ye QH, Wang L, et al. Atypical hepatic focal nodular hyperplasia presenting as acute abdomen and misdiagnosed as hepatocellular carcinoma. Hepatol Res. 2007;37(12):1100–5 [cited

27. Rahili A, Cai J, Trastour C, Juwid A, Benchimol D, Zheng M, et al. Spontaneous rupture and hemorrhage of hepatic focal nodular hyperplasia in lobus caudatus. J Hepatobiliary Pancreat Surg. 2005;12(2):138–42 [cited 2021 Feb 19]. Available from: https://pubmed.ncbi.nlm.nih.gov/15868078/.

28. Kinoshita M, Takemura S, Tanaka S, Hamano G, Ito T, Aota T, et al. Ruptured focal nodular hyperplasia observed during follow-up: a case report. Surg Case Rep. 2017;3(1):44 [cited 2021 Feb 19]. Available from: https://www.ncbi.nlm.nih.gov/pmc/articles/PMC5357241/.

29. Mocchegiani F, Vincenzi P, Coletta M, Agostini A, Marzioni M, Baroni GS, et al. Prevalence and clinical outcome of hepatic haemangioma with specific reference to the risk of rupture: a large retrospective cross-sectional study. Dig Liver Dis. 2016;48(3):309–14 [cited 2021 Feb 19]. Available from: https://pubmed.ncbi.nlm.nih.gov/26514738/.

30. Donati M, Stavrou GA, Donati A, Oldhafer KJ. The risk of spontaneous rupture of liver hemangiomas: a critical review of the literature. J Hepatobiliary Pancreat Sci. 2011;18:797–805 [cited 2021 Feb 5]. Available from: https://pubmed.ncbi.nlm.nih.gov/21796406/.

31. Ribeiro MAF, Papaiordanou F, Gonçalves JM, Chaib E. Spontaneous rupture of hepatic hemangiomas: a review of the literature. World J Hepatol. 2010;2(12):428–33 [cited 2021 Feb 5]. Available from: https://pubmed.ncbi.nlm.nih.gov/21191518/.

32. Reshamwala PA, Kleiner DE, Heller T. Nodular regenerative hyperplasia: not all nodules are created equal. Hepatology. 2006;44(1):7–14 [cited 2021 Feb 20]. Available from: http://doi.wiley.com/10.1002/hep.21258.

33. Soares KC, Arnaoutakis DJ, Kamel I, Anders R, Adams RB, Bauer TW, et al. Cystic neoplasms of the liver: biliary cystadenoma and cystadenocarcinoma. J Am Coll Surg. 2014;218:119–28 [cited 2021 Feb 20]. Available from: https://www.ncbi.nlm.nih.gov/pmc/articles/PMC4106371/.

34. Kawashima A, Fishman EK, Hruban RH, Tempany CM, Kuhlman JE, Zerhouni EA. Biliary cystadenoma with intratumoral bleeding: Radiologic-pathologic correlation. J Comput Assist Tomogr. 1991;15(6):1035–8 [cited 2021 Feb 20]. Available from: https://pubmed.ncbi.nlm.nih.gov/1939756/.

35. Ramacciato G, Nigri GR, D'Angelo F, Aurello P, Bellagamba R, Colarossi C, et al. Emergency laparotomy for misdiagnosed biliary cystadenoma originating from caudate lobe. World J Surg Oncol. 2006;4(1):76 [cited 2021 Feb 20]. Available from: http://wjso.biomedcentral.com/articles/10.1186/1477-7819-4-76.

36. Low SCS, Peh WCG, Muttarak M, Cheung HS, Ng IOL. Imaging features of hepatic angiomyolipomas. J Med Imaging Radiat Oncol. 2008;52:118–23 [cited 2021 Feb 20]. Available from: https://pubmed.ncbi.nlm.nih.gov/18373801/.

37. Huber C, Treutner KH, Steinau G, Schumoelick V. Ruptured hepatic angiolipoma in tuberous sclerosis complex. Langenbecks Arch Chir. 1996;381(1):7–9 [cited 2021 Feb 20]. Available from: https://pubmed.ncbi.nlm.nih.gov/8717168/.

38. Kim SH, Kang TW, Lim K, Joh HS, Kang J, Sinn DH. A case of ruptured hepatic angiomyolipoma in a young male. Clin Mol Hepatol. 2017;23(2):179–83 [cited 2021 Feb 20]. Available from: https://www.ncbi.nlm.nih.gov/pmc/articles/PMC5497672/.

39. Marini P, Vilgrain V, Belghiti J. Management of spontaneous rupture of liver tumours. Dig Surg. 2002;19:109–13 [cited 2021 Feb 5]. Available from: https://pubmed.ncbi.nlm.nih.gov/11978996/.

40. Aoki T, Kokudo N, Matsuyama Y, Izumi N, Ichida T, Kudo M, et al. Prognostic impact of spontaneous tumor rupture in patients with hepatocellular carcinoma: an analysis of 1160 cases from a nationwide survey. Ann Surg. 2014;259(3):532–42 [cited 2021 Feb 20]. Available from: https://pubmed.ncbi.nlm.nih.gov/23478524/.

41. Zhang W, Zhang ZW, Zhang BX, Huang ZY, Zhang WG, Liang HF, et al. Outcomes and prognostic factors of spontaneously ruptured hepatocellular carcinoma. J Gastrointest Surg. 2019;23:1788.

42. Wu J-J, Zhang Z-G, Zhu P, Mba'nbo-koumpa A-A, Zhang B-X, Chen X-P, et al. Comparative liver function models for ruptured hepatocellular carcinoma: a 10-year single center experience. Asian J Surg. 2019;42(9):874–82.

43. Schwarz L, Bubenheim M, Zemour J, Herrero A, Muscari F, Ayav A, et al. Bleeding recurrence and mortality following interventional management of spontaneous HCC rupture: results of a Multicenter European Study. World J Surg. 2018;42(1):225–32 [cited 2021 Feb 5]. Available from: https://pubmed.ncbi.nlm.nih.gov/28799103/.

44. Zou J, Li C, Chen Y, Chen R, Xue T, Xie X, et al. Retrospective analysis of transcatheter arterial chemoembolization treatment for spontaneously ruptured hepatocellular carcinoma. Oncol Lett. 2019;18(6):6423–30 [cited 2021 Feb 20]. Available from: https://pubmed.ncbi.nlm.nih.gov/31807165/.

45. Scioscia M, Noventa M, Vitulo A, Basile F. Spontaneous bleeding of hepatocellular carcinoma during pregnancy. Arch Gynecol Obstet. 2021;303(1):279.

46. Chien CY, Hwang C-C, Yeh C.-N, Chen H.-Y, Wu JT, Cheung CS, et al. Liver angiosarcoma, a rare liver malignancy, presented with intraabdominal bleeding due to rupture—a case report. World J Surg Oncol. 2012;10 [cited 2021 Feb 20]. Available from: https://pubmed.ncbi.nlm.nih.gov/22280556/.

47. Rujeerapaiboon N, Wetwittayakhlang P. Primary hepatic angiosarcoma: a rare liver malignancy-varying manifestations but grave prognosis. Case Rep Gastroenterol. 2020;14(1):137–49 [cited 2021 Feb 20]. Available from: https://www.ncbi.nlm.nih.gov/pmc/articles/PMC7184854/.

48. Pierce DB, Johnson GE, Monroe E, Loggers ET, Jones RL, Pollack SM, et al. Safety and efficacy outcomes of embolization in hepatic sarcomas. Am J Roentgenol. 2018;210(1):175–82 [cited 2021 Feb 20]. Available from: https://pubmed.ncbi.nlm.nih.gov/29090997/.
49. Lau WY, Dewar GA, Li AKC. Spontaneous rupture of hepatic epithelioid haemangio-endothelioma. Aust N Z J Surg. 1989;59(12):972–4 [cited 2021 Feb 20]. Available from: https://pubmed.ncbi.nlm.nih.gov/2597104/.
50. Yang JW, Li Y, Xie K, Dong W, Cao XT, Xiao WD. Spontaneous rupture of hepatic epithelioid hemangioendothelioma: a case report. World J Gastroenterol. 2017;23(1):185–90 [cited 2021 Feb 20]. Available from: https://www.ncbi.nlm.nih.gov/pmc/articles/PMC5221283/.
51. Lai M, Burjonrappa S. Perinatal hemorrhage complicating neonatal hepatoblastoma: case report. J Pediatr Surg. 2012;47(10) [cited 2021 Feb 20]. Available from: https://pubmed.ncbi.nlm.nih.gov/23084227/.
52. Nezami N, Michell H, Georgiades C, Portnoy E. Bland embolization of a ruptured hepatoblastoma with massive intraperitoneal hemorrhage. Radiol Case Rep. 2020;15(11):2367–70 [cited 2021 Feb 20]. Available from: https://www.ncbi.nlm.nih.gov/pmc/articles/PMC7502784/.
53. Lee SC, Chung JW, Kim KH, Kim WK. Successful transumbilical embolization of congenitally ruptured hepatoblastoma. J Pediatr Surg. 1999;34(12):1851–2 [cited 2021 Feb 20]. Available from: https://pubmed.ncbi.nlm.nih.gov/10626871/.
54. Madanur MA, Battula N, Davenport M, Dhawan A, Rela M. Staged resection for a ruptured hepatoblastoma: a 6-year follow-up. Pediatr Surg Int. 2007;23(6):609–11 [cited 2021 Feb 20]. Available from: https://pubmed.ncbi.nlm.nih.gov/17066271/.
55. Ravindra KV, Cullinane C, Lewis IJ, Squire BR, Stringer MD. Long-term survival after spontaneous rupture of a malignant rhabdoid tumor of the liver. J Pediatr Surg. 2002;37(10):1488–90 [cited 2021 Feb 20]. Available from: https://pubmed.ncbi.nlm.nih.gov/12378463/.
56. Kachanov D, Teleshova M, Kim E, Dobrenkov K, Moiseenko R, Usychkina A, et al. Malignant rhabdoid tumor of the liver presented with initial tumor rupture. Cancer Genet. 2014;207(9):412–4 [cited 2021 Feb 20]. Available from: https://pubmed.ncbi.nlm.nih.gov/24894493/.
57. Nguyen H, Stelling A, Kuramoto A, Patel C, Keller J. Malignant rhabdoid tumor of the liver: Findings at US, CT, and MRI, with histopathologic correlation. Radiol Case Rep. 2014;9(1):854 [cited 2021 Feb 20]. Available from: https://www.ncbi.nlm.nih.gov/pmc/articles/PMC4838746/.
58. Mochimaru T, Minematsu N, Ohsawa K, Tomomatsu K, Miura H, Betsuyaku T, et al. Hemoperitoneum secondary to rupture of a hepatic metastasis from small cell lung cancer during chemotherapy: a case with a literature review. Intern Med. 2017;56:695–9 [cited 2021 Feb 20]. Available from: https://www.ncbi.nlm.nih.gov/pmc/articles/PMC5410483/.
59. Liu YH, Ma HX, Ji B, Cao DB. Spontaneous hemoperitoneum from hepatic metastatic trophoblastic tumor. World J Gastroenterol. 2012;18(31):4237–40 [cited 2021 Feb 20]. Available from: https://www.ncbi.nlm.nih.gov/pmc/articles/PMC3422809/.
60. Schoedel KE, Dekker A. Hemoperitoneum in the setting of metastatic cancer to the liver—a report of two cases with review of the literature. Dig Dis Sci. 1992;37(1):153–4 [cited 2021 Feb 20]. Available from: https://pubmed.ncbi.nlm.nih.gov/1728523/.
61. Cimbanassi S, Aseni P, Mariani A, Sammartano F, Bonacina E, Chiara O. Spontaneous hepatic rupture during pregnancy in a patient with peliosis hepatis. Ann Hepatol. 2015;14(4):553–8.
62. Sommacale D, Palladino E, Tamby EL, Diebold MD, Kianmanesh AR. Spontaneous hepatic rupture in a patient with peliosis hepatis: a report of one case. Int J Surg Case Rep. 2013;4(5):508–10 [cited 2021 Feb 20]. Available from: https://pubmed.ncbi.nlm.nih.gov/23562904/.
63. Choi SK, Jin JS, Cho SG, Choi SJ, Kim CS, Choe YM, et al. Spontaneous liver rupture in a patient with peliosis hepatis: a case report. World J Gastroenterol. 2009;15(43):5493–7 [cited 2021 Feb 20]. Available from: https://pubmed.ncbi.nlm.nih.gov/19916182/.
64. Kim EA, Yoon KH, Jeon SJ, Cai QY, Lee YW, Seong EY, et al. Peliosis hepatis with hemorrhagic necrosis and rupture: a case report with emphasis on the multidetector CT findings. Korean J Radiol. 2007;8(1):64–9 [cited 2021 Feb 20]. Available from: https://pubmed.ncbi.nlm.nih.gov/17277565/.
65. Leonard-Murali S, Nasser H, Ivanics T, Woodward A. Spontaneous hepatic rupture due to primary amyloidosis. BMJ Case Rep. 2019;12(10):e232448 [cited 2021 Feb 20]. Available from: https://pubmed.ncbi.nlm.nih.gov/31676504/.
66. Naito KS, Ichiyama T, Kawakami S, Kadoya M, Tabata T, Matsuda M, et al. AL amyloidosis with spontaneous hepatic rupture: successful treatment by transcatheter hepatic artery embolization. Amyloid. 2008;15(2):137–9 [cited 2021 Feb 20]. Available from: https://pubmed.ncbi.nlm.nih.gov/18484340/.
67. Szturz P, Kyclova J, Moulis M, Navratil M, Adam Z, Vanicek J, et al. Extensive AL amyloidosis presenting with recurrent liver hemorrhage and hemoperitoneum: case report and literature review. Klin Onkol. 2013;26(1):49–52 [cited 2021 Feb 20]. Available from: https://pubmed.ncbi.nlm.nih.gov/23528174/.
68. Mells GF, Buckels JA, Thorburn D. Emergency liver transplantation for hereditary lysozyme amyloidosis. Liver Transpl. 2006;12(12):1908–9 [cited 2021 Feb 20]. Available from: http://doi.wiley.com/10.1002/lt.20984.
69. Zhou J, Chen W, Zhu F. Hepatic rupture induced by spontaneous intrahepatic hematoma. Case Rep Surg. 2018;2018:1–3 [cited 2021 Feb 20]. Available from: https://www.ncbi.nlm.nih.gov/pmc/articles/PMC5829334/.

70. Haslock I. Spontaneous rupture of the liver in systemic lupus erythematosus. Ann Rheum Dis. 1974;33(5):482–4 [cited 2021 Feb 20]. Available from: https://www.ncbi.nlm.nih.gov/pmc/articles/PMC1006309/.
71. Cozzi PJ, Morris DL. Two cases of spontaneous liver rupture and literature review. HPB Surg. 1996;9(4):257–60 [cited 2021 Feb 20]. Available from: https://pubmed.ncbi.nlm.nih.gov/8809590/.
72. Battula N, Tsapralis D, Morgan M, Mirza D. Spontaneous liver haemorrhage and haemobilia as initial presentation of undiagnosed polyarteritis nodosa. Ann R Coll Surg Engl. 2012;94(4):e163–5.
73. Senaati S, Cekirge S, Akhan O, Balkanci F. Spontaneous perirenal and hepatic hemorrhage in periarteritis nodosa. Can Assoc Radiol J. 1993;44(1):49–51 [cited 2021 Feb 20]. Available from: https://europepmc.org/article/med/8093852.
74. Kaltofen T, Grabmeier J, Weissenbacher T, Hallfeldt K, Mahner S, Hutter S. Liver rupture in a 28-year-old primigravida with superimposed pre-eclampsia and hemolysis, elevated liver enzyme levels, and low platelet count syndrome. J Obstet Gynaecol Res. 2019;45(5):1066–70 [cited 2021 Feb 20]. Available from: https://pubmed.ncbi.nlm.nih.gov/30854740/.
75. Singh P, Warren K, Collier V. Ruptured subcapsular liver hematoma: a rare complication of HELLP syndrome. Case Rep Hepatol. 2020;2020:1–3 [cited 2021 Feb 20]. Available from: https://www.ncbi.nlm.nih.gov/pmc/articles/PMC7516696/.
76. Escobar Vidarte MF, Montes D, Pérez A, Loaiza-Osorio S, José Nieto Calvache A. Hepatic rupture associated with preeclampsia, report of three cases and literature review. J Matern Fetal Neonatal Med. 2019;32:2767–73 [cited 2021 Feb 20]. Available from: https://pubmed.ncbi.nlm.nih.gov/29478361/.
77. Stevenson JT, Graham DJ. Hepatic hemorrhage and the HELLP syndrome: a surgeon's perspective. Am Surg. 1995;61(9):756–60 [cited 2021 Feb 20]. Available from: https://europepmc.org/article/med/7661469.
78. Kelly J, Ryan D, O'Brien N, Kirwan W. Second trimester hepatic rupture in a 35 year old nulliparous woman with HELLP syndrome: a case report. World J Emerg Surg. 2009;4(1):23.
79. Ko HH, Yoshida EM. Acute fatty liver of pregnancy. Can J Gastroenterol. 2006;20:25–30 [cited 2021 Feb 20]. Available from: https://www.ncbi.nlm.nih.gov/pmc/articles/PMC2538964/.
80. Doumiri M, Elombila M, Oudghiri N, Saoud AT. Hématome sous-capsulaire du foie rompu compliquant une stéatose hépatique aiguë gravidique. Pan Afr Med J. 2014;19:1937–8688 [cited 2021 Feb 20]. Available from: https://www.ncbi.nlm.nih.gov/pmc/articles/PMC4314140/.
81. Pereira SP, O'Donohue J, Wendon J, Williams R. Maternal and perinatal outcome in severe pregnancy-related liver disease. Hepatology. 1997;26(5):1258–62 [cited 2021 Feb 20]. Available from: https://pubmed.ncbi.nlm.nih.gov/9362370/.

# Acute Pancreatitis

**65**

Ari Leppäniemi and Matti Tolonen

## 65.1 Introduction

> **Learning Goals**
> - To be able to stratify acute pancreatitis based on severity.
> - To know when surgical intervention is required.
> - To select the appropriate intervention for each patient.

Acute inflammation of the pancreas—acute pancreatitis—is a common abdominal surgical emergency. Even if the majority of patients with acute pancreatitis do not need surgery, patients with severe form of the disease often require prolonged intensive care and sometimes multiple surgical and other interventions, and therefore in most institutions are managed by surgeons.

A. Leppäniemi (✉)
Abdominal Center, Helsinki University Hospital, Helsinki, Finland

Meilahti Hospital, Helsinki, Finland
e-mail: ari.leppaniemi@hus.fi

M. Tolonen
Abdominal Center, Helsinki University Hospital, Helsinki, Finland
e-mail: matti.tolonen@hus.fi

The main emphasis of this chapter is in the stratification of patients by severity and the management of severe acute pancreatitis (SAP).

### 65.1.1 Epidemiology

The incidence of acute pancreatitis in Europe ranges from 4.6 to 100 per 100.000 population [1]. In Finland, the incidence in 1989 was 73.4 per 100.000 population with an increasing trend [2]. At the Helsinki University Hospital, acute pancreatitis is one of the most common abdominal surgical emergencies with about 400 admissions annually, of which about 25 are classified as SAP [3]. In the United States, acute pancreatitis along with gastrointestinal hemorrhage and gallbladder disease were the three most common discharge diagnoses overall in 2014 [4].

### 65.1.2 Etiology

Gallstone disease and alcohol are two most common etiologies for acute pancreatitis comprising about 70–80% of all cases [5–7]. The list of less common causes is long and includes hypercalcemia, hypertriglyceridemia, trauma, certain drugs, infections, postoperative conditions (e.g., cardiac surgery), endoscopic retrograde cholangiopancreatography (ERCP), developmental anomalies (e.g., pancreas divisum), tumors, hereditary and

**Table 65.1** The proportion of gallstone disease and alcohol as the etiologic factor for acute pancreatitis in selected countries [5–7]

| Country | Cholelithiasis (%) | Alcohol (%) |
|---|---|---|
| Germany | 34.9 | 37.9 |
| Hungary | 24.0 | 60.7 |
| France | 24.6 | 38.5 |
| Greece | 71.4 | 6.0 |
| Italy | 60.3 | 13.2 |
| Finland | 37.6 | 33.4 |
| United States | 21–33 | 16–27 |

autoimmune diseases [7, 8]. In about 10% of the cases, the etiology remains unknown although a significant proportion of these patients have biliary sludge [8]. Pancreatic adenocarcinoma is a rare cause of necrotizing pancreatitis, and in one series accounted for 1% of the patients [9]. Table 65.1 lists the proportions of the two of the most common causes in different countries.

### 65.1.3 Classification

The clinically most useful and basic classification of acute pancreatitis is by severity. The majority of patients have the "one week disease" or acute edematous pancreatitis which is characterized by the absence of organ dysfunctions or infectious complications, and often resolving spontaneously requiring only symptomatic treatment. At the other end of the spectrum is the severe, necrotizing acute pancreatitis that often requires prolonged intensive care and usually multiple interventions. However, to be able to compare results between different institutions and time periods, a more granular severity stratification with commonly agreed criteria is needed.

The 2012 revision of the Atlanta classification and definitions based on international consensus identifies two phases of the disease (early and late) [10]. Severity is classified as mild, moderate, or severe. In the mild form (interstitial edematous pancreatitis), the patient has no organ failure, local or system complications, and in most cases recovers during the first week. In the moderate form, the patient has organ dysfunctions that resolve within 48 h, and no local complications or exacerbation of co-morbid disease.

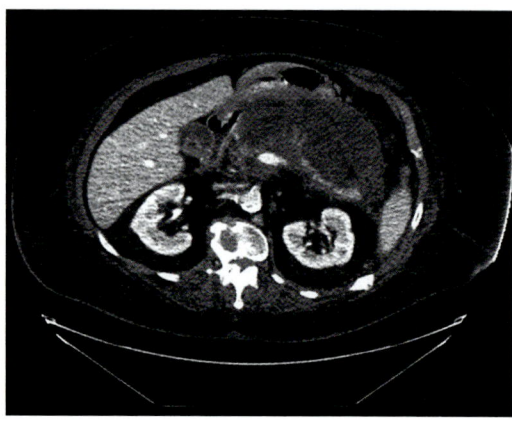

**Fig. 65.1** CT image of acute necrotic collection (ANC)

In the severe form, patients' organ failures are persistent for at least 48 h. The definition of organ dysfunction or failure affects three organ systems (respiratory, cardiovascular, and renal), and a score of two or more using the modified Marshall scoring system or the Sequential Organ Failure Assessment (SOFA) score defines organ failure.

Peripancreatic fluid collections, sterile or infected pancreatic and peripancreatic necrosis, pseudocyst, and sterile or infected walled-off necrosis (WON) are defined as local complications. Acute peripancreatic fluid collections contain mostly liquid and very little solid material, are seen in the early phase, remain usually sterile, and resolve spontaneously. If a localized fluid collection persists beyond 4 weeks, it can sometimes develop to a pancreatic pseudocyst. It is surrounded by a well-defined wall and contains no solid material. A collection seen during the first 4 weeks that contains variable amounts of fluid and necrotic tissue is an acute necrotic collection (ANC) (Fig. 65.1).

In contrast, a walled-off necrosis (WON) is a mature encapsulated collection of pancreatic and/or peripancreatic necrosis with a well-defined inflammatory wall, and typically (and by definition) can be seen more than 4 weeks after the onset of necrotizing pancreatitis. In most cases, the necrotic collection is first homogenous resembling acute fluid collection, becomes heterogeneous for days of even weeks, and finally over several weeks becomes again more liquid-like (Fig. 65.2).

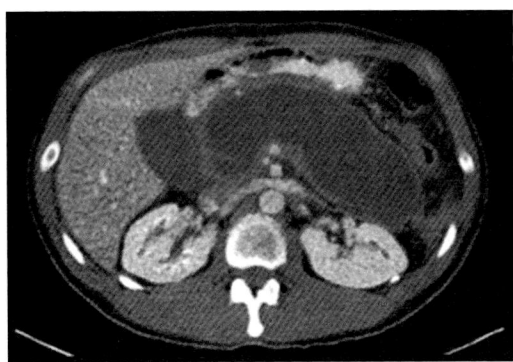

**Fig. 65.2** CT image of walled-off necrotic collection (WON)

Many other classification systems have been published, some historic like the Ranson or Imrie scores, and some based on severity or physiological parameters. It is of note that amylase levels do not correlate with severity. A C-reactive protein (CRP) level of >150 mg/L is a better indication of severity but manifests only 24–48 h later. Other laboratory markers such as procalcitonin are not in clinical use in most institutions.

### 65.1.4 Pathophysiology

The initial step after the condition is triggered by the etiological factors that are acinar cell injury and intrapancreatic activation of the pancreatic proenzymes. Inflammatory cells are activated by the local inflammation and lead to secretion of inflammatory mediators. Sometimes the process is controlled locally, but if not, a systemic inflammatory condition develops. In about 80% of the patients, a self-limiting disease takes place, but in about 20% a more severe condition develops leading to transient or more prolonged dysfunction of several organ systems. In these patients, the pancreas and/or the peripancreatic fat tissue undergo necrosis, hence the term necrotizing pancreatitis. Sometimes the necrotic tissue is invaded by microbes (infected necrosis), although pneumonia and bacteremia are more common infectious complications during the first 2 weeks of the disease.

## 65.2 Diagnosis

### 65.2.1 Clinical Presentation

Important parts of previous medical history should include previous episodes of acute pancreatitis, known gallstone disease, amount of alcohol use especially during the previous 2–3 weeks, metabolic disorders, such as hypercalcemia or hyperlipidemia, and medications that can potentially induce acute pancreatitis. Recent operations, ERCP or other biliary procedures, injuries to the abdominal area, and family history of acute pancreatitis should also be recorded.

Acute onset of upper abdominal pain, often radiating into the back, or a belt-like feeling around the upper abdomen are typical symptoms of acute pancreatitis. Nausea and vomiting are frequent. Fever is more common in patients with biliary pancreatitis and accompanying cholangitis.

On physical examination, abdominal tenderness and distension are common. The discolorations around the umbilicus (Cullen's sign) or in the flanks (Grey-Turner's sign) associated with necrotizing pancreatitis are usually late signs. Because the abdominal tenderness and even guarding are common, it is important to differentiate acute pancreatitis from secondary peritonitis. Percussion can reveal significant amount of ascites and bowel sounds are often absent due to paralytic ileus.

Occasionally, the patient presents with unstable vital signs. While the patient is examined, securing airways and adequate ventilation and starting fluid resuscitation in hypovolemic shock should precede any diagnostic workup. The physical examination should always include assessment of hemodynamic, pulmonary, and renal functions.

### 65.2.2 Tests

Measurement of serum amylase and lipase levels are the most commonly used laboratory tests for diagnosing acute pancreatitis. Plasma amylase levels rise within 6–12 h from the onset of pain and have a half-life of about 10 h. Serum lipase level typically peak at 24 h and stay elevated for a longer time than amylase levels. It should be noted that other conditions, such as parotitis or salpingitis, can increase amylase levels. Therefore, determining serum lipase levels is more sensitive and specific for pancreatitis.

The diagnostic criteria for acute pancreatitis are based on three criteria, of which at least two should be present: typical clinical picture, elevated amylase, or lipase level more than three times of the normal the upper limit, and finding on imaging studies indicative of acute pancreatitis.

A useful marker for the severity of acute pancreatitis is the C-reactive protein level (CRP), but it can be initially normal and elevate only 24–48 h from the onset even of a severe disease. Blood count, electrolyte, liver enzyme, creatinine, and glucose levels should be taken routinely, and in if cellular hypoperfusion is suspected, arterial blood gas analysis and serum lactate measurements are important. Triglyceride levels should be measured if known or suspected to be the cause.

Routine imaging is not needed, if the patient fulfills the two other criteria and the condition is not severe. If the diagnosis is uncertain, it is important to exclude secondary peritonitis or other conditions requiring early surgery, and continue with imaging studies.

Computed tomography (CT) is the most reliable diagnostic method for acute pancreatitis. Oral contrast is not needed. The risk for kidney injury caused by intravenous contrast is probably not as high as previously thought, but it should be used with caution and after confirming adequate circulating volume and urine output. Non-contrast CT is useful in detecting acute pancreatitis. In patients with necrotizing pancreatitis, the contrast enhancement and patency of the pancreas itself can be evaluated using intravenous contrast-enhanced CT scan few days or even weeks after the onset of the disease.

While CT may reveal the presence of gallbladder stones, an ultrasound (US) investigation should always be carried out in patients with acute pancreatitis, even among those with history of alcohol abuse. The presence of dilated common bile duct and/or elevated liver enzymes should prompt a magnetic resonance cholangiopancreatogram (MRCP). It identifies common bile duct stones and occasionally can confirm that a presumed common bile duct stone has passed through to the duodenum, thus saving an unnecessary endoscopic retrograde cholangiopancreatography (ERCP) examination. ERCP is needed when imaging reveals dilated common bile duct and there is a suspicion of a persistent stone or the patient has signs of cholangitis. Endoscopic sphincterotomy with clearance of the common duct from stones or drainage of pus (in cholangitis) is recommended.

> **Differential Diagnosis**
> In patients with acute upper abdominal pain, the differential diagnoses to be concerned with include perforated peptic ulcer, acute calculous cholecystitis or biliary colic, acute hepatitis, reflux esophagitis, acute mesenteric ischemia, intestinal obstruction, and ruptured abdominal aortic aneurysm. Sometimes extra-abdominal conditions, such as inferior myocardial infarction or basal pneumonia, can present with epigastric pain.
>
> The main differential diagnostic problem includes identifying severe secondary peritonitis caused by hollow organ perforation. While early or urgent surgery is needed in these patients, unnecessary early laparotomy in patients with acute pancreatitis is harmful. CT performed in the emergency department is helpful as long as it does not delay the initiation of treatment in critically ill patients, whether having pancreatitis or peritonitis.

## 65.3 Treatment

### 65.3.1 Medical Treatment

In general and with some exceptions, the initial management of acute pancreatitis regardless of severity is nonoperative. Most patients with mild acute pancreatitis require only supportive and symptomatic treatment consisting of moderate fluid resuscitation, medication for pain and nausea, and sedative if the patient is restless. Nasogastric tube is not routinely needed, and oral feeding can be started as soon as it is tolerated. Urine output should be monitored, usually with the placement of a Foley catheter (goal 0.5–1.0 mL/kg/h), and sufficient volume restoration secured. If the patient develops signs of severe pancreatitis (worsening clinical condition, increasing CRP, threatening organ dysfunctions), they should be noted early, and the need to admit the patient to the ICU should be assessed.

The management of patients with severe acute pancreatitis requires more resources and is usually carried out in the ICU. The main components are standard critical care interventions, and include supporting and preventing organ dysfunctions, infection prevention and control, prevention of bedsores, and maintaining adequate nutritional status.

The principles of fluid resuscitation in severe acute pancreatitis have removed toward more conservative and response-based strategies. Over-resuscitation may increase intra-abdominal pressure (IAP) and cause intra-abdominal hypertension (IAH) or even abdominal compartment syndrome (ACS). The main aim is to maintain adequate tissue perfusion which usually requires a mean arterial pressure (MAP) of about 80 mmHg. Depending on the IAP, the abdominal perfusion pressure (APP = MAP-IAP) should be at least 60 mmHg. Monitoring blood lactate levels and base deficit are helpful and the goal is to reach normal values during the first 12–24 h. As soon as the set resuscitation end-points are reached, the infusion rate should be slowed down in order to avoid fluid overloading.

It is not uncommon to see early IAH in patients with severe acute pancreatitis, especially in the early phase and associated with excessive fluid resuscitation. If IAH (IAP $\geq$12 mmHg) develops, nonoperative methods to decrease IAP should be applied to prevent the development of ACS. These include restriction of intravenous fluids if possible, gastrointestinal decompression with naso-gastric and rectal tubes, and drainage of ascites fluid. Abdominal wall compliance can be increased with adequate pain management, and intubation and sedation usually decrease IAP. In some cases, short-term neuromuscular blockade can be used. Removal of fluid by extracorporeal techniques is effective in rapidly removing excess fluid.

Prevention of infections and especially the use of prophylactic antibiotics is controversial. In some institutions, a short (5–7 days) course of prophylactic antibiotics is given for patients with severe acute pancreatitis.

Early enteral feeding has been shown to decrease infectious complications and the only contraindication is poor motility of the gastrointestinal tract. The route of enteral feeding can be either gastric or post-pyloric. Most patients tolerate gastric feeding via a nasogastric tube. If the residuals are high and not relieved with the administration of prokinetics, a nasojejunal feeding type should be inserted either with the help of endoscopy or using self-advancing tubes. Enteral feeding should be started with 10 mL/h for example, and increased gradually until the target volume of enteral nutrition is achieved. Volumes should not exceed 40–60 mL/h to avoid the rare but catastrophic complication of bowel necrosis. If the patient does not tolerate enteral nutrition in sufficient volumes, parenteral nutrition can be combined with enteral nutrition to fulfill the nutritional requirements.

If oxygen supply becomes ineffective in correcting tachypnea and dyspnea, mechanical ventilation should be started. Invasive ventilation is mandatory when bronchial secretion clearance is ineffective and the patient is getting exhausted. Lung-protective strategies should be used.

In addition to percutaneous catheter drainage of pancreatic ascites, and endoscopically inserted nasojejunal feeding tubes, there are many other interventional radiological and endoscopic interventions that are part of medical management and often needed to manage complications. Their indications and techniques are discussed in more detail the prognosis section and in association with complications.

## 65.3.2 Surgical Treatment

In general, the management of acute pancreatitis, even its severe form, is nonoperative. Surgical, endoscopic, or interventional radiological interventions are needed when complications occur, and listed under subtitles below.

The management of **biliary pancreatitis** consists of removal of common bile duct stones and cholecystectomy. Endoscopic retrograde cholangiogram is indicated when imaging reveals dilated common bile duct and there is a suspicion of a persistent stone or the patient has signs of cholangitis. Endoscopic sphincterotomy with clearance of the common duct from stones and/or drainage of pus (in cholangitis) should be performed as soon as feasible. Laparoscopic cholecystectomy during index admission is recommended in mild acute gallstone pancreatitis, whereas in acute gallstone pancreatitis with peripancreatic fluid collections, cholecystectomy should be deferred until fluid collections resolve or stabilize and acute inflammation ceases.

There are some studies showing that cholecystectomy after an episode of **idiopathic acute pancreatitis** reduces the risk of recurrent pancreatitis implicating that current diagnostics are insufficient in excluding a biliary cause [11].

### 65.3.2.1 Infected Pancreatic Necrosis (IPN)

Among patients with necrotizing pancreatitis, in about 75% the necrosis involves both the pancreatic parenchyma and peripancreatic fat, in 20% the peripancreatic fat only and in 5% only the pancreatic parenchyma [10]. While in most patients the necrosis remains sterile, infected necrosis is seen in about 20% of the patients [3, 10]. In the past, ultrasound-guided fine needle aspiration of the necrosis was used more often and it may still be helpful in selected cases. Gas bubbles in the CT-scan are reliable signs of infection, but they are present only in less than 10% of patients with infected necrosis (Fig. 65.3). Clinical signs of sepsis are not reliable criteria infected necrosis, even though a new increase in the CRP-value associated with worsening organ functions (increasing SOFA-score) is an indica-

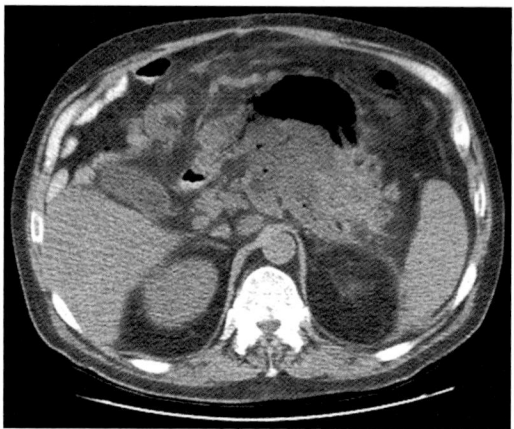

**Fig. 65.3** CT image of infected pancreatic necrosis with gas bubbles

tion to look for potential infection sources and consider the presence of infected necrosis, if no other causes are found.

If an infection of the necrosis is established or strongly suspected, the initial management during the first 1–2 weeks is nonoperative with antibiotics, especially in the absence of organ failures. If organ failures are present, the interventions should be delayed if possible for at least 2 weeks, but ideally 4 weeks from the start of the symptoms. However, according to a systematic review and meta-analysis nonoperative management was successful in about two-thirds of the patients with infected necrosis, and only 26% required surgical intervention [12].

If nonoperative management is inadequate, the preferred first-line treatment is based on the step-up approach. In a multicenter randomized study comparing a step-up approach (percutaneous drainage followed, if necessary, by minimally invasive retroperitoneal necrosectomy) to primary open necrosectomy, 35% of the patients assigned to the step-up approach were treated with percutaneous drainage only. It is of note, however, that there was no difference in the mortality rates (19% vs. 16%) [13]. The site of the insertion of the percutaneous drain depends on the location of the collections, but usually the preferred site is from the left and posterior to the descending colon aiming at the retroperitoneal collection. It can be inserted with either US- or

CT-guidance. Once in place, a bacterial sample is taken. If the sample is sterile and the drain has removed the liquid part of the collection, it can be removed.

If percutaneous drainage is insufficient and the patient is not getting better, a secondary intervention, that is, necrosectomy is required. If possible, the intervention should be postponed until about 4 weeks from the onset of the symptoms so that a well-demarcated WON cavity has developed. There are several surgical and endoscopic methods to perform necrosectomy, such as video-assisted retroperitoneal debridement (VARD), endoscopic or surgical transgastric necrosectomy, and open surgical necrosectomy. The choice of the procedure depends on the location of the necrotic collection, and the institutional and individual experience and skills, but in most cases a less invasive procedure is preferred. Several studies have shown the benefits of less invasive methods [14–16]. In an observational cohort study comparing open surgical necrosectomy with multidisciplinary minimally invasive step-up approach (including percutaneous drainage, endoscopic transgastric necrosectomy, VARD, sinus tract endoscopic necrosectomy or a combination of techniques, and with selective use of open surgical necrosectomy), a fivefold decrease in 90-day mortality from 10% to 2% was seen when the multidisciplinary approach was adopted [17].

However, the results of open surgical necrosectomy are comparable to less invasive methods. In a retrospective study, 394 patients with severe necrotizing pancreatitis underwent either a minimal access retroperitoneal pancreatic necrosectomy or open pancreatic necrosectomy. There was no significant difference in mortality (15% vs. 23%), and increased mortality was independently associated with age, preoperative intensive care, multiple organ failure, operation during earlier study period, and conversion to open necrosectomy [18].

In a retrospective cohort study from a single center with 109 consecutive patients undergoing open necrosectomy, the overall 90-day mortality rate was 23%. The risk factors for mortality

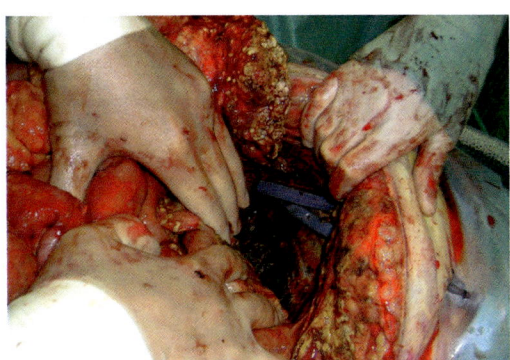

**Fig. 65.4** Open transabdominal necrosectomy

included age over 60 years, pre-existing co-morbidities, early necrosectomy (before 4 weeks), multiple organ failure, leukocytosis over $23 \times 10^9$, and deterioration or prolonged organ failure as an indication for necrosectomy. Among the 52 patients (48%) with one or no risk factors, there was no mortality [19]. It seems that the option for performing open surgical necrosectomy (Fig. 65.4) should not be discarded and can be useful in selected cases, especially if other approaches are not possible due to the anatomic location of the infected collections [20, 21].

### 65.3.2.2 Disconnected Duct Syndrome (DDS)

In some cases, the necrotizing process destroys part of the pancreatic parenchyma dividing the gland in two parts with a viable part of the distal pancreas (Fig. 65.5). It continues to produce pancreatic excretion, and presents itself as a fluid collection and/or pancreatic fistula [22]. This condition is known as disconnected duct syndrome (DDS) or disconnected left pancreatic remnant.

Percutaneous drainage of the collection usually fails [23]. Internal drainage to the stomach via endoscopic or open transgastric route (Fig. 65.6) is the recommended first-line treatment. The other option is to connect the distal pancreatic remnant to a Roux-en-Y pancreaticojejunostomy. In patients with very short pancreatic remnant and splenic vein thrombosis, distal pancreatectomy can be considered.

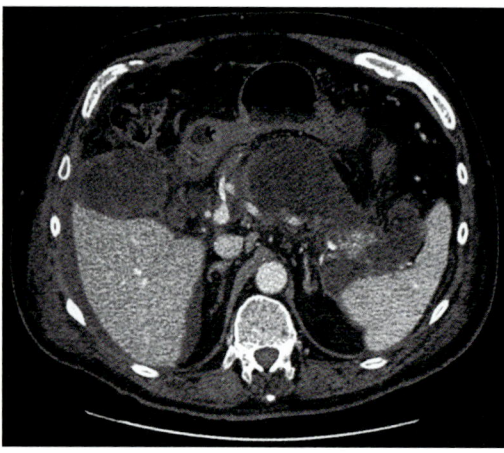

**Fig. 65.5** CT image of disconnected left pancreatic remnant

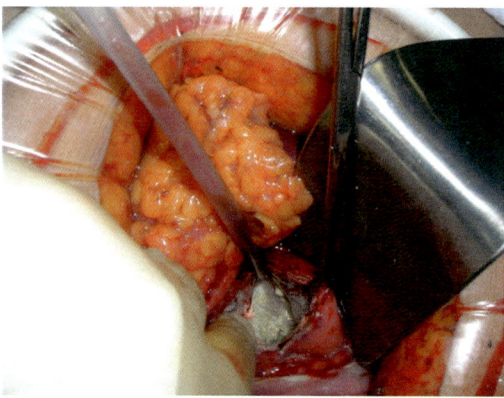

**Fig. 65.6** Open transgastric necrosectomy

### 65.3.2.3 Abdominal Compartment Syndrome (ACS)

Early reports suggested that unrecognized and untreated intra-abdominal hypertension (IAH) and abdominal compartment syndrome (ACS) might contribute to the fatal early multi organ failure (MOF) seen in patients with severe acute pancreatitis [24]. The main reason for IAH in these patients was aggressive fluid resuscitation leading to accumulation of excessive fluid in the tissues. Other contributing factors included paralytic ileus and the accumulation of pancreatic ascites. High intra-abdominal pressure (IAP) decreases perfusion of abdominal organs that may contribute to intestinal ischemia and increased bacterial translocation, increased risk of lung injury, and decreased renal and cardiovascular function.

Every patient with suspected or verified severe acute pancreatitis should have their IAP measured routinely and repeatedly at least every 4 h in critically ill patients. If IAH (IAP ≥12 mmHg) is diagnosed, the first line of treatment (and with the aim of preventing progression to ACS) is nonoperative consisting of restriction of intravenous fluids if possible, gastrointestinal decompression with nasogastric and rectal tubes, and drainage of ascites fluid [25]. Abdominal wall compliance can be increased with adequate pain management, and intubation and sedation usually decrease IAP. Short-term neuromuscular blockade can also be used in selected cases. An effective way to improve fluid balance and prevent ACS is early use of hemofiltration.

Percutaneous catheter drainage is more useful in patients with ACS and significant amount of ascites, but large amounts of ascites develop only in about half of the patients with acute pancreatitis [26, 27]. In one study, successful reduction of IAP with percutaneous drainage predicted better outcome [28].

If nonoperative management fails to decrease IAP and the condition progresses to ACS with increasing organ dysfunctions, surgical decompression should be performed without a delay. If performed early, it has shown to decrease mortality [29]. It is also crucial in detecting mesenteric ischemia in the early phase, since it can be present in more than half of patients with ACS [30]. Midline laparostomy and the use of vacuum-assisted closure with mesh-mediated fascial traction are the preferred methods, and have the highest fascial closure and lowest enteric fistula rates of the temporary abdominal closure techniques [31].

### 65.3.2.4 Gastrointestinal Perforations and Fistulas

The incidence of some part of the gastrointestinal tract developing necrosis and perforation is about 5–15%, colon fistulas being the most common followed by duodenal fistulas [32–34]. They are usually caused by the spread of the necrotic process to nearby organs, and mesenteric thrombosis and iatrogenic factors such as invasive interventions can also contribute to their development.

In a retrospective analysis of 647 patients with necrotizing pancreatitis, colon involvement was seen in 69 patients (11%), and consisted of ischemia in 29, perforation in 18, fistula in 12, inflammatory stricture in 7, and fulminant *Clostridioides difficile* colitis in 3 patients, respectively [35]. Colonic involvement was also associated with increased overall morbidity and mortality. The majority of colonic perforations occur after 2–4 weeks from the onset and can be difficult to diagnose. Ongoing abdominal sepsis or rectal bleeding can be the leading symptoms, and the diagnosis is usually confirmed with a CT scan where gas bubbles in the colonic wall are suggestive of colonic necrosis. The caecum and transverse colon are the most common sites of necrosis, and in most cases resection of the affected part with a colostomy is the safest option.

Most gastric and duodenal fistulas can resolve spontaneously during the disease course. In an analysis of 121 patients with necrotizing pancreatitis and infected pancreatic necrosis, 10 patients (8%) developed duodenal fistula, of whom 9 resolved spontaneously after control of infection [36]. If there is extended necrosis of the duodenum, spontaneous resolution is unlikely. CT scan and upper gastrointestinal (GI) endoscopy can confirm the diagnosis. In most cases, the treatment requires some form of duodenal resection with anastomosis, either a duodeno-duodenostomy or duodeno-jejunostomy. The anastomosis has a high risk of leakage and should be protected with effective decompression (nasoduodenal and nasogastric tubes, often T tube choledochostomy). A feeding jejunostomy and periduodenal drains are also recommended.

### 65.3.2.5 Gangrenous Cholecystitis

Acute gangrenous cholecystitis in patients with severe acute pancreatitis can be a deceiving source of worsening clinical condition, and has been detected in up to 15% of patients with severe acute pancreatitis, although the actual incidence is probably lower. Typical CT findings include enlarged and high-tensioned gallbladder, wall thickening, luminal emphysema, discontinuous and/or irregular enhancement of mucosa, and pericholecystic effusion [37]. It is of note that occasionally the gangrenous wall of the gallbladder can be thin and innocent looking on ultrasound examination. Prompt cholecystectomy is the best treatment.

### 65.3.2.6 Acute Bleeding or Pseudoaneurysm

The incidence bleeding complications associated with acute pancreatitis is about 0.5–1.2%, either in the form of direct arterial bleeding or a bleeding pseudoaneurysm. Among 76 patients with severe acute pancreatitis undergoing digital subtraction angiography, 22 patients had arterial bleeding and 11 pseudoaneurysms [38]. Among 647 patients with necrotizing pancreatitis, the incidence of visceral artery pseudoaneurysm was 4.3%. Splenic artery was the most commonly involved artery, followed by the gastroduodenal artery [39]. If bleeding is suspected by bloody drain output or hemodynamic instability, contrast-enhanced triple phase CT is the most accurate imaging method. Angioembolization is the method of choice to treat arterial pseudoaneurysms and other arterial bleeding complications in acute pancreatitis. Angioembolization using microcoils is successful in 88–100% and the need for re-embolization is rare [40, 41].

### 65.3.2.7 Gastric Outlet Obstruction (GAO)

Gastric outlet obstruction (GAO) is seen in two forms, early and late [42]. The early one is seen during the first 4 weeks, is caused by tissue edema, compression caused by necrotic the collections and poor motility or gastric paralysis. The management is conservative, and sometimes a nasojejunal tube needs to be inserted for enteral feeding.

The late onset GAO is in most cases related to the compression of WON collections. The management is expectant, especially with sterile collections, since most of the collections resolve with time. If the GAO persists over 8 weeks, a gastrojejunostomy can be considered.

## 65.3.3 Prognosis

### 65.3.3.1 Complications

In addition to the complications requiring early intervention discussed above, there are other complications, some of them manifesting themselves later on.

The incidence of splanchnic vein thrombosis (SVT) varies from 1% to 37%, the risk factors include smoking, hypertriglyceridemia, hyperglycemia, IAH, infected walled-off necrosis, and recurrent acute pancreatic, and is often an incidental finding on radiological imaging performed to assess the severity of pancreatitis. Early anticoagulation does not seem to prevent the occurrence [43]. The most commonly involved vessel is the splenic vein followed by isolated portal vein and superior mesenteric vein thrombosis. Even if there is no definitive evidence to support the use of anticoagulation, most institutions treat SVT when diagnosed.

Other complications occurring after pancreatic necrosectomy include pancreatic fistula, biliary stricture and delayed collections, most of them manageable with endoscopic or percutaneous interventions. Late complications include exocrine and endocrine insufficiency, symptomatic chronic pancreatitis, pancreatic duct stricture, duodenal stricture, gastrointestinal fistula, chronic pain and ventral hernia [44, 45].

### 65.3.4 Mortality

Including all patients with acute pancreatitis, the mortality rate currently is about 4% [46]. In severe acute pancreatitis, the mortality rate is about 20% and has changed little over the last decade [3, 47].

Infected necrosis and organ failure are the most important predictors of mortality, and the mortality rate in patients with organ failure is about 30% and in patients with infected necrosis and organ failure about 35% [48, 49]. Different combinations of failed organs are good predictors of mortality, and the mortality rate with two organ failures varies from 50% to 91% with the highest rate attributed to a combined hepatic and renal failure [50]. In addition to respiratory and renal failure, advanced age and history of cardiovascular or anticoagulation medication have prognostic value, and can be used to create a prognostic model [51].

In the long-term, about 13% of patients with severe acute pancreatitis surviving the initial hospitalization period die within a few years. While the quality of life is comparable to those of the control population, patients continuing alcohol abuse after alcohol-induced pancreatitis have a high risk of diabetes, recurrent pancreatitis and shortened life-span [52]. Poor long-term outcome is associated with continuing alcohol use and the mortality rate is about 4 times higher than in the age- and sex-matched control population, with 43% relating to recurrence [53].

**Dos and Don'ts**
- Look for early signs of severe acute pancreatitis—obvious or compensated shock, organ dysfunctions including renal and respiratory failure, altered sensorium, or metabolic derangement.
- Monitor fluid resuscitation, reach goals but don't overdo it, and monitor intra-abdominal pressure regularly.
- Start enteral feeding early.
- Look for infected necrosis, avoid intervention before 4 weeks if possible, start with a step-up approach, and be familiar with different surgical and endoscopic treatment options assessed with a multidisciplinary team.

**Take-Home Messages**
- Most patients with acute pancreatitis require only symptomatic treatment.
- Severe acute pancreatitis is associated with persistent organ failure and require treatment in the intensive care unit.
- Infected necrosis is a serious complication but rarely manifests during the first 2 weeks.
- Severe acute pancreatitis requires prolonged hospitalization, is associated with multiple complications, requires some form of interventions at some stage, and has a good long-term prognosis except when alcohol abuse continues.

**Multiple Choice Questions**

1. In which of the following independent European countries is the proportional cause of acute pancreatitis highest when compared with gallstone etiology?
   A. Finland
   B. France
   C. **Hungary**
   D. Scotland

2. To diagnose acute pancreatitis, you may have typical epigastric pain, elevated amylase levels (three times over upper limit) and typical CT characteristics for acute pancreatitis. To make a diagnosis of acute pancreatitis, you need
   A. One criteria of the three
   B. **Two criteria of the three**
   C. All three criteria
   D. Elevated lipase levels (three times upper limit)

3. According to the 2021 revision of the Atlanta classification of severity of acute pancreatitis, it is divided into mild, moderate and severe forms. The moderate form is defined as
   A. No organ failure
   B. Transient organ failure of less than 24 h
   C. **Transient organ failure of less than 48 h**
   D. Transient organ failure of less than 72 h

4. WON on CT in patients with acute pancreatitis signifies
   A. Without necrosis
   B. With omental necrosis
   C. With ongoing necrosis
   D. **Walled-off necrosis**

5. In mild acute pancreatitis, nasogastric tube
   A. Should always be inserted
   B. Should never be inserted
   C. Should always be inserted if the patient has a pulmonary disease
   D. **Should be inserted if the patient vomits repeatedly**

6. Intra-abdominal hypertension (IAH) in patients with severe acute pancreatitis
   A. Is diagnosed when the intra-abdominal pressure (IAP) exceeds 20 mmHg
   B. Always warrants decompressive laparostomy
   C. **Should prompt nonoperative measures to decrease IAP**
   D. Should prompt the start of antihypertensive medication

7. In patients with severe biliary pancreatitis and verified gallbladder stones
   A. Laparoscopic cholecystectomy should be performed as soon as possible
   B. Open cholecystectomy should be performed as soon as possible
   C. **Laparoscopic cholecystectomy should be performed once the acute inflammation ceases**
   D. Endoscopic sphincterotomy should be performed prophylactically

8. In patients with infected pancreatic necrosis
   A. **The infection seldom manifests during the first 2 weeks**
   B. Gas bubbles on CT are required for diagnosis
   C. The first line of treatment usually involves the step-down approach
   D. One of the management options include VATN (video-assisted transmesenteric necrosectomy)

9. Disconnected duct syndrome in severe acute pancreatitis signifies
   A. **Disconnected left pancreatic remnant**
   B. Disconnection of the papilla Vateri from the rest of the gland
   C. Disconnection of the ducts of Wirsung and Santorini
   D. Bare pancreatic duct with complete necrosis of the surrounding gland

10. The mortality rate of acute pancreatitis in current series is
    A. **About 5%**
    B. About 10%
    C. About 20%
    D. About 30%

# References

1. Roberts SE, Morrison-Rees S, John A, et al. The incidence and aetiology of acute pancreatitis across Europe. Pancreatology. 2017;17:155–65.
2. Jaakkola M, Nordback I. Pancreatitis in Finland between 1970 and 1989. Gut. 1993;34:1255–60.
3. Husu HL, Leppäniemi AK, Lehtonen TM, et al. Short- and long-term survival after severe acute pancreatitis: a retrospective 17 years' cohort study. J Crit Care. 2019;53:81–6.
4. Peery AF, Crockett SD, Murphy CC, et al. Burden and cost of gastrointestinal, liver, and pancreatic diseases in the United States: update 2018. Gastroenterology. 2019;156:254–72.
5. Gullo L, Migliori M, Olah A, et al. Acute pancreatitis in five European countries: etiology and mortality. Pancreas. 2002;2483:223–7.
6. Nikkola A, Nikkola J, Kari E, et al. The incidence and etiology of acute pancreatitis in Finland have changed—a population-based study in 2014-2015. Pancreatology. 2020;20:S80.
7. Mederos MA, Reber HA, Girgis MD. Acute pancreatitis. A review. JAMA. 2021;325:382–90.
8. Seppänen H, Puolakkainen P. Classification, severity assessment, and prevention of recurrences in acute pancreatitis. Scand J Surg. 2020;109:53–8.
9. Lewellen KA, Maatman TK, Heimberger MA, et al. Pancreatic adenocarcinoma causing necrotizing pancreatitis: not as rare as you think? J Surg Res. 2020;250:53–8.
10. Banks PA, Bollen TL, Dervenis C, et al. Classification of acute pancreatitis—2012: revision of the Atlanta classification and definitions by international consensus. Gut. 2013;62:102–11.
11. Uman DS, Hallensleben ND, Verdonk RC, et al. Recurrence if idiopathic acute pancreatitis after cholecystectomy: systematic review and meta-analysis. Br J Surg. 2020;107:191–9.
12. Mouli VP, Sreenivas V, Garg PK. Efficacy of conservative treatment, without necrosectomy, for infected pancreatic necrosis: a systematic review and meta-analysis. Gastroenterology. 2013;144:333–40.
13. van Santvoort HC, Besselink MG, Bakker OJ, et al. A step-up approach or open necrosectomy for necrotizing pancreatitis. N Engl J Med. 2010;362:1491–502.
14. Freeman ML, Werner J, van Santvoort HC, et al. Interventions in necrotizing pancreatitis. Summary of a multidisciplinary consensus conference. Pancreas. 2012;41:1176–94.
15. Tan V, Charachon A, Lescot T, et al. Endoscopic transgastric versus surgical necrosectomy in infected pancreatic necrosis. Clin Res Hepatol Gastroenterol. 2014;38:770–6.
16. Bakker OJ, van Santvoort HC, Brunschot S, et al. Endoscopic transgastric vs surgical necrosectomy for infected pancreatic necrosis. A randomized trial. JAMA. 2012;307:1053–61.
17. Luckhurst CM, El Hechi M, Elsharkawy AE, et al. Improved mortality in necrotizing pancreatitis with a multidisciplinary minimally invasive step-up approach: comparison with modern open necrosectomy cohort. J Am Coll Surg. 2020;230:873–83.
18. Gomatos IP, Halloran CM, Ghanek P, et al. Outcomes from minimal access retroperitoneal and open pancreatic necrosectomy in 394 patients with necrotizing pancreatitis. Ann Surg. 2016;263:992–1001.
19. Husu HL, Kuronen JA, Leppäniemi AK, et al. Open necrosectomy in acute pancreatitis—obsolete or still useful? World J Emerg Surg. 2020;15:21.
20. Maatman TK, Flick KF, Roch AM, et al. Operative pancreatic debridement: contemporary outcomes in changing times. Pancreatology. 2020;20:968–75.
21. Sgaramella LI, Gurrado A, Pasculli A, et al. Open necrosectomy is feasible as a last resort in selected cases with infected pancreatic necrosis: a case series and systematic literature review. World J Emerg Surg. 2020;15:44.
22. Murage KP, Ball CB, Zyromski NJ, et al. Clinical framework to guide operative decision making in disconnected left pancreatic remnant (DLPR) following acute or chronic pancreatitis. Surgery. 2010;148:847–57.
23. Maatman TK, Mahajan S, Roch AM, et al. Disconnected pancreatic duct syndrome predicts failure of percutaneous therapy in necrotizing pancreatitis. Pancreatology. 2020;20:362–8.
24. Keskinen P, Leppäniemi A, Pettilä V, et al. Intra-abdominal pressure in severe acute pancreatitis. World J Emerg Surg. 2007;2:2.
25. Kirkpatrick AW, Roberts DJ, De Waele J, et al. Intra-abdominal hypertension and the abdominal compartment syndrome: updated consensus definitions and clinical practice guidelines from the World Society of the Abdominal Compartment Syndrome. Intensive Care Med. 2013;39:1190–206.
26. Park S, Lee S, Lee HD, et al. Abdominal compartment syndrome in severe acute pancreatitis treated with percutaneous catheter drainage. Clin Endosc. 2014;47:469–72.
27. Samanta J, Rana A, Dhaka N, et al. Ascites in acute pancreatitis: not a silent bystander. Pancreatology. 2019;19:646–52.
28. Singh AK, Samanta J, Dawra S, et al. Reduction of intra-abdominal pressure after percutaneous catheter drainage of pancreatic fluid predicts sur-

vival. Pancreatology. https://doi.org/10.1016/j.pan.2020.04.012.
29. Mentula P, Hienonen P, Kemppainen E, et al. Surgical decompression for abdominal compartment syndrome in severe acute pancreatitis. Arch Surg. 2010;145:764–9.
30. Smit M, Buddingh KT, Bosma B, et al. Abdominal compartment syndrome and intra-abdominal ischemia in patients with severe acute pancreatitis. World J Surg. 2016;40:1454–61.
31. Atema JJ, Gans SL, Boermeester MA. Systematic review and meta-analysis of the open abdomen and temporary abdominal closure techniques in non-trauma patients. World J Surg. 2015;39:912–25.
32. Hua Z, Su Y, Huang X, Zhang K, et al. Analysis of risk factors related to gastrointestinal fistula in patients with severe acute pancreatitis: a retrospective study of 344 cases in a single Chinese center. BMC Gastroenterol. 2017;17:29.
33. Jiang W, Tong Z, Yang D, et al. Gastrointestinal fistulas in acute pancreatitis with infected pancreatic or peripancreatic necrosis: a 4-year single-center experience. Medicine (Baltimore). 2016;95:e3318.
34. Kochhar R, Jain K, Gupta V, et al. Fistulization in the GI tract in acute pancreatitis. Gastrointest Endosc. 2012;75:436–40.
35. Maatman TK, Nicolas ME, Roch AM, et al. Colon involvement in necrotizing pancreatitis. Incidence, risk factors, and outcomes. Ann Surg. 2020; https://doi.org/10.1097/SLA.0000000000004149. [Online ahead of print].
36. Shen D, Ning C, Huang G, Liu Z. Outcomes of infected pancreatic necrosis complicated with duodenal fistula in the era of minimally invasive techniques. Scand J Gastroenterol. 2019;54:766–72.
37. Chen EZ, Huang J, Xu ZW, et al. Clinical features and outcomes of patients with severe acute pancreatitis complicated with gangrenous cholecystitis. Hepatobiliary Pancreat Dis Int. 2013;12:317–23.
38. Ai M, Lu GM, Xu J. Endovascular embolization of arterial bleeding in patients with severe acute pancreatitis. Videosurg Miniinv. 2019;14:401–7.
39. Maatman TK, Heimberger MA, Lewellen KA, et al. Visceral artery pseudoaneurysm in necrotizing pancreatitis: incidence and outcomes. Can J Surg. 2020;63:E272–7.
40. Balthazar EJ, Fisher LA. Hemorrhagic complications of pancreatitis: radiologic evaluation with emphasis on CT imaging. Pancreatology. 2001;1:306–13.
41. Taori K, Rathod J, Disawal A, et al. Endovascular embolization of pseudoaneurysms complicating pancreatitis using microcoils: case series. Open J Radiol. 2013;3:33–40.
42. Qu C, Yu X, Duan Z, et al. Clinical characteristics and management of gastric outlet obstruction in acute pancreatitis. Pancreatology. 2021;21:64–8.
43. Li H, Yang Z, Tian F. Clinical characteristics and risk factors for sinistral portal hypertension associated with moderate and severe acute pancreatitis: a seven-year single-center retrospective study. Med Sci Monit. 2019;25:5969–76.
44. Connor S, Alexakis N, Raraty MGT, et al. Early and late complications after pancreatic necrosectomy. Surgery. 2005;137:499–505.
45. Maatman TK, Roch AM, Ceppa EP, et al. The continuum of complications in survivors of necrotizing pancreatitis. Surgery. 2020;168:1032–40.
46. Sternby H, Bolado F, Canaval-Zuleta HJ, et al. Determinants of severity in acute pancreatitis. A nation-wide multicenter prospective cohort study. Ann Surg. 2019;270:348–55.
47. Halonen KI, Leppäniemi AK, Puolakkainen PA, et al. Severe acute pancreatitis: prognostic factors in 270 consecutive patients. Pancreas. 2000;21:266–71.
48. Petrov MS, Shanbhag S, Chakraborty M, et al. Organ failure and infection of pancreatic necrosis as determinants of mortality in patients with acute pancreatitis. Gastroenterology. 2010;139:813–20.
49. Werge M, Novovic S, Schmidt PN, et al. Infection increases mortality in necrotizing pancreatitis: a systematic review and meta-analysis. Pancreatology. 2016;16:698–707.
50. Halonen K, Pettilä V, Leppäniemi A, et al. Multiple organ dysfunction associated with severe acute pancreatitis. Crit Care Med. 2002;30:1274–9.
51. Halonen KI, Leppäniemi AK, Lundin JE, et al. Predicting fatal outcome in the early phase of severe acute pancreatitis by using novel prognostic models. Pancreatology. 2003;3:309–15.
52. Halonen K, Pettilä V, Leppäniemi A, et al. Long-term health-related quality of life in survivors of severe acute pancreatitis. Intensive Care Med. 2003;29:782–6.
53. Karjula H, Saarela A, Ohtonen P, et al. Long-term outcome and causes of death for working-age patients hospitalized due to acute pancreatitis with a median follow up of 10 years. Ann Surg. 2019;269:932–6.

## Further Reading

Leppäniemi A, Tolonen M, Tarasconi A, et al. 2019 WSES guidelines for the management of severe acute pancreatitis. World J Emerg Surg. 2019;14:27. https://doi.org/10.1186/s13017-019-0247-0.

Mentula P, Leppäniemi A. Position paper: timely interventions in severe acute pancreatitis are crucial for survival. World J Emerg Surg. 2014;9:15.

The Italian Association for the Study of Pancreas (ASIP). Consensus guidelines on severe acute pancreatitis. Dig Liver Dis. 2015;47:532–43.

Working Group IAP/APA Acute Pancreatitis Guidelines. IAP/APA evidence-based guidelines for the management of acute pancreatitis. Pancreatology. 2013;13:e1–e15.

Yokoe M, Takada T, Mayumi T, et al. Japanese guidelines for the management of acute pancreatitis: Japanese guidelines 2015. J Hepatobiliary Pancreat Sci. 2015;22:405–32.

# Acute Appendicitis

Gaetano Gallo, Mauro Podda, Marta Goglia, and Salomone Di Saverio

*A job like any other, a life like any other.* (Leonid Rogozov—April 30, 1961)

## 66.1 Introduction

Acute appendicitis (AA) is one of the most frequent surgical emergencies in Western countries with an estimated lifetime risk of 9% for men and 7% for women and with a recent rising in industrialized countries in our century [1, 2].

G. Gallo
Department of Medical and Surgical Sciences, University of Catanzaro, Catanzaro, Italy
e-mail: gallog@unicz.it

M. Podda
Department of Emergency Surgery, Cagliari University Hospital, University of Cagliari, Cagliari, Italy

M. Goglia
Department of General Surgery, "La Sapienza" University of Rome—Sant'Andrea University Hospital, Rome, Italy

S. Di Saverio (✉)
Department of General Surgery, Ospedale Madonna del Soccorso, AST 5 Ascoli Piceno, San Benedetto del Tronto, Italy

> **Learning Goals**
> - Understanding the extreme diffusion as well as framing the typical clinical scenario of AA, allowing differential diagnosis with other abdominal disorders which may show similar symptoms.
> - The learner should be able to evaluate the pathophysiology of appendicitis and its clinical course, including the various types of classification reported in the current Literature.
> - The learner should be able to understand both the patient selection criteria and the possible complications that could be caused by a delayed or an incorrect management.
> - The learner should be able to understand the economic and social burden caused by AA.

### 66.1.1 Epidemiology

AA occurs mainly in childhood and adolescence, slightly predominant in males, with a greater incidence between 10 and 19 years old. Only 5–10% of cases occur in people over the age of 70.

Interestingly, almost 30% of children with acute abdominal pain who presented to an emergency surgical department, then received a diagnosis of AA [3].

In the United States, the annual incidence is 11 cases per 10,000 patients with approximately 300.000 appendectomies performed each year, and a subsequent healthcare burden of 3 billion dollars per year relating to hospitalizations for AA [4, 5].

According to literature, between 2% and 7% of AA are complicated at onset with the presence of phlegmon or peri-appendicular abscess and the mortality rate ranges between 0.07% and 0.7% and between 0.5% and 2.4% in cases with or without perforation, respectively [6].

Approximately one-third of patients will experience a perforation of their appendix before appendectomy, which leads to higher morbidity, longer hospital stays, and higher economic costs.

Golz et al. [7] recently demonstrated that socioeconomic advantages are associated with a lower incidence of AA but not with a decreased incidence of perforating appendicitis which does not have a strong association with geographic distribution.

In 1886 Reginal Fitz first described AA as an inflammatory condition of the right lower abdominal quadrant, although the first appendectomy was performed by Claudius Amyand in 1735 during the repair of an inguinal hernia in a 11-year-old boy with a fecal fistula [8], which is still called today "Amyand's Hernias" [9].

A few years later, at the end of the nineteenth century, Charles McBurney published a series of studies that definitively framed AA as a surgery-related pathology. In fact, according to his experience, AA was a condition associated with pain in the right lower abdominal quadrant, which would later be referred to as McBurney's point [10, 11].

## 66.1.2 Etiology, Pathophysiology, and Classification

The most common etiopathogenetic cause of AA is the obstruction of the appendiceal lumen which causes distension and increase in intraluminal pressure with a consequent trans-mural inflammation, alteration of the vascular flow of the bowel wall, ischemia, gangrene, and necrosis with bacterial overgrowth [12, 13]. The obstruction can be provoked by a fecalith, foreign body, an incidental neoplasia, or it can be due to other idiopathic origins.

Initially, the inflammation of the appendix is walled off by the surrounding tissues, such as the omentum, forming an inflammatory mass. At this stage, some episodes of mild mucosal inflammation may spontaneously regress.

Subsequently, there is a progression to generalized peritonitis or localized purulent collection with appendix abscess (Table 66.1; Fig. 66.1). In these cases, the finding of *Bacteroides fragili*s, *Escherichia coli* or *Pseudomonas aeruginosa* is very frequent.

Unfortunately, this theory does not support all cases of AA. In fact, during pediatric age lymphoid hyperplasia contributes to the pathogenesis, considering that the vermiform appendix is a component of the immune system and has a specific function in the lymphoid tissue associated with the intestine (GALT, gut-associated lymphoid tissue).

Adenovirus is one of the most common pathogens related to the development of AA. In addition, it has been associated, in pediatric age, with ileal and ileocecal intussusception which could be caused by the induction of lymphoid hyperplasia and a consequent alteration of intestinal motility [14].

**Table 66.1** Stratified disease approach to acute appendicitis

| | Macroscopic appearances | Microscopic appearances | Clinical relevance |
|---|---|---|---|
| *Normal appendix (Fig. 66.1a)* | | | |
| Normal underlying pathology | No visible changes | Absence of any abnormality | Consider other causes |
| Acute intraluminal inflammation | No visible changes | Luminal neutrophils only with no mucosal abnormality | Might be the cause of symptoms, but consider other causes |
| Acute mucosal/submucosal inflammation | No visible changes | Mucosal or submucosal neutrophils and/or ulceration | Might be the cause of symptoms, but consider other causes |
| *Simple, non-perforated appendicitis (Fig. 66.1b)* | | | |
| Suppurative/phlegmonous | Congestion, colour changes, increased diameter, exudate, pus | Transmural inflammation, ulceration, or thrombosis, with or without extramural pus | Likely cause of symptoms |
| *Complex appendicitis (Fig. 66.1c)* | | | |
| Gangrenous | Friable appendix with purple, green, or black colour changes | Transmural inflammation with necrosis | Impending perforation |
| Perforated | Visible perforation | Perforation; not always visible in microscope | Increased risk of postoperative complications |
| Abscess (pelvic/abdominal) | Mass found during examination or abscess seen on preoperative imaging; or abscess found at surgery | Transmural inflammation with pus with or without perforation | Increased risk of postoperative complications |

Modified from the classification system by Carr [6]. Figure 66.1 provides photographic examples of macroscopic pathology
From Bhangu et al. [12]

Other viral pathogens are *cytomegalovirus* (CMV), which is common in patients with AIDS, Epstein-Barr virus, and Rubella virus which has lymphoid hyperplasia and multinucleated giant cells of Warthin–Finkeldey as a characteristic (Table 66.2) [15].

The bacterial species most frequently involved are Yersinia, Salmonella, Shigella, Campylobacter, Clostridia, and Mycobacteria. In particular, Yersinia is the main cause of bacterial enteritis in Western and Northern Europe. The infection is transmitted through food and water especially with cold temperatures and showing a natural affinity for frozen products. The species that affect the gastrointestinal tract in humans are *Yersinia enterocolitica* and *Yersinia pseudotuberculosis* [16]. These gram-negative bacteria have been isolated from granulomatous appendicitis and mesenteric lymphadenitis.

Recent studies have hypothesized a multifactorial origin given by the interaction of genetics, environmental factors, and pathogens [17].

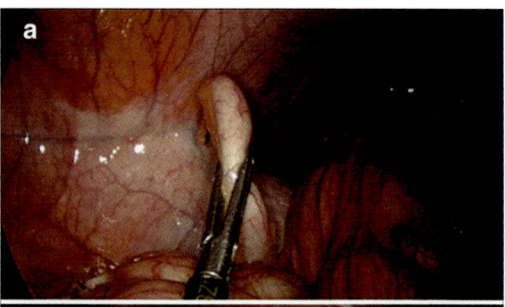
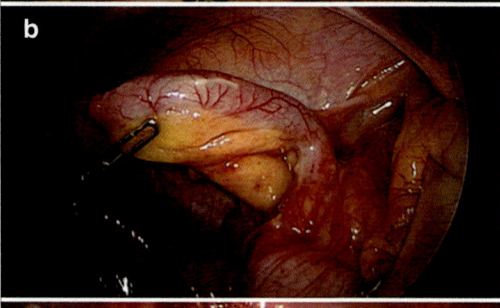
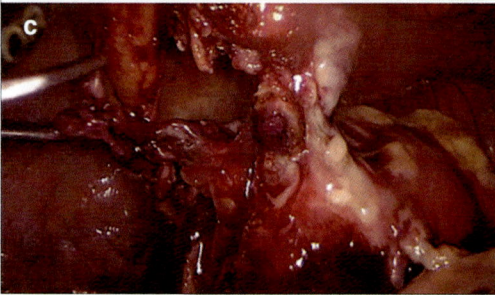

**Fig. 66.1** Macroscopic pathological features of appendicitis. (**a**) Macroscopically normal appendix. (**b**) Simple inflamed appendicitis. (**c**) Complex appendicitis showing perforation with pus formation. (From Bhangu et al. [12])

## 66.2 Diagnosis

### 66.2.1 Clinical Presentation, Tests, and Differential Diagnosis

In most cases, the diagnosis of AA just deserves clinical expertise, indeed a complete medical history and physical examination should be enough if correctly matched with inflammation markers within the context of clinical scores [18].

The most common symptom is abdominal pain followed by nausea (61–92%), anorexia (74–78%), vomiting (75%), and diarrhea or constipation (18%).

Abdominal pain is often crampy, vague, and intermittent, following stimulation of the visceral afferent nerve fibers from T8 to T10, and begins as periumbilical or epigastric pain, before migrating to right lower quadrant (RLQ), when the corresponding parietal peritoneum is inflamed. At this stage, pain becomes stabbing with variable intensity based on the degree of inflammation.

Pain worsens with movement and lasts for less than 48 h in 80% of adults, while it can last longer in the elderly and in those patients with perforation [19]. Painful symptomatology is usually reduced by flexing hips, lying down, and drawing knees.

The point of maximum intensity is defined as McBurney's point (Fig. 66.2) located at one-third of the distance from the right anterior superior iliac spine and the umbilicus.

The clinical scenario may vary depending on the location of the appendix (Fig. 66.3).

**Table 66.2** Summary of infections involving the appendix

| Viruses | Bacteria | Fungi | Parasites |
|---|---|---|---|
| Measles | *Salmonella* sp. (both typhoid and nontyphoid) | Mucormycosis | *Enterobius vermicularis* (pinworm) |
| Adenovirus | *Shigella* sp. | Histoplasmosis | Schistosomes |
| CMV | *Yersinia* (both *Y enterocolitica* and *Y pseudotuberculosis*) | | *Entamoeba histolytica* |
| Epstein-Barr virus | *Actinomyces* sp. | | *Balantidium coli* |
| | *Campylobacter* sp. | | *Strongyloides stercoralis* |
| | *Clostridium*, including *Clostridium difficile* | | *Toxoplasma* |
| | Mycobacteria (tuberculosis and atypical) | | *Cryptosporidium* |
| | *Rickettsia rickettsii* | | *Echinococcus* |
| | | | *Trichuris* sp. (whipworms) |
| | | | *Ascaris* sp. (roundworms) |

From Lamps [15]

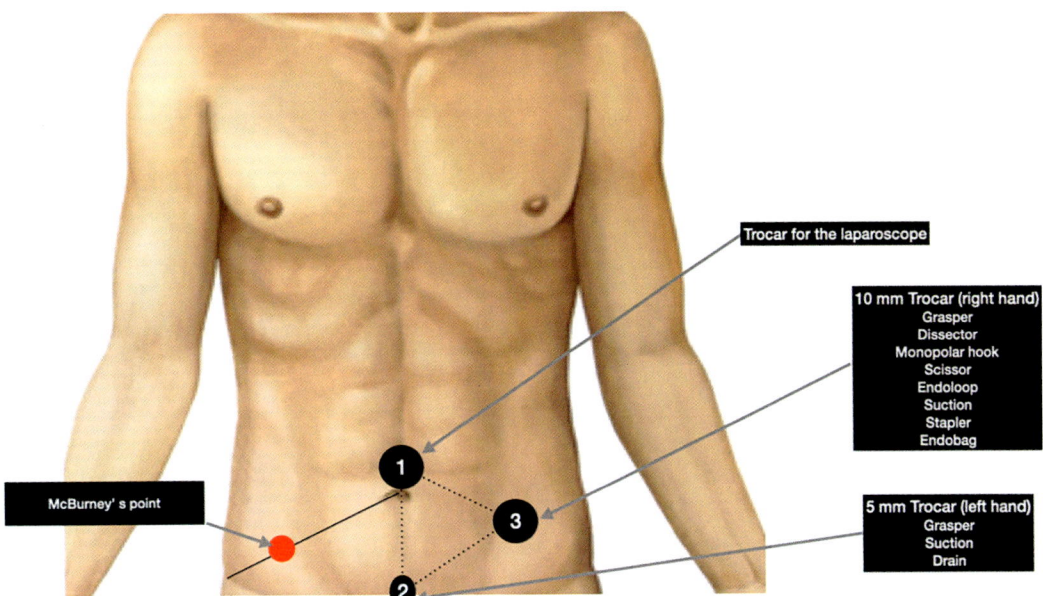

**Fig. 66.2** McBurney's point and Trocar placement during laparoscopic appendectomy. (Adapted by permission from Raul J. Rosenthal et al., Mental Conditioning to Perform Common Operations in General Surgery Training, Springer, 2020)

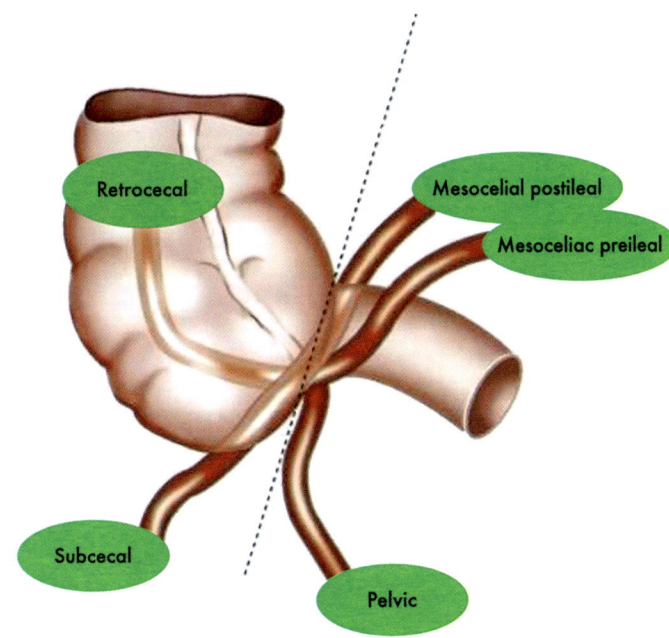

**Fig. 66.3** Different positions of appendix and the related clinical scenario. (Adapted by permission Springer, Emergency Radiology. Appendicitis and beyond: a pictorial review of various appendiceal abnormalities, Andrew K.C. Fenwick et al., 2021)

Ninety-six percent of patients presents with rigidity, tenderness, and guarding in the RLQ. An uncommon but clinically relevant finding of appendix situs inversus may present with left lower quadrant (LLQ) tenderness. During pregnancy, pain and tenderness in the RLQ may be present in the first trimester, while the right upper quadrant is usually involved in the second half of pregnancy, when the appendix may be shifted upwards.

Several physical findings can be helpful in diagnosing AA:

- Rovsing sign is positive when the pain in RLQ is caused by palpation of the LLQ.
- The obturator sign is considered positive when the pain is caused by the internal or external rotation of the flexed right hip and is indicative of irritation of the obturator muscle with pelvic inflammation, that is, appendix located deep in the right pelvis.
- The Markle's sign (or jumping up sign in the Anglo-Saxon Literature) consists in pain in the RLQ elicited by quickly dropping the patients from standing on the toes to the heels with a jarring landing. It suggests localized peritonitis.
- Psoas sign: Pain is elicited with the patient on his/her left side, while the right thigh is flexed backward. It may indicate an inflamed appendix overlying the psoas muscle, in the retrocecal position.
- Rotter sign: Pain induced during rectal or vaginal examination suggesting an endopelvic location of the appendix and the presence of a pelvic abscess.
- Dunphy sign: Pain in the RLQ during a voluntary cough. It suggests a localized peritonitis.

Laboratory tests are not specific for AA, but they can be considered for the differential diagnosis with other pelvic and abdominal diseases (Table 66.3).

In this context, urinalysis could rule out urinary tract infections. In fact, pyuria and microscopic hematuria can be present in case of AA due to irritation of the ureter or bladder, while bacteriuria is rarely associated. Some bacteria that can be isolated in cases of perforated AA are *Bacteroides fragilis*, *Escherichia coli*, *Pseudomonas aeruginosa*, *Peptostreptococcus species*, and *Fusobacteria*. Beta human chorionic gonadotropin (B-hCG) is fundamental for the differential diagnosis to rule out the possibility of an early ectopic pregnancy (Figs. 66.4 and 66.5) [20].

**Table 66.3** Differential diagnosis of acute appendicitis

| |
|---|
| **Surgical etiology** |
| Intestinal obstruction |
| Intussusception |
| Acute cholecystitis |
| Perforated peptic ulcer |
| Meckel's diverticulitis |
| Colonic acute diverticulitis |
| **Medical etiology** |
| Adenomesenteritis |
| Gastroenteritis |
| Right basal pneumonia |
| Terminal ileitis |
| Pancreatitis |
| Hematoma of the right rectus muscle |
| Diabetic ketoacidosis |
| Acute intermittent porphyria |
| Pre-herpetic pain to the 10th and 11th dorsal nerve |
| **Urologic etiology** |
| Right ureteral colic |
| Right pyelonephritis |
| Urinary tract infection |
| **Gynecologic etiology** |
| Ectopic pregnancy |
| Rupture of right ovarian follicle |
| Torsion of right ovarian cyst |
| Pelvic inflammatory disease |

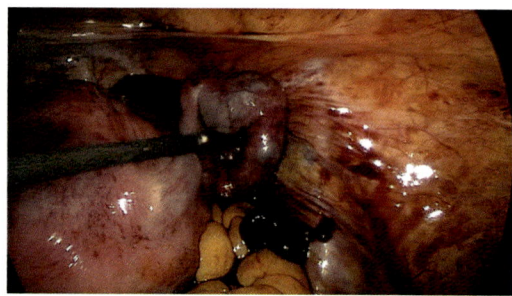

**Fig. 66.4** Ruptured ectopic pregnancy in the right Fallopian tube with surrounding blood clots and fresh blood responsible for the persistent right iliac fossa pain. (From Di Saverio et al. [20])

Less than 4% of patients with AA have a white blood cell count <10,500 mm³. These cases can include the elderly and infants who do not have an adequate immune response. Neutrophilia is present in 75–78% of cases.

Fecal calprotectin and inflammation markers [erythrocyte sedimentation rate (ESR), C-reactive

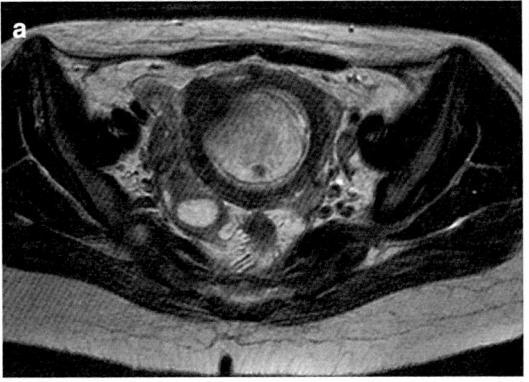
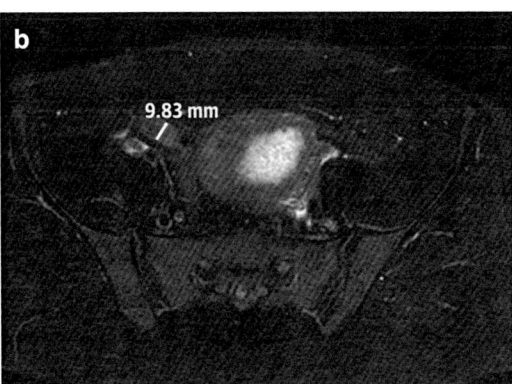

**Fig. 66.5** Magnetic resonance imaging showing the gestational chamber and a normal intrauterine pregnancy as well as the presence of a tubular structure in the right iliac fossa (RIF) (**a**) and what appeared to be an inflamed, thickened appendix (9.83 mm in the proximal appendix) (**b**). (From Di Saverio et al. [20])

protein (CRP)] can help in the differential diagnosis with an ileocecal localization of Crohn's disease, in which an abdominal ultrasound (US) will highlight the thickening of the small bowel wall.

Hyperbilirubinemia (>1.0 mg/dL) may be present in patients with AA, although this finding remains controversial. Several bacterial infections can cause cholestasis and *Escherichia coli* and *Bacteroides fragilis* are among the main pathogens causing AA. *Escherichia coli* causes erythrocyte hemolysis with increased bilirubin load and its endotoxins cause dose-dependent cholestasis. Furthermore, in some cases of severe inflammation, such as in complicated AA, there is an edema of the intestinal wall with increased motility and subsequent cholestasis and hyperbilirubinemia. According to some studies, elevated levels of CRP (>0.5 mg/dL) and bilirubin (>1.2 mg/dL) are associated with gangrenous or perforated AA [21].

To date, several scoring systems have been reported with the attempt to combine subjective complaints with objective physical and laboratory findings in order to facilitate the diagnosis and staging of the AA [22–25] (Table 66.4).

According to a recent meta-analysis of randomized studies, the raja isteri pengiran anak saleha appendicitis (RIPASA) score has a sensitivity of 94% and a specificity of 55%, while the Alvarado score has a sensitivity of 69% and a specificity of 77% [26].

During pregnancy, timing for diagnosis is crucial considering how a diagnostic delay can increase both maternal (1–4%) and fetal (1.5–35%) mortality due to perforation of the appendix [27]. In these cases, the RIPASA score proved to be the most suitable, having a positive predictive value of 94.4%, a negative predictive value of 44%, and a sensitivity and specificity of 78.5% and 78.6%, respectively.

### 66.2.2 Imaging

Abdominal imaging is particularly useful for ruling out other causes of non-specific abdominal pain.

Nowadays, there is a wide variation in the use of imaging modalities. In this context, only 13% of European patients perform pre-operative exams; meanwhile in the United States they are widely used (86%) with computed tomographic (CT) scan as the most frequent modality adopted (91%) [28, 29].

According to Podda et al. [18], abdominal imaging is needed in patients with score-based intermediate probability of AA.

Abdominal ultrasound is an operator-dependent exam and for this reason it has a variable sensitivity (75–90%) and specificity (86–100%). In fact, a recent systematic review and meta-analysis highlighted that its effectiveness is not superior to that of physical examination [30].

However, there is no ionizing radiation exposure associated, and the exam is much more accessible, easy to run, and less time consuming when compared to computed tomography (CT) and magnetic resonance imaging (MRI).

**Table 66.4** Summary of the clinical scoring systems and their interpretation

| AIR score | | | Alvarado score | | | AAS score | | |
|---|---|---|---|---|---|---|---|---|
| Vomiting | No | 0 | Right lower quadrant tenderness | No | 0 | Pain in right lower quadrant | No | 0 |
| | Yes | +1 | | Yes | +2 | | Yes | +2 |
| RIF pain | No | 0 | Elevated temperature (37.3 °C or 99.1 °F) | No | 0 | Pain relocation | No | 0 |
| | Yes | +1 | | Yes | +1 | | Yes | +2 |
| Rebound tenderness | None | 0 | Rebound tenderness | No | 0 | Right lower quadrant tenderness | | |
| | Light | +1 | | | | | | |
| | Medium | +2 | | Yes | +1 | Women, aged 16–49 years | Yes | +1 |
| | Strong | +3 | | | | All other patients | | +3 |
| Temp ≥101.3 °F (38.5 °C) | No | 0 | Migration of pain to the right lower quadrant | No | 0 | Guarding | No | 0 |
| | Yes | +1 | | Yes | +1 | Mild | Yes | +2 |
| | | | | | | Moderate or severe | | +4 |
| Polymorphonuclear leukocytes | <70% | 0 | Anorexia | No | 0 | Blood leukocyte count (×10⁹) | No | 0 |
| | 70–84% | +1 | | Yes | +1 | ≥7.2 and <10.9 | Yes | +1 |
| | ≥85% | +2 | | | | ≥10.9 and <14.0 | | +2 |
| | | | | | | ≥14.0 | | +3 |
| WBC count, ×10⁹/L | <10 | 0 | Nausea or vomiting | No | 0 | Proportion of neutrophils (%) | No | 0 |
| | 10.0–14.9 | +1 | | Yes | +1 | ≥62 and <75 | Yes | +2 |
| | ≥15 | +2 | | | | ≥75 and <83 | | +3 |
| | | | | | | ≥83 | | +4 |
| CRP level, mg/L | <10 | 0 | Leukocytosis >10,000 | No | 0 | CRP (mg/L), symptoms <24 h | No | 0 |
| | 10–49 | +1 | | Yes | +2 | ≥4 and <11 | Yes | +2 |
| | ≥50 | +2 | | | | ≥11 and <25 | | +3 |
| | | | | | | ≥25 and <83 | | +5 |
| | | | | | | ≥83 | | +1 |
| | | | Leukocyte left shift >75% neutrophils | No | 0 | CRP (mg/L), symptoms >24 h | No | 0 |
| | | | | Yes | +1 | ≥12 and <53 | Yes | +2 |
| | | | | | | ≥53 and <152 | | +2 |
| | | | | | | ≥152 | | +1 |

| Interpretation AIR score | Risk | Recommendation | Interpretation Alvarado score | Risk | Recommendation | Interpretation AAS score | Risk | Recommendation |
|---|---|---|---|---|---|---|---|---|
| 0–4 | Low | Outpatient follow-up (if unaltered general condition) | 1–4 | Low | Discharge | ≤10 | Low | Discharge without imaging |
| 5–8 | Intermediate | In-hospital active observation with serial re-exams, imaging, or diagnostic laparoscopy, according to local practice | 5–7 | Intermediate | Monitoring/admission | 11–15 | Intermediate | Imaging |
| 9–12 | High | Surgical exploration | 8–10 | High | Surgical exploration | ≥16 | High | Surgical exploration without preoperative imaging |

Despite the high predictive value, a negative finding sometimes does not exclude the disease and it may be necessary to perform a CT of the abdomen.

On abdominal ultrasound, a normal appendix has a blind tubular structure with a diameter of about 6–7 mm and a wall thickness of <2 mm (Fig. 66.6) [31] while an inflamed appendix is dilated, not compressible and mobile, with a thickened and hyperemic wall on Doppler. The presence of a fecalith (20% of cases in pediatric age) or of a periappendiceal fluid collection can also be indicative of AA (Fig. 66.7). Transvaginal ultrasound can rule out gynecological diseases.

Abdominal CT scan should be used as a second-line examination in patients with negative

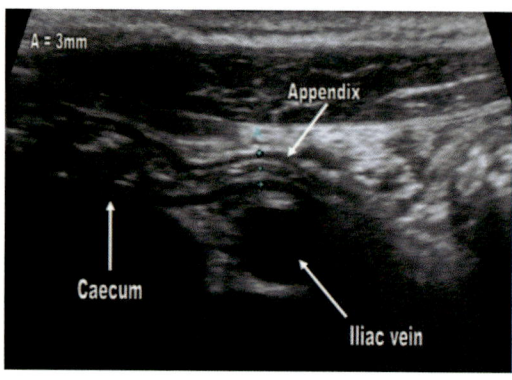

**Fig. 66.6** A normal appendix draped over the iliac vessels in a 10-year-old girl. It is shown a thin-walled appendix, measuring less than 6 mm in diameter (A width of 3 mm). The caecum can be seen in continuity with the appendix superior to it. (From Quigley et al. [31])

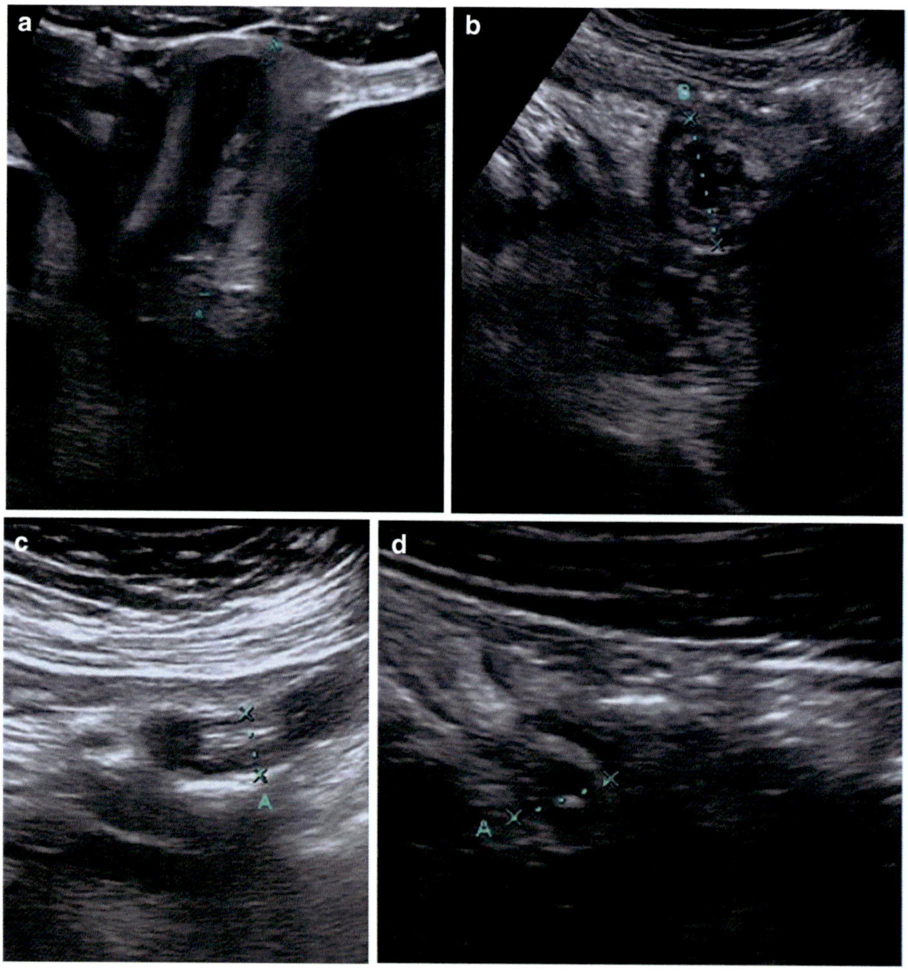

**Fig. 66.7** Ultrasound diagnosis of acute appendicitis. (**a**) Distended appendiceal lumen with thickened wall. (**b**) The "target" sign (a fluid-filled hypoechoic center surrounded by the hyperechoic layer of mucosa/submucosa and the hypoechoic layer of the muscolaris). (**c**, **d**) Acute appendicitis with intra luminal fecalith

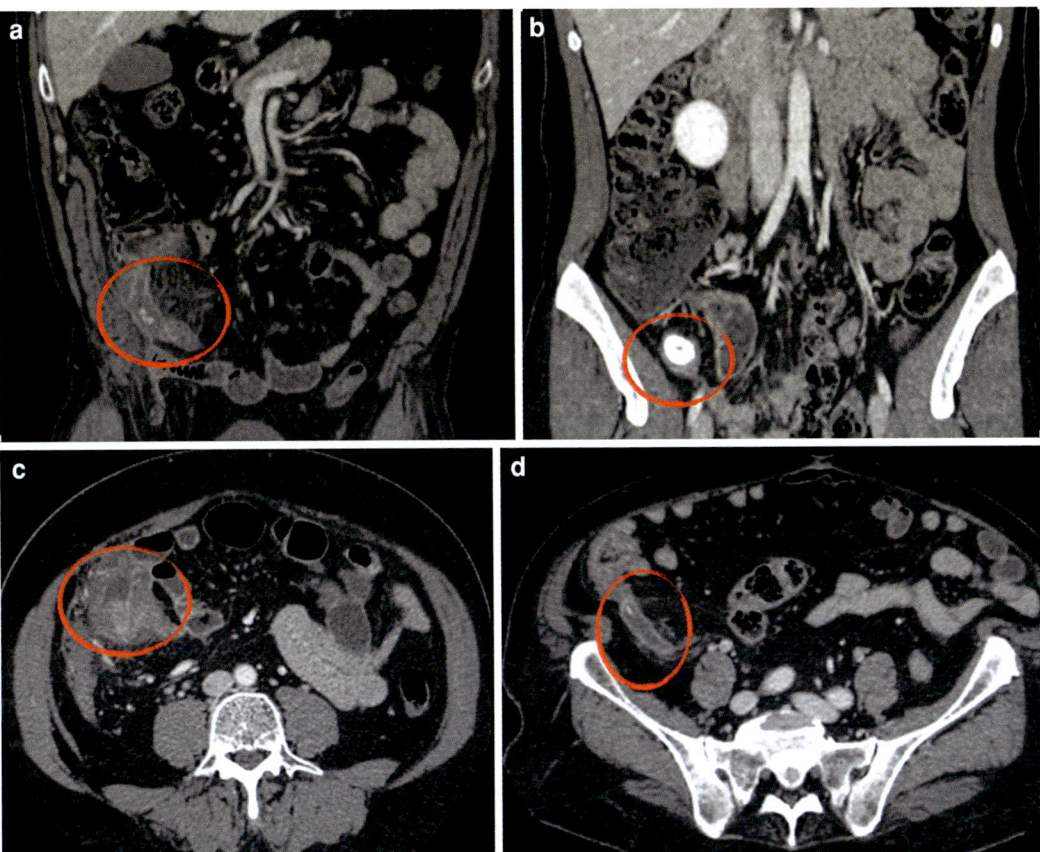

**Fig. 66.8** CT scan diagnosis of acute appendicitis. (**a**) Sub-cecal appendicitis (thickened appendiceal wall, and "Dirty Fat" sign. (**b**) Acute appendicitis with huge intra luminal appendicolith. (**c**) Acute appendicitis with right iliac fossa phlegmon. (**d**) Acute appendicitis with the lumen filled by liquid content

or inconclusive ultrasound in order to increase sensitivity and reduce both exposure to radiation and healthcare costs [32]. Its usefulness is greater in case of suspicion of complicated AA with localized abscess or perforation. The proper use of CT has significantly reduced the negative appendectomy rate. Typical findings are represented by dilation of the appendix (>6 mm) and thickening of its wall (>2 mm) as well as by both a peri-appendiceal fat stranding and the presence of an appendicolith (Fig. 66.8). Free air fluid suggestive of perforated appendicitis can be detected too.

Other imaging methods have no specific indication in AA except for MRI which may be suggested in pregnant women to reduce radiation exposure.

## 66.3 Treatment

### 66.3.1 Nonoperative

A non-operative approach with antibiotic can be considered effective in patients with uncomplicated AA and in the absence of an intra-luminal appendicolith [33]. However, this strategy is associated with a 5-year AA recurrence rate of approximately 40% [34, 35].

A systematic review with meta-analysis of randomized controlled trials, comparing appendectomy and non-operative management, demonstrated how antibiotic therapy is associated with lower efficacy at 1-year follow-up with respect to the surgical approach (75.9% vs. 98.3%; $p < 0.0001$).

Furthermore, patients in the conservative treatment group had a higher rate of peritonitis identified at the time of surgical operation (19.9% vs. 8.5%; p = 0.02) [36].

These results are consistent with those reported by Varadhan and colleagues, in another meta-analysis of randomized controlled trials. They confirmed the role of antibiotics in the management of early uncomplicated appendicitis [37]; in fact, no statistically significant differences in the complication rate between the two groups were demonstrated so far [38].

### 66.3.2 Surgical Treatment

The first laparoscopic appendectomy was reported in 1983 by Semm, a German gynecologist, even though the Dutch surgeon Hans J de Kok performed an assisted laparoscopic procedure 5 years earlier [39, 40].

The introduction of laparoscopy represented a notable change in the treatment of AA, replacing open appendectomy, through the McBurney point, which until then was considered the referral procedure.

Nowadays, laparoscopic appendectomy still remains the gold standard in the treatment of AA (Fig. 66.2) [3], with a superiority over the laparotomy approach in terms of reduced length of hospitalization, early return to work as well as a lower rate of complications and post-operative adhesions [41, 42]. These results were also confirmed in elderly and pregnant patients [1, 43]. Interestingly, the long-term outcomes are equal [44].

In a population-based study, concerning the pediatric population in Denmark, including 24.046 pediatric cases of appendicitis, the surgical approach changed radically from open (97%) to laparoscopic (94%) over 15 years (2000–2015) [45] with a resulting reduction in the length of hospital stay from 41 to 17 h.

Single incision laparoscopic surgery (SILS) has been applied in the treatment of AA [46], but no significant differences were identified with respect to the traditional laparoscopic approach.

Moreover, the operative time of SILS is longer [47] and with a steeper learning curve. The slightly nicer cosmetic result does not justify its use. Ussia et al. [48] demonstrated that, with a proper learning curve, laparoscopic appendectomy can be performed by trainees without affecting the outcomes.

Recently, the updates WSES guidelines (Fig. 66.9) recommended planning laparoscopic appendectomy within 24 h after admission in uncomplicated AA (QoE: Moderate; Strength of recommendation: Strong; 1B), without increasing complications or perforations rate in both adults and children [1].

Other minimally invasive approaches, such as endoscopic retrograde appendicitis therapy (ERAT) [49, 50], transgastric appendectomy (TGAE), and transvaginal appendectomy (TVAE) [51], have been described over time without finding a fertile ground.

In case of abscess, a percutaneous drainage is indicated. In this context, the optimal therapeutic approach is a matter of debate. Currently, there are two therapeutic options: early appendectomy, preferably with a laparoscopic approach, and non-operative management. The latter, concerning the use of antibiotic therapy along with CT or ultrasound-guided percutaneous trans-abdominal drainage of the abscess, is considered an effective therapeutic option as a first-line treatment for AA complicated by localized peritonitis.

However, although surgical treatment is significantly associated with a higher incidence of complications (wound infections, abdominal/pelvic abscesses, ileus/intestinal obstruction, and reoperation), its use can be recommended in expert hands.

### 66.3.3 Prognosis

The most common postoperative complications following appendectomy, such as wound infections, intra-abdominal abscess, and ileus caused by adhesions, vary in frequency between open (overall complication rates 11.1%) and laparoscopic appendectomy (8.7%) [52, 53].

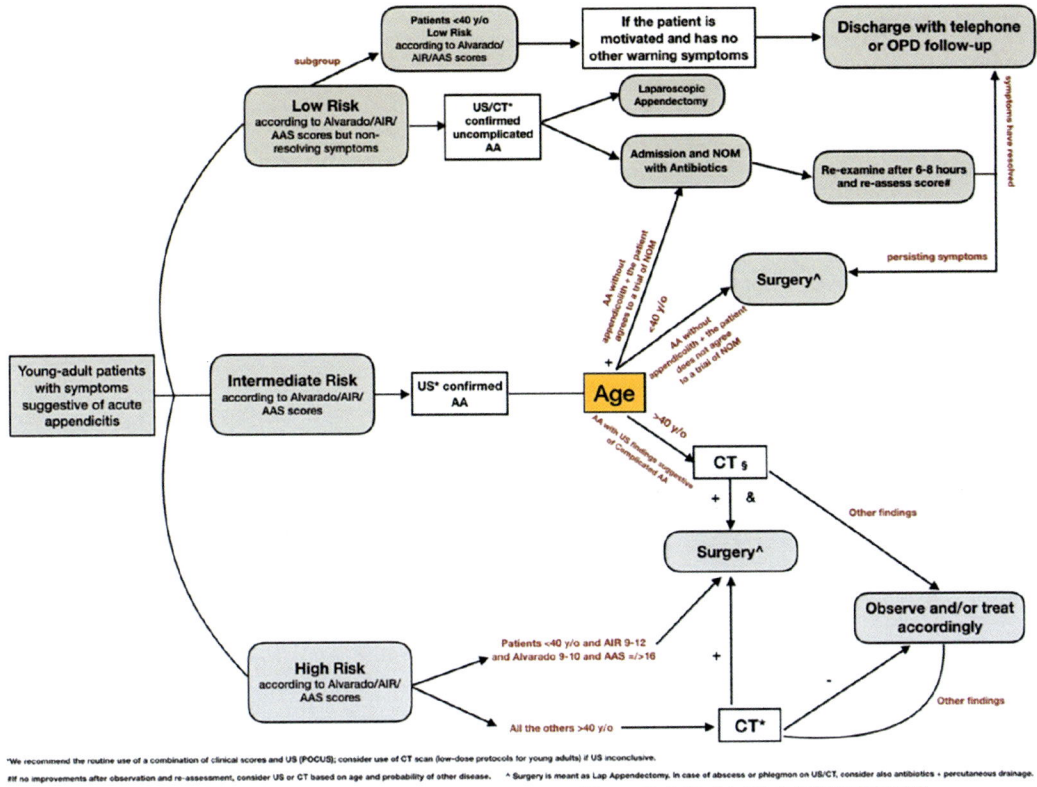

**Fig. 66.9** Practical World Society of Emergency Surgery (WSES) algorithm for diagnosis and treatment of adult patients with suspected acute appendicitis. (From Di Saverio et al. [1])

Despite the possibility of decease exists, appendicitis is rarely responsible for deaths after appendectomy. The 30-day post-appendectomy mortality rate is around 2/1000 patients. Increased mortality is found in patients over 60 years of age, patients who underwent a negative surgical exploration, and those with complicated appendicitis [54].

Elderly patients have a higher risk for morbidity following appendectomy. Morbidity rate is estimated to be around 70% as compared to 1% in the general population [55].

Higher adverse outcomes rates observed in the elderly population can be explained not only by delay in the appropriate diagnosis, more advanced disease, and operative technique, but also by higher number of co-morbidities, such as cognitive impairment and functional dependence, that might complicate the recovery.

**Dos and Don'ts**
- A tailored individualized diagnostic approach for stratifying the risk and disease probability and planning an appropriate stepwise diagnostic pathway should be adopted in all patients with suspected acute appendicitis, depending on age, sex, and clinical signs and symptoms.
- The use of AIR score and AAS score as clinical predictors of acute appendicitis is recommended.
- Cross-sectional imaging (i.e., CT scan) for high-risk patients younger than 40 years old (AIR score 9–12 and AAS ≥16) may be avoided before diagnostic ± therapeutic laparoscopy.

- Point-of-care ultrasonography is suggested as the most appropriate first-line diagnostic tool in both adults and children, if an imaging investigation is indicated based on clinical assessment. Contrast-enhanced low-dose CT scan is preferable over contrast-enhanced standard-dose CT scan in patients with suspected acute appendicitis and negative ultrasonography findings.
- The antibiotic-first strategy can be considered safe and effective in selected patients with uncomplicated acute appendicitis. Patients who wish to avoid surgery must be aware of a risk of recurrence of up to 39% after 5 years.
- Patients with acute appendicitis and the finding of an intra-luminal appendicolith should not be treated non-operatively.
- Laparoscopic appendectomy should be planned for the next available operating list within 24 h in case of uncomplicated acute appendicitis, minimizing the delay wherever possible. Conversely, delaying appendectomy for acute appendicitis over 24 h from the admission is not advisable.

### Take-Home Messages
- Acute appendicitis represents an important burden on our healthcare systems being an extremely frequent pathological condition.
- The use of antibiotics as first-line treatment of acute appendicitis has been discussed for several years without leading to clear recommendations, but results suggest that antibiotic therapy could be a safe alternative to surgery in selected patients with acute uncomplicated appendicitis.
- Clinical assessment has a pivotal role in the suspicion of appendicitis. Abdominal US is the first-line radiological imaging, especially preferred in young and pregnant women. On the other hand, CT scan is considered the second line but also the gold standard.
- Laparoscopic approach is the gold standard among the surgical options in case of complicated acute appendicitis.

### Multiple Choice Questions with Four Answers
1. Among the different location that the appendix can have, the most frequent is
   A. Sub-hepatic
   B. Epigastric
   C. Retrocecal
   D. Pelvic

   **Correct answer: C**

2. In developed countries, acute appendicitis has an incidence rate of
   A. 90–100 patients/100,000 inhabitants/year
   B. 20–30 patients/100,000 inhabitants/year
   C. 200–250 patients/100,000 inhabitants/year
   D. 150/200 patients/100,000 inhabitants/year

   **Correct answer: A**

3. What are the most used clinical scores to guide the diagnostic process in patients with acute appendicitis?
   A. Alvarado score, Helsinki score, AIR score
   B. Atlanta score, Alvarado score, RIPASA score
   C. Alvarado score, Matthew score, AIR score
   D. Alvarado score, AIR score, adult appendicitis score (AAS)

   **Correct answer: D**

4. On US of the abdomen in cross section, the appendix in an acute inflammatory state appears as an image of
   A. Target
   B. Cross
   C. Star
   D. Seashell

**Correct answer: A**

5. The standard setting of laparoscopic appendectomy involves the placement of three trocars
   A. One in the epigastrium, one in the right hypochondrium, one in the left flank
   B. One in the periumbilical area, one in the suprapubic area, one in the left iliac fossa
   C. One in the periumbilical area, one in the epigastrium, one in the right iliac fossa
   D. One in the left hypochondrium, one in the epigastrium, one in the suprapubic area

**Correct answer: B**

6. All of the following clinical conditions or pathologies, except one, must be included in the differential diagnosis of acute appendicitis. Which one does not enter into differential diagnosis?
   A. Biliary colic
   B. Acute perforated cholecystitis
   C. Pyelonephritis
   D. Pelvic inflammatory disease (PID)

**Correct answer: A**

7. Appendiceal abscess can be treated with:
   A. Antibiotic therapy alone
   B. Antibiotic therapy and percutaneous drainage
   C. Upfront laparoscopic surgery
   D. All the listed options are correct

**Correct answer: D**

8. Antibiotic therapy for uncomplicated acute appendicitis is effective in
   A. 40–45% of patients at 1-year follow-up
   B. 65–85% of patients at 1-year follow-up
   C. 61% of patients at 5-year follow-up
   D. B + C

**Correct answer: D**

9. Appendicular or colonic neoplasms should be investigated after conservatively treated appendiceal abscesses, especially in patients older than:
   A. 30 years
   B. 40 years
   C. 50 years
   D. 60 years

**Correct answer: B**

10. The correct option for diagnostic imaging among patients scored at high-risk with the AIR or AAS scores is
    A. Upfront CT scan
    B. Upfront MRI scan
    C. Conditional CT scan after inconclusive US scan
    D. None of the above

**Correct answer: C**

11. Regarding the timing of surgical treatment, delaying the appendectomy up to 24 h from admission is related to
    A. Decreased rate of postoperative mortality
    B. Increased rate of postoperative morbidity
    C. Equivalent rate of postoperative morbidity
    D. Increased rate of postoperative mortality

**Correct answer: C**

# References

1. Di Saverio S, Podda M, De Simone B, Ceresoli M, Augustin G, Gori A, Boermeester M, Sartelli M, Coccolini F, Tarasconi A, De' Angelis N, Weber DG, Tolonen M, Birindelli A, Biffl W, Moore EE, Kelly M, Soreide K, Kashuk J, Ten Broek R, Gomes CA, Sugrue M, Davies RJ, Damaskos D, Leppäniemi A, Kirkpatrick A, Peitzman AB, Fraga GP, Maier RV, Coimbra R, Chiarugi M, Sganga G, Pisanu A, De' Angelis GL, Tan E, Van Goor H, Pata F, Di Carlo I, Chiara O, Litvin A, Campanile FC, Sakakushev B, Tomadze G, Demetrashvili Z, Latifi R, Abu-Zidan F,

1. Romeo O, Segovia-Lohse H, Baiocchi G, Costa D, Rizoli S, Balogh ZJ, Bendinelli C, Scalea T, Ivatury R, Velmahos G, Andersson R, Kluger Y, Ansaloni L, Catena F. Diagnosis and treatment of acute appendicitis: 2020 update of the WSES Jerusalem guidelines. World J Emerg Surg. 2020;15(1):27. https://doi.org/10.1186/s13017-020-00306-3.
2. Lee JH, Park YS, Choi JS. The epidemiology of appendicitis and appendectomy in South Korea: national registry data. J Epidemiol. 2010;20(2):97–105. https://doi.org/10.2188/jea.je20090011.
3. Guaitoli E, Gallo G, Cardone E, Conti L, Famularo S, Formisano G, Galli F, Giuliani G, Martino A, Pasculli A, Patini R, Soriero D, Pappalardo V, Casoni Pattacini G, Sparavigna M, Meniconi R, Mazzari A, Barra F, Orsenigo E, Pertile D. Consensus Statement of the Italian Polispecialistic Society of Young Surgeons (SPIGC): diagnosis and treatment of acute appendicitis. J Investig Surg. 2021;34:1089–103. https://doi.org/10.1080/08941939.2020.1740360.
4. Davies GM, Dasbach EJ, Teutsch S. The burden of appendicitis-related hospitalizations in the United States in 1997. Surg Infect. 2004;5:160–5.
5. Addiss DG, Shaffer N, Fowler BS, Tauxe RV. The epidemiology of appendicitis and appendectomy in the United States. Am J Epidemiol. 1990;132(5):910–25.
6. Bagi P, Dueholm S. Nonoperative management of the ultrasonically evaluated appendiceal mass. Surgery. 1987;101:602–5.
7. Golz RA, Flum DR, Sanchez SE, Liu X, Donovan C, Drake FT. Geographic association between incidence of acute appendicitis and socioeconomic status. JAMA Surg. 2020;155(4):330–8. https://doi.org/10.1001/jamasurg.2019.6030.
8. Fitz RH. Perforating inflammation of the vermiform appendix. Am J Med Sci. 1886;92:321–46.
9. Shaban Y, Elkbuli A, McKenney M, Boneva D. Amyand's hernia: a case report and review of the literature. Int J Surg Case Rep. 2018;47:92–6. https://doi.org/10.1016/j.ijscr.2018.04.034.
10. McBurney C. II. The indications for early laparotomy in appendicitis. Ann Surg. 1891;13(4):233–54.
11. McBurney C. IV. The incision made in the Abdominal Wall in cases of appendicitis, with a description of a new method of operating. Ann Surg. 1894;20(1):38–43.
12. Bhangu A, Soreide K, Di Saverio S, Assarsson JH, Drake FT. Acute appendicitis: modern understanding of pathogenesis, diagnosis, and management. Lancet. 2015;386(10000):1278–87. https://doi.org/10.1016/S0140-6736(15)00275-5.
13. Carr NJ. The pathology of acute appendicitis. Ann Diagn Pathol. 2000;4(1):46–58. https://doi.org/10.1016/s1092-9134(00)90011-x.
14. Guarner J, de Leon-Bojorge B, Lopez-Corella E, et al. Intestinal intussusception associated with adenovirus infection in Mexican children. Am J Clin Pathol. 2003;120:845–50.
15. Lamps LW. Infectious causes of appendicitis. Infect Dis Clin N Am. 2010;24(4):995–1018, ix–x. https://doi.org/10.1016/j.idc.2010.07.012.
16. Natkin J, Beavis KG. Yersinia enterocolitica and Yersinia pseudotuberculosis. Clin Lab Med. 1999;19:523–36.
17. Sadr Azodi O, Andrén-Sandberg A, Larsson H. Genetic and environmental influences on the risk of acute appendicitis in twins. Br J Surg. 2009;96(11):1336–40. https://doi.org/10.1002/bjs.6736.
18. Podda M, Andersson R, Boermeester M, Coccolini F, Sartelli M, Moore EE, Sugrue M, Abu-Zidan F, Tolonen M, Damaskos D, Kluger Y, Soreide K, Pisanu A, Augustin G, Latifi R, Kelly M, Leppaniemi A, Fraga GP, Ten Broek R, Tan E, Van Goor H, Chiara O, Maier RV, Pata F, De Simone B, Ordoñez CA, Ansaloni L, Catena F, Di Saverio S. Do young patients with high clinical suspicion of appendicitis really need cross-sectional imaging? Proceedings from a highly controversial debate among the experts' panel of 2020 WSES Jerusalem guidelines. J Trauma Acute Care Surg. 2021;90(5):e101–7. https://doi.org/10.1097/TA.0000000000003097.
19. Yeh B. Evidence-based emergency medicine/rational clinical examination abstract. Does this adult patient have appendicitis? Ann Emerg Med. 2008;52:301–3. https://doi.org/10.1016/j.annemergmed.2007.10.023.
20. Di Saverio S, Gelmi CAE, Perrone A. Right lower quadrant pain in early pregnancy. JAMA Surg. 2018;153(2):181–2. https://doi.org/10.1001/jamasurg.2017.4936.
21. Eren T, Rombalak E, Ozemir IA, et al. Hyperbilirubinemia as a predictive factor in acute appendicitis. Eur J Trauma Emerg Surg. 2016;42:471–6.
22. Alvarado A. A practical score for the early diagnosis of acute appendicitis. Ann Emerg Med. 1986;15(5):557–64.
23. Andersson M, Andersson RE. The appendicitis inflammatory response score: a tool for the diagnosis of acute appendicitis that outperforms the Alvarado score. World J Surg. 2008;32(8):1843–9.
24. Chong CF, Adi MI, Thien A, Suyoi A, Mackie AJ, Tin AS, et al. Development of the RIPASA score: a new appendicitis scoring system for the diagnosis of acute appendicitis. Singap Med J. 2010;51(3):220–5.
25. Sammalkorpi HE, Mentula P, Leppäniemi A. A new adult appendicitis score improves diagnostic accuracy of acute appendicitis—a prospective study. BMC Gastroenterol. 2014;14:114.
26. Frountzas M, Stergios K, Kopsini D, Schizas D, Kontzoglou K, Toutouzas K. Alvarado or RIPASA score for diagnosis of acute appendicitis? A meta-analysis of randomized trials. Int J Surg. 2018;56:307–14. https://doi.org/10.1016/j.ijsu.2018.07.003.
27. Guttman R, Goldman RD, Koren G. Appendicitis during pregnancy. Can Fam Physician. 2004;50:355–7.
28. Collaborative NSR. Multicentre observational study of performance variation in provision and outcome of emergency appendicectomy. Br J Surg. 2013;100:1240–52.
29. Collaborative SCOAP. Negative appendectomy and imaging accuracy in the Washington State Surgical

30. Quigley AJ, Stafrace S. Ultrasound assessment of acute appendicitis in paediatric patients: methodology and pictorial overview of findings seen. Insights Imaging. 2013;4(6):741–51. https://doi.org/10.1007/s13244-013-0275-3.
31. Giljaca V, Nadarevic T, Poropat G, Nadarevic VS, Stimac D. Diagnostic accuracy of abdominal ultrasound for diagnosis of acute appendicitis: systematic review and meta-analysis. World J Surg. 2017;41(3):693–700. https://doi.org/10.1007/s00268-016-3792-7.
32. Laméris W, van Randen A, van Es HW, et al. Imaging strategies for detection of urgent conditions in patients with acute abdominal pain: diagnostic accuracy study. BMJ. 2009;338:b2431.
33. Talan DA, Di Saverio S.N. Treatment of acute uncomplicated appendicitis. Engl J Med. 2021;385(12):1116–23. https://doi.org/10.1056/NEJMcp2107675.
34. Salminen P, Tuominen R, Paajanen H, Rautio T, Nordström P, Aarnio M, Rantanen T, Hurme S, Mecklin JP, Sand J, Virtanen J, Jartti A, Grönroos JM. Five-year follow-up of antibiotic therapy for uncomplicated acute appendicitis in the APPAC randomized clinical trial. JAMA. 2018;320(12):1259–65. https://doi.org/10.1001/jama.2018.13201. Erratum in: JAMA 2018 Oct 23;320(16):1711.
35. Podda M, Gerardi C, Cillara N, Fearnhead N, Gomes CA, Birindelli A, Mulliri A, Davies RJ, Di Saverio S. Antibiotic treatment and appendectomy for uncomplicated acute appendicitis in adults and children: a systematic review and meta-analysis. Ann Surg. 2019;270(6):1028–40. https://doi.org/10.1097/SLA.0000000000003225.
36. Podda M, Cillara N, Di Saverio S, Lai A, Feroci F, Luridiana G, Agresta F, Vettoretto N, ACOI (Italian Society of Hospital Surgeons) Study Group on Acute Appendicitis. Antibiotics-first strategy for uncomplicated acute appendicitis in adults is associated with increased rates of peritonitis at surgery. A systematic review with meta-analysis of randomized controlled trials comparing appendectomy and non-operative management with antibiotics. Surgeon. 2017;15(5):303–14. https://doi.org/10.1016/j.surge.2017.02.001.
37. Varadhan KK, Neal KR, Lobo DN. Safety and efficacy of antibiotics compared with appendicectomy for treatment of uncomplicated acute appendicitis: meta-analysis of randomised controlled trials. BMJ. 2012;344:e2156. https://doi.org/10.1136/bmj.e2156.
38. Prechal D, Damirov F, Grilli M, Ronellenfitsch U. Antibiotic therapy for acute uncomplicated appendicitis: a systematic review and meta-analysis. Int J Color Dis. 2019;34(6):963–71. https://doi.org/10.1007/s00384-019-03296-0.
39. Semm K. Endoscopic appendectomy. Endoscopy. 1983;15(2):59–64. https://doi.org/10.1055/s-2007-1021466.
40. de Kok HJ. A new technique for resecting the non-inflamed not-adhesive appendix through a mini-laparotomy with the aid of the laparoscope. Arch Chir Neerl. 1977;29(3):195–8.
41. Olmi S, Magnone S, Bertolini A, Croce E. Laparoscopic versus open appendectomy in acute appendicitis: a randomized prospective study. Surg Endosc. 2005;19(9):1193–5. https://doi.org/10.1007/s00464-004-2165-8.
42. Dai L, Shuai J. Laparoscopic versus open appendectomy in adults and children: a meta-analysis of randomized controlled trials. United European Gastroenterol J. 2017;5(4):542–53.
43. Wang D, Dong T, Shao Y, Gu T, Xu Y, Jiang Y. Laparoscopy versus open appendectomy for elderly patients, a meta-analysis and systematic review. BMC Surg. 2019;19(1):54. https://doi.org/10.1186/s12893-019-0515-7.
44. Di Saverio S, Mandrioli M, Sibilio A, Smerieri N, Lombardi R, Catena F, Ansaloni L, Tugnoli G, Masetti M, Jovine E. A cost-effective technique for laparoscopic appendectomy: outcomes and costs of a case-control prospective single-operator study of 112 unselected consecutive cases of complicated acute appendicitis. J Am Coll Surg. 2014;218(3):e51–65. https://doi.org/10.1016/j.jamcollsurg.2013.12.003.
45. Hansen GL, Kleif J, Jakobsen C, Paerregaard A. Changes in incidence and management of acute appendicitis in children-a population-based study in the period 2000-2015. Eur J Pediatr Surg. 2020; https://doi.org/10.1055/s-0040-1714655.
46. Di Saverio S, Mandrioli M, Birindelli A, Biscardi A, Di Donato L, Gomes CA, Piccinini A, Vettoretto N, Agresta F, Tugnoli G, Jovine E. Single-incision laparoscopic appendectomy with a low-cost technique and surgical-glove port: "How To Do It" with comparison of the outcomes and costs in a consecutive single-operator series of 45 cases. J Am Coll Surg. 2016;222(3):e15–30. https://doi.org/10.1016/j.jamcollsurg.2015.11.019. Epub 2015 Nov 24.
47. Feng J, Cui N, Wang Z, Duan J. Bayesian network meta-analysis of the effects of single-incision laparoscopic surgery, conventional laparoscopic appendectomy and open appendectomy for the treatment of acute appendicitis. Exp Ther Med. 2017;14(6):5908–16. https://doi.org/10.3892/etm.2017.5343.
48. Ussia A, Vaccari S, Gallo G, Grossi U, Ussia R, Sartarelli L, Minghetti M, Lauro A, Barbieri P, Di Saverio S, Cervellera M, Tonini V. Laparoscopic appendectomy as an index procedure for surgical trainees: clinical outcomes and learning curve. Updat Surg. 2021;73(1):187–95. https://doi.org/10.1007/s13304-020-00950-z.
49. Costamagna G. Acute appendicitis: will a novel endoscopic "organ-sparing" approach change the treatment

paradigm? Gastrointest Endosc. 2020;92(1):190–1. https://doi.org/10.1016/j.gie.2020.02.044.
50. Podda M, Di Saverio S, Agresta F, Pisanu A. Endoscopic retrograde appendicitis therapy: the true proof of the pudding is in the eating. Gastrointest Endosc. 2020;92(6):1278–9. https://doi.org/10.1016/j.gie.2020.07.016.
51. Bulian DR, Kaehler G, Magdeburg R, et al. Analysis of the first 217 appendectomies of the German NOTES registry. Ann Surg. 2017;265(3):534–8.
52. Nakhamiyayev V, Galldin L, Chiarello M, Lumba A, Gorecki PJ. Laparoscopic appendectomy is the preferred approach for appendicitis: a retrospective review of two practice patterns. Surg Endosc. 2010;24(4):859–64. https://doi.org/10.1007/s00464-009-0678-x.
53. Flum DR, Koepsell T. The clinical and economic correlates of misdiagnosed appendicitis: nationwide analysis. Arch Surg. 2002;137(7):799–804; discussion 804. https://doi.org/10.1001/archsurg.137.7.799.
54. Kotaluoto S, Ukkonen M, Pauniaho SL, Helminen M, Sand J, Rantanen T. Mortality related to appendectomy; a population based analysis over two decades in Finland. World J Surg. 2017;41(1):64–9. https://doi.org/10.1007/s00268-016-3688-6.
55. Poillucci G, Podda M, Pisanu A, Mortola L, Dalla Caneva P, Massa G, Costa G, Savastano R, Cillara N, ERASO (Elderly Risk Assessment and Surgical Outcome) Collaborative Study Group. Risk factors for postoperative morbidity following appendectomy in the elderly: a nationwide prospective cohort study. Eur J Trauma Emerg Surg. 2019; https://doi.org/10.1007/s00068-019-01186-2. Epub ahead of print.

## Suggested Reading

Bhangu A, Soreide K, Di Saverio S, Assarsson JH, Drake FT. Acute appendicitis: modern understanding of pathogenesis, diagnosis, and management. Lancet. 2015;386(10000):1278–87. https://doi.org/10.1016/S0140-6736(15)00275-5.

Costamagna G. Acute appendicitis: will a novel endoscopic "organ-sparing" approach change the treatment paradigm? Gastrointest Endosc. 2020;92(1):190–1. https://doi.org/10.1016/j.gie.2020.02.044.

Di Saverio S, Podda M, De Simone B, Ceresoli M, Augustin G, Gori A, Boermeester M, Sartelli M, Coccolini F, Tarasconi A, De' Angelis N, Weber DG, Tolonen M, Birindelli A, Biffl W, Moore EE, Kelly M, Soreide K, Kashuk J, Ten Broek R, Gomes CA, Sugrue M, Davies RJ, Damaskos D, Leppäniemi A, Kirkpatrick A, Peitzman AB, Fraga GP, Maier RV, Coimbra R, Chiarugi M, Sganga G, Pisanu A, De' Angelis GL, Tan E, Van Goor H, Pata F, Di Carlo I, Chiara O, Litvin A, Campanile FC, Sakakushev B, Tomadze G, Demetrashvili Z, Latifi R, Abu-Zidan F, Romeo O, Segovia-Lohse H, Baiocchi G, Costa D, Rizoli S, Balogh ZJ, Bendinelli C, Scalea T, Ivatury R, Velmahos G, Andersson R, Kluger Y, Ansaloni L, Catena F. Diagnosis and treatment of acute appendicitis: 2020 update of the WSES Jerusalem guidelines. World J Emerg Surg. 2020;15(1):27. https://doi.org/10.1186/s13017-020-00306-3.

Podda M, Gerardi C, Cillara N, Fearnhead N, Gomes CA, Birindelli A, Mulliri A, Davies RJ, Di Saverio S. Antibiotic treatment and appendectomy for uncomplicated acute appendicitis in adults and children: a systematic review and meta-analysis. Ann Surg. 2019;270(6):1028–40. https://doi.org/10.1097/SLA.0000000000003225.

Ussia A, Vaccari S, Gallo G, Grossi U, Ussia R, Sartarelli L, Minghetti M, Lauro A, Barbieri P, Di Saverio S, Cervellera M, Tonini V. Laparoscopic appendectomy as an index procedure for surgical trainees: clinical outcomes and learning curve. Updat Surg. 2021;73(1):187–95. https://doi.org/10.1007/s13304-020-00950-z.

# Acute Left Colonic Diverticulitis

## 67

Massimo Sartelli

**Learning Goals**
- The author schematically presents the principles of diagnosis and treatment of acute left colonic diverticulitis.

## 67.1 Introduction

Acute colonic diverticulitis (ALCD) is one of the most common clinical conditions encountered by surgeons in the acute setting. The sigmoid colon is usually the most commonly involved part, while acute right-sided diverticulitis is rarer but much more common in non-Western populations. In 2020, the World Society of Emergency Surgery (WSES) updated guidelines for the management of acute colonic diverticulitis in the emergency setting [1].

## 67.2 Classifications

ALCD ranges in severity from uncomplicated phlegmonous diverticulitis to complicated diverticulitis including abscess and/or perforation.

For the past three decades, the Hinchey classification has been the most used classification in the international literature [2].

In patients with surgical findings of abscesses and peritonitis, Hinchey et al. classified the severity of acute diverticulitis into four levels:

1. Pericolic abscess
2. Pelvic, intra-abdominal, or retroperitoneal abscess
3. Generalized purulent peritonitis
4. Generalized fecal peritonitis

Computer tomography (CT) imaging has become a primary diagnostic tool in the diagnosis and staging of patients with ALCD, and more detailed information provided by CT scans led to several modifications of the Hinchey classification [3–5].

A proposal for a CT-guided classification of ALCD was published in 2015 by the WSES acute diverticulitis working group [6]. It is a simple classification system of ALCD based on CT scan findings. It may guide clinicians in the management of acute diverticulitis and may be universally accepted for day-to-day practice. The WSES classification divides acute diverticulitis into two groups: uncomplicated and complicated.

In the event of uncomplicated acute diverticulitis, the infection only involves the colon and does not extend to the peritoneum. In the event of complicated acute diverticulitis, the infectious process proceeds beyond the colon. Complicated acute diverticulitis is divided into four stages, based on the extension of the infectious process:

M. Sartelli (✉)
Department of Surgery, Macerata Hospital, Macerata, Italy

**Uncomplicated**

0. Diverticula, thickening of the wall, increased density of the pericolic fat

**Complicated**

1A. Pericolic air bubbles or small amount of pericolic fluid without abscess (within 5 cm from inflamed bowel segment)
   1B. Abscess ≤4 cm
   2A. Abscess >4 cm
   2B. Distant gas (>5 cm from inflamed bowel segment)
3. Diffuse fluid without distant free gas
4. Diffuse fluid with distant free gas

## 67.3 Diagnosis

Clinical findings of patients having ALCD include acute pain or tenderness in the left lower quadrant that may be associated with increased inflammatory markers, including C-reactive protein (CRP) and white blood cell count (WBC). CRP has been identified as a useful biomarker of inflammation, and it may be useful in the prediction of the clinical severity of acute diverticulitis as demonstrated by several studies [7]. Clinical diagnosis of ALCD usually lacks accuracy.

Radiological imaging techniques that are used for diagnosing ALCD in the emergency setting are US and CT. Currently, CT is the established method of choice when compared to US and most guidelines cite the high accuracy and other advantages of CT. This approach is the gold standard for both the diagnosis and the staging of patients with ALCD due to its excellent sensitivity and specificity [8]. CT scan can also rule out other diagnoses such as ovarian pathology, or leaking aortic or iliac aneurysm.

CT findings in patients with ALCD may include diverticulosis with associated colon wall thickening, fat stranding, phlegmon, extraluminal gas, abscess formation, or intra-abdominal free fluid. CT imaging can go beyond accurate diagnosis of ALCD. CT criteria may also be used to determine the grade of severity and may drive treatment planning of patients.

## 67.4 Treatment of Uncomplicated ALCD

The definition of uncomplicated ALCD is often vague and poorly defined. Uncomplicated acute diverticulitis is defined as localized diverticular inflammation without any abscess or perforation. A universally accepted classification divides intra-abdominal infections (IAIs) into complicated and uncomplicated [9]. In uncomplicated IAIs, the infection only involves a single organ and does not extend to the peritoneum, while in complicated IAIs, the infectious process extends beyond the organ, causing either localized or diffuse peritonitis [9]. For a better definition of ALCD, the term complicated and uncomplicated according to the classification of IAIs is used.

CT findings of uncomplicated acute diverticulitis include diverticula, thickening of the wall, and increased density of the pericolic fat (Fig. 67.1). Patients with uncomplicated diverticulitis usually have an indolent course with a low incidence of subsequent complications.

Historically, the treatment of uncomplicated ALCD consisted in antibiotics. In recent years, the utility of antibiotics in acute uncomplicated ALCD has been a point of controversy. Several studies demonstrated that antibiotic treatment was not superior to withholding antibiotic ther-

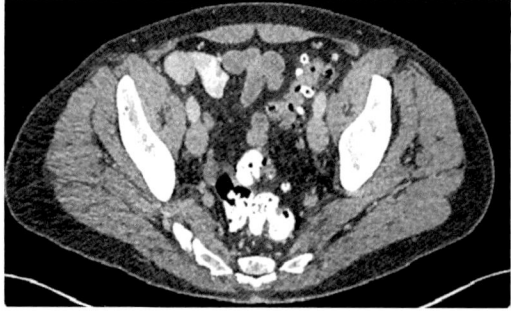

**Fig. 67.1** Slightly thickened sigmoid diverticular disease, without abscess or perforation

apy, in terms of clinical resolution, in patients with mild unperforated diverticulitis [10, 11]. The current consensus is that uncomplicated ALCD may be a self-limiting condition in which local host defenses can manage the inflammation without antibiotics in immunocompetent patients. In this context, antibiotics are not necessary in the treatment of uncomplicated disease in stable patients without serious comorbidities.

Patients with uncomplicated acute diverticulitis symptoms without significant comorbidities, who are able to take fluids orally and manage themselves at home, can be treated as outpatients. They should be re-evaluated within 7 days from the time of the diagnosis. However, if the clinical condition deteriorates, re-evaluation should be carried out earlier. Patients with significant comorbidities and unable to take fluids orally should be treated in hospital with intravenous fluids [1].

## 67.5 Treatment of Diverticular Abscess

Approximately 15–20% of patients admitted with acute diverticulitis have an abscess on CT scan [12] (Fig. 67.2).

The treatment of abscess always requires antibiotic therapy. If the abscess is limited in size, systemic antibiotic therapy alone is considered safe and effective in removing the abscess and solving acute inflammation.

When abscess diameter is larger, antibiotics could fail to reach the adequate concentration inside the abscess leading to an increased failure rate.

The size of 4–5 cm may be a reasonable limit between antibiotic treatment alone, versus percutaneous drainage combined with antibiotic treatment in the management of diverticular abscesses. When the patient's clinical conditions allow it and percutaneous drainage is not feasible, antibiotic therapy alone can be considered. However, careful clinical monitoring is mandatory. A high suspicion for surgical control of the septic source should be maintained and a surgical treatment should be performed if the patient shows a worsening of inflammatory signs or the abscess does not reduce with medical therapy [13–15].

## 67.6 Treatment of Diverticular Peritonitis

The treatment of patients with acute diffuse peritonitis includes three options:

- Laparoscopic peritoneal lavage and drainage
- Hartmann's procedure (HP)
- Primary resection with anastomosis with or without a diverting stoma

A minimally invasive approach using laparoscopic peritoneal lavage and drainage has been debated in recent years as an alternative to colonic resection mainly due to the discrepancy and sometime disappointing results of the latest prospective trials such as SCANDIV, Ladies, and DILALA trials [16–18].

Several controversies remain about laparoscopic lavage and drainage. It may be an acceptable alternative in patients with purulent peritonitis; however, it cannot be considered the first-line treatment in patients with diverticular peritonitis.

Hartmann procedure has been considered the procedure of choice in patients with generalized peritonitis and remains a safe technique for emergency colectomy in diverticular peritonitis, and is especially useful in critically ill patients and in

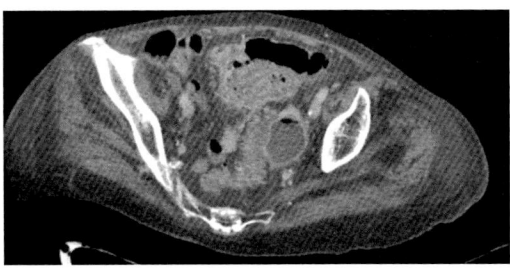

**Fig. 67.2** Sigmoid diverticulitis with associated abscess formation

patients with multiple comorbidities. However, restoration of bowel continuity after a HP is associated with significant morbidity and resource utilization [19]. As a result, many of these patients do not undergo reversal surgery and remain with a permanent stoma [20].

In recent years, some authors have reported the role of primary resection and anastomosis with or without a diverting stoma, in the treatment of acute diverticulitis, even in the presence of diffuse peritonitis. The decision regarding the surgical choice in patients with diffuse peritonitis is generally left to the judgment of the surgeon, who takes into account the clinical condition and the comorbidities of the patient. Studies comparing mortality and morbidity of the HP versus primary anastomosis did not show any significant differences [21, 22].

Laparoscopic sigmoidectomy for diverticulitis had initially been confined to the elective setting. However, in physiologically stable patients, laparoscopic sigmoidectomy may be feasible in the setting of purulent and fecal diverticular peritonitis, if technical skills and equipment are available.

## 67.7 Conclusions

ALCD can be categorized into uncomplicated and complicated disease. Uncomplicated ALCD involves thickening of the colon wall and pericolonic inflammatory changes. Complicated ALCD additionally includes the presence of abscess, peritonitis. The management of diverticulitis depends on the severity of presentation, presence of complications, and concomitant comorbid diseases as discussed in more detail in this chapter Antibiotics have been the mainstay of therapy, although recent studies indicate that select patients with uncomplicated diverticulitis can be safely managed without antibiotics. Patients with diverticular peritonitis require surgical intervention.

**Take-Home Messages**
- Computer tomography imaging has become a primary diagnostic tool in the diagnosis and staging of patients with ALCD.
- The treatment of abscess always requires antibiotic therapy. If the abscess is limited in size, systemic antibiotic therapy alone is considered safe and effective in removing the abscess and solving acute inflammation. When abscess diameter is larger, antibiotics could fail to reach the adequate concentration inside the abscess leading to an increased failure rate.
- The treatment of patients with acute diffuse peritonitis includes three options:
  - Laparoscopic peritoneal lavage and drainage
  - Hartmann's procedure (HP)
  - Primary resection with anastomosis with or without a diverting stoma

**Multiple Choice Questions**
1. Which is the treatment of choice for uncomplicated acute left colonic diverticulitis in patients without comorbidities and stable clinical conditions?
   A. **Clinical observation**
   B. Antibiotic therapy alone
   C. Hartmann's procedure
   D. Percutaneous drainage
2. Which is the treatment of choice for a diverticular abscess smaller than 4 cm in patients without comorbidities and in stable clinical conditions?
   A. Clinical observation
   B. **Antibiotic therapy alone**
   C. Hartmann's procedure
   D. Percutaneous drainage

3. Which is the treatment of choice for a diverticular abscess greater than 5 cm in patients without comorbidities and in stable clinical conditions?
   A. Clinical observation
   B. Antibiotic therapy alone
   C. Hartmann's procedure
   D. **Percutaneous drainage**
4. Which of these statements is correct about the laparoscopic peritoneal lavage and drainage?
   A. **It cannot be considered the first line treatment in patients with diverticular peritonitis**
   B. It can be considered the first line treatment in patients with diverticular peritonitis
   C. It is always recommended in all critically ill patients with acute diverticulitis
   D. It should never be used in patients with acute left colonic diverticulitis

# References

1. Sartelli M, Weber DG, Kluger Y, Ansaloni L, Coccolini F, Abu-Zidan F, et al. 2020 update of the WSES guidelines for the management of acute colonic diverticulitis in the emergency setting. World J Emerg Surg. 2020;15(1):32.
2. Hinchey EJ, Schaal PH, Richards MB. Treatment of perforated diverticular disease of the colon. Adv Surg. 1978;12:85–109.
3. Neff CC, van Sonnenberg E. CT of diverticulitis. Diagnosis and treatment. Radiol Clin N Am. 1989;27:743–52.
4. Ambrosetti P, Becker C, Terrier F. Colonic diverticulitis: impact of imaging on surgical management—a prospective study of 542 patients. Eur Radiol. 2002;12:1145–9.
5. Kaiser AM, Jiang JK, Lake JP, Ault G, Artinyan A, Gonzalez-Ruiz C, et al. The management of complicated diverticulitis and the role of computed tomography. Am J Gastroenterol. 2005;100:910–7.
6. Sartelli M, Catena F, Ansaloni L, Coccolini F, Griffiths EA, Abu-Zidan FM, et al. WSES guidelines for the management of acute left sided colonic diverticulitis in the emergency setting. World J Emerg Surg. 2016;11:37.
7. Mäkelä JT, Klintrup K, Takala H, Rautio T. The role of C-reactive protein in prediction of the severity of acute diverticulitis in an emergency unit. Scand J Gastroenterol. 2015;50:536–41.
8. Laméris W, van Randen A, Bipat S, Bossuyt PM, Boermeester MA, Stoker J. Graded compression ultrasonography and computed tomography in acute colonic diverticulitis: meta-analysis of test accuracy. Eur Radiol. 2008;18:2498–511.
9. Sartelli M, Chichom-Mefire A, Labricciosa FM, Hardcastle T, Abu-Zidan FM, Adesunkanmi AK, et al. The management of intra-abdominal infections from a global perspective: 2017 WSES guidelines for management of intra-abdominal infections. World J Emerg Surg. 2017;12(29). Erratum in: World J Emerg Surg. 2017;12:36.
10. Shabanzadeh DM, Wille-Jørgensen P. Antibiotics for uncomplicated diverticulitis. Cochrane Database Syst Rev. 2012;11:CD009092.
11. Chabok A, Påhlman L, Hjern F, Haapaniemi S, Smedh K, AVOD Study Group. Randomized clinical trial of antibiotics in acute uncomplicated diverticulitis. Br J Surg. 2012;99:532–9.
12. Andersen JC, Bundgaard L, Elbrønd H, Laurberg S, Walker LR, Støvring J, et al. Danish national guidelines for treatment of diverticular disease. Dan Med J. 2012;59:C4453.
13. Ambrosetti P, Chautems R, Soravia C, Peiris-Waser N, Terrier F. Long-term outcome of mesocolic and pelvic diverticular abscesses of the left colon: a prospective study of 73 cases. Dis Colon Rectum. 2005;48:787–91.
14. Brandt D, Gervaz P, Durmishi Y, Platon A, Morel P, Poletti PA. Percutaneous CT scan guided drainage versus antibiotherapy alone for Hinchey II diverticulitis: a case-control study. Dis Colon Rectum. 2006;49:1533–8.
15. Siewert B, Tye G, Kruskal J, Sosna J, Opelka F, Raptopoulos V, et al. Impact of CT-guided drainage in the treatment of diverticular abscesses: size matters. AJR. 2006;186:680–6.
16. Angenete E, Thornell A, Burcharth J, Pommergaard HC, Skullman S, Bisgaard T, et al. Laparoscopic lavage is feasible and safe for the treatment of perforated diverticulitis with purulent peritonitis: the first results from the randomized controlled trial DILALA. Ann Surg. 2016;263:117–22.
17. Schultz JK, Yaqub S, Wallon C, Blecic L, Forsmo HM, Folkesson J, et al. Laparoscopic lavage vs primary resection for acute perforated diverticulitis: the SCANDIV randomized clinical trial. JAMA. 2015;314:1364–75.
18. Vennix S, Musters GD, Mulder IM, Swank HA, Consten EC, Belgers EH, et al. Laparoscopic peritoneal lavage or sigmoidectomy for perforated diver-

ticulitis with purulent peritonitis: a multicentre, parallel-group, randomised, open-label trial. Lancet. 2015;386(10000):1269–77.
19. McCafferty MH, Roth L, Jorden J. Current management of diverticulitis. Am Surg. 2008;74:1041–9.
20. Fleming FJ, Gillen P. Reversal of Hartmann's procedure following acute diverticulitis: is timing everything? Int J Color Dis. 2009;24:1219–25.
21. Cirocchi R, Trastulli S, Desiderio J, Listorti C, Boselli C, Parisi A, et al. Treatment of Hinchey stage III-IV diverticulitis: a systematic review and meta-analysis. Int J Color Dis. 2013;28:447–57.
22. Lee JM, Bai P, Chang J, El Hechi M, Kongkaewpaisan N, Bonde A, et al. Hartmann's procedure vs primary anastomosis with diverting loop ileostomy for acute diverticulitis: nationwide analysis of 2,729 emergency surgery patients. J Am Coll Surg. 2019;229:48–55.

# Acute Mesenteric Ischemia

## 68

Miklosh Bala and Asaf Kedar

## 68.1 Introduction

Acute mesenteric ischemia (AMI) is an infrequent disorder defined as the sudden interruption of the blood supply to the intestine. If left untreated, it will lead to complications and irreversible changes such as necrosis of the intestinal wall and death [1–3]. It is defined as occlusive and nonocclusive types of acute ischemia of the bowel. Occlusive causes of acute mesenteric ischemia include mesenteric artery embolism (50% of cases), mesenteric artery thrombosis (15–25%), and superior mesenteric vein thrombosis (MVT; 5–15%) [4, 5]. Nonocclusive causes of bowel ischemia (NOMI) are more common in elderly and critically ill and thus have worth prognosis. Nonspecific clinical presentation of patients with AMI deters the diagnostic process, often resulting in delays and late therapeutic intervention [6].

Most publications in the available literature regarding the management of AMI are reviews and retrospective case series [4–10]. This chapter is aimed at presenting strategies for the management of AMI based on an analysis of a variety of modern diagnostics and treatments and identifying risk factors that can be used to improve outcomes and simplify decision making during daily clinical practice.

> **Learning Goals**
> - Acute mesenteric ischemia is caused by arterial insufficiency or venous obstruction.
> - The diagnosis is made most reliably with computed tomography (CT) angiography or surgery.
> - In the absence of peritonitis, minimally invasive treatment options can be considered.

### 68.1.1 Epidemiology

AMI only applies to approximately 1% of all patients with an "acute abdomen," its incidence is significantly rising in patients >70 years of age [1]. Nevertheless, younger people who have atrial fibrillation or risk factors for MVT, such as oral contraceptive use or hypercoagulable states, may present with AMI. Various risk factors, among them advanced age, heart failure, atrial fibrillation, coronary heart disease especially recent acute coronary syndrome, arterial hypertension, peripheral vascular disease and intra-abdominal malignancy should be considered for AMI [4, 6, 11, 12].

M. Bala (✉) · A. Kedar
Trauma and Acute Care Surgery Unit,
Hadassah—Hebrew University Medical Center,
Jerusalem, Israel
e-mail: rbalam@hadassah.org.il;
asafk@hadassah.org.il

© The Author(s), under exclusive license to Springer Nature Switzerland AG 2023
F. Coccolini, F. Catena (eds.), *Textbook of Emergency General Surgery*,
https://doi.org/10.1007/978-3-031-22599-4_68

## 68.1.2 Etiology and Classification

AMI refers to the sudden onset of small intestinal hypoperfusion due to factors such as mesenteric arterial embolism (50%), mesenteric arterial thrombosis (15–25%), or mesenteric venous thrombosis (5–15%). A separate type of a functional, nonocclusive mesenteric ischemia (NOMI) can occur in low-flow situations, for example following cardiac surgery or during dialysis (12–20%) [13].

There has been a substantial change in the etiology of AMI. There is a remarkable increase in the proportion of arterial thrombosis, which became the main cause of AMI in recent years. The reduction in mesenteric arterial embolisms could be related to better treatment of atrial fibrillation with modern anticoagulant therapies [14].

NOMI continued to be a diagnostic dilemma, poorly reported [15]. Patients with this diagnosis could have been placed in the unclear or "poorly classified" etiology group.

## 68.1.3 Pathophysiology

AMI is a time-critical emergency resulting in irreversible hypoperfusion of the mesenteric organs within a few hours, leading to a high mortality rate. The large diameter and narrow take-off angle of the superior mesenteric artery (SMA) contribute to its anatomical susceptibility to occlusion. Collateralization between the celiac and inferior mesenteric arteries protected against an acute occlusion of their main trunks.

An acute complete circulatory interruption of the intestine leads to irreversible mucosal ischemia within 6 h [16]. The collapse of the mucosal barrier leads to bacterial translocation resulting peritonitis, ileus, sepsis, and multiorgan failure.

## 68.2 Diagnosis

### 68.2.1 Clinical Presentation

AMI tends to occur in older patients (age >60 years) with the exception of MVT which is seen in patients in their forties. It is classically taught that patients with AMI present with abdominal pain that is out of proportion to the physical exam (due to the lack of initial peritoneal signs). The abdominal findings vary during the course of the illness when the patient is examined. Anything from normal findings to general peritonitis may be found. When peritonitis is established, tenderness with muscular guarding and a lack of bowel sounds due to paralysis are found. The onset of pain varies with the etiology of the AMI; typically both emboli and thrombosis present in an acute setting. NOMI is more of a slowly progressive process, while MVT can fall in either category. Patients also commonly present with nausea, vomiting, diarrhea, and abdominal distention (this last is often late finding). Hematochezia is another potential presentation of AMI.

Because of the nonspecific physical exam findings associated with AMI, clinicians should take a detailed history. A past medical history of previous embolic events or recent myocardial infarction would be concerning for emboli, while a long history of atherosclerotic disease is more indicative of thrombosis.

### 68.2.2 Tests

If classic clinical triad of symptoms was found (severe periumbilical pain, vomiting and possible embolic source), other tests can support the diagnosis but should not delay treatment.

#### 68.2.2.1 Laboratory Diagnosis

The elevated leukocyte count can be found early and together with the clinical triad is pathognomonic for AMI. Values above normal for serum lactate and D-dimer have also been suggested as prognostic markers for patients who need surgery. D-dimer is elevated early in the course of AMI, although the magnitude of elevation does not correlate with severity [6]. The specificity of lactic acid, leukocytosis, and elevated amylase is rather low (around 40%). Metabolic acidosis also occurs late in the course of the disease, and as a diagnostic test it has no value. The acid-base balance as well as lactic acid, however, needs to be monitored and corrected continuously during the course of treatment.

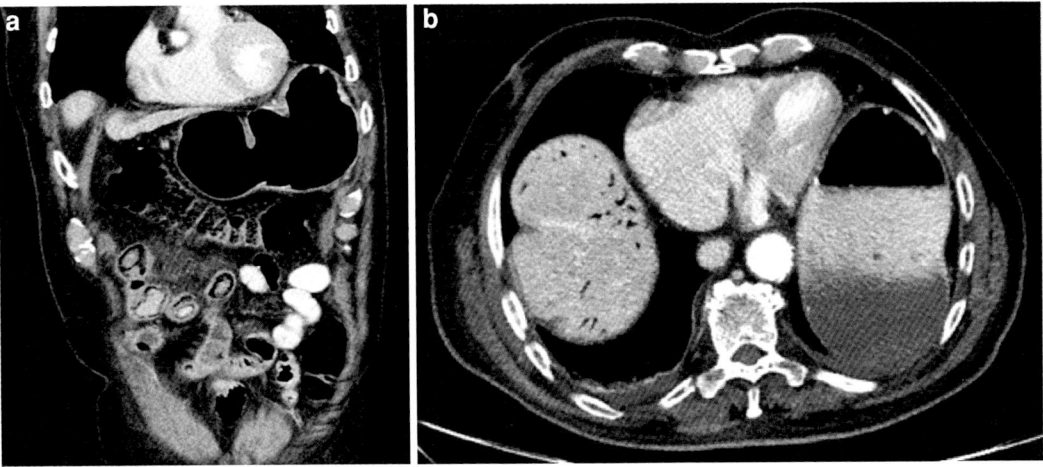

**Fig. 68.1** Contrast-enhanced abdominal CT scans show nonocclusive mesenteric ischemia with bowel wall thickening and pneumatosis intestinalis (**a**). Portal vein gas (**b**). Transmural necrosis was found at pathologic analysis after extensive resection

Potential biomarkers reported to assist in the diagnosis of AMI include intestinal fatty acid binding protein (I-FABP), serum alpha-glutathione S-transferase (alpha-GST), and cobalt-albumin binding assay (CABA) [17–19]. Further research is required to specify their potential use in the future [20, 21].

### 68.2.3 Imaging Techniques

The only radiologic examination that is warranted is computed tomography angiography (CTA). Both angiography and especially plain films have limited value. The resources and expertise available in the hospital should also influence the decision of whether any advanced investigations or tests are performed.

CTA is the gold standard and preferred imaging technique with high sensitivity and specificity. If there is any suspicion of AMI, biphasic contrast-enhanced CT with three dimensional multiplanar reconstruction is the diagnostic tool of choice [22]. In this protocol, there is no need for oral contrast because it does not improve the imaging of intestinal wall but rather contribute to the loss of time during diagnostics. The sensitivity and specificity of multiplanar reconstruction CT are 93% and 100%, respectively; its positive and negative predictive values are between 94% and 100% [23, 24].

CT findings for AMI include SMA or SMV occlusions, intestinal pneumatosis, portal venous gas, lack of bowel-wall enhancement, and ischemia of other organs; less specific findings include distended bowel, thickened bowel wall, mesenteric fat stranding, and ascites, pneumoperitoneum (Fig. 68.1).

Fear of contrast-induced kidney injury should not be a contraindication to contrast use when managing potentially life-threatening conditions such as AMI. Intravenous (IV) hydration is recommended for patients at risk of contrast-induced kidney injury, also hydration is an essential part of AMI management.

Ultrasound is less sensitive than CT, but can be done if MVT is the suspected etiology or CT is contraindicated. MRI is not considered first line for an emergent condition like AMI.

## 68.3 Treatment

The spectrum of AMI is broad, and each type of ischemic injury requires its unique management plan. Most treatment challenges developed on the basis of clinical experience and descriptive studies, not on randomized controlled trials. Progress in imaging and critical care leads to improve survival of this group of surgical critical patients. Clinical aspects of different types of AMI are summarized in Table 68.1 and discussed below.

## 68.3.1 Therapeutic Approaches

The type of therapy needs to be fits with the radiologic findings and the patients' clinical status. Emergency surgery is necessitated for unstable patients and those with signs of peritonitis and obvious signs of intestinal ischemia [11]. If there are no signs of peritonitis or intestinal gangrene, systemic or interventional pharmacotherapy with local fibrinolysis may be considered. The intensive care management includes volume replacement, systemic anticoagulation and antibiotic therapy, as well as close patient monitoring to rule out secondary organ failure. Nonsurgical management should be considered only in specialized centers where operating theater is immediately available.

## 68.3.2 Surgical Options

Clinical signs of peritonitis, any evidence of intestinal gangrene, or failure of endovascular options require an immediate surgical treatment [25]. The goal of surgical treatment is to obtain arterial reperfusion, perform intestinal resection when obviously necrotic bowel was found and provide aggressive resuscitation in order to restore normal physiology. Therefore, surgeon either needs to be trained in vascular surgery techniques of embolectomy and reconstruction of visceral arteries or a vascular surgeon have to be consulted [2, 6, 25]. The damage of the mucosal layer in many cases is much greater than estimated. The underestimation of an ischemic segment that might lead to an anastomotic breakdown further contributes to a high morbidity and mortality [26]. Bowel segments with an "uncertain" reperfusion require a scheduled "second-look" operation usually after 24 h. In case of unavoidable major bowel resections, critical residual length limits must be kept in mind [26]. In elderly comorbid patients with AMI, surgical exploration often comes too late, and palliative care has to be considered [27].

### 68.3.2.1 Surgical Approach to the Superior Mesenteric Artery (SMA)

The SMA is approached in its infra-duodenal, intra-mesenteric portion. The mesocolon is retracted up, while the first jejunal loop is pulled down and to the left and the peritoneum can be incised along the cord. Caution required not to injure the jejunal blanches that take off from the SMA to expose the necessary length of SMA. Once the arterial network is controlled, intra-venous heparin (usually 50 IU/kg) is administered. Embolectomy with Fogarty catheter performed via transverse arteriotomy. After the restoration of blood flow, the SMA repaired primarily or using vein patch.

### 68.3.2.2 SMA Grafting

There are a variety of bypass procedures, providing either antegrade or retrograde flow, with vein (preferably) or synthetic grafts. An antegrade bypass from supraceliac aorta to superior mesenteric trunk is a surgery of choice. However, the most practical option for proximal mesenteric atherosclerotic occlusive disease is a retrograde bypass from common iliac with a vein or synthetic graft (Fig. 68.2).

### 68.3.2.3 Retrograde Stenting in Case of Atheromatous Ostial Disease

Optimal revascularization of the SMA can require retrograde stenting in patients with atheromatous lesions [28]. In this case, the collateral branches of the SMA are identified and looped with vascular tapes. The artery is punctured, and the introducer is inserted, a stiff guide is passed through the obstructing lesion after previous dilation by a small size balloon (3–4 mm). The size of the stent is chosen according to the diameter of the vessel. The flared end is inserted into the aorta, to ensure the best hemodynamics. Arteriography is performed to control the efficacy of the stent placement. This ROMS (Retrograde Open Mesenteric Stenting) technique, first described in

**Table 68.1** Clinical features of acute mesenteric ischemia

| Cause of AMI | Incidence, % | Risk factors | Clinical presentation | Medical therapy | Surgical therapy | Prognosis |
|---|---|---|---|---|---|---|
| Arterial embolism | 40–50 | Recent MI Atrial fibrillation Cardiac thrombi Left ventricular aneurysm Endocarditis Previous embolic disease | The sudden onset of severe pain with spontaneous emptying of the bowel (vomiting and diarrhea) but no significant abdominal physical findings | Fluid resuscitation Heparin 50 U/kg bolus followed by 15 U/kg/h infusion | Laparotomy followed by embolectomy. Bypass if embolectomy fails. Excise dead bowel endovascular treatments, including thrombectomy, thrombolysis, and/or angioplasty and stenting can be considered alongside surgical therapy. Second-look operation should be done between 24 and 48 h after initial procedure | Poor especially in lately diagnosed |
| Arterial thrombosis | 25 | Diffuse atherosclerotic disease Post-pradial pain Weight loss Type B aortic dissection | Prodromal symptoms of mesenteric angina (postprandial abdominal pain, nausea and weight loss) before the acute episode. History of other Vascular events and previous vascular surgery | Fluid resuscitation Heparin 50 U/kg bolus followed by 15 U/kg/h infusion Thrombolytic infusion can be considered if patient has been symptomatic for <8 h | Laparotomy followed by bypass. Excise dead bowel Endarterectomy if bypass is not an option. Endovascular treatments, including thrombectomy, thrombolysis, and/or angioplasty and stenting can be considered alongside surgical therapy. Second-look operation should be done between 24 and 48 h after initial procedure | Poor especially in lately diagnosed |
| NOMI | 20 | Cardiac failure Low flow states Multi-organ dysfunction Vasopressors | Patients with circulatory shock or vasoactive drugs (including amines, cocaine and digitalis) when there is a significant unexpected deterioration in their clinical course. Abdominal pain, bloating, abdominal distension and the presence of occult blood in the stool. | Fluid resuscitation Avoid vasopressors Vasodilators can be used. Papaverine infusion 60 mg/h selectively in the superior mesenteric artery | laparotomy when clinically warrant Excise dead bowel Second-look operation should be done between 24 and 48 h after initial procedure | Very high mortality |

(continued)

**Table 68.1** (continued)

| Cause of AMI | Incidence, % | Risk factors | Clinical presentation | Medical therapy | Surgical therapy | Prognosis |
|---|---|---|---|---|---|---|
| Venous thrombosis | 10 | Thrombophilia History of VTE Oral contraceptives Estrogen use Portal hypertension pancreatitis | Subacute abdominal pain, nausea and vomiting. Although bloating, abdominal distension, fever and occult blood in stool | Heparin 50 U/kg bolus followed by 15 U/kg/h infusion. Heparin monitoring should be performed by trending aPTT TIPS with directed thrombectomy and thrombolysis in very select cases that are refractory to anticoagulation | Laparotomy in very select cases | Good outcome in early diagnosed cases |

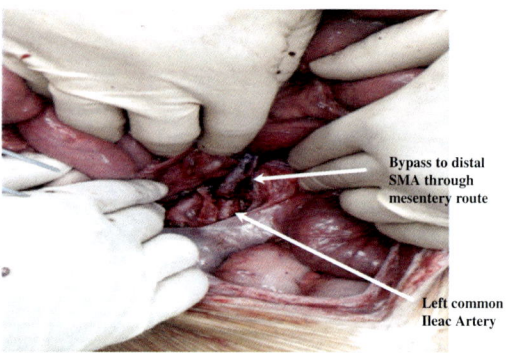

**Fig. 68.2** Patient with acute thrombosis of SMA underwent left ileo–SMA bypass with a common femoral vein graft

2004, should avoid the need for prosthetic bypass material in a potentially septic setting.

Several reports demonstrate its technical success and good long-term results [1–3, 8, 29, 30]. Hybrid operating theater is an ideal option to perform ROMS.

### 68.3.3 Endovascular Techniques

Currently, endovascular techniques for mesenteric arterial occlusion appear to be much more common in cases without clinical signs of peritonitis. Endovascular techniques can be considered for the diagnosis and treatment of AMI. The therapeutic endovascular approach consists of angiographic catheter aspiration, embolectomy and catheter lysis with recombinant tissue plasminogen activator, urokinase, or pharmacotherapy with prostaglandin E1 [31]. The aim is to reopen the main arterial branches of the SMA to allow the remaining occluded segments of intestine to be perfused [1]. In combination with surgery, this also allows retrograde catheterization to obtain access to the central segment [32].

The study of Arthurs et al. [33] represents the largest (70 patients) series of AMI treated with endovascular therapy in one center. The primary technique was thrombolysis infusion, which was used in 48% of the population. Thirty-two percent of patients were treated with primary Percutaneous transluminal angioplasty (PTA) and stenting. Successful endovascular treatment was achieved in 87% of cases, and the mortality rate was 36%, compared with 50% in patients treated with traditional therapy.

Intravascular intervention is controversial due to lack of intestinal viability assessment through direct inspection, such as during laparotomy is absolutely crucial. Intravascular intervention may be a therapeutic alternative for patients with early-stage illness without the characteristics of peritonitis on physical examination. Another perspective option for this narrow group is hybrid therapy combined with exploratory laparoscopy for assessing intra-abdominal ischemia.

## 68.4 Diagnosis and Treatment of NOMI

NOMI is the most lethal form of AMI [34]. Its prevalence is highly dependent on the population studied and ranges from 6% to 47% of all cases of AMI [35]. Low-flow states activate the renin-angiotensin-aldosterone system and cause splanchnic vasoconstriction and SMA resistance, which further decreases mesenteric blood flow. The vasospasm may be reversed if the decrease in flow is rapidly corrected.

Clinical examination in those patients is challenging: they often are intubated and sedated. Abdominal distension, new signs of sepsis, and increased inflammatory parameters need to be considered as suspected for NOMI. Lactate serum levels are frequently increased after surgery with extracorporeal circulation; therefore, increased levels are no proof of mesenteric ischemia but can serve as an additional parameter [36–38]. Contrast-enhanced CT plays an essential role for the diagnosis and differential diagnoses of NOMI. Bowel wall enhancement is an early and suggestive feature in NOMI, while mesenteric artery is narrowed, but not occluded.

Management of NOMI is based on the treatment of the underlying cause. Fluid resuscitation, optimization of cardiac output, and elimination of vasopressors remain important primary measures that greatly impact outcome. Additional treatment may include systemic anticoagulation and the use of angiography-directed infusion of vasodilatory agents, most commonly papaverine hydrochloride [39].

Unstable patients or those with high suspicion of intestinal gangrene require immediate surgery with abdominal exploration and resection of irreversibly damaged ischemic segments. A "second look" operation should be performed if there is any doubt about the remaining intestinal perfusion.

### 68.4.1 Mesenteric Venous Thrombosis (MVT)

MVT can lead to irreversible damage to the intestinal wall. However, an isolated thrombosis of the superior mesenteric vein can be compensated by collateral flow. In contrast, an additional complete thrombosis of the portal vein is associated with venous infarction of small bowel segments [40, 41]. Clinical symptoms are mostly less specific and depend on the extent of thrombosis.

The biphasic contrast-enhanced CT is the imaging of choice for venous thrombosis, revealing thickened intestinal wall, and ascites at the same time (Fig. 68.3). Patients with peritonitis

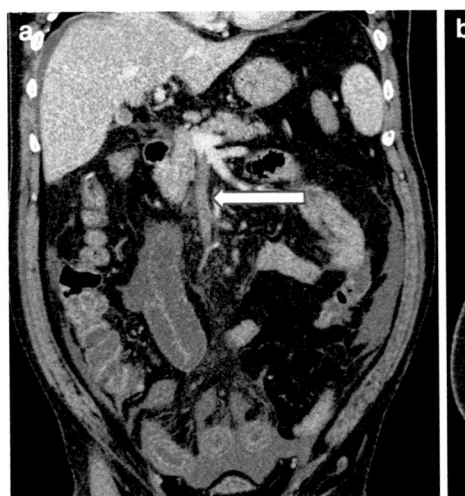 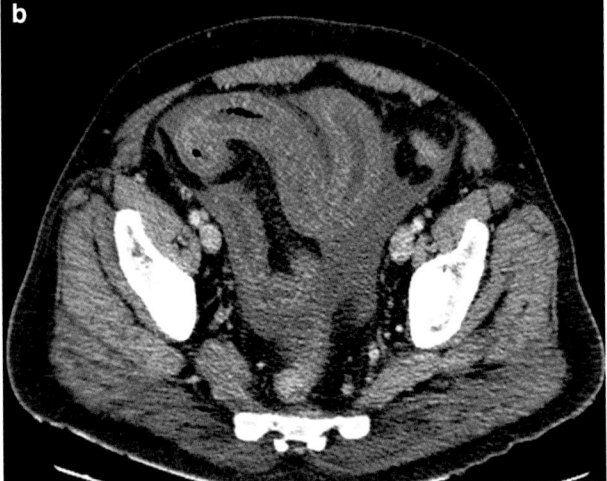

**Fig. 68.3** A 50-year-old male with acute superior mesenteric vein thrombosis (**a**, arrow) and thickened bowel loops and ascites (**b**) due to hypercoagulable state. The patient presented with diffuse peritonitis, resection of 1.2 m of distal ileum performed. Long-term anticoagulation required at postoperative course

require emergency surgery with exploration and resection of infarcted segments. A second-look operation is recommended in patients who show extensive bowel involvement at primary exploration.

The first-line treatment for mesenteric venous thrombosis is anticoagulation. Supportive measures include nasogastric suction, fluid resuscitation, and bowel rest.

The treatment of choice in stable patients without signs of peritonitis is the recanalization via a transjugular transhepatic access, with or without transjugular intrahepatic portosystemic shunt (TIPS) placement [26, 27]. In case of additional involvement of the portal vein, endovascular recanalization is recommended even in clinically compensated patients.

### Take-Home Messages
- Acute mesenteric ischemia (AMI) is a life-threatening condition. Early recognition and treatment are critical for survival.
- CTA is a study of choice for all types of AMI to help determine medical/surgical approaches.
- After diagnosis, initial treatment with anticoagulation, fluid resuscitation, and revascularization is paramount.
- Early laparotomy should be done for patients with overt peritonitis. Planned re-laparotomy is an essential part of AMI management.
- Endovascular therapy is a viable alternative to open surgery in selected cases.

### Dos and Don'ts
- AMI should be suspected in patients with acute abdominal pain disproportional to the physical examination findings and a history of cardiovascular comorbidities.
- In cases of suspected AMI, multidetector computed tomography (MDCT) with intravenous contrast, but not with oral contrast, should be performed immediately.
- Do not start resuscitation with vasopressor drugs in AMI.
- Patients with AMI and signs of peritonitis should undergo immediate surgery.
- When bowel has not been compromised, endovascular techniques should be performed for AMI.
- Anastomosis should be avoided in patients with septic shock or multiple organ failure.
- Anticoagulants and antiplatelets therapy should be started early and continue after recovery.

### Multiple Choice Questions
1. The 72-year-old male brought to the emergency department due to fever, abdominal pain and rectal bleeding. Colonoscopy—Ischemic changes in the mucosa of the colon (splenic flexure) without necrosis. No bleeding. In the background: CABG 5 years ago. What treatment is recommended at this stage?
   A. Angiography with papaverine injection
   B. Left hemicolecomy
   C. Thrombectomy from IMA
   D. Symptomatic treatment and administration of antibiotics
2. The 74-year-old female was referred to the emergency department with severe abdominal pain (started 2 h ago). Preamble, without diarrhea, vomiting or nausea. Yesterday had normal bowel movement. Vitals: 37 °C, BP 140/80, HR 110. Abdomen soft, distended, without peritoneal signs, decreased peristaltic sounds.

Lab: NA 144 mmol/L, CRE 1.3 g/dL, LAC AC 7 mmol/L, HG 13.4, WBC 12,000.

What is the next step in the diagnosis?
A. D-dimer
B. Abdominal X-ray
C. Laparotomy
D. CTA

3. What is the most common cause of an AMI in young patients:
A. Arterial thrombosis
B. Mesenteric venous thrombosis
C. Arteritis
D. Traumatic injury

4. The 82-year-old male was admitted to the emergency department due to severe abdominal pain for several hours. Background: NIDDM, CAD, AF. A month ago he had peptic ulcer bleeding—anticoagulation was stopped.
Fever 37.7 °C, BP 146/80, HR 118 irregular. Abdominal examination—diffuse rigidity (Peritonotis).
What is the next step in treating this patient?
A. IV fluids + labs + administration of antibiotics
B. IV PPI due to ulcer perforation
C. IV MORPHINE for comfort care
D. Endovascular intervention required initially

5. You were called to medical intensive care unit to check a patient who was hospitalized 3 days ago due to cardiac event. He complained of abdominal pain and bloating. He is currently intubated, responding to pain. BP 80/60, HR 70, receiving Noraderenaline and Heparine.
On examination the abdomen is distended, sensitive for palpation in the RLQ.
What is the most likely diagnosis?
A. Gastritis due to ASA treatment
B. Mesenteric vein thrombosis
C. NOMI
D. Abdominal compartment syndrome

**Answers**: 1-D; 2-D; 3-B; 4-A; 5-C

## References

1. Newton WB 3rd, Sagransky MJ, Andrews JS, Hansen KJ, Corriere MA, Goodney PP, Edwards MS. Outcomes of revascularized acute mesenteric ischemia in the American College of Surgeons National Surgical Quality Improvement Program database. Am Surg. 2011;77(7):832–8.
2. Schermerhorn ML, Giles KA, Hamdan AD, Wyers MC, Pomposelli FB. Mesenteric revascularization: management and outcomes in the United States. 1998-2006. J Vasc Surg. 2009;50(2):341–8.
3. Eslami MH, Rybin D, Doros G, McPhee JT, Farber A. Mortality of acute mesenteric ischemia remains unchanged despite significant increase in utilization of endovascular techniques. Vascular. 2016;24(1):44–52.
4. Acosta S. Mesenteric ischemia. Curr Opin Crit Care. 2015;21(2):171–8.
5. Clair DG, Beach JM. Mesenteric ischemia. N Engl J Med. 2016;374(10):959–68.
6. Bala M, Kashuk J, Moore EE, Kluger Y, Biffl W, Gomes CA, Ben-Ishay O, Rubinstein C, Balogh ZJ, Civil I, Coccolini F, Leppaniemi A, Peitzman A, Ansaloni L, Sugrue M, Sartelli M, Di Saverio S, Fraga GP, Catena F. Acute mesenteric ischemia: guidelines of the World Society of Emergency Surgery. World J Emerg Surg. 2017;12:38.
7. Huang HH, Chang YC, Yen DH, Kao WF, Chen JD, Wang LM, Huang CI, Lee CH. Clinical factors and outcomes in patients with acute mesenteric ischemia in the emergency department. J Chin Med Assoc. 2005;68(7):299–306.
8. Kougias K, Lau D, El Sayed FH, Zhou W, Huynh TT, Lin PH. Determinants of mortality and treatment outcome following surgical interventions for acute mesenteric ischemia. J Vasc Surg. 2007;46(3):467–74.
9. Alhan E, Usta A, Çekiç A, Saglam K, Türkyılmaz S, Cinel A. A study on 107 patients with acute mesenteric ischemia over 30 years. Int J Surg. 2012;10(9):510–3.
10. Yıldırım D, Hut A, Tatar C, Dönmez T, Akıncı M, Toptaş M. Prognostic factors in patients with acute mesenteric ischemia. Turk J Surg. 2017;33(2):104–9.
11. Klar E, Rahmanian PB, Bücker A, Hauenstein K, Jauch KW, Luther B. Acute mesenteric ischemia: a vascular emergency. Dtsch Arztebl Int. 2012;109(14):249–56.

12. Luther B, Mamopoulos A, Lehmann C, Klar E. The ongoing challenge of acute mesenteric ischemia. Visc Med. 2018;34(3):217–23.
13. Sise MJ. Mesenteric ischemia: the whole spectrum. Scand J Surg. 2010;99:106–10.
14. Liew A, O'Donnell M, Douketis J. Comparing mortality in patients with atrial fibrillation who are receiving a direct-acting oral anticoagulant or warfarin: a meta-analysis of randomized trials. J Thromb Haemost. 2014;12:1419–24.
15. Acosta-Mérida MA, Marchena-Gómez J, Saavedra-Santana P, Silvestre-Rodríguez J, Artiles-Armas M, Callejón-Cara MM. Surgical outcomes in acute mesenteric ischemia: has anything changed over the years? World J Surg. 2020;44(1):100–7.
16. Udassin R, Vromen A, Haskel Y. The time sequence of injury and recovery following transient reversible intestinal ischemia. J Surg Res. 1994;56(3):221–5.
17. Nuzzo A, Maggiori L, Ronot M, Becq A, Plessier A, Gault N, Joly F, Castier Y, Vilgrain V, Paugam C, Panis Y, Bouhnik Y, Cazals-Hatem D, Corcos O. Predictive factors of intestinal necrosis in acute mesenteric ischemia: prospective study from an intestinal stroke center. Am J Gastroenterol. 2017;112:597–605.
18. Block T, Nilsson TK, Björck M, Acosta S. Diagnostic accuracy of plasma biomarkers for intestinal ischaemia. Scand J Clin Lab Invest. 2008;68:242–8.
19. Kashuk JL, Moore EE, Sabel A, Barnett C, Haenel J, Le T, Pezold M, Lawrence J, Biffl WL, Cothren CC, Johnson JL. Rapid thrombelastography (r-TEG) identifies hypercoagulability and predicts thromboembolic events in surgical patients. Surgery. 2009;146:764–72.
20. Matsumoto S, Sekine K, Funaoka H, Yamazaki M, Shimizu M, Hayashida K, Kitano M. Diagnostic performance of plasma biomarkers in patients with acute intestinal ischaemia. Br J Surg. 2014;101:232–8.
21. Treskes N, Persoon AM, van Zanten ARH. Diagnostic accuracy of novel serological biomarkers to detect acute mesenteric ischemia: a systematic review and meta-analysis. Intern Emerg Med. 2017;12:821–36.
22. Kanasaki S, Furukawa A, Fumoto K, Hamanaka Y, Ota S, Hirose T, Inoue A, Shirakawa T, Hung Nguyen LD, Tulyeubai S. Acute mesenteric ischemia: multidetector CT findings and endovascular management. Radiographics. 2018;38(3):945–61.
23. Aschoff AJ, Stuber G, Becker BW, Hoffmann MH, Schmitz BL, Schelzig H, Jaeckle T. Evaluation of acute mesenteric ischemia: accuracy of biphasic mesenteric multi-detector CT angiography. Abdom Imaging. 2009;34(3):345–57.
24. Yang H, Wang BL. Evaluation of the diagnostic value of multi-slice spiral CT in acute mesenteric ischemic diseases: a meta-analysis of randomized controlled trials. Eur Rev Med Pharmacol Sci. 2019;23(23):10218–25.
25. Duran M, Pohl E, Grabitz K, Schelzig H, Sagban TA, Simon F. The importance of open emergency surgery in the treatment of acute mesenteric ischemia. World J Emerg Surg. 2015;10(1):45.
26. Kesseli S, Sudan D. Small bowel transplantation. Surg Clin North Am. 2019;99(1):103–16.
27. Ritz JP, Germer CT, Buhr HJ. Prognostic factors for mesenteric infarction: multivariate analysis of 187 patients with regard to patient age. Ann Vasc Surg. 2005;19(3):328–34.
28. Blauw JTM, Meerwaldt R, Brusse-Keizer M, Kolkman JJ, Gerrits D, Geelkerken RH. Retrograde open mesenteric stenting for acute mesenteric ischemia. J Vasc Surg. 2014;60:726–34.
29. Milner R, Woo EY, Carpenter JP. Superior mesenteric artery angioplasty and stenting via a retrograde approach in a patient with bowel ischaemia, a case report. J Vasc Surg. 2007;45:269–75.
30. Roussel A, Della Schiava N, Coscas R, et al. Results of retrograde open mesenteric stenting for acute thrombotic mesenteric ischemia. J Vasc Surg. 2019;69:1137–42.
31. Schoots IG, Levi MM, Reekers JA, Lameris JS, van Gulik TM. Thrombolytic therapy for acute superior mesenteric artery occlusion. J Vasc Interv Radiol. 2005;16(3):317–29.
32. Pisimisis GT, Oderich GS. Technique of hybrid retrograde superior mesenteric artery stent placement for acute-on-chronic mesenteric ischemia. Ann Vasc Surg. 2011;25(1):132.e7–11.
33. Arthurs ZM, Titus J, Bannazadeh M, Eagleton MJ, Srivastava S, Sarac TP, Clair DG. A comparison of endovascular revascularization with traditional therapy for the treatment of acute mesenteric ischemia. J Vasc Surg. 2011;53:698–704.
34. Schoots IG, Koffeman GI, Legemate DA, Levi M, van Gulik TM. Systematic review of survival after acute mesenteric ischaemia according to disease aetiology. Br J Surg. 2004;91:17–27.
35. Garzelli L, Nuzzo A, Copin P, Calame P, Corcos O, Vilgrain V, Ronot M. Contrast-enhanced CT for the diagnosis of acute mesenteric ischemia. AJR Am J Roentgenol. 2020;215(1):29–38.
36. Björck M, Wanhainen A. Nonocclusive mesenteric hypoperfusion syndromes: recognition and treatment. Semin Vasc Surg. 2010;23(1):54–64.
37. Miyazawa R, Kamo M. What affects the prognosis of NOMI patients? Analysis of clinical data and CT findings. Surg Endosc. 2019; https://doi.org/10.1007/s00464-019-07321-9. Epub ahead of print.
38. Mangi AA, Christison-Lagay ER, Torchiana DF, Warshaw AL, Berger DL. Gastrointestinal complications in patients undergoing heart operation: an analysis of 8709 consecutive cardiac surgical patients. Ann Surg. 2005;241(6):895–901.
39. Meilahn JE, Morris JB, Ceppa EP, Bulkley GB. Effect of prolonged selective intramesenteric arterial vasodilator therapy on intestinal viability after acute segmental mesenteric vascular occlusion. Ann Surg. 2001;234:107–15.
40. Harnik IG, Brandt LJ. Mesenteric venous thrombosis. Vasc Med. 2010;15(5):407–18.
41. Intagliata NM, Caldwell SH, Tripodi A. Diagnosis, development, and treatment of portal vein thrombosis in patients with and without cirrhosis. Gastroenterology. 2019;156(6):1582–1599.e1.

# Upper Gastrointestinal Bleeding

**69**

Helmut A. Segovia Lohse
and Herald R. Segovia Lohse

## 69.1 Introduction

Upper gastrointestinal bleeding (UGIB) is a potentially life-threatening emergency that remains a common cause of hospitalization around the world. It is defined as bleeding arising from the esophagus, stomach, or duodenum. Patients commonly present with hematemesis and/or melena. Almost all patients who develop acute UGIB are treated in hospital, and this chapter therefore focuses on hospital care.

> **Learning Goals**
> - Know the clinical presentation and treatment options of the upper gastrointestinal bleeding.
> - Apply the best strategy to make the prompt diagnosis, resuscitation, and adequate treatment options in an upper gastrointestinal bleeding.
> - Recognize the upper gastrointestinal bleeding as a potential life-threatening disease.

H. A. Segovia Lohse (✉) · H. R. Segovia Lohse
Hospital de Clínicas, II Cátedra de Clínica Quirúrgica, Facultad de Ciencias Médicas, Universidad Nacional de Asunción,
San Lorenzo, Paraguay
e-mail: hhaassll@fcmuna.edu.py

### 69.1.1 Epidemiology

UGIB is an entity often present for the acute care physician. It comprises the bleeding of the digestive tract up to the ligament of Treitz (foregut: esophagus, stomach, and/or duodenum). It can be presented in outpatient or in-hospital patient, and has an incidence of 100–150 cases per 100,000 population per year [1–3]. These incidence do not account the patients who experience UGIB while hospitalized, a special subset of bleeders with higher mortality [4].

Numerous improvements in treatment and new medications have decreased slightly the incidence of UGIB while increased age and comorbidities of the population have led to increase in incidences of UGIB [2, 3, 5]. The incidence of UGIB is higher in men and patients with lower social economic status [5].

More than 75% of the patients resolve with only supportive measures, but a significant percentage of cases requires further intervention [2, 6]. It is important to remind that UGIB must be managed by many clinicians including emergency room physicians, internists, gastroenterologists, surgeons, interventional radiologists, and hematologists [2].

The mortality including all causes of UGIB is low, lower than 5%, but in different series, it ranges between 2% and 14% [1–3, 5].

## 69.1.2 Etiology

Peptic ulcer bleeding is the most frequent cause of UGIB, responsible for about half of all cases [2–5]. Gastroesophageal varices, Mallory-Weiss syndrome, and acute gastric mucosal lesions (erosions or stress gastritis) are the next more frequent etiologies [4].

Nonsteroidal anti-inflammatory drugs (NSAIDs) and *Helicobacter pylori* (*H. pylori*) are recognized as two important etiologic risk factors for peptic ulcer disease (PUD) and UGIB [5]. A meta-analysis in 2002 found that the risk of PUD and the risk of bleeding with the use of NSAIDs were 3.55/4.88-fold and with *H. pylori* infection 1/1.79-fold. And if both risk factors were present, the risks of PUD and the risk of bleeding were 3.53/6.13-fold [7].

From all NSAIDs users, 1–2% will develop complications such as peptic ulcer bleeding each year [5].

Based on clinical classification (because the certain etiology can be elucidated only with endoscopy), most guidelines separate UGIB into variceal and non-variceal bleeding, whereas management and outcomes are different [2].

## 69.1.3 Classification

The Advanced Trauma Life Support (ATLS) classification for hemorrhagic shock, designed for injured patients, is based on clinical signs and can be used to estimate the volume of blood loss, seen in Table 69.1 [8]. This classification system emphasizes the early signs and pathophysiology of the shock state, but lately several studies showed that the classification is academically and didactical easy to use but does not reflect clinical state accurately [9].

Despite all this, this classification can be used to guide the initial management of a patient with UGIB.

## 69.1.4 Pathophysiology

The pathophysiology of the UGIB depends on the specific etiology.

### 69.1.4.1 Peptic Ulcer Disease (PUD)

Gastric and duodenal ulcer are the most common cause of UGIB, responsible for about 50% of all cases [5]. Duodenal ulcer is common than gastric ulcer. In the last decades, there is a strong fall in the incidence, admission, rebleeding, and principally mortality of PUD. That all was caused by the introduction of H2-receptor antagonist in the seventies, proton pump inhibitor in the eighties, endoscopy as a routine in the last two decades, and the recognition of the *H. pylori* as an important etiologic factor for the development of PUD [5].

*H. pylori* was identified in 1982, which is a gram-negative bacterium that disrupts the mucosal barrier and causes inflammation of the mucosa in the stomach and duodenum. Ninety percent of

**Table 69.1** Classification of hemorrhagic shock

| Parameter | Class I | Class II | Class III | Class IV |
|---|---|---|---|---|
| Blood loss, mL (%) | <750 (15) | 750–1500 (15–30) | 1500–2000 (30–40) | >2000 (>40) |
| Heart rate, beats/min | <100 | 100–120 | 120–140 | >140 |
| Blood pressure | Normal | Normal | Decreased | Decreased |
| Pulse pressure | Normal | Narrowed | Narrowed | Narrowed |
| Respiratory rate, breaths/min | 14–20 | 20–30 | 30–40 | >35 |
| Urinary output, mL/h | >30 | 20–30 | 5–15 | Negligible |
| Mental status | Slightly anxious | Mildly anxious | Anxious, confused | Confused, lethargic |
| Initial management | Crystalloids | Crystalloids | Crystalloids and blood products | Crystalloids and blood products |

Blood loss of total blood volume is for a male patient with a body weight of 70 kg
Committee on Trauma of the American College of Surgeons [8]

duodenal ulcers and 70% of gastric ulcers are associated with *H. pylori* [1].

### 69.1.4.2 Mallory-Weiss Syndrome

The Mallory-Weiss syndrome is characterized by longitudinal tear or the mucosa and submucosa in the gastroesophageal junction, due to the strong involuntary effort to vomit (retching), or event that provokes a sudden rise in the intragastric pressure, including antecedent of transesophageal echocardiography [10]. It is responsible for 1–15% of cases of upper gastrointestinal bleeding [1].

### 69.1.4.3 Stress Gastritis

It is an heterogenous group of gastroduodenal lesions due to pathophysiological stress: misbalance between protective factors (mucus, bicarbonate, prostaglandins, and blood flow) and aggressive factors. When the balance of gastric acid and defenses is disrupted, the acid injures the epithelium, and causes gastritis [1].

There are four principal causes of stress gastritis: shock, sepsis, burns (Curling ulcer), and tumors or trauma of the central nervous system (Cushing ulcer).

### 69.1.4.4 Variceal Bleeding

Gastroesophageal varices are responsible of 9–14% of all cases of UGIB, and up to 60% in cirrhotic patients [5]. Bleeding by gastroesophageal varices has a high morbidity and mortality rate (30%, up to 88% in some series) compared to other causes [11, 12].

Gastroesophageal varices result from decompression of the portal venous system into the systemic circulation, due to portal hypertension: it begins to appear with a pressure gradient of 8–10 mmHg, and rising 12 mmHg bleeding can occur [11].

The primary prevention of bleeding of gastroesophageal varices is based on nonselective beta-blockers (propranolol or nadolol) that reduces portal venous inflow by blocking adrenergic dilatation of mesenteric arterioles [11]. Propranolol is useful in prophylaxis against initial variceal hemorrhage as well as for prevention of recurrent bleeding. Has also demonstrated a reduction in deaths by 20% [1].

### 69.1.4.5 Other Causes of UGIB

Less common causes include Dieulafoy lesion, cancer, fistulas, hemobilia, celiac disease, vascular ectasias, and others.

Dieulafoy lesion is a large tortuous submucosal vessel most often located in the gastroesophageal junction. When protrude through the mucosa, the gastric acid can erode it producing bleeding. Because of that, it has an insidious onset, trend to produce intermittent but severe bleeding, and difficulty of endoscopic diagnosis [1, 13].

Bleeding by gastric cancer represents a late stage in the disease and therefore bad prognosis. Only 3% of all cases of severe UGIB are caused by neoplasms of the upper gastrointestinal tract [13].

Other tumors that can present with UGIB are gastrointestinal stromal tumors (GIST), leiomyomas, lymphomas, esophageal cancer among other tumors. GIST derived from the interstitial cells of Cajal nearly always express c-kit receptor and the stomach is the most common site of occurrence. Leiomyomas are derived from smooth muscle cells, therefore do not express the c-kit receptor, and during the endoscopy appear as a small submucosal mass covered by normal mucosa. It was demonstrated a strong association between chronic *H. pylori* infection and gastric extranodal marginal zone B cell lymphomas (extranodal MZL) [13].

Aortoduodenal or aortoenteric fistula may be primary (caused by arteriosclerosis, aortic aneurysms, aortic infections) or secondary (e.g., after aortic aneurism repair). It clinically manifest with a sentinel (herald) bleeding before exsanguinating hemorrhage [1, 14]. The fistula may originate from the aorta or his branches and if untreated, mortality of bleeding is nearly 100%.

Endoscopic therapy is not an option for a bleeding aortoenteric fistula, although it may be required to confirm the diagnosis or exclude other causes of UGIB [14]. Surgical repair of the aneurysm or pseudoaneurysm and fistula is the standard treatment regardless of the cause (see Fig. 69.1) [13].

Hemobilia is the bleeding into the biliary tract, caused by iatrogenic procedures (liver biopsy,

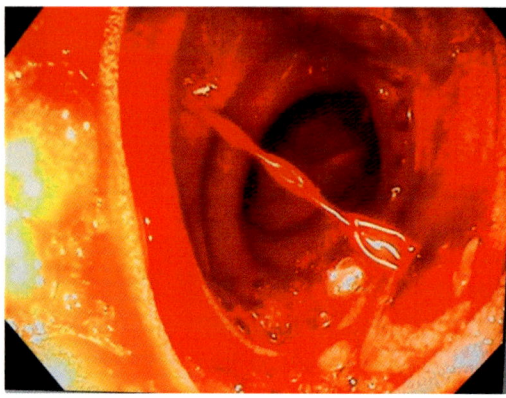

**Fig. 69.1** Active spurting ("jet") hemorrhage in the third part of duodenum, not feasible to treat with endoscopy. The patient goes to laparotomy, and a pseudoaneurysm of the superior mesenteric artery was responsible for the bleeding and fistula. (Picture courtesy of Dr. Rogrido Pérez, with permission)

instrumentation of the biliary tree), trauma, and neoplasms. The classic presentation is known as Quincke's triad: jaundice, right upper quadrant abdominal pain, and UGIB, but present only in one-third of the patients making the diagnosis challenging [15].

UGIB caused by celiac disease is very rare; most frequently, it can lead to iron-deficiency anemia due to malabsorption. Celiac disease affects about 0.5–1% of the Western world in genetically susceptible people [16].

Vascular ectasia, principally gastric antral vascular ectasia exhibits iron-deficiency anemia, sometimes as an incidental finding in endoscopy, and occasionally causes acute UGIB. This disease is associated with scleroderma and chronic renal disease [13].

Gastroesophageal reflux disease (GERD) is a specific disease caused by occurrence of gastroesophageal reflux through the lower esophageal sphincter into the esophagus and causes symptoms and/or injury to esophageal tissue. Physiologic reflux can cause symptoms like heartburn specially after meal, but they disappear quickly. Pathologic refluxes are more frequent and have longer duration, leading to chronic symptoms, inflammation, and esophageal mucosa injury [17].

Despite GERD being a usually non-progressive disease, the range of complications are esophagitis, bleeding, esophageal ulcerations, stricture formations, Barrett's esophagus, and adenocarcinoma of the esophagus [17].

## 69.2 Diagnosis

### 69.2.1 Clinical Presentation

The patients present with hematemesis and/or melena and/or anemia. Rectal bleeding or hematochezia (classic presentation from lower gastrointestinal bleeding) is associated with massive bleeding and hemodynamic instability. Lipothymia and/or altered level of consciousness may occur in these patients.

Hematemesis is vomiting of blood, red or coffee-ground material. Melena is the passage of black and tarry stools. Hematochezia is the passage of fresh blood per anus, usually in or with stools.

Patients with melena present with lower levels of hemoglobin than those with hematemesis, probably because of the chronic non-massive hemorrhage [2]. Because of that the patients with melena have a lower mortality, but moreover require transfusion [2]. Red hematemesis represents more acute and significant blood loss with a worse prognosis [4].

Depending on the cause of the UGIB, the clinical symptoms may vary [18]:

- PUD: nocturnal epigastric distress, right upper quadrant pain.
- Esophagitis: odynophagia, dysphagia, gastroesophageal reflux.
- Mallory-Weiss syndrome: emesis, retching, or coughing before hematemesis.
- Cancer: dysphagia, early satiety, involuntary weight loss, cachexia.
- Variceal hemorrhage: jaundice, weakness, abdominal distention, collateral circulation, ascites.

History of recent trauma should be ruled out, also history of previous surgery: antecedent of aortic aneurism repair provides a clue to possible aortoenteric fistula. As well as history of gastrectomy raises the possibility of marginal ulcer.

It is very important to question specifically if the patient had a prescription use or also use of over-the-counter NSAIDs, dose, and duration? One-third of the patients with Mallory-Weiss will not present history of repetitive retching [4].

After the prompt diagnosis of the UGIB, initial evaluation must immediately address hemodynamic status [4].

## 69.2.2 Test

In must be taken blood samples to test hemoglobin, platelet count, blood type, creatinine, blood urea nitrogen, liver function test, and prothrombin time or INR. Hemoglobin level is a poor initial indicator of severity of UGIB, comparing with heart rate and pressure, but it should be monitored [6].

An electrocardiogram should obtain to exclude myocardial ischemia in patients at risk for coronary disease. Chest radiography is not mandatory and should be used selectively [4].

> **Differential Diagnosis**
> When a patient with bleeding present in the emergency room is a key point to define if it is a UGIB or a lower hemorrhage. Or even if the bleeding comes from the airways (hemoptysis or less frequent swallowed epistaxis).
> Lower gastrointestinal bleeding presents with dark blood mixed with stool or hematochezia, abdominal pain, and unexplained weakness. Sometimes also presents with melena when cecum is bleeding.
> Hemoptysis is the expectoration of blood from the lower airways, alone or with mucus. The most frequent worldwide cause of hemoptysis is tuberculosis. Because the small space in airways is not necessary an excessive amount of bleeding to impair the exchange of gases, that lead to cyanosis, dyspnea, tachypnea, altered level of consciousness, and in massive bleedings death from asphyxia [19]. Rarely naso- or oropharyngeal bleeding presents without classical sign of the underlying pathology [4].

## 69.3 Treatment

### 69.3.1 Workup and Initial Treatment

The guidelines recommend that the initial workup in a patient with UGIB is based on tree steps (performed simultaneously): hemodynamic assessment and resuscitation, blood transfusion, and risk assessment [2, 20, 21].

#### 69.3.1.1 Hemodynamic Assessment and Resuscitation

The initial clinical evaluation of the patients starts with ABC (as in trauma): airway, breathing, and circulation. Hemodynamic assessment implies blood pressure, pulse, and orthostatic hypotension measures [6].

Immediate assessment of the hemodynamic status and begin resuscitative measures as needed is a corner stone of the initial management [20]. There are three goals in hemodynamic resuscitation [22]:

- To correct intravascular hypovolemia
- To restore adequate tissue perfusion
- To prevent multi-organ failure

Two large bore intravenous cannula must be inserted and start monitoring of pulse, blood pressure, and oxygen saturation [2]. By now there are no evidence of which fluid is recommended (crystalloids or colloids) and the volume to be infused [22]. A RCT in patients with trauma hemorrhagic shock suggests that a more restrictive fluid resuscitation may be better than more intensive fluid resuscitation [23].

In patients with severe hematemesis or with high risk of aspiration, the trachea should be intubated to protect the airway [2, 22].

#### 69.3.1.2 Blood Transfusion

Blood transfusion should be given restrictively to maintain hemoglobin level of 7–9 g/dL or 4.34–5.59 mmol/L (higher levels in patients with hypotension and tachycardia or with ongoing bleeding, or with comorbidities) [21, 22]. The Transfusion Requirements in Critical Care, a trial in 838 critically ill patients, suggested lower mortality with hemoglobin levels of 7–9 g/dL than with levels of 10–12 g/dL [21].

Based principally on expert opinion recommendations, a threshold of <50 × 10/L indicates platelets transfusion [24].

### 69.3.1.3 Risk Assessment

The risk assessment is very useful in patients with UGIB to try to determine the level of care (on ward, emergency room, or intensive care unit [ICU] hospitalization), the better timing for endoscopy, and which of them are in higher risk of rebleeding or death [6, 20].

Uncontrolled and/or recurrent hemorrhage is recognized as the major risk factor impacting the outcome in UGIB. Other factors that predict severity are history of malignancy, cirrhosis, presentation with hematemesis, and signs of hypovolemia (including hypotension, tachycardia and shock, and hemoglobin <8 g/dL) [14].

Factors that may prompt admission in ICU include active bleeding, hypotension, coagulopathy, altered mental status, and comorbidities, especially in elderly patients; however clinical judgment must prevail [4].

Risks factors associated with high mortality are advanced age, severe comorbidity, hypotension or shock, rebleeding, and onset of bleeding in in-hospital patients [6, 5]. Several studies show a significant difference in mortality among in-hospital patients who presents UGIB (23–42%) and emergency admissions (3.7–11%) [5].

Several risk assessment scores have been developed for patient with UGIB, including those that can be calculated early after presentation (pre-endoscopy) and those that includes endoscopy findings [2, 14, 21, 22].

The most stablished and commonly used are the Glasgow Blatchford score (GBS), the Rockall "admission" score, and the AIMS65 score [2]. These scores are validated to predict which patients are in low risks that which of them are in high risk, but the GBS seen to be superior to predict clinical outcome, need of intervention, and risk of death [2, 25].

The pre-endoscopic Rockall score (range 0–7) uses only clinical data, and the GBS (range 0–23) and the AIMS65 score (range 0–5) use clinical and laboratory data (Tables 69.2, 69.3, and 69.4).

Patients with Rockall scores of 2 or less (low rate of bleeding, recurrence, and death) should be considered for management in the community. In their study, Phang et al. show that patients with Rockall score of <4 (low risk, mortality rate of 3.2%) could have been managed in a general ward, and when the score rise to ≥4 (high risk, mortality 22.4%), those patients should be admitted to an ICU [26].

There is a group of low-risk patients with UGIB, GBS 0–1: patients without melena, syncope, hepatic disease, and cardiac failure, and

**Table 69.2** Rockall score

|  | 0 | 1 | 2 | 3 |
|---|---|---|---|---|
| Age | <60 years | 60–79 years | >80 years | - |
| Shock | No shock SBP >100, HR <100 | Tachycardia SBP >100, HR >100 | Hypotension SBP <100 | - |
| Comorbidity | - | - | Ischemic heart disease, congestive heart failure, any major comorbidity | Renal/liver failure, disseminated malignancy |
| Diagnosis[a] | Mallory-Weiss tear or no lesion observed | Peptic ulcer disease, erosive esophagitis | Malignancy of UGI tract | - |
| Stigmata of recent hemorrhage[a] | Clean-based ulcer, flat pigmented spot | - | Blood in UGI tract, clot, visible vessel, bleeding | - |

*SBP* systolic blood pressure (in mmHg), *HR* heart rate (in beats/min), *UGI* upper gastrointestinal
[a] Variables not included in the pre-endoscopic Rockall score. Range in the pre-endoscopic Rockall score: 0–7 points. Range in the post-endoscopic Rockall score: 0–11 points

**Table 69.3** Glasgow Blatchford score

|  | 0 | 1 | 2 | 3 | 4 | 6 |
|---|---|---|---|---|---|---|
| BUN | <18.2 | - | ≥18.2 to <22.4 | ≥22.4 to <28 | ≥28 to <70 | ≥70 |
| Hgb in men | ≥13 | ≥12 to <13 | - | ≥10 to <12 | - | <10 |
| Hgb in women | ≥12 | ≥10 to <12 | - | - | - | <10 |
| SBP | ≥110 | ≥100 to <109 | ≥90 to <99 | <90 | - | - |
| Other markers | - | Pulse rate ≥100 bpm, melena | Syncope, hepatic disease, heart failure | - | - | - |

*BUN* blood urea nitrogen (in mg/dL), *Hgb* hemoglobin (in g/dL), *SBP* systolic blood pressure, *bpm* beats per minute

**Table 69.4** AIMS65 score

| | |
|---|---|
| Albumin <3 g/dL | 1 |
| INR >1.5 | 1 |
| Altered mental status | 1 |
| Systolic blood pressure <90 mmHg | 1 |
| Age >65 years | 1 |

systolic blood pressure ≥110 mmHg, pulse <100 beats/min, hemoglobin ≥13.0 g/dL for men or ≥12.0 g/dL for women, blood urea nitrogen <18.2 mg/dL. These patients can be discharged and managed as an outpatient without endoscopy [22].

Patients with a GBS ≥8 should be classified as very high risk, and these patients should be transferred to an ICU as soon as possible.

### 69.3.2 Medical Treatment

#### 69.3.2.1 Pre-endoscopic Medical Treatment

The indication of pre-endoscopic intravenous proton pump inhibitor (PPI) varies substantively between different guidelines [2, 6, 14, 20–22]. A Cochrane meta-analysis of 6 randomized clinical trial shows that the use of PPI before endoscopy reduced high risk stigmata of bleeding and the need for endoscopic therapy, but do not improve clinical outcomes such as further bleeding, surgery, or death [27]. Despite this the use of PPI (e.g., omeprazole 80 mg bolus followed by 8 mg/h infusion) was associated with decreased high-risk endoscopic findings and the need of endoscopic therapy [6, 20]. The European Society of Gastrointestinal Endoscopy (ESGE) recommend intravenous high-dose bolus followed by continuous infusion for patients awaiting endoscopy, extending continuous infusion for 72 h for patients who receive endoscopic hemostasis [22].

A single intravenous dose of 250 mg (or 3 mg/kg) of erythromycin (30–120 min before endoscopy) improves visualization of the gastric mucosa [2, 6, 20, 22].

Some guidelines recommend the use of vasoactive drugs (terlipressin, somatostatin, or its analogs octreotide and vapreotide) as soon as variceal hemorrhage is suspected [2]. These vasoactive drugs cause splanchnic artery vasoconstriction and are recommended as following: terlipressin 2 mg every 4 h, somatostatin 250 μg bolus followed by 250–500 μg/h, and octreotide and vapreotide 50 μg bolus followed by 50 μg/h, for 5 days [28]. Despite the ESGE does not recommend the use of somatostatin or its analogue octreotide [22].

In variceal bleeding, antibiotic prophylaxis for 7 days is recommended, because decreases overall infections, including spontaneous bacterial peritonitis [4]. Intravenous ceftriaxone is preferred although the choice of antibiotic is dependent on local antimicrobial sensitivity patterns [2].

If the patient is taking vitamin K antagonists (anticoagulants), it should withholding and correct coagulopathy with INR control <2.5 (i.e., vitamin K IV, prothrombin complex concentrate, fresh frozen plasma) [21, 22]. New direct oral anticoagulant should temporarily withholding (i.e., dabigatran, rivaroxaban, apixaban). Several studies demonstrate that antiplatelet agents (i.e., aspirin, clopidogrel) lower mortality if there are not discontinued following PUD bleeding [22]. Correction of coagulopathy is recommended but should not delay endoscopy [21].

A meta-analysis and other studies evaluated the role of nasogastric aspiration/lavage: low sensitivity distinguishing UGIB from lower (44%), sensitivity and specificity to identify severe UGIB similar to clinical parameters and laboratory findings (77%), did not improve visualization of the stomach, uncomfortable procedure not well tolerated or desired by patients [22, 29].

A Cochrane review in 2012 comparing tranexamic acid versus placebo or versus cimetidine or lansoprazole found no evidence to support or refute the use of tranexamic acid for UGIB, in terms of mortality, bleeding, surgery, or transfusion requirements [30].

### 69.3.2.2 Endoscopy

Endoscopy is a crucial procedure in both diagnosis and therapy for UGIB: can identify the diseases or lesion and provide intervention to control the bleeding [1, 20–22, 25].

ESGE recommends the following definitions about the timing of upper gastrointestinal endoscopy in acute UGIB: very early <12 h, early ≤24 h, and delayed >24 h [22].

The guidelines recommend that generally all the patients with UGIB should undergo endoscopy within 24 h of admission (early endoscopy) after appropriate resuscitation [2, 20–22]. This early endoscopy is associated with reduced transfusion and decreases length of stay of nonvariceal bleeding in high-risk patients [1]. But studies cannot demonstrate that endoscopy reduces mortality rate [1, 4].

Patients with hemodynamic instability (tachycardia, hypotension) despite resuscitation, in-hospital bloody emesis/nasogastric aspirate, contraindication to the interruption of anticoagulation or with variceal bleeding should undergo endoscopy within 12 h after presentation (very early endoscopy) [2, 20, 22]. But a randomized trial of 516 patients with GBS of 12 or higher, performed in Hong Kong and comparing urgent versus early endoscopy found that in patients with acute UGIB who were at high risk for further bleeding or death, endoscopy performed within 6 h was not associated with lower 30-day mortality than endoscopy performed between 6 and 24 h after consultation [25].

In patients with active bleeding, clinically unstable, and only hematochezia without melena or hematemesis (or even with), endoscopy should be performed (can be an UGIB rather than lower) [4].

In different series, the rate of rebleeding after endoscopic treatment to control bleeding from PUD arises from 15–20%. Patients with recurrent bleeding generally respond favorably to repeat endoscopic therapy [14]. A RCT of 92 patients with recurrent bleeding after first endoscopic control of bleeding PUD compared immediate endoscopic retreatment and surgery and found that endoscopic retreatment reduces the need for surgery without increasing the risk of death and is associated with fewer complications than is surgery, with a successful rate of 73% [31].

Rebleeding is often defined as fresh hematemesis, melena or both with either hemodynamic instability (pulse rate >110 beats/min and systolic blood pressure <90 mmHg) or a decrease in hemoglobin concentration of at least 2 g/dL (1.2 mmol/L) during a 24 h period, with confirmation of recurrent bleeding by endoscopy or surgery.

The ESGE recommends the Forrest classification to be used in all patients with bleeding PUD, to differentiate low- and high-risk endoscopic stigmata [22]. The Forrest classification (Table 69.5) was developed almost half a century ago. It can be useful to stratify the risks of rebleeding or surgery [6]. In high-risk stigmata findings (Forrest Ia, Ib, and IIa), endoscopic hemostasis needs to be performed because these lesions are at high risk for persistent bleeding or rebleeding. In Forrest IIb, the clot needs to be removed endoscopically and if underlying findings are a high-risk stigmata, endoscopic hemostasis should be performed. In patients with low-risk stigmata (Forrest IIc–III), the ESGE does not recumbent endoscopic hemostasis [22].

**Table 69.5** Forrest classification

| Forrest | | Endoscopic appearance | Risk of rebleeding[a] | Stigmata[b] | Surgery rate[b] | Prevalence |
|---|---|---|---|---|---|---|
| I Active hemorrhage | Ia | Spurting hemorrhage | 55–80% | High risk | 35% | 10% |
| | Ib | Oozing hemorrhage | c | High risk | c | c |
| II Signs of recent hemorrhage | IIa | Nonbleeding visible vessel | 43–50% | High risk | 34% | 20% |
| | IIb | Adherent clot | 22% | d | 10% | 20% |
| | IIc | Flat pigmented spot | 10% | Low risk | 6% | 15% |
| III No signs of hemorrhage | III | Clean base ulcer | 5% | Low risk | 0.5% | 30% |

[a] Risk of rebleeding if endoscopic therapy is not performed. Based on a study from Laine and Peterson from articles published in 1980–1990 [6]
[b] Stigmata: risk of persistent bleeding or rebleeding. In high-risk stigmata, endoscopic hemostasis needs to be performed. Low-risk stigmata don't need endoscopic hemostasis
[c] Same as Forrest Ia
[d] In Forrest IIb should considered endoscopic clot removal, and then identify if there are high- or low-risk stigmata to proceed

There are several hemostatic agents [14, 22]:

- Thermal therapies are argon plasma coagulation (non-contact), bipolar electrocoagulation, or heater probe (contact).
- Polidocanol, ethanolamine, and absolute ethanol are sclerosing agent (causing tissue necrosis or fixation).
- Thrombin injection develops clot formation.
- Clips and bands represent mechanical therapy.
- Topical therapy is new agents in powder or spray, used in non-variceal UGIB.
- Epinephrine is alpha- and beta-adrenergic agonists (sympathomimetic).

Epinephrine injection therapy is effective for hemostasis (e.g., 1:10,000 dilution), but inferior to other endoscopic hemostasis monotherapies or combination therapy in preventing ulcer rebleeding. In patients with PUD and active bleeding should be used double therapy (epinephrine + contact thermal/mechanical therapy/or sclerosing agent) [21, 22].

Endoscopic band ligation devices are commonly used in variceal bleeding and Mallory-Weiss syndrome [22]. Other therapeutic options for variceal bleeding are clips, sclerosants, and thrombin injection [1]. When ligation of gastroesophageal varices was not achieved, consider Sengstaken–Blakemore tube for control of immediately life-threatening UGIB [1, 32].

The advent of endoscopic sclerotherapy controls the acute bleeding in 80–95% of patients, reducing the need of surgery [12]. When esophageal varices bleeding recurs, a second attempt at endoscopic treatment is justified in most cases [12].

UGIB from gastric varices or portal hypertensive gastropathy can be treated endoscopically although this is not a long-term option (most common cause of chronic sclerotherapy failure) and surgical or interventional radiology therapy will be required [4, 12].

Balloon tamponade for esophageal variceal bleeding was first described in 1950 [32]. A Sengstaken–Blakemore tube consists of a flexible plastic tube, inserted through the nose or mouth, containing three ports and one end [32, 33]:

- Gastric aspiration port, which removes fluid and air out of the stomach, like a nasogastric tube.
- Gastric balloon port, which inflates a round balloon in the stomach, inflate with 100–300 mL air, and with traction of the tube compresses the cardias.
- Esophageal balloon port, which inflates a small elongated balloon in the esophagus, with 50 mL normal saline, or approximate 35–45 mmHg. The tube needs a sustained traction with 0.5–1 kg (approx. 1–2 pounds) and needs to deflate de esophageal balloon every 12 h to avoid esophageal ischemia.

### 69.3.2.3 Interventional Radiology

Transcatheter angiographic embolization (TAE), an interventional radiology procedure, is the second-line treatment (before surgery) in patients who are unresponsive to medical and endoscopic treatment. The extravasation should be investigated in the following order: celiac artery, superior mesenteric artery, and his branch pancreaticoduodenal artery. If extravasation is founded, superselective angioembolization should be performed [1].

The embolization can be performed with coils or foam pledgets into the artery [4].

Successful rates for patients with PUD bleeding are between 52% and 98%, with recurrent bleeding rates of 10–20%. To be visualized with angiography, the hemorrhage rate of 0.5–1.0 mL/min is required [4, 18].

In patients with variceal bleeding due to portal hypertension after medical and endoscopic failed therapy, the transjugular intrahepatic portosystemic shunt (TIPS) is an option. This minimally invasive procedure decompresses the portal venous by a shunt between the hepatic vein with the portal vein [1].

### 69.3.3 Surgical Treatment

Surgery is the third line treatment for UGIB: surgery should be considered if endoscopy and embolization failed to treat the bleeding, or if embolization is likely to be delayed [1, 21, 22].

Also probably surgery will be the first option in a hemodynamically unstable patient, unresponsive to resuscitation, or when perforated viscus is suspected [1].

Only 1–2% of patients with UGIB will require emergency surgery, a declining rate in recent decades, but in some series goes up to 8% [4, 34]. Possible justification for the decreasing rate may include advances in endoscopic technology, more widespread use of PPI, more aggressive eradication of *H. pylori*, greater awareness of side effects NSAIDs [34]. For this reason, surgery had high mortality rates over 20% [4].

When surgery is the treatment option, transfusion cutoff may vary (to higher) from patient to patient: more important than the quantity is to maintain the goals of resuscitation (see above). The majority of patients requiring emergency surgery are aged over 70 years with pre-existing cardiorespiratory comorbidity [34]. More than a half had ischemic heart disease, one-third had hypertension, and less frequent diabetes, chronic obstructive pulmonary disease, cerebrovascular disease, or rheumatoid arthritis [35].

Emergency surgery in non-variceal UGIB may consist of oversewing the bleeding vessel in the stomach or duodenum (usually preoperatively identified by endoscopy) or partial gastrectomy [1]. Historically vagotomy + antrectomy was also performed, but in the era of PPIs and understanding the pathophysiology of *H. pylori*, the utility of this acid-reducing procedure has greatly diminished or disappear [18].

When an endoscopy was previously performed, the surgeon knows where the bleeding site is. If not, and being the PUD the most frequent cause of UGIB, and duodenal ulcer most frequent than gastric, probably the duodenum and the stomach will be the first organs to explore: a pyloro-duodenotomy and/or gastrotomy with oversewing the ulcer, or even gastrectomy with reconstruction [36]. Duodenal ulcer most commonly presents in the first part of the duodenum eroding posteriorly the gastroduodenal artery, so the approach consist in longitudinal pyloroduodenotomy, inspection of the duodenal bulb and gastric antrum, oversewing the ulcer with three stitches including the pancreatoduodenal artery, and a transverse closure of the duodenum, with Heineke-Mikulicz pyloroplasty, and troncular vagotomy [18].

The gastroduodenal artery is one of the most important sources of UGIB, and if cannot be controlled with stitches through the mucosa (when a pyloro-duodenotomy was performed), must be ligated extraluminally. It run behind to the first part of the duodenum, to the left of the common bile duct. It must be ligated superiorly and inferiorly to the duodenum. Should be taken care to avoid injury to the common bile duct during suture placement [37].

If a bleeding site is not identified, the mucosa should be carefully inspected for an ulcer. When founded, the base must be cleaned to identify a visible vessel and ligate it proximally and distally. Always look for other potential bleeding lesions. If the duodenum is discarded as a source of bleeding, a gastrotomy near the esophageal junction must be opened to explore the stomach. Then closure the stomach, perform pyloroplasty and finally troncular vagotomy.

In variceal bleeding, if medical and endoscopic therapy could not control the bleeding, TIPS was not possible, chronic sclerotherapy failure, surgery is clearly indicated. All operations used to control an acute UGIB caused by variceal hemorrhage can be classified into four groups [12]:

- Non-selective portosystemic shunts (most common operative procedure performed, that is, portacaval shunt, interposition mesocaval shunt, using a prosthetic graft).
- Selective portosystemic shunts (i.e., splenorenal shunt).
- Devascularization procedures (i.e., Sugiura procedure, esophageal transection, which is associated with a higher incidence of late rebleeding rather than shunts).
- Liver transplantation (rarely alternative for the acutely bleeding).

Non-selective shunt completely divert portal flow away from the liver and tend to cause more encephalopathy than devascularization procedures. Distal splenorenal shuts tend to have lower mortality than portacaval shunt. The distal splenorenal shunt preserves the portal perfusion of the liver and maintains intestinal venous hypertension [12].

In 1973, Sugiura and Futagawa described a surgical technique with double approach (thoracic and abdominal) later known as Sugiura procedure (Fig. 69.2) [38]. The thoracic procedure includes extensive paraesophageal devascularization up to the inferior pulmonary vein (12–18 cm or 30–50 shunting veins to be ligated) and esophageal transection and anastomosis, performed through a left lateral thoracotomy entering beneath the sixth rib. The abdominal procedure involves splenectomy, selective vagotomy, devascularization of abdominal esophagus and cardia through the greater and lesser curvature of the stomach, and the cardioesophageal branches of the left gastric vessels, and finally pyloroplasty (because of the division of the gastric vagus nerves) [38, 39].

Due to the complexity and high mobility and mortality of the Sugiura procedure, different authors develop less complex procedures like esophageal transection, with low rates of rebleeding, hepatic coma, and mortality. The most common modification implies a splenectomy as a first step, then devascularization as described previously, and then a longitudinal gastrotomy to perform an esophageal transection with end-to-end anastomosis using a circular stapler (usually 28 mm) 3–5 cm above the gastroesophageal junction. The transaction is performed to achieve complete separation of the azygous vein system from the intramucosal vein [39].

The mortality in patients with UGIB requiring surgery reminds elevated throughout the last decades (34%) with a complication rate of 55%, despite diagnostic and therapeutic advances. This is probably explained by the fact that these cases represent a worst cases with unsuccessful conservative and endoscopic treatment, as well as by the rising and comorbidities of the population [34, 40].

A retrospective study from 91 patients who underwent surgery for UGIB requiring transfusion found that the use of anticoagulants, the need for postoperative ventilation, and an ICU length of stay >7 days were identified as significant risk factors for mortality. Transfusions of more than 10 units of red blood cells, the need for further surgery, a prolonged ICU length of stay, and recurrent bleeding were identified as significant risk factors for postoperative complications (such as pneumonia, sepsis, rebleeding, and anastomotic leakage) [40].

### 69.3.4 Follow-Up

When endoscopy hemostasis was performed (high-risk stigmata) or the patient does not require hemostasis (low-risk stigmata), the inten-

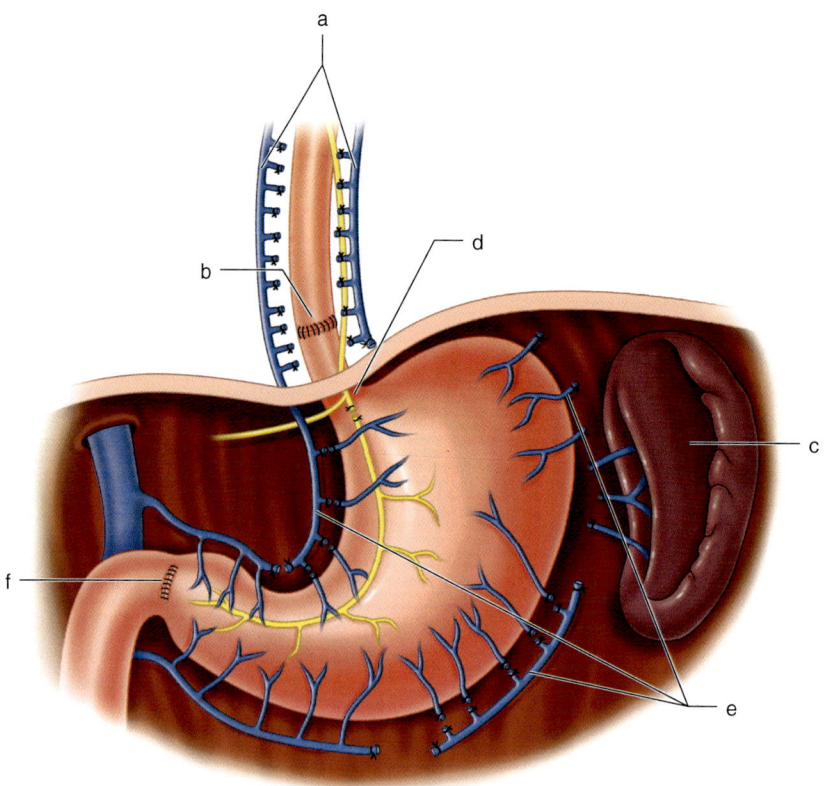

**Fig. 69.2** Sugiura procedure. Thoracotomy and (**a**) paraesophageal devascularization up to the inferior pulmonary vein, (**b**) esophageal transection and anastomosis. Laparotomy and (**c**) splenectomy, (**d**) selective vagotomy, (**e**) devascularization of abdominal esophagus and cardia, and (**f**) pyloroplasty

sity of monitoring is dependent of the rebreeding rate, based on Forrest classification (Table 69.5) [4]. Monitoring should include vital signs, hematocrit, stool frequency, and color. Generally ulcer rebleeding occurs within 72 h.

For patients at low risk of recurrent bleeding, the diet can be liberalized immediately after anesthesia recovery from endoscopy, and early discharged planned with standard PPI therapy (once-daily) [4, 22].

In patients with high-risk stigmata, liquid diet can be started after 24 h later endoscopic therapy, and observation as in-patient for minimally 72 h with a continuous infusion of high-dose intravenous PPI, and then discharged after clinical stabilization with indication of high-dose oral PPI [4, 14, 22].

Oral high-dose PPI recommended are: 80–160 mg daily in divided doses for 3 days, then twice daily oral PPI on days 4–14. Omeprazole or esomeprazole should not be prescribed in patients who are taking clopidogrel [2].

Patients with peptic ulcer bleeding generally receive 4–8 weeks of once-daily oral PPI [2].

In patients with UGIB secondary to PUD, the ESGE recommends investigating for the presence of *H. pylori* in the acute setting and indicates the eradication therapy when *H. pylori* is detected, because numerous studies demonstrated cure of PUD [4, 22]. A re-test for *H. pylori* should be performed in those patients with a negative test in the acute setting, because of the false negative rate is higher when is performed at the time of the bleeding episode as compared to later follow-up [22].

When possible and if are believed causative, NSAIDs should be proscribed. Patients who require long-term conventional NSAIDs therapy will require PPIs, or another strategy that could be discontinued NSAIDs and start cyclooxygenase-2 inhibitors (COX-2) [4, 21].

In patients with UGIB due to variceal bleeding antibiotics and vasoactive drugs should be continued for up to 7 days [2].

Anticoagulation resumption should be assessed on a patient-by-patient basis [22]. The ESGE suggests restarting warfarin from "as soon as hemostasis is established" to 7–15 days after the bleeding event [22].

Survival benefits were demonstrated with several studies that continue or reintroduce antithrombotic drugs after UGIB, because the mortality after bleeding is more often caused by underlying comorbidities rather than rebleeding [2]. The National Institute for Health and Care Excellence suggests continuing aspirin (or reintroducing the drug within 3 days for higher risk endoscopic lesions) once hemostasis is achieved. When an antithrombotic drug is reintroduced, a PPI is usually also administered [2].

> **Dos and Don'ts**
>
> **Dos**
> - Initial and prompt assessment of hemodynamic status in patients who present with UGIB, with early intravascular volume replacement using crystalloids when hemodynamic instability is present.
> - Red blood cell transfusion to target 7 g/dL.
> - Early endoscopy (within 24 h of presentation) is recommended for most patients with acute upper gastrointestinal bleeding.
> - Endoscopic hemostatic therapy is indicated for patients with high-risk stigmata.
> - An intravenous bolus followed by continuous-infusion PPIs therapy should be used to decrease rebleeding and mortality in patients with high-risk stigmata who have undergone successful endoscopic therapy.
> - Patients with low-risk stigmata can be discharged early.
> - A second attempt at endoscopic therapy is generally recommended in cases of rebleeding.
> - Seek surgical consultation for patients for whom endoscopic therapy has failed.
>
> **Don'ts**
> - Don't use one only hemoglobin level to assess risk or stratify patients.
> - Don't use routinely nasogastric or orogastric aspiration/lavage in patients presenting UGIB.
> - Rarely is necessary an urgent endoscopy. In the first hours, the main treatment is resuscitation.
> - Endoscopic hemostatic therapy is not indicated for patients with low-risk stigmata.
> - Epinephrine injection alone provides suboptimal efficacy (should be used in combination with another method).
> - Don't delay endoscopy because of uncorrected coagulopathy.
> - Don't leave without follow-up negative *H. pylori* diagnostic tests obtained in the acute setting: Tests should be repeated.

> **Take-Home Messages**
> - UGIB still remains a severe entity in the emergency room and in in-hospital patients.
> - Initial stabilization and resuscitation are essential and priority in all patients, regardless of the underlying cause.
> - After initial management, most of the patients can be treated conservative.
> - Early endoscopy (within 24 h of presentation) is recommended for most

patients with acute upper gastrointestinal bleeding.
- A second attempt at endoscopic therapy is generally recommended in cases of rebleeding. If it was unsuccessful remain the options for interventional radiology or even surgery.

**Questions**

1. After initial resuscitation, which of the following treatments option may be done acutely for patients with symptoms typical of variceal bleeding?
   A. Balloon tamponage with Sengstaken–Blakemore tube
   B. Upper gastrointestinal endoscopy
   C. Trans arterial embolization
   D. Surgery

2. A middle-aged man with UGIB was admitted to the emergency room. He is taking anticoagulant drugs, and presented hematemesis, hemodynamic instability, and hemoglobin 5.5 g/dL. Which are the next steps?
   A. Fluid resuscitation without red blood cells transfusion, plasma transfusion, endoscopy
   B. Fluid resuscitation, blood transfusion, correct the coagulopathy, endoscopy
   C. Fluid resuscitation, blood transfusion, correct the coagulopathy, surgery
   D. Fluid resuscitation, surgery

3. A Forrest Ia ulcer is found during endoscopy in a patient with UGIB due to PUD. What are the best treatment?
   A. Stops endoscopy and refer to surgery
   B. Hemostasis with epinephrine alone
   C. Hemostasis with epinephrine and other sclerosant agent
   D. Plan a second look endoscopy in 72 h

4. After a hemostasis control endoscopy (Forrest IIa), the patient recurs with a new bleeding episode. What would you do?
   A. Repeat endoscopy
   B. More aggressive resuscitation and transfusion without endoscopy
   C. Sent to interventional radiology department
   D. Open surgery

5. The clinical presentation of the UGIB is, except:
   A. Hematemesis
   B. Hematochezia and hypotension in massive hemorrhage
   C. Altered mental status in non-massive hemorrhage
   D. Melena

6. Initial medical treatment in UGIB includes:
   A. Resuscitation with D5%W
   B. Transfusion up to 10 g/dL hemoglobin
   C. Aggressive and liberal resuscitation with crystalloids
   D. Restrictive transfusion

7. A Sengstaken–Blakemore tube balloon is indicated when:
   A. Unstable patient with UGIB due to PUD
   B. Any variceal bleeding, regardless the hemodynamic status
   C. Life-threatening UGIB due to esophageal varices
   D. UGIB due to gastric cancer

8. The most obvious sign of UGIB is:
   A. Gastroesophageal reflux
   B. Hematemesis
   C. Left upper quadrant pain
   D. Weight loss

9. Which case of UGIB can be managed as an outpatient?
   A. Rockall score <4
   B. Rockall score ≥4
   C. Glasgow Blatchford score ≥8
   D. Glasgow Blatchford score ≤1

10. After an episode of UGIB in a patient taking antiplatelet and/or anticoagulant drugs:
    A. Anticoagulant drugs should be discontinued and start PPI
    B. Antiplatelet drugs should restart early without PPI
    C. Antiplatelet and anticoagulant drugs should be discontinued
    D. Antiplatelet and/or anticoagulant drugs should restart early once hemostasis has been achieved

**Answers**: 1.B, 2.B, 3.C, 4.A, 5.C, 6.D, 7.C, 8.B, 9.D, 10.D

## References

1. Feinman M, Haut ER. Upper gastrointestinal bleeding. Surg Clin North Am. 2014;94(1):43–53. https://doi.org/10.1016/j.suc.2013.10.004.
2. Stanley AJ, Laine L. Management of acute upper gastrointestinal bleeding. BMJ. 2019;364:l536. https://doi.org/10.1136/bmj.l536.
3. Laine L, Yang H, Chang SC, Datto C. Trends for incidence of hospitalization and death due to GI complications in the United States from 2001 to 2009. Am J Gastroenterol. 2012;107:1190–5. https://doi.org/10.1038/ajg.2012.168.
4. Wilcox CM. Upper gastrointestinal bleeding. In: Encyclopedia of gastroenterology. Amsterdam: Elsevier; 2004. p. 557–65. https://doi.org/10.1016/b0-12-386860-2/00707-3.
5. van Leerdam ME. Epidemiology of acute upper gastrointestinal bleeding. Best Pract Res Clin Gastroenterol. 2008;22(2):209–24. https://doi.org/10.1016/j.bpg.2007.10.011.
6. Laine L, Peterson WL. Bleeding peptic ulcer. N Engl J Med. 1994;331(11):717–27. https://doi.org/10.1056/NEJM199409153311107.
7. Huang JQ, Sridhar S, Hunt RH. Role of Helicobacter pylori infection and non-steroidal anti-inflammatory drugs in peptic-ulcer disease: a meta-analysis. Lancet. 2002;359(9300):14–22. https://doi.org/10.1016/S0140-6736(02)07273-2.
8. American College of Surgeons Committee on Trauma. Advanced Trauma Life Support (ATLS) student course manual. 9th ed. Chicago: American College of Surgeons; 2012. p. 69.
9. Mutschler M, Nienaber U, Brockamp T, Wafaisade A, Wyen H, Peiniger S, Paffrath T, Bouillon B, Maegele M, TraumaRegister DGU. A critical reappraisal of the ATLS classification of hypovolaemic shock: does it really reflect clinical reality? Resuscitation. 2013;84(3):309–13. https://doi.org/10.1016/j.resuscitation.2012.07.012. Epub 2012 Jul 24.
10. Cappell MS, Dass K, Manickam P. Characterization of the syndrome of UGI bleeding from a Mallory-Weiss tear associated with transesophageal echocardiography. Dig Dis Sci. 2014;59(10):2381–9.
11. Wright AS, Rikkers LF. Current management of portal hypertension. J Gastrointest Surg. 2005;9(7):992–1005. https://doi.org/10.1016/j.gassur.2004.09.028.
12. Rikkers LF, Jin G. Surgical management of acute variceal hemorrhage. World J Surg. 1994;18:193–9. https://doi.org/10.1007/BF00294400.
13. Acosta RD, Wong RK. Differential diagnosis of upper gastrointestinal bleeding proximal to the ligament of Trietz. Gastrointest Endosc Clin N Am. 2011;21(4):555–66. https://doi.org/10.1016/j.giec.2011.07.014.
14. Hwang JH, Fisher DA, Ben-Menachem T, Chandrasekhara V, Chathadi K, Decker GA, Early DS, Evans JA, Fanelli RD, Foley K, Fukami N, Jain R, Jue TL, Khan KM, Lightdale J, Malpas PM, Maple JT, Pasha S, Saltzman J, Sharaf R, Shergill AK, Dominitz JA, Cash BD, Standards of Practice Committee of the American Society for Gastrointestinal Endoscopy. The role of endoscopy in the management of acute non-variceal upper GI bleeding. Gastrointest Endosc. 2012;75(6):1132–8. https://doi.org/10.1016/j.gie.2012.02.033.
15. Berry R, Han JY, Kardashian AA, LaRusso NF, Tabibian JH. Hemobilia: etiology, diagnosis, and treatment. Liver Res. 2018;2(4):200–8. https://doi.org/10.1016/j.livres.2018.09.007. Epub 2018 Sep 22.
16. Gwiggner M, Patel P. An unusual case of obscure gastrointestinal bleeding in a patient with coeliac disease. Case Rep Gastrointest Med. 2011;2011:634684. https://doi.org/10.1155/2011/634684. Epub 2011 Nov 13.
17. Kahrilas PJ. GERD pathogenesis, pathophysiology, and clinical manifestations. Cleve Clin J Med. 2003;70(Suppl 5):S4–19. https://doi.org/10.3949/ccjm.70.suppl_5.s4.
18. Nelms DW, Pelaez CA. The acute upper gastrointestinal bleed. Surg Clin North Am. 2018;98(5):1047–57. https://doi.org/10.1016/j.suc.2018.05.004. Epub 2018 Jul 29.
19. Ittrich H, Bockhorn M, Klose H, Simon M. The diagnosis and treatment of hemoptysis. Dtsch Arztebl Int. 2017;114(21):371–81.
20. Laine L, Jensen DM. Management of patients with ulcer bleeding. Am J Gastroenterol. 2012;107(3):345–60; quiz 361. https://doi.org/10.1038/ajg.2011.480. Epub 2012 Feb 7.
21. Barkun AN, Bardou M, Kuipers EJ, et al., International Consensus Upper Gastrointestinal Bleeding Conference Group. International consensus recommendations on the management of patients with nonvariceal upper gastrointestinal bleeding. Ann Intern Med. 2010;152:101–13. https://doi.org/10.7326/0003-4819-152-2-201001190-00009.

22. Gralnek IM, Dumonceau JM, Kuipers EJ, Lanas A, Sanders DS, Kurien M, Rotondano G, Hucl T, Dinis-Ribeiro M, Marmo R, Racz I, Arezzo A, Hoffmann RT, Lesur G, de Franchis R, Aabakken L, Veitch A, Radaelli F, Salgueiro P, Cardoso R, Maia L, Zullo A, Cipolletta L, Hassan C. Diagnosis and management of nonvariceal upper gastrointestinal hemorrhage: European Society of Gastrointestinal Endoscopy (ESGE) Guideline. Endoscopy. 2015;47(10):a1–46. https://doi.org/10.1055/s-0034-1393172. Epub 2015 Sep 29.

23. Carrick MM, Morrison CA, Tapia NM, et al. Intraoperative hypotensive resuscitation for patients undergoing laparotomy or thoracotomy for trauma: early termination of a randomized prospective clinical trial. J Trauma Acute Care Surg. 2016;80:886–96. https://doi.org/10.1097/TA.0000000000001044.

24. Razzaghi A, Barkun AN. Platelet transfusion threshold in patients with upper gastrointestinal bleeding: a systematic review. J Clin Gastroenterol. 2012;46:482–6.

25. Lau JYW, Yu Y, Tang RSY, Chan HCH, Yip HC, Chan SM, Luk SWY, Wong SH, Lau LHS, Lui RN, Chan TT, Mak JWY, Chan FKL, Sung JJY. Timing of endoscopy for acute upper gastrointestinal bleeding. N Engl J Med. 2020;382(14):1299–308. https://doi.org/10.1056/NEJMoa1912484.

26. Phang TS, Vornik V, Stubbs R. Risk assessment in upper gastrointestinal haemorrhage: implications for resource utilisation. N Z Med J. 2000;113(1115):331–3.

27. Sreedharan A, Martin J, Leontiadis GI, et al. Proton pump inhibitor treatment initiated prior to endoscopic diagnosis in upper gastrointestinal bleeding. Cochrane Database Syst Rev. 2010;7:CD005415.

28. Garcia-Tsao G, Abraldes JG, Berzigotti A, Bosch J. Portal hypertensive bleeding in cirrhosis: Risk stratification, diagnosis, and management: 2016 practice guidance by the American Association for the Study of Liver Diseases. Hepatology. 2017;65:310–35. https://doi.org/10.1002/hep.28906.

29. Aljebreen AM, Fallone CA, Barkun AN. Nasogastric aspirate predicts high-risk endoscopic lesions in patients with acute upper GI bleeding. Gastrointest Endosc. 2004;59:172–8.

30. Bennett C, Klingenberg SL, Langholz E, Gluud LL. Tranexamic acid for upper gastrointestinal bleeding. Cochrane Database Syst Rev. 2014;(11):CD006640. https://doi.org/10.1002/14651858.CD006640.pub3.

31. Lau JY, Sung JJ, Lam YH, Chan AC, Ng EK, Lee DW, Chan FK, Suen RC, Chung SC. Endoscopic retreatment compared with surgery in patients with recurrent bleeding after initial endoscopic control of bleeding ulcers. N Engl J Med. 1999;340(10):751–6. https://doi.org/10.1056/NEJM199903113401002.

32. Sengstaken RW, Blakemore AH. Balloon tamponage for the control of hemorrhage from esophageal varices. Ann Surg. 1950;131(5):781–9. https://doi.org/10.1097/00000658-195005000-00017.

33. Powell M, Journey JD. Sengstaken-Blakemore tube. In: StatPearls. Treasure Island, FL: StatPearls Publishing; 2021

34. Clarke MG, Bunting D, Smart NJ, Lowes J, MitchellSJ. The surgical management of acute upper gastrointestinal bleeding: a 12-year experience. Int J Surg. 2010;8(5):377–80. https://doi.org/10.1016/j.ijsu.2010.05.008. Epub 2010 Jun 9.

35. Eriksson LG, Ljungdahl M, Sundbom M, Nyman R. Transcatheter arterial embolization versus surgery in the treatment of upper gastrointestinal bleeding after therapeutic endoscopy failure. J Vasc Interv Radiol. 2008;19(10):1413–8. https://doi.org/10.1016/j.jvir.2008.06.019. Epub 2008 Aug 27.

36. Kyaw M, Tse Y, Ang D, Ang TL, Lau J. Embolization versus surgery for peptic ulcer bleeding after failed endoscopic hemostasis: a meta-analysis. Endosc Int Open. 2014;2(1):E6–E14. https://doi.org/10.1055/s--0034-1365235. Epub 2014 Mar 7.

37. Ali A, Ahmed BH, Nussbaum MS. Chapter 59: Surgery for peptic ulcer disease. In: Yeo CJ, editor. Shackelford's surgery of the alimentary tract, vol. 2. 8th ed. Elsevier; 2019. p. 673–701. ISBN: 9780323402323. https://doi.org/10.1016/B978-0-323-40232-3.00059-5.

38. Sugiura M, Futagawa S. A new technique for treating esophageal varices. Thorac Cardiovasc Surg. 1973;66(5):677–85. https://doi.org/10.1016/S0022-5223(19)40560-6.

39. Kurokawa T, Arikawa T, Sano T, Nonami T. Chapter 43: Surgical treatment Sugiura procedure and Hassab's operation. In: Obara K, editor. Clinical investigation of portal hypertension. Singapore: Springer Nature Singapore; 2019. p. 429–37. https://doi.org/10.1007/978-981-10-7425-7_43.

40. Czymek R, Großmann A, Roblick U, Schmidt A, Fischer F, Bruch HP, Hildebrand P. Surgical management of acute upper gastrointestinal bleeding: still a major challenge. Hepatogastroenterology. 2012;59(115):768–73. https://doi.org/10.5754/hge10466.

## Further Reading

Barkun AN, Bardou M, Kuipers EJ, et al., Consensus Upper Gastrointestinal Bleeding Conference Group. International International consensus recommendations on the management of patients with nonvariceal upper gastrointestinal bleeding. Ann Intern Med. 2010;152:101-113. https://doi.org/10.7326/0003-4819-152-2-201001190-00009.

Gralnek IM, Dumonceau JM, Kuipers EJ, Lanas A, Sanders DS, Kurien M, Rotondano G, Hucl T, Dinis-Ribeiro M, Marmo R, Racz I, Arezzo A, Hoffmann RT, Lesur G, de Franchis R, Aabakken L, Veitch A, Radaelli F, Salgueiro P, Cardoso R, Maia L, Zullo A, Cipolletta L, Hassan C. Diagnosis and management of nonvariceal upper gastrointestinal hemorrhage: European Society of Gastrointestinal Endoscopy (ESGE) Guideline. Endoscopy. 2015;47(10):a1–46. https://doi.org/10.1055/s-0034-1393172. Epub 2015 Sep 29.

Laine L, Jensen DM. Management of patients with ulcer bleeding. Am J Gastroenterol. 2012;107(3):345–60; quiz 361. https://doi.org/10.1038/ajg.2011.480. Epub 2012 Feb 7.

Lau JYW, Yu Y, Tang RSY, Chan HCH, Yip HC, Chan SM, Luk SWY, Wong SH, Lau LHS, Lui RN, Chan TT, Mak JWY, Chan FKL, Sung JJY. Timing of endoscopy for acute upper gastrointestinal bleeding. N Engl J Med. 2020;382(14):1299–308. https://doi.org/10.1056/NEJMoa1912484.

Stanley AJ, Laine L. Management of acute upper gastrointestinal bleeding. BMJ. 2019;364:l536. https://doi.org/10.1136/bmj.l536.

# Gastric Outlet Obstruction

Feibo Zheng, Liang Ha, and Yunfeng Cui

## 70.1 Introduction

Gastric outlet obstruction (GOO) means that the passage from the stomach to the small intestine is obstructed. The lesion site can be at the distal stomach (antrum and pylorus) and proximal duodenum. GOO is mainly manifested with nonspecific abdominal pain or dyspepsia. Therefore, it is hard to identify GOO. GOO is generally divided into benign and malignant based on mechanical cause. Additionally, motility disorders and congenital malformation are also important causes of GOO. Consequently, individualized and comprehensive treatments should be considered: proton pump inhibitor, endoscopic techniques, or/and surgery.

> **Learning Goals**
> - Identify how to diagnose gastric outlet obstruction.
> - Determine how to establish the etiology of gastric outlet obstruction.
> - Outline the approach to the treatment of gastric outlet obstruction based on the etiology of the disease.

### 70.1.1 Epidemiology

The incidence of GOO is with precision is unknown [1]. Peptic ulcer disease (PUD) used to account for most cases of GOO. It is still common but has declined in frequency with the use of proton pump inhibitor. Hypertrophic pyloric stenosis (HPS) is the most common cause of GOO in children, strictly speaking, it mostly occurs in infants. Hypertrophic pyloric stenosis is an obstructive idiopathic hypertrophy of the pyloric muscle and the usual demographic is a 2–8 weeks in age; a patient, who presents with forceful nonbilious vomiting [2], rarely later than 3 months of age, with a clear preponderance in boys [3].

In contrast, in recent decades, we have seen a trend toward more cases that were attributable to cancer [4, 5]. Gastric cancer used to be the most common cause of malignant GOO but the morbidity also has declined due to the eradication of *Helicobacter pylori* infection [1]. In the mean-

F. Zheng
Nankai Clinical School of Medicine, Tianjin Medical University, Tianjin, China

Department of Surgery, Tianjin Occupational Diseases Precaution and Therapeutic Hospital, Tianjin, China

L. Ha · Y. Cui (✉)
Department of Surgery, Tianjin Nankai Hospital, Nankai Clinical School of Medicine, Tianjin Medical University, Tianjin, China

time, pancreatic cancer is on the rise, and up to 20% of patients with pancreatic cancer develop gastric outlet obstruction. Now, pancreatic cancer predominates [6]. In addition, as far as gender is concerned, males are more commonly affected than females with a ratio of about 3 to 4:1 for both malignant and benign causes [5, 7].

### 70.1.2 Etiology

#### 70.1.2.1 Mechanical Obstruction
(Table 70.1)

Mechanical obstruction is generally divided into benign and malignant. Pancreatic cancer and gastric cancer are the most common cause of malignant GOO [1, 6, 8] (Figs. 70.1 and 70.2). Other rare causes of malignant gastric outlet obstruction include gastric lymphoma, large tumors of the proximal duodenum and ampulla, local extension of advanced gallbladder or cholangiocarcinoma, metastatic malignancies, retroperitoneal sarcoma, and gastrointestinal stroma tumor.

Peptic ulcer disease is the leading cause of benign GOO (Fig. 70.3). Less common causes have been seen in postsurgical stricture or scarring (Fig. 70.4), pancreatitis and pancreatic pseudocyst [9] (Fig. 70.5), nonsteroidal anti-inflammatory drugs (NSAIDs)-associated stricture (Fig. 70.6a), gastric volvulus (Fig. 70.6b), etc.

#### 70.1.2.2 Motility Disorders
(Table 70.2)

Gastroparesis is a disorder characterized by delayed gastric emptying of solid food in the absence of a mechanical obstruction of the stomach [10]. It is the most common motility disorder that causes GOO. The leading causes of gastroparesis are idiopathic (39.4%) and diabetic gastroparesis (37.5%) [11, 12].

#### 70.1.2.3 Congenital Malformation
(Table 70.2)

Congenital malformations cause a very small amount of gastric outlet obstruction, including infantile hypertrophic pyloric stenosis, duodenal atresia, duodenal web, annular pancreas, malrotation with midgut volvulus, enteric duplication cyst, and other rare anomalies [2].

### 70.1.3 Classification

GOO can be broadly divided into two categories based on etiology as well as development mechanism: mechanical obstruction and motility disorders. Mechanical obstruction is generally divided into benign and malignant [6]. As with any diagnostic classification scheme, there may be overlap between the categories. In terms of obstruction mechanism, GOOs due to congenital malformation pertain to the mechanical obstruction as well.

### 70.1.4 Pathophysiology

Frequent and massive vomiting of gastric contents leads to electrolyte abnormalities—deple-

**Table 70.1** Etiologies of gastric outlet obstruction—mechanical

| Etiologies | Specific diseases |
|---|---|
| Malignant | Pancreatic cancer |
| | Gastric cancer |
| | Duodenal cancer |
| | Gallbladder cancer |
| | Liver/biliary cancer |
| | Ampullary cancer |
| | Gastric lymphoma |
| | Metastases |
| | Retroperitoneal sarcoma |
| | Gastrointestinal stromal tumor |
| Benign | Peptic ulcer disease |
| | Pancreatitis |
| | Postsurgical stricture or scarring |
| | Pancreatic pseudocyst |
| | NSAID-associated stricture |
| | Gastric volvulus |
| | Crohn disease |
| | Tuberculosis |
| | Duodenitis |
| | Caustic ingestion |
| | Benign tumor |
| | Foreign body |
| | Duodenal hematoma |
| | Amyloidosis |
| | Bouveret's syndrome |

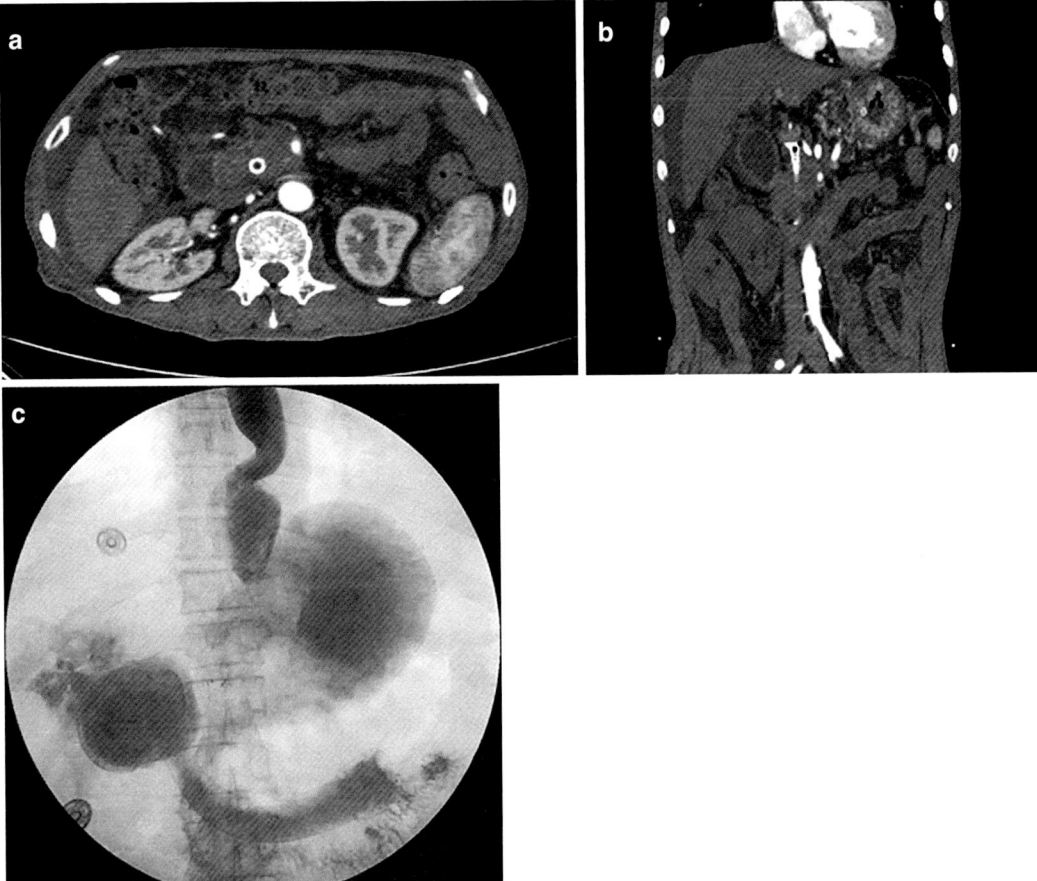

**Fig. 70.1** Pancreatic cancer. A 76-year-old male with experiencing weight loss, abdominal discomfort, and early satiety. Axial (**a**) and coronal (**b**) images CECT show a distended stomach with narrowing of the second portion of the duodenum near the pancreas, duodenal obstruction. The head of pancreas enlarged, the superior mesenteric artery and portal vein were wrapped locally. (**c**) Post duodenal stenting, upper gastrointestinal radiography shows the patency of pylorus and duodenum. (From Tianjin Nankai Hospital, Tianjin, China)

tion of sodium, potassium, chloride, and hydrogen ions, eventually resulting in the classical hypochloremic and/or hypokalemic metabolic alkalosis. The kidney's ability to maintain normal pH by excreting bicarbonate is impaired by chloride depletion [13]. Excess bicarbonate is reabsorbed instead in an attempt to remain electrochemically neutral. This aggravates alkalosis. Furthermore, the kidneys preserve potassium at the expense of hydrogen ions, leading to paradoxical aciduria and further aggravating alkalosis. Metabolic alkalosis can potentially affect the respiratory drive of an infant and has been associated with apneas and extubation difficulties [14].

It has been demonstrated that nitric oxide synthase (NOS) inhibitors can delay gastric emptying and colonic transport [15]. The decreased expression of neuronal NOS is related to the impairment of local NO production (NO is synthesized through the activation of neuronal NOS in the myenteric plexus), which may be the cause of gastrointestinal motility disturbance. NO regulates the muscle tone of the lower esophagus, pylorus, Oddi sphincter, and anal sphincter. The impairment of neuronal NOS synthesis in myenteric plexus seems to be an important pathogenic factor for achalasia, diabetic gastroparesis, and hypertrophic pyloric stenosis in infants.

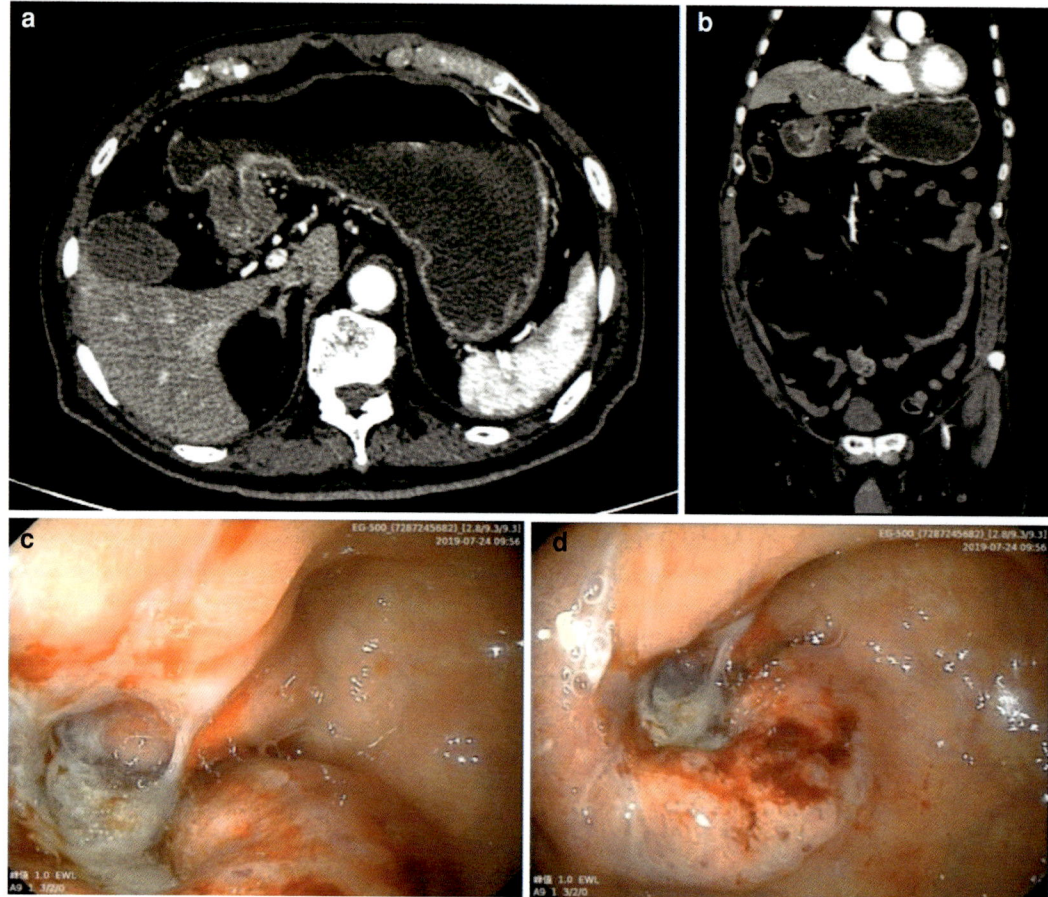

**Fig. 70.2** Gastric cancer. Axial (**a**) and sagittal (**b**) CECT suggest numerous contents can be seen in the stomach, gastric antrum wall thickening, mucosal linear enhancement and gastric outlet obstruction; (**c**, **d**) gastroscope show antrum mucosa is rough, a deep concave ulcer can be seen next to the pyloric canal, covered with white moss, surrounding hyperemia and edema, tissue stiffness, and deformation, pyloric stenosis. (From Tianjin Nankai Hospital, Tianjin, China)

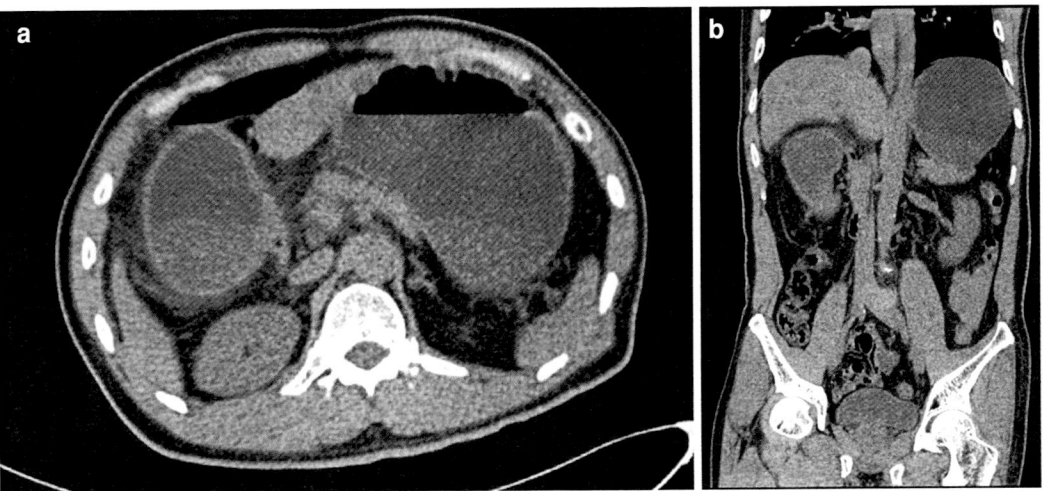

**Fig. 70.3** Pyloric stenosis due to peptic ulcer disease (**a** and **b**). A 56-year-old male who presented with vomiting and epigastric pain. (From Tianjin Nankai Hospital, Tianjin, China)

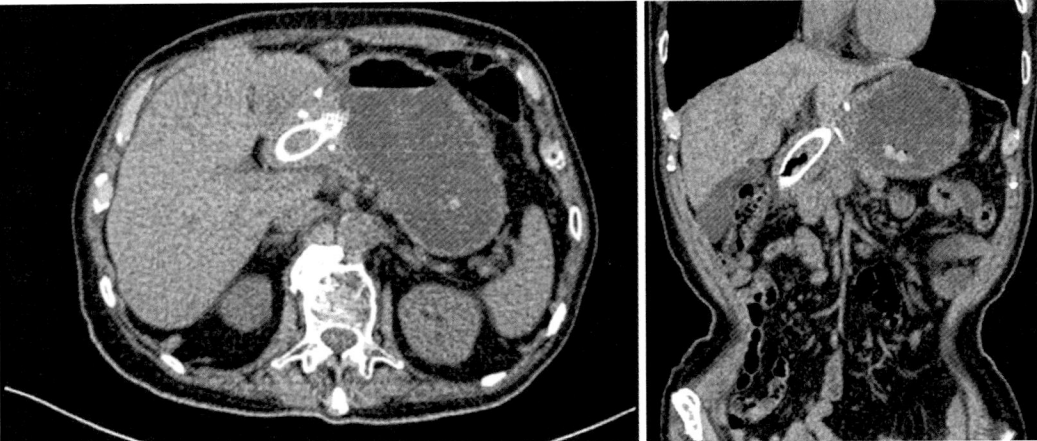

**Fig. 70.4** Gastrointestinal anastomotic obstruction and stent implantation after operation of gastric cancer. (From Tianjin Nankai Hospital, Tianjin, China)

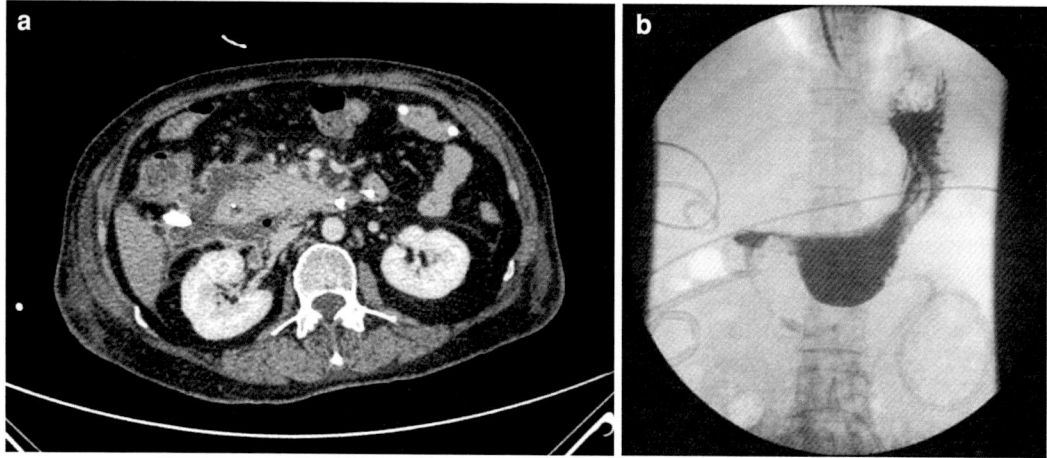

**Fig. 70.5** Severe acute pancreatitis. A 56-year-old female with abdominal pain and vomiting (**a**) CECT shows acute necrotizing pancreatitis with exudation, inflammatory involvement of adjacent stomach and duodenum; (**b**) upper gastrointestinal radiography suggests the contrast medium passes through the pylorus slowly, and after the delay, a little contrast medium can be seen to enter the duodenum, considering duodenal obstruction. (From Tianjin Nankai Hospital, Tianjin, China)

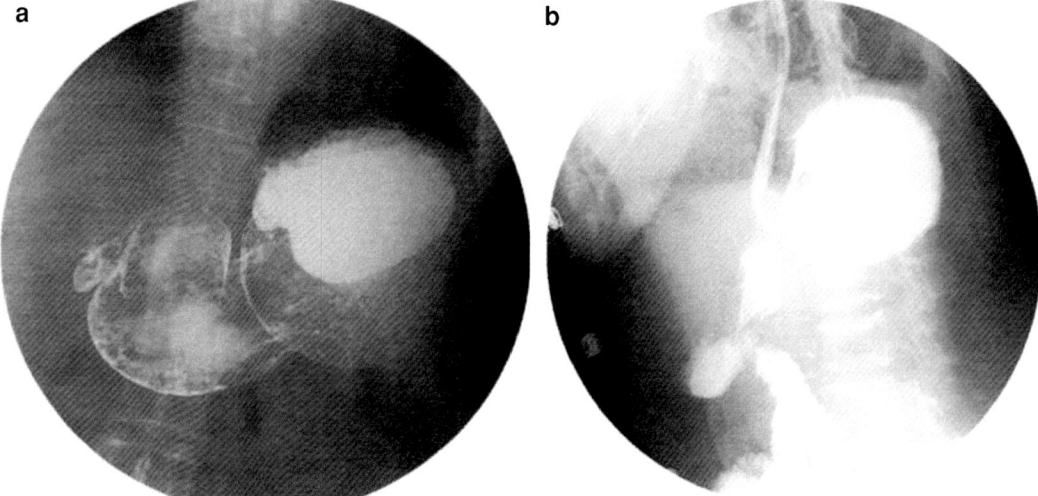

**Fig. 70.6** (**a**) Gastric antrum and duodenal obstruction (oral contrast of meglumine diatrizoate); (**b**) gastric axial semi-volvulus, duodenal diverticulum. (From Tianjin Nankai Hospital, Tianjin, China)

**Table 70.2** Etiologies of gastric outlet obstruction—mobility disorders and congenital malformation

| Etiologies | Specific diseases |
|---|---|
| Mobility disorders-gastroparesis | Idiopathic |
| | Diabetes mellitus |
| | Post-surgical (fundoplication and vagotomy) |
| | Medications (opioids, antibiotics, antiarrhythmics and anticonvulsants) |
| | Neurologic disorders (Parkinson disease, amyloidosis and dysautonomia) |
| | Post-viral infection (norovirus, Epstein–Barr virus, cytomegalovirus and herpesvirus) |
| | Connective tissue disorders (scleroderma and systemic lupus erythematosus) |
| | Renal insufficiency |
| Congenital malformation | Infantile hypertrophic pyloric stenosis |
| | Duodenal atresia |
| | Duodenal web |
| | Annular pancreas |
| | Malrotation |
| | Pyloric stenosis |
| | Enteric duplication cyst |
| | Vascular anomalies |

## 70.2 Diagnosis

### 70.2.1 Clinical Presentation

The patients often present with nausea and vomiting as their chief complaint, others like abdominal pain, abdominal distention, early satiety, and weight loss.

The physical examination may reveal evidence of hypovolemia, malnutrition, and dehydration. Abdominal distension may occur. A succussion splash may suggest gastric outlet obstruction; the test is considered positive if present 3 or more hours after drinking fluids and suggests retention of gastric materials [16, 17].

On top of that, a detailed drugs history pertaining to the use of NSAIDs, aspirin, opioids, anticholinergic medications may contribute to the diagnosis.

### 70.2.2 Tests

#### 70.2.2.1 Laboratory Test

Electrolyte abnormalities and acid-base balance disorder, including hypokalemia, hypochloremic metabolic alkalosis and paradoxical aciduria should be emphasized. Increased serum gastrin levels (400–800 pg/mL range), have to be differentiated with Zollinger-Ellison syndrome [18].

#### 70.2.2.2 Imaging

Upper gastrointestinal radiography with oral barium may reveal an enlarged gastric bubble, and contrast studies may be useful to determine whether the obstruction is partial or complete. Abdominal ultrasonography is still effective and concise tool for the diagnosis. Magnetic resonance imaging (MRI) with magnetic resonance cholangiopancreatography (MRCP) can show the pancreatic duct encircling the duodenum [19]. What needs to be emphasized, contrast-enhanced computer tomography should be first choice of medical imaging [20].

#### 70.2.2.3 Endoscopy

Upper endoscopy is often needed to establish the diagnosis and cause; the findings include retained food and liquid. Endoscopic biopsy is crucial to differentiate whether benign or malignant. Moreover, endoscopic ultrasonography is useful for diagnosis via tissue sampling with fine-needle aspiration and locoregional staging [21].

The diagnosis may not be suspected clinically due to be vague and nonspecific of the presenting symptoms of GOO; therefore, we need to make a comprehensive evaluation in combination with laboratory tests, imaging as well as endoscopy.

> **Differential Diagnosis**
> GOO is not strictly a disease, but the outcome of many diseases and symptoms such as abdominal pain and postprandial vomiting. Its differential diagnosis depends on its etiology, as long as the etiology is ascertained; subsequently the differential diagnosis is clear as well.

## 70.3 Treatment

### 70.3.1 Medical Treatment

#### 70.3.1.1 Endoscopic Balloon Dilation (EBD)

Dilation can be accomplished using endoscopy and a balloon dilator inserted through the working channel of the scope, or by using a balloon placed over a guidewire positioned under fluoroscopic guidance. EBD is often successful in the short term with immediate symptom improvement [22, 23]. Long-term results often require more dilation; however, it is likely to be associated with a higher probability of surgery [24].

#### 70.3.1.2 Self-Expanding Metal Stents (SEMS)

With the assistance of endoscopy and fluoroscopy, a wire passes through the gastroduodenal stricture, and then the metal stent passes over the wire and is released across the stenosis. There are two different types of SEMS, covered and uncovered stents. Uncovered stents are less likely to migrate and more flexible, but the tumor can grow into the stent and result in stent obstruction. Covered stents provide the advantage of low tumor growth, but they are more prone to migration and less flexible [25, 26]. In order to make up for the shortcomings of existing stents, the development of stents continues, and the recent anti-migration design of new covered stents is considered to be superior in terms of stent patency and complications [27].

#### 70.3.1.3 Lumen-Apposing Metal Stents (LAMS)

LAMS is a novel SEMS, and has primarily been used to drain pancreatic fluid collections to good effect [28, 29]. Recently, a growing pool of data has demonstrated that LAMS provide a new option for the effective endoscopic management of benign GOO [30, 31]. One study suggests the utility of stent therapy-less postoperative morbidity than and a similar food intake and equivalent survival times to surgical gastrojejunostomy [32].

### 70.3.2 Surgical Treatment

**Surgical bypass** used to be the standard of care for palliation of malignant gastric obstruction, but that was before endoscopic stenting was developed.

**Laparoscopic gastrojejunostomy** is a feasible option, and presents improved morbidity and mortality rates compared with the open surgical approach [33]. Min et al. [34] show laparoscopic gastrojejunostomy provide better outcomes (better oral intake, better tolerance of chemotherapy, and longer overall survival) than duodenal stenting for patients with malignant GOO.

**Endoscopic ultrasound-guided gastroenterostomy (EUS-GE)** has been developed and proposed an innovative technique that allows the creation of a stable gastrojejunal anastomosis through a EUS-guided procedure in the last years. In the EUS-GE procedure, the small bowel is punctured from the stomach at the level of the distal duodenum or in the proximal jejunum (i.e., gastroduodenostomy or gastrojejunostomy, respectively) under EUS and fluoroscopic guidance, with subsequent placement of a LAMS, thus creating a tight and sealed anastomosis, owing to the lumen-to-lumen apposition effect of the stent [35]. Many data [36–38] propose EUS-GE as a valuable minimal invasive option for patient with malignant GOO. Presently, there are three types of techniques to perform EUS-GE with LAMS [39]: (1) direct EUS-GE; (2) assisted EUS-GE; and (3) EUS-guided double balloon occluded gastrojejunostomy bypass (EPASS). Regardless of the technique adopted, data from several studies reported high technical and clinical success rate for EUS-GE in malignant GOO [36–38].

An algorithm of treatment for benign and malignant GOO is presented in Figs. 70.7 and 70.8.

## 70.3.4 Prognosis

EBD is usually a safe procedure, with few complications of bleeding and perforation with a diameter less than 15 mm. Pain and mild bleeding are common during EBD procedure, but they are self-limited, whereas arterial bleeding is rarely reported. Endoscopic incision could be further performed after endoscopic balloon dilation in pyloric stenosis refractory to EBD.

As to SEMS, tumor ingrowth/overgrowth has been reported in 17.2% of patients receiving uncovered metal stents and in 6.9% of patients with covered stents. This stent obstruction can be managed with a stent-in-stent technique, and stent occlusion rate was reported to be 10–34% after the secondary SEMS insertion [43, 44]. It has been suggested that recent new covered stents with anti-migration designs may improve patency and complications of original stents [27].

Compared to surgery, the advantages of endoscopic stents are shorter procedure time, less time to ingestion, and shorter hospitalization periods, but repeated procedures are often required due to frequent stent failures [41], mainly secondary to stent ingrowth, and, for this reason, they are the first-line strategy in ill patients with short life expectancy (<3 months). Despite these exciting novelties, EUS-GE is still a difficult and not standardized technique, and is currently limited to centers with high experience in therapeutic EUS. Gastrojejunostomy surgery has more benefits and is associated with a longer life expectancy.

For patients with gastric outlet obstruction secondary to chronic PUD, early surgery is recommended. Without surgery, the likelihood of recurrent obstruction, hemorrhage, and perforation remains high. Early treatment of PUD has a good prognosis.

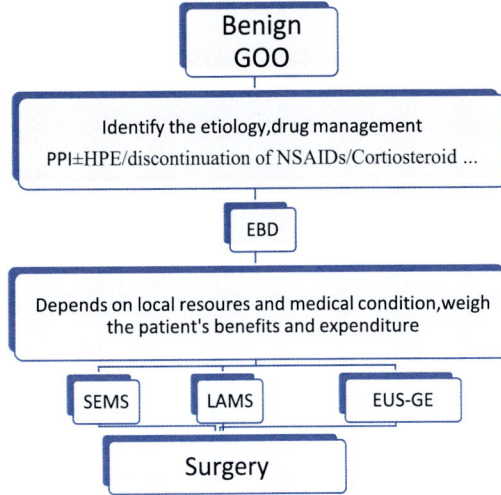

**Fig. 70.7** Treatment algorithm for benign GOO

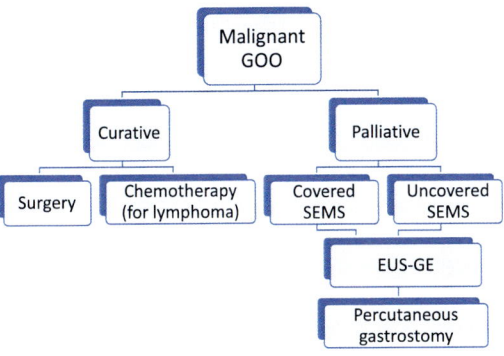

**Fig. 70.8** Treatment algorithm for malignant GOO

## 70.3.3 Chinese Medicine Treatment: Acupuncture

Acupuncture is widely used in the treatment of gastrointestinal disorders, although its role in symptomatic gastroparesis is unclear [40]. Many studies have shown that acupuncture can promote the recovery of gastrointestinal function and relieve the symptoms of obstruction in humans and rats [41, 42], but it is only limited to GOO caused by gastric motility disorder. In any case, acupuncture therapy enriches the treatments for GOO.

## Dos and Don'ts
- First of all, patients with clinical presentation of GOO should be given:
  - Nothing by mouth (NPO).
  - Intravenous fluids to correct electrolyte abnormalities and acid-base balance disorder.
  - A nasogastric tube is essential for gastric decompression and symptom relief if symptoms persist despite being NPO.
  - A parenteral acid inhibitors (proton pump inhibitor) should be used to decrease gastric secretions despite of the cause of obstruction.
  - The stricture seen with Crohn's should be first treated with steroids.
  - Medications for pain and nausea, if needed.
- Second, patients with malignancy that is potentially curable by resection should have the preference of undergoing surgical evaluation.
- Third, surgery is indicated if the obstruction cannot be safely dilated, or if the obstruction persists or recurs despite medical and endoscopic management.
- Fourth, endoscopic therapy is preferred for benign patients when the effect of basic support treatment is not optimal.
- Last, for patients who are not suitable for surgery or endoscopic stent implanting, percutaneous gastrostomy can be considered for gastric decompression and symptom relief.
- Different causes and extent of GOO lead to different treatment or management. Definitive treatment strategies widely vary depending on the underlying etiology, whether benign or malignant, including surgical and/or nonsurgical treatment. We should take into account the balance between clinical benefits and expenditures.

## Take-Home Messages
- GOO should not be ruled out as long as the patient manifested with epigastric pain and postprandial vomiting.
- CT should be first considered in the diagnosis of GOO.
- Treatment depends on etiology, focusing on individual treatment and comprehensive treatment.
- In the early stage of GOO, parenteral nutrition support is of paramount importance in maintaining electrolyte and acid-base homeostasis.
- Weighing the ratio of patients' benefit–cost in the choice of treatment.

Early recognition of the diagnosis, aggressive resuscitation, and early institution of surgical management is crucial if morbidity and mortality associated with gastric outlet obstruction are to be avoided.

## 10 Single Choice Questions with 4 Answers (Only 1 Right Answers)
1. Which is the most common cause of benign GOO? (Answer: A)
   A. Peptic ulcer disease
   B. Pancreatitis
   C. Gastric volvulus
   D. NSAID-associated stricture
2. Which two are the most common malignant cause of GOO? (Answer: B)
   A. Gastric cancer and gallbladder cancer
   B. Pancreatic cancer and gastric cancer
   C. Duodenal cancer and gallbladder cancer
   D. Ampullary cancer and metastases

3. What is the most common symptom of GOO? (Answer: D)
   A. Nausea and dizzy
   B. Diarrhea or constipation
   C. Weight loss
   D. Epigastric pain and postprandial vomiting
4. Which of the following causes cannot result in mechanical GOO? (Answer: A)
   A. Gastroparesis
   B. Cholangiocarcinoma
   C. Pancreatitis and pancreatic pseudocyst
   D. Gastrointestinal stroma tumor
5. Which of the following items does not belong to congenital GOO? (Answer: C)
   A. Duodenal atresia
   B. Infantile hypertrophic pyloric stenosis
   C. Bouveret's syndrome
   D. Annular pancreas
6. What type of electrolyte abnormalities and acid-base balance disorder can be caused by GOO? (Answer: A)
   A. Hypochloremic and/or hypokalemic metabolic alkalosis
   B. Hypochloremic and/or hypokalemic metabolic acidosis
   C. Hyperkalemic metabolic acidosis
   D. Hyperchloremic metabolic alkalosis
7. Which one in the following is the first choice of medical imaging regarding the diagnosis of GOO? (Answer: C)
   A. Ultrasonography
   B. X-ray
   C. CT
   D. MRI
8. Which of the following treatments belongs to traditional Chinese medicine? (Answer: B)
   A. Ultrasonography
   B. Acupuncture
   C. Endoscopic balloon dilation (EBD)
   D. Lumen-apposing metal stents (LAMS)
9. Which of the following complications is rare likelihood of GOO secondary to chronic peptic ulcer disease? (Answer: D)
   A. Perforation
   B. Recurrent obstruction
   C. Hemorrhage
   D. Liver failure
10. Which of the following is a non-invasive treatment? (Answer: B)
    A. Endoscopic balloon dilation (EBD)
    B. Chemotherapy
    C. Percutaneous gastrostomy
    D. Endoscopic ultrasound-guided gastroenterostomy (EUS-GE)

**Conflict of Interest** The authors have no conflict of interest associated with this manuscript.

## References

1. Tringali A, Giannetti A, Adler DG. Endoscopic management of gastric outlet obstruction disease. Ann Gastroenterol. 2019;32(4):330–7.
2. Tantillo K, Dym RJ, Chernyak V, Scheinfeld MH, Taragin BH. No way out: causes of duodenal and gastric outlet obstruction. Clin Imaging. 2020;65:37–46.
3. Tam PKH, Chung PHY, St Peter SD, Gayer CP, Ford HR, Tam GCH, Wong KKY, Pakarinen MP, Davenport M. Advances in paediatric gastroenterology. Lancet. 2017;390(10099):1072–82.
4. Misra SP, Dwivedi M, Misra V. Malignancy is the most common cause of gastric outlet obstruction even in a developing country. Endoscopy. 1998;30(5):484–6.
5. Sukumar V, Ravindran C, Prasad RV. Demographic and etiological patterns of gastric outlet obstruction in Kerala, South India. N Am J Med Sci. 2015;7(9):403–6.
6. Koop AH, Palmer WC, Stancampiano FF. Gastric outlet obstruction: a red flag, potentially manageable. Cleve Clin J Med. 2019;86(5):345–53.
7. Appasani S, Kochhar S, Nagi B, Gupta V, Kochhar R. Benign gastric outlet obstruction—spectrum and management. Trop Gastroenterol. 2011;32(4):259–66.
8. Tringali A, Didden P, Repici A, Spaander M, Bourke MJ, Williams SJ, Spicak J, Drastich P, Mutignani M, Perri V, Roy A, Johnston K, Costamagna G. Endoscopic treatment of malignant gastric and duodenal strictures: a prospective, multicenter study. Gastrointest Endosc. 2014;79(1):66–75.

9. Burke G, Binder S, Barron A, Dratch P, Umlas J. Heterotopic pancreas: gastric outlet obstruction secondary to pancreatitis and pancreatic pseudocyst. Am J Gastroenterol. 1989;84(1):52–5.
10. Camilleri M, Chedid V, Ford AC, Haruma K, Horowitz M, Jones KL, Low PA, Park SY, Parkman HP, Stanghellini V. Gastroparesis. Nat Rev Dis Primers. 2018;4(1):41.
11. Grover M, Farrugia G, Stanghellini V. Gastroparesis: a turning point in understanding and treatment. Gut. 2019;68(12):2238–50.
12. Ye Y, Jiang B, Manne S, Moses P, Almansa C, Bennett D, Dolin P, Ford A. Epidemiology and outcomes of gastroparesis, as documented in general practice records, in the United Kingdom. Gut. 2021;70(4):644–53.
13. Jobson M, Hall NJ. Contemporary management of pyloric stenosis. Semin Pediatr Surg. 2016;25(4):219–24.
14. Pandya S, Heiss K. Pyloric stenosis in pediatric surgery: an evidence-based review. Surg Clin North Am. 2012;92(3):527–39, vii–viii.
15. Takahashi T. Pathophysiological significance of neuronal nitric oxide synthase in the gastrointestinal tract. J Gastroenterol. 2003;38(5):421–30.
16. Lau J, Chung S, Sung J, Chan A, Ng E, Suen R, Li A. Through-the-scope balloon dilation for pyloric stenosis: long-term results. Gastrointest Endosc. 1996;43:98–101.
17. Ray K, Snowden C, Khatri K, McFall M. Gastric outlet obstruction from a caecal volvulus, herniated through epiploic foramen: a case report. BMJ Case Rep. 2009;2009 https://doi.org/10.1136/bcr.05.2009.1880.
18. Chen IF, Liu KW, Tang TQ, Wang WL. An unusual gastric tumour with gastric outlet obstruction. Gut. 2018;67(9):1645–6.
19. Manuel-Vázquez A, Latorre-Fragua R, Ramiro-Pérez C, López-Marcano A, De la Plaza-Llamas R, Ramia JM. Laparoscopic gastrojejunostomy for gastric outlet obstruction in patients with unresectable hepatopancreatobiliary cancers: a personal series and systematic review of the literature. World J Gastroenterol. 2018;24(18):1978–88.
20. Hohmann C, Bizer B, Finnmann I, Arnold J. [Bouveret syndrome: the stone that broke the camel's back (and stomach)]. Dtsch Med Wochenschr. 2020;145(2):100–3.
21. Valero M, Robles-Medranda C. Endoscopic ultrasound in oncology: an update of clinical applications in the gastrointestinal tract. World J Gastrointest Endosc. 2017;9(6):243–54.
22. Solt J, Bajor J, Szabó M, Horváth O. Long-term results of balloon catheter dilation for benign gastric outlet stenosis. Endoscopy. 2003;35(6):490–5.
23. Kozarek R, Botoman V, Patterson D. Long-term follow-up in patients who have undergone balloon dilation for gastric outlet obstruction. Gastrointest Endosc. 1990;36(6):558–61.
24. Perng C, Lin H, Lo W, Lai C, Guo W, Lee S. Characteristics of patients with benign gastric outlet obstruction requiring surgery after endoscopic balloon dilation. Am J Gastroenterol. 1996;91(5):987–90.
25. Woo S, Kim D, Lee W, Park K, Park S, Han S, Kim T, Koh Y, Kim H, Hong E. Comparison of uncovered and covered stents for the treatment of malignant duodenal obstruction caused by pancreaticobiliary cancer. Surg Endosc. 2013;27(6):2031–9.
26. van den Berg M, Walter D, Vleggaar F, Siersema P, Fockens P, van Hooft J. High proximal migration rate of a partially covered "big cup" duodenal stent in patients with malignant gastric outlet obstruction. Endoscopy. 2014;46(2):158–61.
27. Lee H, Min B, Lee J, Shin C, Kim Y, Chung H, Lee S. Covered metallic stents with an anti-migration design vs. uncovered stents for the palliation of malignant gastric outlet obstruction: a multicenter, randomized trial. Am J Gastroenterol. 2015;110(10):1440–9.
28. Zhu H, Lin H, Jin Z, Du Y. Re-evaluation of the role of lumen-apposing metal stents (LAMS) for pancreatic fluid collection drainage. Gut. 2017;66(12):2192.
29. Ryan B, Venkatachalapathy S, Huggett M. Safety of lumen-apposing metal stents (LAMS) for pancreatic fluid collection drainage. Gut. 2017;66(8):1530–1.
30. Irani S, Jalaj S, Ross A, Larsen M, Grimm I, Baron T. Use of a lumen-apposing metal stent to treat GI strictures (with videos). Gastrointest Endosc. 2017;85(6):1285–9.
31. Larson B, Adler D. Lumen-apposing metal stents for gastrointestinal luminal strictures: current use and future directions. Ann Gastroenterol. 2019;32(2):141–6.
32. Haga Y, Hiki N, Kinoshita T, Ojima T, Nabeya Y, Kuwabara S, Seto Y, Yajima K, Takeuchi H, Yoshida K, Kodera Y, Fujiwara Y, Baba H. Treatment option of endoscopic stent insertion or gastrojejunostomy for gastric outlet obstruction due to gastric cancer: a propensity score-matched analysis. Gastric Cancer. 2020;23(4):667–76.
33. Guzman E, Dagis A, Bening L, Pigazzi A. Laparoscopic gastrojejunostomy in patients with obstruction of the gastric outlet secondary to advanced malignancies. Am Surg. 2009;75(2):129–32.
34. Min S, Son S, Jung D, Lee C, Ahn S, Park D, Kim H. Laparoscopic gastrojejunostomy versus duodenal stenting in unresectable gastric cancer with gastric outlet obstruction. Ann Surg Treat Res. 2017;93(3):130–6.
35. Troncone E, Fugazza A, Cappello A, Del Vecchio BG, Monteleone G, Repici A, Teoh AYB, Anderloni A. Malignant gastric outlet obstruction: which is the best therapeutic option? World J Gastroenterol. 2020;26(16):1847–60.
36. Chen Y, Itoi T, Baron T, Nieto J, Haito-Chavez Y, Grimm I, Ismail A, Ngamruengphong S, Bukhari M, Hajiyeva G, Alawad A, Kumbhari V, Khashab M. EUS-guided gastroenterostomy is comparable

to enteral stenting with fewer re-interventions in malignant gastric outlet obstruction. Surg Endosc. 2017;31(7):2946–52.
37. Carbajo A, Kahaleh M, Tyberg A. Clinical review of EUS-guided gastroenterostomy (EUS-GE). J Clin Gastroenterol. 2020;54(1):1–7.
38. Ge P, Young J, Dong W, Thompson C. EUS-guided gastroenterostomy versus enteral stent placement for palliation of malignant gastric outlet obstruction. Surg Endosc. 2019;33(10):3404–11.
39. Itoi T, Baron T, Khashab M, Tsuchiya T, Irani S, Dhir V, Bun Teoh A. Technical review of endoscopic ultrasonography-guided gastroenterostomy in 2017. Dig Endosc. 2017;29(4):495–502.
40. Kim KH, Lee MS, Choi T-Y, Kim T-H. Acupuncture for symptomatic gastroparesis. Cochrane Database Syst Rev. 2018;12:CD009676.
41. Zhuang L, Chen C, Guo Y. [Comparative study on treatment of diabetic gastroparesis by acupuncture and Western medicine]. Zhongguo Zhen Jiu. 2005;25(4):249–51.
42. Sun B, Luo M, Wu S, Chen X, Wu M. Acupuncture versus metoclopramide in treatment of postoperative gastroparesis syndrome in abdominal surgical patients: a randomized controlled trial. Zhong Xi Yi Jie He Xue Bao. 2010;8(7):641–4.
43. Sasaki T, Isayama H, Nakai Y, Takahara N, Hamada T, Mizuno S, Mohri D, Yagioka H, Kogure H, Arizumi T, Togawa O, Matsubara S, Ito Y, Yamamoto N, Sasahira N, Hirano K, Toda N, Tada M, Koike K. Clinical outcomes of secondary gastroduodenal self-expandable metallic stent placement by stent-in-stent technique for malignant gastric outlet obstruction. Dig Endosc. 2015;27(1):37–43.
44. Kim C, Choi I, Lee J, Cho S, Kim S, Kim M, Park S, Park Y. Outcomes of second self-expandable metallic stent insertion for malignant gastric outlet obstruction. Surg Endosc. 2014;28(1):281–8.

# Acute Lower Gastrointestinal Bleeding

**71**

Muhammed A. Khalil Ali, Henry Bergman, Salomone Di Saverio, M. Adil Butt, and Ewen A. Griffiths

## 71.1 Introduction

Lower gastrointestinal (GI) bleeding is caused by luminal bleeding from a source distal to the Ligament of Trietz. It remains a significant health burden worldwide, with an annual incidence of 36 per 100,000 patients. This represents almost 3% of emergency surgical referrals [1]. Of all causes of GI bleeding, about 20% are lower GI in origin but result in the use of half of all red blood cell transfusions for this population [2]. The overall mortality is estimated between 2.3% and 3.9% and is mainly related to advanced age and patient comorbidities [3]. Mortality significantly rises in patients who develop lower GI bleeding and reside in nursing homes or other long-term medical institutions [4, 5]. Mortality in these patients reflects their poor general health and general frailty rather than a consequence of acute bleeding per se [6].

Historically, despite the magnitude of the clinical problem [7], there has been a lack of consensus in the investigation and treatment of this patient group with no clear management guidelines [8]. However, as a consequence of two recent reviews of lower GI bleeding management in the UK, consensus guidelines have now been achieved [9, 10]. The reviews identified large gaps in the care of such patients in the emergency setting, notably in the ability to tailor emergency investigation and treatment to emergent endoscopic and interventional radiologic approaches [11].

This chapter provides an up-to-date clinical review for the practising clinician in the management of lower GI bleeding.

**Learning Goals**
- Identify the principal causes of lower GI bleeding.
- Detail specific management guidance for patients with lower GI bleeding.
- Understand the indications and role interventional radiology, endoscopy and surgery play in the management of lower GI bleeding.
- Understand the latest BSG guidelines and patient algorithm for lower GI bleeding.
- Understand the limited role of surgery in the management of these patients; however when it is required have an understanding and algorithm on what to do in a life-saving emergency scenario.

## 71.1.1 Aetiology of Lower GI Bleeding

Although there are multiple causes for lower GI bleeding (Table 71.1), the majority relate to diverticular disease, inflammatory, infective or ischaemic colitis, anorectal pathology)e.g. haemorrhoids, fissures and rectal ulcers), colonic malignancy and vascular malformations. Figure 71.1 demonstrates the common causes, their frequency and some detail on each cause.

**Table 71.1** Causes of lower GI bleeding

| Cause | Frequency (%) | Comments |
|---|---|---|
| Diverticular disease | 30 | Stops spontaneously in 80%. Typically painless. Bleeding is usually arterial from the neck or dome of the diverticulum. |
| Haemorrhoids | 14 | Anorectal examination and proctoscopy should be included in the initial evaluation. |
| Ischaemic colitis | 12 | Often presents with abdominal pain. Colitis is segmental affecting the splenic flexure. |
| Inflammatory bowel disease (Crohn's or Ulcerative colitis) | 9 | Bloody diarrhoea is the most frequent symptom. |
| Post-polypectomy | 8 | Is frequently self-limiting, but can occur up to 14 days after polypectomy. Risk factors include large polyp size, thick stalk, right colon location and anti-coagulation. |
| Colon cancer/polyp | 6 | Rectal bleeding with change in bowel habit has a 3–5 × increased risk of colorectal cancer. Characteristically low volume bleeding associated with anaemia. Massive bleeding is rare. |
| Rectal ulcer | 6 | Chronic benign ulceration, usually solitary but can be multiple, from 3 to 10 cm from the anal verge. |
| Vascular ectasia or angiodysplasia | 3 | Acute bleeding more frequent in right sided colon and occurs in elderly patients. |
| Radiation colitis/proctitis | 3 | Secondary to collateral radiotherapy damage to the colonic or rectal mucosa; there is an acute phase and a chronic small-vessel injury resulting in ischaemia, fibrosis and neovascularisation of the mucosa. |
| Miscellaneous causes | 6 | Rarer causes of lower GI bleeding include aorto-enteric fistula, endometriosis, Meckel's diverticulum, Jejunal diverticulum, small bowel lymphoma or adenocarcinoma or gastrointestinal stromal tumours. Minor trauma from enemas or self-infliction. |

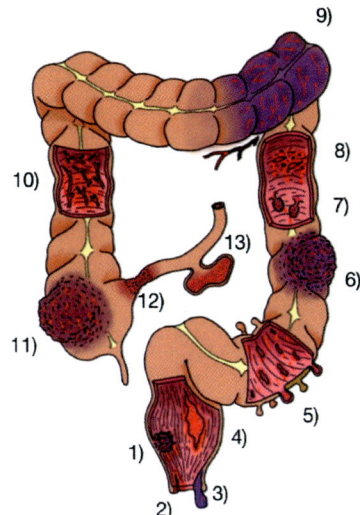

**Fig. 71.1** Causes of lower GI bleeding

1) Rectal Carcinoma
2) Anal Fissure
3) Hemorrhoid
4) Rectal Ulcer
5) Diverticulosis
6) Colonic Carcinoma (Left)
7) Colonic polyps
8) Ulcerative Colitis
9) Ischaemic colitis
10) Vascular ectasia
11) Colonic Carcinoma (Right)
12) Terminal ileitis (Crohn's Disease)
13) Meckel's Diverticulum

## 71.2 Diagnosis

### 71.2.1 Clinical Presentation and History Taking

The presentation of lower GI bleeding can vary according to the underlying cause. It usually presents with overt bleeding in the form haematochezia (the passage of bright red or maroon blood through the rectum), which should be differentiated from melaena (black, tarry stool) that more often relates to an upper GI bleeding though not exclusively. Despite being clinically useful, distinction is not easy to establish. The degree of change in colour of stool varies according to the rate of bleeding and the proximity of the source to the anus. In slow colonic transit states, proximal right colonic pathology may cause melaena. Very brisk upper GI bleedings may conversely present with haematochezia. Importantly, the consequence of bleeding on the haemodynamic stability of the patient usually dictates the way they are managed. It is advisable that in patients with a large GI bleeding, an upper GI source is excluded.

Bleeding varies from being mild and intermittent, to moderate and severe with subsequent associated haemodynamic compromise (pallor, tachycardia, tachypnoea, low blood pressure). Other symptoms may include abdominal pain, dehydration or fever, depending on the aetiology. A history of red flag symptoms such as weight loss, iron deficiency anaemia, change in bowel habit can indicate colonic or rectal malignancy. Recent colonoscopy with or without polypectomy should be sought out as post-procedural bleeding is an important if albeit uncommon complication of this technique with specific management options recommended for it. Any history of pelvic irradiation for previous malignancy (e.g. uterine, prostate or anal cancer) can relate to subsequent acute or chronic radiation proctitis. Patients with inflammatory bowel disease may have a longer period of symptoms with associated constitutional upset such as fatigue, weight loss anaemia from multiple vitamin deficiencies, chronic change in bowel habit but often associated with nocturnal motions, discharge of mucus and a family history of Crohn's or ulcerative colitis. Previous history of AAA surgery could indicate the potential for an aorto-enteric fistula which needs urgent imaging. Blood thinning medications such as dual antiplatelet agents, warfarin, heparin and direct oral anticoagulants should be sought out in the drug history. Anorectal trauma can also cause minor bleedings and may relate to sexual activity, be self-inflicted or related to enema injury in nursing homes for example.

Rectal examination is mandatory in the assessment of patients and can identify anorectal cause for bleeding. The use of a proctoscopy and/or rigid sigmoidoscopy can occur in the assessment unit.

Cardiovascular assessment of the pulse rate and blood pressure allows calculation of the shock index that features centrally in the recent UK lower GI bleeding guidelines. Other signs of severe bleeding should still be sought out, including pallor, cool peripheries, history or evidence of recent collapse, dehydration, poor mental status and reduced urine output.

### 71.2.2 Initial Investigation

In all in-patient's, assessment of full blood count, urea and electrolytes, clotting profile (PT, INR) and group and save is mandatory. Other initial investigations may include fibrinogen if correction with fresh frozen plasma (FFP) is or may be required, crossmatch and ECG for large GI bleeds in older patients or in those with cardiac history and chronic liver disease where the use of Terlipressin may be contemplated.

Most cases of acute colonic bleeding will stop spontaneously, thereby allowing non-urgent evaluation. However, for patients with severe lower GI bleeding, more urgent diagnosis and intervention are required to control the bleeding [12, 13]. These patients can be identified by the following features:

- continued bleeding within the first 24 h of hospitalisation with a drop in the haemoglobin (Hb) of at least 2 g/dL;
- a transfusion requirement of at least 2 units of packed red blood cells;
- pulse >100;
- systolic BP <115 mmHg;
- two serious co-morbidities.

## 71.3 Treatment

### 71.3.1 Medical Treatment

#### 71.3.1.1 Blood Transfusion and Correction of Coagulopathy

GI bleeding patients use 13.8% of all blood transfusions in England. Almost a quarter of patients with lower GI bleeding receive a blood transfusion during their hospital stay [6]. Generally, hospitals in the UK have internal guidance and transfusion protocols, but the consensus is that Hb threshold for transfusion is set at 70 g/L, with the exception of patients with existing cardiovascular disease, where the threshold for transfusion may be lowered to 10 g/L [14–17]. This restrictive trigger for the majority of GI bleeding patients is associated with a better outcome than a liberal strategy of transfusion [16]. There have been reports of increased mortality in those with a history of coronary disease if the haematocrit is more than 25% [18]. In contrast to the use of packed red cells, it is uncommon for patients to require a transfusion of fresh frozen plasma or platelets unless in the context of major haemorrhage. Hospitals have the duty of care to provide acute haemorrhage control and should audit their transfusion practice to ensure appropriate transfusion thresholds are being adhered to.

#### 71.3.1.2 Tranexamic Acid (TXA)

Despite its use in trauma and other forms of bleeding, there is no clear evidence at present to support the use of tranexamic acid (TXA) in the management of acute lower GI bleeding [19]. There has been one large pragmatic randomised controlled trail assessing the outcome of high-dose TXA on the mortality and thromboembolic events with acute GI bleeding (HALT-IT trial). In this double blinded multicentred RCT of 12,009 patients from 164 hospitals in 15 countries, the study concluded that TXA did not reduce death from GI bleeding, but it increased the thromboembolism rates of pulmonary embolism (PE) and deep vein thrombosis (DVT). Therefore, TXA should not be used in clinical practice [20]. However, this trial included upper and lower GI bleeding patients. A smaller randomised controlled trial of TXA specifically in lower GI bleeding patients in 100 patients also showed no meaningful clinical benefit [21].

#### 71.3.1.3 Anticoagulation and Antiplatelet Medications

It is not uncommon that patients presenting with lower GI bleeding would be on multiple medications, considering that a significant subgroup are those with multiple co-morbidities. For any patients on these medications, it is important to understand the reason that they are on them and whether they can be omitted without any untoward consequences. For example, patients who are on them for metallic valvular heart disease, recent myocardial infarction or recent coronary intervention, are at particularly high risk of sequalae if these medications are stopped suddenly.

### 71.3.1.4 Warfarin

The latest BSG guidelines recommendation is the interruption of Warfarin therapy at presentation. In severe GI haemorrhage, anticoagulation should be reversed with prothrombin complex concentrate (PCC; e.g. Beriplex®, Octaplex®) usually in discussion with local haematology expertise and vitamin K. If not available, fresh frozen plasma (FFP) is an alternative reversal agent, however when compared with PCC for major haemorrhage a metanalysis has shown it to be associated with significantly higher all-cause mortality, slower INR correction and higher volume overload but there was no difference in the risk of thromboembolic events [22]. For low thrombotic risk patients, warfarin should be recommenced at 7 days post-haemorrhage. In high thrombotic risk patients (coronary artery stents, prosthetic heart valves, atrial fibrillation, atrial fibrillation and mitral stenosis, <3 months post-venous thromboembolism), consider low molecular weight heparin therapy at 48 h post-haemorrhage.

### 71.3.1.5 Direct Oral Anticoagulants (DOAC)

DOACs such as apixaban, rivaroxaban, dabigatran, edoxaban and betrixaban are increasingly used to prevent thrombosis. They should be paused on presentation and consideration given to the use of reversal inhibitors such as Idarucizumab for dabigatran or andexanet alfa or apixaban and rivaroxaban in life-threatening haemorrhage in discussion with local haematology expertise [23, 24]. For edoxaban reversal has been shown to be effective with PCC in a dose-dependent manner with complete reversal at a dose of 50 IU/kg.

DOACs should be restarted a maximum of 7 days after haemorrhage [25, 26]. When significant co-morbidity warrants treatment earlier, consider anticoagulation after minimum 48 h.

### 71.3.1.6 Aspirin

Aspirin for primary prophylaxis of cardiovascular events can be permanently discontinued. Aspirin for secondary prevention should not be routinely stopped as it is associated with excess cardiovascular mortality with myocardial infarction or stokes. If it is stopped, it should be recommenced as soon as haemostasis is achieved.

### 71.3.1.7 Dual Antiplatelet Therapy (DAPT)

When encountering patients who have coronary stents in-situ and GI bleeding, an early discussion with the cardiology team is recommended. For patients on clopidogrel, ticagrelor or prasugrel with severe or life-threatening GI bleeding requiring emergent endoscopic intervention, discussion of peri-endoscopy platelet transfusion (2–3 adult doses) may be needed in discussion with on call haematology and endoscopy teams [27, 28]. When paused or reversed, DAPT can be re-instated after at least 2 and up to 5 days with Aspirin generally being continued. DAPT is not routinely stopped for minor lower GI bleedings.

### 71.3.1.8 Management Algorithm and Severity Stratification

Acute lower GI bleeding should be urgently assessed and resuscitated whilst stratifying patients into those who are stable and those who are not (Fig. 71.2). In unstable patients the algorithm should follow the management of patients in shock. Priority would be to maintain haemodynamic stability with the transfusion of blood products as required. Increased shock index is associated with an increased mortality stratifying these patients to require urgent treatment [10]. Increased shock index [calculated from heart rate (HR) divided by the Systolic Blood Pressure (SBP)] of more than or equal to 1 can be used to predict extravasation of contrast on angiography [7]. In these patients, once haemodynamic stability is achieved, a computed tomography angiography (CTA) should be performed (Fig. 71.3).

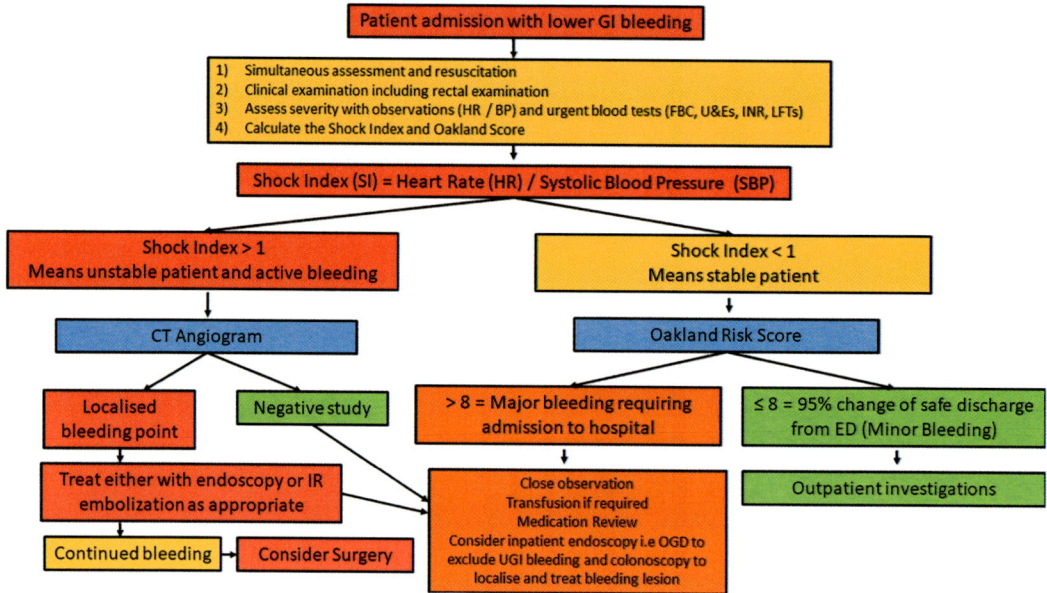

**Fig. 71.2** Management algorithm for lower GI bleeding

Where active extravasation of contrast is identified, this indicates a bleeding point and requires treatment either by interventional radiology or endoscopic techniques [11, 14]. This decision depends on local availability and expertise.

Patients who are stable should be categorised into those who have had a major or minor bleed; the latter may be suitable for discharge for outpatient colonic investigation. Clinicians should err on the side of safety and admission for observation for the following higher risk groups: those with advanced age, large witnessed blood loss, severe cardiovascular or other co-morbidity, history of anticoagulation use and those who living alone with no social support networks.

### 71.3.1.9 Risk Scoring Systems in Lower GI Bleeding

There have recently been a few validated scoring systems for clinical use in lower GI bleeding. Some scoring systems are of limited practical use as they require inpatient colonoscopy first or prolonged inpatient observation [13, 29, 30]. The Oakland and Birmingham Scoring systems are the most useful for clinical management. Whilst helpful on prognosticating, these scoring systems should not replace sound clinical judgement.

Neither system, however, includes any assessment of comorbidities. The more recent ABC (age, blood results, comorbidity) scoring system for any GI bleeding and was developed for use in 3012 patients with upper GI bleeding and validated in 4019 with upper GI bleeding and 2336 with lower GI bleeding. It shows promise as it is relatively simple to calculate and identifies patient's risk of mortality. Patients with lower GI bleeding stratified into low (≤3), medium (4–7) and high (≥8) ABC scores had in-hospital mortality rates of 0.6%, 6.3% and 18%, respectively.

**The Oakland Score**

The Oakland scoring tool (Table 71.2) is recommended to classify stable lower GI bleedings into major or minor categories [6]. Predictors of severe lower GI bleeding on the Oakland score were derived from large prospective study from 143 hospitals across the UK that included 2528 patients [6, 11]. The score compromises seven individual variables: age, gender, previous admission with similar bleed, heart rate, systolic blood pressure, findings on digital rectal examination and Haemoglobin (Hb) level. Patients with a total score of >8 are classified as having a major bleed and require hospital admission and to be consid-

# 71 Acute Lower Gastrointestinal Bleeding

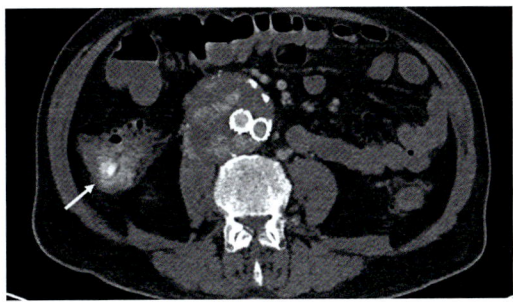

**Fig. 71.3** CT angiogram image of an elderly patient (with previous endovascular AAA repair) with lower GI bleeding showing an arterial blush from the right colon

ered for urgent inpatient investigation. Those patients scoring ≤8 are classified as having a minor bleed and have a 95% chance of being discharged after initial assessment [11]. The Oakland score was found to have a superior ability to identify those who are at low risk to develop adverse outcomes (re-bleeding with 28 days, blood transfusion or need for radiological, endoscopic or surgery intervention) [15]. In this low-risk group, endoscopic colonic assessment can be arranged on an urgent outpatient basis with resultant significant cost saving [17].

## The Birmingham Score

The Birmingham score was developed for use in lower GI bleeding from a database of 469 patients in a derivation cohort and 180 in a validation cohort [31] (Table 71.2). The cohort was developed from three hospitals in the West Midlands, UK from lower GI bleeding admissions between 2010 and 2018. It is simpler that the Oakland score and includes two variables (gender and admission Hb), but has similar accuracy and clinical utility.

The score performs particularly well in predicting adverse outcomes from diverticular disease (AUROC 0.87 [95% CI 0.75–0.98)]. As this is the most common cause of lower GI bleeding it makes it more relevant and applicable in day-to-day practice. A Birmingham Score of <2 (22.3% of patients) had low probability of an adverse

**Table 71.2** Oakland and Birmingham lower GI bleeding scores

| Oakland score | | Birmingham score | |
|---|---|---|---|
| Variable | Value (score) | Variable | Value |
| Age | <40 years (0)<br>40–69 years (1)<br>≥70 years (2) | | |
| Gender | Female (0)<br>Male (1) | Gender | Female (0)<br>Male (1) |
| Previous LGIB admission | No (0)<br>Yes (1) | | |
| DRE findings | No blood (0)<br>Blood (1) | | |
| Heart rate | <70 (0)<br>70–89 (1)<br>90–109 (2)<br>≥110 (3) | | |
| Systolic BP | <90 (5)<br>90–119 (4)<br>120–129 (3)<br>120–159 (2)<br>≥160 (0) | | |
| Admission Hb | <70 (22)<br>70–89 (17)<br>90–109 (13)<br>110–129 (8)<br>130–159 (4)<br>≥160 (0) | Hb | < 3 (6)<br>83–97 (5)<br>97–112 (4)<br>112–116 (3)<br>116–133 (2)<br>133–147 (1)<br>>147 (0) |
| *Clinical usage* | | | |
| An Oakland score of ≤8 and no other reason for admission are suitable for discharge and urgent outpatient investigations | | Probabilities of experiencing adverse outcomes[a] using the Birmingham score<br>Score 6–7; probability 90 (82–95)<br>Score 4–5; probability 38 (30–47)<br>Score 2–3; probability 18 (13–24)<br>Score <2; probability 4 (1–11) | |

*DRE* digital rectal examination, *Hb* haemoglobin, *LGIB* lower GI bleeding
[a] Adverse outcomes defined as the need for blood transfusion, endoscopic intervention, CT angiography, surgical intervention, re-bleeding and mortality

outcome and could be used to define patients for early discharge and outpatient endoscopic assessment, allowing significant healthcare savings.

### 71.3.1.10 Investigations and Treatments

A variety of investigations and techniques can be used to investigate and treat lower GI bleeding.

### 71.3.1.11 Upper GI Endoscopy

In patients with haemodynamic instability, upper GI bleeding may be present in up to 15% cases [17–19]. It is recommended they have an urgent upper GI endoscopy after resuscitation. Suggestive features of upper GI aetiology include a history of haematemesis, past history of peptic ulcers, known portal hypertension, the use of non-steroidal anti-inflammatory drugs (NSAIDs) or antiplatelet medications [32–34]. In low resource settings a nasogastric tube insertion and aspiration may be used to ascertain this, however, this has poor diagnostic accuracy and is not generally recommended [35, 36].

## 71.3.2 Radiology

### 71.3.2.1 Computer Tomography Angiography (CTA)

CTA has revolutionised the management of patients with severe lower GI bleeding. It is indicated in all haemodynamically unstable patients (Shock Index >1) after initial resuscitation for localisation of a bleeding point. It has a sensitivity of 75–95% and specificity approaching 100% [37, 38]. Triple phase CT angiography with no intraluminal contrast is the approach of choice. The short-term risk of re-bleeding following a negative CTA is 10–50%. There is a higher pick-up rate when CTA is used in haemodynamically unstable patients [39, 40], in particular for bleeds of a velocity 0.3–1.0 mL/min [41, 42]. For example, CTA has a sensitivity of 84–87% in 'unstable' patients, but this reduces to 12–15% in stable patients [7, 43, 44]. CTA has the advantage of being able to identify bleeding from the whole GI tract. Figure 71.3 shows a positive CTA image diagnostic of bleeding in a patient with right sided colonic luminal contrast following intravenous contrast injection.

### 71.3.2.2 Role of Interventional Radiology

Patients with a positive CTA should ideally be transferred urgently to an interventional radiology suite resource permitting. This allows the best chance at controlling the source of bleeding with selective embolisation having a high (>90%) success rate. A major benefit of angiography over endoscopy is that bowel preparation is not required. Figure 71.4 shows an interventional radiological embolisation of the right colon bleed using coils to a bleeding branch of the ileo-colic vessel. A delay of >90 min

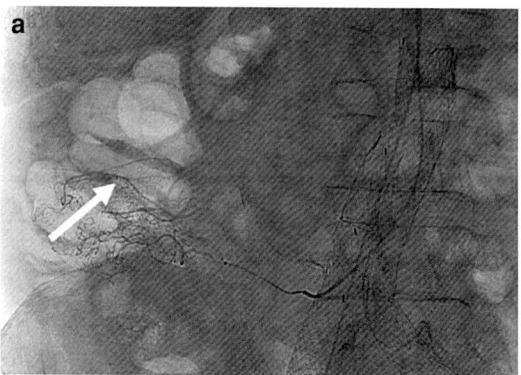
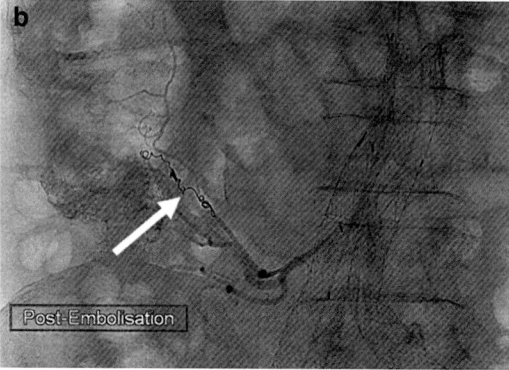

**Fig. 71.4** Interventional radiological embolization of bleeding branch of the ileo-colic vessel (same patient as Fig. 71.3). (**a**) Shows the radiological image prior to embolization and (**b**) shows the coils in the vessel causing haemostasis

between CTA and embolisation reduces success (by factor of 8) as bleeding can resolve rapidly or be intermittent. Higher success rates were found in lower GI bleeding due to diverticular disease.

There are risks with this approach of causing colonic ischaemia in 7–24%, therefore it is recommended that radiologists be supra-selective in their embolisation technique and embolise the most distal bleeding point [41–44]. Patients therefore need to be observed closely for signs of peritonitis or perforation post-embolisation, particularly if they have non-selective embolisation. Trans-arterial embolisation may be of benefit where a bleeding site is not seen on CTA, particularly in the setting of malignancy where the tumour mass and its feeding vessels can be identified. The decision to proceed must be carefully balanced against a possible increased risk of complications.

The latest BSG guidelines recommends that all hospitals that routinely admit lower GI bleeding should have access to 24-h, 7-day interventional radiology service either on site or via a formalised referral pathway for another usually tertiary hospital. In a retrospective analysis of patients bleeding from a diverticular source, the transfer out of the hospital was found to be an indicator of a poorer outcome [39]. Some specialist units have access to Hybrid operating theatre suites where interventional radiology equipment (with built in X-ray facilities) are combined with operating theatre capabilities. Whilst these are mainly used for vascular trauma, they are extremely useful for complex GI bleedings. Close interaction between the surgical and radiological teams allows for rapid and life-saving haemostatic techniques to be deployed.

### 71.3.2.3 Nuclear Scintigraphy

Nuclear scintigraphy also referred to Red Cell Scans and Gastrointestinal Bleeding Scans, involve radiolabelling of red blood cells to detect active GI bleeding at rates as low as 0.1–0.3 mL/min. However, it has a low diagnostic accuracy of 41–82% and is neither immediately available nor easy to arrange quickly in most hospitals [45]. It therefore has no place in the acute management stage, but could be used for occult GI bleedings where a cause is not quickly identified with initial radiologic and/or endoscopic approaches [37]. Whilst this modality alone is not precise enough to guide surgical resection when positive, it can direct further angiographic or endoscopic intervention with gastroscopy, enteroscopy or colonoscopy by pointing towards upper, mid or lower GI bleeding respectively. Even if repeat endoscopic intervention is unsuccessful, these can direct subsequent definitive surgical treatment by placement of endoscopic clips or tattoos at or near the precise bleeding point.

### 71.3.2.4 Video Capsule Endoscopy (VCE) and Small Bowel Enteroscopy

This has become an increasingly common and sophisticated modality to investigate lower GI bleeding and define those with obscure GI bleeding who have negative upper and lower GI endoscopy as neither modality can assess the majority of the small bowel. VCE allows assessment of the entire small bowel in up 90% of patients [46]. Its limitations relate to the lack of therapeutic ability and difficulty in precise location of bleeding (as pathology is identified by set time points beyond visualised landmarks). It further has a risk of retention or obstruction with occult structuring disease, which can be overcome with a patency capsule initially [47].

When positive, VCE is combined with direct small bowel endoscopy with push enteroscopy (when proximal to the ligament of Trietz) or device assisted enteroscopy (DAE). Both push enteroscopy and DAE can allow biopsy and therapeutic intervention of bleeding lesions of the small bowel. They may also facilitate guided surgical resection by either tattooing or clipping to allow the lesion to be identified at operation. However, DAE requires specialist endoscopic equipment and training and is not generally available easily in emergencies [48]. When utilised, DAE has a yield of 60–80% in identifying the underlying small bowel disorder, and 40–73% at successfully treating the underlying small bowel pathology when combined with therapeutic endoscopic approaches [48]. Patients who have had GI bleeding with both negative upper and lower GI endoscopy should have a VCE ± enteroscopy as part of their management.

### 71.3.2.5 Lower GI Endoscopy

The use of lower GI endoscopy (flexible sigmoidoscopy or colonoscopy) in the diagnosis of patients with lower GI bleeding should be used in stable patient with minor bleeding in the context of urgent outpatient assessment in the endoscopy unit. In addition, it can also be used in a diagnostic and therapeutic modality in lower GI bleeding in patients who continue to bleed as inpatients. Those who are admitted because of a major lower GI bleeding should be considered for colonoscopy on the next available list although the optimum timing for that remains uncertain [11] and its use is controversial. All hospitals that routinely admit patients with LGIB should have access to 24/7 on site colonoscopy and facilities to provide endoscopy haemostasis therapy.

A recent systematic review and metanalysis of 12 studies which included two randomised controlled trials showed no advantage to urgent colonoscopy, but an increasing haemostatic therapy demand with no difference in overall rates of rebleeding, transfusions, adverse events or mortality [49]. In addition, urgent endoscopy offered no greater therapeutic value, or reduction in length of stay or need for surgery. Colonoscopy can achieve an accurate diagnosis in 45–100% of patients [50] and allows for the use of therapeutic modalities which include thermal haemostasis, adrenaline injection, haemostatic clipping and band ligation [50–52]. The choice of approach depends on the type of lesion that is bleeding, availability of haemostatic techniques and the training of the endoscopist.

Patients with post-polypectomy bleeding are a unique subgroup in the emergency settling. In these patients, it is recommended that emergent colonoscopy is the modality of choice to investigate and treat the cause if bleeding is severe enough to warrant in-patient admission and management [53].

The advantage of direct endoscopic visualisation of the colon is an immediate diagnosis can be possible and combined with endoscopic therapy in certain scenarios. A major disadvantage is the need for bowel preparation to enable adequate visualisation. Unprepped sigmoidoscopy or colonoscopy is not recommended. In studies of urgent colonoscopy without oral or rectal preparation, caecal intubation rates are low (55–70%) and visualisation poor [50–52]. The best results are obtained with polyethylene glycol (PEG) based bowel preparations (4–6 L over 3–4 h) which can be given orally or via nasogastric tube [54]. During colonoscopy, the colonic mucosa is assessed closely for fresh blood, active bleeding, clots, visible vessels or pathology at high risk of bleeding such as angiodysplastic lesions. To maximise success, it is important to have high quality (HD) colonoscopic equipment and access to powered water irrigation. The terminal ileum should be intubated to assess for signs of small bowel bleeding. Withdrawal times should be slow (>6 min) to fully assess the colon and not miss small bleeding lesions.

## 71.3.3 Surgical Treatment

Previous literature documented between 10–25% of patients with lower GI bleeding eventually required emergency surgery [55, 56] and that this was directly related to bleed severity and the requirement for blood transfusion. These rates have fallen as a consequence of the development of interventional radiological and endoscopic haemostatic techniques which have revolutionised practise in recent years. Emergency surgery is now rarely required and reported in only 0.2% in the UK's lower gastrointestinal bleeding audit of 2781 patients over a 2-month period in June 2015 [6]. The current BSG guidelines recommendations emphasise that no patient should proceed to emergency laparotomy unless every effort has been made to localise and treat bleeding by radiological and/or endoscopic modalities, except under exceptional circumstances [11]. However, although catastrophic and severe recurrent lower GI bleeding is rare, it is important that emergency surgeons have the capabilities to deal with this life-threatening situation should it occur.

In a recent American College of Surgeons National Surgical Quality Improvement Program (NSQIP) database analysis of 1614 colectomies carried out between 2005 and 2017 for colonic bleeding, the post-operative 30-day mortality was 12.2% [57]. This compared with 30-day mortality of <1% for elective surgery. Patients operated for cancer were excluded and there was no data available on pre-operative embolisation or colonoscopy. Mortality was associated with age, co-morbidities, higher INR, lower haematocrit, open surgery and having a subtotal or total colectomy. The authors highlight the need for timely surgical intervention if required.

Indications for surgery include:

1. Life threatening lower GI bleeding which has failed radiological and/or endoscopic management.
2. Life threatening lower GI bleeding in a hospital without access to radiological or endoscopic management and where the patient is too unstable for inter-hospital transfer.
3. Lower GI bleeding caused by lesions not amenable to radiological or endoscopic management, for example, aorto-enteric fistula, small bowel tumours or colorectal malignancies.
4. Ischaemic complications from interventional radiological embolisation used to stop colonic haemorrhage which presents with post-embolisation perforation or peritonitis [58].

Table 71.3 details some tips when proceeding for emergency laparotomy in life-threatening GI bleeding. The surgeon faced with this challenge requires a systematic approach. Proceeding in theatre under a GA allows resuscitation to be performed by an anaesthetist and any endoscopy to be both better tolerated and used to deliver precise surgical intervention to the pathology in question by clearly delineating it on table.

The precise operation required will depend on the intra-operative findings.

- If a bleeding lesion is found; an appropriate colonic segmental resection should be performed with either an anastomosis or stoma formation depending on the patient's intra-

**Table 71.3** Surgical approach and tips for emergency surgery in lower GI bleeding

| Timing | Aspect | Rationale |
| --- | --- | --- |
| Pre-op | WHO checklist | Activation of hospitals massive haemorrhage protocols Group and save Cross match blood, platelets, FFP, etc. |
| Patient positioning | Supine, legs up Arms out on boards Active warming blanket on the chest | To allow access to the anus for on-table rectal examination, rigid sigmoidoscopy or colonoscopy Assess for the Anaesthetic team for large bore IV access, fluids and drug administration Prevent hypothermia |
| On table endoscopy | OGD | Assess the oesophagus, stomach and duodenum for causes of UGI bleeding |
| | Rectal examination and rigid sigmoidoscopy | Assess for anorectal causes of bleeding, such as haemorrhoids, rectal cancer, portal Hypertensive varices, etc. |
| Incision | Long midline laparotomy | |
| Intra-abdominal inspection | Inspect the abdomen systematically for potential causes of bleeding | Small bowel tumours Meckel's diverticulum Colorectal cancer Diverticular disease Sites of intra-luminal blood |
| Mobilisation | Mobilise the hepatic and splenic flexures | To aid in inspection and assessment. Also helps washout of the luminal contents if lavage is required. |

(continued)

**Table 71.3** (continued)

| Timing | Aspect | Rationale |
|---|---|---|
| On table colonoscopy after colonic lavage | Consider on-table colonic lavage via a large foley catheter placed into the Caecum via an appendiectomy | This allows on-table colonoscopy to be performed with better views of the mucosa |
| On table enteroscopy | If small bowel bleeding is suspected on-table small bowel enteroscopy can be performed via small bowel enterotomies | Inspect the small bowel for small bleeding sources, for example angiodysplastic lesions |
| Colonic resection | Decide upon a limited colonic resection versus a subtotal colectomy depending on intra-operative findings | |

*WHO* World health Organisation, *FFP* fresh frozen plasma, *OGD* oesophago-gastro-duodenoscopy, *UGI* upper gastrointestinal

operative physiology and risk for subsequent anastomotic leakage. Segmental colectomy after preoperative localisation is associated with a lower perioperative morbidity and mortality compared to subtotal colectomy [59]. This highlights the need to accurately locate the bleeding point prior to or during surgery.

- If no obvious bleeding lesions are found, the surgeon should consider:

  - **On-table colonic washout and intra-operative colonoscopy.** This can be achieved with washout of the colon to achieve good intra-operative views and may be facilitated via a colotomy to improve views further [60].
  - **Intra-operative small bowel enteroscopy** can via an enterotomy to assess the small bowel for bleeding lesions, such as aorto-venous malformations AVMs or angiodysplasia [61]. Small bowel masses such as gastrointestinal stromal tumours (GIST), lymphoma or adenocarcinoma are usually shown on CTA but must be palpated for during laparotomy.

- Surgical resection will depend on the exact circumstances, but can include:

  - **Right hemicolectomy** with end ileostomy and mucous fistula

    This technique is advocated as the majority of bleeding angio-dysplastic lesions are right sided and right sided diverticular disease has greater propensity for bleeding [62]. However, there is a high re-bleeding risk and it is not generally recommended unless bleeding is definitively localised to be coming from the right colon.

  - **Left hemicolectomy with colostomy ± mucous fistula**

    This is recommended in bleeding diverticular disease and other lesions of the left colon which are not controlled with endoscopy or interventional radiology.

  - **Sub-total colectomy with end ileostomy and mucous fistula.**

    This approach is associated with high morbidity and mortality but can be life-saving [63, 64]. A significant proportion of the morbidity is caused by complications from colonic anastomosis. Defunctioning and subsequent delayed reconstruction is therefore advocated [65]. Resection of the whole colon, sparing the rectum should treat all bleeding colonic lesions and is attractive where pre-operative or intra-operative measures fails to define the precise bleeding point. This is approach may also be preferred for certain patients with Inflammatory Bowel Disease and those with diffuse polyposis syndromes.

### 71.3.4 Damage Control Surgery

In patients with massive haemorrhage, damage control surgery can be performed. In a very unstable patient, medial to lateral vascular pedicle ligation (ileocolic, middle colic pedicle, inferior mesenteric artery pedicles) or clamping can be performed to achieve rapid stability rather than the traditional lateral to medial Line of Toldt's dissection. Damage control involves stapled resection of the bleeding bowel, temporary abdominal closure and returning to intensive care for further resuscitation, warming, correction of acidosis and coagulopathy. After resection, if there is any oozing from the raw dissection planes or pelvis, they can be temporarlity packed. Temporary abdominal closure techniques, such as vacuum assisted closure, are helpful to avoid abdominal compartment syndrome and deal with the resuscitation related bowel oedema. The patient is returned to theatre in 48–72 h for reassessment of the bowel, formation of stomas and abdominal wall closure. In patients who are young and fit with no co-morbidities restoring bowel continuity with an anastomosis can be considered when the patient is stable. This may be delayed or avoided in patients with inflammatory bowel disease who need on going medical management and/or immediate or delayed assessment of the remaining bowel first.

> **Dos and Don'ts**
>
> It is important to be aware of the following pitfalls when dealing with the assessment and management of lower GI haemorrhage patients:
>
> - Don't forget to perform a digital rectal examination in all patients with a lower GI bleeding, this is a must.
> - Don't underestimate the severity of bleeding as this can have dire consequences.
> - Do use the Oakland or Birmingham risk scoring tools to assist in making timely clinical management decisions.
> - Don't forget that up to 15% of patients with fresh PR bleeding will have an upper GI source will require urgent gastroscopy.
> - Don't fail to recognise that haemodynamic instability, particularly following initial resuscitation, indicates a higher risk of significant bleeding, complications and fatality.
> - Don't perform blind emergency surgery without attempting to localise the site of bleeding pre/peri-operatively as this can result in high re-bleeding rates and increased mortality.

## 71.4 Summary of Management

Most patients with lower GI bleeding will settle with conservative management. Of the remaining, there had historically been high rates of surgical intervention with accompanying significant morbidity and mortality. Recent advances in the expertise, technique and availability of interventional radiology and endoscopy to achieve haemostasis have seen the role of surgery diminishing and it is now rarely required. Those who are haemodynamically unstable should receive judicious transfusion of blood and blood products with particular measures used to address anticoagulant and antiplatelet medications. There is no role for the use of Tranexamic but the requirement for emergency surgery remains for the life-threatening patient or where radiological and/or endoscopic measures fail or are not considered appropriate.

> **Take-Home Messages**
> - Low-risk patients with minor colonic bleeds may be discharged after thorough assessment with risk stratification tools.
> - Risk scoring systems, such as the Oakland or the Birmingham scores, should be used in lower GI haemorrhage to aid in clinical management, but they should never replace sound clinical judgement.
> - Diverticular disease accounts for approximately 40% of significant lower GI bleedings.
> - In most cases of lower GI haemorrhage, the bleeding will stop spontaneously allowing further investigation to be carried out either as an in-patient or urgent out-patient basis.

- Although the mortality of acute lower GI bleedings is low (~2–4%), bleeding can be catastrophic with mortality as high as 20% in the case of massive haemorrhage or in patients who are elderly with co-morbid diseases.
- Prompt fluid resuscitation, judicious use of blood products with/without anticoagulant reversal agents, early surgical review and involvement of radiology, endoscopy and critical care are the key pillars to the management of unstable GI bleeds in the emergency department.
- Colonoscopy is relatively safe, effective and useful when combined with risk stratification tools to define whether and when it should be performed.
- Surgical intervention is rarely required but remains indicated when haemodynamic instability persists despite aggressive resuscitation, or bleeding continues or returns despite attempts at definitive therapeutic radiological and/or endoscopic approaches.

**Multiple Choice Questions**

1. The most common cause of severe lower gastrointestinal bleeding is the following:
   A. Angiodysplasia
   B. Diverticular disease (**Correct answer**)
   C. Haemorrhoids
   D. Ischaemic colitis
2. Brisk upper gastrointestinal bleeding can cause fresh red rectal bleeding in what percentage of cases?
   A. 15–30%
   B. 10–15% (**Correct answer**)
   C. 5–10%
   D. <5%
3. One of the following risk scores is a specific risk stratification tool to assess for early discharge and low risk readmission or intervention in patients with lower gastrointestinal tract bleeding?
   A. Glasgow-Blatchford scoring system
   B. The Oakland scoring system (**Correct answer**)
   C. ABC scoring system
   D. Rockall scoring system
4. The shock index is calculated by the following equation:
   A. Heart rate divided by the systolic blood pressure (Correct answer)
   B. Systolic blood pressure divided by the heart rate
   C. Heart rate multiplied by systolic blood pressure and divided by diastolic blood pressure
   D. Diastolic blood pressure multiplied by the heart rate
5. A 79 year old female presents with fresh rectal bleeding, a pulse of 110 and a systolic BP of 90. After resuscitation and stabilisation, she undergoes an upper GI endoscopy which is normal. What is the next most appropriate investigation?
   A. Colonoscopy
   B. CT angiography (**Correct answer**)
   C. Radiolabelled red cell scanning
   D. Interventional radiology ± embolization
6. An 88-year-old man with a history of cardiovascular disease and COPD presents with fresh rectal bleeding and a shock index of 1. A CT angiogram shows an arterial blush in the right colon. The most appropriate procedure to stop the bleeding is the following?
   A. Colonoscopy and endoscopic clipping
   B. Immediate interventional radiology and supra-selective coil embolization (**Correct answer**)
   C. Emergency laparotomy and right hemicolectomy
   D. Emergency laparotomy and subtotal colectomy
7. The following are values make up the Oakland lower GI bleeding severity score?
   A. Age and haemoglobin

B. Age, urea, albumin, creatinine, altered mental status, liver cirrhosis and ASA
C. Age, gender, previous lower GI bleeding admissions, rectal examination findings, heart rate and systolic blood pressure (Correct answer)
D. Urea, haemoglobin, systolic blood pressure, pulse, maelena, syncope, hepatic disease and cardiac failure

8. A 75 year-old patient with PR bleeding and renal disease is booked for colonoscopy to assess for the cause of the bleeding and endoscopic haemostasis. What is the most appropriate bowel preparation?
   A. None/unprepared colon
   B. Enema preparation only
   C. Polyethylene glycol (PEG) based colonic bowel preparation (Correct answer)
   D. Oral sodium phosphate (OSP)

9. An 82-year-old female patient with a pulse of 120 and systolic BP of 90 is resuscitated and sent for CT angiogram for lower GI bleeding. This shows an arterial blush in the left colon. The most appropriate treatment is the following:
   A. Emergency left hemicolectomy
   B. Trans-arterial angiography and selective embolization (Correct answer)
   C. Colonoscopy
   D. IV tranexamic acid

10. In modern hospitals in developed countries with access to interventional radiological techniques (arterial embolization) and endoscopic haemostasis, what is the current percentage of patients who require emergency surgery for lower gastrointestinal bleeding?
    A. <1% (Correct answer)
    B. 2–3%
    C. 4–9%
    D. >10%

## References

1. Lanas A, García-Rodríguez LA, Polo-Tomás M, et al. Time trends and impact of upper and lower gastrointestinal bleeding and perforation in clinical practice. Am J Gastroenterol. 2009;104:1633–41.
2. Hreinsson JP, Gumundsson S, Kalaitzakis E, et al. Lower gastrointestinal bleeding: incidence, etiology, and outcomes in a population-based setting. Eur J Gastroenterol Hepatol. 2013;25:37–43.
3. Newman J, Fitzgerald JE, Gupta S, et al. Outcome predictors in acute surgical admissions for lower gastrointestinal bleeding. Color Dis. 2012;14:1020–6.
4. Strate LL, Ayanian JZ, Kotler G, et al. Risk factors for mortality in lower intestinal bleeding. Clin Gastroenterol Hepatol. 2008;6:1004–10.
5. Wheat CL, Strate LL. Trends in hospitalization for diverticulitis and diverticular bleeding in the United States from 2000 to 2010. Clin Gastroenterol Hepatol. 2016;14:96–103.
6. Oakland K, Guy R, Uberoi R, et al. Acute lower GI bleeding in the UK: patient characteristics, interventions and outcomes in the first nationwide audit. Gut. 2018;67:654–62.
7. Ernst O, Bulois P, Saint-Drenant S, et al. Helical CT in acute lower gastrointestinal bleeding. Eur Radiol. 2003;13:114–7.
8. Parekh PJ, Buerlein RC, Shams R, Vingan H, Johnson DA. Evaluation of gastrointestinal bleeding: update of current radiologic strategies. World J Gastrointest Pharmacol Ther. 2014;5(4):200–8.
9. National Comparative Audit of Blood Transfusion. National comparative audit of lower gastrointestinal bleeding and the use of blood. 2016. www.hospital.blood.co.uk.
10. National Confidential Enquiry into Patient Outcomes and Death. Time to get control? 2015. www.ncepod.org.uk.
11. Oakland K, Chadwick G, East JE, et al. Diagnosis and management of acute lower gastrointestinal bleeding: guidelines from the British Society of Gastroenterology. Gut. 2019;68:776–89.
12. Laine L, Yang H, Chang SC, Datto C. Trends for incidence of hospitalization and death due to GI complications in the United States from 2001 to 2009. Am J Gastroenterol. 2012;107(8):1190–5.
13. Strate LL, Orav EJ, Syngal S. Early predictors of severity in acute lower intestinal tract bleeding. Arch Intern Med. 2003;163(7):838–43.
14. Padhi S, Kemmis-Betty S, Rajesh S, et al. Blood transfusion: summary of NICE guidance. BMJ. 2015;351:h5832.
15. Oakland K, Jairath V, Murphy MF. Advances in transfusion medicine: gastrointestinal bleeding. Transfus Med. 2018;28:132–9.
16. Odutayo A, Desborough MJ, Trivella M, et al. Restrictive versus liberal blood transfusion for gastrointestinal bleeding: a systematic review and meta-

analysis of randomised controlled trials. Lancet Gastroenterol Hepatol. 2017;2:354–60.
17. Docherty AB, O'Donnell R, Brunskill S, et al. Effect of restrictive versus liberal transfusion strategies on outcomes in patients with cardiovascular disease in a non-cardiac surgery setting: systematic review and meta-analysis. BMJ. 2016;352:i1351.
18. Hearnshaw S, Travis S, Murphy M. The role of blood transfusion in the management of upper and lower intestinal tract bleeding. Best Pract Res Clin Gastroenterol. 2008;22(2):355–71.
19. Lee PL, Yang KS, Tsai HW, Hou SK, Kang YN, Chang CC. Tranexamic acid for gastrointestinal bleeding: a systematic review with meta-analysis of randomized clinical trials. Am J Emerg Med. 2021;45:269–79. S0735-6757(20)30755-5.
20. HALT-IT Trial Collaborators. Effects of a high-dose 24-h infusion of tranexamic acid on death and thromboembolic events in patients with acute gastrointestinal bleeding (HALT-IT): an international randomised, double-blind, placebo-controlled trial. Lancet. 2020;395(10241):1927–36.
21. Smith SR, Murray D, Pockney PG, Bendinelli C, Draganic BD, Carroll R. Tranexamic acid for lower GI hemorrhage: a randomized placebo-controlled clinical trial. Dis Colon Rectum. 2018;61(1):99–106.
22. Chai-Adisaksopha C, Hillis C, Siegal DM, Movilla R, Heddle N, Iorio A, Crowther M. Prothrombin complex concentrates versus fresh frozen plasma for warfarin reversal. A systematic review and meta-analysis. Thromb Haemost. 2016;116(5):879–90.
23. https://bnf.nice.org.uk/drug/idarucizumab.html.
24. https://bnf.nice.org.uk/drug/andexanet-alfa.html.
25. Andrade JG, Verma A, Mitchell LB, Parkash R, Leblanc K, Atzema C, Healey JS, Bell A, Cairns J, Connolly S, Cox J, Dorian P, Gladstone D, McMurtry MS, Nair GM, Pilote L, Sarrazin JF, Sharma M, Skanes A, Talajic M, Tsang T, Verma S, Wyse DG, Nattel S, Macle L, CCS Atrial Fibrillation Guidelines Committee. 2018 Focused update of the Canadian Cardiovascular Society Guidelines for the management of atrial fibrillation. Can J Cardiol. 2018;34(11):1371–92.
26. Zahir H, Brown KS, Vandell AG, Desai M, Maa JF, Dishy V, Lomeli B, Feussner A, Feng W, He L, Grosso MA, Lanz HJ, Antman EM. Edoxaban effects on bleeding following punch biopsy and reversal by a 4-factor prothrombin complex concentrate. Circulation. 2015;131(1):82–90. https://doi.org/10.1161/CIRCULATIONAHA.114.013445. Epub 2014 Nov 17.
27. Makris M, Van Veen JJ, Tait CR, Mumford AD, Laffan M, British Committee for Standards in Haematology. Guideline on the management of bleeding in patients on antithrombotic agents. Br J Haematol. 2013;160(1):35–46.
28. Keeling D, Tait RC, Watson H, British Committee of Standards for Haematology. Peri-operative management of anticoagulation and antiplatelet therapy. Br J Haematol. 2016;175(4):602–13.
29. Kollef MH, O'Brien JD, Zuckerman GR, Shannon W. BLEED: a classification tool to predict outcomes in patients with acute upper and lower gastrointestinal hemorrhage. Crit Care Med. 1997;25(7):1125–32.
30. Velayos FS, Williamson A, Sousa KH, Lung E, Bostrom A, Weber EJ, Ostroff JW, Terdiman JP. Early predictors of severe lower gastrointestinal bleeding and adverse outcomes: a prospective study. Clin Gastroenterol Hepatol. 2004;2(6):485–90.
31. Smith SCL, Bazarova A, Ejenavi E, Qurashi M, Shivaji UN, Harvey PR, Slaney E, McFarlane M, Baker G, Elnagar M, Yuzari S, Gkoutos G, Ghosh S, Iacucci M. A multicentre development and validation study of a novel lower gastrointestinal bleeding score-the Birmingham score. Int J Color Dis. 2020;35(2):285–93.
32. Green BT, Rockey DC, Portwood G, et al. Urgent colonoscopy for evaluation and management of acute lower gastrointestinal hemorrhage: a randomized controlled trial. Am J Gastroenterol. 2005;100:2395–402.
33. Laine L, Shah A. Randomized trial of urgent vs. elective colonoscopy in patients hospitalized with lower GI bleeding. Am J Gastroenterol. 2010;105:2636–41.
34. Jensen DM, Machicado GA. Diagnosis and treatment of severe hematochezia. The role of urgent colonoscopy after purge. Gastroenterology. 1988;95:1569–74.
35. Kessel B, Olsha O, Younis A, Daskal Y, Granovsky E, Alfici R. Evaluation of nasogastric tubes to enable differentiation between upper and lower gastrointestinal bleeding in unselected patients with melena. Eur J Emerg Med. 2016;23(1):71–3.
36. Palamidessi N, Sinert R, Falzon L, Zehtabchi S. Nasogastric aspiration and lavage in emergency department patients with hematochezia or melena without hematemesis. Acad Emerg Med. 2010;17(2):126–32.
37. Chan V, Tse D, Dixon S, Shrivastava V, Bratby M, Anthony S, Patel R, Tapping C, Uberoi R. Outcome following a negative CT angiogram for gastrointestinal hemorrhage. Cardiovasc Intervent Radiol. 2015;38(2):329–35.
38. Tabibian JH, Wong Kee Song LM, Enders FB, Aguet JC, Tabibian N. Technetium-labeled erythrocyte scintigraphy in acute gastrointestinal bleeding. Int J Color Dis. 2013;28(8):1099–105.
39. Dao HE, Miller PE, Lee JH, Kermani R, Hackford AW. Transfer status is a risk factor for increased in-hospital mortality in patients with diverticular hemorrhage. Int J Color Dis. 2013;28(2):273–6.
40. Kennedy DW, Laing CJ, Tseng LH, et al. Detection of active gastrointestinal hemorrhage with CT angiography: a 4(1/2)-year retrospective review. J Vasc Interv Radiol. 2010;21:848–55.
41. Ren JZ, Zhang MF, Rong AM, et al. Lower gastrointestinal bleeding: role of 64-row computed tomographic angiography in diagnosis and therapeutic planning. World J Gastroenterol. 2015;21:4030–7.
42. Foley PT, Ganeshan A, Anthony S, et al. Multidetector CT angiography for lower gastrointestinal

bleeding: can it select patients for endovascular intervention? J Med Imaging Radiat Oncol. 2010;54:9–16.
43. Abbas SM, Bissett IP, Holden A, et al. Clinical variables associated with positive angiographic localization of lower gastrointestinal bleeding. ANZ J Surg. 2005;75:953–7.
44. Dobritz M, Engels HP, Schneider A, et al. Evaluation of dual-phase multi-detector-row CT for detection of intestinal bleeding using an experimental bowel model. Eur Radiol. 2009;19:875–81.
45. A systematic review on nuclear and CT imaging for patients with lower GI bleeding center for evidence-based practice. Philadelphia: University of Pennsylvania Health System (UPHS); 2009.
46. Rondonotti E, Villa F, Mulder CJ, et al. Small bowel capsule endoscopy in 2007: indications, risks and limitations. World J Gastroenterol. 2007;13:6140–9.
47. Rezapour M, Amadi C, Gerson LB. Retention associated with video capsule endoscopy: systematic review and meta-analysis. Gastrointest Endosc. 2017;85:1157–68.
48. Gerson LB, Fidler JL, Cave DR, et al. ACG clinical guideline: diagnosis and management of small bowel bleeding. Am J Gastroenterol. 2015;110:1265–87.
49. Kouanda AM, Somsouk M, Sewell JL, Day LW. Urgent colonoscopy in patients with lower GI bleeding: a systematic review and meta-analysis. Gastrointest Endosc. 2017;86(1):107–117.e1.
50. ASGE Standards of Practice Committee, Pasha SF, Shergill A, Acosta RD, Chandrasekhara V, Chathadi KV, Early D, Evans JA, Fisher D, Fonkalsrud L, Hwang JH, Khashab MA, Lightdale JR, Muthusamy VR, Saltzman JR, Cash BD. The role of endoscopy in the patient with lower GI bleeding. Gastrointest Endosc. 2014;79(6):875–85.
51. Setoyama T, Ishii N, Fujita Y. Enodoscopic band ligation (EBL) is superior to endoscopic clipping for the treatment of colonic diverticular hemorrhage. Surg Endosc. 2011;25(11):3574–8.
52. Ohyama T, Sakurai Y, Ito M, Daito K, Sezai S, Sato Y. Analysis of urgent colonoscopy for lower gastrointestinal tract bleeding. Digestion. 2000;61(3):189–92.
53. Hong SP. How do I manage post-polypectomy bleeding? Clin Endosc. 2012;45(3):282–4.
54. Strate LL, Gralnek IM. ACG clinical guideline: management of patients with acute lower gastrointestinal bleeding. Am J Gastroenterol. 2016;111(4):459–74.
55. Hoedema RE, Luchtefeld MA. The management of lower gastrointestinal hemorrhage. Dis Colon Rectum. 2005;48(11):2010–24.
56. McGuire HH Jr. Bleeding colonic diverticula. A reappraisal of natural history and management. Ann Surg. 1994;220(5):653–6.
57. Sue-Chue-Lam C, Castelo M, Baxter NN. Factors associated with mortality after emergency colectomy for acute lower gastrointestinal bleeding. JAMA Surg. 2020;155(2):165–7.
58. Köhler G, Koch OO, Antoniou SA, Mayer F, Lechner M, Pallwein-Prettner L, Emmanuel K. Relevance of surgery after embolization of gastrointestinal and abdominal hemorrhage. World J Surg. 2014;38(9):2258–66.
59. Mohammed Ilyas MI, Szilagy EJ. Management of diverticular bleeding: evaluation, stabilization, intervention, and recurrence of bleeding and indications for resection after control of bleeding. Clin Colon Rectal Surg. 2018;31(4):243–50.
60. Scott HJ, Lane IF, Glynn MJ, Theodorou NA, Lloyd-Davies E, Reynolds KW, Parkins RA. Colonic haemorrhage: a technique for rapid intra-operative bowel preparation and colonoscopy. Br J Surg. 1986;73(5):390–1.
61. Wagner HE, Stain SC, Gilg M, Gertsch P. Systematic assessment of massive bleeding of the lower part of the gastrointestinal tract. Surg Gynecol Obstet. 1992;175(5):445–9.
62. Milewski PJ, Schofield PF. Massive colonic haemorrhage—the case for right hemicolectomy. Ann R Coll Surg Engl. 1989;71(4):253–9.
63. Setya V, Singer JA, Minken SL. Subtotal colectomy as a last resort for unrelenting, unlocalized, lower gastrointestinal hemorrhage: experience with 12 cases. Am Surg. 1992;58(5):295–9.
64. Bender JS, Wiencek RG, Bouwman DL. Morbidity and mortality following total abdominal colectomy for massive lower gastrointestinal bleeding. Am Surg. 1991;57(8):536–40; discussion 540–1.
65. Plummer JM, Gibson TN, Mitchell DI, Herbert J, Henry T. Emergency subtotal colectomy for lower gastrointestinal haemorrhage: over-utilised or underestimated? Int J Clin Pract. 2009;63(6):865–8.

## Further Reading

Gralnek IM, Neeman Z, Strate LL. Acute lower gastrointestinal bleeding. N Engl J Med. 2017;376(11):1054–63.

Moss AJ, Tuffaha H, Malik A. Lower GI bleeding: a review of current management, controversies and advances. Int J Color Dis. 2016;31:175–88.

Oakland K, Jairath V, Uberoi R, Guy R, Ayaru L, Mortensen N, Murphy MF, Collins GS. Derivation and validation of a novel risk score for safe discharge after acute lower gastrointestinal bleeding: a modelling study. Lancet Gastroenterol Hepatol. 2017;2(9):635–43.

# Perforated Peptic Ulcer

72

Delphina Yeo Boon Xue, Ramkumar Mohan, and Vishal G. Shelat

## 72.1 Introduction

**Learning Goals**
- To educate learners that perforated peptic ulcer (PPU) is a surgical emergency and requires early diagnosis, prompt resuscitation, and expeditious intervention to deliver good clinical outcomes.
- To understand the importance of imaging in PPU diagnosis. This chapter enables learners to understand rationale of patient selection for various treatment options, including non-operative management of PPU.
- The chapter enables learners to realize the role of various scoring systems in PPU, and highlights importance of sepsis bundle in surgical care of PPU.

Peptic ulcer disease (PUD) is an insult to the gastric mucosa resulting from an imbalance between stomach acid-pepsin and mucosal defense barriers [1]. Mucosal insult results in ulceration extending beyond the mucosa and submucosal layers. Peptic ulcers are typically located in the stomach or duodenum but can be found in the esophagus or Meckel's diverticulum [2]. Bleeding and perforation are two common complications of PUD. Perforation is a severe complication that warrants early recognition, prompt resuscitation, and operative repair to ensure sound clinical outcomes [3, 4]. This review provides an update incorporating the evidence-based practice for a perforated peptic ulcer (PPU).

### 72.1.1 Epidemiology

PUD affects 4 million people worldwide annually, with an estimated lifetime prevalence of about 5% [5, 6]. Although complications of PUD have decreased with widespread availability and access to proton pump inhibitors (PPIs), PPU remains one of the most severe surgical emergencies that occur in 2–10% of PUD patients, with 30 and 90-day mortality risk of almost 30% [7]. Recognition of *Helicobacter pylori* (*H. pylori*) as a common microbe causing PUD, and its link with gastric carcinogenesis, has impacted global epidemiologic trends.

D. Y. B. Xue · R. Mohan
Ministry of Health Holdings, Singapore, Singapore
e-mail: m.ramkumar@u.nus.edu

V. G. Shelat (✉)
Department of General Surgery, Tan Tock Seng Hospital, Singapore, Singapore

Lee Kong Chian School of Medicine, Nanyang Technology University, Singapore, Singapore

## 72.1.2 Etiology

Etiopathogenesis of PUD is diverse and includes both modifiable and non-modifiable, personal, and population-level risk factors. Seasonal association with PPU risk is reported, but more data is required to prove causation [8, 9]. Young male smokers in developing countries are the typical PPU patient profile. In developed countries, patients tend to be elderly with multiple comorbidities, including the use of nonsteroidal anti-inflammatories (NSAIDs). Other risk factors include *H. pylori* infection, renal dysfunction, and critical illness [10–12]. Despite successful treatment of the ulcer, recurrence is expected in the presence of underlying risk factors. A systemic review of 93 studies has reported ulcer recurrence risk 12.2% (odds ratio [OR]: 95% confidence interval [CI]: 2.4–21.9) [13]. This is important as a minority of gastric ulcers are associated with gastric cancer, and tissue diagnosis is essential to rule out malignancy. Clinicians must be aware that even a malignant ulcer may show signs of healing after a trial of PPI, and thus a high index of suspicion and liberal biopsies of gastric ulcer is essential. In patients where common risk factors cannot be established, a clinician must perform an extended workup to evaluate hypercalcemia (e.g., parathyroid disorders) or hypergastrinemia (e.g., Zollinger Ellison syndrome).

### 72.1.2.1 *Helicobacter pylori*

*H. pylori* is an aerobic, gram-negative flagellated rod commonly transmitted via the oral-fecal route [14]. This includes consumption of contaminated water and food, sharing of utensils, and improper handwashing techniques. *H. pylori* is prevalent in developing countries (95%) as compared to developed countries (30%) [15, 16]. Locally, our prevalence rate of *H. pylori* is 31% [17]. This is comparable to the prevalence rate of the United States (36%) [18]. *H. pylori* causes chronic gastric inflammation due to urease, toxins, and flagella. Urease breaks down urea into ammonia, and thus *H. pylori* can remain viable in the acidic gastric environment. Toxins such as CagA/VacA can also cause host tissue damage. Flagella helps motility and movement towards the gastric epithelium. *H. pylori* is more associated with duodenal ulcers, but it is also linked with gastric ulceration. Studies have shown that *H. pylori* eradication is crucial to prevent PUD recurrence [19]. If unrecognized or untreated, chronic infection can cause perforation. *H. pylori* is detected in 50–80% of patients with PPU [11, 20]. A randomized controlled trial by El-Nakeeb et al., which included 77 patients with PPU, showed that 84.8% of patients had *H. pylori* [21]. Of those who had *H. pylori* infection, they were further divided into the control group (omeprazole alone) and eradication group (triple therapy with amoxicillin, metronidazole, and omeprazole). After 1 year, ulcer recurrence was 6.1% in the eradication group versus 29.6% in the control group ($p = 0.001$). This emphasizes the importance of *H. pylori* eradication after repairing the perforation, so future re-ulceration risk is reduced. We routinely treat all PPU patients with empiric *H. pylori* therapy upon discharge following uneventful recovery following surgical repair.

### 72.1.2.2 Nonsteroidal Anti-inflammatory Drugs

NSAIDs are used mainly for their analgesic, anti-inflammatory, and antipyretic effects. Its inhibition of cyclo-oxygenase 1 (COX-1) in the gastrointestinal tract inhibits prostaglandin secretion and reduces cytoprotective effects in the gastric lining, promoting mucosal injury [22]. NSAIDs increase the PPU risk by six to eight times and are responsible for about a quarter of perforation events in PUD patients [23, 24]. Anti-platelet medications are in widespread global use for prophylaxis of cerebrovascular and cardiovascular disease [25–27]. Although prophylaxis is less used in Asia than in Western countries, anti-platelet use continues to increase [28]. Authors have observed a local trend by primary care physicians prescribing PPI alongside anti-platelets, a practice that is primarily based on personal views about PUD risk reduction. In a prospective study including 2416 Danish adults, though Rosenstock et al. did not find a strong association between NSAIDs and PUD, NSAID consumption was associated with bleeding ulcers in elderly patients (OR: 0.4, 95% CI: 0.1–2.3,

$p < 0.001$) [29]. NSAIDs are widely used for post-operative analgesia. In four patients treated by the Caesarean section, Shirazi et al. reported PPU [30]. As gastrointestinal symptoms following orthopedic or gynecological procedures are infrequent, physicians must have a high index of suspicion if a patient develops abdominal symptoms.

#### 72.1.2.3 Cigarette Smoking

Smoking is a public health nuisance and a population hazard. Smoking is harmful to the upper gastrointestinal tract and negatively impacts global human health and well-being [31]. PUD risk is associated with the quantity and duration of tobacco use, and cigarette smokers are more likely to develop ulcers that are more difficult to heal [32]. Smoking inhibits pancreatic bicarbonate secretion and causes vasoconstriction of the gastric mucosa with resultant ischemia [33, 34]. Thus, the effectiveness of the bicarbonate buffer against acidic gastric juices is reduced, and PUD occurs [35]. In a retrospective study including 168 patients with PPU and 4469 control subjects, Svanes et al. reported that smoking predisposes to perforation and accounts for the majority of perforations in the population aged below 75 years (OR: 9.7, 95% CI: 4.9–15.4, $p < 0.001$) [35]. A study including 110 PPU patients with ulcer size $\geq 2$ cm showed that 35.5% ($n = 39$) of patients smoked [9]. Even in a casual smoker, or second-hand smoker, emergency surgery morbidity risk is high as the active ingredients (nicotine and carbon monoxide) decrease oxygen levels and increase the likelihood of cardiovascular morbidity.

#### 72.1.2.4 Marginal Ulcer

Marginal ulcers can develop at the jejunal side of the gastrojejunal anastomosis, with an incidence rate of 1–16% [36, 37]. Perforation of a marginal ulcer is a rare complication and can be potentially life-threatening [38]. Some risk factors for perforation include local ischemia, anastomotic tension, duodenal reflux, cigarette smoking, NSAIDs, and chronic irritation due to the type of suture material used for anastomosis [39]. With the increasing role of surgery in the management of diabetes and obesity, marginal ulcers are increasingly reported following procedures such as Roux-en-Y reconstruction.

### 72.1.3 Pathogenesis

Peptic ulcer occurs due to an imbalance between the protective and ulcerogenic factors. However, it is still unclear why some perforate and some do not [40]. Prostaglandins are a crucial defense as they inhibit acid secretion and stimulate bicarbonate release [41]. As NSAIDs reduce prostaglandin production, chronic NSAID consumption leads to PUD. Though *H. pylori* infection is associated with PUD, reports mention that half of PPU patients do not have *H. pylori* infection [42, 43]. Multiple other overlapping factors increase the burden of risk for perforation. Once an ulcer occurs, the size and location may predispose to perforation. However, small ulcers may perforate too [44]. Perforations happen in the morning, suggesting the circadian variation in acid secretion [40]. The reportedly increased risk of perforations during Ramadan may be due to prolonged fasting and acid secretion and release [45].

PUD and PPU are also reported in relevance to the ongoing coronavirus disease 2019 (COVID-19) pandemic. The use of corticosteroids and NSAIDs increases this risk [46]. Agnes et al. reported that the severe acute respiratory syndrome coronavirus 2 (SARS-CoV-2) virus causes direct epithelial injury and systemic inflammation resultant cytokine storm may predispose to gastrointestinal bleeding or perforation [47]. In addition, interleukin-6 (IL-6) inhibitors may predispose to perforation. However, to accurately determine whether COVID-19 increases the incidence of PPU, more data is necessary.

## 72.2 Diagnosis

### 72.2.1 Clinical Presentation

Symptoms of PUD include abdominal pain, upper abdominal discomfort, bloatedness, and a feeling of fullness. In 1843 Edward Crisp stated that the symptoms are typical; I hardly believe that anyone can fail to make a diagnosis [1]. As PUD develops, the risk of perforation increases, resulting in extravasation of gastric juices and gas into the peritoneal cavity, causing peritonitis. A patient presenting with a clinical triad of sudden severe epigastric abdominal pain, tachycardia, and abdominal rigidity is the hallmark of PPU [1]. In patients with posterior gastric ulcer perforation, gastric contents leak into the lesser sac and mask peritonitis symptoms [48]. A posterior duodenal ulcer perforation can cause a localized retroperitoneal abscess and occasionally present with right iliac fossa pain (Fig. 72.1). This can masquerade as acute appendicitis and is known as Valentino's syndrome [49]. Therefore, it is essential to have a high clinical suspicion for PPU, especially in patients with risk factors.

PPU can present in three phases [50]. In the first 2 h, epigastric tenderness, tachycardia, and cool and clammy peripheries are characteristic. This phase is then followed by generalized abdominal pain that is exacerbated by movement. Other signs may include involuntary guarding and abdominal rigidity with right iliac fossa tenderness due to fluid accumulating in the right paracolic gutter. Initial local peritonitis becomes generalized, and chemical peritonitis transforms into bacterial peritonitis. In the last phase, abdominal distension, fever, and hemodynamic instability ensue [1]. In rare instances, perforation is sealed off by a tag of omentum or adjacent tissues so that progressive peritonitis does not occur (*forme fruste*), and nonoperative management may be undertaken.

### 72.2.2 Investigations

#### 72.2.2.1 Serum Investigations

Blood and biochemical investigations are not diagnostic for PPU but provide information of physiologic insult. Serologic data are nonspecific and have complementary utility in PPU management [51]. Serum amylase is raised less than four times the normal levels and should be done at the emergency department along with an erect chest radiograph [52]. Full blood count for leukocytosis and raised C-reactive protein (CRP) suggest inflammation or infection [52] and is also associated with PPU [53]. A renal panel helps assess if a contrast computerized tomography (CT) scan is safe. PPU can cause organ dysfunction due to systemic inflammatory response syndrome (SIRS) and pre-renal acute kidney injury [54]. Serum albumin levels provide information beyond the nutritional status of the patient. In a single-institution retrospective study comprising of 537 patients, Seow et al. reported that low serum albumin might predict the need for gastric resection (OR: 5.57, 95% CI: 1.56–19.84, $p < 0.001$) [55]. If other etiologies of PPU are suspected, such as Zollinger Ellison syndrome or parathyroid disorders, serum gastrin and calcium levels may be ordered [1]. Inflammatory ratios like platelet to lymphocyte ratio (PLR) are easy to compute and help predict clinical outcomes. In a retrospective study including 152 patients, Omer et al. reported that patients with high PLR had a length of hospital stay of >1 week ($p = 0.005$) [56]. More evidence is required before any recommendations can be made to include PLR or similar ratios in routine clinical practice. In our opinion, serum lactate is an important marker to assess the physiologic insult

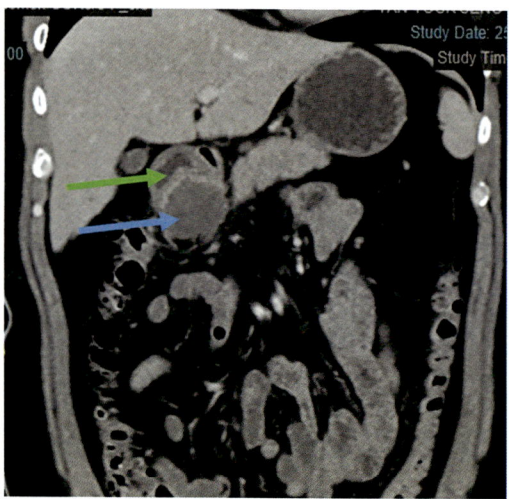

**Fig. 72.1** A computerized tomography scan of an adult patient showing the first part of duodenum (green arrow) and a localized retroperitoneal abscess (blue arrow). Nonoperative management was successful in this patient

from secondary peritonitis, and it not only guides resuscitation but also can predict prognosis. In a single-center retrospective study including 50 PPU patients, serum lactate predicted postoperative morbidity [57].

### 72.2.2.2 Imaging

In a patient with acute upper abdominal pain, the most essential and initial imaging that should be performed is an urgent erect chest X-ray (CXR) [1]. An erect CXR should be ordered to visualize free air under the diaphragm, pneumoperitoneum (Fig. 72.2) [58]. Erect CXR and lateral decubitus radiographs have similar diagnostic accuracy, and should a patient not tolerate an erect CXR due to severe peritonitis; the latter should be done [59]. The free air under the diaphragm is unfortunately only present in about 30–85% of PPU; a negative CXR does not rule out PPU. Thus, an abdominal CT scan [59] is warranted to establish a definite diagnosis. If an abdominal X-ray (AXR) had been performed instead, it might show distinct outlining of the bowel wall due to the appearance of intra and extraluminal air (Rigler's sign) (Fig. 72.3) or a large volume of free gas resulting in a large black area (Football sign). We do not recommend an AXR to be done in the setting of a negative CXR and suggest a CT scan of the abdomen-pelvis. CT scans have a high diagnostic rate of 98% [60]. CT scans are helpful in PPU diagnosis and in excluding other abdominal pathology (like acute pancreatitis). Some findings on the CT scan to note are fluid and air in the peritoneal cavity, thickening of the bowel wall, mesenteric fat stranding, and extravasation of water-soluble contrast. A non-contrast CT scan can be ordered in patients with renal impairment, and visualization of air within the peritoneal cavity is sufficient to diagnose PPU. In patients with no CT scan features of PPU, administering an oral (or via nasogastric tube (NGT)) water-soluble contrast may increase diagnostic yield. Leakage of contrast confirms the diagnosis of PPU. However, the absence of a leak does not eliminate the diagnosis of PPU as the perforation may be sealed off spontaneously [61]. In patients without free air under the diaphragm on the erect CXR and

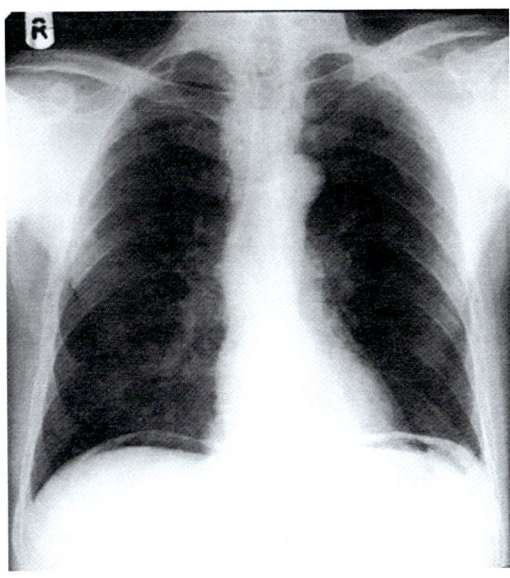

**Fig. 72.2** An erect chest X-ray of an adult patient with sudden onset severe epigastric pain showing free air under the diaphragm, suggestive of perforated peptic ulcer

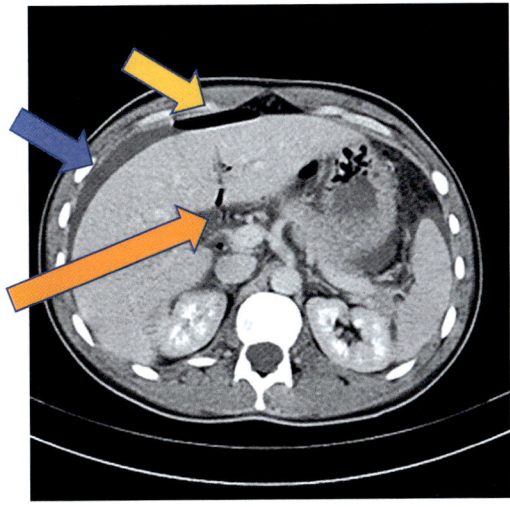

**Fig. 72.3** A computerized tomography scan showing free air along (yellow arrow) with perihepatic free fluid (blue arrow). Air pockets are also seen along the portal triad and first part of duodenum (orange arrow). This is highly suggestive of perforated peptic ulcer

unavailability of CT scan facilities, NG air insufflation may increase diagnostic yield [62]. Ultrasound may detect intraperitoneal free fluid and intestinal paresis and may be used as an adjunct in selected patients.

### Differential Diagnosis

The three categories of differential diagnosis of PPU include: (a) differential diagnosis for epigastric abdominal pain, (b) differential diagnosis of elevated serum amylase, and (c) differential diagnosis of free air under the diaphragm on imaging.

Epigastric or right upper abdominal pain is a common presenting symptom of acute cholecystitis, acute pyogenic cholangitis, pyogenic liver abscess, acute gastroenteritis, and acute colitis. Appropriate history and physical examination would suggest a clinician of foregut versus mid-hindgut pathology. Serology and imaging will aid to narrow down the list of differential diagnosis. Elevated serum amylase can be noticed in PPU patients due to peritoneal reabsorption of leaked contents. Acute pancreatitis should be differentiated as PPU warrants an emergency surgery, while management of acute pancreatitis is largely supportive. Free air under the diaphragm can be evident in other abdominal pathologies like perforated small or large bowel. Appropriate clinical history and demographic profile could assist to achieve diagnosis. In selected stable patients, CT scan of the abdomen could be considered even if chest X-ray detects free air under the diaphragm. A prior knowledge about organ of origin of perforation can alert the duty surgeon and he or she is well prepared rather than caught up with a surprise of sigmoid colon cancer perforation as a cause of free air on chest X-ray.

## 72.3 Management

The management of PPU involves integration of principles of critical care, sepsis bundle, and timely surgical intervention for source control. It is essential that surgical team co-ordinates the care and involve necessary stakeholders (e.g., radiologist or anesthetist) for optimal and timely care to ensure good clinical outcomes. Figure 72.4 shows the flowchart of management principles of PPU.

### 72.3.1 Resuscitation

PPU is frequently associated with peritonitis and septic shock and is thus a medical and surgical emergency requiring rapid evaluation and timely intervention [63]. It is of utmost priority to monitor and recognize sepsis complications and adequately define if a patient is hemodynamically stable or unstable as it impacts management [64, 65]. Symptoms such as altered mental status (low Glasgow coma scale (GCS)) suggest that perforation occurred a few hours ago. Signs such as tachycardia, tachypnea, reduced pulse pressure, reduced urinary output, and laboratory findings of metabolic acidosis and raised creatinine must be promptly evaluated. It is also essential to keep in mind that such findings may be confounded by underlying disease or medications, and thus clinical history must be meticulous [66]. Nil by mouth, nasogastric tube insertion, intravenous PPIs, urinary catheterization, analgesia, and broad-spectrum antibiotics are essential to initial measures along with intravenous fluids and oxygenation. In the "Surviving Sepsis Campaign," it is recommended that in sepsis-induced hypoperfusion, at least 30 mL/kg of IV crystalloids are administered within the first 3 h [65, 67].

Principles of sepsis management include source control and treatment of underlying etiology with antibiotics. Routine microbiologic cultures (two sets of aerobic and anaerobic blood cultures) should be obtained before starting broad-spectrum empirical antibiotics [68]. Antibiotics such as third-generation cephalosporins and metronidazole to cover for gram-negative, gram-positive, and anaerobic species are given pre-operatively to reduce the risk of intraperitoneal bacterial translocation. Antifungals are recommended based on patient factors, such as those who are immunocompromised, of advanced age, with severe co-

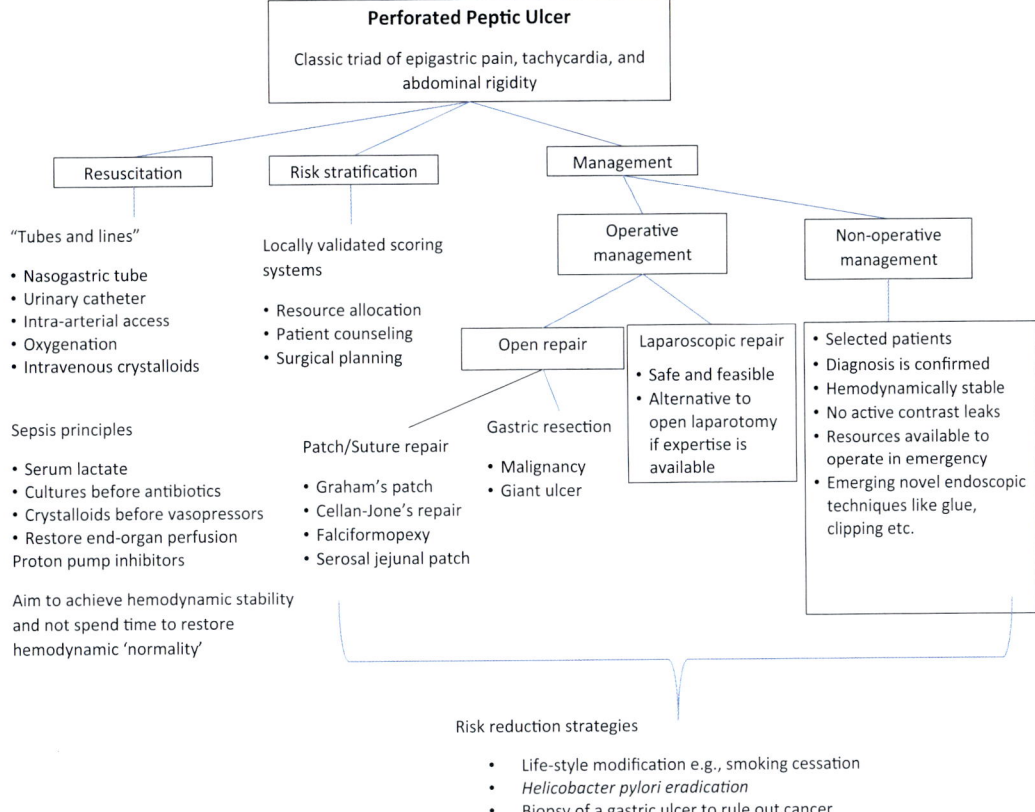

**Fig. 72.4** Flowchart of management principles of perforated peptic ulcer

morbidities, and prolonged ICU-stay or persistent intra-abdominal infections [59, 69]. In a single-center retrospective study including 673 adult patients with perforated gastric and duodenal ulcers over 10 years (January 2004–2014), Kwan et al. reported that on multi-variate analysis, fungal isolates in peritoneal fluid cultures are more likely to occur in older patients who have PPU (OR: 1.031, 95% CI: 1.01–1.047, $p < 0.001$). However, the presence of fungal isolates does not impact perioperative outcomes [70]. Intra-abdominal sepsis management requires a multi-disciplinary team approach involving the general surgeon, radiologist, critical care physician, nurses, microbiologist, and allied health personnel. Continuous assessment of the patient's heart rate, blood pressure, arterial oxygen saturation, respiratory rate, temperature, and urine output are essential. Serum lactate helps to serve as a surrogate marker for tissue perfusion and, monitoring of lactate can help identify improvement or deterioration in septic patients. The possible endpoints of resuscitation include mean arterial pressure (MAP) $\geq 65$ mmHg, urine output $\geq 0.5$ mL/kg/h, and lactate normalization. In practice, source control by prompt surgical intervention is a "part of resuscitation." Thus, the resuscitation goal is not to achieve hemodynamic "normality" but hemodynamic "stability."

### 72.3.2 Scoring Systems in PPU

Scoring systems assist with the prediction of severity or morbidity/mortality outcomes. Knowledge of predicted outcomes can assist in allocating resources, patient and family counseling, and timely evidence-based care. The main scoring systems for PPU are the Boey score, the American Society of Anesthesiologists (ASA) score, the Sepsis score, the Charlson Comorbidity Index, the Mannheim Peritonitis Index (MPI), the Acute Physiology and Chronic Health Evaluation II (APACHE II), the Simplified Acute Physiology Score II (SAPS II), The Physiology and Operative Severity Score for the Enumeration of Mortality and Morbidity Physical Sub-score (POSSUM-phys score), the Mortality Probability Models II (MPM II), Peptic Ulcer Perforation (PULP) score, the Hacettepe score and the Jabalpur score [71]. The most widely used and validated scoring systems are the Boey and ASA scores [54, 72–75]. The other scores are not commonly used due to the lack of validation data or cumbersome to compute. This review focuses on Boey's score, PULP score, and MPI.

Boey's score includes three variables: comorbidity, pre-operative shock (defined as systolic blood pressure <90 mmHg), and time from onset of abdominal pain (≤24 or >24 h). The minimum possible score is zero, and the maximum possible score is three. Boey et al. demonstrated 0%, 10%, 45.5% and 100% mortality for a score of 0, 1, 2 and 3 respectively [4]. Boey score is simple to compute and is still widely utilized [76]. However, as the understanding of comorbidity is varied, and the time from onset of abdominal pain is sometimes not exact, the score is not consistent in the predictive ability for mortality outcomes [73, 77, 78]. The PULP score includes seven clinical and biochemical variables: age, active comorbidities, liver cirrhosis, steroid use, shock on admission, time from perforation to admission, serum creatinine, and ASA score [79]. The minimum possible score is zero, and the maximum possible score is 18. PULP score is regarded as complex and impractical, and more validation studies are required. We could not validate the PULP score due to very few patients with liver cirrhosis and steroid therapy in our cohort. The ASA score is a subjective assessment of a patient's fitness for operation based on five classes (I–V). A patient with a higher ASA score has a higher mortality rate [80, 81]. The MPI score includes eight variables: age >50 years, female sex, presence of organ failure, presence of malignancy, the evolution of peritonitis for >24 h, non-colonic origin, generalized peritonitis, and fecal peritonitis [82]. The maximum possible score is 47 points, and patients are categorized into three risk profiles in increasing order of severity of peritonitis: <21, 21–29, and >29 points. The score is only possible to compute after completion of surgery. In a study involving 332 patients who underwent emergency surgery for PPU, Anbalakan et al. found that all four systems have moderate accuracy of predicting mortality rates, with an area under the receiver operator curve of 72–77.2% [83]. Upon diagnosis, resuscitation, and risk stratification by scoring systems, definite treatment must be done. In general, definitive treatment can be divided into surgical treatment, endoscopic interventions, and nonoperative management. Other novel techniques such as endoscopic clipping, gelatin sponge, and glue sealing will also be discussed.

### 72.3.3 Surgical Treatment

Figure 72.5 shows the perforated duodenal ulcer. Johan Mikuliczradecki stated that every doctor faced with a PPU must consider opening the abdomen, sewing up the hole, and averting a possible inflammation by a careful cleansing of the abdominal cavity [1]. Historically, selective vagotomy was done to prevent gastric acid production from the parietal cells to reduce gastric

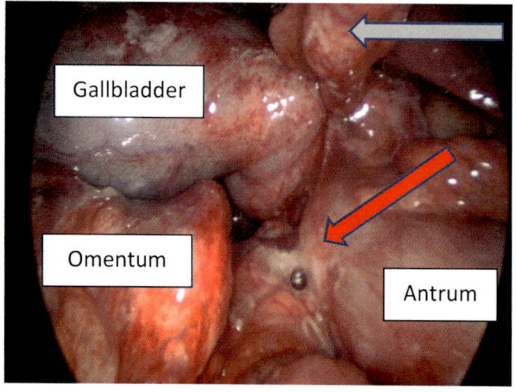

**Fig. 72.5** A laparoscopic view of a patient with perforated duodenal ulcer (red arrow). Grey arrow shows falciform ligament

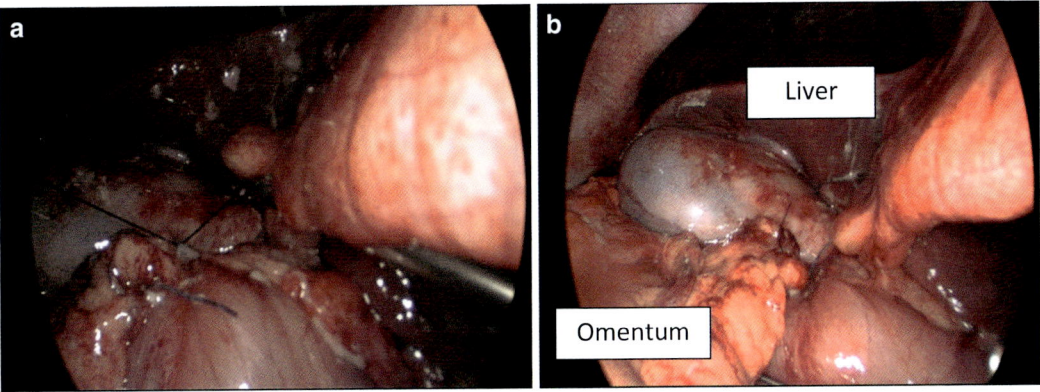

**Fig. 72.6** Laparoscopic omental patch suture repair. (**a**) Shows intracorporeal suturing and (**b**) shows a completed omental patch repair

acid secretion and reduce recurrence rates of PUD [47]. However, with the emergence of histamine receptor antagonists and PPI, vagotomy is obsolete [1]. In surgical treatment, the approaches are broadly divided into open or minimally invasive surgery approaches (MIS), that is, laparoscopic surgery. Figure 72.6a, b shows laparoscopic omental patch repair of perforated duodenal ulcer.

### 72.3.3.1 Open Surgery

The most common techniques for repairing PPU include primary closure by interrupted sutures—Cellan-Jones repair and Graham patch repair. Graham patch involves placement of sutures at a right angle to the long axis of stomach or duodenum, placing a tail of omentum without tension over the ulcer, and tying the sutures snug over to close the ulcer without causing ischemia to omental tissue. Cellan-Jones repair involves tying sutures before placing the omental patch. In addition, some authors have reported using falciform ligament to patch the ulcer. Falciform ligament patch may be helpful in patients with previous omentectomy or omental adhesions following previous abdomino-pelvic surgery. In general, omentopexy and falciformopexy are considered comparable. However, in a retrospective study involving 303 patients, Ölmez et al. reported higher failure rates for falcioformopexy (2.6% and 8.7%, $p = 0.04$) [84]. In a recent report, Tran et al. has reported that falciformopexy was safe and feasible with comparable outcomes to omental patch [85]. However, the authors reported high 30-day mortality (17.5%). Overall, there are less than 100 reported cases of falciformopexy, and more evidence is warranted to establish if falciformopexy has comparable clinical outcomes [85]. Sometimes, it is difficult to identify a healthy omentum or falciform ligament to perform a patch closure. In such instances, a serosal jejunal patch is an option. This can avoid the need for gastrectomy. When deciding between gastrectomy and patch repair, the decision lies in whether there is a suspicion for gastric malignancy, and if so, whether the patient is hemodynamically stable enough to undergo an emergent gastrectomy. Kuwabara et al. compared two techniques and found no significant differences in patient outcomes [86]. However, gastrectomy was associated with higher risks of duodenal stump blowout and anastomotic leak, longer intraoperative time, higher intraoperative blood loss, and longer length of hospital stay [7, 72, 87]. In a study including 601 patients, of which 62 patients had undergone gastrectomy, those who had undergone a gastrectomy had a higher mortality risk of 24.2% than those who did not have a gastrectomy [55]. Thus, one must follow Theodore Kocher's maxim: To do everything necessary and to do nothing unnecessary. The traditional omental patch repair is still considered the gold standard today, as it has lower morbidity and peri/post-operative transfusion rates than gastrectomy [86]. International guidelines and local hospital algorithms advocate gastrectomy beyond a specific ulcer size with variable cut-offs [36]. However, the exact cut-off beyond which omental patch repair is associated with a higher leak rate remains to be determined, and a multicenter prospective randomized study is warranted.

Open surgery can be performed by a smaller wound—minilaparotomy. A minilaparotomy is defined as an abdominal skin incision with a maximum length of 7 cm. In a retrospective review of 87 patients treated for PPU, Ishida et al. reported that patients treated by minilaparotomy ($n = 37$) had 18.4 min shorter mean operative time ($p < 0.01$), lower analgesic requirements ($p = 0.03$), earlier first pass of flatus ($p > 0.01$), and shorter hospital length of stay ($p = 0.04$) [88]. These results need to be validated. In our opinion, an emergency laparotomy is not a "cosmetic procedure," and surgical conduct should never be compromised for the sake of a smaller incision.

### 72.3.3.2 Laparoscopic Surgery

Adoption of minimally invasive surgery to acute care has been slower compared to elective surgery. However, with increasing experience, laparoscopic repair of PPU is widely reported to be safe and feasible, with potentially lower perioperative morbidity [89]. A meta-analysis of seven randomised controlled trials (RCTs) reported that laparoscopic PPU surgery has lower overall postoperative morbidity (OR: 0.54, 95% CI: 0.37–0.79, $p < 0.01$), wound infections (OR: 0.3, 95% CI: 0.16–0.5, $p < 0.01$), as well as shorter duration of hospital stay (6.6 vs. 8.2 days, $p = 0.01$). Although a one-to-one propensity score-matched analysis demonstrated that there is no difference between the 90-day mortality between those who had undergone laparoscopic versus open surgery (7.2% vs. 8.5%, OR: 0.80, 95% CI: 0.56–1.15, $p = 0.23$), Coe et al. demonstrated that over the 4-year study period involving 5253 patients, usage of laparoscopic surgery has increased from 20% to 26% and conversion rates have decreased from 40% to 31% [90]. In addition to comparable or even more superior operative outcomes to open techniques, the laparoscopic repair was reported to be more cost-effective with a decreased length of hospitalization (7.0 vs. 8.0 days, $p < 0.001$) and lower mean hospital bill ($44,095 vs. $52,055, $p = 0.019$). Laparoscopic repair avoids a larger midline laparotomy with potential benefits of reduced pulmonary and wound-related complications, especially in the elderly. This is established by a retrospective analysis carried out using data of the Frailty and Emergency Surgery in Elderly (FRAILESEL) study [91]. The authors reported that out of the 67 patients who fulfilled the inclusion criteria, 47.8% underwent laparoscopic repair. Patients managed by laparoscopic repair had less blood loss and shorter length of hospital stay, but results were not significant likely due to the small sample size. In a propensity score-matched study including 576 patients from the ACS-NSQIP database, Jayaraman et al. has reported that about 10% of patients are treated by laparoscopy, and laparoscopic repair is associated with longer operating time (92 vs. 79 min, $p = 0.003$) and shorter hospital length of stay (8.2 vs. 9.4 days, $p = 0.044$) [92]. Authors also reported that open laparotomy group patients had higher risk of bleeding (14.6% vs. 8%, $p = 0.012$) and pneumonia (8.7% vs. 4.5%, $p = 0.044$).

Many different laparoscopic techniques, including omentopexy alone, suture repair with omentopexy, or falciformopexy, are described [91, 93]. Such techniques require experience and proficiency in intracorporeal suturing skills. With increasing experience of elective laparoscopic procedures, incorporating laparoscopic skills in the residency training curriculum, and widespread availability and accessibility to minimal access surgery, more emergency abdominal procedures are managed by laparoscopy. Patient selection is integral to good outcomes. Patients with severe cardiopulmonary instability should not undergo laparoscopic surgery, as insufflation of the abdomen increases intra-abdominal pressure and worsens hypercarbia [59]. In the learning curve period, surgeons should select their patients to reduce open conversion and leak risk. We suggest that patients with a Boey score of 3, age more than 70 years, and who have been symptomatic for more than 24 h should undergo an open omental patch repair instead as they are at risk of high morbidity and mortality [1]. PPU >9 mm, and duration of pain ≥12.5 h are reported as risk factors for open conversion [94]. Shelat et al. have shown that with the adoption of strict selection criteria during the learning curve of laparoscopic omental patch repair, conversion can be kept low and good outcomes can be achieved [95]. Authors recommended that patients without suspicion of malignancy and with Boey score of 0 or 1, ulcer size of less than 10 mm, ulcer location in the pyloro-duodenal area, hemodynamic stability, no previous abdominal surgeries, ASA score of 2 and below are ideal candidates during the learning curve.

In a retrospective study involving 103 patients, Lau et al. concluded that sutureless repair techniques are faster and have comparable clinical outcomes as suture techniques [96]. In another study involving 43 patients, Wang et al. compared the effectiveness of a sutureless onlay omental patch with sutured omental patch method and reported nil post-operative leaks in both groups. In addition, operating time and length of hospital stay were shorter in the sutureless onlay omental patch group [97].

### 72.3.3.3 Endoscopic Interventions

Novel techniques such as gelatin sponge plug, fibrin glue sealing, polyglycolic acid sheet placement, and endoscopic clipping are reported to be safe and feasible in selected patients with PPU [96]. Endoscopic interventions can be combined with surgical treatment, that is, the laparo-endoscopic hybrid approach. Some authors report that sutureless techniques require strict patient selection and should not be routinely recommended in all PPU patients due to higher post-operative morbidity and mortality [98–100]. In the World Society of Emergency Surgery (WSES) guidelines, endoscopic therapy with clipping, fibrin glue sealing, and stenting is not recommended due to the ineffectiveness of such modalities in fibrotic tissues [59].

Self-expendable metal stents (SEMS) may also be used to treat PPU [101]. SEMS can also be used as a salvage procedure to manage post-operative leaks. In the case series, including eight patients with PPU treated with SEMS, two patients underwent a stent procedure due to post-operative leakage after initial surgical closure. In comparison, the other six patients were treated with SEMS due to extensive co-morbidities. Seven out of eight patients fully recovered without any complications [101]. This was also supported by a RCT including 28 patients with a confirmed perforated duodenal ulcer (stenting, $n = 13$ vs. open repair, $n = 15$). Patients treated by stent had a shorter operating time (68 vs. 92 min, $p = 0.001$). Stents were removed after a median of 3 weeks without complications. These studies show that patients with PPU can be treated with primary stenting if expertise is available. Although endoscopic techniques are not ideal for irrigating the peritoneal cavity and do not permit post-procedure drainage tube placement, the RCT by Vázquez et al. reported that there is no significant difference in mortality and morbidity rates between stent and surgical treatment for PPU [79]. They emphasize that endoscopic intervention for PPU, such as the utilization of SEMS and hybrid laparoscopic lavage plus drainage, is an effective and safe alternative to traditional surgical repair. Most surgeons prefer peritoneal washout with warm saline, although no reports support that irrigation can lower the risk of post-operative sepsis [102, 103]. In our institution, drainage is at the discretion of the primary surgeon as some surgeons believe it prevents intra-abdominal fluid collection, and others believe that it increases skin and soft tissue infections at the drain site and poses a risk of intestinal obstruction [104]. There is a paucity of reports about the success of nonsurgical interventions in special situations like marginal ulcers.

## 72.3.4 Nonoperative Management

Some reports have shown that about 40–80% of PPU are self-resolving and tend to seal off with nonsurgical management spontaneously, and overall outcomes are comparable with surgical repair [61, 105–107]. The protocol for nonsurgical management includes a nasogastric tube, intravenous fluids, antibiotics, PPIs, and repeated clinical assessment [1]. However, before nonsurgical management is decided, patients must undergo a contrast study with gastrografin dye to confirm the absence of free intraperitoneal leakage of dye/gastric contents [1, 59]. Should patients remain clinically stable with progressive signs of improvement, surgery may be avoided. However, surgery must be performed immediately if patients show clinical signs of deterioration. Many authors exclude old patients from nonsurgical management. In a nationwide inpatient database study involving 14,918 patients with PPU, Konishi et al. reported 14,918 patients who underwent nonoperative treatment than prior studies, which only included a total of 107 patients [106–110]. Unlike previous studies, this study included more patients >65 years of age and divided their patients into three distinct groups—young (ages 18–64 years old), old (ages 65–74 years old), and old-old (ages ≥75 years old). Authors reported higher morbidity (15% and 17% vs. 6.6%, $p < 0.001$) and morality (8.3% and 18% vs. 1.4%, $p < 0.001$) in patients >65 years compared to younger age (young group) patients. Nonsurgical treatment is resource-intensive and requires active monitoring of the patient's clinical status, and a surgeon must be available on-demand if the patient deteriorates. Lastly, before nonsurgical management, absolute diagnostic certainty must be ensured as the wrong diagnosis could increase mortality risk [59, 106, 111]. We have summarized the principles of nonoperative management as six R's: radiologically undetected leak; repeated clinical examination; repeated blood investigations; respiratory and renal support; resources for monitoring; and readiness to operate [1].

### 72.3.5 Prognosis

PPU is associated with significant post-operative morbidity and mortality regardless of minimally invasive or open surgery [112]. Common post-operative morbidity includes surgical site infection, intra-abdominal fluid collection/abscess, enterocutaneous fistula, incisional hernia, pneumonia, and ileus. Age >60 years, delayed treatment >24 h, shock (systolic blood pressure <100 mmHg) at presentation with, and co-morbidities predispose to morbidity [105, 113]. Elderly patients experience higher mortality risk (by 3–5 times) due to an atypical presentation or delay diagnosis [114]. To prevent the recurrence, eradication of *H. pylori* infection is important. An upper gastrointestinal endoscopy may be warranted to rule out gastric malignancy. Holistic patient care is essential to optimize the medical comorbidity that is contributory to PUD.

**Dos and Don'ts**
- Do suspect PPU in patients with sudden severe epigastric pain, tachycardia, and abdominal rigidity.
- Do obtain a good quality erect chest X-ray and interpret it promptly.
- Don't delay intervention in pursuit of stabilizing patient's hemodynamics. Resuscitation and intervention for source control must happen concurrent and not sequential.
- Don't embark on laparoscopic PPU repair without proper training and mentoring. In early experience, select your cases well so patient safety is not compromised.
- Don't resort to a routine policy of gastric resections in large or giant gastric ulcers, as outcomes of patients with gastric resections are worse!
- Don't routinely treat all patients with antifungals, as fungus is a commensal, and it is expected in peritoneal fluid samples.
- Don't resort to non-operative management unless your facility has resources and experience to do so.
- Do pay attention towards smoking cessation and *Helicobacter pylori* eradication after patient has recovered from acute illness.

**Take-Home Messages**

- PUD is highly prevalent, and acute care surgical teams must be familiar with the management of PPU.
- The classic triad of sudden onset of epigastric abdominal pain, tachycardia, and abdominal rigidity is the hallmark of PPU.
- Early diagnosis, prompt resuscitation, and surgical repair are the cornerstone to ensure good clinical outcomes.
- Erect chest film may not detect free air, and a computerized tomography scan is warranted if a clinician has a high index of suspicion.
- Laparoscopic omental patch repair is increasingly reported to have lower morbidity compared to open laparotomy.
- Endoscopic interventions have an emerging role, not only for index perforations but also as salvage treatment after surgical complications.
- Selection of patients for non-operative management must be made carefully based on local resources and expertise.

**Multiple Choice Questions**

1. Which of the following is not included in the classic triad of clinical presentation of perforated peptic ulcer?
   A. Abdominal rigidity
   B. **Hypotension**
   C. Sudden severe abdominal pain
   D. Tachycardia
2. The following is not a typical feature of gastric ulcer, in comparison with duodenal ulcer.
   A. Associated with malignancy
   B. **Association with *Helicobacter pylori***
   C. Association with smoking
   D. Epigastric pain is a presenting symptom
3. The primary diagnostic modality for diagnosis of perforated peptic ulcer is?
   A. Computerized tomography scan of abdomen
   B. **Erect chest X-ray**
   C. Gastrograffin dye study
   D. Ultrasonography of abdomen
4. Which of the following patient is an ideal patient for a novice (beginner) to embark on laparoscopic omental patch repair?
   A. 75-year-old gentleman, ASA score 3, about 2 cm anterior gastric ulcer
   B. 30-year-old female, ASA score 2, about 3 cm anterior duodenal ulcer
   C. 40-year-old gentleman, ASA score 3, a pinpoint gastric ulcer
   D. **50-year-old gentleman, ASA score 1, 5 mm duodenal ulcer**
5. Which of the following body tissues can be used to patch the perforated ulcer?
   A. Falciform ligament
   B. Omentum
   C. Jejunum
   D. **All of the above**
6. Which of the following drug is ulcer protective?
   A. Famotidine
   B. Prostaglandin
   C. Rabeprazole
   D. **Sucralfate**
7. Which of the following is true for *Helicobacter pylori*?
   A. Are absent in healthy population
   B. Floats in gastric contents and thus can reach all parts of stomach
   C. **Routine eradication helps reduce ulcer relapse**
   D. Serology tests are most accurate in detection of active infection
8. A 50-year-old gentleman wakes up past midnight with severe upper abdominal pain. He is a chronic smoker. He visits emergency department and has tachycardia and abdomi-

nal rigidity. You suspect he has a perforated peptic ulcer. The chest X-ray is normal. What is your next best course of action?

   A. Manage as per acute pancreatitis
   B. Repeat a chest X-ray after 4 h
   C. Insert a wide bore NG tube, insufflate air, and do an ultrasound abdomen
   D. **Request an urgent computerized tomography scan of abdomen**

9. A 70-year-old female is admitted with a suspected diagnosis of perforated peptic ulcer. She has diabetes, chronic renal impairment, congestive cardiac failure, and previous history of stroke. You calculate Boey's score of 2 and ASA score of 3. A computerized tomography scan shows generalized free fluid and a small pocket of air near duodenum. Your next best course of action is?

    A. Diagnostic laparoscopy and omental patch repair
    B. Endoscopic clipping of the ulcer
    C. **Laparotomy**
    D. Non-operative management

10. With widespread use of proton pump inhibitors, some complications are infrequently encountered in clinical practice. Which of the following complication of peptic ulcer disease is still commonly seen in modern clinical practice?

    A. Gastric outlet obstruction
    B. Hour-glass stomach
    C. **Perforation**
    D. Tea-pot stomach

# References

1. Chung KT, Shelat VG. Perforated peptic ulcer—an update. World J Gastrointest Surg. 2017;9(1):1–12.
2. Lanas A, Chan FKL. Peptic ulcer disease. Lancet. 2017;390(10094):613–24.
3. Rajesh V, Chandra SS, Smile SR. Risk factors predicting operative mortality in perforated peptic ulcer disease. Trop Gastroenterol. 2003;24(3):148–50.
4. Boey J, Choi SK, Poon A, et al. Risk stratification in perforated duodenal ulcers. A prospective validation of predictive factors. Ann Surg. 1987;205(1):22–6.
5. Zelickson MS, Bronder CM, Johnson BL, et al. Helicobacter pylori is not the predominant etiology for peptic ulcers requiring operation. Am Surg. 2011;77(8):1054–60.
6. Søreide KK, Thorsen K, Søreide JA. Strategies to improve the outcome of emergency surgery for perforated peptic ulcer. Br J Surg. 2014;101(1):e51–64.
7. Chan KS, Wang YL, Chan XW, et al. Outcomes of omental patch repair in large or giant perforated peptic ulcer are comparable to gastrectomy. Eur J Trauma Emerg Surg. 2019; https://doi.org/10.1007/s00068-019-01237-8. Epub ahead of print.
8. Svanes C, Sothern RB, Sørbye H. Rhythmic patterns in incidence of peptic ulcer perforation over 5.5 decades in Norway. Chronobiol Int. 1998;15(3):241–64.
9. Gunshefski L, Glancbaum L, Brolin RE, et al. Changing patterns in perforated peptic ulcer disease. Am Surg. 1990;56(4):270–4.
10. Fuccio L, Minardi ME, Zagari RM, et al. Meta-analysis: duration of first-line proton-pump inhibitor based triple therapy for Helicobacter pylori eradication. Ann Intern Med. 2007;147(8):553–62.
11. Gisbert JP, Pajares JM. Helicobacter pylori infection and perforated peptic ulcer prevalence of the infection and role of antimicrobial treatment. Helicobacter. 2003;8(3):159–67.
12. García RLA, Barreales TL. Risk of upper gastrointestinal complications among users of traditional NSAIDs and COXIBs in the general population. Gastroenterology. 2007;132(2):498–506.
13. Lau JY, Sung J, Hill C, et al. Systematic review of the epidemiology of complicated peptic ulcer disease: incidence, recurrence, risk factors and mortality. Digestion. 2011;84(2):102–13.
14. Schwarz S, Morelli G, Kusecek B, et al. Horizontal versus familial transmission of Helicobacter pylori. PLoS Pathog. 2008;4(10):e1000180.
15. Burucoa C, Axon A. Epidemiology of Helicobacter pylori infection. Helicobacter. 2017;22(Suppl):1.
16. Hunt RH, Xiao SD, Megraud F, et al. Helicobacter pylori in developing countries. World Gastroenterology Organisation Global Guideline. J Gastrointestin Liver Dis. 2011;20(3):299–304.
17. Ang TL, Fock KM, Ang D, et al. The changing profile of Helicobacter pylori antibiotic resistance in singapore: a 15-year study. Helicobacter. 2016;21(4):261–5.
18. Smith JG, Li W, Rosson RS. Prevalence, clinical and endoscopic predictors of Helicobacter pylori infection in an urban population. Conn Med. 2009;73(3):133–7.

19. Sebastian M, Chandran VP, Elashaa YI, et al. Helicobacter pylori infection in perforated peptic ulcer disease. Br J Surg. 1995;82(3):360–2.
20. Reinbach DH, Cruickshank G, McColl KE. Acute perforated duodenal ulcer is not associated with Helicobacter pylori infection. Gut. 1993;34(10):1344–7.
21. El-Nakeeb A, Fikry A, Abd El-Hamed TM, et al. Effect of Helicobacter pylori eradication on ulcer recurrence after simple closure of perforated duodenal ulcer. Int J Surg. 2009;7(2):126–9.
22. Brune K, Patrignani P. New insights into the use of currently available nonsteroidal anti-inflammatory drugs. J Pain Res. 2015;8:105–18.
23. Henry D, Dobson A, Turner C. Variability in the risk of major gastrointestinal complications from nonaspirin nonsteroidal anti-inflammatory drugs. Gastroenterology. 1993;105(4):1078–88.
24. García Rodríguez LA, Jick H. Risk of upper gastrointestinal bleeding and perforation associated with individual nonsteroidal anti-inflammatory drugs. Lancet. 1994;343(8900):769–72.
25. Mancia G, Fagard R, Narkiewicz K, et al. 2013 ESH/ESC guidelines for the management of arterial hypertension: the Task Force for the Management of Arterial Hypertension of the European Society of Hypertension (ESH) and of the European Society of Cardiology (ESC). Eur Heart J. 2013;34(28):2159–219.
26. Anderson JL, Adams CD, Antman EM, et al. 2012 ACCF/AHA focused update incorporated into the ACCF/AHA 2007 guidelines for the management of patients with unstable angina/non-ST-elevation myocardial infarction: a report of the American College of Cardiology Foundation/American Heart Association Task Force on Practice Guidelines. J Am Coll Cardiol. 2013;61(23):e179–347.
27. Kristen BD, Christine L, Darren B, et al. Aspirin for the prevention of cardiovascular disease: U.S. Preventive Services Task Force recommendation statement. Ann Intern Med. 2009;150(6):396–404.
28. Sostres C, Gargallo CJ. Gastrointestinal lesions and complications of low-dose aspirin in the gastrointestinal tract. Best Pract Res Clin Gastroenterol. 2012;26(2):141–51.
29. Rosenstock S, Jørgensen T, Bonnevie O, et al. Risk factors for peptic ulcer disesase: a population based prospective cohort study comprising 2416 Danish adults. Gut. 2003;52(2):186–93.
30. Shirazi M, Zaban MT, Gummadi S, et al. Peptic ulcer perforation after cesarean section; case series and literature review. BMC Surg. 2020;20(1):110.
31. Eastwood GL. The role of smoking in peptic ulcer disease. J Clin Gastroenterol. 1988;10:S19–23.
32. Parasher G, Eastwood GL. Smoking and peptic ulcer in the Helicobacter pylori era. Eur J Gastroenterol Hepatol. 2000;12(8):843–53.
33. Nuhu A, Madziga AG, Gali BM. Acute perforated duodenal ulcer in Maiduguri: experience with simple closure and Helicobacter pylori eradication. West Afr J Med. 2009;28(6):384–7.
34. Iwao T, Toyonaga A, Ikegami M, et al. Gastric mucosal blood flow after smoking in healthy human beings assessed by laser Doppler flowmetry. Gastrointest Endosc. 1993;39(3):400–3.
35. Svanes C, Søreide JA, Skarstein A. Smoking and ulcer perforation. Gut. 1997;41(2):177–80.
36. Chung WC, Joen EJ, Lee KM, et al. Incidence and clinical features of endoscopic ulcers developing after gastrectomy. World J Gastroenterol. 2012;18(25):3260–6.
37. Sapala JA, Wood MH, Sapala MA, et al. Marginal ulcer after gastric bypass: a prospective 3-year study of 173 patients. Obes Surg. 1998;8(5):505–16.
38. Patel RA, Brolin RE, Gandhi A. Revisional operations for marginal ulcer after Roux-en-Y gastric bypass. Surg Obes Relat Dis. 2009;5(3):317–22.
39. MacLean LD, Rhode BM, Nohr C, et al. Stomal ulcer after gastric bypass. J Am Coll Surg. 1997;185(1):1–7.
40. Søreide K, Thorsen K, Harrison EM, et al. Perforated peptic ulcer. Lancet. 2015;386(10000):1288–98.
41. Wilson DE. Prostaglandins in peptic ulcer disease. Their postulated role in the pathogenesis and treatment. Postgrad Med. 1987;81(4):309–16.
42. Gisbert JP, Calvet X. Review article: Helicobacter pylori-negative duodenal ulcer disease. Aliment Pharmacol Ther. 2009;30(8):791–815.
43. Malfertheiner P, Chan FK, McColl KE. Peptic ulcer disease. Lancet. 2009;374(9699):1449–61.
44. Søreide K. Current insight into pathophysiology of gastroduodenal ulcers: why do only some ulcers perforate? J Trauma Acute Care Surg. 2016;80(6):1045–8.
45. Gökakın AK, Kury A, Atabey M, et al. The impact of Ramadan on peptic ulcer perforation. Ulus Travma Acil Cerrahi Derg. 2012;18(4):339–43.
46. Curtis JR, Lanas A, John A, et al. Factors associated with gastrointestinal perforation in a cohort of patients with rheumatoid arthritis. Arthritis Care Res (Hoboken). 2012;64(12):1819–28.
47. Agnes A, La GA, Tirelli F, et al. Duodenal perforation in a SARS-CoV-2-positive patient with negative PCR results for SARS-CoV-2 in the peritoneal fluid. Eur Rev Med Pharmacol Sci. 2020;24(23):12516–21.
48. Hasadia R, Kopelman Y, Olsha O, et al. Short- and long-term outcomes of surgical management of peptic ulcer complications in the era of proton pump inhibitors. Eur J Trauma Emerg Surg. 2018;44(5):795–801.
49. Noussios G, Galanis N, Konstantinidis S, et al. Valentino's syndrome (with retroperitoneal ulcer perforation): a rare clinico-anatomical entity. Am J Case Rep. 2020;21:e922647.

50. Silen W, Cope Z. Cope's early diagnosis of the acute abdomen. New York: Oxford University Press; 2005.
51. Di SS, Bassi M, Smerieri N, et al. Diagnosis and treatment of perforated or bleeding peptic ulcers: 2013 WSES position paper. World J Emerg Surg. 2014;9:45.
52. Fakhry SM, Watts DD, Luchette FA. Current diagnostic approaches lack sensitivity in the diagnosis of perforated blunt small bowel injury: analysis from 275,557 trauma admissions from the EAST multi-institutional HVI trial. J Trauma. 2003;54(2):295–306.
53. Malhotra AK, Fabian TC, Katsis SB, et al. Blunt bowel and mesenteric injuries: the role of screening computed tomography. J Trauma. 2000;48(6):991–8; discussion 998–1000.
54. Thorsen K, Søreide JA, Søreide K. What is the best predictor of mortality in perforated peptic ulcer disease? A population-based, multivariable regression analysis including three clinical scoring systems. J Gastrointest Surg. 2014;18(7):1261–8.
55. Seow JG, Lim YR, Low V. Serum albumin may predict the need for gastric resection in patients with perforated peptic ulcer. Eur J Trauma Emerg Surg. 2017;43(3):293–8.
56. Al-Yahri O, Saafan T, Abdelrahman H, et al. Platelet to lymphocyte ratio associated with prolonged hospital length of stay postpeptic ulcer perforation repair: an observational descriptive analysis. Biomed Res Int. 2021;2021:6680414.
57. Sugase T, Michiura T, Urabe S, et al. Optimal treatment and complications of patients with the perforated upper gastrointestinal tract. Surg Today. 2021;51:1446–55.
58. Grassi R, Romano S, Pinto A, et al. Gastro-duodenal perforations: conventional plain film, US and CT findings in 166 consecutive patients. Eur J Radiol. 2004;50(1):30–6.
59. Tarasconi A, Antonio C, Federico B, Walter L, et al. Perforated and bleeding peptic ulcer: WSES guidelines. World J Emerg Surg. 2020 Jan;7(15):3. https://doi.org/10.1186/s13017-019-0283-9.
60. Kim HC, Yang DM, Kim SW, et al. Gastrointestinal tract perforation: evaluation of MDCT according to perforation site and elapsed time. Eur Radiol. 2014;24(6):1386–93.
61. Donovan AJ, Berne TV, Donovan JA. Perforated duodenal ulcer: an alternative therapeutic plan. Arch Surg. 1998;133(11):1166–71.
62. Upadhye A, Dalvi A, Nair H. Nasogastric air insufflation in early diagnosis of perforated peptic ulcer. J Postgrad Med. 1986;32(2):82–4.
63. Ross JT, Matthay MA, Harris HW. Secondary peritonitis: principles of diagnosis and intervention. BMJ. 2018;361:k1407.
64. Sartelli M, Kluger Y, Asaloni L, et al. Raising concerns about the Sepsis-3 definitions. World J Emerg Surg. 2018;13:6.
65. Seymour CW, Gesten F, Prescott HC, et al. Time to treatment and mortality during mandated emergency care for sepsis. N Engl J Med. 2017;376(23):2235–44.
66. Cecconi M, Evans L, Levy M, et al. Sepsis and septic shock. Lancet. 2018;392(10141):75–87.
67. Levy MM, Rhodes A, Phillipis GS, et al. Surviving Sepsis Campaign: association between performance metrics and outcomes in a 7.5-year study. Crit Care Med. 2015;43(1):3–12.
68. Weinstein MP, Rellers LB, Murphy JR, et al. The clinical significance of positive blood cultures: a comprehensive analysis of 500 episodes of bacteremia and fungemia in adults. I. Laboratory and epidemiologic observations. Rev Infect Dis. 1983;5(1):35–53.
69. Solomkin JS, Mazuski JE, et al. Diagnosis and management of complicated intra-abdominal infection in adults and children: guidelines by the Surgical Infection Society and the Infectious Diseases Society of America. Clin Infect Dis. 2010;50(2):133–64.
70. Kwan JR, Lim M, Ng F, et al. Fungal isolates in peritoneal fluid culture do not impact perioperative outcomes of peptic ulcer perforation. Surg Infect (Larchmt). 2019;20(8):619–24.
71. Knudsen NV, Møller MH. Association of mortality with out-of-hours admission in patients with perforated peptic ulcer. Acta Anaesthesiol Scand. 2015;59(2):248–54.
72. Menekse E, Kocer B, Topcu R, et al. A practical scoring system to predict mortality in patients with perforated peptic ulcer. World J Emerg Surg. 2015;10:7.
73. Thorsen K, Søreide JA, Søreide K. Scoring systems for outcome prediction in patients with perforated peptic ulcer. Scand J Trauma Resusc Emerg Med. 2013;21:25.
74. Knaus WA, Drape EA, Wagner DP, et al. APACHE II: a severity of disease classification system. Crit Care Med. 1985;13(10):818–29.
75. Fitz-Henry J. The ASA classification and perioperative risk. Ann R Coll Surg Engl. 2011;93(3):185–7.
76. Lohsiriwat V, Prapasrivorakul S, Lohsiriwat D. Perforated peptic ulcer: clinical presentation, surgical outcomes, and the accuracy of the Boey scoring system in predicting post-operative morbidity and mortality. World J Surg. 2009;33(1):80–5.
77. Mishra A, Sharma D, Raina VK. A simplified prognostic scoring system for peptic ulcer perforation in developing countries. Indian J Gastroenterol. 2003;22(2):49–53.
78. Møller MH, Engebjerg MC, Adamsen S, et al. The Peptic Ulcer Perforation (PULP) score: a predictor of mortality following peptic ulcer perforation. A cohort study. Acta Anaesthesiol Scand. 2012;56(5):655–62.
79. Vázquez A, Khodakaram K, Bergström M, et al. Stent treatment or surgical closure for perforated duodenal ulcers: a prospective randomized study. Surg Endosc. 2020; https://doi.org/10.1007/s00464-020-08158-3.
80. Mäkelä JT, Klviniemi H, Ohtonen P, et al. Factors that predict morbidity and mortality in

patients with perforated peptic ulcers. Eur J Surg. 2002;168(8–9):446–51.
81. Kujath P, Schwandner O, Bruch HP. Morbidity and mortality of perforated peptic gastroduodenal ulcer following emergency surgery. Langenbecks Arch Surg. 2002;387(7-8):298–302.
82. Hunt RH, Xiao SD, Megraud F, et al. World Gastroenterology Organisation Global Guideline: Helicobacter pylori in developing countries. J Clin Gastroenterol. 2011;45(5):383–8.
83. Anbalakan K, Chua D, Pandya GJ, et al. Five year experience in management of perforated peptic ulcer and validation of common mortality risk prediction models—are existing models sufficient? A retrospective cohort study. Int J Surg. 2015;14:38–44.
84. Ölmez A, Cicek E, Aydin C, et al. Omentopexy versus falciformopexy for peptic ulcer perforation. Ulus Travma Acil Cerrahi Derg. 2019;25(6):580–4.
85. Son TQ, Soc TH, Huong TT, et al. Outcomes of surgical management of peptic ulcer perforation using the falciform ligament: a cross-sectional study at a single centre in Vietnam. Ann Med Surg. 2021;67:102477.
86. Kuwabara K, Matsuda S, Fushimi K, et al. Reappraising the surgical approach on the perforated gastroduodenal ulcer: should gastric resection be abandoned? J Clin Med Res. 2011;3(5):213–22.
87. Gupta S, Kaushik R, Sharma R, et al. The management of large perforations of duodenal ulcers. BMC Surg. 2005;5:15.
88. Ishida H, Ishiguoro T, Kumamoto K, et al. Minilaparotomy for perforated duodenal ulcer. Int Surg. 2011;96(3):194–200.
89. Song KY, Kim TH, Kim SN, et al. Laparoscopic repair of perforated duodenal ulcers: the simple "one-stitch" suture with omental patch technique. Surg Endosc. 2008;22(7):1632–5.
90. Coe PO, Lee MJ, Boyd-Carson H, et al. Open versus laparoscopic repair of perforated peptic ulcer disease: a propensity-matched study of the national emergency laparotomy audit. Ann Surg. 2020; https://doi.org/10.1097/SLA.0000000000004332.
91. Agresta F, Michelet I, Coluci G, et al. Emergency laparoscopy: a community hospital experience. Surg Endosc. 2000;14(5):484–7.
92. Jayaraman SS, Allen R, Feather C, et al. Outcomes of laparoscopic vs open repair of perforated peptic ulcers: an ACS-NSQIP study. J Surg Res. 2021;265:13–20.
93. Khoursheed M, Fuad M, Safar H, et al. Laparoscopic closure of perforated duodenal ulcer. Surg Endosc. 2000;14(1):56–8.
94. Kim JH, Chin HM, Bae YJ, et al. Risk factors associated with conversion of laparoscopic simple closure in perforated duodenal ulcer. Int J Surg. 2015;15:40–4.
95. Shelat VG, Ahmed S, Chia CL, et al. Strict selection criteria during surgical training ensures good outcomes in laparoscopic omental patch repair (LOPR) for perforated peptic ulcer (PPU). Int Surg. 2015;100(2):370–5.
96. Lau WY, Leung KL, Kwong KH, et al. A randomized study comparing laparoscopic versus open repair of perforated peptic ulcer using suture or sutureless technique. Ann Surg. 1996;224(2):131–8.
97. Wang YC, Hsieh CH, Lo HC, et al. Sutureless onlay omental patch for the laparoscopic repair of perforated peptic ulcers. World J Surg. 2014;38(8):1917–21.
98. Lee FY, Leung KL, Lai PB, et al. Selection of patients for laparoscopic repair of perforated peptic ulcer. Br J Surg. 2001;88(1):133–6.
99. Ishiguro T, Nagawa H. Inadvertent endoscopic application of a hemoclip to the splenic artery through a perforated gastric ulcer. Gastrointest Endosc. 2001;53(3):378–9.
100. Hashiba K, Carvalho AM, Diniz G, et al. Experimental endoscopic repair of gastric perforations with an omental patch and clips. Gastrointest Endosc. 2001;54(4):500–4.
101. Bergström M, Vázquez A, Park PO. Self-expandable metal stents as a new treatment option for perforated duodenal ulcer. Endoscopy. 2013;45(3):222–5.
102. Schein M, Gecelter G, Freinkel W, et al. Peritoneal lavage in abdominal sepsis. A controlled clinical study. Arch Surg. 1990;125(9):1132–5.
103. Whiteside OJ, Tytherleigh MG, Thrush S, et al. Intra-operative peritoneal lavage—who does it and why? Ann R Coll Surg Engl. 2005;87(4):255–8.
104. Pai D, Sharma A, Kanungo R, et al. Role of abdominal drains in perforated duodenal ulcer patients: a prospective controlled study. Aust N Z J Surg. 1999;69(3):210–3.
105. Zittel TT, Jehle EC, Becker HD. Surgical management of peptic ulcer disease today—indication, technique and outcome. Langenbecks Arch Surg. 2000;385(2):84–96.
106. Crofts TJ, Park KG, Steele RJ, et al. A randomized trial of nonoperative treatment for perforated peptic ulcer. N Engl J Med. 1989;320(15):970–3.
107. Bucher P, Oulhaci W, Morel P, et al. Results of conservative treatment for perforated gastroduodenal ulcers in patients not eligible for surgical repair. Swiss Med Wkly. 2007;137(23–24):337–40.
108. Cao F, Li J, Li A, et al. Nonoperative management for perforated peptic ulcer: who can benefit? Asian J Surg. 2014;37(3):148–53.
109. Lay PL, Huang HH, Chang WK, et al. Outcome of nonsurgical intervention in patients with perforated peptic ulcers. Am J Emerg Med. 2016;34(8):1556–60.
110. Konishi T, Fujiogi M, Michihata N, et al. Outcomes of nonoperative treatment for gastroduodenal ulcer perforation: a nationwide study of 14,918 inpatients in Japan. J Gastrointest Surg. 2021;25:2770.
111. Truscott BM, Withycombe JF. Perforated peptic ulcer; an assessment of the value of nonoperative treatment. Lancet. 1950;1(6611):894–6.
112. Lunevicius R, Morkevicius M. Management strategies, early results, benefits, and risk factors of lapa-

roscopic repair of perforated peptic ulcer. World J Surg. 2005;29(10):1299–310.
113. Sarosi GA, Jaiswal KR, Nwariaku FE, et al. Surgical therapy of peptic ulcers in the 21st century: more common than you think. Am J Surg. 2005;190(5):775–9.
114. Feliciano DV, Bitondo CG, Burch JM, et al. Emergency management of perforated peptic ulcers in the elderly patient. Am J Surg. 1984;148(6):764–7.

## Further Reading

Chan KS, Wang YL, Chan XW, et al. Outcomes of omental patch repair in large or giant perforated peptic ulcer are comparable to gastrectomy. Eur J Trauma Emerg Surg. 2019; https://doi.org/10.1007/s00068-019-01237-8. Epub ahead of print.

Chung KT, Shelat VG. Perforated peptic ulcer—an update. World J Gastrointest Surg. 2017;9(1):1–12.

Shelat VG, Ahmed S, Chia CL, et al. Strict selection criteria during surgical training ensures good outcomes in laparoscopic omental patch repair (LOPR) for perforated peptic ulcer (PPU). Int Surg. 2015;100(2):370–5.

Tarasconi A, Antonio C, Federico B, Walter L, et al. Perforated and bleeding peptic ulcer: WSES guidelines. World J Emerg Surg. 2020 Jan;7(15):3. https://doi.org/10.1186/s13017-019-0283-9.

# Diagnosis and Management of Acute Small Bowel Obstruction

## 73

Pepijn Krielen and Richard ten Broek

## 73.1 Introduction

Small bowel obstruction (SBO) is a major contributor to morbidity and mortality in emergency abdominal surgery. In the most recent update of the national emergency laparotomy audit (NELA) report, bowel obstruction made up for almost half of all emergency laparotomies in the United Kingdom [1]. An inconvenient truth about SBO is that approximately 70% of cases is caused by adhesions [2]. Adhesions, a form of internal scar tissue, essentially are the footprint of previous abdominal surgical procedures. In the NELA cohort, the 30- and 90-day mortality rates after emergency laparotomy for adhesive SBO were 7% and 9.8%, respectively, which is comparable with the mortality from an anastomotic leakage [1]. A national study of emergency abdominal surgery in the USA showed similar results, between 2008 and 2011 SBO and adhesiolysis was among the top five of emergency surgical procedures ranked by morbidity and mortality [3].

P. Krielen (✉) · R. ten Broek
Department of Surgery, Radboud University Medical Center, Nijmegen, The Netherlands
e-mail: Pepijn.krielen@radboudumc.nl;
Richard.tenbroek@radboucum.nl

In the past decade, a paradigm shift in the treatment of SBO in patients with previous abdominal surgery has been implemented. "Never let the sun rise or set on a small bowel obstruction" was the old adage, implicating that most cases of SBO require emergency surgical exploration. Today, the majority of small bowel obstructions are successfully managed non-operatively, with bowel decompression, water-soluble contrast agents, and fluid resuscitation. Non-operative management has been found safe and efficacious in 70% of SBOs caused by adhesions [4].

Nevertheless, there are still many important questions and clinical challenges related to adhesive small bowel obstruction (ASBO). How long is a trial of non-operative management appropriate? There is evidence that prolonged delays in surgery increase mortality [1, 5]. How can we select patients that will require surgery at an early stage? Can we also apply a conservative treatment in patients with "virging abdomen" (i.e., no history of previous surgery)? How to manage SBO in the elderly frail patients and patients with polypharmacy? Further, laparoscopy is increasingly used as the surgical approach in patients with an SBO.

In this chapter, we will review the evidence on the optimal diagnostic and therapeutic approach to the patient with SBO and make evidence-based recommendations.

> **Learning Goals**
> - Implementation of laparoscopy and the use of adhesion barriers are useful to reduce the risk of adhesive small bowel obstruction.
> - The most important goal in diagnostic workup of patients with SBO is to establish the etiology and the need for emergency surgery. Computed tomography (CT) scan is very useful to establish these goals.
> - Non-operative management can safely be continued for up to 72 h in most patient. Patients with comorbidities and diabetes in particular might require more early operative intervention.
> - Laparoscopic adhesiolysis might reduce morbidity in patients with SBO that need surgery, but only in selected cases.

## 73.1.1 Epidemiology

Small bowel obstruction is one of the most common pathologies of the small bowel. Approximately one in ten adults and elderly patients with abdominal pain presenting at the emergency department are diagnosed with SBO [6–8]. SBO is predominantly diagnosed in patients with a history of abdominal surgery, which results from the fact that most cases of SBO are caused by post-operative adhesions. Incidence rates of ASBO vary, depending on the anatomical location of the index surgery. Overall, approximately 2–3% of all patient will be admitted to a hospital with a case of ASBO in the first 5 years after surgery. The risk of ASBO is the highest after lower gastrointestinal tract and pediatric surgery (3–4%) and the lowest after abdominal wall or upper gastrointestinal tract surgery (0.5–1%) [2]. Mean length of stay for an episode of ASBO ranges from 4 to 13 days, depending on the type of treatment [2].

After open surgery as many as 89–93% of patients develop adhesions, incidence rates of adhesion formation are lower after minimally invasive surgery, 45–62% [9–11]. Observational studies have shown that the lower incidence of adhesions following laparoscopy also results in a lower incidence of ASBO [12]. In the surgical and clinical adhesions research (SCAR) update study, the number of readmissions definitively related to adhesions dropped by 32% after laparoscopy, and readmissions possibly related to adhesions by 11% [12]. Nevertheless, the morbidity related to adhesions remains substantial. Within 5 years following laparoscopic colon surgery, 2.4% of patients are readmitted for a definitively adhesion-related complication, rising to 7% following laparoscopic rectal surgery.

## 73.1.2 Etiology

Causes of SBO can be mechanical or functional. Mechanical obstructions can be caused by external compression, intrinsic bowel disease, or an intraluminal mass, resulting in partial or complete blockage of the lumen of the bowel, preventing normal passage of bowel contents. Symptoms for SBO are abdominal pain, bloating, nausea, vomiting, and constipation.

The most common cause for small bowel obstruction is external compression, most often caused by post-operative adhesions [2]. Other causes of adhesion formation are radiotherapy, and abdominal infection [13]. Despite adhesions, SBO can be caused by abdominal hernias, or peritoneal metastases. Intrinsic bowel diseases resulting in obstruction are much more rare. Examples of intrinsic bowel diseases causing SBO include strictures secondary to inflammatory bowel disease, and small bowel malignancies [14]. Intraluminal masses are among the most rare causes of bowel obstruction and can be ingested (bezoars, corpora aliena) or indigenous such as gall stones.

The etiology of the SBO can have important implications for the treatment. Whereas conservative treatment might be effective for most cases of ASBO, it might not be appropriate for many of the other causes.

### 73.1.2.1 Etiology in the Virgin Abdomen

The term "virgin abdomen" refers to the abdomen of a patient without prior surgery, radiotherapy, or known peritoneal inflammatory disease in history. SBO is much less common in patients with a virgin abdomen (VA). In three cohort studies, SBO-VA accounted for 5–16% of all cases of SBO [15–17]. The true proportion of SBO-VA might even be lower as good epidemiological studies and population-based data are lacking. The included cohorts have a sample size ranging between only 60–100 patients with SBO; moreover, most studies were single-center studies.

Many authors suggest that surgical exploration is still mandatory in the case of SBO in the virgin abdomen, based on the assumption that SBO-VA is usually caused by other etiologies than adhesions, such as malignancy, internal hernia, and bezoars [18, 19]. Recent studies, however, demonstrated a high incidence of adhesions also in patients with SBO-VA [15, 20]. Several recent studies retrospectively analyzed the etiology in patients undergoing surgical treatment for SBO-VA; adhesions were the cause of SBO-VA in 26–100% [15, 17, 20–23]. In two studies, 75–100% of patients conservatively treated were diagnosed with adhesions [15, 20]. Overall, adhesions were reported to be the cause of bowel obstruction in 134/280 (47.9%) patients in six studies with known etiology. Fukami et al. reported one a cohort of 44 patients with SBO-VA, treated by non-operative management. In this cohort, conservative treatment only failed in one patient [17]. In conclusion, recent papers suggest that most cases of SBO in the virgin abdomen are caused by adhesions and that guidelines for SBO in general can also be applied to cases with a virgin abdomen.

## 73.1.3 Classification

Different classes of scoring systems are in use in the field of SBO surgery and research, with different purposes. The first class is scoring system to assess severity of adhesions during reoperations. There is wide variation in the clinical appearance of adhesions in SBO, ranging from a single adhesive strand to wide and extensive adhesions as seen in the "frozen abdomen." It is not difficult to imagine that such differences in adhesions can impact clinical outcome, impacting operative time, and risk of inadvertent organ injuries. A limitation of this type of scoring is that they are only applicable to operatively treated cases, and have little predictive value for clinical outcomes.

The oldest and still frequently used severity score in general surgery is the Zühlke score (Table 73.1) [24]. The score is based on the tenacity of adhesions and their morphologic aspects, but it does not include the extent of adhesions. Also, this score does not account for potential differences in the tenacity of adhesions in different parts of the abdomen.

To overcome these limitations, the ASBO working group of the world society of emergency surgery developed the peritoneal adhesion index (Fig. 73.1) [25]. Using the peritoneal adhesion index the tenacity of adhesions is measured at 10 predefined anatomical areas. Thus, the total score integrates both the tenacity and the extent of adhesions. However, similarly to the score by Zühlke, it does not correlate to the clinical burden of adhesions.

Another newly developed class of scoring system is the adhesion-related morbidity score. Adhesions do not only cause SBO but also cause a whole range of long-term complications including difficulties during (elective) reoperations, chronic abdominal pain, and female infertility [2, 26]. The CLinical Adhesion Score (CLAS) integrates all four domains of adhesion-related complications, as well as the likelihood that symptoms

**Table 73.1** Zühlke classification

| Grade | Description |
|---|---|
| 0 | No adhesions or insignificant adhesions |
| I | Adhesions that are filmy and easy to separate by blunt dissection |
| II | Adhesions with beginning vascularization that can be dissected blunt but some sharp dissection is necessary |
| III | Adhesions with clear vascularization that can only be dissected using sharp dissection |
| IV | Adhesions which strongly attached organs, dissection is only possible by sharp dissection, damage of organs is hardly preventable |

Table adapted from original publication: Langenbecks Arch Chir Suppl II Verh Dtsch Ges Chir, 1990: p. 1009–16

**Fig. 73.1** Peritoneal adhesion index. (Figure originally published: World J Emerg Surg, 2013. 8(1): p. 6)

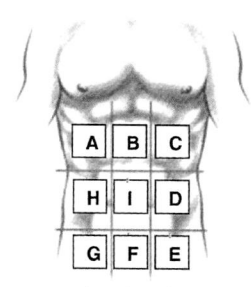

**PERITONEAL ADHESION INDEX:**

| Regions: | Adhesion grade: | Adhesion grade score: |
|---|---|---|
| **A** Right upper | ___ | 0 No adhesions |
| **B** Epigastrium | ___ | 1 Filmy adhesions, blunt dissection |
| **C** Left upper | ___ | 2 Strong adhesions, sharp dissection |
| **D** Left flank | ___ | 3 Very strong vascularized adhesions, sharp |
| **E** Left lower | ___ | dissection, damage hardly preventable |
| **F** Pelvis | ___ | |
| **G** Right lower | ___ | |
| **H** Right flank | ___ | |
| **I** Central | ___ | |
| **L** Bowel to bowel | ___ | |

**PAI** ☐

are truly caused by adhesions [27]. The CLAS is the first score in its kind, and can be used to monitor and compare long-term outcomes related to adhesions between operative techniques and strategies.

Finally, there is a clinical demand for predicting the need of emergency surgery in patients with SBO. Although conservative treatment is often successful, prolonged conservative treatment is associated with an increased risk of mortality [5, 28, 29]. Therefore, it is important to recognize cases early in which further continuation of conservative treatment is unlike to result in resolving the symptoms. Clinical and radiological signs can be used for this purpose. Zielinski developed a simple score based on three radiological and clinical parameters: mesenteric edema, absence of small bowel feces sign, and constipation. In 100 cases, the score predicted the need for surgery with a concordance index of 0.77 [30]. This research group continued to develop not only a more accurate but also more sophisticated, scoring system. The scoring system published by Baghdadi et al. comprises radiological findings, sepsis criteria, and comorbidity index. Although the score is somewhat complex to assess, it correlates with an area under the curve of 0.80 in a validation study of 351 cases [31].

## 73.2 Diagnosis

### 73.2.1 Clinical Presentation

Although small bowel obstruction is a relative common diagnosis, delayed clinical diagnosis is a frequent issue, especially in elderly patients [32]. In a large cohort study, SBO was initially not diagnosed in more than half of elderly patients, and in 45% of younger adult patients [33]. A possible cause for delays in diagnosis is that patients with SBO might present to a wide variety of physicians, including surgeons, but also internal medicine physicians, gastroenterologists, general practitioners, and geriatricians. Not all of these specialties have frequent exposure to SBO patients.

Typical clinical symptoms of SBO include abdominal pain, bloating, nausea and absence of stool, and flatus. It is important to note that patients that only recently developed an episode SBO can still have passage of stools due to feces still present in the large bowel. Also patients with an incomplete obstruction might present themselves with watery diarrhea or normal stool passage in the first few days after the onset of symptoms. This factor is often a pitfall for physician with infrequent exposure to SBO. A pitfall in the elderly patient is that abdominal pain is often much less prominent [32].

The diagnostic workup of a SBO patient is concentrated on the need for emergency surgery, the etiology of obstruction, and signs and symptoms related to dehydration and starvation. Medical history taking should include previous intra-abdominal tumors, abdominal surgeries, inflammatory bowel disease, and a family history of abdominal tumors and inflammatory bowel diseases. History taking should further include undesirable weight loss, intermittent colicky or continues abdominal pain, nausea, vomiting, urinary production, and absence of stool or flatus.

Physical examination should focus on palpable abdominal masses, abdominal distention, scars of previous surgeries, and abdominal wall hernias including groin hernias. Digital rectal examination should be performed when patients present with rectal blood loss to search for palpable rectal masses. When patients did undergo previous surgery and have a colo- or ileostomy, gentle digital examination of colo- or ileostomy should be performed to check for fascial strictures obstructing fecal passage. Physical examination should look out for ischemia and strangulation of the bowel requiring emergent surgical exploration. However, the sensitivity of the detection of such even in experienced hands is only 48% [34].

## 73.2.2 Investigations and Imaging

Mandatory laboratory test includes blood count, C-reactive protein (CRP), electrolytes, creatinine, and lactate. When a CRP above 75 or a white blood cell count of above 10.000/mm$^3$ is found, peritonitis or ischemia should be suspected and further radiological imaging is required. The preferred imaging technique in SBO is an abdominal computed tomography (CT) scan. CT scans can accurately determine the cause of the SBO. Adhesions cannot be visualized on a CT scan. However, ruling out of other options such as tumors and abdominal wall hernia has high predictive value of adhesions as the cause of the SBO. Furthermore, a CT scan is the preferred technique to identify patients who might require emergent surgical exploration [4]. Radiological findings on CT that might require emergent surgical exploration are free intraperitoneal air or fluid, perforation, strangulation, closed loop obstruction, mesenteric edema or engorgement, pneumatosis intestinalis, decreased or lack of bowel enhancement indicating bowel ischemia, mesenteric swirling, and thickened bowel wall [30, 35, 36]. Water-soluble contrast might enhance the diagnostic accuracy of CT scans. Water-soluble contrast images are also useful in evaluating the effects of conservative treatment. Passage of the contrast to the colon after 24–48 h of administration is predictive for relief of symptoms with conservative treatment [4]. Plain abdominal X-rays can not only support diagnosis of SBO but also add little diagnostic information on the cause of obstruction and the need for emergency surgery and has now become largely obsolete [4].

## 73.3 Treatment

### 73.3.1 Non-operative Treatment

Non-operative treatment is successful in over 70% of all cases of ASBO [2]. Treatment includes a nil per os policy and decompression of the gastrointestinal tract by naso-gastric tube. Care should be taken to monitor urine production and resuscitate patients with intravenous fluids taking in to account possible electrolyte disturbances. Furthermore, management should include anti-emetic medication, analgesia, nutritional support and prevention of aspiration. When the SBO has an inflammatory origin targeted intravenous antibiotics might be needed. When patients deteriorate or no clinical and/or biochemical progression is seen over the course of the non-operative treatment, operative treatment should be discussed. The optimal duration of non-operative treatment is debated, current guidelines suggest that prolonged non-operative management of more than 72 h has been associated with adverse outcomes and increased mortality [5, 28, 29, 37, 38]. Water soluble contrast studies might be helpful in the discussion on whether or not to operate, if contrast has not reached the colon in 24–48 h after administration, non-operative treatment is likely to fail and surgical management should be considered. Figure 73.2 presents an algorithm in the diagnosis and treatment of SBO based on the Bologna Guidelines for ASBO 2017.

In the elderly patients and patients with comorbidity nil per os can conflict with concurrent treatment of co-morbidities and multiple drug intake [5, 39–42]. There are roughly three options to deal with medication; discontinuing the medication, exempting medication from the starvation regimen, or administering the same or similar drug via other routes, for example, rectal or intravenously. It is generally accepted that medication taken for long-term risk management can safely be discontinued during the course of treatment for small bowel obstruction [40]. Oral medications can be administered while shortly clamping the decompression tube. Care should be taken while clamping the tube in elderly patients with pre-existing dysphagia or neurologic conditions with risk of aspiration of medication. Even though oral ingestion or administering drugs via a tube is often feasible, the uptake of medication is questionable in small bowel obstruction [42]. There is marked paucity in evidence from literature to guide the optimal strategy to medication use during nil per os.

### 73.3.2 Surgical Treatment

There is increasing evidence for a potential benefit of the laparoscopic approach versus open surgery for SBO [43, 44]. Nevertheless, it is important to note that laparoscopic surgery for SBO is challenging and demanding procedure. Laparoscopy in an abdomen with multiple extensive adhesions and distended loops of bowel, provides little working space and the distended bowel is more prone to injury. Indeed, some authors have reported bowel injuries in 6.3–26.9% of patients treated with laparoscopic adhesiolysis for ASBO [37, 45, 46]. Careful selection of patients for this procedure and correctly evaluating your laparoscopic skills is therefore of key importance.

Provided that proper selection has been applied, a recent systematic review showed that the laparoscopic approach is associated with lower post-operative mortality (relative risk [RR], 0.36; 95% CI, 0.29 to 0.45), reduced length of post-operative hospital stay (mean difference [MD], −4.19; 95% CI, −4.43 to −3.95), earlier time to flatus (MD, −0.98; 95% CI, −1.28 to −0.68), and lower severe post-operative complications (RR, 0.51; 95% CI, 0.4 to −0.56) [43].

The exact criteria for attempting a laparoscopic approach are subject to debate. Farinella et al. described an very reasonable and easy to apply set of criteria: ≤2 laparotomies in history, appendectomy as the operation in history, no previous median laparotomy incision, and an expected single adhesive band [47].

Potentially, a laparoscopic approach could also reduce the risk of future recurrences, by inducing less aggressive adhesion reformation. However, this has not been investigated.

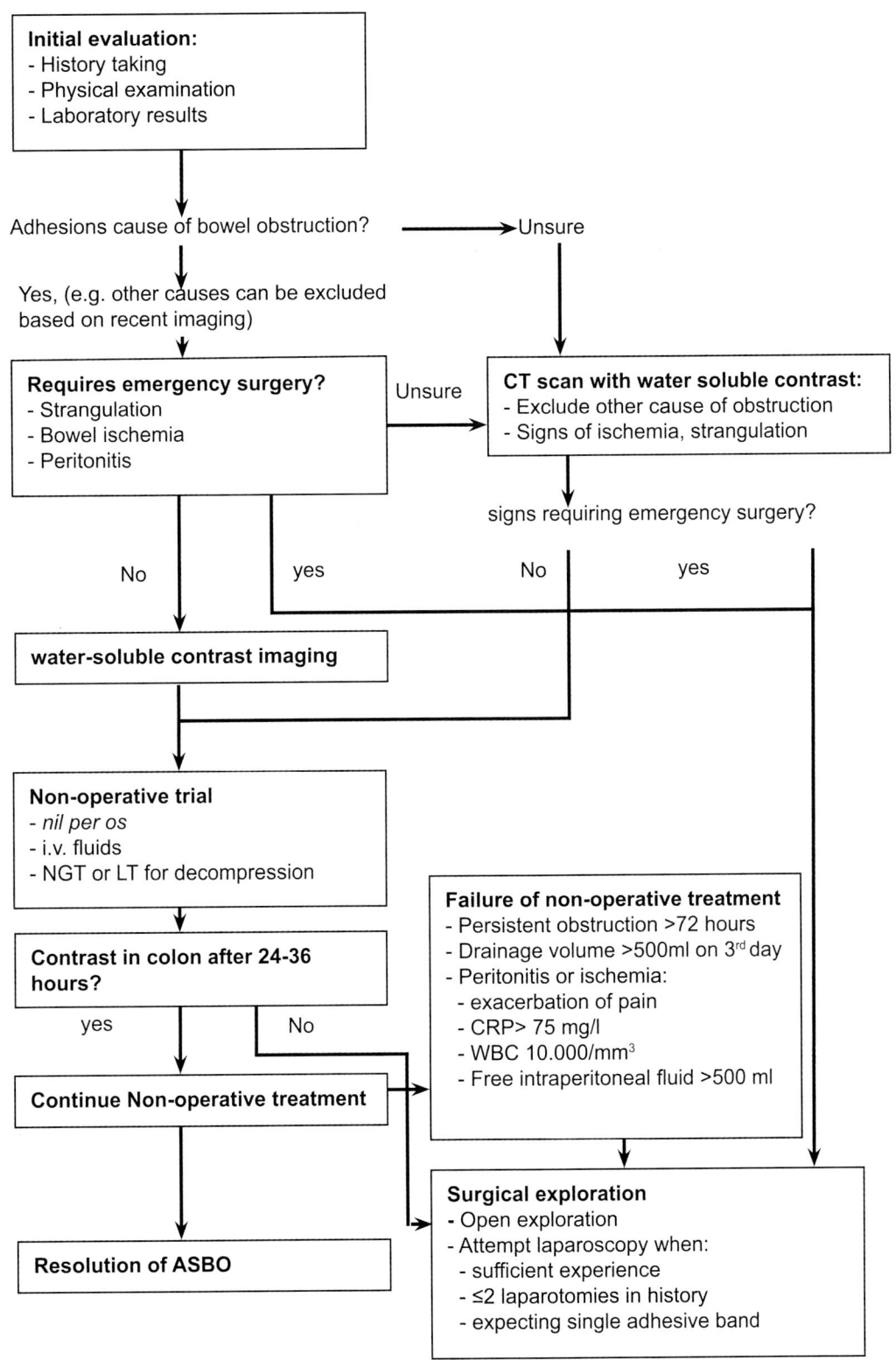

**Fig. 73.2** Algorithm for the diagnosis and treatment of ASBO. (Figure originally published: World J Emerg Surg, 2018. 13: p. 24)

### 73.3.3 Prognosis

It is important to establish that SBO is a serious surgical emergency. Overall, mortality of an episode of ASBO is estimated at 3% [4]. Mortality rises in patients requiring an emergency reoperation. In the NELA cohort the 30 and 90-day mortality rates after emergency laparotomy for adhesive SBO were 7% and 9.8% respectively, which is comparable to the mortality from an anastomotic leakage [1].

Another important aspect of the prognosis following SBO is the long-term risk of recurrence, especially in patients with adhesions as the etiology of obstruction. Risk of recurrence is high after both conservative and surgical treatment. In conservative treatment the adhesions that caused obstruction are still in place. Following operative treatment adhesions might reform. Epidemiological data shows that 12% of non-operatively treated patients are readmitted within 1 year, rising to 20% after 5 years. The risk of recurrence is slightly lower after operative treatment: 8% after 1 year and 16% after 5 years [28].

The use of adhesions barriers might reduce risk of future recurrences in patients requiring operative treatment. In the P.O.P.A. trial, patients were randomized to a liquid 4% icodextrin adhesion barrier or standard operative treatment without an adhesion barrier. The ASBO recurrence rate was 2.19% (2/91) in the icodextrin groups versus 11.11% (10/90) in the control group after a mean follow-up period of 41.4 months ($p < 0.05$) [48]. In this trial, the barrier was applied in patients treated for ASBO by laparotomy. However, the icodextrin 4% adhesion barrier can also be administered in laparoscopic surgery.

Icodextrin might, however, not even be the most potent adhesion barrier that is currently on the market [2]. More potent adhesion barriers might also further reduce recurrence risk; however, these have not been investigated in a setting for SBO and some not even in general surgery.

> **Dos and Don'ts**
> - Not all patients with small bowel obstruction need operative treatment, even if there is no history of previous surgery.
> - CT scans can provide crucial information on the etiology of obstruction and the need to perform emergency surgical exploration.
> - Minimally invasive surgery is useful in reducing morbidity from surgical exploration, but only in selected cases.
> - Use of adhesion barriers might reduce long-term recurrence risk.

> **Take-Home Messages**
> - Adhesions are the most common cause of small bowel obstruction.
> - Small bowel obstruction in virgin abdomen is relative rare but is also most frequently caused by adhesions.
> - Most patients can be treated conservatively, but timely recognition of the need for surgery is key to prevent mortality.
> - Laparoscopic surgery has favorable outcomes in selected patients.
> - Recurrence of small bowel obstruction is high; adhesion barriers can be used to reduce risk of recurrence.

## References

1. Sixth Patient Report of the National Emergency Laparotomy Audit December 2018 to November 2019. London: The Royal College of Anaesthetists, NELA Project Team; 2020.
2. ten Broek RP, et al. Burden of adhesions in abdominal and pelvic surgery: systematic review and metanalysis. BMJ. 2013;347:f5588.
3. Scott JW, et al. Use of national burden to define operative emergency general surgery. JAMA Surg. 2016;151(6):e160480.

4. Ten Broek RPG, et al. Bologna guidelines for diagnosis and management of adhesive small bowel obstruction (ASBO): 2017 update of the evidence-based guidelines from the world society of emergency surgery ASBO working group. World J Emerg Surg. 2018;13:24.
5. Keenan JE, et al. Trials of nonoperative management exceeding 3 days are associated with increased morbidity in patients undergoing surgery for uncomplicated adhesive small bowel obstruction. J Trauma Acute Care Surg. 2014;76(6):1367–72.
6. Spangler R, et al. Abdominal emergencies in the geriatric patient. Int J Emerg Med. 2014;7:43.
7. Bugliosi TF, Meloy TD, Vukov LF. Acute abdominal pain in the elderly. Ann Emerg Med. 1990;19(12):1383–6.
8. Sikirica V, et al. The inpatient burden of abdominal and gynecological adhesiolysis in the US. BMC Surg. 2011;11:13.
9. Menzies D, Ellis H. Intestinal obstruction from adhesions—how big is the problem? Ann R Coll Surg Engl. 1990;72(1):60–3.
10. Stommel MWJ, et al. Multicenter observational study of adhesion formation after open-and laparoscopic surgery for colorectal cancer. Ann Surg. 2018;267(4):743–8.
11. Polymeneas G, et al. A comparative study of postoperative adhesion formation after laparoscopic vs open cholecystectomy. Surg Endosc. 2001;15(1):41–3.
12. Krielen P, et al. Adhesion-related readmissions after open and laparoscopic surgery: a retrospective cohort study (SCAR update). Lancet. 2020;395(10217):33–41.
13. Stommel MW, Strik C, van Goor H. Response to pathological processes in the peritoneal cavity—sepsis, tumours, adhesions, and ascites. Semin Pediatr Surg. 2014;23(6):331–5.
14. Hoilat GJ, Rentea RM. Crohn disease stricturoplasty. In: StatPearls. Treasure Island, FL: StatPearls Publishing; 2021.
15. Beardsley C, et al. Small bowel obstruction in the virgin abdomen: the need for a mandatory laparotomy explored. Am J Surg. 2014;208(2):243–8.
16. Collom ML, et al. Deconstructing dogma: nonoperative management of small bowel obstruction in the virgin abdomen. J Trauma Acute Care Surg. 2018;85(1):33–6.
17. Fukami Y, et al. Clinical effect of water-soluble contrast agents for small bowel obstruction in the virgin abdomen. World J Surg. 2018;42(1):88–92.
18. Zielinski MD, Bannon MP. Current management of small bowel obstruction. Adv Surg. 2011;45:1–29.
19. McCloy C, et al. The etiology of intestinal obstruction in patients without prior laparotomy or hernia. Am Surg. 1998;64:19–22; discussion 22.
20. Ng YY, Ngu JC, Wong AS. Small bowel obstruction in the virgin abdomen: time to challenge surgical dogma with evidence. ANZ J Surg. 2018;88(1–2):91–4.
21. Tavangari FR, et al. Small bowel obstructions in a virgin abdomen: is an operation mandatory? Am Surg. 2016;82(10):1038–42.
22. Strajina V, Kim BD, Zielinski MD. Small bowel obstruction in a virgin abdomen. Am J Surg. 2019;218(3):521–6.
23. Skoglar A, Gunnarsson U, Falk P. Band adhesions not related to previous abdominal surgery - A retrospective cohort analysis of risk factors. Ann Med Surg (Lond). 2018;36:185–90.
24. Zuhlke HV et al. [Pathophysiology and classification of adhesions]. Langenbecks Arch Chir Suppl II Verh Dtsch Ges Chir. 1990;1009–16.
25. Coccolini F, et al. Peritoneal adhesion index (PAI): proposal of a score for the "ignored iceberg" of medicine and surgery. World J Emerg Surg. 2013;8(1):6.
26. ten Broek RP, et al. Epidemiology and prevention of postsurgical adhesions revisited. Ann Surg. 2016;263(1):12–9.
27. Lier EJ, et al. Clinical adhesion score (CLAS): development of a novel clinical score for adhesion-related complications in abdominal and pelvic surgery. Surg Endosc. 2021;35:2159–68.
28. Foster NM, et al. Small bowel obstruction: a population-based appraisal. J Am Coll Surg. 2006;203(2):170–6.
29. Sakakibara T, et al. The indicator for surgery in adhesive small bowel obstruction patient managed with long tube. Hepatogastroenterology. 2007;54(75):787–90.
30. Zielinski MD, et al. Prospective, observational validation of a multivariate small-bowel obstruction model to predict the need for operative intervention. J Am Coll Surg. 2011;212(6):1068–76.
31. Baghdadi YMK, et al. Validation of the anatomic severity score developed by the American Association for the Surgery of Trauma in small bowel obstruction. J Surg Res. 2016;204(2):428–34.
32. Ozturk E, et al. Small bowel obstruction in the elderly: a plea for comprehensive acute geriatric care. World J Emerg Surg. 2018;13:48.
33. Laurell H, Hansson LE, Gunnarsson U. Acute abdominal pain among elderly patients. Gerontology. 2006;52(6):339–44.
34. Sarr MG, Bulkley GB, Zuidema GD. Preoperative recognition of intestinal strangulation obstruction. Prospective evaluation of diagnostic capability. Am J Surg. 1983;145(1):176–82.
35. Millet I, et al. Assessment of strangulation in adhesive small bowel obstruction on the basis of combined CT findings: implications for clinical care. Radiology. 2017;285(3):798–808.
36. Millet I, et al. Value of CT findings to predict surgical ischemia in small bowel obstruction: a sys-

tematic review and meta-analysis. Eur Radiol. 2015;25(6):1823–35.
37. Wullstein C, Gross E. Laparoscopic compared with conventional treatment of acute adhesive small bowel obstruction. Br J Surg. 2003;90(9):1147–51.
38. Fevang BT, et al. Early operation or conservative management of patients with small bowel obstruction? Eur J Surg. 2002;168(8–9):475–81.
39. Haider SI, et al. Trends in polypharmacy and potential drug-drug interactions across educational groups in elderly patients in Sweden for the period 1992–2002. Int J Clin Pharmacol Ther. 2007;45(12):643–53.
40. Leder SB, Lerner MZ. Nil per os except medications order in the dysphagic patient. QJM. 2013;106(1):71–5.
41. Hovstadius B, et al. Increasing polypharmacy—an individual-based study of the Swedish population 2005-2008. BMC Clin Pharmacol. 2010;10:16.
42. Gubbins PO, Bertch KE. Drug absorption in gastrointestinal disease and surgery. Clinical pharmacokinetic and therapeutic implications. Clin Pharmacokinet. 1991;21(6):431–47.
43. Krielen P, et al. Laparoscopic versus open approach for adhesive small bowel obstruction, a systematic review and meta-analysis of short term outcomes. J Trauma Acute Care Surg. 2020;88(6):866–74.
44. Sallinen V, et al. Laparoscopic versus open adhesiolysis for adhesive small bowel obstruction (LASSO): an international, multicentre, randomised, open-label trial. Lancet Gastroenterol Hepatol. 2019;4(4):278–86.
45. Grafen FC, et al. Management of acute small bowel obstruction from intestinal adhesions: indications for laparoscopic surgery in a community teaching hospital. Langenbecks Arch Surg. 2010;395(1):57–63.
46. Johnson KN, et al. Laparoscopic management of acute small bowel obstruction: evaluating the need for resection. J Trauma Acute Care Surg. 2012;72(1):25–30; discussion 30–1; quiz 317.
47. Farinella E, et al. Feasibility of laparoscopy for small bowel obstruction. World J Emerg Surg. 2009;4:3.
48. Catena F, et al. P.O.P.A. study: prevention of postoperative abdominal adhesions by icodextrin 4% solution after laparotomy for adhesive small bowel obstruction. A prospective randomized controlled trial. J Gastrointest Surg. 2012;16(2):382–8.

## Further Reading

ten Broek RP, et al. Burden of adhesions in abdominal and pelvic surgery: systematic review and met-analysis. BMJ. 2013;347:f5588.

ten Broek RPG, et al. Bologna guidelines for diagnosis and management of adhesive small bowel obstruction (ASBO): 2017 update of the evidence-based guidelines from the world society of emergency surgery ASBO working group. World J Emerg Surg. 2018;13:24.

# Small Bowel Perforation

# 74

Dimitrios Damaskos, Anne Ewing, and Judith Sayers

## 74.1 Introduction

> **Learning Goals**
>
> - Summarize causes of small bowel perforation.
> - Analyse the pathophysiology of different mechanisms of small bowel perforation.
> - Discuss diagnosis and treatment options.

### 74.1.1 Epidemiology

Small bowel perforation can be initially differentiated into traumatic and non-traumatic.

In blunt trauma, small bowel injury is mainly associated with the seatbelt sign [1] and is the third most common injury associated with blunt abdominal trauma [2]. Due to its location in the abdomen the small bowel is the organ most commonly injured in penetrating trauma (30–83%). In stab wounds in particular, a higher body mass index (BMI) seems to be a protective factor [3].

Iatrogenic injuries are a less common cause of traumatic perforation.

Non-traumatic small bowel perforation is a common cause of peritonitis in Western countries, where it is mainly is related to ischaemia of the bowel from obstruction due to adhesions and hernias. *It has a significant peri-operative and long-term mortality, which can be as high as 32.8% at 3 years, as recently demonstrated in the National Emergency Laparotomy Audit (an ongoing quality improvement project in the United Kingdom*, www.nela.org.uk*).* In low- and middle-income countries (LMICs), small bowel perforations caused by infectious conditions are more common and a major challenge for local health care systems, with a mortality rate of up to 60% [4].

### 74.1.2 Aetiology

The causes of small bowel perforation are summarized in Table 74.1. We will focus our chapter on the general management of small bowel perforation.

### 74.1.3 Classification

Small bowel perforations can be classified according to anatomy (duodenal/jejunal/ileal), aetiology (traumatic versus non-traumatic) and

D. Damaskos (✉) · A. Ewing · J. Sayers
Royal Infirmary of Edinburgh, Edinburgh, UK
e-mail: dimitrios.damaskos@nhslothian.scot.nhs.uk; anne.ewing@nhslothian.scot.nhs.uk; Judith.sayers@nhslothian.scot.nhs.uk

**Table 74.1** Causes of small bowel perforation

| Causes of small bowel perforation | |
|---|---|
| Traumatic | Blunt trauma<br>Penetrating trauma<br>Iatrogenic injuries<br>Foreign bodies |
| Non-traumatic | Ischaemia (obstruction due to adhesions and hernias, vascular occlusion from atherosclerosis or autoimmune disorders affecting the vasculature of the small bowel)<br>Inflammatory (Crohn's disease, celiac disease, collagenous sprue)<br>Infectious (*Salmonella paratyphi*, *Mycobacterium tuberculosis*, cytomegalovirus [CMV], *Entamoeba histolytica*, *Ascaris lumbricoides*)<br>Meckel's diverticulum/jejunal and ileal duplications<br>Drugs (non-steroidal anti-inflammatory drugs [NSAIDs], chemotherapy ± radiotherapy, monoclonal antibodies, potassium chloride)<br>Neoplasms (either primary or secondary) |

type of perforation (free vs. contained). A very proximal position of the perforation has implications regarding the ability to perform diversion in case of patients in extremis, due to inevitably high gastrointestinal (GI) losses. Certain aetiologies can have even poorer prognosis than the already significant mortality related to peritonitis (perforated malignancy, patients on chemotherapy/radiotherapy, typhoid perforations in LMICs). Contained perforations of the small bowel are uncommon, due to the organ's predominantly intraperitoneal anatomy, with the exception of the retroperitoneal duodenum, which is covered in another chapter.

### 74.1.4 Pathophysiology

The mechanisms behind the perforation are inherently related to the aetiology. In trauma, they usually are related to direct penetrating injury, crush injury between internal and external structures, acceleration/deceleration injuries and low perfusion state from haemorrhagic shock or direct vascular trauma. Small bowel obstruction due to adhesions or hernias, which is not relieved, will lead to proximal bowel dilation, venous outflow obstruction and eventually bowel wall ischaemia and perforation. The progressive transmural inflammatory process related to Crohn's disease and its complications (abscess and fistulas in this case) is responsible for spontaneous bowel perforations. Other autoimmune processes, like celiac disease and celiac disease related lymphoma, create histopathologic bowel changes that predispose to ulcerations [5]. In typhoid perforations, the mechanism is hyperplasia and necrosis of Peyer's patches of the terminal ileum [6]. Drug-related direct mucosal injury seems to be the insult leading to full-thickness defects of the bowel [7] on a lot of cases, but also chemotherapy and radiotherapy can cause enterocolitis leading to a perforation [8]. T- and B-cell lymphomas have been reported to have perforation as the first presentation leading to their diagnosis, with a rate that can reach 34% [9–11].

## 74.2 Diagnosis

### 74.2.1 Clinical Presentation

The clinical presentation of small bowel perforation is largely associated with the underlying aetiology, as outlined above.

In the majority of cases, patients will present with pain, peritonism and sepsis in the later stages. Further symptoms will be related to underlying causes:

- Obstruction—vomiting, reduced bowel movements, abdominal distension
- Ischaemia—significant abdominal pain, atrial fibrillation or coagulopathy
- IBD—may be known Crohn's, or new presentation with loose stools with blood and mucous
- Infection—diarrhoea
- Meckel's—pain, bleeding
- Neoplasms—weight loss, fatigue, night sweats
- Coeliac disease—known Coeliac, bloating, iron-deficiency anaemia
- Iatrogenic—recent procedure, for example, ERCP, laparoscopic surgery
- Foreign body—recent ingestion

For those presenting following abdominal trauma, concerning features in blunt injuries are widespread peritonism and significant bruising. Following penetrating trauma, any pain or peritonism distant from the site of injury warrants further investigation.

### 74.2.2 Tests

As with all patients, a thorough history and clinical examination are essential parts of the assessment process.

All patients presenting with suspected small bowel perforation should have a routine blood screen performed, including inflammatory markers, albumin and clotting. Arterial blood gas analysis is useful in those who are unwell on presentation, or in those where ischemic bowel is a suspected as an underlying cause.

Erect chest X-ray may show presence of sub-diaphragmatic free air. Abdominal X-ray can show non-specific signs such as Rigler's or the football sign.

Urinalysis may be useful to exclude underlying urinary tract infection. Urinary beta-HCG should be performed in all females of child-bearing age.

The mainstay of investigation in most sites is the abdominal computed tomography (CT), with intravenous contrast. Oral contrast may be used and can be helpful in assessing more proximal perforations. In the United Kingdom, the majority of patients will undergo CT scanning prior to ongoing management.

Where the underlying aetiology is small bowel obstruction, CT may show hyperaemic small bowel wall with or without pneumatosis. While a small volume of extraluminal fluid may be the only sign of perforation, extraluminal gas is more diagnostic [12]. Walled-off collections may be present, particularly in those with underlying inflammatory conditions such as Crohn's disease.

For those in whom small bowel perforation is suspected, but CT is non-diagnostic, a diagnostic laparoscopy is the next step. The same follows for victims of both blunt and penetrating trauma.

> **Differential Diagnosis**
>
> Differential diagnoses for small bowel perforation include other sites of perforation:
>
> - Gastric
> - Duodenal
> - Colonic
>
> Abdominal aortic aneurysm (AAA) rupture may cause significant and widespread peritonism, along with cardiovascular instability and collapse. Any concern of AAA rupture should prompt immediate investigation.
>
> Similarly, ruptured ectopic pregnancies can cause significant pain and collapse. Pregnancy should be excluded in all females of child-bearing age presenting with abdominal pain.
>
> Significant and widespread peritonism may also be present in acute pancreatitis. Other causes of intra-abdominal sepsis should also be considered:
>
> - Cholangitis
> - Cholecystitis
> - Appendicitis
> - Diverticulitis
> - Tubo-ovarian pathology

## 74.3 Treatment

### 74.3.1 Medical Treatment

The mainstay of treatment for small bowel perforation is surgical. In a small group of patients where the perforation has been contained by surrounding structures and signs of generalized peritonism are absent, a non-operative approach may be appropriate. This is more common in duodenal perforation (which is covered in another chapter) but rare in small bowel perforation.

Key management steps for small bowel perforation are

- Timely diagnosis
- Resuscitation
- Initiation of broad-spectrum antibiotics
- Early and definitive source control

The investigation and diagnosis of small bowel perforation has been discussed. Initial medical management involves resuscitation and treatment of sepsis. Broad spectrum antibiotic therapy (which should cover both aerobic and anaerobic organisms) should be initiated promptly. Resuscitation with intravenous fluids is also critical in patients with intra-abdominal sepsis. The Surviving Sepsis Campaign (SSC) has led to the development of guidelines for the management of patients with sepsis [13] with specific bundles of care which should be implemented.

## 74.3.2 Surgical Treatment

The goals of surgical treatment are to correct the underlying anatomic problem, remove the source of contamination and prevent persistent or recurrent infection. In most cases this will be achieved through a laparotomy.

Some debate exists regarding the benefit of peritoneal lavage at time of laparotomy. While the need to remove obvious contamination is not questioned, there is some debate about the role of more aggressive intra-abdominal lavage in peritonitis with limited clinical evidence to support this [14]. Indeed, it has been shown that routine use of intra-operative irrigation for appendicectomies does not prevent abscess formation [15]. However, in cases of small bowel perforation there is often significant contamination and lavage of the abdominal cavity removing all enteric content and pus should be performed, with careful attention to common sites of intra-abdominal abscess including the pelvis, paracolic gutters and subphrenic space. There is no evidence to support lavage solutions containing antibiotics in patients who are already receiving systemic antibiotics [14].

Operative strategy for control of the bowel depends on the underlying aetiology and the clinical state of the patient. For stable patients with limited contamination primary small bowel repair or resection and anastomosis is recommended [16]. However in those who are clinically unstable or with delayed presentations where the bowel is significantly inflamed and oedematous, proximal diversion/ileostomy should be considered. This scenario is more challenging and more consideration is given when the perforation is very proximal to the ligament of Treitz, as a proximal stoma will result in significant gastrointestinal losses and electrolyte disturbances.

The aetiology, size of defect and presence of associated mesenteric injury will determine whether the defect can be primarily closed or a small bowel resection is required. Primary repair is associated with lower complication rates [17], which likely reflects smaller injuries with less tissue damage. Those with large perforations (involving more than 50% circumference of the bowel), multiple contiguous perforations, malignancy, ischaemia, or mesenteric disruption should undergo a small bowel resection.

Standard principles of bowel resection and anastomosis are important; excising the entire diseased segment, ensuring adequate blood supply, lack of tension and approximation of the resected ends with meticulous technique.

Studies have suggested a higher rate of anastomotic leak with stapled compared to hand sewn anastomosis in the trauma setting [18]. However, a systematic review and meta-analysis [19] found no evidence to favour hand sewn over stapled technique in emergency laparotomy. The choice of anastomotic technique is therefore determined by surgeon's preference.

While laparoscopy has gained acceptance in the management of perforated appendicitis and diverticulitis, there are no studies comparing outcomes for laparoscopic and open surgery for small bowel perforation. Reports suggest that laparoscopic techniques can be used safely with low post-operative wound infection rates [20] but should be used selectively in centres with experienced surgeons.

Where there is severe contamination and inflammation, haemodynamic instability, or concern regarding viability of the bowel, anastomosis should not be performed. Options are formation of a stoma or planned re-laparotomy with deferred primary anastomosis [21]. This latter approach is in keeping with the principles of damage control surgery, which are now established for trauma management, and allows anastomosis to be created when the patient's physiology and local conditions are more favourable.

### 74.3.3 Prognosis

Prognosis following small bowel perforation is variable depending on the clinical situation and underlying aetiology. The morbidity and mortality rates are probably less affected by surgical technique than general condition of the patient, nature of underlying disease and duration of perforation prior to surgical intervention (Table 74.2).

**Table 74.2** Complications of small bowel perforation

| Early complications | Late complications |
|---|---|
| Sepsis | Delayed wound healing |
| Multi-organ failure | Fistula formation |
| Wound infection | Adhesions |
| Anastomotic leak | Hernia |
| Intra-abdominal abscess | |

> **Dos and Don'ts**
> - **Do** initiate antibiotic therapy and fluid resuscitation promptly.
> - **Do** involve critical care team early.
> - **Don't** delay theatre. Small bowel perforations require surgical management.
> - **Don't** perform primary closure or anastomosis in if any concerns about patient stability or bowel viability—either plan for relook laparotomy with delayed anastomosis or stoma formation.

> **Take-Home Messages**
> - Small bowel perforation is a surgical emergency.
> - The aetiology is varied, but it is useful to classify into traumatic and non-traumatic causes.
> - Abdominal CT is the most useful investigation, as this allows localization of the of perforation and can identify the underlying cause.

> - The mainstay of treatment, after resuscitation and administration of antibiotics, is surgical.
> - Principles of surgical management are removal of enteric contamination, correction of the anatomic problem causing the perforation and restoration of bowel continuity or formation of a stoma.

**Multiple Choice Questions**

1. Which of the following findings on plain abdominal X-ray raises suspicion of small bowel perforation?
   A. **Gas outlining both sides of the bowel wall**
   B. Colonic faecal loading
   C. Dilated small bowel loops
   D. A 'lead pipe' featureless colon
2. Which of the following is the most useful investigation for suspected small bowel perforation?
   A. **Abdominal CT with IV and oral contrast**
   B. Chest X-ray
   C. Abdominal X-ray
   D. Abdominal ultrasound
3. Which of the following does not form part of the mainstay management of small bowel perforation?
   A. Broad spectrum antibiotics
   B. Resuscitation with intravenous fluids
   C. Surgery
   D. **Watch and wait**
4. Which of the following are not components of the management of sepsis in small bowel perforation?
   A. Use of sepsis care bundles
   B. Administration of broad-spectrum antibiotics
   C. Early source control with removal of pus and enteric content
   D. **Abdominal lavage with antibiotic containing solutions**

5. Choose the most appropriate management option in the following scenario. An 18-year-old female stabbed in the abdomen. At laparotomy, there is a small (2 cm) defect in the wall of the proximal ileum with limited intra-abdominal contamination.
   A. **Primary small bowel repair**
   B. Small bowel resection and anastomosis
   C. Small bowel resection and end ileostomy
   D. Small bowel resection, re-look laparotomy ± deferred primary anastomosis
6. Choose the most appropriate management option in the following scenario. A 66-year-old female presents with a strangulated femoral hernia. There is a knuckle of ischemic small bowel with localized perforation within the hernia sac. There is no intra-abdominal contamination and the patient is stable.
   A. Primary small bowel repair
   B. **Small bowel resection and primary anastomosis**
   C. Small bowel resection and end ileostomy
   D. Small bowel resection, re-look laparotomy ± deferred primary anastomosis
7. A 76-year-old male with multiple co-morbidities presents with small bowel perforation secondary to closed loop adhesional obstruction. At laparotomy, there is a 50 cm segment of necrotic distal and terminal ileum with multiple perforations. There is significant intra-abdominal contamination. The patient is in septic and on vasopressors.
   A. Primary small bowel repair
   B. Small bowel resection and anastomosis
   C. **Small bowel resection and end ileostomy**
   D. Small bowel resection, re-look laparotomy ± deferred primary anastomosis
8. Choose the most appropriate management option in the following scenario. A 29-year-old male has suffered blunt abdominal trauma during a road traffic accident. At laparotomy, he is found to have a small bowel perforation with associated mesenteric injury, as well as other intra-abdominal injuries. After initial resuscitation and control of bleeding he remains acidotic and coagulopathic.
   A. Primary small bowel repair
   B. Small bowel resection and anastomosis
   C. Small bowel resection and end ileostomy
   D. **Small bowel resection, re-look laparotomy ± deferred primary anastomosis**
9. Choose the most appropriate management option in the following scenario. A 72-year-old lady presents with small bowel perforation secondary to small bowel obstruction, with widespread peritoneal metastases. The primary tumour could not be identified at time of laparotomy.
   A. Primary small bowel repair
   B. Small bowel resection and anastomosis
   C. **Small bowel resection and end ileostomy**
   D. Small bowel resection, re-look laparotomy ± deferred primary anastomosis
10. Which of the following is <u>not</u> an important operative factor in determining outcome of small bowel anastomosis?
    A. Adequate blood supply to bowel ends
    B. Correct bowel orientation with lack of tension
    C. **Stapled vs handsewn anastomosis**
    D. Good approximation with accommodation for any size discrepancy

# References

1. Chandler CF, Lane JS, Waxman KS. Seatbelt sign following blunt trauma is associated with increased incidence of abdominal injury. Am Surg. 1997;63(10):885–8.
2. Iaselli F, Mazzei MA, Firetto C, D'Elia D, Squitieri NC, Biondetti PR, Danza FM, Scaglione M. Bowel and mesenteric injuries from blunt abdominal trauma: a review. Radiol Med. 2015;120(1):21–32.
3. Bloom MB, Ley EJ, Liou DZ, Tran T, Chung R, Melo N, Margulies DR. Impact of body mass index on injury in abdominal stab wounds: implications for management. J Surg Res. 2015;197(1):162–6.
4. Gupta S, Kaushik R. Peritonitis—the Eastern experience. World J Emerg Surg. 2006;1:13. https://doi.org/10.1186/1749-7922-1-13.
5. Freeman HJ. Free perforation due to intestinal lymphoma in biopsy-defined or suspected celiac disease. J Clin Gastroenterol. 2003;37:299–302.
6. Chalya PL, Mabula JB, Koy M, et al. Typhoid intestinal perforations at a University teaching hospital in Northwestern Tanzania: a surgical experience of 104 cases in a resource-limited setting. World J Emerg Surg. 2012;7:4.
7. Zeino Z, Sisson G, Bjarnason I. Adverse effects of drugs on small intestine and colon. Best Pract Res Clin Gastroenterol. 2010;24:133–41.
8. Davila ML. Neutropenic enterocolitis: current issues in diagnosis and management. Curr Infect Dis Rep. 2007;9:116–20.
9. Vaidya R, Habermann TM, Donohue JH, Ristow KM, Maurer MJ, Macon WR, Colgan JP, Inwards DJ, Ansell SM, Porrata LF, et al. Bowel perforation in intestinal lymphoma: incidence and clinical features. Ann Oncol. 2013;24:2439–43.
10. Sager GF. Primary malignant tumors of the small intestine. A twenty-two year experience with thirty patients. Am J Surg. 1978;135:601–3.
11. Sun J, Lu Z, Yang D, Chen J. Primary intestinal T-cell and NK-cell lymphomas: a clinicopathological and molecular study from China focused on type II enteropathy-associated T-cell lymphoma and primary intestinal NK-cell lymphoma. Mod Pathol. 2011;24:983–92.
12. Singh JP, Steward MJ, Booth TC, Mukhtar H, Murray D. Evolution of imaging for abdominal perforation. Ann R Coll Surg Engl. 2010;92(3):182–8.
13. Levy MM, Evans LE, Rhodes A. The surviving sepsis campaign bundle: 2018 update. Crit Care Med. 2018;46(6):925–8.
14. Platell C, Papadimitriou JM, Hall JC. The influence of lavage on peritonitis. J Am Coll Surg. 2000;191(6):672–80.
15. Moore CB, et al. Does use of intraoperative irrigation with open or laparoscopic appendectomy reduce post-operative intra-abdominal abscess? Am Surg. 2011;77(1):78–80.
16. Sartelli M, et al. The management of intra-abdominal infections from a global perspective: 2017 WSES guidelines for management of intra-abdominal infections. World J Emerg Surg. 2017;12:29.
17. Kirkpatrick AW, et al. Intra-abdominal complications after surgical repair of small bowel injuries: an international review. J Trauma. 2003;55(3):399–406.
18. Brundage SI, et al. Stapled versus sutured gastrointestinal anastomoses in the trauma patient: a multicenter trial. J Trauma. 2001;51(6):1054–61.
19. Naumann DN, et al. Stapled versus handsewn intestinal anastomosis in emergency laparotomy: a systemic review and meta-analysis. Surgery. 2015;157(4):609–18.
20. Sinha R, Sharma N, Joshi M. Laparoscopic repair of small bowel perforation. J Soc Laparoendosc Surg (JSLS). 2005;9(4):399–402.
21. Ordoñez CA, Puyana JC. Management of peritonitis in the critically ill patient. Surg Clin North Am. 2006;86(6):1323–49.

# Small Bowel Diverticular Disease

**75**

Carlos Yánez Benítez

## 75.1 Introduction

> **Learning Goals**
> - The reader should get acquainted with the epidemiology, characteristics, and anatomical location of small bowel diverticular (SBD).
> - The reader should be able to diagnose SBD and differentiate SBD complications: diverticulitis, perforation, obstruction, or gastrointestinal (GI) bleeding.
> - Finally, the reader should understand the principles of non-operative and surgical treatment options for this rare entity.

This chapter addresses the epidemiology, diagnosis, and treatment of small bowel diverticular (SBD) disease, based on a review of current literature. SBD disease is an uncommon entity, with a prevalence of 1–2% of the general population [1]. SBD can be classified depending on their etiology, configuration, location, presence of symptoms, and complications. According to the tissues involved they are identified as true or false, congenital, or acquired, and duodenal or jejunoileal. They are often asymptomatic, and discovered incidentally during imaging or endoscopic studies, surgery, or when complications arise, which can be in the form of diverticulitis, perforation, obstruction, or gastrointestinal bleeding [2, 3]. Multi-detector CT (MDCT) scans with intravenous contrast are the preferred imaging modality, due to their accuracy to detect complications [4]. Additionally, MDCT image quality allows for conservative management in selected cases when diffuse peritonitis or abdominal sepsis are absent. However, surgical intervention must not be delayed when conservative management fails or the patient manifests signs of diffuse peritonitis, intestinal occlusion, or severe hemorrhage. Surgery can be either open or minimally invasive, tailored to the patient's condition and surgical team expertise. Diverticulectomy, wedge resection, or segmental small bowel resection with primary anastomosis are the preferred options.

### 75.1.1 Epidemiology

With the advances in imaging technology, incidental diagnosis of SBD among the general population has increased. Currently, the incidence of both congenital and acquired SBD is between 2% and 4% [4, 5] (Fig. 75.1). These can be encountered as either an isolated diverticulum or clusters

C. Yánez Benítez (✉)
San Jorge University Hospital, SALUD, Huesca, Spain
e-mail: cjyanezb@salud.aragon.es

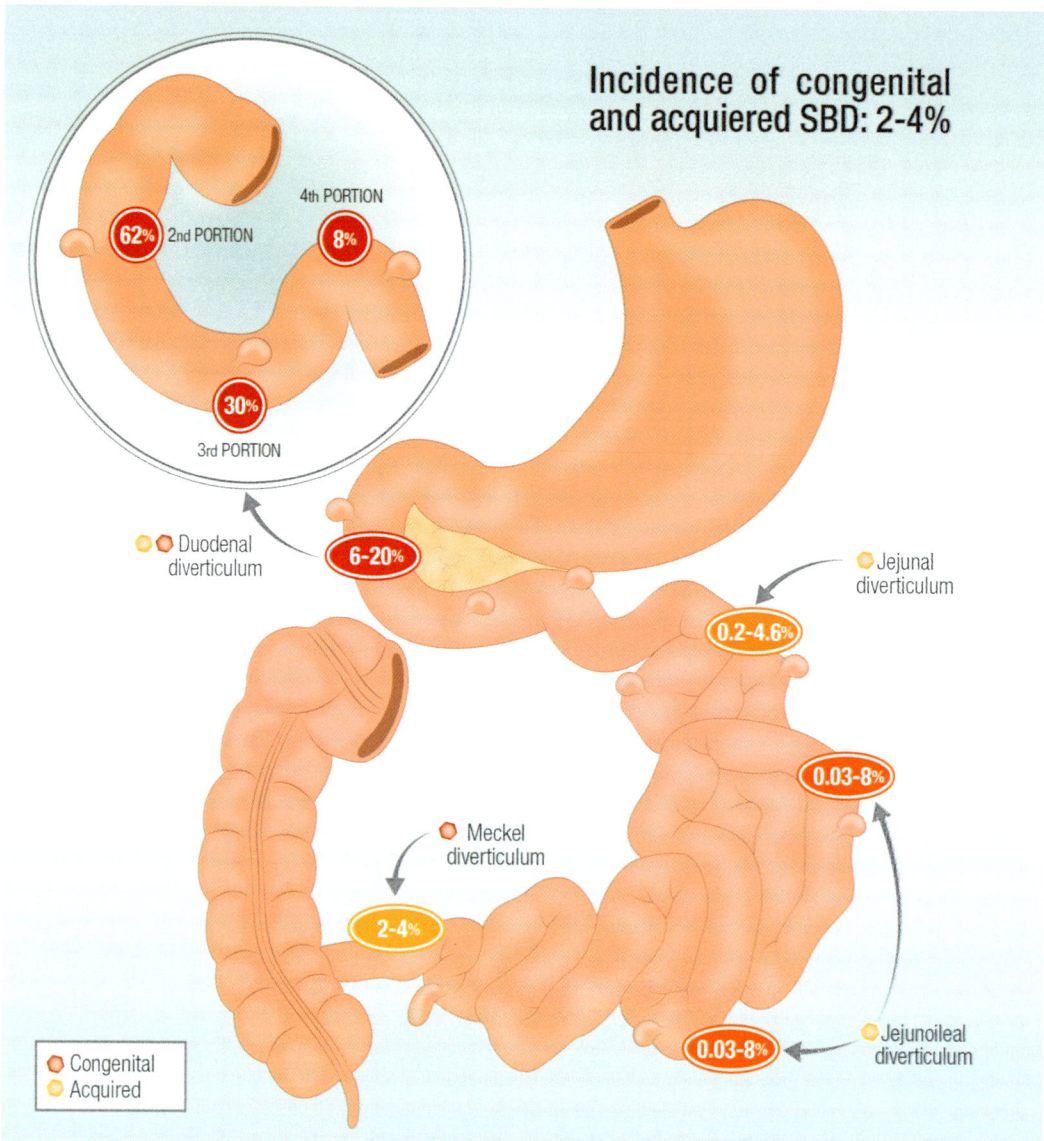

**Fig. 75.1** Incidence of both congenital and acquired SBD by location in the small bowel. (Illustration by Ilaria Bondi)

of multiple lesions throughout the small bowel. The acquired form is the more frequent, and the duodenum the most common location. Autopsy reports have described duodenal diverticula (DD) in close to 20% of the population, and 6% have been reported on upper GI imaging studies [6, 7]. The presence of DD is even higher in patients undergoing endoscopic retrograde cholangiopancreatography (ERCP), where up to 25% of the patients have these findings [7, 8]. They are mostly located in the second portion of the duodenum in over 62% of the cases, followed by the third portion with 30% and the fourth portion only 8% [9]. DD has no difference in frequency by gender and is diagnosed more frequently between the third and seventh decades [7].

In contrast, acquired jejunal or ileal diverticulum (JID) is less common, described on autopsy between 0.2% and 4.6% in the jejunum [8], and 0.03–8% as a jejunoileal disease [10, 11]. JID is predominantly diagnosed in the male population with a ratio of 2:1 and in patients over 40 years old [12]. Diverticulum size may vary depending on its location; when located more proximal in the jejunum, they tend to be located on the mesenteric side of the bowel, multiple and larger, in contrast to those found in the ileum, usually fewer in number and smaller in size [4].

Regarding congenital SBD, the Meckel diverticulum (MD) is the most common congenital anomaly of the gastrointestinal tract, affecting 2–4% of the general population [13]. Other congenital forms of the small bowel diverticulum have been described in the duodenum; however, there is limited data available due to their rarity, and their incidence among the general population has not been described [14, 15].

## 75.1.2 Etiology

The Meckel diverticulum (MD), first described by Johann Friedrich Meckel in 1809, is a true diverticulum of the distal ileum, with an embryonic origin [16, 17]. It originates as an incomplete obliteration of the vitelline or omphalomesenteric duct (OMD) that connects the yolk sac with the developing midgut during fetal life. It is formed by all the walls of the ileum on the anti-mesenteric side of the distal ileum (Fig. 75.2), 40–100 cm from the ileocecal valve. Meckel diverticulum may contain ectopic mucosa, most frequently gastric (50–60%), pancreatic, duodenal, and on rare occasions colonic mucosa has also been described [18].

A common mnemonic can be useful to remember Meckel diverticulum common characteristics (Box 75.1) [1, 13, 19].

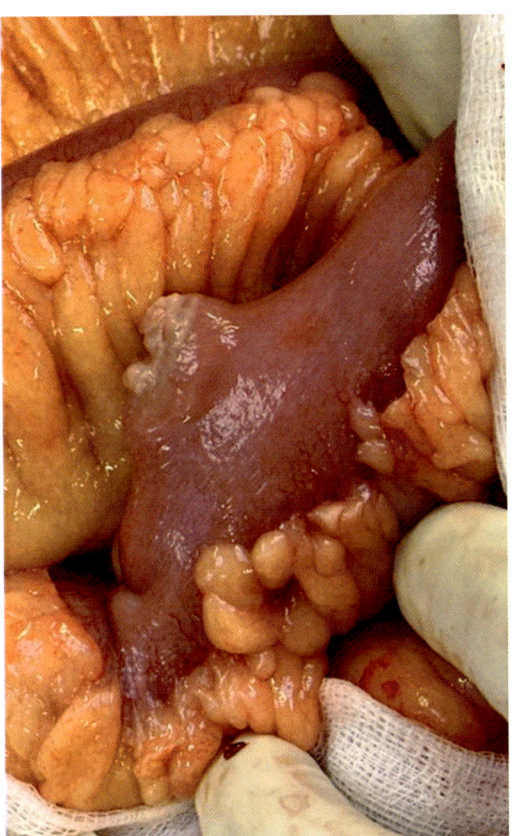

**Fig. 75.2** Small broad based non complicated Meckel diverticulum (MD) with apparent ectopic tissue on its tip

---

**Box 75.1 Rule of 2's for Meckel Diverticulum**

**2%** of the population
**2%** can develop symptoms
**2:1** male-to-female ratio
**2** ft from the ileocecal valve
**2** in. in diameter
**2** cm in length
Almost half of the patients with Meckel diverticulum become symptomatic at age 2 or before

---

Regarding acquired SBD disease, the etiology is unclear, and a multifactorial explanation is commonly accepted. Intestinal dyskinesis generates high intraluminal pressure, is associated with the bowel's smooth muscle weakness, and is considered to be the main contributing factor [20]. Additionally, some forms of SBD have been associated with rare genetic diseases, including Fabry's disease, Cronkhite-Canada syndrome, Marfan's disease, cystic fibrosis, and familial visceral myopathy [21].

## 75.1.3 Classification

SBD can be classified by etiology, configuration, location, presence of symptoms, and complications. Considering their etiologic origin, SBD can be classified as acquired or congenital.

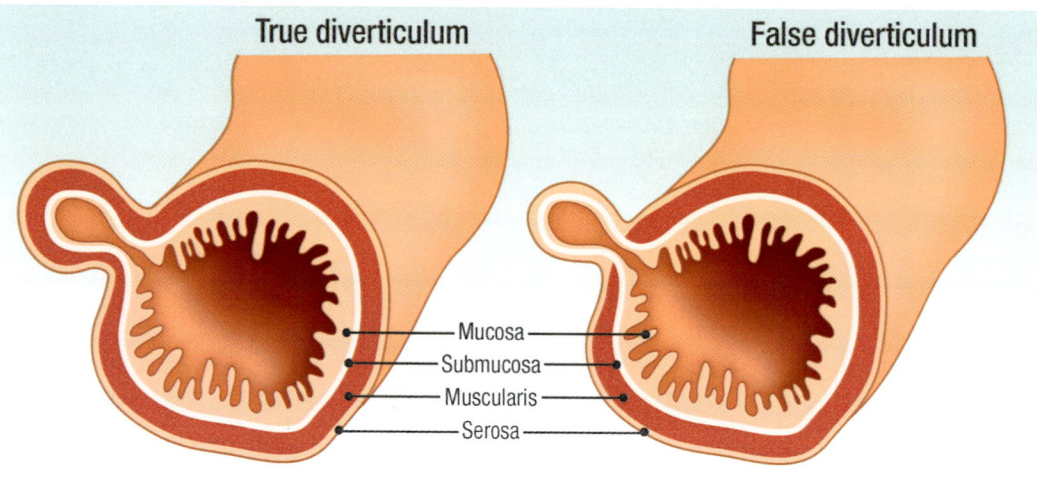

**Fig. 75.3** Differences in the layers that form true and false SBD. (Illustration by Ilaria Bondi)

Depending on their configuration they are known either as false or true. A true diverticulum is a protrusion which involves all the layers of the gastrointestinal tract, while in false ones only the mucosa and submucosa protrude into the peritoneum through a defect in the muscular wall (Fig. 75.3).

Depending on their location, SBD can be either duodenal (DD) or jejunoileal (JID).

Because most SBDs are asymptomatic, they are found incidentally while conducting imaging or endoscopic studies, during surgeries or when complication arise. They can manifest with chronic and unspecific symptoms (colicky pain, malabsorption, anemia) or as an acute complication, such as a perforated peritonitis (Fig. 75.4), GI bleeding, or mechanical intestinal obstruction.

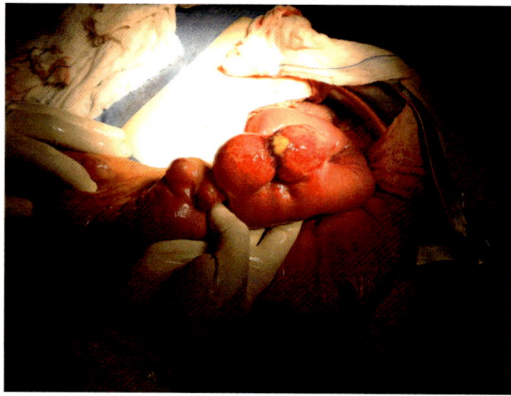

**Fig. 75.4** Perforated jejunal diverticulum. (Notice the cluster distribution on the mesenteric side of the jejunum and the diverticulum's wall ischemic appearance with a small perforation)

### 75.1.4 Pathophysiology

SBD consists of mucosa and submucosal layers that bulge through a muscular layer's weakness, creating a regular and thin-walled false diverticulum. Acquired DD can be primary or secondary; the first are idiopathic, nearly all found on the second and third portion of the duodenum on the medial wall, and only 5% are located on the duodenum's lateral aspect [7]. Secondary DD result from the healing process of peptic ulcers that create an outpouching of the duodenal wall [22]. The congenital variant of DD, less common, is a true diverticulum that contains mucosa, submucosa, and muscularis. The factors that influence its formation are unclear and it may be associated with other congenital anomalies in the upper GI tract.

Even though the cause or causes of acquired JID are unknown, some investigators relate them to dietary fiber deficiencies, which can cause elevated intraluminal pressures. This by itself or in association with a weak bowel smooth muscle wall along the mesenteric border results in a pulsion effect of mucosa and submucosa, which are irrigated by blood vessels [3, 23]. Other theories focus their attention on potential abnormalities of the myenteric plexus that generate a lack of coordination in the small bowel peristalsis, responsible for the high intraluminal pressure and consequently, for diverticular formation [24]. The existing evidence is insufficient to establish the real cause.

## 75.2 Diagnosis

### 75.2.1 Clinical Presentation

Clinical diagnosis of both MD and non-Meckelian SBD can be challenging because there are no specific pathognomonic symptoms, and SBD disease is commonly asymptomatic. When symptoms are present, these can be mild and unspecific, making clinical-based diagnosis difficult. The diagnosis is commonly the result of evaluating an acute complication, and the clinical presentation will vary depending on the type of complication observed (Box 75.2).

When diverticular inflammation occurs, acute onset of abdominal pain is the most common. If the inflammatory process is severe and has led to diverticulum wall necrosis or perforation, the patient would complain of severe diffuse abdominal pain, abdominal wall guarding, and present fever and toxicity signs [25, 26]. Mechanical intestinal occlusion manifests as diffuse colicky abdominal pain along with abdominal distension, nausea, and vomiting. Intraluminal bleeding leads to GI hemorrhage, and the clinical presentation will depend on its intensity, where small amounts of blood loss will generate anemia, and copious bleeding will manifest as hematochezia, often associated with signs of hypovolemia. On rare occasions a Meckel diverticulum can become incarcerated within an inguinal hernia, this is termed Littre's hernia; however, this is extremely uncommon.

### 75.2.2 Tests

#### 75.2.2.1 Labs
Laboratory findings will depend on the type of presentation. Inflammation, obstruction, or perforation will show elevated white blood cell (WBC) count, neutrophilia, and C-reactive protein (CRP). Hemorrhage can lead to choric anemia or acute decrease in hemoglobin and hematocrit levels.

#### 75.2.2.2 Conventional Radiology
Conventional abdominal radiology studies can occasionally show pneumoperitoneum, but this finding is uncommon and rarely diagnostic [4, 12]. SBD radiographic diagnoses are classically made by means of contrast series or enteroclysis study.

#### 75.2.2.3 Ultrasound (US)
Abdominal ultrasound (US), as described for colonic diverticulitis, can help to identify free fluid in cases of perforated SBD disease. However, it has lower sensitivity than computer tomography (CT), and image quality may be compromised by free abdominal gas [27]. CTs demonstrated high sensitivity for colonic diverticulitis (almost 95%) and specificity (99%) suggesting that similar results could be expected for SBD. Additionally, multi-detector CT (MDCT) widespread accessibility, speed, and diagnostic accuracy have made it the imaging study option of choice for SBD [28, 29].

**Box 75.2 Clinical Presentation in Complicated SBD Disease**

| | |
|---|---|
| Diverticulitis | Acute onset of focalized abdominal pain |
| Perforation | Focalized or diffuse peritonitis (fever, abdominal pain, guarding and peritoneal irritation) with or without septic response |
| Intestinal occlusion | Abdominal distension, nauseas and vomits |
| Gastrointestinal hemorrhage | Hematochezia with or without signs of hypovolemia |

Even though there is a lack of specific imaging protocols for complicated SBD disease, most authors recommend evaluation with contrast-enhanced MDCT with a portal venous phase without oral contrast.

### 75.2.2.4 MDCT Scans

MDCT scans with intravenous contrast are considered the preferred imaging modality, both for its accuracy which enables to detect acute complications [4]. MDCT of non-complicated SBD disease frequently show clusters, and even isolated round and regular duodenal or jejunoileal outpouchings with air-fluid levels, debris, or enteric content [30]. Normal small vowel wall will have its characteristic and uniform concentric thickness (close to 3 cm) when not distended, but on diverticulum it will be reduced to 1 or 2 mm depending on the degree of bowel distension. Occasionally, the thin and smooth diverticulum wall, lacking valvulae conniventes, can be challenging to identify [30]. Inflammatory acute diverticulitis complications are characterized by irregular bowel wall thickening of close or neighboring bowels and peri-diverticular fat stranding [31]. In cases of asymmetric wall thickening, differential diagnosis of small bowel malignancy must also be considered. To help distinguish inflammation from malignancy, three elements can help: bowel enhancement patterns, mesentery characteristics, and regional lymph node patterns. In acute diverticulitis, a normal bowel wall enhancement (high inner attenuation, the middle layer of low attenuation, and a highly attenuated outer layer) suggests diverticulitis rather than malignancy [29]. The presence of mesentery engorgement and fluid also suggests an inflammatory process. Last, reactive, and small nodes are seen in diverticulitis, where large or solitary lymphadenopathy close to a segmental wall thickening is more suggestive of malignancy.

In perforated SBD disease there are marked mesenteric abnormalities, extraluminal air, free fluid, or peri-diverticular abscess. In severe cases, the abundance of local inflammatory changes, fluid, and gas can sometimes obscure the diverticulum's localization. Though uncommon, additional findings in perforated diverticulitis are abscess formation between small bowel loops or close to the abdominal wall, hepatic abscess, and even portal vein thrombosis.

### 75.2.2.5 MRI Findings

The use of magnetic resonance imaging (MRI) is increasing for the assessment of the small bowel, especially in patients for whom ionization radiation is to be avoided.

However, there is limited availability when compared to MDCT, and literature describing its findings for SBD is lacking. The most common techniques for small bowel imaging are magnetic resonance (MR) enterography and MR enteroclysis [32, 33]. With the aid of spasmolytic agents like glucagon, the T2-weighed sequences can provide remarkable intraluminal and extraluminal contrast images. The findings, wall asymmetric thickening of the mesenteric border, wall and mesenteric enhancement enclosed by mesenteric edema, resemble those described for colonic diverticulitis.

### 75.2.2.6 Scintigraphy

The use of scintigraphy for the study of patients with lower GI hemorrhage due to bleeding MD can be useful when the diverticulum contains ectopic gastric mucosa. $^{99m}$Tc-pertechnetate is taken up by the mucin-secreting cells in gastric mucosa, so delayed abdominal uptake, after the gastric, suggests ectopic gastric mucosa within the diverticulum. Even though this study has a higher sensitivity in the pediatric population (>85%), it can be also useful in adults with GI hemorrhage and suspicion of MD as the potential origin for the bleeding [34]. Its sensitivity in adults is near 60%, and can be increased with the administration of pentagastrin, glucagon, or $H_2$ antagonists [35] Patients with MD without ectopic gastric mucosa will have a negative scan.

> **Differential Diagnosis**
> The differential diagnosis of complicated SBD disease is challenging to establish and should be related to other causes of acute abdominal pain, particularly in the right

lower quadrant (RLQ). The most common differential diagnosis should be with acute appendicitis [36, 37]. The clinical presentation of both entities may be very similar, and diagnosis based only on clinical evaluation challenging, so imaging techniques should be employed. Inflammatory bowel disease, infectious enteritis, or colitis should be considered in patients with history of recurrent colicky abdominal pain, chronic diarrhea, or chronic nutritional deficits. Intense pain that irradiates to the pelvis of the genitourinary tract should raise suspicion for right ureteric stones. Other less frequent diagnoses to be considered are enteric duplication cyst, intussusception secondary to small bowel lipomas, or small bowel polyps. When the abdominal pain, and the clinical presentation is of generalized peritoneal irritation, non-small bowel perforation should be ruled out. Among the potential diagnosis are colonic diverticulitis, perforated gastric or duodenal peptic ulcer disease, and extremely infrequently perforated primary or secondary small GI tumors with enteric spillage.

## 75.3 Treatment

The low incidence of SBD disease has limited the development of treatment modality's guidelines based on large patient series. Most are about individual clinical cases or small case series. Even though surgical procedures are commonly described in complicated SBD disease, controversy surrounds the best treatment modality for incidentally detected cases. Some authors consider applicable, to some degree, the guidelines for complicated colonic diverticular disease [4, 38, 39]. Even though they could be of help for diagnosing SBD disease, the author considers it as a different entity, whose management should be tailored individually for each patient, based on patient's overall condition, comorbidities, physiological reserve, presence of sepsis, multi-organ dysfunction. In general, surgical removal is the recommended management option for surgically fit patients with symptomatic MD and non-Meckelian SBD, but excluding those in high risk, such as the elderly or frail, with uncontrolled diabetes, on immunosuppressive or chronic steroids treatment.

### 75.3.1 Medical Treatment

High-quality US and MDCT scans allow for better patient selection for conservative management and are a priceless resource and allow for performing percutaneous drainage of accessible and walled abscesses in high-risk surgical patients. Conservative or non-operative approach for small perforations walled off by omentum, mesentery, or adjacent tissues is an option [40, 41]. This type of management will require close follow-up of the patient's condition, bowel rest, nasogastric suction in cases of DD, parenteral nutritional support, broad-spectrum intravenous antibiotics and, rarely, peri-diverticular percutaneous abscess drainage. Percutaneous drainage procedures (PDP) are frequently described for colonic diverticulitis, and only in selected cases is described as applied to SBD disease. In case of non-operative management close follow-up and risk assessment discussion with the patient should be considered, and differed elective surgery discussed.

#### 75.3.1.1 Percutaneous Drainage

Percutaneous drainage procedures (PDP) are frequently described for colonic diverticulitis and most of the experience comes from the treatment of colonic rather the SBD. PDP's utility in SBD is more limited and described in selected cases. Image-guided PDP of well-organized fluid collections are considered for selected patients without diffuse peritonitis [42]. Case selection will depend on the patient's general condition, location of the abscess, accessibility for safe puncture, resources and expertise of the interventional radiology team. Single catheter drainage procedures can yield clinical success in over 80% of the cases [43]. Causes for single catheter drainage procedure failure include multiloculation, abscesses fistulized to a hollow viscus, phlegmon, and inadequate catheter position. Additionally, complex abscesses with thick content, debris, intestinal content, or blood clots can be difficult to drain with conventional percutaneous technique. For such cases, a paired drainage catheter technique, described by Ballard et al. [44], which consists of the placement of two or more catheters into the same abscess. This technique requires the positioning of catheter's tips closely to create an irrigation-aspiration channel that enhances debris removal and adequate drainage. Several episodes of controlled isovolumetric irrigation and aspiration with saline solution generate a constant flow and washout of high viscosity fluid and promote mechanical debridement for these complex abscesses.

In cases managed by PDP, serial images, physical exploration, and lab tests should be part of the patient's follow-up, despite their good clinical evolution. When conservative management fails, surgical exploration should not be delayed.

## 75.3.2 Surgical Treatment

Patients with complicated MD and non-Meckelian SBD disease in which acute peritonitis, GI bleeding with hemodynamic instability, signs of systemic toxicity, mechanical small bowel obstruction are best treated by early surgical approach, performing either an open or laparoscopic surgical exploration [45–47]. Delay in surgical treatment can lead to life-threatening complications. The patient should be approached in a systematic fashion with treatment bundles, addressing first hemodynamic instability and sepsis, followed by MDCT and multidisciplinary consultant evaluation. Prompt source control is essential when free abdominal perforation is identified.

Regarding the surgical approach, both laparotomy or laparoscopic access can be employed. The decision will be conditioned by the patient's hemodynamic conditions, the surgical team's experience, and resources available. However, laparoscopy is preferred in stable patients because of lower complication rates and improved patient comfort. Advances in laparoscopic equipment (cauterizing energy devices and endostaplers) and techniques allow safe and equivalent outcomes to the traditional open approach. Surgical DD treatment should avoid large resections in emergency situations. Limit surgery to drainage procedures and hemostatic sutures for hemorrhage cannot be controlled endoscopically. Complex surgical resections should be avoided in the acutely ill due to the duodenum's high risk for fistulas formation and associated mortality [9]; instead, they can often be treated with percutaneous or open drainage procedures. Feeding jejunostomy can be helpful in selected cases, and complex duodenal resections, though seldomly performed, are occasionally necessary.

For complicated JID (free perforation with diffuse peritonitis, hemorrhage or obstruction) the type of procedure performed will depend on patients' general status, age, the number and location of the diverticulum, the integrity of the diverticulum's base, the condition of adjacent tissue, and the presence of ectopic tissue within the diverticulum. Meckel diverticulum is currently treated, preferably with a three-trocar laparoscopic approach with a 12 mm umbilical optic trocar, a 5 mm suprapubic trocar, and a 12 mm working left flank trocar that will allow the use of an endo-stapler (Fig. 75.5).

For those patients with uncomplicated non-perforated diverticulitis there is ongoing debate: while some advocate for no treatment [48] other recommend selective resection in healthy adults under 50 years, with diverticulum size longer than 2 cm, broad base (>2 cm) and suspicion of heterotopic tissue [49, 50]. The height-to-diameter ratio (H-D-R) can help predict the ectopic tissue distribution within the diverticulum. Long diverticulum with an H-D-R >2 tends to have ectopic tissue distributed both in the body and tip. In contrast, wide and short diverticulum tend have a wider distribution of ectopic tissue, including the diverticulum base. Two methods of resection can be performed, diverticulectomy (Fig. 75.6) for long diverticulum with a small base, and wedge resections for short diverticulum

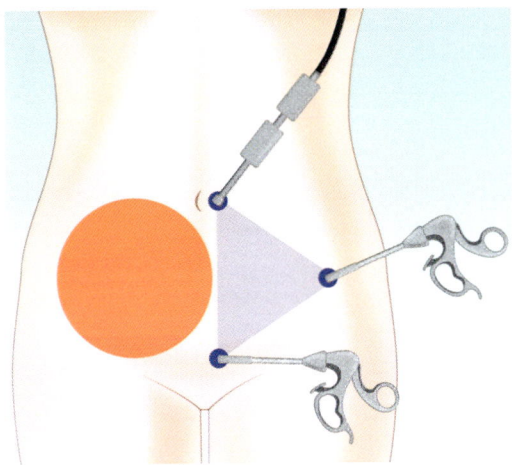

**Fig. 75.5** Trocar positioning for a Meckel diverticulum is currently treated, preferably three-trocar approach. The working zone is highlighted with a red dot. (Illustration by Ilaria Bondi)

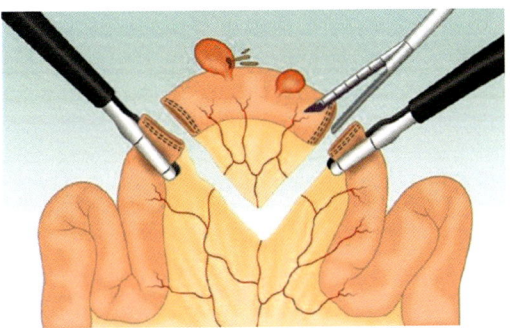

**Fig. 75.7** Laparoscopic segmental small bowel resection containing isolated or clusters of perforated SBDs. (Illustration by Ilaria Bondi)

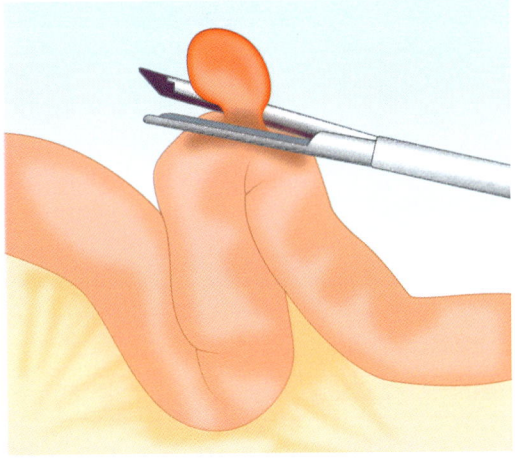

**Fig. 75.6** Laparoscopic endostapler diverticulectomy. (Illustration by Ilaria Bondi)

with a broad base. When the diverticulum is associated with perforation, GI bleeding, intestinal obstruction, or signs of potential malignancy, segmental resection is the preferred option (Fig. 75.7).

Primary anastomosis is achieved with a side-to-side endostapler on the anti-mesenteric border of the small bowel and the common enterotomy site closed with barbed or non-barbed absorbable suture. Laparoscopic diverticulectomy can be easily extracted using an endobag that will avoid spillage and wound infection. In cases of segmental small bowel resections both extra and intracorporal anastomosis are safe; however, a mini-laparotomy may be necessary for specimen extraction. In these cases, care must be taken to use wound protective devices to avoid infection.

Treatment of perforated non-Meckelian clusters of JID should be treated with segmental resection of the small bowel. The resection should include the perforated diverticulum and only those in close vicinity, followed by diverticular free bowel primary anastomosis (Figs. 75.8 and 75.9). Prophylactic resection in uncomplicated SBD is not recommended in most cases.

In summary treatment of SBD should be tailored individually for each patient, based on patient's surgical risk, physiological reserve, type of complication.

> **Dos and Don'ts**
> **Dos**
> - Do an early surgical laparoscopic approach with surgical removal as the first management option for most complicated Meckelian and symptomatic non-Meckelian SBD.
> - Do a diverticulectomy when the diverticulum's base is <2 cm, and there is no suspicion of ectopic tissue. In contrast do a segmental resection of the SBD when there is a broad base (>2 cm) or a

height-to-diameter ratio (H-D-R) >2, since these SBD tend to have ectopic tissue.
- Do a segmental resection when encountered with perforation, bleeding, intestinal obstruction, or signs of malignancy.

**Don'ts**
- Do not delay in surgical treatment in patients with acute complication, sepsis, organ disfunction or severe GI bleeding; unnecessary explorations and efforts to manage these cases medically can be life-threatening.
- Do not delay definitive surgical treatment if the patient does no improve with initial medical or non-operative management.
- Do not delay conversion to open surgery if the laparoscopic approach results unsuccessful to perform the surgical management necessary.
- Do not perform procedures for which the surgical team lacks the necessary equipment or expertise.

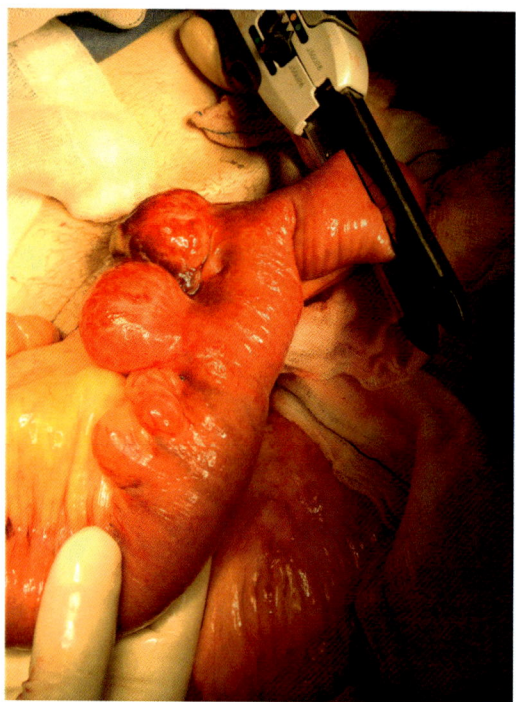

**Fig. 75.8** Stapler resection of clusters of complicated jejunal SBD

### 75.3.3 Prognosis

Diverticulitis is the most common cause of JID, present in up to 2–6% of the cases [4]. Infection may be caused either by stasis of the intestinal content or by obstruction at the neck of the diverticulum, creating bacterial growth and increment in diverticular wall pressure. Most of these inflammatory processes are mild, but some can be severe and lead to persistent inflammation with increments in intraluminal pressure and an increase in the diverticular wall's tension leading to perforation.

Between 2% and 7% of SBD diverticulitis crisis can lead to perforation caused by the necrotizing inflammatory reaction in the thin diverticular wall. When perforation occurs, and there is spillage of enteric content, mortality can be as high as 40% [25]. Surgical procedures should not be

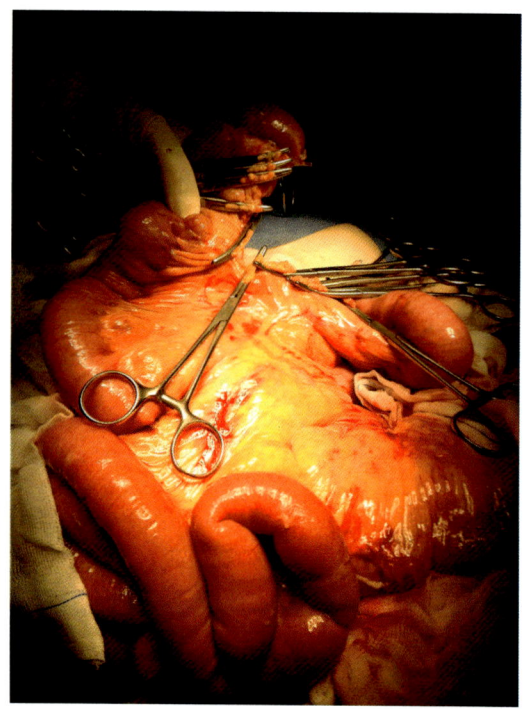

**Fig. 75.9** Open segmental small bowel resection

delayed for patients with signs of diffuses peritonitis, sepsis, or hemodynamic instability. Prognosis will be influenced by age, comorbidities, focalized or diffuse peritonitis, time to diagnosis, and the onset of treatment [51]. Delaying surgery in perforated BBD disease with peritonitis will contribute to a dimmer prognosis with higher morbidity, prolonged length of stay in the hospital, and higher mortality rate. Early patient risk assessment by a multidisciplinary team of surgical consultant, anesthetist, and intensivist will help identify those with high-risk.

Emergency laparotomy or abdominal laparoscopic exploration treatment pathways and bundles of care will help reduce overall mortality. Do not delay surgical exploration in patients with hemodynamically instability. In septic, the patient early blood cultures and broad-spectrum antibiotics should be administered within the first hour of the patient's arrival to the emergency department.

**Take-Home Messages**
- SBD is usually asymptomatic and uncomplicated, found incidentally during imaging studies or surgical procedures.
- MDCT scan is the preferred diagnostic imaging modality that allows not only the presence and location of SBD but also can diagnose complications (inflammation, perforation, and bleeding).
- Meckel diverticulum is present in close to 2% of the general population and is the most common congenital anomaly of the gastrointestinal tract.
- Non-operative management with bowel rest, IV antibiotics, parenteral nutrition support, localized abscess percutaneous drainage, and close follow-up are acceptable options in selected surgical high-risk cases without diffuse peritonitis. However, surgery should not be delayed when in presence of diffuse peritonitis, toxic general condition, or failure of non-operative management occur.
- Both open or minimally invasive laparoscopic approaches can be suitable, depending on proper patent selection, resources available, and level of expertise of the attending team.
- All symptomatic MD should be surgically resected either by diverticulectomy or by segmental small bowel resection with primary anastomosis.

**Questions**
1. Where is the acquired small bowel diverticular disease more frequently found?
   A. The ileum
   B. The jejunum
   **C. The duodenum**
   D. There is currently no available data
2. Duodenal diverticula are mostly located in?
   A. The first portion of the duodenum
   **B. The second portion of the duodenum**
   C. The third portion of the duodenum
   D. The fourth portion of the duodenum
3. Most small bowel diverticula are:
   **A. Acquired, asymptomatic, and incidentally found**
   B. Acquired and symptomatic
   C. Congenital, asymptomatic, and incidentally found
   D. Congenital and symptomatic
4. Which of the following SBD definitions is correct according to the layers that conform them?
   **A. False SBD are those in which the mucosa and submucosa protrude through a muscular wall defect**

B. True SBD are those in which the mucosa and submucosa protrude through a muscular wall defect
C. In false SBD when the protrusion involves all the gastrointestinal layers tract
D. In true SBD when only the mucosa protrudes through a muscular wall defect

5. What is the predominant ratio for male to female jejunum-ileal diverticulum?
   A. **2:1**
   B. 4:1
   C. 6.1
   D. 10:1

6. Meckel diverticulum is the most common congenital anomaly of the gastrointestinal tract, affecting what percentage of the general population?
   A. 0.5–1%
   B. **2–4%**
   C. 5–6%
   D. 6–8%

7. The most frequent type of ectopic mucosa encountered in Meckel diverticulum is?
   A. Pancreatic mucosa
   B. **Gastric mucosa**
   C. Duodenal mucosa
   D. Colonic mucosa

8. What is the current imaging modality of choice for small bowel diverticulum?
   A. Abdominal X-ray
   B. Abdominal point of care US
   C. **MDCT scans**
   D. MRI

9. Patients with complicated SBD and peritonitis are best treated by?
   A. Medically with systemic antibiotics
   B. Endoscopically
   C. With percutaneous drainage procedures
   D. **With early surgical approach**

10. Regarding percutaneous drainage procedures in complicated SBD disease.
    A. **Image-guided percutaneous drainage procedures are most useful in organized fluid collections without diffuse peritonitis**
    B. Image-guided percutaneous drainage procedures are most useful in non-organized fluid collections without diffuse peritonitis
    C. Image-guided percutaneous drainage procedures are most useful in diffuse peritonitis
    D. The paired drainage catheter technique is preferred to the single catheter drainage procedures

**Acknowledgments** The author extends his acknowledgments to Mercedes Muñoz and Visitación Ortega Riba, information specialists, for the assistance with the literature search; to Carlos Yánez Sr., PhD, for his proofreading; and to Ilaria Bondi, the medical illustrator.

# References

1. Sinclair A. Diverticular disease of the gastrointestinal tract. Prim Care. 2017;44(4):643–54. https://doi.org/10.1016/j.pop.2017.07.007.
2. Kassahun WT, Fangmann J, Harms J, Bartels M, Hauss J. Complicated small-bowel diverticulosis: a case report and review of the literature. World J Gastroenterol. 2007;13(15):2240–2.
3. Ferreira-Aparicio FE, Gutiérrez-Vega R, Gálvez-Molina Y, Ontiveros-Nevares P, Athie-Gútierrez C, Montalvo-Javé EE. Diverticular disease of the small bowel. Case Rep Gastroenterol. 2012;6(3):668–76. https://doi.org/10.1159/000343598. Epub 2012 Oct 25.
4. Transue DL, Hanna TN, Shekhani H, Rohatgi S, Khosa F, Johnson JO. Small bowel diverticulitis: an imaging review of an uncommon entity. Emerg Radiol. 2017;24(2):195–205. https://doi.org/10.1007/s10140-016-1448-4. Epub 2016 Nov 4.
5. Gayer G, Zissin R, Apter S, Shemesh E, Heldenberg E. Acute diverticulitis of the small bowel: CT findings. Abdom Imaging. 1999;24(5):452–5. https://doi.org/10.1007/s002619900538.
6. Fatoides CIKI, Papandreou I, Pillichos C, Zografos G, Mahairasi A. Current diagnostic and treatment aspects of duodenal diverticula: report of two polar

cases and review of the literature. Ann Gastroenterol. 2005;18(4):441.
7. Pearl MS, Hill MC, Zeman RK. CT findings in duodenal diverticulitis. AJR Am J Roentgenol. 2006;187(4):W392–5. https://doi.org/10.2214/AJR.06.0215.
8. Makris K, Tsiotos GG, Stafyla V, Sakorafas GH. Small intestinal nonmeckelian diverticulosis. J Clin Gastroenterol. 2009;43(3):201–7. https://doi.org/10.1097/MCG.0b013e3181919261.
9. Oukachbi N, Brouzes S. Management of complicated duodenal diverticula. J Visc Surg. 2013;150(3):173–9. https://doi.org/10.1016/j.jviscsurg.2013.04.006.
10. Maglinte DD, Chernish SM, DeWeese R, Kelvin FM, Brunelle RL. Acquired jejunoileal diverticular disease: subject review. Radiology. 1986;158(3):577–80. https://doi.org/10.1148/radiology.158.3.3080802.
11. Cunningham SC, Gannon CJ, Napolitano LM. Small-bowel diverticulosis. Am J Surg. 2005;190(1):37–8. https://doi.org/10.1016/j.amjsurg.2005.03.024.
12. Coulier B, Maldague P, Bourgeois A, Broze B. Diverticulitis of the small bowel: CT diagnosis. Abdom Imaging. 2007;32(2):228–33. https://doi.org/10.1007/s00261-006-9045-8. Epub 2006 Sep 12.
13. Pepper VK, Stanfill AB, Pearl RH. Diagnosis and management of pediatric appendicitis, intussusception, and Meckel diverticulum. Surg Clin North Am. 2012;92(3):505–26, vii. https://doi.org/10.1016/j.suc.2012.03.011.
14. Mantas D, Kykalos S, Patsouras D, Kouraklis G. Small intestine diverticula: Is there anything new? World J Gastrointest Surg. 2011;3(4):49–53. https://doi.org/10.4240/wjgs.v3.i4.49.
15. Longo WE, Vernava AM 3rd. Clinical implications of jejunoileal diverticular disease. Dis Colon Rectum. 1992;35(4):381–8. https://doi.org/10.1007/BF02048119.
16. Opitz JM, Schultka R, Göbbel L. Meckel on developmental pathology. Am J Med Genet A. 2006;140(2):115–28. https://doi.org/10.1002/ajmg.a.31043.
17. Edmonson JM. Johann Friedrich Meckel the younger: Meckel's diverticulum. Gastrointest Endosc. 2001;54(1):19A–20A. https://doi.org/10.1053/ge.2001.v54.054101.
18. St-Vil D, Brandt ML, Panic S, Bensoussan AL, Blanchard H. Meckel's diverticulum in children: a 20-year review. J Pediatr Surg. 1991;26(11):1289–92. https://doi.org/10.1016/0022-3468(91)90601-o.
19. Morris G, Kennedy A Jr, Cochran W. Small bowel congenital anomalies: a review and update. Curr Gastroenterol Rep. 2016;18(4):16. https://doi.org/10.1007/s11894-016-0490-4.
20. Krishnamurthy S, Kelly MM, Rohrmann CA, Schuffler MD. Jejunal diverticulosis. A heterogenous disorder caused by a variety of abnormalities of smooth muscle or myenteric plexus. Gastroenterology. 1983;85(3):538–47.
21. Meagher AP, Porter AJ, Rowland R, Ma G, Hoffmann DC. Jejunal diverticulosis. Aust N Z J Surg. 1993;63(5):360–6.
22. Jayaraman MV, Mayo-Smith WW, Movson JS, Dupuy DE, Wallach MT. CT of the duodenum: an overlooked segment gets its due. Radiographics. 2001;21 Spec No:S147–60. https://doi.org/10.1148/radiographics.21.suppl_1.g01oc01s147.
23. De Peuter B, Box I, Vanheste R, Dymarkowski S. Small-bowel diverticulosis: imaging findings and review of three cases. Gastroenterol Res Pract. 2009;2009:549853. https://doi.org/10.1155/2009/549853. Epub 2009 Aug 2.
24. Liu CY, Chang WH, Lin SC, Chu CH, Wang TE, Shih SC. Analysis of clinical manifestations of symptomatic acquired jejunoileal diverticular disease. World J Gastroenterol. 2005;11(35):5557–60. https://doi.org/10.3748/wjg.v11.i35.5557.
25. Lebert P, Millet I, Ernst O, Boulay-Coletta I, Corno L, Taourel P, Zins M. Acute jejunoileal diverticulitis: multicenter descriptive study of 33 patients. AJR Am J Roentgenol. 2018;210(6):1245–51. https://doi.org/10.2214/AJR.17.18777. Epub 2018 Apr 9.
26. Horesh N, Klang E, Gravetz A, Nevo Y, Amiel I, Amitai MM, Rosin D, Gutman M, Zmora O. Jejunal diverticulitis. J Laparoendosc Adv Surg Tech A. 2016;26(8):596–9. https://doi.org/10.1089/lap.2016.0066. Epub 2016 May 16.
27. van Randen A, Laméris W, van Es HW, van Heesewijk HP, van Ramshorst B, Ten Hove W, Bouma WH, van Leeuwen MS, van Keulen EM, Bossuyt PM, Stoker J, Boermeester MA, OPTIMA Study Group. A comparison of the accuracy of ultrasound and computed tomography in common diagnoses causing acute abdominal pain. Eur Radiol. 2011;21(7):1535–45. https://doi.org/10.1007/s00330-011-2087-5. Epub 2011 Mar 2.
28. Urban BA, Fishman EK. Tailored helical CT evaluation of acute abdomen. Radiographics. 2000;20(3):725–49. https://doi.org/10.1148/radiographics.20.3.g00ma12725. Erratum in: Radiographics 2000 Sep-Oct;20(5):1494.
29. Purysko AS, Remer EM, Filho HM, Bittencourt LK, Lima RV, Racy DJ. Beyond appendicitis: common and uncommon gastrointestinal causes of right lower quadrant abdominal pain at multidetector CT. Radiographics. 2011;31(4):927–47. https://doi.org/10.1148/rg.314105065.
30. Fintelmann F, Levine MS, Rubesin SE. Jejunal diverticulosis: findings on CT in 28 patients. AJR Am J Roentgenol. 2008;190(5):1286–90. https://doi.org/10.2214/AJR.07.3087.
31. Hoeffel C, Crema MD, Belkacem A, Azizi L, Lewin M, Arrivé L, Tubiana JM. Multi-detector row CT: spectrum of diseases involving the ileocecal area. Radiographics. 2006;26(5):1373–90. https://doi.org/10.1148/rg.265045191.
32. Mansoori B, Delaney CP, Willis JE, Paspulati RM, Ros PR, Schmid-Tannwald C, Herrmann KA. Magnetic resonance enterography/enteroclysis in acquired small bowel diverticulitis and small bowel diverticulosis. Eur Radiol. 2016;26(9):2881–91. https://doi.org/10.1007/s00330-015-4098-0. Epub 2015 Nov 23.

33. Fidler JL, Guimaracs L, Einstcin DM. MR imaging of the small bowel. Radiographics. 2009;29(6):1811–25. https://doi.org/10.1148/rg.296095507.
34. Poulsen KA, Qvist N. Sodium pertechnetate scintigraphy in detection of Meckel's diverticulum: is it usable? Eur J Pediatr Surg. 2000;10(4):228–31. https://doi.org/10.1055/s-2008-1072364.
35. Ford PV, Bartold SP, Fink-Bennett DM, Jolles PR, Lull RJ, Maurer AH, Seabold JE. Procedure guideline for gastrointestinal bleeding and Meckel's diverticulum scintigraphy. Society of Nuclear Medicine. J Nucl Med. 1999;40(7):1226–32.
36. Khandelwal A, Virmani V, Ryan J, Kielar A, Fraser-Hill M, Sheikh A. Solving the mystery of Meckel diverticulum. Vancouver: American Roentgen Ray Society; American Journal of Roentgenology; 2012.
37. Kusumoto H, Yoshida M, Takahashi I, Anai H, Maehara Y, Sugimachi K. Complications and diagnosis of Meckel's diverticulum in 776 patients. Am J Surg. 1992;164(4):382–3. https://doi.org/10.1016/s0002-9610(05)80909-2.
38. Veen M, Hornstra BJ, Clemens CH, Stigter H, Vree R. Small bowel diverticulitis as a cause of acute abdomen. Eur J Gastroenterol Hepatol. 2009;21(1):123–5. https://doi.org/10.1097/MEG.0b013e328303bfdb.
39. Sartelli M, Weber DG, Kluger Y, Ansaloni L, Coccolini F, Abu-Zidan F, Augustin G, Ben-Ishay O, Biffl WL, Bouliaris K, Catena R, Ceresoli M, Chiara O, Chiarugi M, Coimbra R, Cortese F, Cui Y, Damaskos D, De' Angelis GL, Delibegovic S, Demetrashvili Z, De Simone B, Di Marzo F, Di Saverio S, Duane TM, Faro MP, Fraga GP, Gkiokas G, Gomes CA, Hardcastle TC, Hecker A, Karamarkovic A, Kashuk J, Khokha V, Kirkpatrick AW, Kok KYY, Inaba K, Isik A, Labricciosa FM, Latifi R, Leppäniemi A, Litvin A, Mazuski JE, Maier RV, Marwah S, McFarlane M, Moore EE, Moore FA, Negoi I, Pagani L, Rasa K, Rubio-Perez I, Sakakushev B, Sato N, Sganga G, Siquini W, Tarasconi A, Tolonen M, Ulrych J, Zachariah SK, Catena F. 2020 update of the WSES guidelines for the management of acute colonic diverticulitis in the emergency setting. World J Emerg Surg. 2020;15(1):32. https://doi.org/10.1186/s13017-020-00313-4.
40. Costa Simões V, Santos B, Magalhães S, Faria G, Sousa Silva D, Davide J. Perforated duodenal diverticulum: surgical treatment and literature review. Int J Surg Case Rep. 2014;5(8):547–50. https://doi.org/10.1016/j.ijscr.2014.06.008. Epub 2014 Jun 19.
41. Levack MM, Madariaga ML, Kaafarani HM. Nonoperative successful management of a perforated small bowel diverticulum. World J Gastroenterol. 2014;20(48):18477–9. https://doi.org/10.3748/wjg.v20.i48.18477.
42. Levin DC, Eschelman D, Parker L, Rao VM. Trends in use of percutaneous versus open surgical drainage of abdominal abscesses. J Am Coll Radiol. 2015;12(12 Pt A):1247–50. https://doi.org/10.1016/j.jacr.2015.06.015.
43. Ballard DH, Flanagan ST, Griffen FD. Percutaneous versus open surgical drainage: surgeon's perspective. J Am Coll Radiol. 2016;13(4):364. https://doi.org/10.1016/j.jacr.2016.01.012. Epub 2016 Feb 26.
44. Ballard DH, Flanagan ST, Brown RW, Vea R, Ahuja C, D'Agostino HB. Paired drainage catheter insertion: feasibility of placing two catheters within the same complex abscess cavity as a primary and salvage percutaneous drainage technique. Acad Radiol. 2020;27(2):e1–9. https://doi.org/10.1016/j.acra.2019.03.010. Epub 2019 Apr 26.
45. Leigh N, Sullivan BJ, Anteby R, Talbert S. Perforated jejunal diverticulitis: a rare but important differential in the acute abdomen. Surg Case Rep. 2020;6(1):162. https://doi.org/10.1186/s40792-020-00929-3.
46. Ghrissi R, Harbi H, Elghali MA, Belhajkhlifa MH, Letaief MR. Jejunal diverticulosis: a rare case of intestinal obstruction. J Surg Case Rep. 2016;2016(2):rjv176. https://doi.org/10.1093/jscr/rjv176.
47. Tenreiro N, Moreira H, Silva S, Marques R, Monteiro A, Gaspar J, Oliveira A. Jejunoileal diverticulosis, a rare cause of ileal perforation—case report. Ann Med Surg (Lond). 2016;6:56–9. https://doi.org/10.1016/j.amsu.2016.01.089.
48. Zani A, Eaton S, Rees CM, Pierro A. Incidentally detected Meckel diverticulum: to resect or not to resect? Ann Surg. 2008;247(2):276–81. https://doi.org/10.1097/SLA.0b013e31815aaaf8.
49. Park JJ, Wolff BG, Tollefson MK, Walsh EE, Larson DR. Meckel diverticulum: the Mayo Clinic experience with 1476 patients (1950-2002). Ann Surg. 2005;241(3):529–33. https://doi.org/10.1097/01.sla.0000154270.14308.5f.
50. Żyluk A. Management of incidentally discovered unaffected Meckel's diverticulum—a review. Pol Przegl Chir. 2019;91(6):41–6. https://doi.org/10.5604/01.3001.0013.3400.
51. Spasojevic M, Naesgaard JM, Ignjatovic D. Perforated midgut diverticulitis: revisited. World J Gastroenterol. 2012;18(34):4714–20. https://doi.org/10.3748/wjg.v18.i34.4714.

# Large Bowel Obstruction

# 76

Tiffany Paradis, Tarek Razek, and Evan G. Wong

**Learning Objectives**
- To recognize the clinical signs, symptoms, and pathophysiology of large bowel obstruction.
- To select the appropriate imaging modality for investigation and recognize characteristic radiologic findings of large bowel obstruction and bowel compromise.
- To understand the indications for emergent operative management in large bowel obstruction.
- To select the appropriate treatment and surgical option based on underlying pathology and clinical setting.

## 76.1 Introduction

Abdominal pain represents a significant proportion of emergency department visits annually. Approximately 15–20% of all hospital admissions in the United States are the result of both small and large bowel obstructions (LBOs) [1, 2]. Although small bowel obstruction is more common, large bowel obstruction (LBO) comprises 25% of all intestinal obstructions [3]. Despite guidelines and screening protocols, colorectal cancer (CRC) remains the most frequent cause of LBOs followed by diverticular disease and volvulus [4].

Obstruction occurs when there is an interruption in the propagation of enteric contents through the colon. LBOs are classified as mechanical or functional. Mechanical obstructions can be further divided into intrinsic—processes taking place within the colon or intramural—and extrinsic being other abdominal pathologies leading to colonic compression. Non-mechanical obstructions are characterized by the absence of intestinal contractility associated with decreased colonic motility (Table 76.1). The proximal colon becomes dilated with fluid secondary to poor absorption and gas. Significant distension of the bowel will eventually compress venous return resulting in further congestion. As this cycle progresses, there is a loss in the pressure gradient in addition to compression of the arterial supply to the bowel. The lack of blood supply results in ischemia,

T. Paradis · T. Razek
Division of Trauma and General Surgery, McGill University Health Centre, Montreal General Hospital Site, Montreal, QC, Canada
e-mail: tiffany.paradis@mail.mcgill.ca; tarek.razek@muhc.mcgill.ca

E. G. Wong (✉)
Division of Trauma and General Surgery, McGill University Health Centre, Montreal General Hospital Site, Montreal, QC, Canada

Division of General Surgery, Jewish General Hospital, Montreal, QC, Canada
e-mail: evan.wong@mcgill.ca

**Table 76.1** Differential diagnosis for large bowel obstruction including mechanical (intrinsic, extrinsic) and non-mechanical etiologies. Adapted from Current Surgical Therapy [34]

| Intrinsic | Extrinsic | Functional |
|---|---|---|
| Colon cancer | Malignancy (ovarian, sarcoma, carcinomatosis) | Chronic constipation |
| Rectal cancer | | Ogilvie's syndrome |
| Inflammatory bowel disease stricture | Endometriosis | Narcotic-induced adynamic ileus |
| Diverticular stricture | Pelvic collection/inflammation | |
| Ischemia | Hernia | Toxic megacolon |
| Radiation | Volvulus | Hirschsprung's |
| Intussusception | Congenital band | |
| Fecal impaction | Adhesions | |
| Foreign body | | |

necrosis, and eventual perforation [5]. An acute interruption in vascular flow can occur with a mechanical obstruction and a competent ileocecal valve, volvulus, and strangulated hernias. This is referred to as a closed-loop obstruction and poses a surgical emergency. While functional causes of LBO may not present as an abrupt closed loop, progressive untreated dilatation can result in vascular compromise. The location of perforation will depend on the location of ischemia, although the cecum has been identified as a common place of perforation due to its thin wall [6].

Despite population-based screening protocols, colorectal cancer remains the leading cause of LBO in North America. Approximately 20% of patients with colorectal cancer (CRC) will have a primary presentation of obstruction [7]. The most common location of a new colonic mass is the sigmoid colon and the splenic flexure [8]. However, less frequent, rectal and right sided-colonic masses can also result in obstruction. While a large proportion of individuals presenting with obstructing colon and rectal cancers are above the age of 70, there is a significant rise among those younger than 50 [9].

Diverticular disease is common in Western populations and approximately 25% of patient with diverticulosis will have an episode of diverticulitis [10]. Chronic repetitive inflammation can result in stricture formation and sequentially LBO. While not as common as CRC, diverticular disease remains the second most common cause of LBO followed by acute volvulus.

Acute sigmoid volvulus occurs when there is a torsion of the sigmoid colon mesentery resulting in acute obstruction of the intestinal lumen and vascular compromise. Sigmoid volvulus is more common than cecal volvulus and accounts for less than 10% of all large bowel obstructions [11]. Risk factors include a long redundant sigmoid with a short mesentery, chronic constipation, and fecal loading. Colonic dysmotility has also been described as a risk factor for sigmoid volvulus. These factors are highly present in the elderly population and patients with neuropsychological comorbidities [11].

While the above clinical presentations have an underlying mechanical obstruction, non-mechanical LBO can also present with significant colonic distension. Acute colonic pseudo-obstruction (ACPO) occurs when patients present with signs and symptoms of colonic obstruction without a clear transition point or an anatomic lesion on imaging. Typically, ACPO is a chronic issue presenting over a period of 7–10 days; however, it can also occur acutely in hospitalized or chronically ill patients within 24–48 h [12]. ACPO is commonly seen in elderly patients, those with chronic neurodegenerative diseases (Parkinson's, diabetes), hospitalized or institutionalized patients, patients with electrolyte imbalances, and significant opiate usage [13, 14]. If the distension is not managed, the patient is at risk of colonic ischemia and perforation.

## 76.2 Diagnosis

All patients should undergo a thorough history including bowel habits, family history of colon cancer, inflammatory bowel disease, and recent colonoscopy. Presenting symptoms often include nausea, vomiting, inability to tolerate oral intake, progressive abdominal distension, and obstipation. Depending on the duration of symptoms, patients may present with dehydration, electrolyte abnormalities, acute kidney injury, and significant hypovolemia. In the context of a slow growing colonic mass, patients may report a gradual change in their bowel function, occasional post-prandial discomfort, weight loss, melena, or blood in stool. Patients with a diverticular stricture will likely report recent episodes of diverticulitis. Cecal or sigmoid volvulus results in acute abdominal pain, distension, and obstipation. ACPO will also present with significant constipation and progressive abdominal distension and is commonly seen in those with chronic condition [13].

Examination should focus on signs of peritonitis, inspection for hernias, and a digital rectal exam. Standard blood work should be performed on all patients. As patients typically present with poor oral intake and vomiting, it is crucial to evaluate for electrolyte imbalances and elevated creatinine levels. Ischemic bowel may result in significant leukocytosis. A venous blood gas should be done to evaluate lactate and pH levels as a monitor of end-organ perfusion. Elevated lactate can suggest intestinal ischemia; however, the specificity is low [15]. Other preoperative lab work should be performed including coagulation profile, type and screen, and beta-chorionic gonadotropin, if applicable.

An abdominal radiograph is typically the primary imaging modality used due to its rapid availability. The large colon will appear dilated proximally, with air fluid levels and collapsed loops or absence of air distal to the obstruction. In cases of bowel perforation, pneumoperitoneum can be identified beneath the diaphragm. A characteristic finding of sigmoid volvulus is the Bird's Beak sign, whereas the coffee bean sign is indicative of cecal volvulus. While these plain film signs support the diagnosis of a bowel obstruction, the specificity remains low; further investigations should be pursued to identify the underlying cause [16].

Computed tomography (CT) is a reliable imaging modality for the evaluation of a bowel obstruction and has been recommended as the primary imaging modality by the World Society of Emergency Surgery [17]. CT typically demonstrates distended colonic loops with air-fluid levels proximal to the obstruction and decompressed loops distally. In the context of an incompetent ileocecal valve dilatation may involve the small bowel and stomach, while a competent valve will limit dilatation to the colon. The key radiologic findings to look for on CT are a transition point, the etiology of the obstruction, competency of the ileocecal valve, and signs of ischemia or perforation. Findings of bowel compromise include pneumatosis intestinalis, wall thickening, portovenous gas, and, in cases of necrosis and perforation, pneumoperitoneum [18].

In fact, patients should undergo CT of the abdomen and pelvis with intravenous contrast as to better identify complications related to inflammation and ischemia [19]. Some centers have incorporated oral contrast as part of their imaging algorithm for all patients presenting with abdominal pain. While oral and rectal contrast can be used to evaluate acute abdominal pain, omission of this step in the emergency setting has resulted in reduced length of stay and time to CT scan [20]. Moreover, administration of oral contrast in an already obstructed patient presents a risk of aspiration [21]. Therefore, in the acute setting, we do not advocate for the administration of oral contrast.

The etiology of the obstruction can be elucidated based on certain signs. With colorectal cancer, CT findings include colonic wall thickening, luminal narrowing, enhancing soft-tissue mass, and advanced lesions may present with a necrotic center. The presence of metastases should favor a malignant process. Some cases of colorectal cancer may imitate diverticulitis on CT especially if there is a significant amount of pericolonic

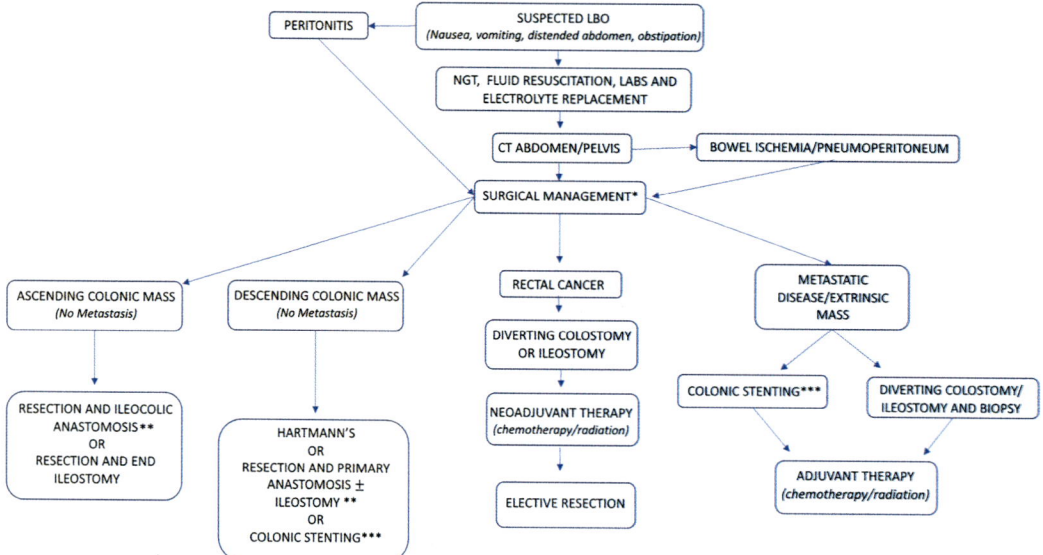

**Fig. 76.1** Flow diagram for the management of mechanical large bowel obstruction. *Surgical management will depend on disease location and patient physiology. **Anastomosis to be performed in clinically appropriate settings. ***Colonic stenting to be considered in technically feasible cases

spread, mimicking inflammatory changes. For patients with diverticulitis, as chronic inflammation leads to fibrosis and wall thickening, imaging findings may be difficult to distinguish stricture from malignancy. While cecal and sigmoid volvulus have characteristic findings on plain film, CT remains the principal method of evaluation. Sigmoid volvulus on CT typically projects to the right upper quadrant, with two transition points, twisting along its mesentery [22]. In contrast, cecal volvulus projects to the left supper quadrant as it distends following twisting along its mesentery. Classical findings of ACPO can also be diagnosed on CT imaging including diffuse colonic dilatation without a transition point [23].

While magnetic resonance imaging (MRI) is not commonly used, this may be an option to consider in children or pregnant women. MRI is associated with a high specificity and sensitivity in the diagnosis of bowel obstruction [24]. However, due to the feasibility, time constraints, and accessibility, MRIs have limited utility in the acute setting (Fig. 76.1).

## 76.3 Management

The initial management for all patients with presumed bowel obstruction is similar. Nasogastric (NGT) decompression should be attempted. Many patients, particularly those with delayed presentations, are dehydrated at the time of presentation; therefore, proper resuscitation is crucial. Electrolytes should be monitored and corrected daily. Those presenting with clinical signs of sepsis should be started on broad-spectrum antibiotics and pan cultured immediately. Surgical intervention will vary based on the underlying obstructive pathology. For most patients, emergency surgery for LBO be performed through a mid-line laparotomy incision. Although some case series show favorable results, laparoscopic surgery should not be attempted on patients presenting with significant distension as there is a high risk of iatrogenic bowel injury and poor visualization [17].

Patients presenting with an acute sigmoid volvulus, without peritonitis on examination or concerns for ischemia, are candidates for endoscopic decompression. Post decompression, patients deemed to be surgical candidates should undergo sigmoidectomy within 24–48 h as the rate of recurrence is approximately 50–60% [25]. There is still much debate regarding the number of endoscopic decompression attempts prior to surgical intervention as recurrent volvulus and perforation are procedural risks [26]. In circumstances where decompression is unsuccessful, patients may undergo resection and primary anastomosis (RPA) versus Hartmann's procedure (HP). A recent retrospective study examining outcomes between the two procedures identified <5% leak rate, and no difference in postoperative complications or mortality [27]. HP is associated with a significant morbidity including stomal related complications such as parastomal hernias, skin irritation, and significant lifestyle alterations. The rate of colostomy reversal has been reported as low as 25% secondary to adhesions and failure to locate the rectal stump [28]. For these reasons, resection and primary anastomosis are the favored method of treatment in the appropriate clinical setting.

Patients presenting with a cecal volvulus should undergo surgical management, as decompression has been shown to be ineffective [11]. Ileocecectomy and primary anastomosis versus detorsion and suture fixation are the two surgical options. The former has been associated with a <5% leak rate, whereas the latter has the potential for recurrence [29]. Therefore, resection and primary anastomosis is the favored method of surgical intervention in patients presenting with a physiologic status favorable for anastomotic survival.

ACPO is usually managed conservatively including NGT insertion, rectal tube decompression, serial abdominal examination, and radiographs. These patients in particular should undergo daily electrolyte measurement, correction, and intravenous hydration as these are often correctable contributing factors. Opioid and anticholinergic medications should be limited when possible [30]. Patients, without cardiovascular risk factors, who fail conservative management may undergo medical treatment with neostigmine. Medical therapy with neostigmine should occur in a monitored setting due to the potential risk of symptomatic bradycardia and is contraindicated in patients with bradyarrhythmia's, bronchospasm, and pregnancy [31]. Endoscopic decompression can also be attempted in those who fail medical management, however, poses a risk of perforation [32, 33]. In patients who fail the above therapy, surgical intervention can be considered. A laparotomy is recommended to identify the integrity of the bowel. If the colon does not appear ischemic, a colostomy or ileostomy is recommended. If a segment of colon appears ischemic, it should be resected with a diverting stoma and mucus fistula. Primary anastomosis is not recommended in unstable patients, due to the increased risk of anastomotic leak. Medical management should not be attempted in patients presenting with sepsis, perforation, or peritonitis; these patients should immediately be managed surgically [34] (Fig. 76.2).

Surgical management of patients presenting with an obstructing colonic mass will depend on the location, extent of disease, and the patient's physiologic status. Stable patients with an isolated left-sided colonic mass should undergo surgical resection. HP remains one of the most common surgical interventions in emergency colonic surgery [35]. Recently there has been a trend towards performing RPA with or without a diverting ileostomy in properly selected patients. In fact, more recent evidence supports a single-staged procedure as a significant proportion of stomas are not reversed following a HP [36]. However, candidates must be chosen judiciously. Anastomotic leak is a feared complication as it is associated with significant morbidity, mortality, and prolonged hospital stay. Yet, there are important differences between the elective and emergent patient population presenting with LBO that place emergency patients at increased risk of leak. Emergency patients typically present dehydrated, malnourished, and without appropriate bowel preparation. Patients may be in shock, requiring vasopressor support, or there may be

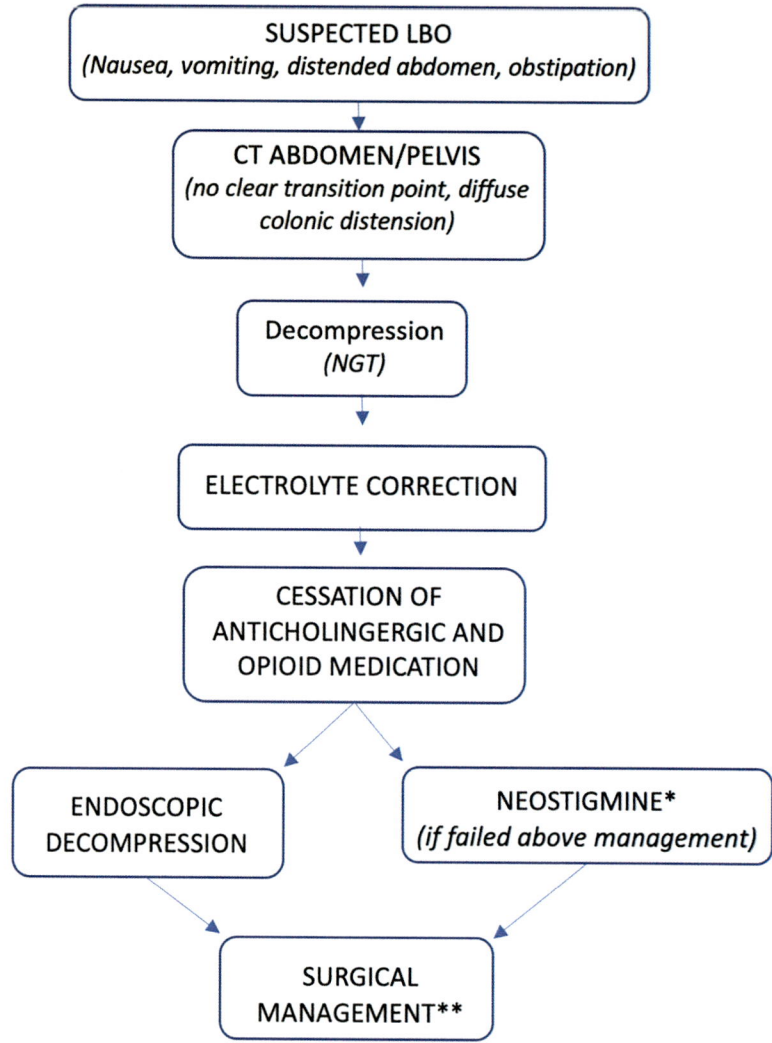

**Fig. 76.2** Flow diagram for the management of pseudo-obstruction. *Neostigmine should be given in a monitored setting as patients are at risk of symptomatic bradycardia. **Surgical management is indicated in the presence of perforation, ischemia or refractory disease

extensive contamination from a proximal perforation. Patient factors including older age and increased body mass index (BMI) (>30) have been associated with higher rates of anastomotic leak [37, 38]. Preoperative poor nutritional status has also been linked with increased postoperative complications including anastomotic leak and intraabdominal collections [39]. These factors must be taken into consideration when deciding between a HP or RPA. Furthermore, if performing a RPA, there has been a movement towards adding a diverting ileostomy. While its use has shown a significantly reduced rates of anastomotic leak in patients undergoing a low-anterior resection for rectal cancer, the evidence support-

ing its application in left-sided obstructing colon cancers is limited [40]. Therefore, the decision to perform a diverting ileostomy remains at the surgeon's discretion. Nevertheless, in patients presenting with uncomplicated left-sided colonic mass, RPA is preferred over HP as this avoids a second major operation [17]. Patients with a high surgical risk or in circumstances where the treating surgeon is not comfortable performing an RPA, HP remains a safe option.

Although less common, it is recommended that patients with right-sided or transverse colonic mass undergo resection with ileocolic anastomosis in a single-staged procedure. If the patient's physiologic status is deemed unfavorable for an anastomosis as delineated previously, a terminal ileostomy with a mucus fistula can be used as a substitute. End ileostomies are associated with a degree of morbidity secondary to significant dehydration, electrolyte imbalance, and acute kidney injury requiring hospitalization [17]. Therefore, these risks as well as those associated with primary anastomosis should be discussed with the patient pre-operatively if possible and taken into account in the intra-operative decision-making.

Patients with left sided colon cancers may be candidates for endoscopic stenting with a self-expanding metallic stent (SEMS). Stenting of colonic malignancies was initially introduced as a palliative measure to relieve obstructed patients [41]. Emergency surgery, especially at centers without access to a colorectal specialist, has been associated with higher rates of morbidity and mortality. Therefore, endoscopic stenting is used as a bridging method to avoid the morbidity and mortality associated with emergency surgery and the risk of stoma formation [42]. While stent placement is user dependent, the literature has reported a 92% success rate of colonic decompression within 72 h of stent placement. A systematic review investigating stent placement in patients with malignant LBO demonstrated that the majority of patients with stents as a bridge to elective intervention underwent surgery within 2–12 days [43]. A retrospective study comparing patients undergoing stent insertion and elective surgery with those undergoing an emergency resection identified a higher number of HPs in patients undergoing emergency surgery. Only 42% of patients in the emergency group underwent a single-staged procedure as compared to 87% of patients in the stented group. Moreover, among all patients undergoing a HP, those in the emergency group had a lower stomal conversion rate in comparison to the previously stented group [44]. As stated previously, stoma-related complications account for a high percentage of morbidity, especially among patients undergoing emergency surgery, as often stoma marking and teaching have not occurred preoperatively [45].

However, there is also concern surrounding the safety of SEMS and the associated risk of perforation, which would prompt an emergency operation and result in upstaging of the disease. Perforation, bowel ischemia, and robust inflammatory findings on CT are contraindications to stent insertion as they are associated with a high complication rate. Tumors located at the splenic flexure, those occupying a long segment of colon, and proximal tumors can be technically challenging which may contribute to a higher failure rate [46]. A systematic review on the safety of SEMS reported a perforation rate of approximately 4.5% and a migration rate of 11% [43]. A multicenter randomized controlled trial comparing stenting versus emergency surgery identified similar complication rates, and no oncologic difference between the two groups. However, the median length of stay was found to be longer in the stented group in comparison to the emergency surgery group [47]. In summary, the ability to stent a patient is based on their physiologic status and the underlying malignant process. If technically feasible, the use of stents as a bridge to elective surgery allows for preoperative optimization including nutrition status, electrolyte replacement, resuscitation following dehydration, and surgical planning. Furthermore, the use of stents is well accepted in the palliative setting, which avoids emergency surgery in poor operative candidates.

Obstructing rectal cancer poses its own challenges. The decision for an abdominal perineal resection versus a low anterior resection should not be a discussion for the emergency setting. Furthermore, an obstructing rectal tumor can be considered locally advanced and as such, is better treated with a multimodal approach. Therefore, according to the World Society of Emergency Surgery, acute obstruction from rectal cancer should be treated with diversion only as to permit a more appropriate evaluation and treatment in an elective setting [17]. A loop ileostomy or colostomy can be considered. There is evidence that loop ileostomies are associated with less complications; however, in obstructed patients with competent ileocecal valves, a colostomy is preferred to facilitate decompression of the distended colon [48].

As the majority of patients undergo CT imaging during initial evaluation, advanced metastatic disease can be diagnosed preoperatively. In patients presenting with a large bowel obstruction with metastatic disease, systemic therapy is the preferred treatment to prolong life expectancy. Therefore, the goal of surgical intervention is not curative, but focused on symptomatic relief and managing complications, without causing undue morbidity and mortality. Patients presenting with hemodynamic stability and minimal physiologic derangements should undergo palliative stent placement if technically feasible. In these situations, stents are preferred over diverting colostomy as stents are associated with a shorter hospital stay and similar morbidity rates. Patients with significant intraabdominal tumor burden who are not candidates for stenting should undergo a diverting stoma with biopsies of potential peritoneal metastatic disease if deemed safe and feasible [17]. Similarly, patients with an extracolonic malignancy resulting in compressive obstruction should undergo a diverting stoma as stenting would not be an option [17]. Palliative bypass or stent insertion provides patients with the best opportunity to begin or resume systemic treatment as soon as possible [47, 49].

Patients presenting in shock with significant physiologic derangements including acidosis, coagulopathy, hypothermia, and hypotension should undergo a damage control laparotomy. The surgical procedure will depend on the patient's physiologic status and the underlying disease. The ultimate goal in the critical setting is source control, decompression, and correction of physiologic derangements. The anastomotic leak rate in patients undergoing emergency surgery ranges from 4% to 13% with a significant increase in severely ill patients [50]. Therefore, the decision to perform an anastomosis is not recommended. Patients with right sided obstruction can be treated with a right hemicolectomy and terminal ileostomy. Unstable patients with left-sided colonic mass should undergo a HP. However, for patients who present with severe physiologic derangement, a loop ileostomy or colostomy for decompression should be the treatment option of choice [17]. If there is concern for the development of abdominal compartment syndrome, progression of ischemia, or extensive contamination secondary to perforation, source control should be achieved with resection and the patient should be left in discontinuity with an open abdomen. Patients should then return to the operating room for definitive management once physiologically normalized.

### Dos and Don'ts

- Patients presenting with an acute abdomen, perforation, or signs of bowel ischemia should be managed surgically.
- Cecal volvulus should not be reduced endoscopically as surgical management is the treatment of choice.
- In the absence of worrisome features, sigmoid volvulus should initially be managed endoscopically prior to definitive surgical management.
- For right-sided obstructions, a single-staged procedure with resection and primary anastomosis should be performed if the risk of leak is minimal.
- For left-sided obstructions, a single-staged procedure with resection and primary anastomosis with or without proximal diversion should strongly be considered; however, a Hartmann's procedure is a safer alternative in certain settings.
- Patients with advanced colon cancer or obstructing rectal cancer should undergo diversion in the emergency setting.
- Stents can be considered as a bridge to definitive management or in palliative settings.

## Take-Home Messages

- Individuals presenting with peritonitis, free air, or signs of bowel ischemia should be taken to the operating room immediately.
- Patients should be evaluated clinically prior to attempting a primary anastomosis as poor nutritional status and hemodynamic instability are associated with higher leak rates.
- In the case of a left-sided obstruction, the preferred management is resection and primary anastomosis with or without proximal diversion; however, a Hartmann's procedure is an acceptable alternative in certain clinical contexts.
- Stenting may also be an option for left-sided colon masses as a bridge to surgery or in the palliative setting.
- Right-sided colonic masses are similarly managed through resection and primary anastomosis if clinically safe; however, an end ileostomy should be performed in high-risk patients.
- Patients with metastatic disease or rectal cancer presenting with an obstruction should undergo proximal diversion; definitive management should not be attempted in an emergency setting.
- For patients presenting with a sigmoid volvulus, endoscopic decompression is the initial method of treatment, and surgery should subsequently be considered as the recurrence rate is high.
- Cecal volvulus requires immediate surgical resection and primary anastomosis.
- Pseudo-obstruction can mimic an LBO, especially in the elderly population or those with significant opioid use. These patients should be managed medically, and surgical intervention should be considered as a rescue option.

## Multiple Choice Questions

1. A 56-year-old male presents to the emergency department with a 1-week history of abdominal pain, distension, and constipation. Computed tomography of the abdomen demonstrates a large rectal mass and local lymphadenopathy. What is the best next step for management of this patient's large bowel obstruction?
    A. Colonoscopy, biopsy, and stent insertion
    B. Emergency laparotomy and low anterior resection
    C. Emergency laparotomy and abdominal perineal resection
    D. Diverting colostomy

**Answer: D**

2. A 78-year-old man with poorly controlled diabetes, hypertension, and coronary artery disease presents with significant abdominal distension and tenderness. The patient describes a history of recent weight loss, poor oral intake, constipation, and a 24-hour history of worsening abdominal pain. Vital signs on presentation are as follows: blood pressure 90/60, heart rate 140, and temperature 38.9. His bloodwork reveals a white blood cell count of 24 and a lactate of 8. The patient is fluid resuscitated, and computed tomography of the abdomen demonstrates a large sigmoid mass, a distended colon ~8 cm and a competent ileocecal valve. What is the best next step for management of this patient's large bowel obstruction?
    A. Emergency total colectomy
    B. Emergency sigmoidectomy and primary anastomosis
    C. Emergency sigmoidectomy, primary anastomosis and diverting ileostomy
    D. Emergency sigmoidectomy and end colostomy

**Answer: D**

3. The same patient in question two now presents with normal hemodynamics and bloodwork. Once again, computed tomography of the abdomen demonstrates a large sigmoid mass, a distended colon ~8 cm and a competent ileocecal valve. What is the best next step for management of this patient's large bowel obstruction?
    A. Conservative management
    B. Emergency total colectomy
    C. Emergency sigmoidectomy and primary anastomosis
    D. Emergency sigmoidectomy and end colostomy

**Answer: C**

4. A 98-year-old man from a nursing home known for diabetes, hypertension, and severe dementia presents with a 24-h history of abdominal distension, pain, and constipation. Vitals signs and bloodwork are unremarkable. An abdominal film shows distended loops with the largest projecting to the right-upper-quadrant. A computed tomography of the abdomen demonstrates a large sigmoid volvulus, with no pneumatosis, nor perforation. What is the best next step for management of this patients' large bowel obstruction?
    A. Endoscopic decompression
    B. Emergency laparotomy and sigmoidectomy with primary anastomosis
    C. Emergency laparotomy and sigmoidectomy with end colostomy
    D. Emergency laparotomy and sigmoidopexy

**Answer: A**

5. The same patient in question four presents with a computed tomography of the abdomen demonstrating a cecal volvulus without signs of bowel compromise. What is the best next step for management of this patients' large bowel obstruction?
    A. Endoscopic decompression
    B. Emergency laparotomy, right hemicolectomy and primary anastomosis
    C. Emergency laparotomy, right hemicolectomy and end ileostomy
    D. Emergency laparotomy and cecopexy

**Answer: B**

6. A 62-year-old man, previously healthy, presents to the emergency department with gradual abdominal distension and constipation. Physical examination is within normal limits and no mass is palpable on rectal examination. Lab results demonstrate a microcytic anemia. Computed tomography of the abdomen shows a distended colon >6 cm and a large sigmoid mass with three liver lesions suspicious for metastatic disease. What is the best next step for management of this patient's large bowel obstruction?
    A. Emergency laparotomy and sigmoidectomy with primary anastomosis
    B. Colonic stent insertion
    C. Emergency laparotomy, sigmoidectomy with primary anastomosis and synchronous resection of liver metastases
    D. Emergency laparotomy, sigmoidectomy and end colostomy

**Answer: B**

7. A 75-year-old woman known for smoking and rheumatoid arthritis on prednisone, underwent a left hemicolectomy and primary anastomosis for a sigmoid cancer. On postoperative day one the patient suffered from a myocardial infarction resulting in cardiogenic shock. The patient was immediately intubated, started on dobutamine, and admitted to the intensive care unit. Which of the following factors will have a major effect on the survivability of the patient's anastomosis?

A. Smoking
B. Steroids
C. Hypotension
D. All of the above

**Answer: D**

8. An 89-year-old woman with Parkinson's disease and diabetes presents to the emergency department from her nursing home with abdominal distension and tenderness. Upon presentation her vitals are within normal limits, and her abdomen is distended with minimal tenderness. Computed tomography of the abdomen demonstrates pan-colonic distension with no clear transition point. What is the best next step for management of this patient's large bowel obstruction?
   A. Endoscopic decompression
   B. Laparotomy, total colectomy and end ileostomy
   C. Nasogastric tube and electrolyte replacement
   D. Neostigmine

**Answer: C**

9. The above patient from question eight presents with a similar scenario; however, she is tachycardic on admission (150) and has a significant leukocytosis (24). Plain film of the abdomen shows a large distended colon >11 cm and free air under the diaphragm. What is the best next step for management of this patient's large bowel obstruction?
   A. Endoscopic decompression and observation
   B. Total colectomy and ileorectal anastomosis
   C. Total colectomy and end ileostomy
   D. Neostigmine

**Answer: C**

10. A 75-year-old patient known for urothelial cancer treated with a radical cystectomy presents to the emergency department with gradual abdominal distension and constipation. On examination the patient's abdomen is distended with minimal tenderness. Computed tomography of the abdomen demonstrates a large pelvic mass, suspicious for recurrence, compressing the rectum resulting in a transition point. What is the best next step for management of this patients' large bowel obstruction?
    A. Stent insertion
    B. Exploratory laparotomy and debulking of pelvic mass
    C. Diverting colostomy
    D. Observation

**Answer: C**

# References

1. Townsend CM Jr, et al. Sabiston textbook of surgery: the biological basis of modern surgical practice. 17th ed. Philadelphia: Elsevier Saunders; 2004.
2. Gore RM, Silvers RI, Thakrar KH, Wenzke DR, Mehta UK, Newmark GM, et al. Bowel obstruction. Radiol Clin N Am. 2015;53(6):1225–40.
3. Markogiannakis H, Messaris E, Dardamanis D, Pararas N, Tzertzemelis D, Giannopolous P, Larentzakis A, Lagoudianakis E, Manouras A, Bramis I. Acute mechanical bowel obstruction: Clinical presentation, etiology, management and outcome. World J Gastroenterol. 2007;3(13):432–7.
4. Biondo S, Pares D, Frago R, Marti-Rague J, Kreisler E, De Oca J, et al. Large bowel obstruction: predictive factors for postoperative mortality. Dis Colon Rectum. 2004;47(11):1889–97.
5. Frago R, Ramirez E, Millan M, Kreisler E, del Valle E, Biondo S. Current management of acute malignant large bowel obstruction: a systematic review. Am J Surg. 2014;207(1):127–38.
6. Yeo HL, Lee SW. Colorectal emergencies: review and controversies in the management of large bowel obstruction. J Gastrointest Surg. 2013;17(11):2007–12.
7. Luca Ansaloni REA, Bazzoli F, Catena F, Cennamo V, Di Saverio S, Fuccio L, Jeekel H, Leppäniemi A, Moore E, Pinna AD, Pisano M, Repici A, Sugarbaker PH, Tuech J-J. Guidelines in the management of obstructing cancer of the left colon: consensus conference of the World Society of Emergency Surgery (WSES) and Peritoneum and Surgery (PnS) Society. World J Emerg Surg. 2010;5:29.
8. Verheyden C, Orliac C, Millet I, Taourel P. Large-bowel obstruction: CT findings, pitfalls, tips and tricks. Eur J Radiol. 2020;130:109155.

9. Myers EA, Feingold DL, Forde KA, Arnell T, Jang JH, Whelan RL. Colorectal cancer in patients under 50 years of age: a retrospective analysis of two institutions' experience. World J Gastroenterol. 2013;19(34):5651–7.
10. Matrana MR, Margolin DA. Epidemiology and pathophysiology of diverticular disease. Clin Colon Rectal Surg. 2009;22(3):141–6.
11. Swenson BR, Kwaan MR, Burkart NE, Wang Y, Madoff RD, Rothenberger DA, et al. Colonic volvulus: presentation and management in metropolitan Minnesota, United States. Dis Colon Rectum. 2012;55(4):444–9.
12. Rex DK. Colonoscopy and acute colonic pseudo-obstruction. Gastrointest Endosc Clin N Am. 1997;7(3):499–508.
13. De Giorgio R, Sarnelli G, Corinaldesi R, Stanghellini V. Advances in our understanding of the pathology of chronic intestinal pseudo-obstruction. Gut. 2004;53(11):1549–52.
14. Vanek VW, Al-Salti M. Acute pseudo-obstruction of the colon (Ogilvie's syndrome). An analysis of 400 cases. Dis Colon Rectum. 1986;29(3):203–10.
15. Werner J, Preotle J. Atypical obstructions: what do emergency providers need to know about incarcerated and strangulated hernia, closed loop obstruction, volvulus, and internal hernia? What is the prognostic value of a lactate? In: Graham A, Carlberg DJ, editors. Gastrointestinal emergencies: evidence-based answers to key clinical questions. Cham: Springer International Publishing; 2019. p. 179–82.
16. Cappell MS, Batke M. Mechanical obstruction of the small bowel and colon. Med Clin N Am. 2008;92(3):575–97.
17. Pisano M, Zorcolo L, Merli C, Cimbanassi S, Poiasina E, Ceresoli M, et al. 2017 WSES guidelines on colon and rectal cancer emergencies: obstruction and perforation. World J Emerg Surg. 2018;13(1):36.
18. Angelelli G, Scardapane A, Memeo M, Stabile Ianora AA, Rotondo A. Acute bowel ischemia: CT findings. Eur J Radiol. 2004;50(1):37–47.
19. Vernuccio F, Picone D, Scerrino G, Midiri M, Lo Re G, Lagalla R, et al. Intravenous contrast agent in abdominal CT: is it really needed to identify the cause of bowel obstruction? Proof of concept. Gastroenterol Res Pract. 2019;2019:2350948.
20. Levenson RB, Camacho MA, Horn E, Saghir A, McGillicuddy D, Sanchez LD. Eliminating routine oral contrast use for CT in the emergency department: impact on patient throughput and diagnosis. Emerg Radiol. 2012;19(6):513–7.
21. Thompson JS. Contrast radiography and intestinal obstruction. Ann Surg. 2002;236(1):7–8.
22. Levsky JM, Den EI, DuBrow RA, Wolf EL, Rozenblit AM. CT findings of sigmoid volvulus. Am J Roentgenol. 2010;194(1):136–43.
23. Choi JS, Lim JS, Kim H, Choi J-Y, Kim M-J, Kim NK, et al. Colonic pseudoobstruction: CT findings. Am J Roentgenol. 2008;190(6):1521–6.
24. Beall DP, Fortman BJ, Lawler BC, Regan F. Imaging bowel obstruction: a comparison between fast magnetic resonance imaging and helical computed tomography. Clin Radiol. 2002;57(8):719–24.
25. Ifversen AK, Kjaer DW. More patients should undergo surgery after sigmoid volvulus. World J Gastroenterol. 2014;20(48):18384–9.
26. Lou Z, Yu E-D, Zhang W, Meng R-G, Hao L-Q, Fu C-G. Appropriate treatment of acute sigmoid volvulus in the emergency setting. World J Gastroenterol. 2013;19(30):4979–83.
27. Kazem Shahmoradi M, Khoshdani Farahani P, Sharifian M. Evaluating outcomes of primary anastomosis versus Hartmann's procedure in sigmoid volvulus: a retrospective-cohort study. Ann Med Surg. 2021;62:160–3.
28. Rosen MJ, Cobb WS, Kercher KW, Sing RF, Heniford BT. Laparoscopic restoration of intestinal continuity after Hartmann's procedure. Am J Surg. 2005;189(6):670–4.
29. Atamanalp SS. Comments on 'Colectomy for caecal and sigmoid volvulus: a national analysis of outcomes and risk factors for postoperative complications'. Color Dis. 2020;22(3):346.
30. Johnson CD, Rice RP, Kelvin FM, Foster WL, Williford ME. The radiologic evaluation of gross cecal distension: emphasis on cecal ileus. AJR Am J Roentgenol. 1985;145(6):1211–7.
31. Kahi CJ, Rex DK. Bowel obstruction and pseudo-obstruction. Gastroenterol Clin N Am. 2003;32(4):1229–47.
32. Weinstock LB, Chang AC. Methylnaltrexone for treatment of acute colonic pseudo-obstruction. J Clin Gastroenterol. 2011;45(10):883–4.
33. Vantrappen G. Acute colonic pseudo-obstruction. Lancet. 1993;341(8838):152–3.
34. Cameron JL, Cameron AM. Current surgical therapy. 11th ed. London: Royal College of Surgeons; 2015.
35. Trompetas V. Emergency management of malignant acute left-sided colonic obstruction. Ann R Coll Surg Engl. 2008;90(3):181–6.
36. Desai DC, Brennan EJ Jr, Reilly JF, Smink RD Jr. The utility of the Hartmann procedure. Am J Surg. 1998;175(2):152–4.
37. Bakker IS, Grossmann I, Henneman D, Havenga K, Wiggers T. Risk factors for anastomotic leakage and leak-related mortality after colonic cancer surgery in a nationwide audit. Br J Surg. 2014;101(4):424–32; discussion 32.
38. Nugent TS, Kelly ME, Donlon NE, Fahy MR, Larkin JO, McCormick PH, et al. Obesity and anastomotic leak rates in colorectal cancer: a meta-analysis. Int J Color Dis. 2021;36:1819–29.
39. Tokunaga R, Sakamoto Y, Nakagawa S, Miyamoto Y, Yoshida N, Oki E, et al. Prognostic nutritional index predicts severe complications, recurrence, and poor prognosis in patients with colorectal cancer undergoing primary tumor resection. Dis Colon Rectum. 2015;58(11):1048–57.

40. Mrak K, Uranitsch S, Pedross F, Heuberger A, Klingler A, Jagoditsch M, et al. Diverting ileostomy versus no diversion after low anterior resection for rectal cancer: a prospective, randomized, multicenter trial. Surgery. 2016;159(4):1129–39.
41. Dohmoto M. New method-endoscopic implantation of rectal stent in palliative treatment of malignant stenosis. Endosc Dig. 1991;3:1507–12.
42. Morris EJ, Taylor EF, Thomas JD, Quirke P, Finan PJ, Coleman MP, et al. Thirty-day postoperative mortality after colorectal cancer surgery in England. Gut. 2011;60(6):806–13.
43. Watt AM, Faragher IG, Griffin TT, Rieger NA, Maddern GJ. Self-expanding metallic stents for relieving malignant colorectal obstruction: a systematic review. Ann Surg. 2007;246(1):24–30.
44. Lee GJ, Kim HJ, Baek J-H, Lee W-S, Kwon KA. Comparison of short-term outcomes after elective surgery following endoscopic stent insertion and emergency surgery for obstructive colorectal cancer. Int J Surg. 2013;11(6):442–6.
45. Martinez-Santos C, Lobato RF, Fradejas JM, Pinto I, Ortega-Deballón P, Moreno-Azcoita M. Self-expandable stent before elective surgery vs. emergency surgery for the treatment of malignant colorectal obstructions: comparison of primary anastomosis and morbidity rates. Dis Colon Rectum. 2002;45(3):401–6.
46. de Gregorio MA, Mainar A, Rodriguez J, Alfonso ER, Tejero E, Herrera M, et al. Colon stenting: a review. Semin Intervent Radiol. 2004;21(3):205–16.
47. Arezzo A, Balague C, Targarona E, Borghi F, Giraudo G, Ghezzo L, et al. Colonic stenting as a bridge to surgery versus emergency surgery for malignant colonic obstruction: results of a multicentre randomised controlled trial (ESCO trial). Surg Endosc. 2017;31(8):3297–305.
48. Geng HZ, Nasier D, Liu B, Gao H, Xu YK. Meta-analysis of elective surgical complications related to defunctioning loop ileostomy compared with loop colostomy after low anterior resection for rectal carcinoma. Ann R Coll Surg Engl. 2015;97(7):494–501.
49. Malakorn S, Stein SL, Lee JH, You YN. Urgent management of obstructing colorectal cancer: divert, stent, or resect? J Gastrointest Surg. 2019;23(2):425–32.
50. Lee YM, Law WL, Chu KW, Poon RT. Emergency surgery for obstructing colorectal cancers: a comparison between right-sided and left-sided lesions. J Am Coll Surg. 2001;192(6):719–25.

## Further Reading

Frago R, Ramirez E, Millan M, Kreisler E, del Valle E, Biondo S. Current management of acute malignant large bowel obstruction: a systematic review. Am J Surg. 2014;207(1):127–38.

Luca Ansaloni REA, Bazzoli F, Catena F, Cennamo V, Di Saverio S, Fuccio L, Jeekel H, Leppäniemi A, Moore E, Pinna AD, Pisano M, Repici A, Sugarbaker PH, Tuech J-J. Guidelines in the management of obstructing cancer of the left colon: consensus conference of the World Society of Emergency Surgery (WSES) and Peritoneum and Surgery (PnS) Society. World J Emerg Surg. 2010;5:29.

Malakorn S, Stein SL, Lee JH, You YN. Urgent management of obstructing colorectal cancer: divert, stent, or resect? J Gastrointest Surg. 2019;23(2):425–32.

Pisano M, Zorcolo L, Merli C, Cimbanassi S, Poiasina E, Ceresoli M, et al. 2017 WSES guidelines on colon and rectal cancer emergencies: obstruction and perforation. World J Emerg Surg. 2018;13(1):36.

Watt AM, Faragher IG, Griffin TT, Rieger NA, Maddern GJ. Self-expanding metallic stents for relieving malignant colorectal obstruction: a systematic review. Ann Surg. 2007;246(1):24–30.

Yeo HL, Lee SW. Colorectal emergencies: review and controversies in the management of large bowel obstruction. J Gastrointest Surg. 2013;17(11):2007–12.

# Large Bowel Perforation

**77**

V. Khokha

**Learning Goals**

- Main causes of large bowel perforation.
- Useful diagnostic tools.
- Principles of surgical treatment depending on the etiology and course of large bowel perforation.

## 77.1 Introduction

Large bowel perforation is a violation of the integrity of the intestinal wall, accompanied by the release of intestinal contents into the abdominal cavity. It is an urgent condition requiring emergency surgery, diagnosed on the basis of clinical symptoms and data from instrumental examination methods. Morbidity and mortality in these patients depend on age, preoperative health status, operating surgeon, time of surgical intervention, and type of surgical procedure. Large bowel perforation continues to carry a high risk despite several major changes in the provision of emergency surgery. Further developments are needed to improve postoperative outcomes in these patients.

### 77.1.1 Epidemiology

Large bowel perforation is the second most common cause of free gas in the abdomen after perforation of the stomach and duodenum [1]. Because of the large number of bacteria in the large intestine, colon perforation is rapidly complicated by the development of bacterial peritonitis. The mortality rate for perforations of this anatomical part of the intestine reaches 50%. Especially often a poor prognosis is observed in the elderly. Colon perforations subdivided into non-traumatic and traumatic.

### 77.1.2 Etiology

The first place in terms of prevalence among the causes of non-traumatic perforations is occupied by acute diverticulitis (45–50% of the total number of cases). Approximately 12% of patients with diverticulitis present with complicated disease [2].

The overall incidence of perforated diverticular disease is 2.66 per 100,000 person-years and 6.11 per 100,000 person-years in those over the age of 45 years [3]. Inflammatory complications, when they occur, usually result from inflammation around a single diverticulum. This may lead to the formation of a pericolic or pelvic abscess. Free perforation of these leads to purulent peritonitis. The original communication with the lumen

V. Khokha (✉)
City Hospital, Mozyr, Belarus

of the bowel usually is obliterated. More rarely, with either rapid evolution or failure of the diverticular neck to obliterate, a free communication develops between the bowel lumen and the peritoneal cavity, leading to fecal peritonitis [4].

Large bowel obstruction represents almost 80% (15–30% of colorectal cancer [CRC]) of the emergencies related to colorectal cancer (CRC), while perforation accounts for the remaining 20% (1–10% of CRC) [5]. The prevalence of perforation in colon cancer patients is reported to be 3–10%. CRC patients with perforation exhibit a greater frequency of recurrence and poorer overall survival compared with those without perforation [6]. Perforation occurs at the tumor site in almost 70% of cases and proximal to the tumor site in around 30% of cases [7–9], occurring most commonly in the sigmoid colon (47.3%) and cecum (24.8%). Two mechanisms are recognized: (1) tumor necrosis and subsequent perforation at the tumor site, usually causes a small amount of free gas; (2) diastatic—occurs proximal to the malignancy, as a result of bowel distension secondary to obstruction, frequently occurs at the cecum, and usually leads to massive pneumoperitoneum or pneumo-retroperitoneum.

In toxic megacolon, as a result of paralysis of the colonic smooth muscle, leading to dilatation and subsequent ischemic necrosis, the diameter of the transverse colon ranges from 6 to 15 cm. Colonic perforation occurs in 30–50% of cases and is associated with a high mortality rate [10].

Perforation of the bowel caused by pressure necrosis from a fecal mass (stercoral perforation) is a rare entity, first reported by Berry at the Pathological Society of London in 1894. There appears to be an equal incidence in men and women and the median age for these patients is 60 years. Predisposing factors have included chronic constipation, megacolon, scleroderma, hypercalcemia, renal failure, and renal transplantation. Medications associated with stercoral perforation include narcotics, postoperative analgesia, antacids, calcium channel blockers, and antidepressants. Only 11% of cases are accurately diagnosed prior to operation. Perforations usually occur on the antimesenteric border, with the majority occurring in the sigmoid colon and rectosigmoid region [11]. Zhang et al. report about spontaneous perforation of the colon, defined as a sudden perforation of the normal colon in the absence of diseases such as tumors, diverticulosis, or external injury [12]. In the description the authors indicate that spontaneous colonic perforation caused by compression of the colonic wall with the solid feculent mass, what leads to ischemia and necrosis of colonic mucosa. Consequently, the authors interpret stercoral perforation as spontaneous.

The most usual type of intestinal ischemia is ischemic colitis. It is an insult to the colonic wall resulting from diminished blood flow. This can range from superficial injury of the mucosa and submucosal layer to full thickness necrosis of the colonic wall. Most attacks are transient and resolve spontaneously, whereas others may result to gangrene and necrosis of the colon with resultant perforation and feculent peritonitis. It mostly occurs in old patients (80%) and mainly occurs among debilitated elderly women [13].

Colon injuries are subdivided into nondestructive and destructive that involve 50% or greater of the colon wall circumference or occur with segmental devascularization. Traumatic large bowel injury occurs in approximately 51% of patients with penetrating hollow viscus injuries, and the transverse colon is the most commonly injured segment. Perforation is found in approximately 0.5% of patients with major blunt trauma and is diagnosed in approximately 10% of patients undergoing laparotomy. The right colon is the most commonly injured segment followed by the transverse colon or the sigmoid colon, and the left colon. The massive deceleration force may result in mesenteric tears and ischemic necrosis of the colon. In rare settings, a colonic wall contusion may cause delayed perforation several days after the injury [14].

Iatrogenic perforations are most likely to occur in diseased rather than in healthy bowel. They comprise 20% of colorectal perforations, usually occurring post-colonoscopy and most commonly involving the sigmoid (40.7%), followed by the rectum and cecum. Globally, the incidence is estimated to be 0.016–0.8% for diagnostic colonoscopies and 0.02–8% for therapeutic colonoscopies [15]. The mechanisms of perforation associated with colonoscopy are as follows: (1) direct mechanical trauma caused by the forward movement of the tip of the colonoscope, (2) lateral pressure against the bowel wall caused by bowing of a loop of the scope, (3) passage of the endoscope through areas of pathology (e.g., strictures, tumors, and diverticula), (4) barotrauma caused by excessive air insufflation, and (5) application of electrosurgical current during therapeutic procedures [16–18].

The perforation risk in colorectal stenting for colorectal cancer obstruction is 7.4%; almost 70% of perforations occur in the first week after stent placement. The risk of perforation influences the type of stent. Van Halsema et al. in meta-analysis showed that of the nine most frequently used stent types, the WallFlex, the Comvi, and the Niti-S D-type had a perforation rate >10%, while Hanarostent and the Niti-S covered stent <5%. The authors also found the perforation rate in stented patients treated without concomitant therapies, with chemotherapy with bevacizumab and without it 9.0%, 12.5%, and 7.0%, respectively [19].

Large bowel perforation is a rare complication of percutaneous renal surgery, reported in <1% of cases. Patients at higher risk for colonic injury include those with congenital anomalies such as horseshoe kidney and other forms of renal fusion and ectopia, as well as those with colonic distention resulting from jejunoileal bypass, partial ileal bypass, neurologic impairment, and "institutional" bowel. Other proposed risk factors are lower pole puncture, left-sided procedure, previous colonic surgery, older age, and female sex [20].

Colonic perforation occasionally may be due to foreign bodies. Over 300 cases of bowel perforation caused by foreign bodies have been reported in the literature, with fish bones, chicken bones, and dentures being the commonest objects, followed by toothpicks and cocktail sticks. Foreign body-associated perforation commonly occurs at the point of acute angulation and narrowing [21].

**Table 77.1** Classification by the etiology of perforation

| |
|---|
| *1. Non-traumatic* |
| Diverticulitis |
| Cancer |
| Perforated toxic megacolon |
| Stercoral perforation |
| Ischemic colon perforation |
| *2. Traumatic* |
| Open (stab wound, gunshot) |
| Blunt (nondestructive, destructive) |
| Iatrogenic (colonoscopy, stenting, percutaneous renal surgery, during laparoscopic operations, abortion) |
| Foreign bodies |

### 77.1.3 Classification (Table 77.1)

Depending on the cause and localization, there can be following types of colon perforation: extraperitoneal, confined (sealed-off) intraperitoneal, and free intraperitoneal. Accordingly, the clinical variants may be retroperitoneal abscess or phlegmon, intraperitoneal abscess, purulent peritonitis (due to abscess breakthrough into the abdominal cavity), fecal peritonitis. When tumor of the colon or a diverticulum due to inflammation ingrows to adjacent bladder an intestinal-bladder fistula forms, accompanied by the release of gases and intestinal contents from the urethra. Rarely, the colon perforates into the abdominal wall and patients may present with extensive cellulitis and an enterocutaneous fistula.

## 77.2 Diagnosis

### 77.2.1 Clinical Presentation

Rapid diagnosis and treatment of these conditions are essential to reduce the high morbidity and mortality. The type and degree of peritoneal contamination depend on the site, size, and duration of the perforation and on the physiologic state, including the time from the last meal, administration of a mechanical bowel preparation before the perforation, coexistent diseases, and the presence or absence of an ileus or bowel obstruction with accompanying bacterial overgrowth. Colonic perforations may present without immediate perforation-associated pain and tend to have a slower clinical progression, with the development of a secondary bacterial peritonitis or localized abscess formation.

A thorough history and physical examination are crucial. It should be obtained from the patient, family, or bystanders when possible and should focus on the history of the present condition, symptoms, time course of events, pain, type, evolution, medication, allergies, past history (cancer, abdominal surgery), and obstruction (last bowel movement, vomiting), colonoscopy (when, why). General signs and symptoms include sudden onset of abdominal pain and abdominal distention, nausea, vomiting, obstipation, fever, decreased or absent bowel sounds, loss of liver dullness on right upper quadrant percussion. The vital signs provide clues regarding disease severity, volume status, pain severity, systemic inflammatory response syndrome (SIRS), and sepsis. Tachycardia, hypoxia, tachypnea, and hypotension suggest a compromised physiologic state consistent with shock.

## 77.2.2 Tests

Laboratory tests typically include a complete blood cell count, coagulation, and electrolyte panel, liver function tests, arterial blood gas, and serum lactate level, and infections markers such as procalcitonin and C-reactive protein (CRP).

Despite the low sensitivity, accuracy and a negative predictive value an upright chest radiograph, and in severely ill latero-lateral supine abdominal radiographs are an inexpensive and rapid test of patients who have a high suspicion for hollow viscus perforation [22]. The mainstream radiologic sign of the colon perforation is pneumoperitoneum. However, nearly 50% of patients who had hollow viscus perforation at laparotomy failed to demonstrate pneumoperitoneum on plain abdominal radiographs [23]. It is mandatory that plain abdominal X-ray includes both subdiaphragmatic regions. Moreover, the finding of pneumoperitoneum in patients who have acute abdominal pain is not always associated with the need for surgery for hollow viscus perforation. Commonly reported nonsurgical causes of pneumoperitoneum include (a) thoracic (positive pressure ventilation, pulmonary bleb rupture, cardiopulmonary resuscitation); (b) abdominal (recent laparoscopy or laparotomy, peritoneal dialysis, spontaneous bacterial peritonitis); (c) gynecologic (pelvic inflammatory disease, vaginal douching or insufflation, sexual intercourse).

Ultrasonography (US) is an excellent tool to rapidly evaluate pneumoperitoneum, free intra-abdominal fluid, and gynecologic pathology. US is widely available and frequently used to evaluate patients with acute abdominal pain. Bedside abdominal US has a higher sensitivity and same specificity with abdominal plain X-ray; moreover, it allows environmental stress reduction to an acutely ill patient [24]. US has the advantage of a real-time dynamic examination and this characteristic conveys dynamic information about bowel motility and depicted blood flow, suggesting a variety of pathologies, including perforated viscus. A perforation can be diagnosed at US when echogenic lines or spots with comet-tail reverberation artefacts representing free intraperitoneal air are seen adjacent to the abdominal wall in a supine patient. A sensitivity of 92% and a specificity of 53% have been reported for the detection of perforation with US and constitute an overall accuracy of 88% [25, 26]. One of the limitations of the abdominal US and of the abdominal plain X-ray is the risk of false negatives of pneumoperitoneum, when a small amount of intraperitoneal free air is present, such as in the case of early perforation at the tumor site [27].

The diagnosis of colon perforation relies heavily on computed tomographic (CT) evaluation. The sensitivity and specificity of triple-contrast (oral, rectal, and intravenous) CT scan are found to be 97 and 98%, respectively, albeit lower for blunt colonic trauma. The intravenous contrast-only CT scan also shows high sensitivity and specificity, 91% and 96%, respectively. CT findings include critical bowel diameter for perforation (cecal—10 cm, transverse—8 cm, descending—6 cm), extraluminal gas, visible bowel wall discontinuity, extraluminal contrast, bowel wall thickening, abnormal mural enhancement, localized fat stranding and/or free fluid, as well as localized phlegmon or abscess in confined perforations [28].

Digital rectal exams (DRE) routinely used on trauma patients and the presence of gross blood on DRE can be significant for a colorectal injury. However, the sensitivity of the DRE for the diagnosis of colon injury is poor and the DRE is not recommended as a screening tool for traumatic colon injuries.

## 77.3 Treatment

### 77.3.1 Medical Treatment

The treatment of colonic perforation includes fluid resuscitation, antibiotics, source control, organ system support, and nutrition. The overall clinical state of the patient dictates the treatment. Patients in extremis from diffuse peritonitis require rapid resuscitation, initiation of antibiotics, and emergency surgery. Relatively stable patients undergo a similar therapeutic approach but with a greater focus on preoperative optimization of the patient's physiologic status with vigorous resuscitation and correction of any concurrent coagulopathy, acidosis, and electrolyte disturbances [29].

The choice of antimicrobials depends on the general condition of the patient, severity of infection, the pathogens presumed to be involved, local epidemiological data and resistance profiles. Considering intestinal microbiota of large bowel acute diverticulitis requires antibiotic coverage for Gram-positive and Gram-negative bacteria, as well as for anaerobes. Most of the colonic perforations is mainly a community-acquired infection. The main resistance threat in IAIs is posed by extended-spectrum beta-lactamase (ESBL)-producing Enterobacteriaceae, which are becoming increasingly common in community-acquired infections worldwide [30]. Candida species frequently contribute to polymicrobial infections in patients with gastroduodenal perforation or anastomotic leaks after bowel surgery. However, according to the study of de Ruiter et al., Candida was not at all isolated in appendicular perforation. This suggests that Candida is not an important pathogen in large bowel perforation. Hence, the routine use of empiric antifungal agents in these patients is unnecessary [31]. Further studies could help to identify subpopulations of patients who might benefit from antifungal therapy.

Fluid therapy to improve microvascular blood flow and increase cardiac output is an essential part of the treatment of patients with large bowel perforation and sepsis. Crystalloid solutions should be the first choice because they are well tolerated and cheap [32]. They should be infused rapidly to induce a quick response and should be interrupted when no improvement of tissue perfusion occurs in response to volume loading. Basal lung crepitations may indicate fluid overload or impaired cardiac function. Recently, measuring inferior vena cava (IVC) diameter by ultrasound was suggested as a novel outcome measure to guide this resuscitative approach [33] avoiding fluid overload.

### 77.3.2 Surgical Treatment

The general principles of surgical treatment of colon perforations include suture, resection of the involved bowel segment, colostomy or primary anastomosis with or without defunctioning ileostomy, debridement of necrotic tissue. The laparoscopic approach is feasible for many emergency conditions and it possible only if the patient has stable vital parameters. It has the advantage to allow, at the same time, an adequate diagnosis and appropriate treatment with a less invasive abdominal approach [34].

A careful revision of the abdominal cavity, the colonic disease and physiological status of the patient are cornerstone in choosing of the surgical tactics. However, no uniform surgical strategy exists worldwide for patients with generalized peritonitis from colon perforation. Depending on the etiology of perforation, surgical treatment has its own peculiarities.

### 77.3.2.1 Non-traumatic Perforations

*Source control of acute left and right-sided diverticulitis.* The abscess size of 4–5 cm has been found as a reasonable limit between antibiotic treatment alone, versus percutaneous drainage combined with antibiotic treatment in the management of diverticular abscesses. When percutaneous drainage is not feasible and the patient's clinical conditions allow it, antibiotic therapy alone can be considered. In case of worsening of inflammatory signs or when the abscess does not reduce with medical therapy a surgical treatment should be performed. Hartmann's procedure (HP) has been considered the procedure of choice in patients with generalized diverticular peritonitis, and is especially useful in critically ill patients and in patients with multiple comorbidities [35]. In 2019, the results of the LADIES study [36] demonstrated that in hemodynamically stable, immunocompetent patients younger than 85 years, primary anastomosis is preferable to the HP. In the setting of purulent or fecal diverticular peritonitis (Hinchey III or Hinchey IV disease) in physiologically stable patients laparoscopic sigmoidectomy with primary anastomosis may be feasible [37]. A viable alternative is the association of a defunctioning ileostomy. This alternative doesn't reduce the rate of anastomosis leakage but allows to manage conservatively the eventual anastomotic complication. Colonic intraoperative lavage through cecal enterotomy and washing catheter insertion may help in reducing anastomosis related complications.

### Colorectal Cancer

The priority is immediate patient safety and control of the source of sepsis, but principles of oncologic resection should be followed. For right-sided perforation, a right colectomy should be performed. In case of poor general or adverse local conditions, a resection without anastomosis and terminal ileostomy should be performed. For transverse/left-sided perforation: resection with anastomosis, with or without ileostomy, should be attempted. Hartmann's procedure might be considered, keeping in mind the low rate of stoma reversal. In case of diastatic perforation a subtotal colectomy should be attempted. Postoperative diarrhea is less common with resection of less than 10 cm of terminal ileum and a distant colon remnant above the peritoneal reflection of at least 10 cm of length [27].

### Ischemic Colitis

Colon resection is required in case of gangrenous bowel in ischemic colitis and is usually performed with open laparotomy but it can be performed also laparoscopically. Severe ischemia is usually limited to the mucosa and the submucosa, so the extent of bowel resection can be scheduled preoperatively on colonoscopy or contrast CT imaging. Right hemicolectomy with ileostomy is usually performed for right-sided colonic ischemia and necrosis, respectively a HP for left-sided. More extensive ischemia in the large bowel with massive bleeding may urge for subtotal colectomy and end ileostomy. The decision for anastomosis depends on the patient's general condition and trend for ongoing ischemia.

### Ulcerative Colitis

The threshold for surgical intervention in ulcerative colitis must be extremely low. The emergent indications for surgery include perforation, uncontrolled hemorrhage, fulminant disease failure of medical therapy, and toxic megacolon. Clinical deterioration, increasing colonic dilation, colonic "thumb printing", or pneumatosis intestinalis on imaging studies are indications for emergent surgery. The most common surgical procedure in the emergent setting of fulminant colitis or toxic megacolon is total abdominal colectomy (TAC) with end ileostomy. Proctectomy should not be performed in the emergent setting as it increases the procedural time, risk of injury to pelvic nerves, risk of bleeding, and negatively affects the future ileal pouch-anal anastomosis [38, 39].

### 77.3.2.2 Stercoral Perforations

Successful management depends on early diagnosis as the mortality is high—34%. If peritonitis is recognized, an emergency laparotomy is indicated. Although there are a few reports of successful primary repair, the usual procedure is a HP with resection of the site of perforation. A primary repair may be justified where peritoneal contamination is minimal and the patient is stable [39].

### 77.3.2.3 Traumatic Perforations

Patients who undergo surgery within 12 h are more appropriate candidates for less invasive techniques, such as primary suturing of the defect or linear wedge resection. When edges of perforation are healthy, well vascularized and can be approximated without tension and narrowing, the bowel lumen primary repair can be done [40]. Fundamental in deciding surgical approach in traumatic perforations are the patient general conditions. Unstable patients should be considered for damage control procedures. Wullstein et al. determined the size of the defect suitable for laparoscopic suturing 1 cm, 2.5 cm for marginal resection, above 2.5 cm for segmental resection. Both sutured and stapled repair techniques seem to be safe and feasible to repair defects of up to 4 cm [41]. The defect should be free of significant inflammation and the colon mobilized well enough to perform a tension-free repair. In case of colon perforation during colonoscopy the European Society of Gastrointestinal Endoscopy guidelines recommend considering endoscopic closure if the bowel is clean and within the first 4 h [42]. It can be done with metal or hemoclips, over or through the scope, band-ligation, fully covered self-expanded metal stent. Colonic resection may be indicated if the traumatic perforation edges are devitalized, or an avulsion of the adjacent mesocolon is seen. The severity of peritonitis and condition of the bowel seem to be more important than the size of the defect. In the setting of diffuse peritonitis in clinically stable patients without comorbidities primary resection and anastomosis with or without a diverting stoma is indicated. In critically ill patients and/or in patients with multiple major comorbidities HP is preferable [43].

In cases of delayed surgery (>24 h), extensive peritoneal contamination, major comorbidities, or a deterioration of the general status of the patient (i.e., sepsis), a staged repair or colostomy by exteriorization of the perforation (e.g., double-barreled colostomy) must also be considered. Patient with traumatic colonic perforation should be considered decompensated, who will benefit from the damage control (DC) if at least one of the following items is present: pH <7.2, core temperature <35 °C, BE <−8, laboratory/clinical evidence of coagulopathy, any signs of sepsis/septic shock, the necessity of inotropic support [44]. Becher et al. [45] added to the aforementioned conditions age ≥70 years and multiple comorbidities.

Timing of source control interventions has not yet been studied adequately. Delayed operation is recognized as a contributor to adverse outcome in many fields of emergency surgery. While an intestinal perforation on its own leads to a mortality of about 14%, a septic clinical progress is associated with an increase in mortality to 30%. Over the first 24 h after admission, each hour of surgical delay is associated with a 2% decrease in patient survival [46].

The phases of peritonitis are often separated. Initially, the perforation leads to chemical peritonitis, with or without contamination with microorganisms. The contamination phase lasts 3–6 h and is characterized by increased vascular permeability and influx of protein-rich fluid and white cells into the peritoneal cavity, resulting in the release of mediators of inflammation. The exact time point in which the contaminating microorganisms become invasive-infective is unknown. Therefore, one should consider any perforation operated upon with a delay of more than 12 h as infection rather than contamination [47].

Guidelines of the Surviving Sepsis Campaign advises a time-to-intervention of 12 h from diagnosis to source control [48]. A wide range of different biomarkers were tested concerning their predictive value on patients with abdominal sepsis. Most markers show peak values within 12 h of septic progress [49] (Table 77.2).

The surgical management of colon perforation has changed significantly over time. Some of the non-resectional approaches were associated with inadequate source control, so the Hartmann's procedure became a gold standard especially in severely sick patients. The shift toward resection with primary anastomosis is based on the fact that

**Table 77.2** Summary of surgical treatment depending on timing and clinical scenario

| Type of perforation, patient's condition | General management strategies |
|---|---|
| *Non-traumatic* | |
| Localized/mild peritonitis Stable patient | |
|   Without abscess | Antibiotic therapy |
|   Abscess <5 cm | Antibiotic therapy |
|   Abscess >5 cm | Antibiotic therapy + drainage |
| Generalized peritonitis Stable patient | Laparoscopic/open lavage + drainage (in diverticulitis but rarely indicated) Resection open/laparoscopic with primary anastomosis with/without protective ileostomy |
| Generalized peritonitis or Unstable patient | Hartmann procedure, colostomy, exteriorization/damage control surgery |
| Ischemic colitis + perforation | Hemicolectomy with or without ileostomy, resection with or without colostomy, Hartmann procedure |
| Toxic megacolon + perforation | Extremely rare—total abdominal colectomy without proctectomy |
| *Traumatic* | |
| Non-destructive | Laparoscopic/open suturing, lineal wedge resection |
| Destructive | Laparoscopic/open resection with primary anastomosis |
| Non-destructive, destructive Stabile patient | Suturing, resection with primary anastomosis with/without protective ileostomy |
| Non-destructive, destructive Unstable patient | Resection + ileostomy or colostomy, Hartmann procedure/damage control surgery |
| *Other types* | |
| Extraperitoneal perforation | Antibiotic therapy + drainage, resection with/without defunctioning ileostomy |

HP reversal is associated with significant morbidity and mortality and a large number of patients never had closure of their colostomy. Stoma-related complications after HP also play a role.

### Dos and Don'ts

**Dos**

- Do decide the emergency surgery based on individual case-by-case basis, considering general status of the patient, type, and localization of the perforation, severity of the peritonitis.
- Do primary suturing of the traumatic colon defect or linear wedge resection if edges of perforation are healthy, well vascularized, and can be approximated without tension and narrowing the bowel lumen.
- Do consider Hartmann's procedure in patients with severe perforation-related generalized peritonitis, in critically ill patients and in patients with multiple comorbidities.
- Do consider primary anastomosis in hemodynamically stable, immunocompetent patients younger than 85 years.
- Do the damage control surgery if at least one of the following items is present: pH <7.2, core temperature <35 °C, BE <−8, laboratory/clinical evidence of coagulopathy, any signs of sepsis/septic shock, the necessity of inotropic support.

**Don'ts**

- Don't use the laparoscopic approach in patient with unstable vital parameters.
- Don't ignore the principles of oncological resection in perforated colon cancer patients.
- Don't perform proctectomy in the emergent setting of fulminant colitis or toxic megacolon.

## Take-Home Messages

- Perforation is a life-threatening complication which may develop in a row of the diseases and trauma of a large bowel.
- Absence of free gas on X-ray does not rule out perforation, as well as free gas not always the indication for laparotomy.
- Hartmann procedure is a standard procedure in the setting of generalized peritonitis on the ground of large bowel perforation. In selected cases, resection (including laparoscopic) with primary anastomosis with or without protective ileostomy is feasible.

## Multiple Choice Questions

1. Which part of the colon is usually the most commonly involved in diverticulitis in Eastern populations: Sigmoid; Descending; Ascending; Transverse
   Correct answer: Ascending
2. The cause of pneumoperitoneum can't be: Cardiopulmonary resuscitation; Positive pressure ventilation; Recent laparotomy/scopy; Pneumothorax
   Correct answer: Pneumothorax
3. Patients who have hollow viscus perforation failed to demonstrate pneumoperitoneum on plain abdominal radiographs in: Nearly 50%; 40%; About 30%; 10%
   Correct answer: Nearly 50%
4. Which part of the colon injuries most common during blunt trauma: Right colon; Left colon; Transverse; Sigmoid
   Correct answer: Right colon
5. Mechanisms of perforation during colonoscopy include, but: Direct mechanical trauma; Lateral pressure against the colon wall; Application electrosurgical current; Insufficient air inflation
   Correct answer: Insufficient air inflation
6. Which of the following is not recommended as a screening tool for traumatic colon injuries: Ultrasound; CT; X-ray; Digital rectal examination
   Correct answer: Digital rectal examination
7. In diverticulitis and localized peritonitis and abscess >5 cm most appropriate is: Hartmann's procedure; Laparoscopic resection with ileostoma; Open resection and ileostoma; Antibacterial therapy and drainage
   Correct answer: Antibacterial therapy and drainage
8. In stable patient with diverticulitis and generalized peritonitis not indicated: Hartmann's procedure; Laparoscopic or open resection with ileostoma; Laparoscopic or open resection with primary anastomosis; Damage control surgery
   Correct answer: Damage control surgery
9. In unstable patient with large bowel perforation and generalized peritonitis contraindicated: Hartmann's procedure; Laparoscopic resection with primary anastomosis; Damage control surgery; Exteriorization
   Correct answer: Laparoscopic resection with primary anastomosis
10. Primary suturing of the traumatic colon defect or linear wedge resection not appropriate if edges of perforation: Healthy; Well vascularized; Can be approximated with tension; Can be approximated without narrowing the bowel lumen
    Correct answer: Can be approximated with tension

# References

1. Kumar A, Muir MT, Cohn SM, Salhanick MA, Lankford DB, Katabathina VS. The etiology of pneumoperitoneum in the 21st century. J Trauma Acute Care Surg. 2012;73(3):542–8. https://doi.org/10.1097/TA.0b013e31825c157f.
2. Kaiser AM, Jiang JK, Lake JP, Ault G, Artinyan A, Gonzalez-Ruiz C, et al. The management of complicated diverticulitis and the role of computed tomography. Am J Gastroenterol. 2005;100(4):910–7.
3. Hume DJ. A population-based study of perforated diverticular disease incidence and associated mortality. Gastroenterology. 2009;136:1198–205. https://doi.org/10.1053/j.gastro.2008.12.054.
4. Hinchey EJ, Schaal PG, Richards GK. Treatment of perforated diverticular disease of the colon. Adv Surg. 1978;12:85–109.
5. Alvarez JA, Baldonedo RF, Bear IG, Truan N, Pire G, Alvarez P. Presentation, treatment, and multivariate analysis of risk factors for obstructive and perforative colorectal carcinoma. Am J Surg. 2005;190(3):376–82. https://doi.org/10.1016/j.amjsurg.2005.01.045.
6. Gunnarsson H, Holm T, Ekholm A, Olsson LI. Emergency presentation of colon cancer is most frequent during summer. Color Dis. 2011;13(6):663–8. https://doi.org/10.1111/j.1463-1318.2010.02270.x.
7. Zielinski MD, Merchea A, Heller SF, You YN. Emergency management of perforated colon cancers: how aggressive should we be? J Gastrointest Surg. 2011;15(12):2232–8. https://doi.org/10.1007/s11605-011-1674-8.
8. Biondo S, Kreisler E, Millan M, Fraccalvieri D, Golda T, Marti Rague J, Salazar R. Differences in patient postoperative and long-term outcomes between obstructive and perforated colonic cancer. Am J Surg. 2008;195(4):427–32. https://doi.org/10.1016/j.amjsurg.2007.02.027.
9. Anwar MA, D'Souza F, Coulter R, Memon B, Khan IM, Memon MA. Outcome of acutely perforated colorectal cancers: experience of a single district general hospital. Surg Oncol. 2006;15(2):91–6. https://doi.org/10.1016/j.suronc.2006.09.001.
10. Messmer JM. Gas and soft tissue abnormalities. In: Textbook of gastrointestinal radiology. 3rd ed. Philadelphia, PA: Elsevier; 2008.
11. Fudin HR, Ray SD. Side effects of drugs annual, vol. 40. Amsterdam: Elsevier; 2018. p. 29–89.
12. Zhang MJ, Wu JB. Treatment of spontaneous perforation of the large intestine: a report of 9 cases. Zhongguo Putong Waike Zazhi. 2002;32:836–9.
13. Misiakos EP, Tsapralis D, Karatzas T, et al. Advents in the diagnosis and management of ischemic colitis. Front Surg. 2017;4:47. https://doi.org/10.3389/fsurg.2017.00047. Published 2017 Sep 4.
14. Sharpe JP, Magnotti LJ, Weinberg JA, Shahan CP, Cullinan DR, Fabian TC, Croce MA. Applicability of an established management algorithm for colon injuries following blunt trauma. J Trauma Acute Care Surg. 2013;74(2):419–24; discussion 424–5.
15. Luning TH, Keemers-Gels ME, Barendregt WB, Tan AC, Rosman C. Colonoscopic perforations: a review of 30,366 patients. Surg Endosc. 2007;21:994–7.
16. Jovanovic I, Zimmermann L, Fry LC, Mönkemüller K. Feasibility of endoscopic closure of an iatrogenic colon perforation occurring during colonoscopy. Gastrointest Endosc. 2011;73:550–5.
17. Cotton PB, Eisen GM, Aabakken L, et al. A lexicon for endoscopic adverse events: report of an ASGE workshop. Gastrointest Endosc. 2010;71:446–54.
18. Avgerinos DV, Llaguna OH, Lo AY, Leitman IM. Evolving management of colonoscopic perforations. J Gastrointest Surg. 2008;12:1783–9.
19. Van Halsema EE, van Hooft JE, Small AJ, Fockens P, Dijkgraaf M, Repici A. Perforation in colorectal stenting: a meta-analysis and a search for risk factors. Clin Endosc. 2014;79(6):970–82.
20. Lipkin M, Shah O. Complications of urologic surgery (Colon). 4th ed. Philadelphia, PA: Elsevier; 2010.
21. Akhtar S, McElvanna N, Gardiner KR, Irwin ST. Bowel perforation caused by swallowed chicken bones—a case series. Ulster Med J. 2007;76:37–8.
22. Sureka B, Bansal K, Arora A. Pneumoperitoneum: What to look for in a radiograph? J Family Med Prim Care. 2015;4(3):477–8. https://doi.org/10.4103/2249-4863.161369.
23. Yamamoto R, Logue AJ, Muir MT. Colon trauma: evidence-based practices. Clin Colon Rectal Surg. 2018;31(1):11–6. https://doi.org/10.1055/s--0037-1602175. Epub 2017 Dec 19.
24. Chen SC, Yen ZS, Wang HP, Lin FY, Hsu CY, Chen WJ. Ultrasonography is superior to plain radiography in the diagnosis of pneumoperitoneum. Br J Surg. 2002;89(3):351–4. https://doi.org/10.1046/j.0007-1323.2001.02013.x.
25. Chen SC, Wang HP, Chen WJ, Lin FY, Hsu CY, Chang KJ, Chen WJ. Selective use of ultrasonography for the detection of pneumoperitoneum. Acad Emerg Med. 2002;9(6):643–5.
26. Mazzei MA, Guerrini S, CioffiSquitieri N, et al. The role of US examination in the management of acute abdomen. Crit Ultrasound J. 2013;5:S6.
27. Pisano M, Zorcolo L, Merli C, et al. 2017 WSES guidelines on colon and rectal cancer emergencies: obstruction and perforation. World J Emerg Surg. 2018;13:36. https://doi.org/10.1186/s13017-018-0192-3.
28. Pouli S, Kozana A, Papakitsou I, Daskalogiannaki M, Raissaki M. Gastrointestinal perforation: clinical and MDCT clues for identification of aetiology. Insights Imaging. 2020;11(1):31. https://doi.org/10.1186/s13244-019-0823-6.
29. Blot S, DeWaeleJJ. Critical issues in the clinical management of complicated intra-abdominal infections. Drugs. 2005;65(12):1611–20.
30. Sartelli M, Weber DG, Kluger Y, et al. 2020 update of the WSES guidelines for the management of acute colonic diverticulitis in the emergency setting. World J Emerg Surg. 2020;15:32.

31. de Ruiter J, Weel J, Manusama E, Kingma WP, van der Voort PH. The epidemiology of intra-abdominal flora in critically ill patients with secondary and tertiary abdominal sepsis. Infection. 2009;37(6):522–7.
32. Vincent JL, De Backer D. Circulatory shock. N Engl J Med. 2013;369:1726–34.
33. Abu-Zidan FM. Optimizing the value of measuring inferior vena cava diameter in shocked patients. World J Crit Care Med. 2016;5:7–11.
34. Agresta F, Ciardo LF, Mazzarolo G, Michelet I, Orsi G, Trentin G, et al. Peritonitis: laparoscopic approach. World J Emerg Surg. 2006;24:1–9.
35. Sartelli M, et al. 2020 Update of the WSES guidelines for the management of acute colonic diverticulitis in the emergency setting. World J Emerg Surg. 2020;15(1):32. https://doi.org/10.1186/s13017-020-00313-4.
36. Lambrichts DPV, Vennix S, Musters GD, Mulder IM, Swank HA, Hoofwijk AGM, Belgers EHJ, Stockmann HBAC, Eijsbouts QAJ, Gerhards MF, van Wagensveld BA, van Geloven AAW, Crolla RMPH, Nienhuijs SW, Govaert MJPM, di Saverio S, D'Hoore AJL, Consten ECJ, van Grevenstein WMU, Pierik REGJM, Kruyt PM, van der Hoeven JAB, Steup WH, Catena F, Konsten JLM, Vermeulen J, van Dieren S, Bemelman WA, Lange JF, LADIES Trial Collaborators. Hartmann's procedure versus sigmoidectomy with primary anastomosis for perforated diverticulitis with purulent or faecal peritonitis (LADIES): a multicentre, parallel-group, randomised, open-label, superiority trial. Lancet Gastroenterol Hepatol. 2019;4(8):599–610.
37. Vennix S, Boersema GS, Buskens CJ, Menon AG, Tanis PJ, Lange JF, Bemelman WA. Emergency laparoscopic sigmoidectomy for perforated diverticulitis with generalised peritonitis: a systematic review. Dig Surg. 2016;33(1):1–7.
38. Gajendran M, Loganathan P, Jimenez G, Catinella AP, Ng N, Umapathy C, Ziade N, Hashash JG. A comprehensive review and update on ulcerative colitis. Dis Mon. 2019;65(12):100851. https://doi.org/10.1016/j.disamonth.2019.02.004. Epub 2019 Mar 2.
39. Chakravartty S, Chang A, Nunoo-Mensah J. A systematic review of stercoral perforation. Color Dis. 2013;15(8):930–5. https://doi.org/10.1111/codi.12123.
40. Paspatis GA, Dumonceau JM, Barthet M, et al. Diagnosis and management of iatrogenic endoscopic perforations: European Society of Gastrointestinal Endoscopy (ESGE) position statement. Endoscopy. 2014;46:693–711.
41. Wullstein C, Koppen M, Gross E. Laparoscopic treatment of colonic perforations related to colonoscopy. Surg Endosc. 1999;13:484–7.
42. Hansen AJ, Tessier DJ, Anderson ML, Schlinkert RT. Laparoscopic repair of colonoscopic perforations: indications and guidelines. J Gastrointest Surg. 2007;11:655–9.
43. de'Angelis N, Di Saverio S, Chiara O, et al. 2017 WSES guidelines for the management of iatrogenic colonoscopy perforation. World J Emerg Surg. 2018;13:5. https://doi.org/10.1186/s13017-018-0162-9.
44. Weber DG, Bendinelli C, Balogh ZJ. Damage control surgery for abdominal emergencies. Br J Surg. 2014;101(1):e109–18.
45. Becher RD, Peitzman AB, Sperry JL, Gallaher JR, Neff LP, Sun Y, Miller PR, Chang MC. Damage control operations in non-trauma patients: defining criteria for the staged rapid source control laparotomy in emergency general surgery. World J Emerg Surg. 2016;11:10.
46. Fang JF, Chen RJ, Lin BC, Hsu YB, Kao JL, Kao YC, Chen MF. Small bowel perforation: is urgent surgery necessary? J Trauma. 1999;47(3):515–20. https://doi.org/10.1097/00005373-199909000-00014.
47. Dart AJ, Chapman H-S. Robinson's current therapy in equine medicine. 7th ed. St. Louis: Elsevier; 2015.
48. Dellinger RP, Levy MM, Rhodes A, Annane D, Gerlach H, Opal SM, et al. Surviving sepsis campaign: international guidelines for management of severe sepsis and septic shock. Crit Care Med. 2012;41(2):580–637.
49. Hecker A, Uhle F, Schwandner T, et al. Diagnostics, therapy and outcome prediction in abdominal sepsis: current standards and future perspectives. Langenbecks Arch Surg. 2014;399:11–22. https://doi.org/10.1007/s00423-013-1132-z.

## Further Reading

De Simone B, Sartelli M, Coccolini F, Ball CG, Brambillasca P, Chiarugi M, Campanile FC, Nita G, Corbella D, Leppaniemi A, Boschini E, Moore EE, Biffl W, Peitzmann A, Kluger Y, Sugrue M, Fraga G, Di Saverio S, Weber D, Sakakushev B, Chiara O, Abu-Zidan FM, Ten Broek R, Kirkpatrick AW, Wani I, Coimbra R, Baiocchi GL, Kelly MD, Ansaloni L, Catena F. Intraoperative surgical site infection control and prevention: a position paper and future addendum to WSES intra-abdominal infections guidelines. World J Emerg Surg. 2020;15(1):10. https://doi.org/10.1186/s13017-020-0288-4.

de'Angelis N, Di Saverio S, Chiara O, Sartelli M, Martínez-Pérez A, Patrizi F, Weber DG, Ansaloni L, Biffl W, Ben-Ishay O, Bala M, Brunetti F, Gaiani F, Abdalla S, Amiot A, Bahouth H, Bianchi G, Casanova D, Coccolini F, Coimbra R, de'Angelis GL, De Simone B, Fraga GP, Genova P, Ivatury R, Kashuk JL, Kirkpatrick AW, Le Baleur Y, Machado F, Machain GM, Maier RV, Chichom-Mefire A, Memeo R, Mesquita C, Salamea Molina JC, Mutignani M, Manzano-Núñez R, Ordoñez C, Peitzman AB, Pereira BM, Picetti E, Pisano M, Puyana JC, Rizoli S, Siddiqui M, Sobhani I, Ten Broek RP, Zorcolo L, Carra MC, Kluger Y, Catena F. 2017 WSES guidelines for the management of iatrogenic colonoscopy perforation. World J Emerg Surg. 2018;13:5. https://doi.org/10.1186/s13017-018-0162-9.

Pisano M, Zorcolo L, Merli C, Cimbanassi S, Poiasina E, Ceresoli M, Agresta F, Allievi N, Bellanova G, Coccolini F, Coy C, Fugazzola P, Martinez CA, Montori G, Paolillo C, Penachim TJ, Pereira B, Reis T, Restivo A, Rezende-Neto J, Sartelli M, Valentino M, Abu-Zidan FM, Ashkenazi I, Bala M, Chiara O, De'Angelis N, Deidda S, De Simone B, Di Saverio S, Finotti E, Kenji I, Moore E, Wexner S, Biffl W, Coimbra R, Guttadauro A, Leppäniemi A, Maier R, Magnone S, Mefire AC, Peitzmann A, Sakakushev B, Sugrue M, Viale P, Weber D, Kashuk J, Fraga GP, Kluger I, Catena F, Ansaloni L. 2017 WSES guidelines on colon and rectal cancer emergencies: obstruction and perforation. World J Emerg Surg. 2018;13:36. https://doi.org/10.1186/s13017-018-0192-3.

Sartelli M, Chichom-Mefire A, Labricciosa FM, Hardcastle T, Abu-Zidan FM, Adesunkanmi AK, Ansaloni L, Bala M, Balogh ZJ, Beltrán MA, Ben-Ishay O, Biffl WL, Birindelli A, Cainzos MA, Catalini G, Ceresoli M, Che Jusoh A, Chiara O, Coccolini F, Coimbra R, Cortese F, Demetrashvili Z, Di Saverio S, Diaz JJ, Egiev VN, Ferrada P, Fraga GP, Ghnnam WM, Lee JG, Gomes CA, Hecker A, Herzog T, Kim JI, Inaba K, Isik A, Karamarkovic A, Kashuk J, Khokha V, Kirkpatrick AW, Kluger Y, Koike K, Kong VY, Leppaniemi A, Machain GM, Maier RV, Marwah S, McFarlane ME, Montori G, Moore EE, Negoi I, Olaoye I, Omari AH, Ordonez CA, Pereira BM, Pereira Júnior GA, Pupelis G, Reis T, Sakakhushev B, Sato N, Segovia Lohse HA, Shelat VG, Søreide K, Uhl W, Ulrych J, Van Goor H, Velmahos GC, Yuan KC, Wani I, Weber DG, Zachariah SK, Catena F. The management of intra-abdominal infections from a global perspective: 2017 WSES guidelines for management of intra-abdominal infections. World J Emerg Surg. 2017;12:29. https://doi.org/10.1186/s13017-017-0141-6. Erratum in: World J Emerg Surg. 2017 Aug 2;12:36.

Sartelli M, Weber DG, Kluger Y, et al. 2020 Update of the WSES guidelines for the management of acute colonic diverticulitis in the emergency setting. World J Emerg Surg. 2020;15:32. https://doi.org/10.1186/s13017-020-00313-4.

# Emergency Management of Abdominal Wall Hernia

## 78

M. M. J. van Rooijen, J. F. Lange, and J. Jeekel

## 78.1 Introduction

**Learning Goals**

- Recognize the importance of abdominal wall hernias with regard to their epidemiology, burden for patients and society, and know the etiology and risk factors for hernias.
- Being able to define the clinical significance of incarcerated and strangulated abdominal wall hernias, their diagnostic trajectory, and their (emergency) management.
- Being able to outline the indications, surgical options, normal postoperative course, possible complications, and prognosis of abdominal wall hernia repair.

### 78.1.1 The (Societal) Problem of Abdominal Wall Hernia

The general definition of an abdominal wall hernia (AWH) is a protrusion of abdominal fat tissue, the greater omentum or the intestines through the abdominal wall. AWHs come in different types and sizes, occurring at naturally weakened spots (Fig. 78.1). These can be either already present from birth, such as hiatal, umbilical, or femoral (especially females) and inguinal hernias (especially males), or created due to surgery, being incisional or parastomal hernias. The size of a hernia can vary from smaller than 1 cm to over 20 cm in width. However, regardless the type or size, AWHs pose a problem to both patients, surgeons, and society. First of all, patients may experience discomfort, pain, and reduced quality of life due to an AWH [1]. Second, surgeons face challenges in closing giant AWHs, but must also act decisively despite scientific uncertainties in the management of (very) small AWHs. Third, on a larger societal level, AWHs are problematic with regard to costs of care due to their incidence. AWHs occur frequently: men have a 25% life-time risk of developing an inguinal hernia [2], umbilical hernias show an incidence of 2% in the adult population, and up to 20% in cirrhotic patients [3], and the risk of an incisional hernia remains 10–20% after midline incision laparotomy [4–6]. This results in high costs, with nearly 350,000 performed incisional hernia repairs on a yearly basis in the United States alone, costing approximately 3 billion dollars [7]. Inguinal hernia repair is even more common, with 800,000 surgeries in the United States annually [8].

M. M. J. van Rooijen · J. F. Lange · J. Jeekel (✉)
Department of Surgery, Erasmus University Medical Center, Rotterdam, The Netherlands
e-mail: m.vanrooijen@erasmusmc.nl;
j.lange@erasmusmc.nl; j.jeekel@erasmusmc.nl

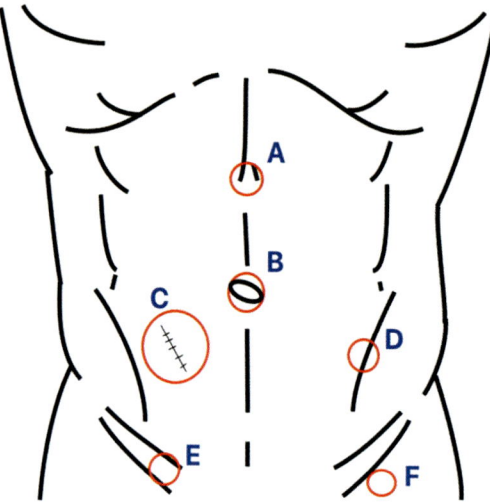

**Fig. 78.1** Types of abdominal wall hernias. A: epigastric, B: umbilical, C: incisional, D: Spigelian, E: inguinal, F: femoral

**Table 78.1** Classification of primary abdominal wall hernias according to the EHS

| Classification | | Diameter | | |
|---|---|---|---|---|
| Hernia location | | Small (<2 cm) | Medium (≥2–4 cm) | Large (≥4 cm) |
| Midline | Epigastric | | | |
| | Umbilical | | | |
| Lateral | Spigelian | | | |
| | Lumbar | | | |

## 78.1.2 Classification

Many types of AWH exist. Inguinal hernias are usually subdivided in direct and indirect inguinal hernias, in which the inguinal canal is the weak spot through which protrusion of tissue occurs. At the posterior wall of the femoral canal a weak spot can occur too, caudally to the inguinal ligament and medially to the femoral vein, which is a femoral hernia. In a sportsman's hernia, true herniation is not present, but the main symptomatology is marked by chronic pain in the groin area.

Ventral hernias can be at any point on the abdominal wall and can be primary or incisional. For these ventral hernias, the European Hernia Society (EHS) has created separate classifications [9]. In the classification for primary AWH, the division is between epigastric or umbilical (both at the midline), or Spigelian or lumbar (both lateral) (Table 78.1). Also dorsal hernias (such as Petit's hernia and Grynfeltt-Lesshaft hernia) can occur. These primary hernias are either small when they are less than 2 cm large in diameter, medium with a size of 2–4 cm, and large when they are over 4 cm in diameter. Incisional hernias are divided as either being at the midline, such as subxiphoidal, epigastric, umbilical, infraumbilical, or suprapubic hernias; or lateral at various heights (subcostal, flank, iliac, lumbar hernias). Incisional hernias are only considered large in the EHS classification when they are over 10 cm in width. Incisional hernias may be difficult to treat when there is a potentially infected (VWHG grade 3) or infected environment (VHWG grade 4). The VWHG classification should be mentioned here.

### 78.1.2.1 Incarcerated and Strangulated Hernias

Special cases are incarcerated or strangulated AWHs. In an incarcerated AWH, tissue becomes trapped in the hernia sac and cannot be reduced back easily. Approximately 5–15% of operated AWHs are incarcerated [10]. Thereafter, the herniated tissue in an incarcerated AWH can become strangulated, which is a medical emergency. Strangulation is a complication of the AWH in which the greater omentum or a fold of bowel or mesentery remains trapped in the hernia sac and the blood supply is cut off. The risk of an inguinal hernia becoming strangulated is estimated at roughly 5% within 2 years [11]; for other AWHs, research on strangulation incidence is scarce, but strangulation is reported frequently as a complication. For all three stakeholders mentioned above (patient, surgeon, and society), strangulation results in additional burden. Strangulated tissue causes extreme pain and can release hazardous toxins, with the potential of causing sepsis or even death. Surgeons will need to act quickly, are less prepared, and must perform emergency surgery [12], which is associated with higher risks of morbidity and mortality compared to elective surgery [13–16]. For society, emergency surgery is more expensive and generates less profit in the form of full-quality life years gained [17].

### 78.1.3 Etiology and Hernia Risk Factors

AWHs occur at anatomically weak spots of the abdomen, *id est* at the linea alba between the rectus muscles, at the umbilicus, at the epigastric region, or at the inguinal canal. In addition, incisional hernia may occur at the site of a surgical incision, as dysregulation of collagen type 1 and 3 in scar tissue might occur [18]. Obesity and Abdominal aneurysm are therefore a serious risk factor for incisional hernia, as it might impair the synthesis of mature collagen, due to hypoxia that occurs due to reduced vascularization of adipose tissue [19, 20]. Current literature further indicates high age as risk factor for the development of AWHs [5]. Also, conditions that lead to high intraabdominal pressure are suggested to be AWH risk factors, such as heavy lifting, strenuous activity, chronic coughing, chronic obstructive pulmonary disease, and pregnancy [21]. However, most important factors for AWH development are: obesity with BMI > 27, abdominal aneurysm, and smoking [22, 23]. Level-1 evidence exists that closure with the routine large bites will lead to significant more incisional hernias than closing with small bites of 5- 5mm. It can also be hypothesized that—in line with collagen weakness—muscle weakness or muscle wasting, such as sarcopenia, could increase the risk of developing an AWH. However, current literature lacks sufficient evidence for a definitive conclusion with regard to sarcopenia [24].

Incarceration of AWH has been associated with defect sizes of 3–4 cm compared to smaller defect sizes, and occurs more often at the peri- and infraumbilical region. Higher age and increasing body mass index also seem to be associated with incarceration [25]. A strangulated AWH can be a consequence of incarceration; however, no specific risk factors for strangulation of AWHs are known. Incarceration and strangulation seem less likely to occur in larger AWHs, where hernia content can easier slide in and out of the hernia. Moreover, the largest risk of strangulation exists in the first few months of AWH presence [11].

## 78.2 Diagnosis

### 78.2.1 Clinical Presentation

An incarcerated AWH shows visible bulging at the location of the hernia, with the hernia content being non-reducible, yet the content does usually not feel tense and the overlying skin appears normal. In the case of a strangulated AWH, clinical characteristics could be (increased) acute pain (with onset in a window of minutes), tenderness and/or erythema around the hernia, and irritation or even necrosis of the overlying skin [26]. In addition, symptoms of obstruction of the strangulated bowel can occur: constipation, nausea, vomiting, bloody stools, and the inability to pass gas. As the hypoxic tissue in the hernia produces toxins and might sometimes release bacteria in the abdomen [27], sepsis might occur, with possible symptoms of fatigue, fever, and inflammation.

> **Differential Diagnosis**
>
> The differential diagnosis is relatively short:
> – Symptoms in the inguinal region: lymphadenopathy, abscess, undescended testicle, lipoma, and a vascular aneurysm.
> – Scrotal symptoms: hydrocele, testicular tumor, varicocele, or torsio testis.
> – Abdominal symptoms: omphalocele, seroma, abscess, diastasis recti, or a hematoma.

### 78.2.2 Diagnostics

At the clinical examination, the surgeon or resident should always palpate the AWH in lying and standing position, while the patient is performing the Valsalva maneuver. First, manual reduction of the hernia can be attempted. AWH—also when incarcerated or strangulated—is diagnosed clinically. However, when strangulation is suspected, bowel ischemia should be ruled out, among others through a blood screening for leukocytosis and metabolic abnormalities [28]. Lactate only has a limited clinical utility in the acute setting after the blood supply is compromised [29]. To determine the size of the hernia and the presence of bowel obstruction, an abdominal or inguinal ultrasound or a computed tomography (CT) scan can be performed. Both appear to have additional value in the detection of AWH, yet a CT scan seems more accurate [30]. There is general consensus for the preference of a CT scan, as it allows for adequate, examiner-independent visualization of the abdomen with anatomic detail, fast imaging acquisition, and conversion of data from the axial plane to other planes [31]. These favorable characteristics of CT scans may also help in detecting subtle signs of complication within the hernia sac, such as wall thickening, abnormal mural hypo- or hyperattenuation and enhancement, distention of mesenteric vessels, mesenteric haziness and ascites, which are findings often associated with ischemia [31]. In the acute setting of a strangulated AWH in which small bowel obstruction or acute mesenteric ischemia is present, magnetic resonance imaging (MRI) is of little to no additional value [28, 32].

## 78.3 Treatment

### 78.3.1 Medical Treatment

AWHs cannot be resolved by medical treatment alone, yet a conservative approach in the form of "watchful waiting" can be a valid option in asymptomatic or mild symptomatic inguinal hernias. Despite common arguments that the risk of incarceration is a reason to operate asymptomatic AWHs, current literature does not support this view [33–35]. The rate of incarceration of inguinal hernia at 4 years is relatively low: at approximately 0.55% [36]. A conservative approach does not seem to lead to significant more complaints of pain [34] and in addition, after 10 years of follow-up in one randomized controlled trial, 30% of patients in the watchful waiting group remained without having undergone inguinal hernia surgery [37].

Also, asymptomatic incisional hernia and umbilical hernia can be (and currently are) managed conservatively in clinical practice [38–40].

However, in most (symptomatic) patient groups and especially high-risk patient groups, surgical hernia repair is the preferred treatment option [39, 41–43].

In incarcerated AWH, taxis can be attempted. Taxis ("reduction en masse") is represented by the manual reduction of the AWH under analgesia or sedation, sometimes performed with the patient in Trendelenburg position to let gravity aid the hernia reduction in inguinal hernia cases. Taxis is a much-debated technique: some surgeons view it as an effective way to prevent morbidity and mortality associated with emergency herniorrhaphy in the elderly population, whereas other surgeons discourage the use of taxis due to the risk of reduction of necrotic bowel. Current—yet limited—evidence suggests that taxis is safe in younger children [44, 45], and seemingly too in adults [46, 47]. Taxis therefore might be performed when signs of strangulation are absent, to delay definitive hernia repair surgery.

### 78.3.2 Surgical Treatment

Despite options for conservative treatment, AWH in general often requires surgical elective repair when the patient experiences complaints. The aim of AWH surgery is to relieve symptoms, to prevent complications, or to resolve acute complications. Many surgical techniques and options are available for AWH repair, including simple suture repair, mesh repair with synthetic or biological products, repair with relaxing incisions like component separation techniques, and use of musculofascial flaps. There is ample evidence that mesh repair is superior to suture repair. Repair can be approached open or laparoscopically. Several choices should be made in preparation of, and during AWH repair: how quickly should repair take place? Should the intervention be open or laparoscopic? And what techniques and which products like meshes, sutures, tackers and glues should be used during repair?

#### 78.3.2.1 Timing and Access

When there are no signs of incarceration or strangulation, the patient should be offered elective repair. This can often take place laparoscopically, as this is less invasive for the patient and, with regard to inguinal hernia surgery, associated with less chronic pain [48, 49]. However, an incarcerated AWH requires urgent surgery, and a strangulated AWH is an emergency complication that necessitates surgical intervention as soon as possible. Faster access to the abdomen can be gained through an open approach, which—in an emergency setting—also lowers the risk of injury compared to laparoscopic AWH repair [48]. However, recent studies into laparoscopic repair of strangulated AWH have shown mildly positive results [50]. Nonetheless, surgical consensus exists that laparoscopic relief of incarcerated or strangulated AWH should be restricted to surgeons with maximum expertise [51]. If bowel obstruction is present, as a rule, a nasogastric tube will be placed for decompression. When bowel perforation or necrosis is suspected, broad-spectrum antibiotics should be administered.

The first step during the surgical procedure is to reduce the incarcerated or strangulated AWH. In case of necrotic tissue, resection of this affected tissue has to take place. Only after these necessary steps, AWH repair can commence. Inguinal hernia can be repaired via Lichtenstein procedure or through an endoscopic/laparoscopic technique (TEP, TAP) if the surgeon has the necessary expertise. In ventral hernia such as incisional, umbilical and epigastric hernia, either open or laparoscopic excision of the hernia sac can take place, after which fascial closure should be achieved. In the case of bowel resection, higher morbidity and mortality have been reported [10, 52–54].

### 78.3.2.2 Use of Mesh

Synthetic mesh repair procedures, either open or laparoscopic, lead to fewer recurrences compared to primary suture repair, both in inguinal hernia [55], umbilical hernia [56], epigastric hernia, and primary abdominal wall or incisional hernia [57, 58]. This is also applicable for acute AWH repair procedures. Improved outcomes are believed to be related to reduced tension on the fascial edges and sutures when mesh is used in AWH repair procedures. Therefore, the use of mesh has been recommended in the guidelines of the European Hernia Society (EHS) and Americas Hernia Society [40].

However, synthetic mesh use has been associated with complications in approximately 17% of patients, such as pain, infection, adhesions, fistula, and foreign body reaction [59, 60]. Also, in the case of bowel necrosis or bowel resection—with any contamination of the operative field—surgeons are cautious with placing synthetic mesh as they foresee a risk of bacterial invasion of the mesh [61]. Therefore, medical device companies decided to further innovate their products, and biological meshes became available on the market. These biological products are hypothesized to be relatively infection resistant and therefore useful in contaminated wound sites [62]. In addition, slowly resorbable "biosynthetic" meshes have become more widely available, which are less costly and are thought to cause abdominal wall remodeling as a result of gradual mesh resorption [63]. Early studies suggest safe use of biosynthetic mesh in potentially contaminated AWH sites [64]. Despite these developments, permanent synthetic mesh has also been shown to be safe in clean-contaminated environments [65] and in the case of bowel resection during repair of incarcerated AWHs [10]. Insufficient evidence is currently available to definitely recommend the use of one mesh product over another.

### 78.3.2.3 Preoperative Preparation

As stated above, incarcerated and strangulated AWHs require emergency surgery, which means time is limited and preoperative patient optimalization cannot take place. However, in the case of elective AWH repair, patients can benefit from preoperative preparation, sometimes also described as "prehabilitation" or "better in is better out" [66]. The goal would be to reduce operative risk factors, through the cessation of smoking, weight reduction, or exercise [67]. Patients could also obtain advantages from gaining muscle mass, as decline of muscle mass has been associated with an increased number of postoperative complications and increased long-term mortality after abdominal surgery [68].

In addition, the preoperative use of botulinum toxin A injections has been researched. Several authors suggest positive results from preoperative botulinum toxin A injections in the three lateral abdominal muscle layers with regard to fascial closure, without being associated with severe complications [69–72]. Therefore, botulinum toxin A might become more common in the near future in the standard clinical practice of AWH repair.

### 78.3.3 Prognosis

Hernia surgery is associated with a relatively good prognosis, though some factors are associated with less favorable outcomes. Hernia width is an important measurement to determine the difficulty of successfully repairing the AWH [9, 73], meaning that very large AWHs can be more challenging for surgeons and therefore result in more postoperative complications [74]. Furthermore repair in infected environment VWHG grade 3 and 4 is a risk factor. Examples of postoperative complications that might occur are wound infection, acute and chronic seroma formation, hematoma, superficial or deep infection (also of mesh), skin necrosis, wound dehiscence, recurrence, and pain.

In particular, recurrences remain a significant problem. Inguinal hernias have a reported recurrence rate of 3–8% [2], umbilical hernias have a large variety in reported recurrence rates but are estimated between 5% and 10% [56], whereas incisional hernias have reported recurrence rates of up to 40% [75]. To prevent recurrence, closing of the fascia after hernia reduction requires special attention. Most authors agree on the use of at least a 4:1 suture-length to wound-length ratio during fascia closure at the midline [76], and this might best be achieved through the use of small stitch bites [77]. Furthermore mesh repair should be used.

A more seldomly occurring, yet serious complication after open surgery is burst abdomen. This is a postoperative separation of the musculoaponeurotic layers, also called acute postoperative hernia, fascial dehiscence, or—in a more visual term by German surgeons—Platzbauch. This complication most often occurs around 1 week after surgery, marked by renewed bulging of the wound. Whereas superficial wound dehiscence can be managed conservatively through daily saline dressings or negative pressure wound therapy, (deep) fascial dehiscence requires urgent operative care, especially in the presence of evisceration. Its operative management can be primary closure of the wound, closure with relaxing incisions, or closure with mesh products or tissue flaps. The preferred treatment option includes the use of mesh [78], except in the presence of abdominal infection or abscesses [79]. The treatment of burst abdomen is usually associated with unsatisfactory surgical outcomes [80]. Therefore, tension-free fascia closure should be pursued in AWH repair.

In elective AWH repair, postoperative complications are frequent, yet manageable; and therefore, the prognosis is favorable although recurrence rates are still too high, up to 60% in obese patients with BMI> 27 and in patients with abdominal aneurysm. However, as also noted above, incarcerated and strangulated AWHs require emergency surgery, which several studies have shown is generally associated with higher risks of morbidity; and mortality can be increased up to seven times when AWH operation is carried out as an emergency [52]. This underlines the importance of acting quickly when incarceration or strangulation of an AWH is suspected, and adequate postoperative care should be provided. This comprises of leaving a nasogastric tube in place until ileus is resolved, monitoring of bowel function, and advising the patient to refrain from heavy lifting temporarily. Adequate analgesic care should be provided, yet surgeons should be cautious with prescribing narcotics, as these might contribute to constipation and lead to delay of hospital discharge.

**Dos and Don'ts** (Table 78.2)

**Table 78.2** List with dos and don'ts for treatment of incarcerated and strangulated hernias

| Do | Don't |
|---|---|
| Perform emergency surgery if strangulation is suspected | Waste time through superfluous diagnostics |
| Resect necrotic tissue if present | Perform taxis in case of suspected strangulation |
| Use mesh products in AWH repair | Primary closure under circumstances without fecal contamination |

**Take-Home Messages**

- Incarceration and strangulation are acute complications of an abdominal wall hernia, in which organ tissue can be cut off from its blood supply and can cause sepsis or even death.
- The diagnosis of incarcerated or strangulated hernias can be made clinically, through the presence of extreme pain, possible accompanying symptoms of obstruction, and the impossibility of manual reduction of hernia contents.
- An incarcerated or strangulated hernia requires emergency surgery, in which both an open or laparoscopic approach can be used, yet timely resection of necrotic tissue should be achieved.
- Abdominal wall hernia repair should take place after the incarceration or strangulation has been resolved, with the use of mesh.
- As morbidity and mortality after emergency abdominal surgery are increased, adequate postoperative care should be provided.

**Ten Multiple Choice Questions**

1. What is the incidence of incarceration of abdominal wall hernias?
    A. Less than 1% of all operated abdominal wall hernias
    B. Roughly 1% to 5% of all operated abdominal wall hernias
    C. Roughly 5% to 20% of all operated abdominal wall hernias
    D. Over 20% of all operated abdominal wall hernias
2. Which type of abdominal wall hernia is most likely to incarcerate?
    A. Inguinal hernias
    B. Femoral hernias
    C. Umbilical hernias
    D. Incisional hernias
3. What causes tissue to become necrotic when strangulation occurs?
    A. Due to obstruction of bowel in the hernia sac, intestinal perforation takes place causing septicemia and subsequent necrosis of tissue
    B. Due to clamping of hernia sac content, the hernia becomes non-reducible and the blood supply is cut off, causing necrosis of tissue
    C. Due to the inflammation of bowel in the hernia sac, the overlying skin becomes necrotic
    D. Due to the hernia content remaining outside of the abdomen, the natural environment is disturbed, causing non-viable conditions for the hernia content
4. What are emergency symptoms of an abdominal wall hernia, in which the surgeon should suspect strangulation?
    A. Mild pain and hindrance in daily activities, itch around the hernia, and tingling sensation in flanks
    B. Coughing, shortness of breath, pain on the chest, and vomiting
    C. Sharp or severe pain, stomach ache, nausea, and dizziness
    D. Sharp or severe pain, vomiting, and tenderness of the hernia
5. Ileus can be a symptom of:
    A. Inguinal hernia
    B. Incisional hernia
    C. Umbilical hernia
    D. Incarcerated hernia
6. What medical imaging is indicated in case of suspected strangulation?
    A. Usually none, abdominal wall hernia strangulation is a clinical diagnosis, which requires emergency surgery
    B. An abdominal ultrasound should be made to assess type and volume of hernia content

C. A computed tomography scan should always be made for the detection of subtle signs of ischemia
D. Magnetic Resonance Imaging should be performed as it renders superior images of hernia content without radiation exposure

7. Taxis ("reduction en masse") of incarcerated hernia:
   A. Can be performed safely in every patient and therefore reduce the risk of morbidity and mortality related to surgical herniorrhaphy—especially in the elderly
   B. Can only be performed safely in children
   C. Can be performed to delay surgical herniorrhaphy when no signs of strangulation are present, yet should not be standard practice
   D. Should never be performed due to the risk of reduction of necrotic bowel

8. Two statements on burst abdomen are:
I. Burst abdomen is an open wound due to dehiscence of abdominal fascia
II. Burst abdomen usually occurs within 2 weeks of the postoperative trajectory after laparotomy
   A. Only statement I is correct
   B. Only statement II is correct
   C. Both statement I and II are correct
   D. Both statement I and II are incorrect

9. Which of the 4 statements below on the use of mesh in abdominal wall hernia repair is or are correct?
   A. Mesh should always be used to reduce recurrence rates, except when simultaneous bowel resection takes place
   B. In strangulated hernia cases, mesh should never be used as the risk of infection is too high
   C. In strangulated hernia cases, only resorbable mesh can be used, as the risk of infection of permanent synthetic mesh is too high
   D. Both synthetic and resorbable biosynthetic mesh can be used in clean-contaminated settings

10. Two statements on abdominal wall hernias are:
I. Hernia sac content can exist of abdominal fat tissue, the greater omentum, mesentery, and/or intestines
II. The larger the hernia, the larger is the risk of incarceration and strangulation
   A. Only statement I is correct
   B. Only statement II is correct
   C. Both statement I and II are correct
   D. Both statement I and II are incorrect

**Correct answers**: 1C; 2B; 3B; 4D; 5D; 6A; 7C; 8C; 9D; 10A

# References

1. van Ramshorst GH, Eker HH, Hop WC, Jeekel J, Lange JF. Impact of incisional hernia on health-related quality of life and body image: a prospective cohort study. Am J Surg. 2012;204(2):144–50.
2. Jensen KK, Henriksen NA, Jorgensen LN. Inguinal hernia epidemiology. In: Hope WW, Cobb WS, Adrales GL, editors. Textbook of hernia. Cham: Springer International Publishing; 2017. p. 23–7.
3. Chapman CB, Snell AM, Rowntree LG. Decompensated portal cirrhosis: report of one hundred and twelve cases. JAMA. 1931;97(4):237–44.
4. van't Riet M, Steyerberg EW, Nellensteyn J, Bonjer HJ, Jeekel J. Meta-analysis of techniques for closure of midline abdominal incisions. Br J Surg. 2002;89(11):1350–6.
5. Bosanquet DC, Ansell J, Abdelrahman T, et al. Systematic review and meta-regression of factors affecting midline incisional hernia rates: analysis of 14,618 patients. PLoS One. 2015;10(9):e0138745.
6. Itatsu K, Yokoyama Y, Sugawara G, et al. Incidence of and risk factors for incisional hernia after abdominal surgery. Br J Surg. 2014;101(11):1439–47.
7. Poulose BK, Shelton J, Phillips S, et al. Epidemiology and cost of ventral hernia repair: making the case for hernia research. Hernia. 2012;16(2):179–83.
8. Hammoud M, Gerken J. Inguinal hernia. In: StatPearls [Internet]. Treasure Island, FL: StatPearls Publishing; 2022.

9. Muysoms FE, Miserez M, Berrevoet F, et al. Classification of primary and incisional abdominal wall hernias. Hernia. 2009;13(4):407–14.
10. Venara A, Hubner M, Le Naoures P, Hamel JF, Hamy A, Demartines N. Surgery for incarcerated hernia: short-term outcome with or without mesh. Langenbecks Arch Surg. 2014;399(5):571–7.
11. Gallegos NC, Dawson J, Jarvis M, Hobsley M. Risk of strangulation in groin hernias. Br J Surg. 1991;78(10):1171–3.
12. Pastorino A, Alshuqayfi AA. Strangulated hernia [updated 2020 Mar 14]. In: StatPearls. Treasure Island, FL: StatPearls Publishing; 2020.
13. Mullen MG, Michaels AD, Mehaffey JH, et al. Risk associated with complications and mortality after urgent surgery vs elective and emergency surgery: implications for defining "Quality" and reporting outcomes for urgent surgery. JAMA Surg. 2017;152(8):768–74.
14. Ozturk E, Yilmazlar T. Factors affecting the mortality risk in elderly patients undergoing surgery. ANZ J Surg. 2007;77(3):156–9.
15. Schumpelick V, Treutner KH, Arlt G. Inguinal hernia repair in adults. Lancet. 1994;344(8919):375–9.
16. Primatesta P, Goldacre MJ. Inguinal hernia repair: incidence of elective and emergency surgery, readmission and mortality. Int J Epidemiol. 1996;25(4):835–9.
17. Haider AH, Obirieze A, Velopulos CG, et al. Incremental cost of emergency versus elective surgery. Ann Surg. 2015;262(2):260–6.
18. Klinge U, Binnebosel M, Mertens PR. Are collagens the culprits in the development of incisional and inguinal hernia disease? Hernia. 2006;10(6):472–7.
19. Larsen OA, Lassen NA, Quaade F. Blood flow through human adipose tissue determined with radioactive xenon. Acta Physiol Scand. 1966;66(3):337–45.
20. Crandall DL, Goldstein BM, Huggins F, Cervoni P. Adipocyte blood flow: influence of age, anatomic location, and dietary manipulation. Am J Phys. 1984;247(1 Pt 2):R46–51.
21. Simons MP, Aufenacker T, Bay-Nielsen M, et al. European Hernia Society guidelines on the treatment of inguinal hernia in adult patients. Hernia. 2009;13(4):343–403.
22. Sorensen LT, Hemmingsen UB, Kirkeby LT, Kallehave F, Jorgensen LN. Smoking is a risk factor for incisional hernia. Arch Surg. 2005;140(2):119–23.
23. Tubre DJ, Schroeder AD, Estes J, Eisenga J, Fitzgibbons RJ Jr. Surgical site infection: the "Achilles Heel" of all types of abdominal wall hernia reconstruction. Hernia. 2018;22(6):1003–13.
24. van Rooijen MMJ, Kroese LF, van Vugt JLA, Lange JF. Sarcomania? The inapplicability of sarcopenia measurement in predicting incisional hernia development. World J Surg. 2019;43(3):772–9.
25. Sneiders D, Yurtkap Y, Kroese LF, et al. Risk factors for incarceration in patients with primary abdominal wall and incisional hernias: a prospective study in 4472 patients. World J Surg. 2019;43(8):1906–13.
26. Bittner JGt. Incarcerated/strangulated hernia: open or laparoscopic? Adv Surg. 2016;50(1):67–78.
27. Guo Y, Tan J, Miao Y, Sun Z, Zhang Q. Effects of microvesicles on cell apoptosis under hypoxia. Oxidative Med Cell Longev. 2019;2019:5972152.
28. Oldenburg WA, Lau LL, Rodenberg TJ, Edmonds HJ, Burger CD. Acute mesenteric ischemia: a clinical review. Arch Intern Med. 2004;164(10):1054–62.
29. Evennett NJ, Petrov MS, Mittal A, Windsor JA. Systematic review and pooled estimates for the diagnostic accuracy of serological markers for intestinal ischemia. World J Surg. 2009;33(7):1374–83.
30. Kroese LF, Sneiders D, Kleinrensink GJ, Muysoms F, Lange JF. Comparing different modalities for the diagnosis of incisional hernia: a systematic review. Hernia. 2018;22(2):229–42.
31. Aguirre DA, Santosa AC, Casola G, Sirlin CB. Abdominal wall hernias: imaging features, complications, and diagnostic pitfalls at multi-detector row CT. Radiographics. 2005;25(6):1501–20.
32. Chang KJ, Marin D, Kim DH, et al. ACR Appropriateness Criteria® suspected small-bowel obstruction. Revised 2019. https://acsearch.acr.org/docs/69476/Narrative/. Accessed 23 Jan 2021.
33. Fitzgibbons RJ Jr, Giobbie-Hurder A, Gibbs JO, et al. Watchful waiting vs repair of inguinal hernia in minimally symptomatic men: a randomized clinical trial. JAMA. 2006;295(3):285–92.
34. de Goede B, Wijsmuller AR, van Ramshorst GH, et al. Watchful waiting versus surgery of mildly symptomatic or asymptomatic inguinal hernia in men aged 50 years and older: a randomized controlled trial. Ann Surg. 2018;267(1):42–9.
35. Reistrup H, Fonnes S, Rosenberg J. Watchful waiting vs repair for asymptomatic or minimally symptomatic inguinal hernia in men: a systematic review. Hernia. 2020; https://doi.org/10.1007/s10029-020-02295-3.
36. Mizrahi H, Parker MC. Management of asymptomatic inguinal hernia: a systematic review of the evidence. Arch Surg. 2012;147(3):277–81.
37. Fitzgibbons RJ Jr, Ramanan B, Arya S, et al. Long-term results of a randomized controlled trial of a nonoperative strategy (watchful waiting) for men with minimally symptomatic inguinal hernias. Ann Surg. 2013;258(3):508–15.
38. Nieuwenhuizen J, Kleinrensink GJ, Hop WC, Jeekel J, Lange JF. Indications for incisional hernia repair: an international questionnaire among hernia surgeons. Hernia. 2008;12(3):223–5.
39. de Goede B, van Rooijen MMJ, van Kempen BJH, et al. Conservative treatment versus elective repair of umbilical hernia in patients with liver cirrhosis and ascites: results of a randomized controlled trial (CRUCIAL trial). Langenbecks Arch Surg. 2020; https://doi.org/10.1007/s00423-020-02033-4.
40. Henriksen NA, Montgomery A, Kaufmann R, et al. Guidelines for treatment of umbilical and epigastric hernias from the European Hernia Society and Americas Hernia Society. Br J Surg. 2020;107(3):171–90.
41. Miserez M, Peeters E, Aufenacker T, et al. Update with level 1 studies of the European Hernia Society

guidelines on the treatment of inguinal hernia in adult patients. Hernia. 2014;18(2):151–63.
42. Eker HH, van Ramshorst GH, de Goede B, et al. A prospective study on elective umbilical hernia repair in patients with liver cirrhosis and ascites. Surgery. 2011;150(3):542–6.
43. Khorgami Z, Hui BY, Mushtaq N, Chow GS, Sclabas GM. Predictors of mortality after elective ventral hernia repair: an analysis of national inpatient sample. Hernia. 2019;23(5):979–85.
44. Linzer JF. Chapter 47: Inguinal hernia. In: Sharieff G, Schafermeyer R, editors. Strange and Schafermeyer's pediatric emergency medicine. 4th ed. New York: McGraw-Hill Education; 2014.
45. Puri P, Guiney EJ, O'Donnell B. Inguinal hernia in infants: the fate of the testis following incarceration. J Pediatr Surg. 1984;19(1):44–6.
46. East B, Pawlak M, de Beaux AC. A manual reduction of hernia under analgesia/sedation (Taxis) in the acute inguinal hernia: a useful technique in COVID-19 times to reduce the need for emergency surgery-a literature review. Hernia. 2020;24(5):937–41.
47. Harissis HV, Douitsis E, Fatouros M. Incarcerated hernia: to reduce or not to reduce? Hernia. 2009;13(3):263–6.
48. O'Reilly EA, Burke JP, O'Connell PR. A meta-analysis of surgical morbidity and recurrence after laparoscopic and open repair of primary unilateral inguinal hernia. Ann Surg. 2012;255(5):846–53.
49. Eklund A, Montgomery A, Bergkvist L, Rudberg C, Swedish Multicentre Trial of Inguinal Hernia Repair by Laparoscopy (SMIL) Study Group. Chronic pain 5 years after randomized comparison of laparoscopic and Lichtenstein inguinal hernia repair. Br J Surg. 2010;97(4):600–8.
50. Sgourakis G, Radtke A, Sotiropoulos GC, et al. Assessment of strangulated content of the spontaneously reduced inguinal hernia via hernia sac laparoscopy: preliminary results of a prospective randomized study. Surg Laparosc Endosc Percutan Tech. 2009;19(2):133–7.
51. Sauerland S, Agresta F, Bergamaschi R, et al. Laparoscopy for abdominal emergencies: evidence-based guidelines of the European Association for Endoscopic Surgery. Surg Endosc. 2006;20(1):14–29.
52. Nilsson H, Stylianidis G, Haapamaki M, Nilsson E, Nordin P. Mortality after groin hernia surgery. Ann Surg. 2007;245(4):656–60.
53. Martinez-Serrano MA, Pereira JA, Sancho JJ, et al. Risk of death after emergency repair of abdominal wall hernias. Still waiting for improvement. Langenbecks Arch Surg. 2010;395(5):551–6.
54. Derici H, Unalp HR, Bozdag AD, Nazli O, Tansug T, Kamer E. Factors affecting morbidity and mortality in incarcerated abdominal wall hernias. Hernia. 2007;11(4):341–6.
55. EU Hernia Trialists Collaboration. Repair of groin hernia with synthetic mesh: meta-analysis of randomized controlled trials. Ann Surg. 2002;235(3):322–32.
56. Kaufmann R, Halm JA, Eker HH, et al. Mesh versus suture repair of umbilical hernia in adults: a randomised, double-blind, controlled, multicentre trial. Lancet. 2018;391(10123):860–9.
57. Luijendijk RW, Hop WC, van den Tol MP, et al. A comparison of suture repair with mesh repair for incisional hernia. N Engl J Med. 2000;343(6):392–8.
58. Mathes T, Walgenbach M, Siegel R. Suture versus mesh repair in primary and incisional ventral hernias: a systematic review and meta-analysis. World J Surg. 2016;40(4):826–35.
59. Burger JW, Luijendijk RW, Hop WC, Halm JA, Verdaasdonk EG, Jeekel J. Long-term follow-up of a randomized controlled trial of suture versus mesh repair of incisional hernia. Ann Surg. 2004;240(4):578–83; discussion 83–5.
60. Markar SR, Karthikesalingam A, Alam F, Tang TY, Walsh SR, Sadat U. Partially or completely absorbable versus nonabsorbable mesh repair for inguinal hernia: a systematic review and meta-analysis. Surg Laparosc Endosc Percutan Tech. 2010;20(4):213–9.
61. Choi JJ, Palaniappa NC, Dallas KB, Rudich TB, Colon MJ, Divino CM. Use of mesh during ventral hernia repair in clean-contaminated and contaminated cases: outcomes of 33,832 cases. Ann Surg. 2012;255(1):176–80.
62. Ventral Hernia Working Group, Breuing K, Butler CE, et al. Incisional ventral hernias: review of the literature and recommendations regarding the grading and technique of repair. Surgery. 2010;148(3):544–58.
63. Cavallaro A, Lo Menzo E, Di Vita M, et al. Use of biological meshes for abdominal wall reconstruction in highly contaminated fields. World J Gastroenterol. 2010;16(15):1928–33.
64. van Rooijen M, Jairam A, Tollens T, et al. Outcomes of a new slowly resorbable biosynthetic mesh (Phasix) in potentially contaminated incisional hernias: a prospective, multi-center, single-arm trial. Int J Surg. 2020;83:31–6.
65. Carbonell AM, Criss CN, Cobb WS, Novitsky YW, Rosen MJ. Outcomes of synthetic mesh in contaminated ventral hernia repairs. J Am Coll Surg. 2013;217(6):991–8.
66. Liang MK, Bernardi K, Holihan JL, et al. Modifying risks in ventral hernia patients with prehabilitation: a randomized controlled trial. Ann Surg. 2018;268(4):674–80.
67. Hughes MJ, Hackney RJ, Lamb PJ, Wigmore SJ, Christopher Deans DA, Skipworth RJE. Prehabilitation before major abdominal surgery: a systematic review and meta-analysis. World J Surg. 2019;43(7):1661–8.
68. Hasselager R, Gogenur I. Core muscle size assessed by perioperative abdominal CT scan is related to mortality, postoperative complications, and hospitalization after major abdominal surgery: a systematic review. Langenbecks Arch Surg. 2014;399(3):287–95.
69. Nielsen MØ, Bjerg J, Dorfelt A, Jørgensen LN, Jensen KK. Short-term safety of preoperative administration

of botulinum toxin A for the treatment of large ventral hernia with loss of domain. Hernia. 2020;24(2):295–9.
70. Rodriguez-Acevedo O, Elstner KE, Jacombs ASW, et al. Preoperative Botulinum toxin A enabling defect closure and laparoscopic repair of complex ventral hernia. Surg Endosc. 2018;32(2):831–9.
71. Yurtkap Y, van Rooijen MMJ, Roels S, et al. Implementing preoperative Botulinum toxin A and progressive pneumoperitoneum through the use of an algorithm in giant ventral hernia repair. Hernia. 2020; https://doi.org/10.1007/s10029-020-02226-2.
72. van Rooijen MMJ, Yurtkap Y, Allaeys M, Ibrahim N, Berrevoet F, Lange JF. Fascial closure in giant ventral hernias after preoperative botulinum toxin a and progressive pneumoperitoneum: a systematic review and meta-analysis. Surgery. 2021;170:769–76.
73. Chevrel JP, Rath AM. Classification of incisional hernias of the abdominal wall. Hernia. 2000;4(1):7–11.
74. Lindmark M, Strigard K, Lowenmark T, Dahlstrand U, Gunnarsson U. Risk factors for surgical complications in ventral hernia repair. World J Surg. 2018;42(11):3528–36.
75. Flum DR, Horvath K, Koepsell T. Have outcomes of incisional hernia repair improved with time? A population-based analysis. Ann Surg. 2003;237(1):129–35.
76. Millbourn D, Cengiz Y, Israelsson LA. Effect of stitch length on wound complications after closure of midline incisions: a randomized controlled trial. Arch Surg. 2009;144(11):1056–9.
77. Deerenberg EB, Harlaar JJ, Steyerberg EW, et al. Small bites versus large bites for closure of abdominal midline incisions (STITCH): a double-blind, multicentre, randomised controlled trial. Lancet. 2015;386(10000):1254–60.
78. Lopez-Cano M, Garcia-Alamino JM, Antoniou SA, et al. EHS clinical guidelines on the management of the abdominal wall in the context of the open or burst abdomen. Hernia. 2018;22(6):921–39.
79. van't Riet M, de Vos van Steenwijk PJ, Bonjer HJ, Steyerberg EW, Jeekel J. Mesh repair for postoperative wound dehiscence in the presence of infection: is absorbable mesh safer than non-absorbable mesh? Hernia. 2007;11(5):409–13.
80. van Ramshorst GH, Eker HH, Harlaar JJ, Nijens KJ, Jeekel J, Lange JF. Therapeutic alternatives for burst abdomen. Surg Technol Int. 2010;19:111–9.

## Further Reading

Burger JW, Luijendijk RW, Hop WC, Halm JA, Verdaasdonk EG, Jeekel J. Long-term follow-up of a randomized controlled trial of suture versus mesh repair of incisional hernia. Ann Surg. 2004;240(4):578–83.

Henriksen NA, Montgomery A, Kaufmann R, et al. Guidelines for treatment of umbilical and epigastric hernias from the European Hernia Society and Americas Hernia Society. Br J Surg. 2020;107(3):171–90.

Jairam AP, Timmermans L, Eker HH, et al. Prevention of incisional hernia with prophylactic onlay and sublay mesh reinforcement versus primary suture only in midline laparotomies (PRIMA): 2-year follow-up of a multicentre, double-blind, randomised controlled trial. Lancet. 2017;390(10094):567–76.

Sartelli M, Coccolini F, van Ramshorst GH, Campanelli G, Mandalà V, Ansaloni L, Moore EE, Peitzman A, Velmahos G, Moore FA, Leppaniemi A, Burlew CC, Biffl W, Koike K, Kluger Y, Fraga GP, Ordonez CA, Di Saverio S, Agresta F, Sakakushev B, Gerych I, Wani I, Kelly MD, Gomes CA, Faro MP Jr, Taviloglu K, Demetrashvili Z, Lee JG, Vettoretto N, Guercioni G, Tranà C, Cui Y, Kok KY, Ghnnam WM, Ael-S A, Sato N, Marwah S, Rangarajan M, Ben-Ishay O, Adesunkanmi AR, Segovia Lohse HA, Kenig J, Mandalà S, Patrizi A, Scibé R, Catena F. WSES guidelines for emergency repair of complicated abdominal wall hernias. World J Emerg Surg. 2013;8(1):50.

# Emergency Management of Internal Hernia

**79**

David Czeiger, Julia Vaynshtein, Ivan Kukeev, and Gad Shaked

## 79.1 Introduction

Internal hernias (IHs; alternative plural: herniae) are protrusions of the viscera through the peritoneum or mesentery but remaining within the abdominal cavity. The most common presentation is an acute obstruction of small bowel loops that are incarcerated in normal or abnormal apertures. The affected loops in internal hernias are prone to strangulation and ischemia making this condition a potentially life threatening which makes it a surgical emergency.

In contemporary practice, virtually all patients undergo computed tomography (CT), which is the gold-standard imaging modality for the assessment of bowel obstruction and suspected internal hernias. Traditionally, barium studies were performed and may still on occasion be used in niche circumstances. Abdominal wall, inguinal, and femoral hernias can usually be detected on clinical examination. On the contrary, small incisional hernias, hernias in obese individuals, and internal hernias—the objective of this chapter, may not be clinically evident but can usually be identified on CT scan.

Intestinal obstruction is a common disorder requiring emergency treatment. Diagnosis is usually straightforward, based upon history of vomiting and difficulty to pass gases. Physical findings of a distended abdomen and hypovolemia, with abnormal roentgenograms, show air and fluid filled loops of intestine. Internal hernia (IH) is one of the rare causes of intestinal obstruction. The protrusion of abdominal viscera, most commonly small bowel loops, may occur through a congenital or acquired peritoneal or mesenteric opening into a compartment in the abdominal or the pelvic cavity. Congenital IH orifices are either normal foramina or the result of abnormal peritoneal bands and internal rotation during the embryologic development. Acquired openings may develop due to inflammation, trauma, or surgery [1]. Surgical procedures cause internal hernia by two mechanisms—First, mesenteric defects that develop secondary to anastomosis of the digestive tract during gastrointestinal tract reconstruction; second, a small bowel that enters a closed space through adhesive peritoneal bands or the omentum. A herniated intestine often becomes strangulated and distended if the hernia orifice compresses its mesentery. In occasions, the clinical presentation is mild and vague diagnosis may be difficult and delayed. Abdominal CT scan with oral contrast material would usually provide the correct diagnosis [2].

---

D. Czeiger · J. Vaynshtein · G. Shaked (✉)
Department of General Surgery, Soroka University Medical Center, Ben Gurion University, Beer Sheva, Israel
e-mail: czeiger@bgu.ac.il

I. Kukeev
Department of General Surgery, Soroka University Medical Center, Beer Sheva, Israel

> **Learning Goals**
> - To increase the awareness to the diagnosis of internal hernia which is relatively a rare etiology for intestinal obstruction.
> - To understand the management of internal hernia.

## 79.2 Epidemiology

IHs cause 0.6–6.0% of small bowel obstructions [3, 4] and 1–4% of intestinal obstructions attributed to hernias [5].

## 79.3 Etiology

IH can be categorized as congenital (herniation through normal foramina or recesses or from developmental anomalies of peritoneal attachments) or acquired defects in the abdominal cavity (Table 79.1). Acquired internal hernia is attributed to inflammation, trauma, or previous surgical procedure. Acquired IHs have been reported subsequent open surgeries and laparoscopic procedures and currently correspond for higher incidence than the congenital cases [6].

**Table 79.1** Classification of internal hernias

| Name | Etiology | Incidences (%) |
|---|---|---|
| Paraduodenal | | 53 |
| Foramen of Winslow | | 8 |
| Sigmoid mesocolon | | 6 |
| Pericecal | | 13 |
| Supravesical and pelvic | | 6 |
| Transmesenteric | Roux-en-Y procedures | 8 |
| Transomental | | 3 |
| Retroanastomotic | Postoperative | 3 |

## 79.4 Pathophysiology

The pathophysiology that leads to intestinal obstruction and ischemia resembles that of other conditions of bowel herniation. Following incarceration of a bowel segment, the draining mesenteric veins are occluded, thus creating severe congestive changes in the bowel wall and its mesentery. Increased venous and capillary pressure leads to fluid-filled dilatation of the closed loop, edema, rupture of small vessels, and the formation of intramural and mesenteric hematoma. Thrombosis within the mesenteric vein may occur with ongoing congestive changes. Finally, severe congestion may lead to elevated inner-tissue pressure high enough to obstruct small arteries blood flow, which ends in necrosis and eventually perforation of the intestinal wall [2].

## 79.5 Classification and Types

1. IHs can be categorized as congenital versus acquired. Another categorization is according to the type of hernia orifice: herniation through a normal foramen, an unusual peritoneal fossa or site of weakness into the retroperitoneal space, or an abnormal opening in the omentum, pelvic floor, or mesentery.
2. *Paraduodenal hernias (PDH)*—This is the most common type of internal hernia accounting for 53% of all cases. There are several fossae in the area of the duodenum. The fossa of Landzert is the site of left PDH results from failure of fusion of the inferior mesentery to the parietal peritoneum. The fossa of Waldeyer is site of right PDH occurs most frequently in cases of a nonrotated small intestine and a normally or incompletely rotated colon.
3. *Pericecal hernias*—These hernias account for 13% of internal hernias. The pericecal fossa is located behind the cecum and

ascending colon. Most commonly, ileal loops herniate through a defect in the cecal mesentery and extending into the right paracolic gutter.

4. *Foramen of Winslow*—The greater and lesser sacs of the peritoneal cavity communicate through the foramen of Winslow. Hernias involving the foramen of Winslow account for 8% of all internal hernias. The small bowel is the most common intestinal segment involved. Predisposing factors include an enlarged foramen of Winslow and excessively mobile intestinal loops due to a long mesentery.

5. *Transmesenteric hernias*—Transmesenteric hernias account for 8% of all internal hernias. However, transmesenteric hernias are the most common type in children occurring in 35% of the cases of internal hernia [7]. The small bowel mesentery is a broad fold of peritoneum that suspends the loops of the small intestine from the posterior abdominal wall. The two layers of peritoneal reflection form the mesentery, which extends from its origin at the ligament of Treitz to the right toward the ileocecal valve. The defect in the mesentery is usually 2–5 cm in diameter and is located close to the ligament of Treitz or the ileocecal valve. Usually, transmesenteric hernias are congenital in the pediatric group of patients. In contrast, in adults transmesenteric hernias result mainly from surgery.

6. *Sigmoid-related hernias*—The sigmoid mesocolon is a peritoneal fold attaching the sigmoid colon to the pelvic wall. Sigmoid-related hernias account to 6% of all internal hernias. It typically develops when herniated bowel, mainly ileum, protrudes into the intersigmoid fossa, formed between two adjacent sigmoid segments and their respective mesenteries.

7. *Supravesical and pelvic hernias*—Supravesical and pelvic internal hernias account for approximately 6% of all IHs. Broad ligament hernia is the most common type of pelvic internal hernia. The rest of this group are hernias through the perirectal fossa and fossa of Douglas. Usually, small intestine protrudes through an abnormal aperture in the broad ligament of the uterus. Herniation of colon, ovary, and ureter has also been described [8]. In internal supravesical hernias, the intestine protrudes downward into a space around the bladder through supravesical fossa.

8. *Transmesenteric hernias*—Most of the transmesenteric hernias in adults are associated with previous gastrointestinal surgery, abdominal trauma, and intraperitoneal inflammation. Creation of mesenteric defect or retroanastomotic space leads to postoperative transmesenteric or retroanastomotic internal herniation, which develops primarily after gastrectomy or Roux-en-Y bypass surgery [9]. Three main types of postoperative transmesenteric internal hernias are seen. The most common is the postoperative transmesenteric hernia that occurs through the transverse mesocolon, which has been documented to occur mainly in patients after laparoscopic Roux-en-Y gastric bypass surgery [6]. Less commonly occurs when bowel prolapses through a defect in the small-bowel mesentery [10]. Finally, the third type, known as the Peterson type, involves the herniation of small bowel behind the Roux loop before the small bowel eventually passes through the defect in the transverse mesocolon.

9. *Retroanastomotic hernias*—Retroanastomotic hernias occur when small bowel loops herniate posteriorly through a defect related to a surgical anastomosis. These hernias have been most commonly associated with the Roux-en-Y formation and Billroth II reconstruction, and are increasing in incidence as gastric bypasses for bariatric surgeries continue to become more frequent and widespread. If the surgery is of the retrocolic type, a Petersen's space created posterior to the Roux limb, extending from the root of the Roux limb mesentery to the level of the transverse colon [11]. The most common herniated loop is the efferent jejunal segment. Less commonly, a very long afferent limb, ileum, cecum, or omentum can herniate into the retroanastomotic space. However,

if antecolic surgery is done, the afferent loop will be the most commonly involved segment [12].
10. *Perineal hernia*—This is a rare complication after conventional abdominoperineal resection, perineal prostatectomy, cystourethrectomy, or hysterectomy. Perineal hernia is defined by the protrusion of the intraabdominal viscera through a defect in the pelvic floor at an incision site. Perineal hernias mostly occur in females and are usually discovered within 1 year of surgery [13].

## 79.6 Diagnosis

### 79.6.1 Clinical Presentation

The most common manifestation of an internal hernia is strangulating small bowel obstruction. However, IH can be asymptomatic or cause significant symptoms ranging from constant vague epigastric pain to intermittent colicky abdominal pain. Additional symptoms include nausea, vomiting, and recurrent intestinal obstruction. The severity of symptoms depends on the presence or absence of incarceration and strangulation. Since these hernias tend to spontaneously reduce, patients are best imaged when they are symptomatic [12, 14].

### 79.6.2 Diagnostic Studies

Imaging studies play an important role in the diagnosis of internal hernias because they are often difficult to identify clinically. In the past, these hernias were most frequently assessed with small-bowel oral contrast studies. General radiographic features with barium studies include apparent encapsulation of distended bowel loops in an abnormal location, arrangement or crowding of small-bowel loops within the hernial sac, evidence of obstruction with segmental dilatation and stasis, with additional features of apparent fixation and reversed peristalsis during fluoroscopic evaluation [12].

Since the interval between intestinal obstruction and ischemia may be short, a time-consuming diagnostic workup prior surgery, may be dangerous for an acutely ill patient [15]. Multidetector computed tomography (MDCT), has become the first-line imaging technique in these patients [8] because of its availability, speed, and multiplanar reformatting (MPR) capabilities. In the evaluation of small bowel obstruction, it is important to perform the CT scan pre- and postintravenous contrast material injection. Precontrast CT scan can delineate intramural hematoma and intramesenteric hematoma. Intravenous contrast material enhancement allows better delineation of the small bowel and its mesenteric vessels [2].

Currently, with the possibility of using high-quality three-dimensional reformation techniques such as MPR, maximum intensity projection (MIP), and volume rendering (VR), CT provides important advantages in evaluation of small bowel and surrounding structure, increasing the diagnostic confidence in the localization of the transition zone [1].

The following factors may be helpful in preoperative diagnosis of internal hernias with CT: (a) knowledge of the normal anatomy of the peritoneal cavity and the characteristic anatomic location of each type of internal hernia; (b) observation of a saclike mass or cluster of dilated small bowel loops at an abnormal anatomic location in the presence of small bowel obstruction (SBO); (c) observation of an engorged, stretched, and displaced mesenteric vascular pedicle and of converging vessels at the hernia orifice [16]. IH may present itself for the first time as strangulated gangrenous bowel. One should search supportive hints for this condition in the scan.

> **Differential Diagnosis**
>
> The clinical presentation and the plain abdominal X-ray may resemble in the different types of bowel obstruction. Thus, the managing surgeon should take into consideration all the etiologies.

## 79.7 Treatment

### 79.7.1 Medical Treatment

Patients with bowel obstruction with multiple episodes of vomiting lasting for several days and with large-volume intraluminal fluid sequestration can have severe volume depletion, metabolic acidosis or alkalosis, and electrolyte abnormalities.

- *Fluid therapy*—Upon admission, isotonic crystalloid fluid such as Lactated Ringer's solution or normal saline may be appropriate for initial intravenous fluid therapy if the patient is dehydrated. Aggressive potassium repletion may be needed, but it is important to be certain the patient does not have acute renal failure, in which case potassium supplementation should be halted until renal function is improved.
- Even for patients who require immediate surgery, fluid resuscitation and repletion of electrolytes must be completed prior to surgery, to minimize complications related to induction of anesthesia.
- *Gastrointestinal decompression*—The need for gastrointestinal decompression in the setting of IH may vary from patient to patient and remains a matter of clinical judgment. Nasogastric tube decompression of the distended stomach improves patient comfort and minimizes the passage of swallowed air. These patients are made nil per os (NPO).
- *Role of antibiotics*—For most patients with IH, administering broad-spectrum antibiotics is practiced because of concerns for bacterial translocation due to suspected bowel compromise (ischemia, necrosis, or perforation). Standard perioperative prophylactic antibiotics should be administered to those who undergo operative exploration, depending upon the expected wound classification [17].

### 79.7.2 Surgical Treatment

The most serious manifestation of internal hernias is ischemia of the bowel, which occurs because of the tendency to create closed-loop obstruction and strangulation. Therefore, in patients suspected to have internal hernias, early surgical intervention is indicated to reduce the high morbidity and mortality rates.

In patients suspected to have strangulation or perforation based on clinical or imaging findings, it is prudent to perform a laparotomy. In others, diagnostic laparoscopy should be carried out with a plan to progress, if needed, to laparoscopic repair of the IH [18]. Operative success depends on knowledge and accurate intraoperative appreciation of the anatomy.

The surgical procedures for the management of internal hernias include reduction in the herniated loop, resection of ischemic bowel segment, and repair of the hernial opening. Slight traction may be the only maneuver to reduce the herniated intestinal segment, though in difficult situations dilation of the hernial sac opening may be inevitable. Frequently, mild ischemia of the herniated loop reverses a few minutes after its reduction. Resection is indicated for necrosis, perforation, and severe ischemia of the intestinal segment. The hernial orifice must be closed to prevent recurrent herniation. This procedure can be performed by laparoscopy, with lower morbidity and mortality [19].

> **Dos and Don'ts**
> 
> **Dos**
> - Early management of intestinal obstruction should include the insertion of a nasogastric tube and a urinary catheter, and calculated water balance.
> - The presence of systemic inflammation signs supports the inclusion of broad-spectrum antibiotics in the treatment plan.
> - Remember solutions with potassium to replenish water balance should be used in the absence of signs of renal failure.

**Don'ts**
- Do not postpone surgery if the patient demonstrates peritoneal signs.
- Do not delay surgery for more than 12 hours in patients with SBO and no previous abdominal surgery.

## 79.7.3 Prognosis

Prognosis is excellent in cases of internal hernia operated upon as an elective or semi elective surgery. Rapid diagnosis and surgery are essential to ensure good outcome in cases of intestinal obstruction and incarceration. If the situation has progressed to ischemia, necrosis, and perforation of bowel the required operative procedure is more complicated and necessarily might followed by a less favorable outcome.

**Take-Home Messages**
- Internal hernia is not a common cause of abdominal emergencies.
- High index of suspicion is required for correct diagnosis.
- Prompt management is mandatory for good recovery from this condition.

**Questions**

1. What is the name of hernia's mesentery defect after Roux-En-Y reconstruction?
   A. Littre hernia
   B. Amyand's hernia
   C. Richter hernia
   D. **Petersen hernia**
2. What is the most common type of congenital internal hernia?
   A. Supravesical hernia
   B. **Paraduodenal hernia**
   C. Pericecal hernia
   D. Foramen of Winslow hernia
3. What is an Landzert hernia?
   A. **Herniation through left paraduodenal fossa**
   B. Herniation through right iliac fossa
   C. Herniation through right paraduodenal fossa
   D. Herniation through intersigmoid fossa
4. What is the best method for internal hernia detection?
   A. Magnetic resonance imaging
   B. Ultrasound scan
   C. **Computed tomography**
   D. Physical examination
5. Which is structure of mesentery occluded first following bowel segment incarceration?
   A. Fat
   B. **Veins**
   C. Arteries
   D. Lymph nodes
6. What is a congenital internal hernia?
   A. **Herniation through a natural orifice formed as a result of normal embryological development**
   B. Herniation through an orifice because of traumatic incident
   C. Herniation as a result of post-surgery adhesions
   D. Herniation through postoperative wound
7. What is the most common type of congenital internal hernia in children group?
   A. Perineal hernia
   B. **Transmesenteric hernia**
   C. Supravesical hernia
   D. Paraduodenal hernia
8. What is the most common herniated organ in retroanastomotic hernia (retrocolic type)?
   A. **Efferent jejunum**
   B. Herniated cecum
   C. Herniated ileum
   D. Herniated omentum

9. What type of surgery is predisposing to perineal hernia development?
   A. Sigmoidectomy
   B. **Hysterectomy**
   C. Low anterior resection
   D. Oophorectomy
10. What are predisposition factors for foramen of Winslow hernia development?
    A. **Enlargement of Winslow foramen and long mesentery of intestinal loops**
    B. Liver surgery
    C. Obesity
    D. Cirrhosis

## References

1. Lanzetta MM, Masserelli A, Addeo G, et al. Internal hernias: a difficult diagnostic challenge. Review of CT signs and clinical findings. Acta Biomed. 2019;90(5-S):20–37. https://doi.org/10.23750/abm.v90i5-S.8344.
2. Hongo N, Mori H, Matsumoto S, Okino Y, Takaji R, Komatsu E. Internal hernias after abdominal surgeries: MDCT features. Abdom Imaging. 2011;36(4):349–62. https://doi.org/10.1007/s00261-010-9627-3.
3. Newsom BD, Kukora JS. Congenital and acquired internal hernias: unusual causes of small bowel obstruction. Am J Surg. 1986;152(3):279–85. pii: S0002-9610(86)90258-8.
4. Bergstein JM, Condon RE. Obturator hernia: current diagnosis and treatment. Surgery. 1996;119(2):133–6. pii: S0039-6060(96)80159-0.
5. Kulkarni GV, Salgaonkar HP, Sharma PC, Chakkarvarty NR, Katara AN, Bhandarkar DS. Laparoscopic repair of left paraduodenal hernia: report of two cases and review of the literature. Asian J Endosc Surg. 2016;9(2):157–60. https://doi.org/10.1111/ases.12270.
6. Higa KD, Ho T, Boone KB. Internal hernias after laparoscopic Roux-en-Y gastric bypass: incidence, treatment and prevention. Obes Surg. 2003;13(3):350–4. https://doi.org/10.1381/096089203765887642.
7. Mathieu D, Luciani A, GERMAD Group. Internal abdominal herniations. AJR Am J Roentgenol. 2004;183(2):397–404. pii: 183/2/397.
8. Doishita S, Takeshita T, Uchima Y, et al. Internal hernias in the era of multidetector CT: correlation of imaging and surgical findings. Radiographics. 2016;36(1):88–106. https://doi.org/10.1148/rg.2016150113.
9. Filip JE, Mattar SG, Bowers SP, Smith CD. Internal hernia formation after laparoscopic Roux-en-Y gastric bypass for morbid obesity. Am Surg. 2002;68(7):640–3.
10. Renvall S, Niinikoski J. Internal hernias after gastric operations. Eur J Surg. 1991;157(10):575–7.
11. Bauman RW, Pirrello JR. Internal hernia at Petersen's space after laparoscopic Roux-en-Y gastric bypass: 6.2% incidence without closure—a single surgeon series of 1047 cases. Surg Obes Relat Dis. 2009;5(5):565–70. https://doi.org/10.1016/j.soard.2008.10.013.
12. Martin LC, Merkle EM, Thompson WM. Review of internal hernias: radiographic and clinical findings. AJR Am J Roentgenol. 2006;186(3):703–17. pii: 186/3/703.
13. Skipworth RJ, Smith GH, Anderson DN. Secondary perineal hernia following open abdominoperineal excision of the rectum: report of a case and review of the literature. Hernia. 2007;11(6):541–5. https://doi.org/10.1007/s10029-007-0234-3.
14. Blachar A, Federle MP, Dodson SF. Internal hernia: clinical and imaging findings in 17 patients with emphasis on CT criteria. Radiology. 2001;218(1):68–74. https://doi.org/10.1148/radiology.218.1.r01ja5368.
15. Fan HP, Yang AD, Chang YJ, Juan CW, Wu HP. Clinical spectrum of internal hernia: a surgical emergency. Surg Today. 2008;38(10):899–904. https://doi.org/10.1007/s00595-007-3756-5.
16. Takeyama N, Gokan T, Ohgiya Y, et al. CT of internal hernias. Radiographics. 2005;25(4):997–1015. pii: 25/4/997.
17. O'Hara LM, Thom KA, Preas MA. Update to the Centers for Disease Control and Prevention and the Healthcare Infection Control Practices Advisory Committee Guideline for the Prevention of Surgical Site Infection (2017): a summary, review, and strategies for implementation. Am J Infect Control. 2018;46(6):602–9. pii: S0196-6553(18)30063-4.
18. Matsunami M, Kusanagi H, Hayashi K, Yamada S, Kano N. Broad ligament hernia successfully treated by laparoscopy: case report and review of literature. Asian J Endosc Surg. 2014;7(4):327–9. https://doi.org/10.1111/ases.12119.
19. Talebpour M, Habibi GR, Bandarian F. Laparoscopic management of an internal double omental hernia: a rare cause of intestinal obstruction. Hernia. 2005;9(2):195–7. https://doi.org/10.1007/s10029-004-0288-4.

# Emergency Management Hiatal Hernia and Gastric Volvulus

## 80

Imtiaz Wani, G. M. Naikoo, and Nisar Hamdani

**Take-Home Messages**
- Acute gastric volvulus secondary to paraesophageal hernia is a rare surgical emergency.
- A high index of suspicion is required for diagnosing acute gastric volvulus with paraesophageal hernia in the presence of gastroesophageal obstructive symptoms.
- Prompt management of acute gastric volvulus secondary to paraesophageal hernia is necessary to prevent complications associated with high morbidity and mortality.
- Surgical approach is open, laparoendoscopic or laparoscopic.
- Abdominal wall gastropexy in open as well as laparoscopy surgery prevents recurrent gastric volvulus.

I. Wani (✉)
Department of Minimal Access and General Surgery,
Government Gousia Hospital,
Srinagar, Jammu and Kashmir, India

G. M. Naikoo
Department of Minimal Access and General Surgery,
Government Medical College,
Srinagar, Jammu and Kashmir, India

N. Hamdani
Department of Surgical Gastroenterology,
Superspeciality Hospital, Shireen Bagh,
Srinagar, Jammu and Kashmir, India

## 80.1 Introduction

**Learning Goals**
- Acute gastric volvulus is a true surgical emergency.
- Acute gastric volvulus secondary to the paraesophageal hernia is a rare.
- Diagnosis of acute volvulus requires high index of clinical suspicion.
- Ideally should be managed by experts in upper gastrointestinal surgery.

Acute gastric volvulus associated with paraesophageal hernia has a mortality rate of 30–50%, with major sequelae being gastric obstruction, strangulation, gastric wall necrosis, perforation, and hypovolemic shock [1]. The clinical manifestations of acute gastric volvulus mimics as those of strangulated paraesophageal hernia. The cardinal symptoms are severe epigastric pain, lower chest pain, intractable vomiting, or there may be only retching. The only 4% of hiatal hernias are complicated by gastric volvulus [2]. Emergency surgery for paraesophageal hernia is required in patients complicated with gastric volvulus, uncontrolled bleeding, strangulation, perforation, obstruction, or respiratory compromise [3]. Acute gastric volvulus and strangulated paraesophageal hernia represent a surgical emergency and should be managed as an acute emergency [4].

## 80.2 Paraesophageal Hernia

Hiatal hernia is simply the protrusion of the stomach into the thoracic cavity [5]. The etiology of hiatal hernia is still obscure. Most likely causes implicated in the development of hiatal hernias are elevated intra-abdominal pressure, congenital or acquired widening of the diaphragmatic hiatus, trauma, congenital malformations, and iatrogenic factors [6, 7].

### 80.2.1 Classification

Hiatal hernia is classified into four types. This classification is based on anatomic location of the gastroesophageal junction in relation to the diaphragmatic hiatus and by the contents of the sac of hernia [8]. In type I or sliding hiatal hernia, a portion of the gastric cardia herniates upward into thorax through diaphragmatic hiatus. Type II or rolling hernia, also known as "true paraesophageal hernia" has the gastric fundus herniating into the thorax, but the gastroesophageal junction remains at its normal position. Type III hiatal hernia is the association of type II with the migration of the gastroesophageal junction into the thorax (Figs. 80.1 and 80.2). This type III represents the 90% of all paraesophageal hernias [9]. Type IV is associated with presence of the abdominal viscera in the thoracic cavity. Most common viscera present in type IV hiatal hernia is the colon, but there may spleen or small bowel, omentum, and transverse colon [10]. There is type of hiatal hernia known as giant hiatal hernia or giant gastric hernia where there is migration of one third or more of stomach into the thorax.

### 80.2.2 Clinical Presentation and Diagnosis

Paraesophageal hernias are diagnosed in one of three scenarios [11]:

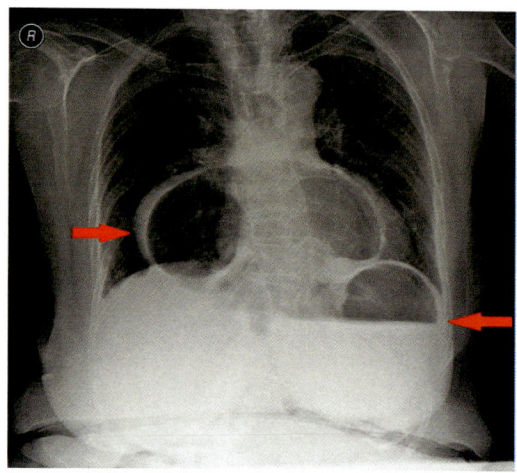

**Fig. 80.1** Chest X-ray showing hiatal hernia. The right arrow shows a stomach portion within the thoracic cavity and the left arrow shows another stomach portion within the abdominal cavity. (Reproduced from Rodrigues C, Taveira I, Deus A, et al. (February 11, 2021) Gastric Volvulus: A Multidisciplinary Approach and Conservative Treatment. Cureus 13(2): e13285. https://doi.org/10.7759/cureus.1328)

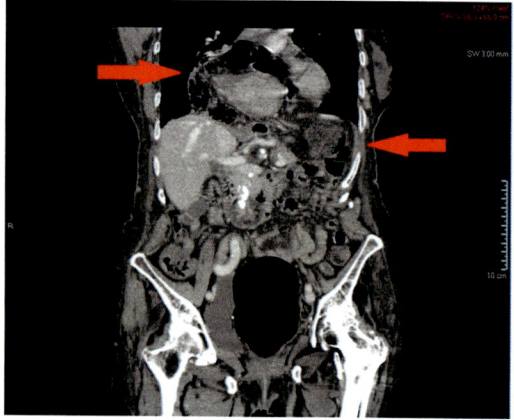

**Fig. 80.2** CT scan in coronal view showing a distended stomach, with a major portion in the intrathoracic segment. The right arrow shows a stomach portion within the thoracic cavity and the left arrow shows another stomach portion within the abdominal cavity. (Reproduced from Rodrigues C, Taveira I, Deus A, et al. (February 11, 2021) Gastric Volvulus: A Multidisciplinary Approach and Conservative Treatment. Cureus 13(2): e13285. https://doi.org/10.7759/cureus.1328)

I. The patient is asymptomatic and the Paraesophageal (PEH) is discovered after performing imaging for an unrelated reason;

II. The patient is symptomatic but not acute; or
III. The patient presents with features of acute obstruction or incarceration of stomach and/or involved organs, which may include ischemia, gangrene, and sepsis.

These paraesophageal hernias especially type I are often asymptomatic or there may vague, intermittent symptoms of gastroesophageal reflux disease (GERD), epigastric pain, heartburn, postprandial fullness, regurgitation, and dysphagia. An upsurge of occurrence of paraesophageal hernia is being recently observed in the population. Complications of paraesophageal hernias are rare and are usually related to reflux, gastric volvulus, bleeding from ulcerations, and erosions of the herniated organs with the respiratory complications seen [12]. Large hiatal hernias, especially in obese patient, may cause compression of the heart and reduce coronary blood flow sufficiently to cause dyspnea, tachycardia, angina, and syncope [13]. Barium swallow, upper endoscopy, computed tomography scan, and esophageal manometry are utilized in the diagnosis.

## 80.3 Gastric Volvulus

Berti in 1866 first described gastric volvulus in autopsy of a female patient and first treated surgically in 1897 by Berg in a patient with traumatic diaphragmatic rupture [14, 15]. Gastric volvulus is characterized by rotation of the stomach along its long or short axis leading to variable degrees of gastric outlet obstruction [16].

### 80.3.1 Etiology

According to etiology of an underlying cause, gastric volvulus can be classified into primary or secondary type. Primary gastric volvulus (type I) occurs due to laxity of the ligaments supporting the stomach, thereby allowing the stomach to twist along its mesentery. Normally stomach is fixed to the abdominal wall by four ligaments: the gastrocolic, gastrohepatic, gastrophrenic, and gastrosplenic. These supportive ligaments along with the pylorus and the gastroesophageal junction act as an anchorage and prevent its malrotation. Laxity of these supportive mechanisms as a consequence of agenesis, elongation, or disruption of the gastric ligaments may predispose to primary gastric volvulus. Secondary gastric volvulus (type II) occurs due to a number of factors including intraabdominal adhesions, eventration of diaphragm, splenic abnormalities, phrenic nerve palsy, traumatic rupture diaphragm or an intrinsic gastric pathology, like tumors, acting as a lead point for gastric volvulus [17]. Paraesophageal hiatal hernia has been documented as the most common predisposing factor for gastric volvulus. Fixity of gastroesophageal junction in the abdomen, enlarged hernia ring with laxity of supporting ligaments displace greater curvature into the thorax in type II, III, and IV paraesophageal hernia, leading to the herniated stomach to twist around its longitudinal axis [18].

### 80.3.2 Classification

This gastric volvulus may be of acute or chronic type. In the acute type, the rotation of the stomach is more than 180°, whereas in chronic form a partial volvulus occurs. This chronic form may progress to a closed-loop obstruction, progressive dilatation of the stomach, and eventually ischemia of the stomach. Chronic gastric volvulus affects 30% of gastric volvulus [4]. Gastric volvulus classification proposed by Von Haberer and Singleton modified by Carter in 1978 [19] described three types of gastric volvulus on the basis of the axis of rotation (Figs. 80.3 and 80.4). Organoaxial volvulus is the most common form occurring in approximately 60% of cases [20]. There is a rotation of the stomach around a longitudinal axis passing through the cardia and the pylorus. In mesenteroaxial volvulus, which comprises 29% of cases, rotation occurs along a transverse, midgastric axis, passing through the midpoints of the small and the great curvature [21]. Third type is the combination-unclassified volvulus type [22].

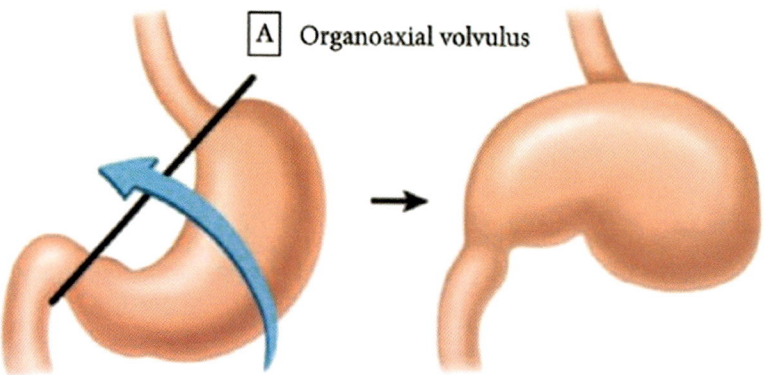

**Fig. 80.3** Organoaxial gastric volvulus. (Reproduced from Yana Cavanagh, Neal Carlin, Ruhin Yuridullah, Sohail Shaikh, "Acute Gastric Volvulus Causing Splenic Avulsion and Hemoperitoneum", Case Reports in Gastrointestinal Medicine, vol. 2018, Article ID 2961063, 5 pages, 2018. https://doi.org/10.1155/2018/2961063)

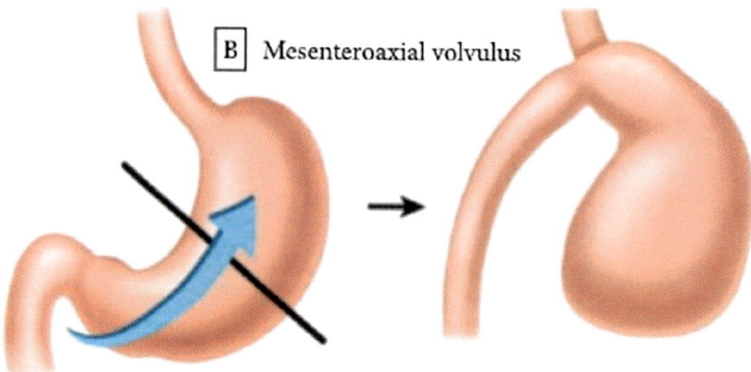

**Fig. 80.4** Mesenteroaxial gastric volvulus. (Reproduced from Yana Cavanagh, Neal Carlin, Ruhin Yuridullah, Sohail Shaikh, "Acute Gastric Volvulus Causing Splenic Avulsion and Hemoperitoneum", Case Reports in Gastrointestinal Medicine, vol. 2018, Article ID 2961063, 5 pages, 2018. https://doi.org/10.1155/2018/2961063)

### 80.3.3 Clinical Picture

The incidence peaks after the fifth decade with adults constituting 80–90% of cases [18]. Regarding gender, there is no predilection but a slight predominance of women is reported. Gastric volvulus presents in classical form of the Bortchardt's triad, only in 70% of cases [23]. The triad has intractable retching, sudden epigastric pain, and an inability to pass a nasogastric tube into the stomach [16]. Clinical picture depends on the degree of rotation, gastric obstruction, and diaphragmatic position of stomach whether subdiaphragmatic or supradiaphragmatic.

Chronic or subacute gastric volvulus usually causes vague or subclinical symptoms such as mild upper abdominal discomfort, dysphagia, and heartburn. These functional signs often correlate with gastric emptying abnormality. Delayed gastric emptying with postprandial fullness, often after meals, induces early satiety gets relieved by vomiting. The intermittent or subacute gastric volvulus is the prerogative of partial volvulus of mesenteroaxial type, with the acute gastric volvulus often the prerogative of complete volvulus which occurs especially in the elderly [23]. Cardiopulmonary signs may be present. The sudden onset dyspnea in a patient with a chronic history of digestive symptoms makes up the bulk of the clinical picture. Clinical findings on examination depend on the severity of the obstruction and presence of any ischemia. Mild tachycardia or hypovolemic shock may be present depending on the fluid deficit. Abdominal distension is sole sign of volvulus having gastric outlet obstruction with fluid filled stomach and resultant distension. Onset of severe abdominal pain and peritonitis signifies gastric ischemia and necrosis [24]. Computed tomography may show esophagus and stomach rotating around one another. This sign is demonstrated best in the transverse plane [25]. The acute gastric volvulus is associated with mortality rates ranging from 30% to 50% [26].

## 80.4 Treatment

Management of asymptomatic paraesophageal hernia require medical management and symptomatic paraesophageal hernia is recommended for repair. Asymptomatic hiatal hernia is usually due to gastroesophageal reflux disease (GERD) and medical management of GERD is the mainstay of therapy [27]. The aim of treatment is to reduce gastric acid secretion. A slew of measures is required to be incorporated. Altered lifestyle is primary line of treatment and includes decreasing body weight, avoiding precipitating foods such as high spicy foods, carbonated drinks, alcohol, caffeine, chocolate, and citrus foods. Keeping the head end of the bed elevated during sleep and to avoid meals 2–3 h before bedtime is to be practiced. An 8-week course of PPI (proton pump inhibitors) starting from minimal dose is therapy of choice for symptom relief in GERD. A twice-daily PPI therapy may be recommended for patients with mild relief on single daily PPI therapy; this is usually suffice to control symptomatology. There are no significant differences in the efficacy between the different types of PPIs. Patients presenting with moderate symptoms may use these treatments on demand, while those with persistent symptoms despite PPI treatment should use them as an add-on treatment. Other alternatives include $H_2$ receptor antagonists and antacids.

The prophylactic correction of asymptomatic paraesophageal hernias remains controversial as the annual risk of developing acute symptoms requiring emergency surgery is less than 2% [28]. This risk decreases exponentially after 65 years, and the mortality rate from elective paraesophageal hernia repair is approximately 1.4% [29]. The data from the National Surgical Quality Improvement Program database shows emergency repair is associated with a nearly tenfold increase in perioperative mortality compared to elective repair [30]. Additionally, mortality is lowest in elective laparoscopic repair group. Many patients with an incidental finding of volvulus or PEH being asymptomatic have significant symptoms on extracting careful and meticulous history. The final decision to provide empiric operative management for incidental gastric volvulus should be based on a patient's desire to undergo repair and assessment of risks of repair to be weighed against risks of developing acute volvulus requiring emergency repair. Latest recommendation is that emergency or delayed emergency surgical intervention is required even in long-standing asymptomatic chronic forms as there is permanent and unpredictable risk of strangulation [31].

### 80.4.1 Preoperative Management

Light et al. present a useful and comprehensive management algorithm for acute gastric volvulus in surgical endoscopy in 2016 [32]. Once the diagnosis is confirmed, initial management for acute gastric volvulus includes resuscitation with intravenous fluids, placement of a nasogastric tube, gastric decompression, and resting in the prone position. Fluid therapy for resuscitation is to be done with isotonic crystalloid, correction of electrolyte imbalance and blood transfusion for bleeding or anemia. The use of broad-spectrum antibiotics as soon as clinical diagnosis is made is important. Nasogastric tube insertion for urgent gastric decompression is highly recommended. Gastric decompression provides quick symptomatic relief and rarely leads to spontaneous reduction of this volvulus. Enhanced perfusion of gastric wall post nasogastric decompression allows more optimized medical resuscitative measures as increased window period for surgery is permissible.

## 80.4.2 Endoscopic Therapy

Endoscopic gastric decompression is recommended for failed nasogastric decompression. Early endoscopy is done to assess ischemia of the gastric wall. This increasing application of technique of endoscopic reduction of gastric volvulus is yielding more and more success in patients [33]. This endoscopic gastric decompression is ideal in patients having airway secured via endotracheal tube intubation. Minimal insufflation should be used during the endoscopy. Once the endoscope is successfully placed in the stomach, gastric contents are suctioned to provide decompression and nasogastric tube is then inserted. Abdominal radiography study is to be repeated to confirm placement of tube and assess status of decompression of the stomach. The nasogastric tube is kept in stomach to prevent repeated distension of the stomach by accumulation of gastric secretions.

Endoscopic untwisting is often used as first-line therapy to manage patients with idiopathic or primary gastric volvulus and in patients who are poor surgical candidates with secondary (paraesophageal hernia-related) gastric volvulus [31]. Endoscopic reduction is done by the alpha-loop maneuver. The maneuver is performed by advancing the endoscope into the second portion of the duodenum by gently advancing through the narrowed and twisted gastric folds, then pulling back the endoscope while twisting. This is to be performed under X-ray guidance to confirm the reduction. Symptoms usually resolve with successful reduction of the volvulus.

## 80.4.3 Anterior Abdominal Wall Gastropexy

Anterior abdominal wall gastropexy is the fixation of the stomach to the left hemidiaphragm and anterior abdominal wall in its normal anatomic configuration to prevent recurrent gastric volvulus. In two scenarios, gastropexy is used as an alternative to PEH repair: first, in patients who are at prohibitively high operative risk to undergo prolonged abdominal surgery; and second, when surgeons lack sufficient experience in gastroesophageal surgery to perform a complex PEH repair [34]. There are three minimally invasive approaches to gastropexy—endoscopic, laparoscopic, and laparoendoscopic.

Endoscopic gastropexy is performed with the placement of one or more percutaneous endoscopic gastrostomy (PEG) tubes. The initial step of endoscopic gastropexy is to reduce the gastric volvulus by gastric insufflations, often reduces the stomach volvulus [35] by the alpha loop technique. After reduction of the volvulus, a first PEG tube is placed on the body of the stomach along the greater curvature, and a second gastrostomy site is then selected on the gastric antrum, at least 12 cm from the first site [33]. It is important to separate these two tubes to prevent creating a fulcrum around which recurrent volvulus might occur. In addition to providing points of fixation for the stomach, PEG tubes provide enteral access for nutritional support and administration of critical enteral medications [36].

## 80.4.4 Laparoscopy Gastropexy

If the volvulus cannot be reduced by purely endoscopic intervention, a laparoendoscopic technique can be used. With this technique, a 5 mm port is placed in the umbilicus and one or two additional 5 mm ports are placed in the upper abdomen. These ports allow for laparoscopic reduction of the volvulus, and the PEG tubes are then placed under direct laparoscopic visualization [37]. This technique has advantage when purely endoscopic gastrostomy tube placement is contraindicated as in the morbid obese patient preventing adequate transabdominal illumination, the colon is adherent to the stomach, if there is apprehension for gastric ischemia and the diagnostic laparoscopy is indicated.

### 80.4.5 Laparoscopic Sutured Gastropexy

Laparoscopic anterior abdominal wall gastropexy using multiple sutures along the greater curvature of the stomach is new technique to provide durable fixation for prevention of recurrent volvulus. This technique is performed to manage high operative risk patients with obstructive gastric volvulus. In laparoscopic sutured gastropexy, the volvulus is reduced, the stomach is sutured to the left hemidiaphragm and anterior abdominal wall. A one or two point sutured gastropexy with or without concomitant gastrostomy tube placement is done [38]. The use of one or two points of fixation may be inadequate to prevent recurrent volvulus [39], besides these fixation points may even act as an axis around which subsequent volvulus can occur.

A modified technique, where once the volvulus is reduced and the stomach is in its normal anatomic position, 2-0 silk sutures are placed every 2–3 cm to attach the stomach to the diaphragm and anterior abdominal wall. The first sutures are placed high on the greater curvature and anchor the stomach to the left crus. Subsequent sutures are placed between the greater curvature and the left hemidiaphragm and finally between the antrum and the anterior abdominal wall. However, performing gastropexy endoscopically using a PEG tube has its own limitations due to the risk of recurrence consequent to inadequate fixation, persistence of predisposing factors such as hernias and adhesions from other surgeries, and the potential that the fixation point will act as an axis for further rotations [4, 39].

## 80.5 Surgery for Gastric Volvulus with Paraesophageal Hernia

### 80.5.1 Open Surgery

Immediate surgical decompression should be performed when nasogastric tube placement or endoscopy fails to achieve gastric decompression. Surgical options for management include open surgery or laparoscopy. Although the operative steps are the same whether they are performed open or laparoscopically. The laparotomy is mostly used in case of acute volvulus allowing broad access to the abdominal cavity [40]. Emergency surgery is done via an upper midline laparotomy. The stomach is reduced from the hernia sac. This reduction is ideally done initially by gentle downward traction of the stomach starting anteriorly. Lysis of adhesions between the stomach/omentum and the hernia sac is often necessary prior to delivery of the stomach into the abdomen where it is then manually derotated. Any obvious ischemic areas of the stomach necessitate gastric resection in the form of partial or rarely subtotal gastrectomy. The hernia sac is to be completely excised and the distal esophagus is mobilized. Repair of the defect, with or without mesh, is performed. Regardless of approach, the principles of surgical repair of PEH remain the same and vary by incision of choice, body cavity approach, and order in which they are performed gastric fixation is done at the end.

A staged approach is an alternative modality for the patient with severe metabolic derangements who might not be fit for definitive repair gastric volvulus secondary to PEH repair. The desperate measures to relieve sepsis incorporate at least a few of the initial principles of surgical management: reduction of the hernia contents, untwisting of the twisted stomach, and resection of nonviable tissue. Surgical sepsis control measures completed to be followed by decision to be made whether patient can tolerate definitive repair or not. Alternatively, leaving the patient in temporary discontinuity with nasogastric decompression in place, abdominal packing on raw surface and temporary abdominal closure devices is a useful alternative. After abbreviated "damage control" operation in which the source of sepsis is controlled, the patient can be taken to the intensive care unit (ICU) for hemodynamic and metabolic optimization as well as the recruitment of experts for definitive repair if required.

## 80.5.2 Laparoscopy Surgery

Laparoscopic repair of hiatal hernia gives adequate magnified visualization, quick postoperative recovery with improved quality of life [41]. This is important to recognize that laparoscopic PEH repair requires advanced laparoscopic skills, only to be performed by the experienced gastric surgeons [42, 43]. In addition, laparoscopic PEH to be done under general anesthesia and repair takes several hours to perform. Because gastric volvulus frequently occurs in old age patients with concomitant comorbidities, having already high risk of occurrence of gastric volvulus with unavoidable intrinsic perioperative risk in prolonged operation under general anesthesia [44]. Referral of patients having acute obstructive gastric volvulus to center with inexperienced surgeon, reluctant to take risk in operating such cases is a high possibility. An urgent referral to tertiary care with unit experienced in operating laparoscopic acute gastric volvulus secondary to paraesophageal hernia is best for patient outcome.

Laparoscopic surgery has proved its advantage in elective surgery for chronic gastric volvulus but also in some cases of acute volvulus. Koger and Stone [45] in 1993 achieved the first laparoscopic success in the treatment of acute gastric volvulus by performing reduction and gastropexy. Untwisting the stomach and repair of secondary defects such as hiatus hernia has been treated successfully using a laparoscopic approach. Performing antireflux surgery in the same sitting, when repairing the paraesophageal defect, may be attempted [46]. Laparoscopic PEH repair in the management of gastric volvulus should follow the basic tenets of this operation Laparoscopic repair of PEH is associated with overall low morbidity and mortality and an estimated 10% recurrence rate [47, 48].

## 80.5.3 Postoperative Management

An optimum level of intensive care unit is required for managing patients in postoperative period. Nasogastric tube is to be kept in postoperative period to maintain persistent gastric decompression. Adequate analgesia and antiemetic are to be given. A barium swallow should be done in 24–48 h to assess any leak, gastric emptying, and status of hernia repair. On confirmation of normal postoperative barium swallow, clear oral liquid diet is started, if well tolerated and allowed to take low residue diet. Those having laparoscopic repair can typically be discharged earlier than having emergency open surgery. There are reports of having recurrence of unrepaired PEH in gastric volvulus. Faulty anatomic repair or inadequate fixation of the stomach to the abdominal wall is factors in recurrence of previously operated gastric volvulus [49].

> **Dos and Don'ts of Treatment**
> - Never forget nasogastric tube insertion for urgent gastric decompression.
> - Open or laparoscopy surgery is option available option for emergency surgery.
> - Do not forget to do gastropexy in emergency surgery whether open or laparoscopically.

## 80.6 Conclusion

Gastric volvulus secondary to paraesophageal hernia may remain obscure, present with subclinical symptoms or as an acute surgical emergency. Paraesophageal hiatal hernia is the most common predisposing factor for gastric volvulus. The type of volvulus may be mesenteroaxial or organoaxial type. Acute gastric volvulus associated with paraesophageal hernia may pursue course as a strangulated hernia, gastric outlet obstruction, gastric perforation, or stomach gangrene. Computed tomography is useful adjunct in diagnosis. Open or laparoscopy surgery is option available for managing acute gastric volvulus. Laparoscopy needs expertise to manage acute gastric volvulus associated with paraesophageal hernia. Surgery in elderly for acute gastric volvulus is associated with high morbidity and mortality.

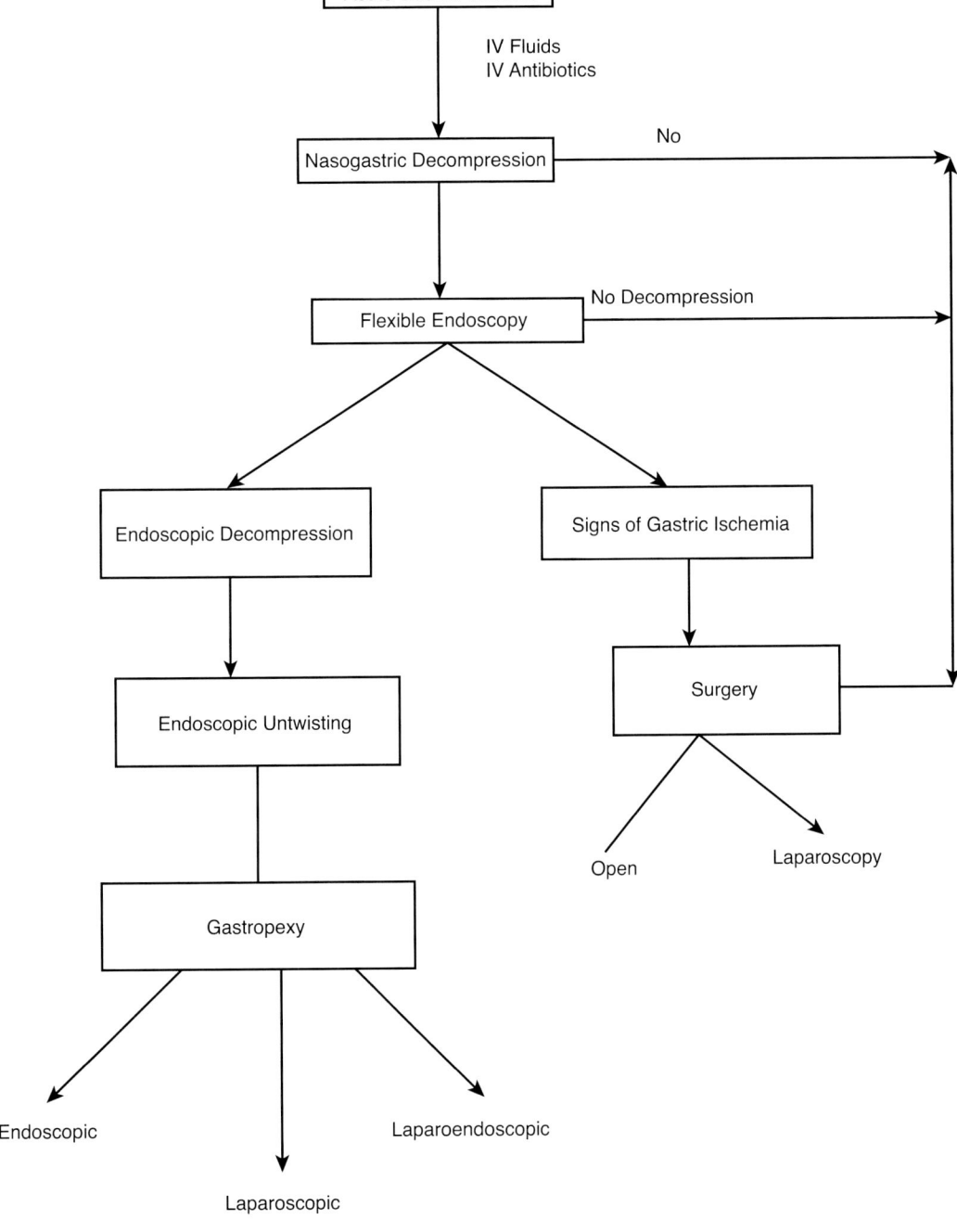

Flow diagram showing treatment options of acute gastric volvulus

**Take-Home Messages**

Gastric volvulus secondary to paraesophageal hernia may remain obscure, present with subclinical symptoms or as an acute surgical emergency. Paraesophageal hiatal hernia is the most common predisposing factor for gastric volvulus. The type of volvulus may be mesenteroaxial or organoaxial type. Acute gastric volvulus associated with paraesophageal hernia may pursue course as a strangulated hernia, gastric outlet obstruction, gastric perforation, or stomach gangrene. Computed tomography is useful adjunct in diagnosis. Open or laparoscopy surgery is option available for managing acute gastric volvulus. Laparoscopy needs expertise to manage acute gastric volvulus associated with paraesophageal hernia. Surgery in elderly for acute gastric volvulus is associated with high morbidity and mortality.

**Multiple Choice Questions**

1. Most common cause of gastric volvulus
   A. Trauma
   B. Idiopathic
   C. Paraesophageal hernia
   D. Adhesions
2. Types of hiatal hernia is
   A. Two
   B. One
   C. Three
   D. Four
3. Which of the following is known as true paraesophageal hernia
   A. Type II
   B. Type III
   C. Type I
   D. Type IV
4. Paraesophageal hernia presents as
   A. Acute obstruction
   B. Symptomatic cardiopulmonary symptoms
   C. Asymptomatic
   D. All of above
5. Gastric volvulus occurs along
   A. Short axis
   B. Long axis
   C. Both A and B
   D. None of above
6. The Bortchardt's triad in acute gastric volvulus is present approximately in
   A. 100%
   B. 20%
   C. <10%
   D. 70%
7. Who suggested algorithm comprehensive management for acute gastric volvulus
   A. Koh YX
   B. Nunes G
   C. DeMeester
   D. Light D
8. Which of following is true
   A. Emergency or delayed emergency surgical intervention is required even in long-standing asymptomatic chronic forms of gastric volvulus
   B. Only acute gastric volvulus needing surgical intervention
   C. There is no need of gastropexy in acute gastric volvulus surgery
   D. None of above
9. Which is type of technique is used for gastropexy in stomach fixation in gastric volvulus
   A. Laparoendoscopic
   B. Laparoscopic
   C. Endoscopic
   D. All of the above
10. Who achieved the first laparoscopic success in the treatment of acute gastric volvulus?
    A. Koger and Stone
    B. K Conley Coleman and Daniel Graboo

C. Lopez PP and Megha R
D. Auyang and Pellegrini

11. Which of the following radiological investigations is done post-surgery to confirm success of surgery?
    A. MRI
    B. Barium swallow
    C. Computed tomography scan
    D. None of the above

**Answers**: 1-C; 2-D; 3-A; 4-D; 5-C; 6-C; 7-D; 8-A; 9-D; 10-A; 11-B

# References

1. Koh YX, Ong LW, Lee J, Wong AS. Para-oesophageal and parahiatal hernias in an Asian acute care tertiary hospital: an underappreciated surgical condition. Singap Med J. 2016;57(12):669–75.
2. Marini L, Azarian R, Gagnadoux F, Brion N, Petitpretz P. Gastric volvulus associated with Zenker's diverticulum: a rare cause of recurrent pneumopathy. Rev Mal Respir. 2000;17(1):121–3.
3. Akhtar A, Siddiqui FS, Sheikh AAE, Sheikh AB, Perisetti A. Gastric volvulus: a rare entity case report and literature review. Cureus. 2018;10(3):e2312.
4. Coleman KC, Graboo D. Paraesophageal hernia and gastric volvulus. In: Brown VR, et al., editors. Emergency general surgery. Cham: Springer International Publishing AG; 2019. https://doi.org/10.1007/978-3-319-96286-3_15.
5. Sfara A, Dumitrascu DL. The management of hiatal hernia: an update on diagnosis and treatment. Med Pharm Rep. 2019;92(4):321–5.
6. Weber C, Davis CS, Shankaran V, Fisichella PM. Hiatal hernias: a review of the pathophysiologic theories and implication for research. Surg Endosc. 2011;25(10):3149–53.
7. Oude Nijhuis RAB, Hoek MV, Schuitenmaker JM, Schijven MP, Draaisma WA, Smout AJPM, Bredenoord AJ. The natural course of giant paraesophageal hernia and long-term outcomes following conservative management. United European Gastroenterol J. 2020;8(10):1163–73.
8. Hyun JJ, Bak YT. Clinical significance of hiatal hernia. Gut Liver. 2011;5(3):267–77.
9. Migaczewski M, Grzesiak-Kuik A, Pędziwiatr M, Budzyński A. Laparoscopic treatment of type III and IV hiatal hernia—authors' experience. Wideochir Inne Tech Maloinwazyjne. 2014;9(2):157–63.
10. Kasper D, Fauci A, Hauser S, Longo D, Larry Jameson J, Loscalzo J. Harrison's principles of internal medicine. 19th ed. New York: McGraw-Hill Global Education; 2015. p. 1902. ISBN: 978-0071802154.
11. Baison GN, Ralph W. Aye complex and acute paraesophageal hernias—type IV, strangulated, and irreducible. Ann Laparosc Endosc Surg. 2020; https://doi.org/10.21037/ales-20-7.
12. Nunes G, Patita M, Fernandes V, Fonseca J. Paraesophageal hernia and gastric volvulus: an uncommon etiology of vomiting and upper gastrointestinal bleeding. Rev Esp Enferm Dig. 2017;109(4):294–5.
13. Schummer W. Hiatal hernia mimicking heart problems. BMJ Case Rep. 2017;2017:bcr2017220508.
14. Berti A. Sgolare attortigliamento dell esofago con duodeno seguito da rapidita morte. Gazz Med Ital. 1886;9:139–41.
15. Hamby W. The case reports and autopsy records of Ambroise Pare. Springfield, IL: Charles C Thomas; 1960.
16. Chau B, Dufel S. Gastric volvulus. Emerg Med J. 2007;24(6):446–7.
17. Rashid F, Thangarajah T, Mulvey D, Larvin M, Iftikhar SY. A review article on gastric volvulus: a challenge to diagnosis and management. Int J Surg. 2010;8(1):18–24.
18. Diko S, Elaasa M, Russell C, Zuberi J, Christian D. First described case of gastric volvulus following open cholecystectomy. J Curr Surg N Am. 2020;10:17–20. Available at: https://www.currentsurgery.org/index.php/jcs/article/view/403. Accessed 8 May 2021.
19. Jacob CE, Lopasso FP, Zilberstein B, Bresciani CJC, Kuga R, Cecconello I, Gama-Rodrigues JJ. Gastric volvulus: a review of 38 cases. ABCD. Arquivos Brasileiros de Cirurgia Digestiva (São Paulo). 2009;22(2):96–100.
20. Al Daoud F, Daswani GS, Perinjelil V, Nigam T. Acute organoaxial gastric volvulus: a massive problem with a twist-case report. Int J Surg Case Rep. 2017;41:366–9. https://doi.org/10.1016/j.ijscr.2017.11.016.
21. Van der Merwe DJ, Louw HB, Dekker G. Gastric volvulus—an explanation through imaging. S Afr J Radiol. 2007;11(4):105.
22. Chafke N, Wihlm JM, Massard G, Morand G, Witz JP. La hernie retro-costo-xyphoïdienne. Proble` mes de diagnostic et de traitement. A propos de huit observations. Ann Chir. 1988;42:467–73.
23. Teague WJ, Ackroyd R, Watson DI, Devitt PG. Changing patterns in the management of gastric volvulus over 14 years. Br J Surg. 2000;87(3):358–61.
24. Patel AV, Senatore FJ, Bhurwal A. Epigastric pain due to acute gastric volvulus. J Emerg Med. 2019;57:e185–6.
25. Mazaheri P, Ballard DH, Neal KA, Raptis DA, Shetty AS, Raptis CA, Mellnick VM. CT of gastric volvulus: interobserver reliability, radiologists' accuracy, and imaging findings AJR. Am J Roentgenol. 2019;212:103–8.
26. Lopez PP, Megha R. Gastric volvulus [updated 2020 Nov 19]. In: StatPearls. Treasure Island, FL: StatPearls Publishing; 2021. Available from: https://www.ncbi.nlm.nih.gov/books/NBK507886/.

27. Kohn GP, Price RR, Demeester SR, et al. Guidelines for the management of hiatal hernia. Available at: http://www.sages.org/publications/guidelines/guidelines-for-the-management-of-hiatal-hernia/. Accessed 21 Oct 2014.
28. Stylopoulos N, Gazelle GS, Rattner DW. Paraesophageal hernias: operation or observation? Ann Surg. 2002;236(4):492–501.
29. Lamberg JJ, Farbaniec M, Kuperman EF. Massive paraesophageal hernia mimicking pulmonary embolus. J Gen Intern Med. 2013;28(9):1241.
30. Kaplan JA, Schecter S, Lin MY, Rogers SJ, Carter JT. Morbidity and mortality associated with elective or emergency paraesophageal hernia repair. JAMA Surg. 2015;150(11):1094–6.
31. Zuiki T, Hosoya Y, Lefor AK, et al. The management of gastric volvulus in elderly patients. Int J Surg Case Rep. 2016;29:88–93. https://doi.org/10.1016/j.ijscr.2016.10.058.
32. Light D, Links D, Griffin M. The threatened stomach: management of the acute gastric volvulus. Surg Endosc. 2016;30(05):1847–52.
33. Tsang TK, Walker R, Yu DJ. Endoscopic reduction of gastric volvulus: the alpha-loop maneuver. Gastrointest Endosc. 1995;42:244–8.
34. Kissane NA, Rattner DW. Chapter 41—Paraesophageal and other complex diaphragmatic hernias. In: Yeo CJ, editor. Shackelford's surgery of the alimentary tract. 7th ed. W.B. Saunders; 2013. p. 494–508. https://doi.org/10.1016/B978-1-4377-2206-2.00041-5. ISBN: 9781437722062. https://www.sciencedirect.com/science/article/pii/B9781437722062000415.
35. Kercher KW, Matthews BD, Ponsky JL, Goldstein SL, Yavorski RT, Sing RF, Heniford BT. Minimally invasive management of paraesophageal herniation in the high-risk surgical patient. Am J Surg. 2001;182(5):510–51.
36. Yates RB, Hinojosa MW, Wright AS, Pellegrini CA, Oelschlager BK. Laparoscopic gastropexy relieves symptoms of obstructed gastric volvulus in high operative risk patients. Am J Surg. 2015;209(5):875–80.
37. Xenos ES. Percutaneous endoscopic gastrostomy in a patient with a large hiatal hernia using laparoscopy. JSLS. 2000;4(3):231–3.
38. Eckhauser ML, Ferron JP. The use of dual percutaneous endoscopic gastrostomy (DPEG) in the management of chronic intermittent gastric volvulus. Gastrointest Endosc. 1985;31(5):340–2.
39. Toyota K, Sugawara Y, Hatano Y. Recurrent upside-down stomach after endoscopic repositioning and gastropexy treated by laparoscopic surgery. Case Rep Gastroenterol. 2014;8(1):32–8.
40. Alamowitch B, Christophe M, Bourbon M, Porcheron J, Balique JG. Para-esophageal hiatal hernia with acute gastric volvulus. Gastroenterol Clin Biol. 1999;23(2):271–4.
41. Mungo B, Molena D, Stem M, Feinberg RL, Lidor AO. Thirty-day outcomes of paraesophageal hernia repair using the NSQIP database: should laparoscopy be the standard of care? J Am Coll Surg. 2014;219(2):229–36.
42. DeMeester SR. Laparoscopic paraesophageal hernia repair: critical steps and adjunct techniques to minimize recurrence. Surg Laparosc Endosc Percutan Tech. 2013;23:429–35.
43. Auyang ED, Pellegrini CA. How I do it: laparoscopic paraesophageal hernia repair. J Gastrointest Surg. 2012;16(7):1406–11.
44. Gourgiotis S, Vougas V, Germanos S, Baratsis S. Acute gastric volvulus: diagnosis and management over 10 years. Dig Surg. 2006;23(3):169–72.
45. Koger KE, Stone JM. Laparoscopic reduction of acute gastric volvulus. Am Surg. 1993;59(5):325–8.
46. Smith CD, McClusky DA, Rajad MA, Lederman AB, Hunter JG. When fundoplication fails: redo? Ann Surg. 2005;241(6):861–71. https://doi.org/10.1097/01.sla.0000165198.29398.4b.
47. Morrow EH, Oelschlager BK. Laparoscopic paraesophageal hernia repair. Surg Laparosc Endosc Percutan Tech. 2013;23(5):446–8.
48. Wolf PS, Oelschlager BK. Laparoscopic paraesophageal hernia repair. Adv Surg. 2007;41:199–210.
49. Cáterin A, Rubén L, Jaspe-L CA, Felipe B, Segura B, Bernardo A. Literature review: a surgeons view of recurrent hiatal hernia. Rev Colomb Gastroenterol. 2015;30(4):447–55.

## Further Reading

Falk GW, Katzka DA. 140—Diseases of the esophagus. In: Goldman L, Schafer AI, editors. Goldman's Cecil medicine. 24th ed. W.B. Saunders; 2012. p. 874–86. https://doi.org/10.1016/B978-1-4377-1604-7.00140-8. ISBN: 9781437716047. https://www.sciencedirect.com/science/article/pii/B9781437716047001408.

Jalilvand A, Dimick JB, Fisichella PM. Treatment of paraesophageal hernias. In: Fisichella P, Allaix M, Morino M, Patti M, editors. Esophageal diseases. Cham: Springer; 2014. https://doi.org/10.1007/978-3-319-04337-1_6.

Podolsky DK, Camilleri M, Fitz JG, Kalloo AN, Shanahan F, Wang TC. Yamada's textbook of gastroenterology. Hoboken, NJ. First published: 27 Nov 2015. ISBN: 9781118512067 (print). ISBN: 9781118512074 (online): Wiley. https://doi.org/10.1002/9781118512074.

Rodriguez-Garcia HA, Wright AS, Yates RB. Managing obstructive gastric volvulus: challenges and solutions. Open Access Surg. 2017;10:15–24. https://doi.org/10.2147/OAS.S91357.

Schlottmann F, Di Corpo M, Patti MG. Management of paraesophageal hernia. In: Patti M, Di Corpo M, Schlottmann F, editors. Foregut surgery. Cham: Springer; 2020. https://doi.org/10.1007/978-3-030-27592-1_17.

# Stoma-Related Surgical Emergencies

## 81

Arda Isik and Rajesh Ramanathan

## 81.1 Introduction

**Learning Goals**
- To differentiate stoma-related surgical and medical emergencies.
- To treat stoma-related surgical emergencies.
- To differentiate early and late stoma-related surgical emergencies.

## 81.2 Diagnosis and Treatment

Stoma is a frequent surgical necessity in both elective and emergency general surgery, including colon, rectal surgery, and in cancer conditions. Stoma complications are common; they usually occur at a rate of 40–90% in ileostomy and 30–70% in colostomy [1–3]. In a retrospective review of 1616 stomas, a 34% rate of complications was reported with early complications in 28% and late complications in 6% [4]. Furthermore, it is possible that most data we have on stoma complications is actually underaccounted, given that peristomal skin irritation is rarely reported as a complication.

Primarily, we divide complications as medical (cutaneous irritation, fluid, and electrolyte imbalance) and surgical (stoma prolapse, ostomy stenosis, parastomal hernia, ostomy retraction, obstruction/ileus, ostomy ischemia/necrosis, hemorrhage/hematoma, fistula).

A variety of factors have been suggested to contribute to stoma complications. Emergency surgery is one of the risk factors for stoma complications [5, 6]. In a report by Duchesne et al. [7], malignant disease was not associated with stoma complications, although contrasting evidence exists [8]. In addition, older age, colorectal surgery, type of stoma, and preoperative stoma site determination were independent risk factors for complications [4]. A review of over 1000 cases found that loop ileostomy had the highest rate of stoma complications, while end colostomies had the highest rate of early complications (skin irritation in 12% and inappropriate choice of stoma site in 7%) [4].

An older report in 1987 by Rutegard et al. found conflicting results with similar rates of complications between ileostomies and colostomies, and that same study found more serious complications occurring after ileostomy [9]. Subsequent studies have echoed the higher incidence and severity of complications in ileostomies. In a retrospective evaluation of 464 patients, Köckerling et al. [10] reported more

A. Isik (✉)
Division of General Surgery, School of Medicine, Istanbul Medeniyet University, Istanbul, Turkey

R. Ramanathan
Division of Surgical Oncology, UPMC, Pittsburgh, PA, USA

**Table 81.1** Various factors decreasing the rate of stoma complications

| |
|---|
| Good selection of the stoma location |
| Proper stoma and fascial defect diameter |
| Tension free |
| Appropriate stoma vascularization |
| Smoking cessation |
| Stoma protrusion less than 1 cm over the skin |
| Control of co-morbidities |
| Fixation of intestinal mesentery to parietal peritoneum |
| Stoma created through the rectus muscle |
| No curling of intestine |
| Stoma appliance fixation and application in the operating room |
| Systemic infection control |

complications requiring surgical treatment in the ileostomy group. In randomized multicenter study conducted by Gooszen et al. [11], overall complications were more common in the ileostomy group with skin irritation being the most common; prolapse was found to be more frequent in the colostomy group. In most studies on stoma complications, the risk of complications is higher in patients with ileostomy [1, 8, 12].

Technical considerations in stoma creation and management include the type of stoma applied, the mouthed bowel cut postoperative stoma care. Qualified stoma therapists and high-quality stoma devices have decreased the complication rates in recent years. Most stoma complications can significantly be reduced by considering various factors shown in Table 81.1.

In this chapter, early and late stoma-related complications will be addressed with discussion of methods to mitigate such complications.

## 81.3 Early Complications Needing for Emergency Surgery

Early complications are defined as those complications that occur within the first 15 days after surgery.

### 81.3.1 Evisceration

Evisceration occurs as a result of the dehiscence of laparotomy incision suture or the too wide opening of the stoma. This is a technical complication requiring urgent reoperation with recreation of the stoma and attention given to the use of internal or external retention sutures.

### 81.3.2 Ischemia and Stoma Necrosis

Stoma ischemia usually occurs early after surgery; for this reason, the change in stoma color should be closely monitored within the first 24–72 h. Healthy stomas should normally be bright pink in color, like the mucosa of the inside of the mouth. Some darkening of color around stoma is common and conservative management is sufficient. If the mucosa appears blue or violaceous, it is presumably ischemic, but can still be observed. However, when the stoma mucosa turns black, urgent intervention is necessary (Fig. 81.1a, b).

Necrosis may be localized only in the exteriorized stoma or in multiple other loops of intraperitoneal intestine. It must be attentively differentiated if ischemia is generalized to the whole intestine or limited to the stoma. Stoma ischemia may occur due to arterial insufficiency, or because the intestine is taken out through a too-narrow opening. Emergency surgery, obesity, and inflammatory bowel disease (i.e., Crohn's disease) have been identified as an independent risk factor for the development of stomal necrosis, and it is approximately 3–17% in series [13, 14]. In contrast, transient ischemic injury may be due to venous circulation impairment and often it resolves spontaneously without turning into necrosis. It usually occurs due to tension-related venous congestion.

In cases where progression to necrosis is suspected, parietal isolation or debridement of the necrosis may be necessary. If the color change plus associated ischemia only extends to the fascia, the stoma can be renewed locally without entering the abdominal cavity in order to prevent further peritoneal contamination [15]. Such end ischemia may be more common after end sigmoid colostomy because there may be insufficient supply of marginal arteries. Strategies to prevent stoma necrosis are shown in Table 81.2.

# 81 Stoma-Related Surgical Emergencies

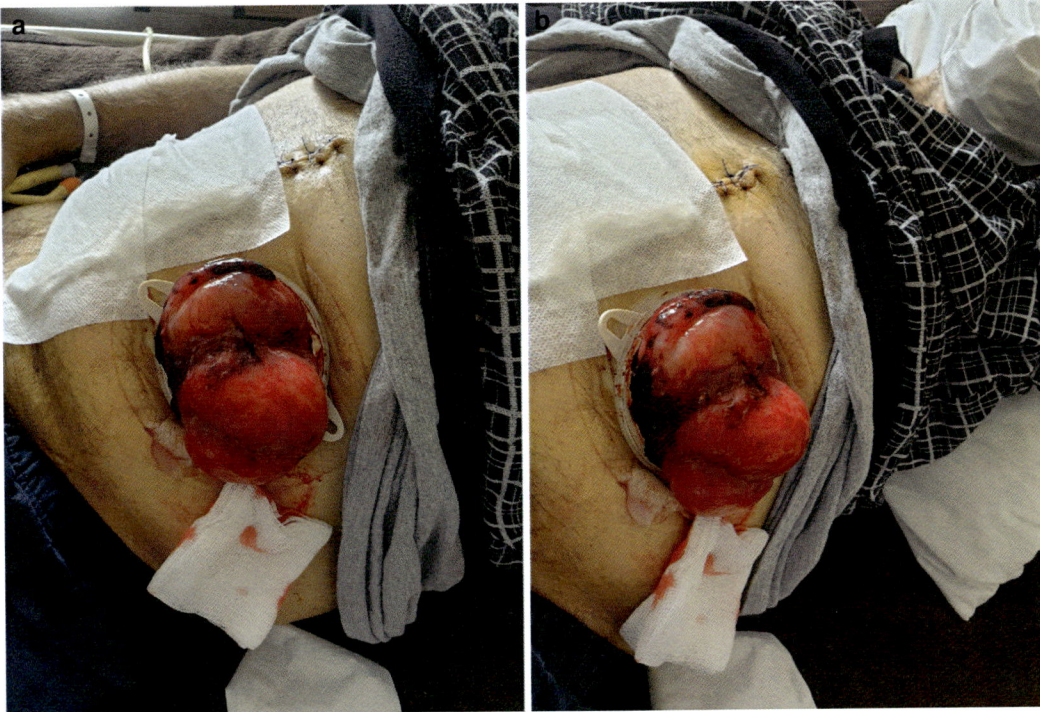

**Fig. 81.1** (**a**, **b**) Partial necrotic stoma

**Table 81.2** Requirements for prevention of stoma necrosis

Avoid tight stitches
Avoid tight fitting bags around edematous stomas
Avoid excessive freeing of the terminal part of the stoma from the mesentery
Avoid tight fascial opening

**Table 81.3** The causes of stoma retraction

Poor stoma fixation to the skin
Careless stoma exploration or irrigation
Short mesentery
Premature removal of the support in loop ostomies
Insufficient release of the intestine
Healing impairing disease or therapies (i.e., Crohn's disease)
Thick abdominal wall

## 81.3.3 Bleeding

Most instances of bleeding at the ostomy site are attributable to bleeding caused during stoma formation and are generally not clinically significant. Such bleeding typically responds to conservative measures such as application of direct pressure or simple sutures. Nontechnical causes of clinically significant stoma bleeding include sclerosing cholangitis or portal hypertension. In such cases, treatment of the underlying causes should be pursued, such as beta-blockers and injection of sclerotherapy.

## 81.3.4 Stoma Retraction

Retraction of the stoma back towards the fascia is one of the most important complications in the early period. Typically, retraction to below 0.5 cm over skin is clinically significant and occurs 1–8% of the time [16]. The causes of stoma retraction are shown in Table 81.3. The most commonly affected ostomies include transverse colon stomas and end sigmoid ostomies.

In loop stomas, use of plastic or other supports below the loop ostomy can help prevent retraction. Supports should left in place approximately 7 days, unless there is evidence of good seal prior that time at the mucocutaneous border. Finger exploration and irrigation in loop stoma without supports are two of the major contributors to retraction in the early postoperative period.

The primary effects of retraction are difficulties in maintaining the application, leakage and peristomal skin problems. Professional stomatherapy is often very helpful in the management of retracted stomas through the use of skin protection agents and utilizing different stoma appliances. In cases where the stomatotherapists cannot improve control and pouching of the ostomy, surgical revision is required.

For revision, if there is no significant tension in the mucosa, the mucocutaneous line can be separated and the intestine advanced out of the abdomen. After removing the dead tissue (if any), it should be affixed to the skin with Brooke style stitches. The best method to prevent retraction is to create a stoma at a sufficient height from the skin level (at least 1 cm in the colon, 2–3 cm in the ileum).

If this local revision is not technically possible, laparotomy and full revision may be necessary. Complete retraction into the abdomen is uncommon and requires urgent surgical intervention.

## 81.3.5 Parastomal Infection

Parastomal abscess is a rare complication. Causes include technical errors whereby the sutures are passed too deeply during the maturation of the stoma and unintentionally pass into the intestinal lumen in eversion. Crohn's disease recurrence may also result in parastomal abscesses. Additionally, in cases of mucocutaneous separation, backflow of the stoma and contamination of subcutaneous tissue with feces may lead to abscess (Table 81.4). Improper irrigation technique may lead to damage of the intestine and abscess.

**Table 81.4** The reasons leading to parastomal infection

| |
|---|
| Ischemia |
| Intestinal content reaching the parastomal area |
| Bowel retraction |
| Stoma opening very close to the incision |
| Peristomal infected hematomas |
| Damage of the intestinal wall during stoma care |

Symptoms usually include abdominal pain that starts suddenly and discomfort that persists. Sepsis may develop with signs of abdominal wall cellulitis. If the event spreads into the peritoneal cavity or begins inside the abdomen, it can lead to extensive peritonitis. Preventing contamination of the tissues around the stoma with the appropriate surgical technique may reduce the rate of infection.

The treatment of parastomal infections without systemic sepsis is usually conservative. The infection is treated by dressing frequent change, cleaning the necrotic tissues and wrapping antiseptic gauze around the intestine. After the infection heals, necessary precautions should be taken to prevent stenosis.

In patients with systemic infection, urgent surgery is typically required with debridement, drainage, stoma replacement, and in some cases a proximal colostomy or ileostomy.

## 81.3.6 Mucocutaneous Separation

Mucocutaneous separation is separation of the stoma where it meets the skin. Causes are insufficient stitching, tightness of stitches, bad formation of stoma, and insufficient tissue perfusion (diabetes, radiation, aging, steroid, immunosuppressive therapy). It happens quite commonly, with reports suggesting an incidence of 12–24% [1–5]. Mucocutaneous separation can be superficial or deep, partial or complete. Problems such as retraction, stenosis, prolapse, and peritonitis may develop following separation.

Management of separation requires evaluation of the depth of separation. Limited separations can be treated by filling the defect with absorbable material (such as calcium alginate, paste-powders, hydrofiber). If a large amount of drainage coming from the separation area causes poor appliance of sealing devices, the defect may be enlarged to include the separation area. Separations extending to the fascia usually require surgical correction.

### 81.3.7 Early Obstruction

Early obstruction may develop due to stoma torsion or edema. If it does not resolve spontaneously, surgical revision may be required. The probability of developing parastomal herniation and bowel obstruction in the early postoperative period is reported to be 4.6–13% [15–17]. Acute parastomal herniation is generally due to a fascial defect larger than necessary. Clinical presentation of early obstruction may be with sudden onset of intestinal occlusion symptoms as nausea, vomiting, abdominal distension, and the eventual detection of a painful mass around the stoma.

In those cases with failure of conservative measures, like herniation manual reduction or medical treatment aiming to reduce edema, surgery may be required to correct the underlying cause. In any case, correction of the early parastomal abdominal wall defect before patient discharge should be taken into consideration.

## 81.4 Late Complications Requiring Emergency Surgery

Complications developing 2 weeks after the index operation are considered as late stoma complications.

### 81.4.1 Parastomal Hernias

Parastomal hernias are hernias that develop through the stoma opening. Its incidence has been reported 2–20% [15, 17]. Parastomal hernia are important because they carry the risk of intestinal obstruction and strangulation. Herniated sacs typically contain intestine and/or omentum. There are four types of hernias: the most common type is subcutaneous, and the others are interstitial, peristomal, and intrastomal. Parastomal fascial weakness and laxity are seen in many patients and are not considered as true hernia.

Nontechnical factors affecting the formation of parastomal hernia are excessive enlargement of the fascia opening, stoma brought out through the abdominal index surgical incision, weight gain, old age, emergency surgeries, weak abdominal wall, increased intra-abdominal pressure (i.e., chronic cough, chronic obstructive pulmonary disease [COPD]), steroid therapy, peristomal infection, postoperative sepsis, and malnutrition. In addition, collagen metabolism and an intrinsic defect in wound healing may be responsible for hernia formation.

The most important technical factor in the development of parastomal hernia is that the stoma is located pararectally. In recent studies, the incidence of this complication has been reported to be 2.8% in those passed through the rectus muscle, and 21.6% in those located laterally [17].

Parastomal hernias often require surgical treatment. Elective operation is recommended for patients presenting:

(a) Growing hernia
(b) Peristomal skin dehiscence
(c) Intermittent mechanical obstruction attacks
(d) Skin leakage and poor application of the appliance
(e) Chronic abdominal and/or back pain
(f) Stoma serious dysfunction

Most patients with asymptomatic parastomal hernias and those with mild symptoms can be managed nonoperatively. Several devices may be suggested to patients as stomal support belts, skin protective sealants, and a flexible appliance.

There are various degrees of hernia recurrence rate with the different surgical techniques; an ideal method has not been definitively identified. Methods to repair the parastomal hernia include: (a) relocate the stoma, (b) direct repair of the facial defect, and (c) repair of the defect with a mesh that can be synthetic, biological, or biosynthetic. Meshes typically have higher rates of success compared to direct tissue repair. However, studies on this topic are generally nonrandomized, involving a small number of patients, and have different techniques and follow-up periods. The recurrence rate after patch repair varies between 4% and 30%; the high recurrence rate after repair as well as patient comorbidities must be strongly considered in deciding and planning repair. The type of surgical approach usually may variate depending on defect size; it can either be laparoscopic or laparotomic. Simple fascial repair is associated with a very high recurrence rate and should be limited only to urgent situations whenever a more definitive prosthetic repair cannot be performed and in those patients unfitting for complex procedures. Whenever possible, it should always be preferred to use the patient's own tissues for parastomal hernia repair. However, a prosthetic material is often required to repair large hernias. The most utilized are synthetic prosthesis such as polypropylene and expanded polytetrafluoroethylene (ePTFE). Several data showed good results associated to the use of biological and biosynthetic materials; For hernia repair, especially in colostomies, some surgeons prefer to wrap the "mesh" around the stoma [15], others to pass the intestine through the middle of the "mesh". Mesh positioning in fascial onlays have been described and are generally utilized in very high-risk patients; sublay techniques may results in better outcomes in regard to recurrence. Placing prosthetic material in a contaminated area is likely to result in mesh infection. However, several data such as Sugarbaker technique (Fig. 81.2) exist about the safety of mesh mediated parastomal hernia repairing [17]; moreover, the use of biological and biosynthetic materials gave promising results even from the infectious point of view.

Given the relatively common occurrence of parastomal hernia, there have been interest in applying mesh at the time of the initial stoma cre-

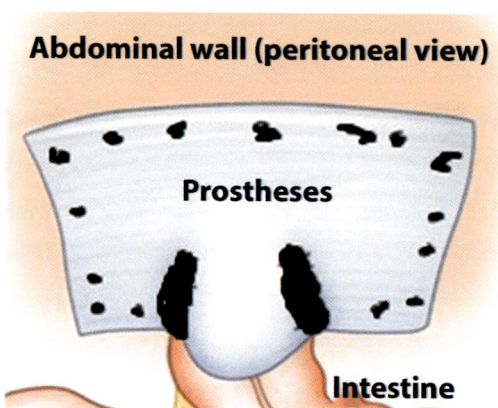

**Fig. 81.2** Sugarbaker technique

ation. In a randomized study of 54 patients on the prevention of hernias, a group of patients undergoing abdominoperineal resection were treated with a stoma patch at the time of stoma creation (Sublay technique), and the other group without a patch. The development of hernia was found to be significantly lower (41% to 15%) in the patch applied group [18].

### 81.4.2 Stoma Prolapse

Prolapse is the excessive protrusion of the intestine from the stoma opening (Fig. 81.3a, b). It may develop in the late period after surgery. Its incidence is approximately 5–15%; it is more common in patients with colostomy than patients with ileostomy; In addition, it is more common in patients with loop colostomy than end colostomy [19]. In loop colostomy or ileostomy, both loops may prolapse; however, prolapse of the proximal loop is more common. Stoma prolapse is more common in: infants and elderly patients who have weak abdominal fascia, in stoma opened through laparotomy incision, in patients affected by paraplegia, during pregnancy, in transverse colostomy, in the event of high intra-abdominal pressure (constipation, cough, heavy lifting, challenging exercises), in case of wide stoma opening, in case of nonfixation of the stoma to the abdominal wall and in long intestinal segment stoma.

In mild prolapse, simple reduction with manual pressure and hyperosmolar agents is suffi-

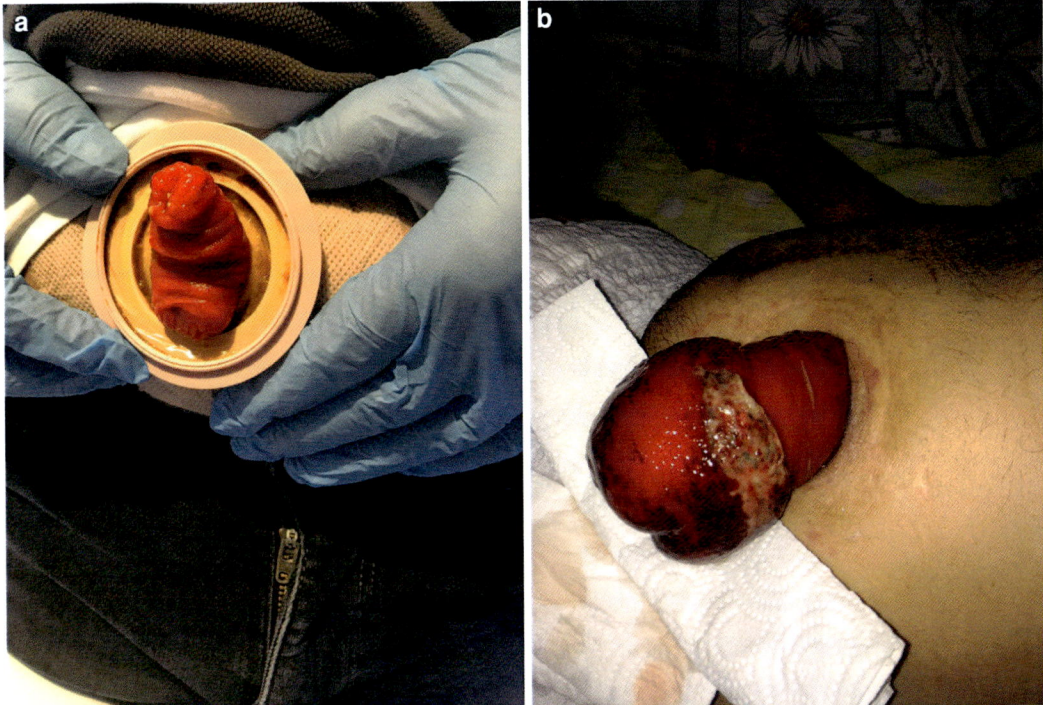

**Fig. 81.3** (**a**, **b**) Stoma prolapse

cient; however, such measures have a 60–65% failure rate [1–5]. In more advanced cases, surgical treatment may be required; the recommended approaches are colopexy, mucoparietal fixation, and reconstruction of the skin mucosa line after excision of the prolobulated intestine. All of these procedures can be performed without the necessity of general anesthesia. However, if prolapse recurs after the repair, laparotomy is required and the stoma should be relocated. Some technical advices such as fixation of the stomal mesentery to the peritoneum and fixation of the intestinal wall to the fascia may be adopted in preventing prolapse [20–22].

### 81.4.3 Stoma Stenosis

Stoma stenosis is a rare complication that develops in the late period (Fig. 81.4a–c). Its incidence is around 5–7% [1–5]. Causes include shrinkage due to malnutrition of the stoma margins, increase in peripheral connective tissue, a very narrow stoma opening, inadequately mobilized bowel, an increase in fibrous tissue due to infection around the stoma, Crohn's disease, primary and recurrent malignancies. For many patients, simple treatment methods such as stool softeners, dilation with a finger or spark plugs and evacuation of the stool are sufficient. In addition, if the stenosis is at the fascia level, fasciotomy can be performed with local anesthesia through small incisions made above and below the stoma (5–6 cm from the stoma). If mechanical obstruction cannot be resolved, surgery must be done to resolve it. In the case of impossibility to solve the obstruction with less invasive approaches, the stoma may need to be rebuilt or relocated.

### 81.4.4 Stoma Fistula

Causes of stoma fistulas such as perforation of the intestinal loop by stitching, trauma, or malignant disease or Crohn's disease, may lead to

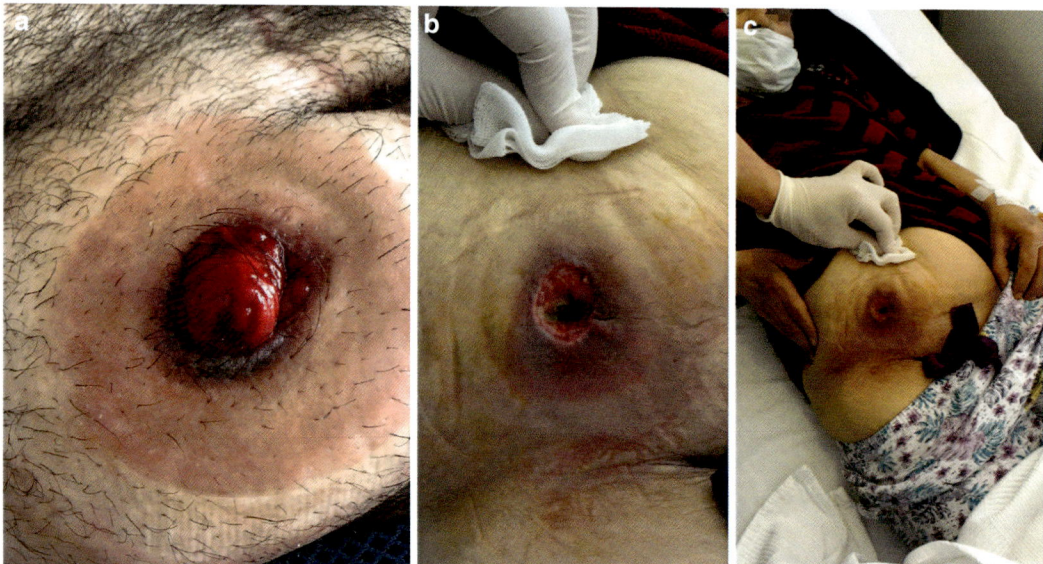

**Fig. 81.4** (a–c) Stoma stenosis

abscesses and fistulas around the stoma. There are three types of stoma fistulae: trans-stomal, blind peristomal and viscerocutaneous. The trans-stoma fistula is usually seen in ileostomies; It occurs due to traumas that develop during the application and maintenance of stoma bags and adapters and it requires surgical treatment. Surgically trans-stoma fistula can be corrected by removing the intestinal section containing the fistula and re-fix the skin and mucosa. Blind peristomal fistula is usually due to stitches fixing the intestine to the fascia; an abundant secretion is seen without presence of the intestinal contents. It requires surgical treatment. Generally, the blind peristomal fistula is usually corrected by removing stitches and fix the defect. Stitches that cause fistula are removed and the defect corrected. A viscerocutaneous fistula may occur when the stoma fixation sutures to the fascia or peritoneum cause a damage to the bowel wall, or an erosion of the intestinal wall caused by other such as mesh; abundant intestinal contents are discharged from the fistula opening and due to this discharge, peristomal dermatitis develops which also makes the appliance of stoma bag difficult. Viscerocutaneous fistulas also requires surgical treatment by detaching the stoma from the skin and possibly the intestine exteriorized through the stoma orifice, up to discover the bowel wall defect, resected below the defect and finally, reconstruct the stoma [17]. Whenever this procedure is not feasible, the stoma rebuilding or relocation must be approached through laparotomy or laparoscopy.

## 81.4.5 Intestinal Obstruction in the Late Period

Another complication seen in people with stoma is bowel obstruction. Its incidence is around 13–15% [4]. Adhesions in the intestinal wall, volvulus, stoma stenosis are causes of late ostomy obstruction. In ostomy, food obstruction is most common in the third and sixth months postoperatively (corn, nuts, citrus fruits, uncooked fibrous vegetables, and fruit peels). Ostomy obstruction may also be due to hernia, tumor recurrence, and stool hardening [23, 24]. Emergency surgery must be done if the status cannot be solved through conservative treatment within 48–72 h.

### Dos and Don'ts

- Whenever possible mark the stoma site preoperatively with the help of professional stomatherapist.
- Be careful in stoma positioning and preparation.
- Transrectal muscles stoma creation reduces the risk of stoma-related complications.
- Consider the more appropriate stoma in relation to the anatomical and clinical patient condition.
- Stoma relocation has a high complications recurrence rate, both at the old and the new ostomy site; for his reason this should be considered as the very last option.
- Emergency surgery must be done if stoma-related intestinal occlusion does not resolve in 48–72 h.

## 81.5 Conclusion

In summary, colostomies and ileostomies are necessary procedures that carry risk of complications. Being aware of the complications that may occur, and using strategies to decrease their risk, may help in preventing development of early and late complications (Fig. 81.5a, b).

### Questions

1. What is the duration of early stoma complications?
   A. 1 week after operation
   B. 2 weeks after operation
   C. 3 weeks after operation
   D. 4 weeks after operation
2. Which one is not important to prevent of stoma necrosis?
   A. Avoid tight stitches
   B. Avoid tight fitting bags around edematous stomas
   C. Avoid emergency operations
   D. Avoid overly tight fascial openings
3. Which one is not a reason leading to parastomal infection?
   A. Ischemia
   B. Bowel retraction
   C. Intestinal content reaching the parastomal area
   D. Gender
4. What is the rate of mucocutaneous separation?
   A. 1%
   B. 5%
   C. 15%
   D. 25%
5. Which one is not clinical sign of early obstruction?
   A. Sudden onset of nausea
   B. Vomiting
   C. Detection of a painful mass around the stoma
   D. Cachexia
6. What is the most important technical factor in the development of parastomal hernia?
   A. Pararectally located stoma
   B. Median located stoma
   C. Laterally located stoma
   D. Upper quadrant located stoma
7. Which one is not a type of stoma fistulae?
   A. Intra-abdominal
   B. Trans-stoma
   C. Blind peristoma
   D. Viscerocutaneous
8. What is the most common type of parastomal hernias?
   A. Subcutaneous
   B. Interstitial
   C. Perstomal
   D. Intrastomal

9. At intestinal obstruction in the late period emergency surgery must be done if the status does not resolve in…
    A. 12–24 h
    B. 24–48 h
    C. 48–72 h
    D. 72–96 h
10. The risk of complications is higher in patients with…
    A. Ileostomy
    B. Colostomy
    C. End colostomy
    D. Loop colostomy

**Answers**: 1B; 2C; 3D; 4C; 5D; 6A; 7A; 8A; 9C; 10A

a **FLOW CHART OF EARLY STOMA COMPLICATIONS MANAGEMENT**

| Evisceration | Ischemia and stoma necrosis | Bleeding | Stoma Retraction | Parastomal Infection and Puncture | Mucocutaneous Separation | Early Obstruction |
|---|---|---|---|---|---|---|
| Urgent reoperation | Conservative/delayed reoperation | Conservative | Conservative/delayed reoperation | Conservative | Conservative/delayed reoperation | Conservative/delayed reoperation |

b **FLOW CHART OF LATE STOMA COMPLICATIONS MANAGEMENT**

| Parastomal Hernias | Stoma Prolapse | Stoma Stenosis | Stoma Fistula | Intestinal Obstruction in the Late Period |
|---|---|---|---|---|
| Conservative/delayed reoperation | Conservative/delayed reoperation | Conservative/delayed reoperation | Conservative/delayed reoperation | Conservative/delayed reoperation |

**Fig. 81.5** (**a**, **b**) Flow chart of stoma complications management

**Acknowledgement** Thank you very much to Dr. Shukri M. Dahir for English language editing.

# References

1. Pearj RK, Prasad ML, Orsay CP, Abcarian H, Tan AB, Melz MT. Early local complications from intestinal stomas. Arch Surg. 1985;120:1145–7.
2. Rullier E, Le Toux N, Laurent C, Garreleon JL, Parneix M, Saric J. Loop ileostomy versus loop colostomy for defunctioning low anastomoses during rectal cancer surgery. World J Surg. 2001;25:274–8.
3. Moscowitz DA, Kirschner JB. İleostomy in ulcerative colits. Am J Surg. 1994;141:727–9.
4. Park JJ, Del Pino A, Orsay CP, et al. Stoma complications: the Cook County Hospital experience. Dis Colon Rectum. 1999;42:1575–80.
5. Stothert JC Jr, Brubacher L, Simonowitz DA. Complications of emergency stoma formation. Arch Surg. 1982;117(3):307–9.
6. Del Pino A, Cintron JR, Orsay CP, Pearl RK, Tan A, Abcarian H. Enterostomal complications are emergently created enterostomas at greater risk? Am Surg. 1997;63(7):653–6.
7. Duchesne JC, Wang YZ, Weintraub SI, Boyle M, Hunt JP. Stoma complications: a multivarite analysis. Am Surg. 2002;68:961–6.
8. Porter IA, Salvati PA, Rubin RI, Eisenstat TE. Complications of colostomies. Dis Colon Rectum. 1998;32:299–303.
9. Rutegard J, Dahlgren S. Transvers colostomy or loop ileostomy as diverting stoma in colorectal surgery. Acta Chir Scand. 1986;153:229–32.
10. Köckerling F, Parth R, Meisner M, Hohenberger W. Ileostomie-Koecafistel-Kolostomie-Welches ist das gecignetste vorgeschaltete Stuhlableitungsverfahren unter Berücksichtigung von Angle, Funktion, Komplikationen und Ruckverlagerung? Zentalb, Chir. 1997;122:34–8.
11. Gooszen AW, Geelgerken RH, Hermans J, Lagxay MB, Gooszen HG. Temporary decompression after colorectal surgery: randomized comparison of loop ileostomy and colostomy. Br J Surg. 1998;85:76–9.
12. Daly JM, De Cosse II. Complications in surgery of the colon and rectum. Surg Clin North Am. 1983;63:1215–31.
13. Leenen LP, Kuypers JH. Some factors influencing the outcome of stoma surgery. Dis Colon Rectum. 1989;32:500–4.
14. Tucker SB, Smith DB. Dermatologic conditions and complications of ostomy care. In: Smith DB, Johnson DE, editors. Ostomy and the cancer patients. Orlando: Grune & Stratton; 1986.
15. Bayer I, Kyzer S, Chaimoff CH. A new approach to primary strengthening of colostomy with Marlex mesh to prevent paracolostomy hernia. Surg Gynecol Obstet. 1986;163:579–80.
16. Akgün ZE, Yoldaş T. İntestinal Stoma Kolon Rektum Hastalıkları Dergisi. 2012;22:133–46.
17. Catoldo PA. Ostomy complications. In: American College of Surgeons, 85th annual clinical congress, San Francisco, 10–15 Oct 1999.
18. Serra-Aracil X, Bombardo-Junca J, Moreno-Matias J, et al. Randomized, controlled, prospective trial of the use of a mesh to prevent parastomal hernia. Ann Surg. 2009;249:583–7.
19. Alemdaroğlu K, Akçal T, Buğra D. Kolon Rektum ve Anal Bölge Hastalıkları. İstanbul: Tasarım, Ofset Hazırlık ve Baskı; 2003. p. 488–92.
20. Maeda K, Maruta M, Utsumi T, et al. Pathophysiology and prevention of loop stomal prolapse in the transverse colon. Tech Coloproctol. 2003;7:108–11.
21. Husain SG, Cataldo TE. Late stomal complications. Clin Colon Rectal Surg. 2008;21:31–40.
22. Beraldo S, Titley G, Allan A, et al. Use of W-plasty in stenotic stoma: a new solution for an old problem. Color Dis. 2006;8:715–6.
23. Hill GL. The operation. Preoperative and postoperative care. In: Hill GL, editor. Ileostomy: surgery physiology and management. New York: Grune Stratton Co.; 1972. p. 13–39.
24. Charles Brunicardi F, Andersen DK, Billiar TR, Dunn DL, Kao LS, Hunter JG, Matthews JB, Pollock RE. Schwartz's principles of surgery. 11th ed. McGraw Hill; 2019.

# Inflammatory Bowel Disease

82

Jeremy Meyer and Justin Davies

## 82.1 Introduction

Inflammatory bowel disease (IBD) constitutes a group of chronic immune diseases affecting the gastrointestinal (GI) tract, most commonly presenting as Crohn's disease and ulcerative colitis.

The prevalence of inflammatory bowel disease has increased over the last decades and is now of 84.3 per 100,000, with the highest prevalence reported in the United States of America and in the United Kingdom [1].

Inflammatory bowel disease has an important impact on society and quality of life, as it bears an age-standardized disability-adjusted life-years of 23.2 per 100,000 individuals [1]. Its etiology appears multifactorial, including genetic predisposition, intestinal microbiota, and environmental factors [2–10].

Crohn's disease is a chronic inflammatory bowel disease which causes focal and skipped transmural inflammation of the entire gastrointestinal tract, ultimately leading to perforation and fistulizing disease, with around half of patients having typical granulomas on biopsies [11].

Ulcerative colitis affects the large bowel mucosa in continuity from the rectum, characterized by relapses, and remissions, and without granulomas found on biopsies [12].

In approximately 10% of patients, it is not possible to distinguish between Crohn's and ulcerative colitis. These patients are considered to have IBD-unclassified colitis [11].

> **Learning Goals**
> - To review the basic knowledge regarding management of patients suffering from inflammatory bowel disease (IBD).
> - To adequately diagnose and manage complications related to inflammatory bowel disease in the emergency setting.
> - To know the indications for emergency surgery in patients with inflammatory bowel disease.
> - To perform optimal surgical treatment in patients with inflammatory bowel disease who require emergency surgery.

J. Meyer
Cambridge Colorectal Unit, Addenbrooke's Hospital, Cambridge University Hospitals NHS Foundation Trust, Cambridge, UK

J. Davies (✉)
Cambridge Colorectal Unit, Addenbrooke's Hospital, Cambridge University Hospitals NHS Foundation Trust, Cambridge, UK

University of Cambridge, Cambridge, UK

## 82.2 Diagnosis

### 82.2.1 Clinical Presentation

Chronic diarrhea associated with weight loss is a typical symptom of inflammatory bowel disease. Abdominal pain, anorexia and fever are

© The Author(s), under exclusive license to Springer Nature Switzerland AG 2023
F. Coccolini, F. Catena (eds.), *Textbook of Emergency General Surgery*,
https://doi.org/10.1007/978-3-031-22599-4_82

common in Crohn's disease, which can also manifest itself with fistulizing and perianal symptoms. Patients with ulcerative colitis usually present with diarrhea, urgency, tenesmus, and lower gastrointestinal bleeding. If the symptoms of inflammatory bowel disease are long-lasting, poor nutrition or growth retardation in children can be evident.

One-fifth of patients have extra-intestinal manifestations, such arthropathy, erythema nodosum, pyoderma gangrenosum, primary sclerosing cholangitis or inflammation of the different compartments of the eye.

### 82.2.2 Diagnostic Management

For a first presentation or a suspicion of flare of inflammatory bowel disease, blood tests should include hemoglobin, hematocrit, inflammatory markers such as C-reactive protein (CRP) and erythrocyte sedimentation rate (ESR), electrolytes, renal and liver function tests, albumin, vitamin B12, folic acid, and ferritin. Fecal calprotectin should be obtained and feces should be screened for infection, including *Clostridium difficile*. Serologic panels can be performed to help in the diagnosis, but the evidence supporting their use is of low quality [13].

Where Crohn's disease is suspected, ileocolonoscopy should be performed to assess the extent of the disease and obtain biopsies. Gastroscopy can be obtained if upper gastrointestinal involvement is suspected. Imaging can include computed tomography (CT), magnetic resonance imaging (MRI) enterography or video-capsule [14]. Diagnosis is usually based on a combination of clinical, radiological, endoscopic, and histologic elements [15]. The phenotype of Crohn's disease, which describes the areas of the gastrointestinal tract involved and the disease behavior (non-stricturing and non-penetrating, stricturing, penetrating, perianal) can be classified according to the Vienna score or the Montreal classification system [12]. Crohn's disease activity can be quantified according to an important number of clinical and/or endoscopic severity scores [16]. The most commonly used is the Crohn's disease activity index (CDAI).

In case of suspicion of ulcerative colitis, an initial flexible sigmoidoscopy can be obtained during the acute phase, but a full ileocolonoscopy should be performed within 1 year of diagnosis [11]. Rectal sparing can be observed in less than 5% of patients, and backwash ileitis in around 20%. The proximal extent of inflammation can also be demonstrated by CT scan.

Ulcerative colitis phenotype is usually classified according to the Montreal classification system [12]. The extent of the inflammation influences the risk of future colectomy [17]. Disease activity is preferentially quantified by the Truelove and Whitts score, by the Ulcerative Colitis Endoscopic Index of Severity (UCEIS) and by the modified Mayo scores [18].

## 82.3 Treatment

### 82.3.1 Medical Treatment

The main objective of medical treatment for inflammatory bowel disease is to obtain and maintain remission.

Treatment for patients with Crohn's disease should include smoking cessation and correction of nutritional deficiencies supervised by a dietician and intestinal failure team where indicated. Remission is usually obtained with oral corticosteroids or, if the disease is limited to the ileocecum, using oral budesonide. Exclusive enteral nutrition using polymeric, elemental, or semi-elemental feeds can serve as an alternative or as an adjunct in motivated patients. In case of moderate-to-severe episodes, treatment relies on intravenous steroids or, as a second line, immunotherapy. Once remission is obtained, thiopurines are usually used for maintenance. In case of failure, immunotherapy (e.g., anti-tumor necrosis factor-alpha [TNF-alpha] therapy) can be used in association with thiopurine [11, 19].

In Crohn's disease, elective surgery is most commonly indicated in patients suffering from complications not responding to medical treatment, such as chronic obstructive symptoms due to stricturing disease, symptomatic intra-abdominal fistula (Figs. 82.1 and 82.2), entero-cutaneous

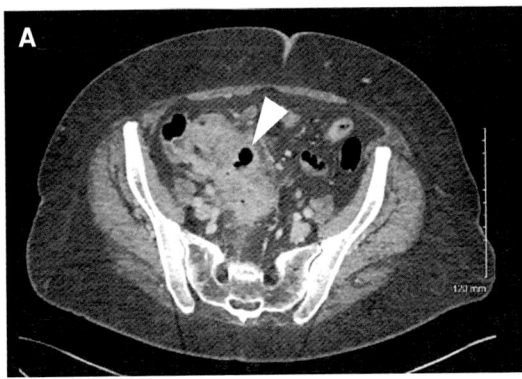
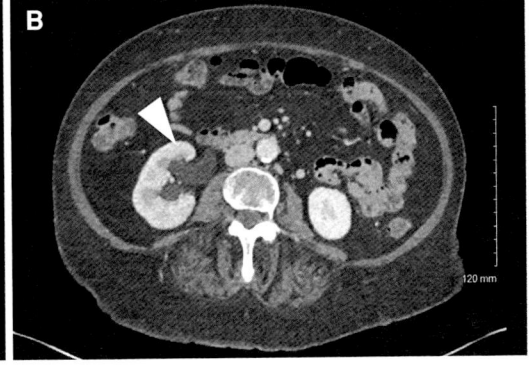

**Fig. 82.1** A 60-year-old female patient, known for Crohn's disease with poor response to immunotherapy, who presented to the emergency department with an acute abdomen and raised inflammatory markers. Computed tomography showed an inflammatory mass in the right iliac fossa (**a**, arrow) with multiple entero-enteric fistulae. There was no collection amenable to drainage. In addition, computed tomography showed a moderate right hydro-ureteronephrosis (**b**, arrow) due to involvement of the right ureter in this inflammatory process and a non-occlusive left common femoral vein thrombus. The patient initially underwent a defunctioning loop ileostomy and ureteric JJ stent, with definitive surgery to be planned subsequently on an elective basis

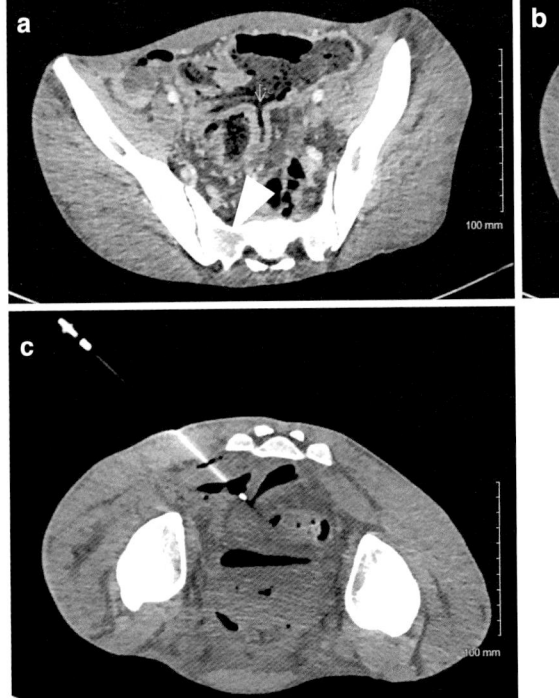
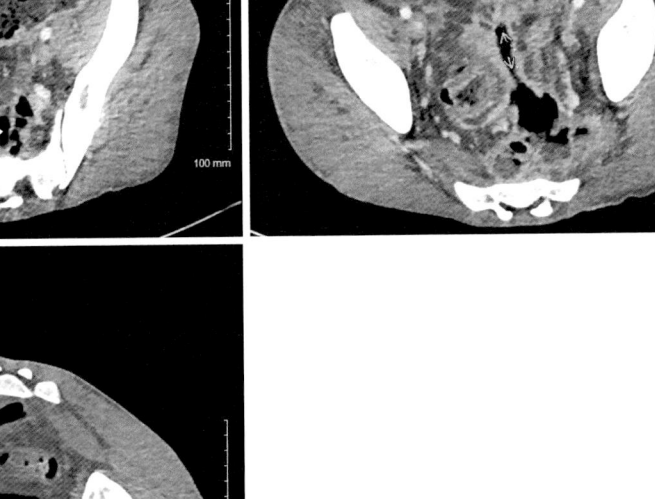

**Fig. 82.2** A 24-year-old male patient, known for Crohn's disease but with poor medical compliance, who presented to the emergency department because of lower abdominal pain and cloudy urine. Computed tomography found an extended pre-sacral collection with a large fistula tract (**a**, **b**, small arrows) arising from the distal sigmoid colon and extending toward the bladder (colovesical fistula) and towards the pre-sacral space. A computed tomography drainage of the posterior collection was performed (**c**), antibiotics were given and the patient underwent an initial defunctioning loop ileostomy with definitive surgery to be planned subsequently on an elective basis

fistula, and perianal disease. Elective surgery in these patients requires careful surgical planning with particular attention to nutrition and medication management.

Patients with ulcerative colitis are usually treated with oral and topical 5-ASA therapy. Oral corticoids constitute the second line of treatment for moderate-to-severe episodes. In case of recurrence requiring repeated administrations of corticoids, or of cortico-dependence, escalation can be performed using thiopurines or immunotherapy [11, 20].

Patients with ulcerative colitis should be considered for elective surgery if they experience persistent symptoms despite maximal medical management, if they cannot tolerate the medical treatment, or if they present with dysplasia, non-endoscopically resectable sporadic adenomas or colorectal cancer [21]. The initial surgical treatment for failure of medical therapy is subtotal colectomy and ileostomy, with subsequent discussions around the role and timing of completion proctectomy, with or without restoration of intestinal continuity (most commonly in the form of an ileoanal pouch).

### 82.3.2 Indications for Emergency Surgery

General surgeons providing emergency care encounter a significant number of patients with inflammatory bowel disease during their clinical practice. Patients with Crohn's disease and ulcerative colitis are exposed to several complications that require hospital admission and emergency life-saving surgery (Tables 82.1 and 82.2).

Patients with Crohn's disease have an annual incidence of hospitalization of 20% [22]. More than half of patients with Crohn's disease will experience bowel resection after 10 years of follow-up [23].

Emergency surgery represents 3.8% of admissions for ulcerative colitis [24]. The risk of having a colectomy is approximately 8%, 10% and 15% after 5, 10, and 20 years of follow-up [25].

**Table 82.1** Indications for emergency surgery in ulcerative colitis

| Life-threatening emergencies |
| --- |
| • Massive colorectal hemorrhage |
| • Toxic megacolon |
| • Colonic perforation |
| Delayed emergency |
| • Severe acute colitis refractory to medical treatment |

**Table 82.2** Indications for emergency surgery in Crohn's disease

| Life-threatening emergencies |
| --- |
| • Massive colorectal hemorrhage |
| • Toxic megacolon |
| • Gastrointestinal tract perforation |
| Delayed emergency |
| • Penetrating disease refractory to non-surgical management |
| • Obstruction refractory to non-surgical management |

**Table 82.3** Definition of severe acute ulcerative colitis

| ≥6 bloody stools per day | |
| --- | --- |
| At least one of the following: | Fever >37.8 °C |
| | Heart rate >90 beats/min |
| | Erythrocyte sedimentation rate (ESR) >30 mm/h |
| | Hemoglobin <105 g/L |

#### 82.3.2.1 Acute Severe Colitis

Severe ulcerative colitis, previously known as fulminant colitis, is usually associated with ulcerative colitis and defined by the Truelove and Witts classification as more than 6 bloody stools per day associated with at least one systematic sign of toxicity (Table 82.3) [26].

Management includes insertion of at least one intravenous cannula, administration of intravenous fluids, complete bloods comprising full blood count, CRP, electrolytes, renal function, and lactate. Polymerase chain reaction (PCR) of the stools should eliminate any infectious cause (notably *Clostridium difficile*) to the clinical presentation, and a CT can to confirm the extent of inflammation of the colon and the absence of complications (toxic megacolon, perforation) is indicated. Flexible sigmoidoscopy confirms the diagnosis with histology aiding this process, as well as excluding cytomegalovirus (CMV) colitis [18]. A gastroenterology team should be principally involved in care with regular multidisciplinary review with the surgical team.

First-line treatment consists of intravenous corticosteroids and second-line with cyclosporin or anti-TNF-alpha therapy [18, 21]. If no improvement is observed within several days of joint medical and surgical care, stoma nurses should be asked to counsel the patient and if the patient deteriorates further, surgery should be performed (subtotal colectomy with end ileostomy).

Patients with Crohn's disease can present with an episode of severe acute colitis which is indistinguishable from that of ulcerative colitis. Its management is initially the same as previously outlined for ulcerative colitis, although second-line therapy tends to favor anti-TNF-alpha therapy [27].

### 82.3.2.2 Toxic Megacolon

Toxic megacolon refers to the acute dilatation of the colon due to dysfunction of the autonomic nervous system in the context of an acute segmental or total colitis. Toxic megacolon, also sometimes named toxic colitis (in the absence of pathologic dilatation of the colon), is by definition associated with signs of systematic inflammation and/or sepsis (Table 82.3).

Toxic megacolon was first described by Marshak and Lester in 1950 as a complication of ulcerative colitis [28]. Since then, several etiologies of toxic megacolon have been reported, including inflammatory bowel disease, infectious colitis due to *Clostridium difficile*, *Salmonella* spp., *Shigella* spp., *Campylobacter* spp., *Escherichia coli* spp., *Entamoeba* spp., *Aspergillus*, or CMV in immunosuppressed patients [29–31]. Inflammatory bowel disease represents about half of the etiologies of toxic megacolon [32].

Pathogenic mechanisms leading to toxic megacolon probably involve significant mucosal inflammation, leading to the release of inflammatory mediators and nitric oxide, as well as transmural inflammation with direct injury to the smooth muscle layer and the myenteric plexus. Progress to toxic megacolon can be worsened by rapid withdrawal of immunomodulators in the context of inflammatory bowel disease, electrolyte disturbances, and medications slowing bowel motility.

Patients with toxic megacolon usually complain of diarrhea, malaise, abdominal pain, and abdominal distension. Many have signs of hemodynamic instability, such as tachycardia and hypotension [33].

Initial management of patients with suspected toxic megacolon should include insertion of two large gauge venous cannulae, volume resuscitation using crystalloids (as these patients are by definition hypovolemic), insertion of a nasogastric tube, insertion of a urinary catheter, analgesia, and empirical broad-spectrum antibiotics according to local guidelines. Vital signs and urine output should be carefully monitored. Blood tests should look for inflammatory markers, electrolyte disturbance, and signs of organ failure. They should include full blood count, prothrombin time, electrolytes, renal function, liver function, and lactate. Arterial blood gas and insertion of an arterial line can be useful adjuncts. Fluid resuscitation should be undertaken to correct any defects and stabilize the patient [34].

If the patient remains unstable, an initial abdominal X-ray should be performed to look for colonic dilatation and potential free air suggestive of perforation. If found, the patient should be directed to surgery.

If the patient is hemodynamically stable, a CT scan with intravenous contrast is the modality of choice as it allows to confirm the extent of dilatation, to look for evidence of perforation and also to rule out any alternative diagnosis. Administration of rectal contrast or endoscopy should be avoided due to the risk of perforation. In patients who remain stable, a trial of medical therapy should be considered. Medical management of toxic megacolon was initially shown to avoid surgery in half of patients, but improved over the last decade so nowadays only 11.5–21.6% of patients require emergency surgery [35, 36].

Stool samples should be taken to exclude *Clostridium difficile* infection and other pathogens reported to be causative pathogens for toxic megacolon. Then, the patient should be directed to an intensive care unit or intermediate care unit for monitoring of vital signs. Total parenteral nutrition should be started, and medications slowing down bowel movement should be avoided. Some authors recommend to roll the patient to redistribute the intestinal gas, but the evidence supporting this maneuver is of low quality and thus it is not generally recommended [37]. If the episode of toxic megacolon is related to inflammatory bowel disease, intravenous steroids should be administered, according to the local gastroenterology team preference. Serial abdominal X-ray should be obtained to monitor colonic dilatation and surgical review arranged. In case of failure of steroid therapy after 2–3 days, anti-TNF-alpha therapy should be started. Cyclosporine might constitute an alternative in patients with known ulcerative colitis.

Absolute indications for surgery are perforation, intraluminal colonic hemorrhage and septic shock. Progression of colonic dilatation on serial abdominal X-ray during second-line therapy, or failure of medical treatment using anti-TNF therapy should also prompt surgical intervention.

Surgery consists of subtotal colectomy with end ileostomy for both ulcerative colitis and Crohn's disease, removing the diseased colon which is the source of inflammatory mediators and bacterial translocation. In general, no attempt should be made to remove the rectum in the emergency setting. In very selected cases where the patient is not fit for major abdominal surgery, colonic decompression using ultrasound (US)- or CT-guided cecostomy or loop transverse colostomy can be considered as an alternative treatment [32].

Mortality rate is estimated to range between 7.9% and 16% [32, 35] but can rise as high as 44% in case of perforation [38].

### 82.3.2.3 Bowel Obstruction

Bowel obstruction is more common in patients suffering from Crohn's disease than in those with ulcerative colitis [39]. Intestinal obstruction due to Crohn's disease may either be the consequence of active inflammation or the consequence of fibrotic stricture of the bowel lumen due to chronic inflammation, and can occur anywhere in the gastrointestinal tract. Areas of previous anastomosis are at increased risk. Approximately half of patients with Crohn's disease will experience bowel obstruction after 10 years of follow-up [23, 40], and adhesions from previous abdominal surgery can also be a cause of obstruction in some patients.

Bowel obstruction is less common in ulcerative colitis and represents 5% of admissions in these patients [41]. By definition, the area most commonly affected is the colon. An important differential diagnosis is colonic obstruction due to colorectal cancer, which represents one quarter of colonic strictures in patients with ulcerative colitis [41].

Depending on the level of obstruction, patients complain of abdominal pain, nausea and vomiting, abdominal distension, impaired evacuation of flatus and stools.

Management includes insertion of a nasogastric tube to avoid vomiting and broncho-aspiration, insertion of at least one venous cannula, and intravenous fluids to compensate for the lack of reabsorption due to the obstruction. Blood tests should include full blood count, CRP, electrolytes, renal, and liver function and lactate to check for tissue hypoperfusion. We do not recommend initial abdominal X-ray as it does not give a detailed anatomical picture of the bowel obstruction, does not allow assessment of bowel perfusion and also does not look for the cause of obstruction. Abdominal CT scan with intravenous contrast is the gold standard to look for the level of obstruction, to exclude complications such as perforation, to assess bowel perfusion and to rule out any alternative diagnosis. Of note, the CT images should be carefully analyzed to look for colorectal cancer that may change the therapeutic strategy.

In a patient with fever, if the bowel distension is significant (to avoid bacterial translocation), if the bowel wall is thickened on CT or in case of elevated inflammatory parameters, broad-spectrum antibiotics covering the gastrointestinal flora should be added.

Prolonged abdominal pain, clinical signs of peritonitis, hypoperfusion of the bowel on CT, or evidence for bowel perforation should prompt for emergency surgery. Colonic dilatation >6 cm, the absence of a transition point and signs of systematic inflammation should orientate towards toxic megacolon.

Small bowel obstruction is much more common in patients with Crohn's disease. In these patients, initial conservative management should be favored [42]. This is of importance to avoid multiple and repeated bowel resections that could lead to short bowel syndrome (defined as a bowel length <100 cm [43]). Initial CT scan of the abdomen is important to aid in the diagnosis, cause, and level of obstruction, to guide whether the stricture(s) is fibrotic or inflammatory in nature (if present) and to look for any evidence of fistula/collection. Conservative management consists of bowel rest, aspiration on the nasogastric tube, correction of electrolytes disorders and avoidance of medications slowing down bowel motility. Intravenous fluids should be continued, but should be switched to parenteral nutrition as soon as is feasible. If adhesions are a suggested cause of obstruction, gastrografin should be administered through the nasogastric tube, which is then clamped for 2 h. An abdominal X-ray is obtained after 4–6 h to check if the contrast product has reached the colon. Further, this procedure may be therapeutic through an osmolar effect and lead to bowel opening. Bowel obstruction in patients with Crohn's disease might also be related or be caused by a flare of the disease. Therefore, if the stenotic area appears inflamed on CT and suggests a flare, the gastroenterology team should be involved and consider changes to medical therapy.

In case of failure of conservative management, the strategy will mostly depend on the level and the extent of obstruction. If the stenosis is localized in an area accessible to endoscopy, either enteroscopy or colonoscopy can be considered [44, 45]. Careful balloon dilatation of the stenotic area can be performed, keeping in mind that these procedures might lead to perforation and prompt for surgery. Placement of a stent, even resorbable, is not recommended. If the stenosis is not accessible to balloon dilatation, either due to its localization or its extent, careful surgical planning should be undertaken.

If emergency surgery is required, the, treatment of choice is resection of the stenotic small bowel segment, removing the inflamed area with minimal margins. In cases where the stenotic segment is the terminal ileum, as it is often the case, an ileocecal resection should be performed. If the nutritional status allows and there is absence of sepsis and steroids, a wide side-to-side anastomosis is most commonly performed, although there is no particular benefit over an end-to-end anastomosis. If the patient is cachectic or at high risk for anastomotic leak, resection with formation of a double barrel stoma is preferred, allowing to close the stoma later without entering the abdominal cavity, although an end ileostomy with potential mucous fistula can be considered too and often leads to a stoma that is more easily managed. If the stricturing disease affects several bowel loops (skip lesions), resection of these loops might expose the patient to short bowel syndrome, and strictureplasty should therefore be favored if strictures are fibrotic and short (generally than 10 cm for a Heineke-Mikulicz strictureplasty [42, 44, 46]). A relative contraindication to strictureplasty is the presence of active Crohn's disease. Controlling the inflammation, if present, and involving the gastroenterology team is therefore of paramount importance. Whatever the surgical procedure, remaining bowel length should be precisely measured and reported in the operative note. If possible, a drawing should be made, depicting the resections and anastomoses/stomas.

In case the patient is hemodynamically unstable, and might benefit from an anastomosis instead of a stoma after hemodynamic stabilization (for example if the affected segment is close to the duodeno-jejunal flexure and creating a stoma might lead to high-output stoma), damage control surgery is possible, leaving the divided stapled bowel ends in the open abdomen equipped with a vacuum assisted closure (VAC) system, and performing the anastomosis during a second look surgery after 48–72 h when the hemodynamic status and bowel perfusion are improved.

For patients with ulcerative colitis presenting with large bowel obstruction due to a colonic stricture, subtotal colectomy and creation of an end ileostomy are the procedure of choice, although a bridge to surgery with a colonic stent may be considered if there is no evidence of active colitis and the stricture is malignant.

#### 82.3.2.4 Gastrointestinal Hemorrhage

The first case of gastrointestinal hemorrhage related to a regional enteritis was reported in 1941 [47].

In ulcerative colitis, bloody diarrhea is a cardinal symptom of the disease. Bleeding is usually diffuse and caused by multiple ulcerations of the colonic and rectal mucosa. In Crohn's disease, hemorrhage can occur anywhere in the gastrointestinal tract as the consequence of transmural inflammation and direct injury to a vessel [48].

There is no strict definition that allows to distinguish between a low intensity bleed due to a flare of ulcerative colitis, for example, and a life-threatening hemorrhage. Therefore, clinical assessment should prevail and any drop in hemoglobin associated with active gastrointestinal bleeding or hemodynamic instability should be considered as an inflammatory bowel disease life-threatening hemorrhage and promptly addressed.

The incidence of severe hemorrhage varies, but represents approximately 0.1% of admissions for ulcerative colitis and 1.2% of admissions for Crohn's disease. It represents up to 10% of urgent colectomies for patients with ulcerative colitis [49].

Initial management includes insertion of two large gauge venous cannulae, a urinary catheter, and volume resuscitation including blood products. If hematemesis is suggested, a nasogastric tube should be inserted. Vital signs and urine output should be carefully monitored. Blood tests should look for hemoglobin concentration, hematocrit, prothrombin time, and platelets. Further, electrolytes, renal function, liver function, and lactate should also be determined. A quick way to obtain the hemoglobin concentration is to perform arterial or venous blood gas determination. In case of hemodynamic instability, insertion of an arterial line can be a useful adjunct [34].

Transfusion with red blood cells, platelets, and plasma should be performed as required. Considering that these patients are most often malnourished, and associated liver disease might be present, correction of coagulation factors should be considered.

In both ulcerative colitis and Crohn's disease, hemorrhage occurs most often in the lower GI tract and is associated with inflammation [49]. Even in Crohn's disease, the upper gastrointestinal tract is rarely involved [48].

A CT scan with arterial phase (CT angiography) should be the imaging of choice and quickly obtained to localize the source of the bleeding. If an active arterial bleed is identified, the patient should be directed immediately to interventional radiology for angiography and selective embolization of the causative vessel [50, 51]. After successful embolization, the patient should be monitored in an intensive care unit or intermediate care unit for 48 h to ensure there is no rebleeding and look for potential complications of embolization, such as bowel ischemic necrosis and perforation. If ischemia is a consideration, a further CT scan or a diagnostic laparoscopy and simultaneous sigmoidoscopy/colonoscopy can be performed. Peroperative fluorescence angiography can be used in case of doubt to identify ischemic areas.

If the source of bleeding is not identified, as is the case in two-thirds of patients [50], usual rules of management of gastrointestinal bleeding should be applied.

If an upper gastrointestinal hemorrhage is suspected (above the duodeno-jejunal junction), gastroscopy is the modality of choice. In case of lower gastrointestinal hemorrhage (below the duodeno-jejunal junction), the patient should undergo colonoscopy. In patients with ulcerative colitis and colonic bleeding, complete hemostasis using clips at different sites has been reported [52, 53]. However, when the inflammation is severe, full colonoscopy is not recommended in patients with ulcerative colitis due to the risk of perforation but flexible sigmoidoscopy should be performed to confirm the diagnosis and be sure there is no significant source of bleeding in the rectum.

In patients with ulcerative colitis, failure to control the hemorrhage with non-surgical techniques should prompt for subtotal colectomy, which often constitutes the only efficient treatment especially since bleeding is usually diffuse [54]. Bleeding from the rectum after subtotal colectomy can be controlled by adding local hemostatic products, preferentially leaving a rectal catheter in place to monitor the volume of bleeding which can accumulate in the rectal stump without being noticed. In the rare case where the rectal stump is the source of significant bleeding, proctectomy might be necessary.

In patients with Crohn's disease, medical management can aim at reducing the causative inflammation and controlling the disease, but has a failure rate of approximately 40% [48, 55, 56]. In addition, emergency video capsule endoscopy can be performed. If the bleeding cannot be controlled and has an identified source, surgical treatment can be performed, keeping in mind that surgery might be difficult in these patients and expose them to the risk of short gut syndrome. Surgery is, however, the fate of around one third of patients with Crohn's disease presenting with significant bleeding [55].

### 82.3.2.5 Penetrating Crohn's Disease

A significant proportion of patients with Crohn's disease will develop penetrating disease, characterized as inflammatory transmural ulceration communicating with adjacent organs or the skin (fistula) [57]. After 10 years of follow-up, approximately a third will also have perianal disease, and a quarter will have internal fistulae [23].

### Perianal Disease

Crohn's disease was first reported in 1938 based on the description of a perianal fistula [58]. Perianal disease is a very common finding in patients with Crohn's disease and will be encountered on many occasions by emergency general surgeons.

Perianal Crohn's disease leads to chronic inflammatory changes in the perianal region leading to perianal fistulae, abscesses, ulceration, fissures, skin tags, and stenosis [59]. Anal incontinence can also be reported.

History of the disease should be carefully taken, and attention should be given to disease activity and signs of sepsis. The activity can be measured by the Perianal Disease Activity Index (PDAI). Blood tests should at least include inflammatory markers. Clinical examination should look for any discharge or mass suggesting an abscess. If the patient is stable and there is no suspicion of sepsis requiring emergency surgery, MRI of the perineum constitutes an excellent imaging technique to guide more elective surgical decision making. In the emergency setting, examination under general anesthesia, often in lithotomy position, should be performed, looking also for any sign of proctitis that would mandate discussing appropriate medical treatment. Any abscess should be drained, and any very obvious fistula should be treated with a loose, draining, low-profile seton. However, if no very obvious fistula is found, forced cannulation of blind orifices should not be attempted due to the significant risk of creating an iatrogenic fistula, and abscess drainage alone should be performed.

Antibiotics should be added in case of localized cellulitis, but no evidence supports their use in the long-term for fistula closure [60]. When the sepsis is addressed, thiopurine and biologic therapy should be introduced by the gastroenterology team before reassessment with endoscopy after 3 months, and definitive treatment if needed [61].

If the perianal disease is very extensive, diverting stoma constitutes an option to improve quality of life and decrease local sepsis, but is rarely indicated in the emergency setting [42].

### Intra-abdominal Fistula, Abscess, and Perforation

Fistulizing Crohn's disease can manifest itself by gastrointestinal perforation leading to abscess or peritonitis. An important cohort study showed that 11.4% of patients with Crohn's disease experienced an intra-abdominal abscess and 6.5% a disseminated intra-abdominal perforation [62].

Septic Crohn's patients with suspected penetrating complication should initially be managed with insertion of two large bore venous catheters, volume resuscitation, and delivery of broad-spectrum antibiotics. Vital signs and urine output should be monitored. Blood tests should include full blood count, prothrombin time, CRP, electrolytes, renal function, liver function and lactate. In case of hemodynamic instability, arterial blood gas and insertion of an arterial line are useful adjuncts. A CT scan should be performed, with intravenous contrast if the renal function allows for it. The objective is to identify the source of sepsis and to look for an associated intra-abdominal abscess or fistula.

The main objective is to control the sepsis with non-surgical measures if feasible [42]. Intra-abdominal abscesses should be drained using US- or CT-guided percutaneous drainage. Samples should be sent for microbiological analysis as antibiotic resistance is frequent in these patients who have often been hospitalized. Of note, it was shown that percutaneous drainage led to lower rate of stoma creation, fewer complications, and shorter hospital stay when compared to emergency surgery [63]. The patient may benefit from initial parenteral nutrition and a repeat CT should be performed after a week or so to assess treatment response.

If the abscess is not accessible to drainage, antibiotics alone, and associated parenteral nutrition can constitute an option but have a higher rate of failure.

In case of failure of medical management, surgical exploration should be performed [42], preceded by nutritional optimization and careful surgical planning (unless the patient has a free perforation and signs of peritonitis, whereby emergency surgery will be needed without time for significant optimization). In this setting, surgical exploration is most commonly performed as an open procedure, although laparoscopy may be feasible in appropriately trained teams, with abscess drainage and abdominal lavage, resection of the perforated segment of bowel and stoma formation, although defunctioning stoma proximal to the pathology may also be considered in selected cases. If a stoma is performed after resection, exteriorization of the two ends is preferable, as it allows to perform stoma closure through a local access after a minimum of 6 months.

**Table 82.4** Definition of toxic megacolon

| | |
|---|---|
| Radiographic evidence of colonic distension | >6 cm |
| At least three of the following: | Fever >38 °C |
| | Heart rate >120 beats/min |
| | Leukocytosis >10,500/μL |
| | Anemia |
| At least one of the following: | Dehydration |
| | Altered sensorium |
| | Electrolyte disturbances |
| | Hypotension |

**Table 82.5** Management of entero-cutaneous fistula

| | |
|---|---|
| S | Sepsis and skin |
| N | Nutrition |
| A | Anatomy |
| P | Procedure |

### Enterocutaneous Fistula

Entero-cutaneous fistulas are feared complications of Crohn's disease, as they expose the patient to severe complications [64]. The management of enterocutaneous fistula can be summarized by the acronym SNAP (Table 82.4) [64, 65]. Briefly, priority should be given to address the sepsis and to protect the skin. This step also includes volume resuscitation and correcting the complications induced by the fistula output. This requires the emergency general surgery team to pay attention to these details. Afterwards, adequate nutritional support should be provided, the fistula anatomy should be defined using appropriate imaging and the definitive surgical procedure should be planned. Principles of management of entero-cutaneous fistula are summarized in Table 82.5.

History taking should look for history of disease, previous interventions, history of the fistula and stoma output. Entero-cutaneous fistulas are classified as high-output if the volume of output is >500 mL/day [66]. Clinical examination should describe the external anatomy of the fistula and look for skin damage. Blood tests should include inflammatory markers, electrolytes, renal and liver function tests as well as trace elements.

Further, detailed nutritional screening can be performed to facilitate future involvement of an intestinal failure team [65]. A CT scan can be obtained as a first step to evaluate the gastrointestinal tract anatomy and exclude eventual intra-abdominal abscess or other complications of Crohn's disease. Administration of oral and/or rectal contrast might be useful adjuncts. At least one peripheral large bore venous catheter should be inserted, which can be later changed for a peripherally inserted central catheter (PICC) for parenteral nutritional support. Intravenous fluids can be administered to compensate for fistula output, and correct eventual electrolytes and renal function disorders. The skin around the fistula should be adequately protected and a specialized stoma nurse team should be actively involved.

Fistula output mainly depends on the level of the fistula in the gastrointestinal tract. The output can be reduced by hypotonic fluid oral restriction, administration of oral rehydration solution, proton pump inhibitor (PPI), loperamide, codeine, and occasionally somatostatin analogues [67]. Some centers also advocate the consumption of dry water-absorbing biscuits or the administration of GLP-2 analogues [68].

As a second step, the anatomy of the enterocutaneous fistula can be determined using MRI entero- or fistulography. Once any eventual accompanying sepsis is addressed, anti-TNF-alpha therapy can be considered with some success reported in entero-cutaneous fistula closure [64, 69]. Surgery usually constitutes the definitive treatment.

### 82.3.2.6 Appendicitis in Patients with Inflammatory Bowel Disease

Some patients with inflammatory bowel disease might present with typical symptoms for appendicitis. History taking should be detailed and investigate whether the patient has a flare or not. In addition, an abdominal CT scan should be performed to provide a complete picture of the gastrointestinal tract and areas of potential inflammation.

In case of inflammation of the lower gastrointestinal tract outside the appendix, the episode should be considered as a flare of inflammatory bowel disease and treated as such. If the radiological findings confirm uncomplicated acute appendicitis, treatment can be conservative with broad-spectrum antibiotics and close follow-up. In case of clinical or biological deterioration or radiological evidence of complicated appendicitis and/or the presence of an appendicolith(s), laparoscopic appendectomy should be performed and consideration given to stapling the appendix base across an area of non-inflamed cecal pole.

Moreover, there has been long-lasting controversy about the role of appendicectomy in protecting against flares of ulcerative colitis. The evidence is not strong enough to conclude [70, 71], and the results of the ACCURE trial are awaited [72].

## 82.3.3 Basic Principles of Emergency Surgery for Inflammatory Bowel Disease

### 82.3.3.1 Principles of Emergency Surgery for Crohn's Disease

In patients with Crohn's disease, emergency surgery should constitute the final therapeutic option after failure of conservative management or as a life-saving procedure. Indeed, these patients are at risk of repeated operations during the course of their life, which may expose them to multiple resections and potential risk of short bowel syndrome. A prospective observational cohort study showed that emergency surgery for Crohn's disease resulted in longer bowel resection and higher rate of stoma formation than elective surgery [73]. Further, chronic malnutrition due to malabsorption associated with chronic transmural inflammation adds to the potential risk of anastomotic leak and fistula.

When surgery is necessary, steroids, if present, should be preferentially weaned off or at least reduced to as minimum a level as safely possible. Although there are some conflicting data, anti-TNF-alpha treatment appears not to increase the risk of infectious complications [27]. However, many surgeons will still prefer to operate following the washout period of the medication if possible. Careful surgical planning, including CT, MRI enterography, and ileocolonoscopy is advised when possible, although not always feasible in the emergency setting.

Laparoscopy should be favored over laparotomy when possible, but open surgery is preferred if the patient has a history of multiple abdominal operations, if the patient is not hemodynamically stable or in cases of significant bowel distention [27].

If a bowel resection is performed, vascular control of the mesentery can be difficult due to chronic inflammation. Repeated use of electrocautery devices is advised before mesentery division and suture transfixion or vascular stapler is recommended on large-caliber vessels, according to preference.

The decision to perform an anastomosis should be carefully weighed with the risk of anastomotic leak. In patients with hemodynamic instability, poor nutrition, sepsis, or significant collection/abscess and/or steroids, a stoma should be preferred. The risk of anastomotic leak increases with each of these risk factors, and as such decision making needs to be individualized for each patient. If an anastomosis is not performed, a double barrel stoma or, alternatively, a terminal stoma with a mucous fistula of the colonic segment for example, should be preferred as it potentially allows for stoma closure through the stoma site. If an anastomosis is performed, a side-to-side stapled technique is most commonly performed, but the surgeon preference in terms of configuration and material (suture vs. stapled) should be taken into account. If the anastomosis is ileocolic, some advocate an iso-peristatic configuration, to facilitate future easier colonoscopy intubation.

The length and localization of resected bowel should be reported in detail in the operation note along with accurate measurement of the remaining small bowel length, if possible with a detailed schematic representation of the procedure.

### 82.3.3.2 Principles of Emergency Surgery for Ulcerative Colitis

Delaying surgery in patients with ulcerative colitis who require emergency surgery is not recommended. A retrospective matched analysis from the American College of Surgeons National Surgical Quality Improvement Program database showed that early surgery (1 day) was associated with a lower mortality rate (4.9% vs. 20.3%, $p < 0.001$) and lower complication rate (64.5% vs. 72.0%, $p = 0.052$) than delayed surgery (6 days). Regression of morbidity on preoperative risk factors demonstrated that early surgery is associated with a 35% decrease in the odds of a complication with delayed surgery ($p = 0.034$) [74]. However, early surgery only represents 20.4% of patients who undergo surgery during an emergency admission [24], leaving room for improvement.

When emergency surgery is needed, subtotal colectomy and end ileostomy with preservation of the rectum is the procedure of choice. The procedure can be preferentially performed by laparoscopy, but laparotomy should be favored in case of hemodynamic instability, life-threatening hemorrhage, and toxic megacolon. In the absence of associated colorectal cancer, it is appropriate to dissect the mesocolon and the mesentery close to the colon, notably at the level of the ileocecal valve, in order to preserve the ileocolic vessels for a potential future ileorectal or ileoanal (pouch) anastomosis, and to retain the inferior mesenteric artery in order to facilitate safe future surgical planes for completion proctectomy. The so-called "rectal stump" should generally be divided in the distal sigmoid colon, leaving options for either a formal mucous fistula (possible at the ileostomy site or in the left iliac fosa) or subcutaneous placement below the midline or Pfannenstiel incision, which might help constitute a directed colocutaneous fistula in case of a leak from the stump ("blow out"). At the completion of the surgical procedure, the rectal stump should be irrigated to remove its content, and a rectal catheter should be considered for 2–3 days to decrease the pressure on the staple line.

In hospital mortality in patients having surgery for acute colitis is as high as 8% in some series, and the 30-day mortality is 5.2% [36].

As a second step, and after a minimum of 3 months when the patient has recovered from the emergency surgery, the rectal stump can be addressed, with discussions around surveillance and future completion proctectomy with or without restoration of intestinal continuity with an ileoanal pouch. In carefully selected patients, there may be a role for future rectal preservation and ileorectal anastomosis [75].

### 82.3.3.3 Prevention of Venous Thromboembolism

Prophylaxis against venous thromboembolism is of crucial importance in patients suffering from inflammatory bowel disease. Patients with inflammatory bowel disease have increased risk for venous thromboembolism, which is approximately twice the risk of the general population. Among patients ≤20 years, this risk if sixfold the risk of the general population [76]. After surgery for ulcerative colitis, the 30-day incidence of venous thromboembolism is 3.8% [77].

Therefore, the American Association of Gastroenterology recommends thromboprophylaxis in hospitalized patients suffering from inflammatory bowel disease without active bleeding or with active non-severe bleeding, as well as in outpatients with moderate-to-severe active flare and positive history for venous thromboembolism [78]. Extended post-discharge prophylaxis should be standard of care for patients following emergency surgery for IBD, for a minimum of 28 days post-surgery [79].

### 82.3.3.4 Risk of Colorectal Cancer

Colorectal cancer should always be taken into account in the differential diagnosis when performing decision-making in patients with inflam-

> **Dos and Don'ts**
> - Do involve the gastroenterology team when assessing patients with inflammatory bowel disease.
> - Do not perform non-life-saving surgery in patients suffering from inflammatory bowel disease without complete preoperative planning and nutritional optimization.
> - Do not rush decisions around surgery in patients suffering from Crohn's disease who do not have a free perforation, as you will expose these patients to the risk of short bowel syndrome and sepsis. Emergency surgery should constitute the final therapeutic option after failure of conservative management or as a life-saving procedure.
> - Do preserve the inferior mesenteric artery when performing subtotal colectomy for ulcerative colitis.
> - Do prescribe extended post-discharge prophylaxis against venous thromboembolism for patients who underwent emergency surgery for inflammatory bowel disease.

> **Take-Home Messages**
> - Patients suffering from inflammatory bowel disease pose complex problems, often with disease-associated comorbidities, and the potential for significant psychological impact. Their management should be cautious and multidisciplinary. Surgical indication should be discussed in accordance with the gastroenterology team, and wider IBD multidisciplinary team when feasible.
> - Indications for emergency surgery in patients with inflammatory bowel disease include severe colitis refractory to medical treatment, gastrointestinal hemorrhage not amenable to or not responding to interventional radiology, toxic megacolon not responding to medical management and non-contained gastrointestinal perforation. In the context of Crohn's disease, penetrating disease refractory to non-surgical management and obstruction refractory to non-surgi-

cal management should be referred to specialized teams when possible.
- Improvement in intensive care medicine and widespread availability of interventional radiology have decreased the need for emergency surgery in patients suffering from toxic megacolon, hemorrhage related to inflammatory bowel disease, and penetrating Crohn's disease. Similarly, balloon dilatation can be considered to manage accessible, short, fibrotic small bowel strictures.
  – Management of penetrating Crohn's disease is mostly conservative and should be focused on controlling the sepsis, nutrition and fluid balance.
  – When performing emergency surgery for Crohn's disease, attention should be given to preserve the small bowel length, and the total length of the bowel remaining should be documented.
  – When performing emergency surgery for inflammatory bowel disease, the patient should always be informed about the risk of extended gastrointestinal resection and of stoma. If possible, the potential stoma site should be marked by a specialized stoma therapist/nurse (but this should not delay the procedure).

**Multiple Choice Questions**
1. What laboratory exams should be obtained in a patient with a suspected flare of inflammatory bowel disease?
   A. Inflammatory markers in the blood
   B. Fecal calprotectin
   C. Nutritional status
   D. PCR for *Clostridium difficile*

   **Answer: A, B, C and D**

2. What are the indications for emergency surgery in patients with ulcerative colitis?
   A. Acute severe colitis
   B. Gastrointestinal hemorrhage not responding to medical management
   C. Toxic megacolon
   D. Obstructive colorectal cancer

   **Answer: B, D**

3. What are the indications for emergency surgery in patients with Crohn's disease?
   A. Perianal abscess
   B. Entero-cutaneous fistula
   C. Toxic megacolon not responding to medical management
   D. Bowel obstruction

   **Answer: A, C**

4. What are the correct propositions regarding the management of severe ulcerative colitis?
   A. Severe ulcerative colitis is defined as one sign of toxicity associated with the passage of 6 bloody stools per day
   B. Microbiological examination of the stools should be performed
   C. Flexible sigmoidoscopy is at high risk of perforation and should not be performed
   D. Management is always surgical due to the risk of perforation

   **Answer: A, B**

5. What propositions are correct regarding the management of Crohn's perianal disease?
   A. Antibiotics should be the rule due to the extent of local penetrating disease
   B. Identification of fistula tract is key for treatment success
   C. An anoscopy should be performed
   D. Anti-TNF-alpha treatment leads to perianal abscesses

   **Answer: C**

6. During management of entero-cutaneous fistulas, what does the acronym SNAP stand for?
   A. Support—Norfloxacin—Anterograde enema—Proctoscopy

B. Support—Nutrition—Antibiotics—Planning
   C. Sepsis and skin—Nutrition—Anatomy—Planning
   D. Sepsis—Norfloxacin—Anatomy—Proctoscopy

**Answer: C**

7. What is correct regarding emergency surgery for Crohn's disease?
   A. Emergency surgery and elective surgery for Crohn's disease have the same surgical outcomes
   B. Steroids should be discontinued within 7 days of surgery
   C. Anti-TNF-alpha should be stopped at least 3 days before surgery
   D. For obstructing disease, surgery should be performed as early as possible due to better outcomes

**Answer: None of the above**

8. What is correct regarding emergency subtotal colectomy for ulcerative colitis?
   A. Surgery should be delayed as much as possible in order to let the medical treatment have an effect
   B. The ileocolic pedicle should be preserved
   C. When possible, an anastomosis should be performed
   D. A proctectomy should be performed to definitely cure the disease

**Answer: B**

9. Which ones of the following are risk factors for anastomotic leak in Crohn's patients undergoing emergency surgery?
   A. Poor nutritional status
   B. Presence of an abscess
   C. High dose steroids
   D. Smoking

**Answer: A, B, C and D**

10. In which categories of patients suffering from inflammatory bowel disease should prophylaxis against thromboembolism be administered?
    A. All patients with active inflammatory bowel disease who are hospitalized
    B. All inpatients and outpatients with inflammatory bowel disease
    C. Inpatients and outpatients who underwent surgery for inflammatory bowel disease within the past month
    D. Inpatients with inflammatory bowel disease-related hemorrhage

**Answer: A, C**

matory bowel disease. Population-based studies estimated the incidence of colorectal cancer to be of 0.82 per 1000 person-years in Crohn's disease (corresponding to a 1.4-fold more important risk than the reference population) [80], and 1.29 per 1000 person-years in those with ulcerative colitis (corresponding to a 1.7-fold increased risk) [81]. In case a colorectal cancer is found, and surgery performed, the extent of lymphadenectomy should respect oncological standards. Of note, in the case of a subtotal colectomy, oncologic resection should be performed on all parts of the colon due to the risk of synchronous lesions [21].

## References

1. Collaborators GBDIBD. The global, regional, and national burden of inflammatory bowel disease in 195 countries and territories, 1990-2017: a systematic analysis for the Global Burden of Disease Study 2017. Lancet Gastroenterol Hepatol. 2020;5(1):17–30. https://doi.org/10.1016/S2468-1253(19)30333-4.
2. Basso PJ, Camara NOS, Sales-Campos H. Microbial-based therapies in the treatment of inflammatory bowel disease—an overview of human studies. Front Pharmacol. 2018;9:1571. https://doi.org/10.3389/fphar.2018.01571.
3. Eck A, de Groot EFJ, de Meij TGJ, Welling M, Savelkoul PHM, Budding AE. Correction for Eck et al., "Robust microbiota-based diagnostics for inflammatory bowel disease". J Clin Microbiol. 2017;55(9):2871. https://doi.org/10.1128/JCM.00958-17.

4. Wright EK, Kamm MA, Teo SM, Inouye M, Wagner J, Kirkwood CD. Recent advances in characterizing the gastrointestinal microbiome in Crohn's disease: a systematic review. Inflamm Bowel Dis. 2015;21(6):1219–28. https://doi.org/10.1097/MIB.0000000000000382.
5. Putignani L, Del Chierico F, Vernocchi P, Cicala M, Cucchiara S, Dallapiccola B, Dysbiotrack Study Group. Gut microbiota dysbiosis as risk and premorbid factors of IBD and IBS along the childhood-adulthood transition. Inflamm Bowel Dis. 2016;22(2):487–504. https://doi.org/10.1097/MIB.0000000000000602.
6. Knoll RL, Forslund K, Kultima JR, Meyer CU, Kullmer U, Sunagawa S, Bork P, Gehring S. Gut microbiota differs between children with inflammatory bowel disease and healthy siblings in taxonomic and functional composition: a metagenomic analysis. Am J Physiol Gastrointest Liver Physiol. 2017;312(4):G327–39. https://doi.org/10.1152/ajpgi.00293.2016.
7. Giaffer MH, Holdsworth CD, Duerden BI. The assessment of faecal flora in patients with inflammatory bowel disease by a simplified bacteriological technique. J Med Microbiol. 1991;35(4):238–43. https://doi.org/10.1099/00222615-35-4-238.
8. Sepehri S, Kotlowski R, Bernstein CN, Krause DO. Microbial diversity of inflamed and noninflamed gut biopsy tissues in inflammatory bowel disease. Inflamm Bowel Dis. 2007;13(6):675–83. https://doi.org/10.1002/ibd.20101.
9. Walker AW, Sanderson JD, Churcher C, Parkes GC, Hudspith BN, Rayment N, Brostoff J, Parkhill J, Dougan G, Petrovska L. High-throughput clone library analysis of the mucosa-associated microbiota reveals dysbiosis and differences between inflamed and non-inflamed regions of the intestine in inflammatory bowel disease. BMC Microbiol. 2011;11:7. https://doi.org/10.1186/1471-2180-11-7.
10. Guyen LH, Ortqvist AK, Cao Y, Simon TG, Roelstraete B, Song M, Joshi AD, Staller K, Chan AT, Khalili H, Olen O, Ludvigsson JF. Antibiotic use and the development of inflammatory bowel disease: a national case-control study in Sweden. Lancet Gastroenterol Hepatol. 2020;5(11):986–95. https://doi.org/10.1016/S2468-1253(20)30267-3.
11. Lamb CA, Kennedy NA, Raine T, Hendy PA, Smith PJ, Limdi JK, Hayee B, Lomer MCE, Parkes GC, Selinger C, Barrett KJ, Davies RJ, Bennett C, Gittens S, Dunlop MG, Faiz O, Fraser A, Garrick V, Johnston PD, Parkes M, Sanderson J, Terry H, IBD Guidelines eDelphi Consensus Group, Gaya DR, Iqbal TH, Taylor SA, Smith M, Brookes M, Hansen R, Hawthorne AB. British Society of Gastroenterology consensus guidelines on the management of inflammatory bowel disease in adults. Gut. 2019;68(Suppl 3):s1–s106. https://doi.org/10.1136/gutjnl-2019-318484.
12. Silverberg MS, Satsangi J, Ahmad T, Arnott ID, Bernstein CN, Brant SR, Caprilli R, Colombel JF, Gasche C, Geboes K, Jewell DP, Karban A, Loftus EV Jr, Pena AS, Riddell RH, Sachar DB, Schreiber S, Steinhart AH, Targan SR, Vermeire S, Warren BF. Toward an integrated clinical, molecular and serological classification of inflammatory bowel disease: report of a Working Party of the 2005 Montreal World Congress of Gastroenterology. Can J Gastroenterol. 2005;19(Suppl A):5A–36A. https://doi.org/10.1155/2005/269076.
13. Long MD, Sands BE. What is the role of the inflammatory bowel disease panel in diagnosis and treatment? Clin Gastroenterol Hepatol. 2018;16(5):618–20. https://doi.org/10.1016/j.cgh.2018.02.010.
14. Baumgart DC, Sandborn WJ. Crohn's disease. Lancet. 2012;380(9853):1590–605. https://doi.org/10.1016/S0140-6736(12)60026-9.
15. Gomollon F, Dignass A, Annese V, Tilg H, Van Assche G, Lindsay JO, Peyrin-Biroulet L, Cullen GJ, Daperno M, Kucharzik T, Rieder F, Almer S, Armuzzi A, Harbord M, Langhorst J, Sans M, Chowers Y, Fiorino G, Juillerat P, Mantzaris GJ, Rizzello F, Vavricka S, Gionchetti P, ECCO. 3rd European evidence-based consensus on the diagnosis and management of Crohn's disease 2016: part 1: diagnosis and medical management. J Crohns Colitis. 2017;11(1):3–25. https://doi.org/10.1093/ecco-jcc/jjw168.
16. Lee JS, Kim ES, Moon W. Chronological review of endoscopic indices in inflammatory bowel disease. Clin Endosc. 2019;52(2):129–36. https://doi.org/10.5946/ce.2018.042.
17. Fumery M, Singh S, Dulai PS, Gower-Rousseau C, Peyrin-Biroulet L, Sandborn WJ. Natural history of adult ulcerative colitis in population-based cohorts: a systematic review. Clin Gastroenterol Hepatol. 2018;16(3):343–56. e343. https://doi.org/10.1016/j.cgh.2017.06.016.
18. Dignass A, Eliakim R, Magro F, Maaser C, Chowers Y, Geboes K, Mantzaris G, Reinisch W, Colombel JF, Vermeire S, Travis S, Lindsay JO, Van Assche G. Second European evidence-based consensus on the diagnosis and management of ulcerative colitis part 1: definitions and diagnosis. J Crohns Colitis. 2012;6(10):965–90. https://doi.org/10.1016/j.crohns.2012.09.003.
19. Torres J, Bonovas S, Doherty G, Kucharzik T, Gisbert JP, Raine T, Adamina M, Armuzzi A, Bachmann O, Bager P, Biancone L, Bokemeyer B, Bossuyt P, Burisch J, Collins P, El-Hussuna A, Ellul P, Frei-Lanter C, Furfaro F, Gingert C, Gionchetti P, Gomollon F, Gonzalez-Lorenzo M, Gordon H, Hlavaty T, Juillerat P, Katsanos K, Kopylov U, Krustins E, Lytras T, Maaser C, Magro F, Marshall JK, Myrelid P, Pellino G, Rosa I, Sabino J, Savarino E, Spinelli A, Stassen L, Uzzan M, Vavricka S, Verstockt B, Warusavitarne J, Zmora O, Fiorino G. ECCO guidelines on therapeutics in Crohn's disease: medical treatment. J Crohns Colitis. 2020;14(1):4–22. https://doi.org/10.1093/ecco-jcc/jjz180.
20. Harbord M, Eliakim R, Bettenworth D, Karmiris K, Katsanos K, Kopylov U, Kucharzik T, Molnar T, Raine T, Sebastian S, de Sousa HT, Dignass A, Carbonnel F, European Crohn's and Colitis Organisation

(ECCO). Third European evidence-based consensus on diagnosis and management of ulcerative colitis. Part 2: current Management. J Crohns Colitis. 2017;11(7):769–84. https://doi.org/10.1093/ecco-jcc/jjx009.
21. Oresland T, Bemelman WA, Sampietro GM, Spinelli A, Windsor A, Ferrante M, Marteau P, Zmora O, Kotze PG, Espin-Basany E, Tiret E, Sica G, Panis Y, Faerden AE, Biancone L, Angriman I, Serclova Z, de Buck van Overstraeten A, Gionchetti P, Stassen L, Warusavitarne J, Adamina M, Dignass A, Eliakim R, Magro F, D'Hoore A, European Crohn's and Colitis Organisation (ECCO). European evidence based consensus on surgery for ulcerative colitis. J Crohns Colitis. 2015;9(1):4–25. https://doi.org/10.1016/j.crohns.2014.08.012.
22. Peyrin-Biroulet L, Loftus EV Jr, Colombel JF, Sandborn WJ. The natural history of adult Crohn's disease in population-based cohorts. Am J Gastroenterol. 2010;105(2):289–97. https://doi.org/10.1038/ajg.2009.579.
23. Cleynen I, Gonzalez JR, Figueroa C, Franke A, McGovern D, Bortlik M, Crusius BJ, Vecchi M, Artieda M, Szczypiorska M, Bethge J, Arteta D, Ayala E, Danese S, van Hogezand RA, Panes J, Pena SA, Lukas M, Jewell DP, Schreiber S, Vermeire S, Sans M. Genetic factors conferring an increased susceptibility to develop Crohn's disease also influence disease phenotype: results from the IBDchip European Project. Gut. 2013;62(11):1556–65. https://doi.org/10.1136/gutjnl-2011-300777.
24. Leeds IL, Truta B, Parian AM, Chen SY, Efron JE, Gearhart SL, Safar B, Fang SH. Early surgical intervention for acute ulcerative colitis is associated with improved postoperative outcomes. J Gastrointest Surg. 2017;21(10):1675–82. https://doi.org/10.1007/s11605-017-3538-3.
25. Targownik LE, Singh H, Nugent Z, Bernstein CN. The epidemiology of colectomy in ulcerative colitis: results from a population-based cohort. Am J Gastroenterol. 2012;107(8):1228–35. https://doi.org/10.1038/ajg.2012.127.
26. Truelove SC, Witts LJ. Cortisone in ulcerative colitis; final report on a therapeutic trial. Br Med J. 1955;2(4947):1041–8. https://doi.org/10.1136/bmj.2.4947.1041.
27. Bemelman WA, Warusavitarne J, Sampietro GM, Serclova Z, Zmora O, Luglio G, de Buck van Overstraeten A, Burke JP, Buskens CJ, Colombo F, Dias JA, Eliakim R, Elosua T, Gecim IE, Kolacek S, Kierkus J, Kolho KL, Lefevre JH, Millan M, Panis Y, Pinkney T, Russell RK, Shwaartz C, Vaizey C, Yassin N, D'Hoore A. ECCO-ESCP consensus on surgery for Crohn's disease. J Crohns Colitis. 2018;12(1):1–16. https://doi.org/10.1093/ecco-jcc/jjx061.
28. Marshak RH, Lester LJ. Megacolon a complication of ulcerative colitis. Gastroenterology. 1950;16(4):768–72.
29. Hommes DW, Sterringa G, van Deventer SJ, Tytgat GN, Weel J. The pathogenicity of cytomegalovirus in inflammatory bowel disease: a systematic review and evidence-based recommendations for future research. Inflamm Bowel Dis. 2004;10(3):245–50. https://doi.org/10.1097/00054725-200405000-00011.
30. Autenrieth DM, Baumgart DC. Toxic megacolon. Inflamm Bowel Dis. 2012;18(3):584–91. https://doi.org/10.1002/ibd.21847.
31. McGregor A, Brown M, Thway K, Wright SG. Fulminant amoebic colitis following loperamide use. J Travel Med. 2007;14(1):61–2. https://doi.org/10.1111/j.1708-8305.2006.00096.x.
32. Ausch C, Madoff RD, Gnant M, Rosen HR, Garcia-Aguilar J, Holbling N, Herbst F, Buxhofer V, Holzer B, Rothenberger DA, Schiessel R. Aetiology and surgical management of toxic megacolon. Color Dis. 2006;8(3):195–201. https://doi.org/10.1111/j.1463-1318.2005.00887.x.
33. Trudel JL, Deschenes M, Mayrand S, Barkun AN. Toxic megacolon complicating pseudomembranous enterocolitis. Dis Colon Rectum. 1995;38(10):1033–8. https://doi.org/10.1007/BF02133974.
34. Gomes CA, Podda M, Veiga SC, do Vale Cabral T, Lima LV, Miron LC, de Lucas Oliveira V, Aranha GL. Management of inflammatory bowel diseases in urgent and emergency scenario. J Coloproctol. 2020;40(1):83–8. https://doi.org/10.1016/j.jcol.2019.10.012.
35. Doshi R, Desai J, Shah Y, Decter D, Doshi S. Incidence, features, in-hospital outcomes and predictors of in-hospital mortality associated with toxic megacolon hospitalizations in the United States. Intern Emerg Med. 2018;13(6):881–7. https://doi.org/10.1007/s11739-018-1889-8.
36. Teeuwen PH, Stommel MW, Bremers AJ, van der Wilt GJ, de Jong DJ, Bleichrodt RP. Colectomy in patients with acute colitis: a systematic review. J Gastrointest Surg. 2009;13(4):676–86. https://doi.org/10.1007/s11605-008-0792-4.
37. Present DH, Wolfson D, Gelernt IM, Rubin PH, Bauer J, Chapman ML. Medical decompression of toxic megacolon by "rolling". A new technique of decompression with favorable long-term follow-up. J Clin Gastroenterol. 1988;10(5):485–90. https://doi.org/10.1097/00004836-198810000-00004.
38. Greenstein AJ, Sachar DB, Gibas A, Schrag D, Heimann T, Janowitz HD, Aufses AH Jr. Outcome of toxic dilatation in ulcerative and Crohn's colitis. J Clin Gastroenterol. 1985;7(2):137–43. https://doi.org/10.1097/00004836-198504000-00007.
39. Katsanos K, Tsianos VE, Maliouki M, Adamidi M, Vagias I, Tsianos EV. Obstruction and pseudo-obstruction in inflammatory bowel disease. Ann Gastroenterol. 2010;23(4):243–56.
40. Yamamoto T, Watanabe T. Surgery for luminal Crohn's disease. World J Gastroenterol. 2014;20(1):78–90. https://doi.org/10.3748/wjg.v20.i1.78.
41. Gumaste V, Sachar DB, Greenstein AJ. Benign and malignant colorectal strictures in ulcerative colitis.

Gut. 1992;33(7):938–41. https://doi.org/10.1136/gut.33.7.938.
42. Adamina M, Bonovas S, Raine T, Spinelli A, Warusavitarne J, Armuzzi A, Bachmann O, Bager P, Biancone L, Bokemeyer B, Bossuyt P, Burisch J, Collins P, Doherty G, El-Hussuna A, Ellul P, Fiorino G, Frei-Lanter C, Furfaro F, Gingert C, Gionchetti P, Gisbert JP, Gomollon F, Gonzalez Lorenzo M, Gordon H, Hlavaty T, Juillerat P, Katsanos K, Kopylov U, Krustins E, Kucharzik T, Lytras T, Maaser C, Magro F, Marshall JK, Myrelid P, Pellino G, Rosa I, Sabino J, Savarino E, Stassen L, Torres J, Uzzan M, Vavricka S, Verstockt B, Zmora O. ECCO guidelines on therapeutics in Crohn's disease: surgical treatment. J Crohns Colitis. 2020;14(2):155–68. https://doi.org/10.1093/ecco-jcc/jjz187.
43. Nightingale J, Woodward JM, Small B, Nutrition Committee of the British Society of Gastroenterology. Guidelines for management of patients with a short bowel. Gut. 2006;55(Suppl 4):iv1–12. https://doi.org/10.1136/gut.2006.091108.
44. Goldstein ES, Rubin PH. Endoscopic therapy for inflammatory bowel disease. Curr Treat Options Gastroenterol. 2003;6(3):237–43. https://doi.org/10.1007/s11938-003-0005-x.
45. Solt J, Hertelendy A, Szilagyi K. Long-term results of balloon catheter dilation of lower gastrointestinal tract stenoses. Dis Colon Rectum. 2004;47(9):1499–505. https://doi.org/10.1007/s10350-004-0619-7.
46. Ambe R, Campbell L, Cagir B. A comprehensive review of strictureplasty techniques in Crohn's disease: types, indications, comparisons, and safety. J Gastrointest Surg. 2012;16(1):209–17. https://doi.org/10.1007/s11605-011-1651-2.
47. Fallis LS. Massive intestinal hemorrhage in regional enteritis: report of a case. Am J Surg. 1941;53:512–3.
48. Podugu A, Tandon K, Castro FJ. Crohn's disease presenting as acute gastrointestinal hemorrhage. World J Gastroenterol. 2016;22(16):4073–8. https://doi.org/10.3748/wjg.v22.i16.4073.
49. Pardi DS, Loftus EV, Tremaine WJ, Sandborn WJ, Alexander GL, Balm R, Gostout CJ. Acute major gastrointestinal hemorrhage in inflammatory bowel disease. Gastrointest Endosc. 1999;49(2):153–7.
50. Kim M, Shin JH, Kim PH, Ko G, Yoon HM, Ko H. Efficacy and clinical outcomes of angiography and transcatheter arterial embolization for gastrointestinal bleeding in Crohn's disease. Int J Gastrointest Interv. 2019;8(2):92–7. https://doi.org/10.18528/ijgii170025.
51. Mallant-Hent R, van Bodegraven AA, Meuwissen SG, Manoliu RA. Alternative approach to massive gastrointestinal bleeding in ulcerative colitis: highly selective transcatheter embolization. Eur J Gastroenterol Hepatol. 2003;15(2):189–93. https://doi.org/10.1097/00042737-200302000-00014.
52. Oshima T, Joh T, Kataoka H, Sasaki M, Fujita F, Togawa S, Wada T, Iio E, Itoh M. Endoscopic treatment for repeated arterial bleeding with ulcerative colitis. Dig Dis Sci. 2007;52(6):1434–7. https://doi.org/10.1007/s10620-006-9552-z.
53. Yoshida Y, Kawaguchi A, Mataki N, Matsuzaki K, Hokari R, Iwai A, Nagao S, Itoh K, Miura S. Endoscopic treatment of massive lower GI hemorrhage in two patients with ulcerative colitis. Gastrointest Endosc. 2001;54(6):779–81. https://doi.org/10.1067/mge.2001.119601.
54. Miranda-Bautista J, Dieguez L, Rodriguez-Rosales G, Marin-Jimenez I, Menchen L. Cases report: severe colonic bleeding in ulcerative colitis is refractory to selective transcatheter arterial embolization. BMC Gastroenterol. 2019;19(1):55. https://doi.org/10.1186/s12876-019-0970-8.
55. Papi C, Gili L, Tarquini M, Antonelli G, Capurso L. Infliximab for severe recurrent Crohn's disease presenting with massive gastrointestinal hemorrhage. J Clin Gastroenterol. 2003;36(3):238–41. https://doi.org/10.1097/00004836-200303000-00011.
56. Belaiche J, Louis E. Severe lower gastrointestinal bleeding in Crohn's disease: successful control with infliximab. Am J Gastroenterol. 2002;97(12):3210–1. https://doi.org/10.1111/j.1572-0241.2002.07143.x.
57. Randall CW, Vizuete JA, Martinez N, Alvarez JJ, Garapati KV, Malakouti M, Taboada CM. From historical perspectives to modern therapy: a review of current and future biological treatments for Crohn's disease. Ther Adv Gastroenterol. 2015;8(3):143–59. https://doi.org/10.1177/1756283X15576462.
58. Penner A, Crohn BB. Perianal fistulae as a complication of regional ileitis. Ann Surg. 1938;108(5):867–73. https://doi.org/10.1097/00000658-193811000-00007.
59. Adegbola SO, Sahnan K, Twum-Barima C, Iqbal N, Reza L, Lung P, Warusavitarne J, Tozer P, Hart A. Current review of the management of fistulising perianal Crohn's disease. Frontline Gastroenterol. 2020; https://doi.org/10.1136/flgastro-2020-101489.
60. Lee MJ, Parker CE, Taylor SR, Guizzetti L, Feagan BG, Lobo AJ, Jairath V. Efficacy of medical therapies for fistulizing Crohn's disease: systematic review and meta-analysis. Clin Gastroenterol Hepatol. 2018;16(12):1879–92. https://doi.org/10.1016/j.cgh.2018.01.030.
61. Kotze PG, Shen B, Lightner A, Yamamoto T, Spinelli A, Ghosh S, Panaccione R. Modern management of perianal fistulas in Crohn's disease: future directions. Gut. 2018;67(6):1181–94. https://doi.org/10.1136/gutjnl-2017-314918.
62. Jeong SH, Choi JS, Kim JW, Kim HM, Kim HS, Im JP, Kim JS, Kim YS, Cheon JH, Kim WH, Ye BD, Kim YH, Han DS. Clinical features of intra-abdominal abscess and intestinal free-wall perforation in Korean patients with Crohn's disease: results from the CONNECT study. J Clin Med. 2020;10(1) https://doi.org/10.3390/jcm10010116.
63. He X, Lin X, Lian L, Huang J, Yao Q, Chen Z, Fan D, Wu X, Lan P. Preoperative percutaneous drainage of spontaneous intra-abdominal abscess in patients with Crohn's disease: a meta-analysis. J

Clin Gastroenterol. 2015;49(9):e82–90. https://doi.org/10.1097/MCG.0000000000000219.

64. Papa A, Lopetuso LR, Minordi LM, Di Veronica A, Neri M, Rapaccini G, Gasbarrini A, Papa V. A modern multidisciplinary approach to the treatment of enterocutaneous fistulas in Crohn's disease patients. Expert Rev Gastroenterol Hepatol. 2020;14(9):857–65. https://doi.org/10.1080/17474124.2020.1797484.

65. Klek S, Forbes A, Gabe S, Holst M, Wanten G, Irtun O, Damink SO, Panisic-Sekeljic M, Pelaez RB, Pironi L, Blaser AR, Rasmussen HH, Schneider SM, Thibault R, Visschers RGJ, Shaffer J. Management of acute intestinal failure: a position paper from the European Society for Clinical Nutrition and Metabolism (ESPEN) Special Interest Group. Clin Nutr. 2016;35(6):1209–18. https://doi.org/10.1016/j.clnu.2016.04.009.

66. Gribovskaja-Rupp I, Melton GB. Enterocutaneous fistula: proven strategies and updates. Clin Colon Rectal Surg. 2016;29(2):130–7. https://doi.org/10.1055/s-0036-1580732.

67. Rahbour G, Siddiqui MR, Ullah MR, Gabe SM, Warusavitarne J, Vaizey CJ. A meta-analysis of outcomes following use of somatostatin and its analogues for the management of enterocutaneous fistulas. Ann Surg. 2012;256(6):946–54. https://doi.org/10.1097/SLA.0b013e318260aa26.

68. Billiauws L, Bataille J, Boehm V, Corcos O, Joly F. Teduglutide for treatment of adult patients with short bowel syndrome. Expert Opin Biol Ther. 2017;17(5):623–32. https://doi.org/10.1080/14712598.2017.1304912.

69. Amiot A, Setakhr V, Seksik P, Allez M, Treton X, De Vos M, Laharie D, Colombel JF, Abitbol V, Reimund JM, Moreau J, Veyrac M, Flourie B, Cosnes J, Lemann M, Bouhnik Y. Long-term outcome of enterocutaneous fistula in patients with Crohn's disease treated with anti-TNF therapy: a cohort study from the GETAID. Am J Gastroenterol. 2014;109(9):1443–9. https://doi.org/10.1038/ajg.2014.183.

70. Frisch M, Johansen C, Mellemkjaer L, Engels EA, Gridley G, Biggar RJ, Olsen JH. Appendectomy and subsequent risk of inflammatory bowel diseases. Surgery. 2001;130(1):36–43. https://doi.org/10.1067/msy.2001.115362.

71. Felice C, Armuzzi A. Therapeutic role of appendectomy in ulcerative colitis: a tangible perspective? J Crohns Colitis. 2019;13(2):142–3. https://doi.org/10.1093/ecco-jcc/jjy151.

72. Gardenbroek TJ, Pinkney TD, Sahami S, Morton DG, Buskens CJ, Ponsioen CY, Tanis PJ, Lowenberg M, van den Brink GR, Broeders IA, Pullens PH, Seerden T, Boom MJ, Mallant-Hent RC, Pierik RE, Vecht J, Sosef MN, van Nunen AB, van Wagensveld BA, Stokkers PC, Gerhards MF, Jansen JM, Acherman Y, Depla AC, Mannaerts GH, West R, Iqbal T, Pathmakanthan S, Howard R, Magill L, Singh B, Htun Oo Y, Negpodiev D, Dijkgraaf MG, Ram D'Haens G, Bemelman WA. The ACCURE-trial: the effect of appendectomy on the clinical course of ulcerative colitis, a randomised international multicenter trial (NTR2883) and the ACCURE-UK trial: a randomised external pilot trial (ISRCTN56523019). BMC Surg. 2015;15:30. https://doi.org/10.1186/s12893-015-0017-1.

73. Celentano V, O'Leary DP, Caiazzo A, Flashman KG, Sagias F, Conti J, Senapati A, Khan J. Longer small bowel segments are resected in emergency surgery for ileocaecal Crohn's disease with a higher ileostomy and complication rate. Tech Coloproctol. 2019;23(11):1085–91. https://doi.org/10.1007/s10151-019-02104-9.

74. Leeds IL, Sundel MH, Gabre-Kidan A, Safar B, Truta B, Efron JE, Fang SH. Outcomes for ulcerative colitis with delayed emergency colectomy are worse when controlling for preoperative risk factors. Dis Colon Rectum. 2019;62(5):600–7. https://doi.org/10.1097/DCR.0000000000001276.

75. Landerholm K, Abdalla M, Myrelid P, Andersson RE. Survival of ileal pouch anal anastomosis constructed after colectomy or secondary to a previous ileorectal anastomosis in ulcerative colitis patients: a population-based cohort study. Scand J Gastroenterol. 2017;52(5):531–5. https://doi.org/10.1080/00365521.2016.1278457.

76. Kappelman MD, Horvath-Puho E, Sandler RS, Rubin DT, Ullman TA, Pedersen L, Baron JA, Sorensen HT. Thromboembolic risk among Danish children and adults with inflammatory bowel diseases: a population-based nationwide study. Gut. 2011;60(7):937–43. https://doi.org/10.1136/gut.2010.228585.

77. McKenna NP, Behm KT, Ubl DS, Glasgow AE, Mathis KL, Pemberton JH, Habermann EB, Cima RR. Analysis of postoperative venous thromboembolism in patients with chronic ulcerative colitis: is it the disease or the operation? Dis Colon Rectum. 2017;60(7):714–22. https://doi.org/10.1097/DCR.0000000000000846.

78. Nguyen GC, Bernstein CN, Bitton A, Chan AK, Griffiths AM, Leontiadis GI, Geerts W, Bressler B, Butzner JD, Carrier M, Chande N, Marshall JK, Williams C, Kearon C. Consensus statements on the risk, prevention, and treatment of venous thromboembolism in inflammatory bowel disease: Canadian Association of Gastroenterology. Gastroenterology. 2014;146(3):835–48. e836. https://doi.org/10.1053/j.gastro.2014.01.042.

79. Brown SR, Fearnhead NS, Faiz OD, Abercrombie JF, Acheson AG, Arnott RG, Clark SK, Clifford S, Davies RJ, Davies MM, Douie WJP, Dunlop MG, Epstein JC, Evans MD, George BD, Guy RJ, Hargest R, Hawthorne AB, Hill J, Hughes GW, Limdi JK, Maxwell-Armstrong CA, O'Connell PR, Pinkney TD, Pipe J, Sagar PM, Singh B, Soop M, Terry H, Torkington J, Verjee A, Walsh CJ, Warusavitarne JH, Williams AB, Williams GL, Wilson RG, Collaboration AISC. The Association of Coloproctology of Great Britain and Ireland consensus guidelines in sur-

gery for inflammatory bowel disease. Color Dis. 2018;20(Suppl 8):3–117. https://doi.org/10.1111/codi.14448.
80. Olen O, Erichsen R, Sachs MC, Pedersen L, Halfvarson J, Askling J, Ekbom A, Sørensen HT, Ludvigsson JF. Colorectal cancer in Crohn's disease: a Scandinavian population-based cohort study. Lancet Gastroenterol Hepatol. 2020; https://doi.org/10.1016/S2468-1253(20)30005-4.
81. Olen O, Erichsen R, Sachs MC, Pedersen L, Halfvarson J, Askling J, Ekbom A, Sorensen HT, Ludvigsson JF. Colorectal cancer in ulcerative colitis: a Scandinavian population-based cohort study. Lancet. 2020;395(10218):123–31. https://doi.org/10.1016/S0140-6736(19)32545-0.

## Further Reading

Adamina M, Bonovas S, Raine T, Spinelli A, Warusavitarne J, Armuzzi A, Bachmann O, Bager P, Biancone L, Bokemeyer B, Bossuyt P, Burisch J, Collins P, Doherty G, El-Hussuna A, Ellul P, Fiorino G, Frei-Lanter C, Furfaro F, Gingert C, Gionchetti P, Gisbert JP, Gomollon F, Gonzalez Lorenzo M, Gordon H, Hlavaty T, Juillerat P, Katsanos K, Kopylov U, Krustins E, Kucharzik T, Lytras T, Maaser C, Magro F, Marshall JK, Myrelid P, Pellino G, Rosa I, Sabino J, Savarino E, Stassen L, Torres J, Uzzan M, Vavricka S, Verstockt B, Zmora O. ECCO guidelines on therapeutics in Crohn's disease: surgical treatment. J Crohns Colitis. 2020;14(2):155–68. https://doi.org/10.1093/ecco-jcc/jjz187.
Baumgart DC, Sandborn WJ. Crohn's disease. Lancet. 2012;380(9853):1590–605. https://doi.org/10.1016/S0140-6736(12)60026-9.
Bemelman WA, Warusavitarne J, Sampietro GM, Serclova Z, Zmora O, Luglio G, de Buck van Overstraeten A, Burke JP, Buskens CJ, Colombo F, Dias JA, Eliakim R, Elosua T, Gecim IE, Kolacek S, Kierkus J, Kolho KL, Lefevre JH, Millan M, Panis Y, Pinkney T, Russell RK, Shwaartz C, Vaizey C, Yassin N, D'Hoore A. ECCO-ESCP consensus on surgery for Crohn's disease. J Crohns Colitis. 2018;12(1):1–16. https://doi.org/10.1093/ecco-jcc/jjx061.
Brown SR, Fearnhead NS, Faiz O, Abercrombie J, Acheson A, Arnott R, Clark SK, Clifford S, Davies RJ, Davies M, Douie W, Dunlop MG, Epstein J, Evans M, George B, Guy R, Hargest R, Hawthorne AB, Hill J, Hughes G, Limdi J, Maxwell-Armstrong C, O'Connell PR, Pinkney T, Pipe J, Sagar P, Singh B, Soop M, Terry H, Torkington J, Verjee A, Walsh CJ, Warasuvitarne J, Williams A, Williams G, Wilson RG, ACPGBI IBD Surgery Consensus Collaboration. Association of Coloproctology of Great Britain and Ireland consensus guidelines in surgery for inflammatory bowel disease. Colorectal Dis. 2018;20(Suppl 8):3–117.
Kotze PG, Shen B, Lightner A, Yamamoto T, Spinelli A, Ghosh S, Panaccione R. Modern management of perianal fistulas in Crohn's disease: future directions. Gut. 2018;67(6):1181–94. https://doi.org/10.1136/gutjnl-2017-314918.
Lamb CA, Kennedy NA, Raine T, Hendy P, Smith PJ, Limdi JK, Hayee B, Lomer M, Parkes GC, Selinger CP, Barrett KJ, Davies RJ, Bennett C, Gittens S, Dunlop M, Faiz O, Fraser A, Garrick V, Johnston PD, Parkes M, Sanderson JD, Terry H, BD Guidelines eDelphi Consensus Group, Gaya DR, Iqbal T, Taylor SA, Smith M, Brookes MJ, Hansen R, Hawthorne AB. British Society of Gastroenterology consensus guidelines on the management of inflammatory bowel disease in adults. Gut. 2019;68(Suppl 3):s1–s106.
Oresland T, Bemelman WA, Sampietro GM, Spinelli A, Windsor A, Ferrante M, Marteau P, Zmora O, Kotze PG, Espin-Basany E, Tiret E, Sica G, Panis Y, Faerden AE, Biancone L, Angriman I, Serclova Z, de Buck van Overstraeten A, Gionchetti P, Stassen L, Warusavitarne J, Adamina M, Dignass A, Eliakim R, Magro F, D'Hoore A, European Crohn's and Colitis Organisation (ECCO). European evidence based consensus on surgery for ulcerative colitis. J Crohns Colitis. 2015;9(1):4–25. https://doi.org/10.1016/j.crohns.2014.08.012.

# Fulminant/Toxic Colitis

Sanjay Marwah, Rajesh Godara, and Shouvik Das

## 83.1 Introduction

There is no precise definition of fulminant colitis and the terms like toxic colitis and acute severe colitis are its synonyms. The term toxic megacolon may be misleading since the colon may or may not be dilated in toxic state. Thus, the patients may develop toxicity without megacolon or megacolon without severe toxic signs. The most common cause of fulminant colitis is ulcerative colitis (UC) apart from other causes like Crohn's colitis, infective colitis (*Clostridium difficile, Salmonella, Cytomegalovirus, Entamoeba histolytica*) and ischemic colitis. Although development of fulminant colitis is less common in *C. difficile infection* (CDI), the incidence of CDI is significantly rising all over the world. In recent times, there is much advancement in the medical management of fulminant colitis, but surgical treatment has remained the same for the last several years. The definite indications for surgical intervention are colonic perforation, ongoing hemorrhage, and failure of response to medical therapy. Although failure of medical treatment is the commonest indication for surgery, there are no definite guidelines deciding the timing of surgical intervention. However, timely surgical intervention decides the final outcome of these cases. This chapter discusses the diagnosis and management of fulminant colitis.

> **Learning Goals**
> - To know the criteria for labelling toxic/fulminant colitis, understand its pathophysiology, and to correlate it with clinical manifestations.
> - To understand the value of investigations in diagnosis as well as in differentiating various etiologies.
> - To learn the role of supportive care, specific medical management, indications, and timing of surgical intervention.
> - To evaluate and compare currently available surgical options.

### 83.1.1 Epidemiology

The precise data on the epidemiology of toxic colitis is not very well documented. The incidence of toxic colitis depends on its etiology; commonest being ulcerative colitis (UC) followed by Crohn's disease (CD), and *Clostridium difficile* infection (CDI) with reported incidence of 10%, 1–5%, and 5–10%, respectively. The mortality rates range from 40% to 80% depending on the disease severity as well as underlying comorbidities [1]. Among patients presenting with UC for the first time, the incidence of toxic

S. Marwah (✉) · R. Godara · S. Das
Department of Surgery, Pandit Bhagwat Dayal Sharma Post Graduate Institute of Medical Sciences, Rohtak, India

colitis is only 5–8% [2]. The toxic colitis in UC is more likely to develop in young and non-smokers, who have not undergone appendicectomy in the past, presenting with extensive disease, having deep ulcers on colonoscopy and highly raised inflammatory markers.

In recent years, the epidemiology of toxic colitis has shifted more towards CDI due to overuse of broad-spectrum antibiotics as well as emergence of hypervirulent strain of CDI (BI/NAP1/027) having 16–23 times more toxicity than common strains [3]. Moreover, demographic change of CDI in recent years has also affected the epidemiology of toxic colitis. More cases of community-acquired CDI are being reported among pediatric patients and peripartum women, previously categorized as low-risk group. The disease in such patients has been found to be more fulminant as well as refractory to the treatment.

In amoebic colitis, a common infectious disease in tropical countries, fulminant colitis may rarely occur in <0.5% cases. However, these cases have very high incidence of colonic perforation (30.4%) as well as mortality (55–100%) [4].

### 83.1.2 Etiology

The commonest causes of toxic colitis are inflammatory bowel disease (IBD; UC and CD) and infective colitis. Among flared up cases of inflammatory bowel disease, superadded intestinal infections (CDI and cytomegalovirus [CMV]) seem to play a role in causing toxic colitis especially in patients using immunosuppressant drugs.

Inflammatory causes:

- Ulcerative colitis
- Crohn colitis

Infectious causes:

- *Clostridium difficile*
- *Salmonella, Shigella, Campylobacter, Yersinia* species
- *Entamoeba histolytica, Cryptosporidium*
- Cytomegalovirus and rotavirus
- Invasive aspergillosis

Rare causes:

- Radiation and ischemic colitis
- Nonspecific colitis secondary to chemotherapy
- Complication of collagenous colitis, Behçet syndrome and Kaposi's sarcoma [5]
- Toxic colitis may also be associated with the hemolytic-uremic syndrome due to *Escherichia coli* O157 [6]
- Iatrogenic causes: Diagnostic and therapeutic procedures like barium enema or colonoscopy may lead to bowel distention and impaired blood supply that may exacerbate a microperforation and cause subsequent toxemia

### 83.1.3 Classification

Proper classification and assessment of disease severity in colitis have a definite bearing on deciding management as well as outcome prediction. For UC, more than ten severity indices have been described using clinical profile, laboratory parameters, and endoscopic findings that include toxic/fulminant colitis (Table 83.1). In Crohn's

**Table 83.1** Toxic/fulminant ulcerative colitis classification by various authors

| Classification | Criteria for toxic/fulminant colitis |
|---|---|
| Truelove and Witts classification [7] | Bloody diarrhea >10 times/day, pulse >90/min, temperature >37.5 °C, ESR >30 mm/h, requiring blood transfusion, abdominal distension and tenderness, dilated colon on imaging |
| Montreal classification [8] | ≥6 bloody stools/day, severe abdominal pain, systemic toxicity++, ESR ≥30 mm/h, Hb <10.5 g/dL |
| Baron et al.: endoscopic grading [9] | Severe exudates, visible ulceration, severely hemorrhagic: spontaneous bleeding and bleed to light touch |
| Le'mann et al.: endoscopic grading [10] | Spontaneous hemorrhage, visible ulcers |
| Feagan et al.: endoscopic grading [11] | Friable mucosa, bleeding spontaneously |

**Table 83.1** (continued)

| Classification | Criteria for toxic/fulminant colitis |
|---|---|
| Ulcerative Colitis Endoscopic Index of Severity (UCEIS) [12] | Obliterated vascular pattern, moderate to severe luminal bleeding, deep mucosal ulcers with slightly raised edge |
| Mayo scoring system: clinical parameters with endoscopic findings [13] | >5 stools/day more than normal, passing blood alone per rectum, severe disease on endoscopic findings and severe disease on physician's global assessment |
| Proposed American College of Gastroenterology Ulcerative Colitis Activity Index: Patient reported outcomes, laboratory- and endoscopy-based values [14] | >10 stools/day, continuous blood in stools, continuous urgency, transfusion required, ESR >30, elevated CRP, FC >150–200 μg/g, endoscopic Mayo subscore 3, Ulcerative Colitis Endoscopic Index of Severity 7–8 |
| Neumann et al.: histological grading [15] | Severe inflammation with heavy infiltrates, crypt abscess, ulceration, purulent exudates, FC Faecal calprotectin |

Abbreviations: *CRP* C-reactive protein, *ESR* erythrocyte sedimentation rate, *Hb* hemoglobin, *FC* Faecal calprotectin

**Table 83.2** CDI severity scoring system for toxic colitis (adapted from Surawicz et al. [17])

| Severe disease | Serum albumin <3 g/dL plus ONE of the following: WBC ≥15,000 cells/mm$^3$ Abdominal tenderness |
|---|---|
| Severe and complicated disease | Any of the following attributable to CDI: Admission to intensive care unit for CDI Hypotension with or without required use of vasopressors Fever ≥38.5 °C Ileus or significant abdominal distention Mental status changes WBC ≥35,000 cells/mm$^3$ or <2000 cells/mm$^3$ Serum lactate levels >2.2 mmol/L End organ failure (mechanical ventilation, renal failure, etc.) |

Abbreviation: *WBC* white blood cell

disease, no classification for toxic colitis has been suggested and clinicians have been using the same criteria as described for UC.

In CDI cases, Dallal et al. [16] have defined fulminant colitis as fulfilling following criteria: heart rate >120/min, >30% band forms, respiratory status: mechanical intubation, severe oliguria, and hypotension requiring vasopressor support.

Another severity score for toxic colitis in CDI has been given to classify severe and complicated disease (Table 83.2).

The main aim of classification of toxic colitis is to timely diagnose the case regardless of its etiology, early surgical consultation, and surgery if indicated. The early surgical intervention has shown to decrease the mortality in such cases (4% in non-perforated and 20% in perforated toxic colitis) [1].

### 83.1.4 Pathophysiology

The term toxic/fulminant indicates the most severe form of colitis and is a part of the spectrum of disease that has been called acute severe colitis. It may or may not be associated with megacolon. The precise pathophysiology of fulminant colitis is not clear but several factors may contribute to its development, progression, and precipitation. In uncomplicated form of colitis inflammatory response is confined to the mucosa, while microscopic hallmark of toxic colitis is extension of inflammation beyond the mucosa into muscularis propria and beyond. This seromuscular extension thus paralyzes the colonic smooth muscle leading to variable extent of colonic dilatation correlated with depth of inflammation and ulceration. The release of proteolytic enzymes, cytokines, leukotriene B4 by neutrophils, and macrophages directly impair smooth muscle cell functioning leading to colonic dilatation, and further systemic absorption of these inflammatory mediators leads to fever, tachycardia and hypotension. Myenteric plexus involvement and electrolyte disturbances probably do not contribute to dilatation in most patients [18]. Inflammation and upregulated nitric oxide synthetase probably increase local nitric oxide levels that inhibits colonic smooth muscle contraction and causes dilatation [19]. The advent of toxic/fulminant colitis must be recognized before progression to the stage of toxic megacolon.

UC is known to result from deregulated intestinal immune response acting against intraluminal antigens and unknown environmental factors in a genetically predisposed host. There is complex interplay between the host genotype and commensal bacteria or other pathogens present in the colon leading to breakdown of homeostatic balance. It results in an aberrant immune response against the gut microflora, leading to the initiation of inflammatory process. The factors responsible for the flare up of inflammation in UC leading to fulminant colitis are [20]:

1. Genetic factors:
   (a) HLA on chromosome 6p encodes the major antigen-presenting proteins leading to the development of fulminant colitis.
   - TNFSF15 (TL1A) locus, implicated in the differentiation and activation of T helper TH1 and TH17 lymphocyte subsets.
   - Single nucleotide polymorphisms (SNPs) in the MDR1gene that contributes to proper intestinal epithelial barrier function and codes for multi-drug resistance protein 1.
2. Microbial factors:
   (a) Low microbial diversity
   - Superimposed infections in UC with organisms such as *C. difficile*, cytomegalovirus, *Escherichia coli*, and *Campylobacter*.

**CD** is a chronic granulomatous inflammatory disease that predominantly involves terminal ileum and adjoining colon but may affect any part of the gastrointestinal (GI) tract. It begins with cryptitis and abscess formation and then progresses to focal aphthoid ulcers. It further progresses to deep ulcer formation with edema of intervening mucosa giving characteristic "cobblestone appearance." CD is now considered to be multifactorial inflammatory disease.

The most accepted hypothesis is that CD is an immune-mediated disease in genetically susceptible individuals having altered immune response to the intestinal flora. The onset of the disease is triggered by various environmental factors and when the epithelial mucosal barrier is invaded by food or bacterial antigens, the mucosal immune system gets activated [21]. It promotes the migration of leukocytes to the site of inflammation enhancing the TH1 lymphocytic response, through production of cytokines like interleukin-12 (IL-12), IL-34, IL-23, and tumor necrosis factor-alpha (TNF-α). The enhanced migration to the sites of inflammation is also determined by a reshaping of the extracellular matrix through the action of metalloproteins (MMP-1 and MMP-3) and the overexpression of adhesion molecules such as MAcCAM-1 and integrin α4β4. Innate immunity also plays a role by variants of the Mut2 or the FUT2 genes that alter the barrier interaction with both pathogenic bacteria and harmful substances [22].

**In colitis caused by CDI,** overgrowth of *C. difficile* occurs in susceptible individuals due to suppression of normal colonic flora following use of antibiotics. *C. difficile* produces two high molecular weight exotoxins, namely toxin A (enterotoxin) and toxin B (cytotoxin) within GI tract. The cytotoxic effect of toxin B is 1000 times more potent in comparison to toxin A. Both these toxins bind with specific receptors located in the colonic mucosa and gain entry into the intercellular space causing systemic symptoms. These toxins are responsible for the release of inflammatory mediators namely interleukin 8, substance P, tumor necrosis factor alpha, and macrophage inflammatory protein 2 that are responsible for systemic toxicity leading to septic shock and multi-organ failure. At the local level, cytokines released due to these toxins incite an intense inflammatory response resulting in fluid shift leading to diarrhea, mucosal ulcerations, inflammatory exudates, and formation of pseudomembranes. The patients having low anti-toxin A IgG levels have severe disease and are more likely to develop fulminant colitis. In recent years, a hypervirulent strain of *C. difficile* namely North American pulse-field gel electrophoresis type 1 (NAP1) has been found to be responsible for the increasing severity of CDI. The loss of toxin regulatory gene (tcdC) allows this strain to increase the production of exotoxins by 16–23 times. Moreover, this strain has high spore-forming capacity and is more resistant to fluoroquinolones. The cases infected with this strain are more likely to have fulminant colitis requiring emergency colectomy with higher mortality (17%) [23].

## 83.2 Diagnosis

### 83.2.1 Clinical Presentation

Patients with fulminant colitis typically have symptoms suggestive of acute colitis such as diarrhea, abdominal pain, rectal bleeding, tenesmus, vomiting, fever, and dehydration that may be refractory to treatment. A detailed history should be taken and thorough clinical examination is done. History of drug intake such as antibiotics, immunosuppressants, chemotherapy, nonsteroidal anti-inflammatory drugs (NSAIDs), proton pump inhibitors, and oral contraceptives should be specifically noted. History of parasitic infestation, foreign travel, and contact with cases of diarrhea are other potential causes for fulminant colitis. The patients with long-standing vascular disease are likely to have ischemic colitis.

The vital signs in a patient with fulminant colitis generally reveal tachycardia, fever, hypotension, or tachypnoea depending on severity. In patients with inflammatory bowel disease, physical findings may be minimal, because high-dose steroids are routinely used. The abdomen may be distended and bowel sounds are usually decreased. Peritoneal signs like rebound tenderness and rigidity that indicate perforation may also be masked by high-dose steroids.

The flare up of **UC** is considered to be fulminant if one or more of the following features are seen: severe malaise, high grade fever, tachycardia, oliguria, dehydration, anemia requiring blood transfusion, and profound leukocytosis with a shift to left [23].

In fulminant **Crohn's colitis**, the cases may present as massive lower GI bleed, internal fistulization, abscess formation, and sealed perforation. There may be associated extraintestinal manifestations like hepatobiliary, ocular, bone, and cutaneous involvement. On examination, there is fever, toxic look, tachycardia, abdominal distension, and tenderness.

In inflammatory bowel disease (IBD), fulminant colitis may occur in a previously established case of IBD or may present as de novo idiopathic IBD. The latter is difficult to differentiate from other causes like ischemic colitis and severe infectious colitis [24].

**CDI cases** present with pain abdomen, fever with chills, bloating and diarrhea (occasionally bloody) usually occurring 2–3 days after starting antibiotics. The decrease in the frequency of diarrhea due to severe colonic dysmotility could be the first warning sign of fulminant colitis in such cases. Hypotension is a late finding and can be resistant to vasopressor support. On abdominal examination, there is marked tenderness and distension.

Although only 1–3% cases of CDI progress to fulminant colitis, but the mortality in this group of patients remain relatively high due to rapid progress to ileus, toxic megacolon, gut perforation, renal shut down and multi-organ failure [16, 25]. However, contrary to the literature, gut perforation is a rare phenomenon in these cases and mortality usually occurs before the intestine perforates. Hence the possibility of fulminant CDI must always be kept in mind in the high-risk population for early diagnosis.

Osman et al. [26] have described the clinical features and investigations in documented cases of fulminant CDI that persist despite maximum anti-clostridial therapy (Table 83.3).

**Table 83.3** Clinical, laboratory, and radiological features of fulminant CDI (adapted from Osman et al. [26])

| Clinical (symptoms and signs) | Laboratory and radiological features |
|---|---|
| History of diarrhea following antibiotic use | Increasing leukocytosis >16 × 10$^9$/L |
| Systemic toxicity | Lactate >2.2 mmol/L |
| Pyrexia ≥38 °C | Hypoalbuminemia <30 g/L |
| Tachycardia >100 beats/min | Radiological evidence of toxic megacolon (abdominal X-ray or CT) |
| Hypotension BP <90 mmHg | Free air under diaphragm |
| Abdominal signs of peritonitis | |
| Generalized abdominal pain | |
| Tenderness | |
| Abdominal distension (increasing abdominal girth) | |
| Rebound tenderness | |
| Organ failure and requirement for vasopressor therapy | |

## 83.2.2 Tests

### 83.2.2.1 Laboratory Investigations

Patients with fulminant colitis develop leukocytosis with a left shift and anemia due to bloody diarrhea but abnormally low or normal count does not rule out toxic colitis because of immunosuppression. Electrolyte disturbances are very common secondary to inflammatory diarrhea and steroid use. A nutritional panel, coagulation profile, liver function tests, and kidney function tests are helpful in determining treatment options. Erythrocyte sedimentation rate and C-reactive protein levels, although non-specific, are usually elevated.

Stool tests for *C. difficile*, CMV, ova and parasites help in differentiating between infectious and non-infectious etiologies of fulminant colitis. A positive stool culture for *C. difficile* indicates the presence of bacteria, whereas a positive stool toxin indicates clinically significant disease. At least three stool samples for *C. difficile* toxin should be obtained to rule out superimposed pseudo-membranous colitis. ELISA test detects both toxin A and toxin B with 92–94.5% sensitivity and 100% specificity; the test is less expensive and can be performed within 2–6 h [27]. However, ELISA tests can be negative in patients with fulminant CDI. The polymerase chain reaction (PCR) test for the detection of *C. difficile* toxin genes is a relatively new modality and is becoming popular as it is faster and more reliable in the diagnosis [28].

### 83.2.2.2 Imaging

**Plain abdominal radiographs** help in the diagnosis and management of fulminant colitis. Radiographic findings indicative of fulminant colitis include colonic distension, air fluid levels, pneumoperitoneum, and presence of mucosal islands. Repeated abdominal plain films are necessary to evaluate efficacy and progress of treatment. Any clinical deterioration during management of fulminant colitis warrants urgent plain X-ray of the abdomen. Daily abdominal X-rays are also indicated in patients with megacolon until the colonic diameter regresses to an acceptable level or surgical intervention is done.

A **computed tomography scan** in patients with diagnosis of toxic colitis may identify a local or contained perforation (Fig. 83.1) [29]. This may be helpful if the diagnosis remains unclear or the cause of toxicity is thought to be an abscess. However, CT scan has low sensitivity (52–85%) as well as specificity (48–92%) in diagnosing fulminant colitis and approximately

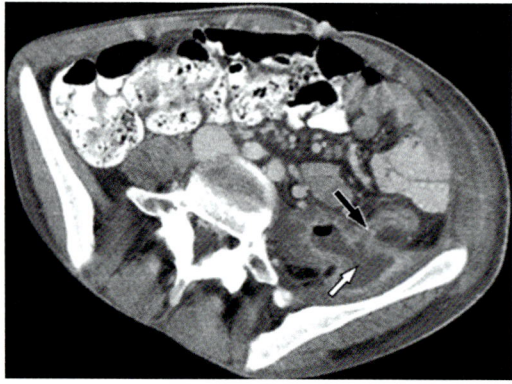

**Fig. 83.1** CT scan of fulminant colitis due to CD. Abscess cavity containing gas marked by white arrow and communication between the bowel and abscess cavity marked by black arrow. (Adapted from Futaba et al. [29])

40% of the patients have normal CT scans. CT findings of fulminant colitis include colonic wall thickening and enhancement, submucosal edema, mesenteric fat stranding, air-filled colonic distension (>6 cm), abnormal haustral pattern, gas in mesenteric veins, pneumatosis intestinalis, free air in the peritoneal cavity, and ascites [1]. Additional studies in form of virtual colonoscopy may help to further define the role of CT scan in diagnosing and deriving a prognosis for toxic colitis.

In fulminant colitis due to CDI, although CT findings are non-specific, but the typical findings are colonic dilatation and wall thickening, "accordion sign" (high-attenuation contrast material trapped in the colonic lumen alternating with low-attenuation thickened mucosal folds) (Fig. 83.2), "double-halo" or "target sign" (high-attenuation mucosa is separated by a ring of low-attenuation submucosal edema), mesenteric stranding and ascites [29, 30]. The CT scan findings are also helpful in categorizing the severity of the colitis when compared with clinical scenario. Moreover, in a seriously ill case not having clear indications of surgical intervention, CT scan and endoscopy are very helpful in early diagnosis of fulminant colitis due to CDI. Early diagnosis is vital since these cases may have mortality as high as 47% [31].

### 83.2.2.3 Endoscopy

If the diagnosis of toxic colitis is in doubt and the patient's condition is not unstable, endoscopy may be attempted by trained personnel. It helps in assessment of endoscopic severity of colitis as well as biopsies are taken to diagnose CMV infection. Flexible unprepared endoscopy (sigmoidoscopy or colonoscopy) with minimal air insufflation should be performed. If clinical concern of toxic colitis exists, the examination should preferably not progress beyond sigmoidoscopy. The scope should be advanced only as far as is needed for diagnosis with minimum air insufflations. Perforation is an obvious potential complication of this approach. Hence a post colonoscopy plain abdominal film should be done routinely.

The endoscopic findings seen in the majority of CDI cases having fulminant colitis are ulcers and pseudomembranes (elevated yellow-white plaques) (Fig. 83.3) [29]. Although less common, the pseudomembranous colitis may also be seen in CMV infection.

In **UC**, the classic endoscopic findings are confluent erythema, bowel wall edema, loss of vascular markings, friable mucosa, ulceration and pseudopolyp formation. The findings in fulminant UC include severe inflammation, hemorrhagic and sloughed mucosa with deep ulceration, mucosal detachment on the edge of these ulcerations, and well like ulcerations (Fig. 83.4) [32]. In a classical case, the colitis is most fulminant in

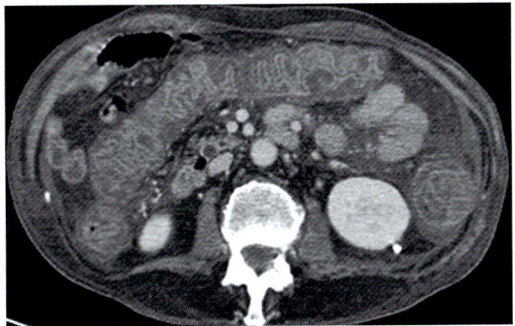

**Fig. 83.2** CT scan of fulminant colitis due to CDI showing typical colonic wall thickening known as the accordion sign with pericolic fluid. (Adapted from Futaba et al. [29])

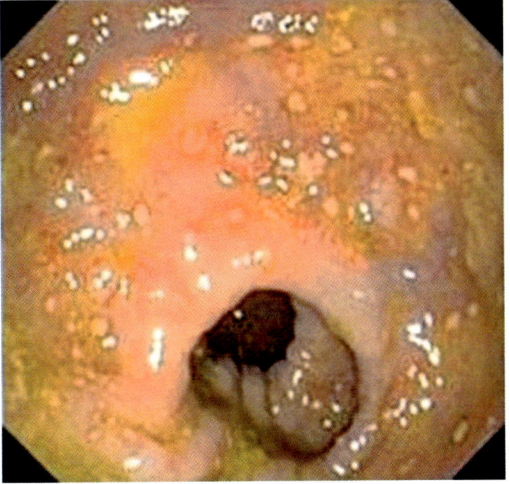

**Fig. 83.3** Colonoscopy showing typical appearance of pseudomembranous colitis. (Adapted from Futaba et al. [29])

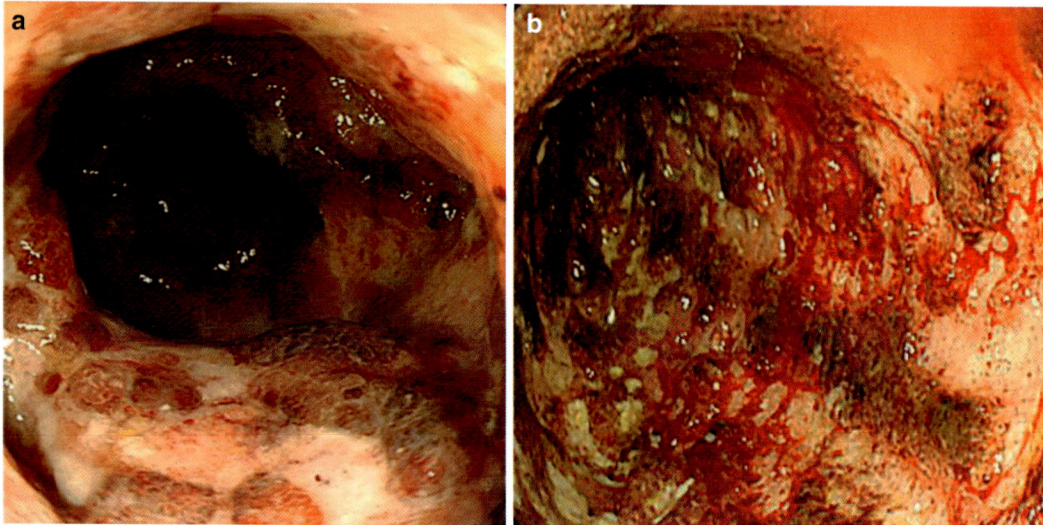

**Fig. 83.4** Colonoscopy in fulminant UC showing, (**a**) severe inflammation and extensive ulceration of the mucosa, (**b**) sloughed mucosa and pseudopolyps in the rectum. (Adapted from Mohri et al. [32])

the rectum and regresses proximally in a contiguous fashion. However, the distal rectum may sometimes appear normal due to the topical use of steroid suppositories.

In **CD**, the classic findings are cobblestone appearance, skip lesions, patchy erythema, mucosal bridging, ulceration and stricture formation. Colonoscopy and biopsy can often differentiate UC from CD, but treatment of severe attacks is presently similar in both which may no longer hold true in the future if novel therapies specific for one of the two conditions are introduced.

## 83.3 Treatment

All patients with clinical profile of fulminant colitis should be hospitalized and carefully evaluated. Communication with patient and family at all times is imperative as toxic colitis can be fatal at times and that should be clearly informed. Treatment includes following main goals: reduce colectasia to prevent perforation, fluid and electrolyte correction, treat toxemia and precipitating factors. Careful and frequent monitoring of the patient is of paramount importance. Frequent blood counts, electrolytes and abdominal radiographs are must and in case patient is malnourished, nutritional support is given. Enteral feeding can be initiated as soon as patient shows signs of improvement to promote gut motility. The enteral nutrition is preferred over parenteral route since it has significantly fewer complications. The parenteral nutrition should be given only when patient doesn't tolerate oral feeds.

### 83.3.1 Medical Treatment

In fulminant colitis due to any etiology, the primary aim of medical treatment is to hemodynamically stabilize the patient and then treat the underlying pathology. The patient should be kept in ICU for intensive monitoring of vital signs and input/output charting. All medications that may affect colonic motility such as narcotics, NSAIDs, antidiarrheals and anticholinergic agents must be stopped. The patient should be put on bowel rest, nasogastric, or long intestinal tube is inserted to assist gastrointestinal decompression and indwelling urethral catheter is inserted for urine output monitoring. During initial phase of resuscitation, fluid replacement, electrolyte repletion, albumin and blood transfusion should be aggressive. One of the initial challenges is to decide whether we are dealing with fulminant colitis due to IBD or infective colitis. In the former situation, the mainstay of treatment is immunosuppressive therapy, whereas it can be counterproductive in the latter. Apart from the cases of infective colitis, the role of antibiotics is controversial. The use of broad-spectrum intravenous antibiotics is justified by some authors to take care of bacteremia, transmural extension of infection, and microperforations. Since patients are mostly bed ridden, hence preventive measures for venous thrombosis such as leg exercises, elastic stocking and early ambulation must be implemented. Low molecular weight heparin injection for thromboprophylaxis is considered but risk of intestinal bleeding must be assessed before starting it. The response to medical treatment should be monitored by stool chart (frequency, liquid versus solid stool, presence or absence of bleeding), vital signs, abdominal examination, blood count, serum electrolytes and CRP levels.

In cases of **fulminant colitis due to IBD (UC and CD)**, steroids are the mainstay of treatment except in patients having colonic ischemia, perforation or progressive dilatation. Early use of IV steroids in high dosage (hydrocortisone 100 mg 6 hourly or methylprednisolone 16–20 mg 8 hourly) has overall response rate of 67% and has shown to avoid colectomy in up to 25% cases [1]. Methyl prednisolone is preferred since it has greater anti-inflammatory potency and lesser mineralocorticoid potency. The parenteral steroids should be given for only 7–10 days and then shifted to oral form such as prednisolone. These are not to be used for long-term maintenance therapy due to the side effects like weight gain, osteoporosis and diabetes. Therefore, steroids are gradually tapered and then withdrawn, and maintenance should be done with thiopurines, immunosalicylates or biologics. However, reactivation of disease occurs following tapering of the steroids in some cases due to drug dependence. Such patients that can't be managed without steroids over a period of 3–6 months are candidates for colectomy. The cases of IBD having co-existing *C. difficile* infection require addition of vancomycin or metronidazole since they have higher morbidity and mortality.

Almost 30% of the patients do not show any improvement with 3–5 days of steroid therapy and are labeled as non-responders [33]. Such cases are the candidates for initiation of rescue therapy with drugs like cyclosporine, infliximab or tacrolimus. Some studies have shown that cyclosporine has similar efficacy to steroids in cases with fulminant colitis, but it should be given as primary therapy only in cases where steroids are contraindicated [34].

In non-responders, another possibility of **cytomegalovirus** superinfection should always be considered. It is diagnosed on sigmoidoscopic biopsy and requires antiviral treatment with ganciclovir [35].

In non-responders, the addition of IV cyclosporine A (4 mg/kg/day) to steroids as rescue therapy has been found to be very effective. Various trials have shown 76–85% response rate with IV cyclosporine in median time of 4 days [34]. Clinically, the patient has decreased frequency of motions and bleeding per rectum, and biochemical parameters also start improving. The cyclosporine is given by IV route for 7–10 days and thereafter it is administered orally 6–8 mg/kg/day in two divided doses. However, it should be stopped if there is no improvement in 7 days. Cyclosporine therapy in responders may obviate the need for urgent colectomy allowing an elective subtotal colectomy or proctocolectomy under more controlled circumstances. However, cyclosporine also has significant adverse effects, including immunosuppression and opportunistic infections, hypertension, cardiac arrhythmia, renal toxicity and neurologic complications. Therefore, calibration of its dosage and monitoring becomes difficult and it is advisable to have long-term maintenance therapy with purine derivatives (Azathioprine [AZA]/6-Mercaptopurine [6-MP]). But, the cases of fulminant UC who are already on purine derivatives have less favorable results with cyclosporine and have high chances of requiring subsequent colectomy [36].

In cases of Crohn's disease having fulminant colitis with internal fistulae formation that is refractory to steroid therapy, cyclosporine has been found to be effective. It is given as IV infusion in dosage of 2–4 mg/kg/day for up to 2 weeks and then given orally.

Infliximab, an anti-TNF-alpha monoclonal antibody, given as 5 mg/kg/dose in three infusions (0, 2, and 6 weeks), is as effective as cyclosporine in treating fulminant colitis. However, the choice between cyclosporine and infliximab as rescue therapy is difficult and the treatment decision depends on clinician's experience as well as clinical condition of the patient. The advantage of infliximab over cyclosporine is that previous treatment with thiopurine doesn't affect the outcome of infliximab therapy [37]. However, drawback is that infliximab has longer half-life than cyclosporine and remains active in the circulation for many weeks. This difference becomes important since it may be a risk factor for surgical complications in case a need for urgent life-saving colectomy arises [2]. In general, cyclosporine is preferred in cases of severe fulminant colitis because of its faster action, shorter half-life and good clinical response. It is specifically recommended for the cases that have not previously received azathioprine/6-MP and are likely candidates for colectomy. On the other hand, infliximab is recommended for moderate fulminant colitis cases that have been previously given azathioprine/6-MP. Infliximab should not be given in patients with poor cardiac reserve, hepatitis B infection, acute sepsis and tuberculosis.

Tacrolimus is another drug used for rescue therapy. It is a calcineurin inhibitor and has mechanism of action similar to that of cyclosporine. It can be given through IV (0.01–0.02 mg/kg) as well as oral route (0.1–0.2 mg/kg) [38].

Additional therapy such as **leukocytapheresis** has shown variable results in cases of fulminant colitis. In this technique, white blood cells are selectively removed from the circulation via an extracorporeal circuit. Presently, this therapy doesn't have formal recommendation for treatment in these cases.

In **fulminant colitis due to CDI**, the inciting antibiotics should be withdrawn immediately and steroids are contraindicated. The proton pump inhibitors should be discontinued since they are associated with an increased risk of CDI. The measures for infection control should be strictly implemented such as patient isolation, surface cleaning with sodium hypochlorite solution, using soap and water for hand scrubbing and wearing gown and gloves. Oral vancomycin is the drug of choice and is given in high dosage (500 mg 6 hourly) for 10 days. IV vancomycin is not effective and should not be given in these cases. In cases with paralytic ileus, vancomycin retention enema (500 mg in 100 mL saline 6 hourly) or administration through nasogastric tube is an alternative option. In addition, IV metronidazole (500 mg 8 hourly) should be given since there is erratic absorption of enteral vancomycin in cases having ileus. In fulminant CDI, the clinical success rate for metronidazole and vancomycin is 66.3 and 78.5%, respectively [1].

In refractory cases of fulminant CDI, other treatment modalities having variable results are [39, 40]:

- Intravenous immunoglobulins
- Alternative antibiotics (fidaxomicin, rifaximin, ramoplanin, nitazoxanide, and tigecycline)
- Monoclonal antibodies
- Fecal microbiota transplantation

The outlines of medical management and decision for surgical intervention in non-responders are given in the flow chart below (Fig. 83.5).

In **infectious fulminant colitis**, definitive diagnosis is based on culture report that identifies the pathogen and antibiotic treatment is given accordingly. However, in *E. coli* O157 infection, antibiotics have no role and can rather enhance bloody diarrhea and cause mortality. Hence antibiotics should not be given in E. coli O157 induced fulminant colitis [41].

### 83.3.2 Surgical Treatment

Apart from emergency indications, the surgical intervention is usually reserved for the non-responders to medical treatment. But its possibility should be discussed with the patient and relatives right from the time of admission. Since the surgical treatment of fulminant colitis requires an ostomy, the pros and cons of the operative pro-

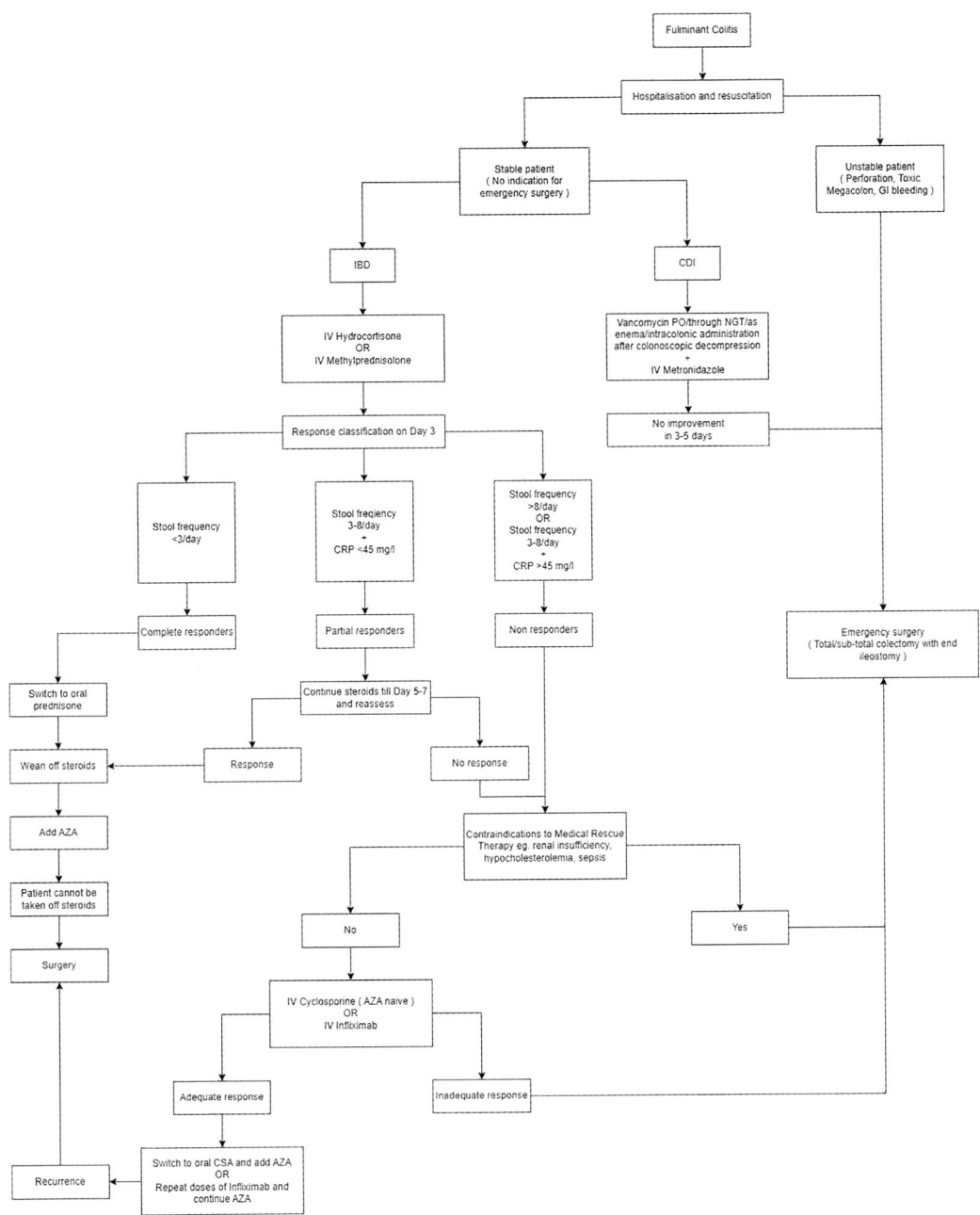

**Fig. 83.5** Algorithm for treatment decisions in fulminant colitis

cedure should be well informed and the consent for the stoma should be obtained that might remain permanent. In planning surgery, important points that need consideration are general condition of the patient, underlying cause of fulminant colitis and condition of the colon seen at the time of surgery. The patients on steroids must continue it in post-operative period to prevent adrenal insufficiency.

The timing of surgery in fulminant colitis is still a matter of controversy and varies with underlying etiology. In cases of UC, indications for operative intervention include perforation, peritonitis, massive hemorrhage and lack of response to medical treatment. The last indication is the commonest reason for surgical treatment but timing of intervention is hard to define in such cases. The patients are initially given IV steroids. In case of non-responders after 3 days or partial responders after 7 days therapy, the patients are put on rescue therapy with cyclosporine or infliximab. If rescue therapy also fails to show improvement, the patient is taken up for surgical intervention. In non-responders, earlier recommendations were in favor of continuing conservative treatment for up to 1 week. But most authors now recommend surgery in cases that fail to respond to the medical management in 2–3 days time. The rationale for early intervention is based on a fivefold increase in mortality after free perforation. Infliximab and cyclosporine do not increase postoperative complications of colectomy, and surgery should not be deferred based on this exposure.

In cases of fulminant colitis due to CDI, surgical intervention is indicated if there is no clinical improvement or worsening after 3–5 days of diagnosis and medical management. However, there are no definitive clinical and laboratory parameters predicting response to medical therapy; hence deciding the timing of surgical intervention in refractory cases is very difficult. The predictive parameters in support of surgical treatment are: perforation peritonitis, organ failure, systemic sepsis, vasopressor requirement, unexplained clinical deterioration, altered sensorium, TLC count $\geq 50 \times 10^9$ µL and serum lactate $\geq 5$ mmol/L.

In cases of fulminant ischemic colitis, it should be managed as a part of systemic vascular disease. Therefore, apart from managing the ischemic colon, the precipitating factors such as poor cardiac functions must also be taken care of adequately. The definitive indications of surgical intervention are perforation peritonitis, worsening sepsis, onset of multi-organ failure, colonoscopic findings of irreversible necrosis and CT findings suggestive of colonic necrosis such as pneumoperitoneum, pneumatosis intestinalis and air in portal venous system. During surgery, it is very difficult to decide the extent of colonic resection since serosa looks normal until occurrence of transmural necrosis. In such situation, intra-operative assessment of bowel wall integrity can be done with IV fluorescein, intraoperative colonoscopy, intraoperative photo-plethysmography and Color Doppler examination. Every effort should be made to preserve the rectal stump. Due to progressive ischemia, primary intestinal anastomosis should be avoided following resection of gangrenous gut and end ileostomy with closure of distal rectal stump is preferred. In cases with doubtful gut viability, second look laparotomy is advisable and further resection is done.

Various operative options for surgical management of fulminant colitis are as follows:

(a) **Subtotal colectomy with end ileostomy.** It is the gold standard in the surgical management of fulminant colitis [1]. It safely removes the pathology, allows resolution of toxemia, gives time for nutritional improvement and permits elective stoma closure on a later date. The primary anastomosis should not be done in emergency since patients are unstable and are on immunosuppressant, thus having high chances of anastomotic leak and pelvic sepsis. The surgery can be performed both by laparoscopic as well as by open technique. In a clinically stable, young patient, laparoscopic resection is advisable due to cosmetic reasons. It also helps in quick recovery, early discharge and less postoperative adhesions that makes the restorative procedure much easier. Based on available resources and condition of the patient, various laparoscopic approaches can be total laparoscopic, laparoscopic assisted or hand assisted laparoscopic technique. In a clinically unstable patient having friable and grossly distended colon, open approach is preferred due to its safety and shorter operative time. In such a case, the laparoscopic instruments are likely to perforate fragile, thin-walled colon while grasping the bowel. However, the cases of Crohn's colitis are more suitable for laparoscopic colonic resection due to thick bowel wall.

On exposure, the colon in cases of UC is usually found to be edematous, fragile with microperforations covered with omentum. The colon is first mobilized from lateral to medial side and adherent omentum is excised en bloc with colon so as to avoid iatrogenic perforations. The mesenteric vessels are then ligated and divided. Terminal ileum is divided near ileocecal valve and colon is divided at rectosigmoid junction or distal sigmoid colon based on the condition of colonic wall (Fig. 83.6a) [42]. In cases of UC, the dissection of inflamed and fragile rectum should not be done to prevent its perforation and to avoid iatrogenic injury to the pelvic nerves that can lead to urinary incontinence and sexual dysfunction. Some authors recommend that colonic mobilization should be done as last step because of the risk of perforations and fecal soiling. Thus, in case of contamination, the deceased colon can be quickly removed from the abdomen. Since, there is a risk of blow out of the distal rectal stump; it can be closed with a staple and then reinforced with sutures. Further, distal pouch can be brought in the subcutaneous plane at the lower end of midline laparotomy wound so that suture line remains above the fascial level (Fig. 83.6b) [42]. Thus, in case of leak, it will produce a controlled fistula. In stapled rectal stump, keeping a rectal tube per anum for 2–3 days also helps in decompression and reduces the incidence of rectal stump blowout. In case, the rectal stump is too friable to hold sutures, then it can be exteriorized as mucus fistula. The divided ileal end is exteriorized as end ileostomy through rectus muscle in the right iliac fossa with a 2–3 cm spout.

In cases of fulminant colitis due to CDI, the peritoneal cavity contains sterile inflammatory fluid. The colon appears boggy and edematous with paracolic inflammation and contains several liters of fluid in its lumen. In delayed cases, the colonic wall may appear friable, necrotic with micro-perforations. Even if the external appearance of colon apparently looks healthy, segmental colectomy should not be considered since disease is invariably found to be pancolonic. Hence total colectomy with end ileostomy should be performed with closure of rectal stump at peritoneal reflection.

The ileostomy closure is planned once clinical condition of the patient improves so that the risk of anastomotic leak is minimized and it usually takes 3–6 months time. Special precaution should be taken in cases of UC getting infliximab since its immunosuppressive effect lasts for 3–4 months after the last dose.

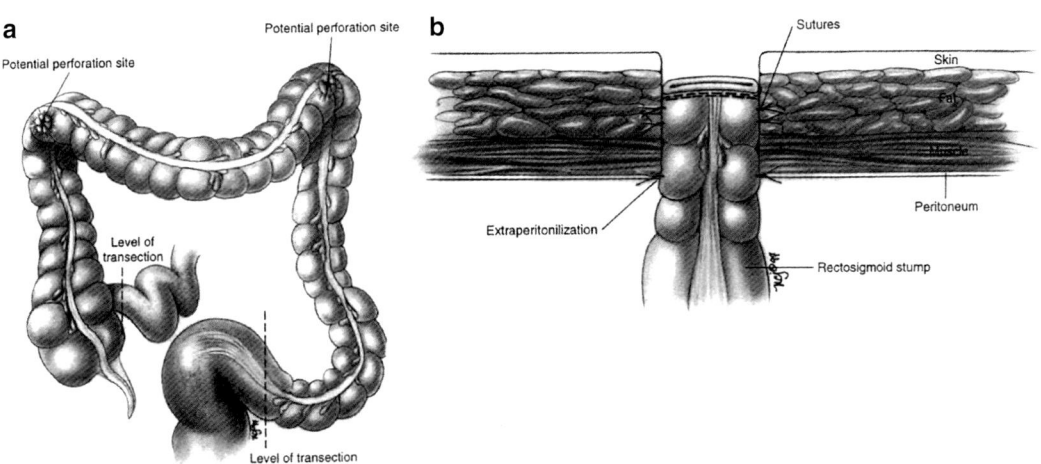

**Fig. 83.6** (**a**) Abdominal colectomy and preservation of rectal stump. (**b**) The retained rectosigmoid stump protrudes beyond the fascia in the subcutaneous fat. (Adapted from Tjandra [42])

In case of CDI and non-active Crohn's disease, ileo-rectal anastomosis is performed [1]. However, in cases with active Crohn's disease involving ano-rectum, stoma reversal is not recommended. In case of UC, recommended procedure is completion proctectomy with ileal J-pouch anal anastomosis. Although it improves the quality of life, but is associated with complications like pouchitis, diarrhea, fecal incontinence and reduced fertility in young females.

(b) **Total proctocolectomy with ileal pouch-anal anastomosis and loop ileostomy**. It is no more preferred technique for fulminant colitis because performing a total proctocolectomy in a toxic patient who is acutely ill and on high-dose immunosuppressant increases the risk of complications and mortality [2].

(c) **Total proctocolectomy and end ileostomy**. It is also not performed any more in fulminant UC because excision of acutely inflamed rectum is technically challenging and is associated with complications such as massive bleed, pelvic nerve damage, sepsis and intestinal obstruction. At a later date, ileal pouch-anal anastomosis is also very difficult due to dense pelvic adhesions. However, the procedure can be considered in cases with very fulminant proctocolitis that have multiple comorbidities and anal incontinence. Such patients are not fit for restorative surgery. The other indications for this surgical procedure are in cases with rectal perforations or ongoing rectal bleed. However, even in such cases, the rectum should be excised only up to a level just distal to the problem site so that future restoration remains possible [2].

(d) **Partial or segmental colectomy** is no longer advocated due to higher mortality and reoperation rate. It is not useful since fulminant colitis involves whole of the colon and intra-operative serosal appearance can't predict the underlying mucosal involvement in UC and CDI. Some authors have performed partial colonic resection with diversion stoma in cases of segmental fulminant colitis with perforation due to Crohn's disease, but the long-term results are not available [1]. In cases of fulminant amoebic colitis, segmental colonic resection can be done as this is a reversible condition and the healed colon is good for subsequent intestinal anastomosis. In these cases, primary intestinal anastomosis should be avoided since tissues contain amoebae and there is a high risk of suture breakdown [43].

(e) **Diverting ileostomy** alone for fulminant colitis was being practiced during mid-twentieth century but was also found to be associated with poor results due to retained diseased colon that was likely to perforate causing high morbidity and mortality [2].

(f) **Diverting loop ileostomy with intra-operative colonic lavage** as an alternative surgical intervention has been proposed in some studies with low mortality rates. The technique has shown good results in cases of fulminant colitis due to CDI [1]. The diverting loop ileostomy can be performed laparoscopically and distal limb of ileostomy is utilized for on table antegrade colonic lavage with warm polyethylene glycol solution. In post-operative period, antegrade vancomycin enemas are given through the distal ileostomy limb along with metronidazole through IV route. This technique helps in rapid recovery, preservation of colon and high chances of stoma reversal.

(g) **Blow-Hole Colostomy and loop ileostomy (Turnbull procedure)** is recommended in selected patients with hugely dilated colon where there is very high chance of perforations and fecal soiling during colonic mobilization. In such cases, colonic decompression can be done by a skin level colostomy and fecal stream can be diverted with proximal loop ileostomy (Fig. 83.7) [42]. The definitive colonic resection can be performed in a couple of months' time when toxemia settles and general condition of the patient improves. However, this procedure is contraindicated in cases of perforation peritonitis, ongoing hemorrhage and pericolic abscess.

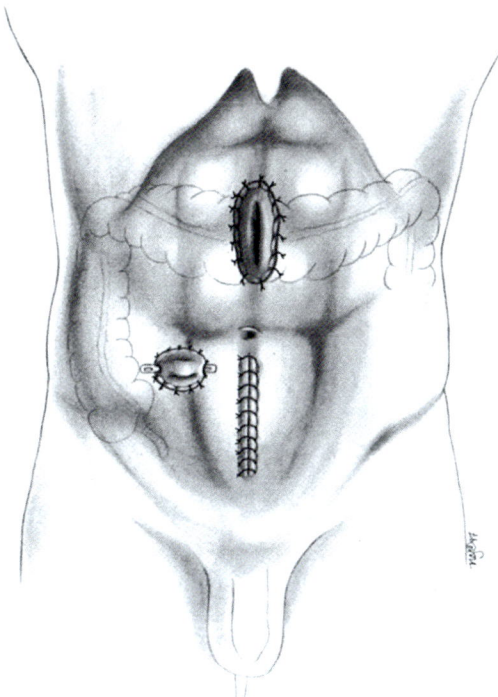

**Fig. 83.7** Diverting loop ileostomy and decompressive "Blowhole" colostomy at skin level. (Adapted from Tjandra [42])

## 83.3.3 Prognosis

The final outcome in cases of fulminant colitis depends upon multiple factors including underlying pathology, timing of surgery, co-morbidities and nutritional status. Prolonged waiting period and continued medical treatment should be discouraged because once patient becomes clinically unstable, there is significant rise in mortality even after surgical intervention. The patients with colonic perforation and massive bleed also have poor outcome.

In IBD, predictive factors for poor prognosis following prolonged medical management are:

- After 3 days of IV steroids, stool frequency >8/day and CRP levels >45 mg/L
- Fever (temperature >37.5 °C), tachycardia (pulse >90 bpm), hypoalbuminemia <3 mg/dL
- Anemia, malnutrition, need for blood transfusion and total parenteral nutrition
- Abdominal X-ray showing mucosal islands or transverse colonic diameter of >5.5 cm
- Colonoscopy showing deep extensive ulcerations has less than 10% chances of responding to medical management
- Lack of mucosal healing after steroid therapy

In fulminant CDI, 30-day mortality is reported to be 58% in medically treated patients in comparison to 34% managed surgically [44]. The need for vasopressors is an important prognostic factor. Once vasopressor requirement arises, the perioperative mortality rises >4 times compared with patients who undergo colectomy before vasopressors are required [16]. Other prognostic factors are old age (>70 years), mental status changes, cardiorespiratory instability, multi organ failure, severe infection (WBC count ≥35,000/μL or <4000/μL or neutrophil bands ≥10%) and rising lactate level (>5 mmol/L). The patients infected with NAP1 strain of *C. difficile* have poorer prognosis with approximately 17% mortality [45].

### Dos and Don'ts

**Dos**

- Hospitalize the patient and manage in ICU (monitoring and resuscitation).
- Do counseling of the family regarding need for stoma, morbidity and mortality.
- Establish the cause of fulminant colitis (IBD or CDI) based on history, clinical examination and investigations.
- Give IV steroids in fulminant colitis due to IBD and in case of no response put on rescue therapy with cyclosporine or infliximab.
- Give enteral vancomycin with IV metronidazole in fulminant colitis due to CDI.
- Monitor the response of treatment by stool chart, vital signs, abdominal examination, blood count, serum electrolytes and CRP levels.
- Do surgical intervention if patients don't respond to medical management in

3–5 days time or with suspected toxicity.
- Do emergency surgery in patients with perforation peritonitis and ongoing bleeding per rectum.
- Do gentle handling of the friable bowel.
- Do ileostomy for fecal diversion with or without colonic resection.
- Do second look laparotomy in patients of ischemic colitis having doubtful gut viability.
- Do ileostomy closure after 3–6 months when condition of the patient is stable.

**Don'ts**
- Don't give narcotics, NSAIDs, opioids, antidiarrheals and anticholinergic agents.
- Don't give antibiotics in *E. coli* O157 infection.
- Don't give steroids in fulminant colitis due to CDI.
- Don't delay surgical intervention in cases with definite indications.
- Don't defer surgery in cases on infliximab or cyclosporine.
- Don't perform primary intestinal anastomosis.
- Don't perform stoma closure before 3–4 months in cases of UC getting infliximab.
- Don't perform stoma closure in cases with active Crohn's disease involving ano-rectum.

**Take-Home Messages**

- Fulminant colitis is a life-threatening medical emergency that usually fails to respond to aggressive medical therapy requiring surgical intervention in many cases.
- Modern medical management can delay surgery in a critically ill patient, but an early surgical intervention should be done whenever indicated.
- Prefer open laparotomy in a toxic and unstable patient. Laparoscopic surgery should be performed only by the experienced surgeons in a clinically stable patient.
- Total/subtotal colectomy with end ileostomy is the surgery of choice in majority of the cases. The primary anastomosis should not be done in emergency due to high chances of leak.
- In fulminant colitis due to CDI, loop ileostomy with colonic lavage that can be performed laparoscopically, is an alternative to colectomy resulting in reduced morbidity and preservation of the colon.

**Multiple Choice Questions**
1. Which of the following is recommended in fulminant *C. difficile* infection?
   A. Oral metronidazole
   B. Intravenous fidaxomicin
   C. Intravenous vancomycin
   D. Oral vancomycin
2. In a case of fulminant colitis with underlying long standing inflammatory bowel disease, there is usually minimal abdominal tenderness with no guarding. This is because of
   A. Immunocompromised status
   B. Use of high dose steroids
   C. Prolonged ileus
   D. Multi-organ failure
3. In a case of CDI, the initial warning sign suggestive of fulminant colitis is
   A. Resistant hypotension
   B. Abdominal distension and tenderness
   C. Decrease in frequency of diarrhea
   D. Renal shut down
4. A 70 years old male, known case of UC for the last 6 years having hepatitis B

infection, develops features of fulminant colitis. He is put on IV hydrocortisone for 5 days but fails to show improvement. Which of the following drugs should **NOT** be used for rescue therapy in this patient?
   A. Infliximab
   B. Cyclosporine
   C. Azathioprine
   D. Tacrolimus
5. A 40 years old male, known case of Crohn's disease for the last 4 years develops fulminant colitis that requires surgical intervention due to the failure of medical management. Which of the following options is BEST suited for this patient?
   A. Laparoscopic segmental colectomy
   B. Laparoscopic subtotal colectomy with end ileostomy
   C. Open proctocolectomy with end ileostomy
   D. Laparoscopic diverting loop ileostomy with intra-operative colonic lavage
6. A 30 years old female, known case of ulcerative colitis for the last 5 years presents with >10 bloody stools/day for the last 2 weeks requiring multiple transfusions. Due to failure of response to medical treatment she is planned for open colectomy with end ileostomy. Which of the following procedure is NOT recommended for prevention of rectal stump blow out in this case?
   A. Staple closure of rectal stump with suture reinforcement
   B. Subcutaneous placement of closed rectal stump
   C. Rectal stump exteriorized as mucus fistula
   D. Proctocolectomy with end ileostomy
7. Antibiotics are contraindicated in fulminant colitis due to:
   A. Ulcerative colitis
   B. *E. coli* O157
   C. Crohn's disease
   D. CDI
8. Which of the following statements regarding management of fulminant colitis is correct:
   A. Patients of fulminant colitis due to CDI are to be taken up for laparotomy straightaway since steroids are contraindicated.
   B. When possible, do an anastomosis after resection of gut in fulminant colitis since it avoids a second surgery.
   C. Surgery should be delayed in patients receiving infliximab and cyclosporine as they increase postoperative complications.
   D. In fulminant colitis due to CDI, loop ileostomy with colonic lavage performed laparoscopically has good results.
9. Which of the following statements regarding management of fulminant colitis is correct:
   A. Antivirals have no role in fulminant colitis
   B. Steroid non-responders should be taken up for surgery
   C. Cyclosporine has a longer half-life than infliximab
   D. Cyclosporine can be given as primary therapy in fulminant colitis
10. In recent years, more cases of community-acquired CDI are being reported among which of the following groups leading to rise in incidence of fulminant colitis?
    A. Elderly males
    B. Immunocompromised patients
    C. Pediatric patients
    D. Young females

**Answers**: 1D; 2B; 3C; 4A; 5B; 6D; 7B; 8D; 9D; 10C

# References

1. Fong C, Abbadessa B. Colonic conditions: toxic colitis. In: Steele SR, Maykel JA, Wexner XD, editors. Clinical decision making in colorectal surgery. 2nd ed. Cham: Springer Nature Switzerland AG; 2020. p. 423–9.
2. Strong SA. Management of acute colitis and toxic megacolon. Clin Colon Rectal Surg. 2010;23:274–84.
3. Loo VG, Poirier L, Miller MA, Oughton M, Libman MD, Michaud S, et al. A predominantly clonal multi-institutional outbreak of Clostridium difficile associated diarrhea with high morbidity and mortality. N Engl J Med. 2005;353:2442–9.
4. Beg MY, Bains L, Mahajan R, Lal P, Choudhury S, Kumar NP, et al. Fulminant necrotising amoebic colitis of whole of large bowel: a rare complication of a common infectious disease. Case Rep Infect Dis. 2020;2020:8845263.
5. Adorian C, Khoury G, Tawil A, Sharara A. Behçet's disease complicated by toxic megacolon. Dig Dis Sci. 2003;48:2366–8.
6. Carter AO, Borczyk AA, Carlson JA, Harvey B, Hockin JC, Karmali MA, et al. A severe outbreak of Escherichia coli O157:H7-associated hemorrhagic colitis in a nursing home. N Engl J Med. 1987;317:1496–500.
7. Truelove SC, Witts LJ. Cortisone in ulcerative colitis; final report on a therapeutic trial. Br Med J. 1955;2:1041–8.
8. Satsangi J, Silverberg MS, Vermeire S, Colombel JF. The Montreal classification of inflammatory bowel disease: controversies, consensus, and implications. Gut. 2006;55:749–53.
9. Baron JH, Connell AM, Lennard-Jones JE. Variation between observers in describing mucosal appearances in proctocolitis. Br Med J. 1964;1:89–92.
10. Lémann M, Galian A, Rutgeerts P, Heuverzwijn RV, Cortot A, Viteau JM, et al. Comparison of budesonide and 5-aminosalicylic acid enemas in active distal ulcerative colitis. Aliment Pharmacol Ther. 1995;9:557–62.
11. Feagan BG, Greenberg GR, Wild G, Fedorak RN, Paré P, McDonald JW, et al. Treatment of ulcerative colitis with a humanized antibody to the alpha4beta7 integrin. N Engl J Med. 2005;352:2499–507.
12. Travis SP, Schnell D, Krzeski P, Abreu MT, Attman DG, Colombel JF, et al. Developing an instrument to assess the endoscopic severity of ulcerative colitis: the Ulcerative Colitis Endoscopic Index of Severity (UCEIS). Gut. 2012;61:535–42.
13. Schroeder KW, Tremaine WJ, Ilstrup DM. Coated oral 5-aminosalicylic acid therapy for mildly to moderately active ulcerative colitis, a randomised study. N Engl J Med. 1987;317:1625–9.
14. Rubin DT, Ananthakrishnan AN, Siegel CA, Sauer BG, Long MD. ACG clinical guideline: ulcerative colitis in adults. Am J Gastroenterol. 2019;114:384–413.
15. Neumann H, Vieth M, Günther C, Neufert C, Kiesslich R, Grauer M, et al. Virtual chromoendoscopy for prediction of severity and disease extent in patients with inflammatory bowel disease: a randomized controlled study. Inflamm Bowel Dis. 2013;19:1935–42.
16. Dallal RM, Harbrecht BG, Boujoukas AJ, Sirio CA, Farkas LM, Lee KK, et al. Fulminant Clostridium difficile: an underappreciated and increasing cause of death and complications. Ann Surg. 2002;235:363–72.
17. Surawicz CM, Brandt LJ, Binion DG, Ananthakrishnan AN, Curry SR, Gilligan PH, et al. Guidelines for diagnosis, treatment, and prevention of Clostridium difficile infections. Am J Gastroenterol. 2013;108:478–98.
18. Sheth SG, LaMont JT. Toxic megacolon. Lancet. 1998;351:509–13.
19. Mourelle M, Casellas F, Guarner F, Salas A, Riveros-Moreno V, Moncada S, et al. Induction of nitric oxide synthase in colonic smooth muscle from patients with toxic megacolon. Gastroenterology. 1995;109:1497–502.
20. Hindryckx P, Jairath V, D'Haens G. Acute severe ulcerative colitis: from pathophysiology to clinical management. Nat Rev Gastroenterol Hepatol. 2016;13:654–64.
21. Boyapati R, Satsangi J, Ho GT. Pathogenesis of Crohn's disease. F1000Prime Rep. 2015;7:44.
22. Petagna L, Antonelli A, Ganini C, Bellato V, Campanelli M, Divizia A, et al. Pathophysiology of Crohn's disease inflammation and recurrence. Biol Direct. 2020;15:23.
23. Halaweish I, Alam HB. Surgical management of severe colitis in the intensive care unit. J Intensive Care Med. 2015;30:451–61.
24. Sands BE. Fulminant colitis. J Gastrointest Surg. 2008;12:2157–9.
25. Flegel W, Muller F, Daubener W, Fisher HG, Hadding U, Northoff H. Cytokine response by human monocytes to Clostridium difficile toxin A and toxin B. Infect Immun. 1991;59:3659–66.
26. Osman KA, Ahmed MH, Hamad MA, Mathur D. Emergency colectomy for fulminant Clostridium difficile colitis: striking the right balance. Scand J Gastroenterol. 2011;46:1222–7.
27. Aldeen WE, Bingham M, Aiderzada A, Kucera J, Jense S, Caroll KC. Comparison of TOX A/B test to a cell culture cytotoxicity assay for the detection of Clostridium difficile in stools. Diagn Microbiol Infect Dis. 2000;36:211–3.
28. Novak-Weekley SM, Marlowe EM, Miller JM, Cumpio J, Nomura JH, Vance PH, et al. Clostridium difficile testing in the clinical laboratory by use of multiple testing algorithms. J Clin Microbiol. 2010;48:889–93.
29. Futaba K, Mak T, Morton D. Surgery for fulminant colitis. In: Brown SR, Hartley JE, Hill J, Scott N, Williams JG, editors. Contemporary coloproctology. London: Springer-Verlag; 2012. p. 261–78.
30. Kirkpatrick ID, Greenberg HM. Evaluating the CT diagnosis of Clostridium difficile colitis: should CT guide therapy? Am J Roentgenol. 2001;176:635–9.

31. Ali SO, Welch JP, Dring RJ. Early surgical intervention for fulminant pseudomembranous colitis. Am Surg. 2008;74:20–6.
32. Mohri K, Hiramatsu K, Shibata Y, Aoba T, Fujii M, Arimoto A, et al. Total proctocolectomy with end ileostomy for acute onset of ulcerative colitis during chemoradiotherapy for lung adenocarcinoma (successfully treated by surgery): a case report. Surg Case Rep. 2020;6:121.
33. Rosenberg W, Ireland A, Lewell DP. High-dose methylprednisolone in the treatment of active ulcerative colitis. J Clin Gastroenterol. 1990;12:40–1.
34. D'Haens G, Lemmens L, Geboes K, Vandeputte L, Van Acker F, Mortelmans L, et al. Intravenous cyclosporine versus intravenous corticosteroids as a single therapy for severe attacks of ulcerative colitis. Gastroenterology. 2001;120:1323–9.
35. Cottone M, Pietrosi G, Martorana G, Casà A, Pecoraro G, Oliva L, et al. Prevalence of cytomegalovirus infection in severe refractory ulcerative and Crohn's colitis. Am J Gastroenterol. 2001;96:773–5.
36. Moskovitz DN, Van Assche G, Maenhout B, Arts J, Ferrante M, Vermeire S, et al. Incidence of colectomy during long-term follow-up after cyclosporine-induced remission of severe ulcerative colitis. Clin Gastroenterol Hepatol. 2006;4:760–5.
37. Järnerot G, Hertervig E, Friis-Liby I, Blomquist L, Karlén P, Grännö C, et al. Infliximab as rescue therapy in severe to moderately severe ulcerative colitis: a randomized, placebo-controlled study. Gastroenterology. 2005;128:1805–11.
38. Fellermann K, Tanko Z, Herrlinger KR, Witthoeft T, Homann N, Bruening A, et al. Response of refractory colitis to intravenous or oral tracolimus (FK506). Inflamm Bowel Dis. 2002;8:317–24.
39. Lao D 2nd, Chiang T, Gomez E. Refractory clostridium difficile infection successfully treated with tigecycline, rifaximin, and vancomycin. Case Rep Med. 2012;2012:702910.
40. van Nood E, Vrieze A, Nieuwdorp M, Fuentes S, Zoetendal EG, de Vos WM, et al. Duodenal infusion of donor feces for recurrent Clostridium difficile. N Engl J Med. 2013;368:407–15.
41. Papaconstantinou HT, Thomas JS. Bacterial colitis. Clin Colon Rectal Surg. 2007;20:18–27.
42. Tjandra JJ. Toxic colitis and perforation. In: Michelassi F, Milsom JW, editors. Operative strategies in inflammatory bowel disease. New York: Springer-Verlag; 1999. p. 234–45.
43. Park SC, Jeon HM, Kim JS, Kim WW, Kim KW, Oh ST, et al. Toxic amebic colitis coexisting with intestinal tuberculosis. J Korean Med Sci. 2000;15:708–11.
44. Lamontagne F, Labbe AC, Haeck O, Lesur O, Lalancette M, Patino C, et al. Impact of emergency colectomy on survival of patients with fulminant Clostridium difficile colitis during an epidemic caused by a hypervirulent strain. Ann Surg. 2007;245:267–72.
45. Pépin J, Valiquette L, Cossette B. Mortality attributable to nosocomial Clostridium difficile-associated disease during an epidemic caused by a hypervirulent strain in Quebec. CMAJ. 2005;173:1037–42.

## Further Reading

De Simone B, Davies J, Chouillard E, et al. WSES-AAST guidelines: management of inflammatory bowel disease in the emergency setting. World J Emerg Surg. 2021;16:23.

Hurst R, Stein SL, Michelassi F. Fulminant ulcerative colitis. Gastrointestinal tract and abdomen. Scientific American Surgery. Decker Intellectual Properties Inc.; 2009. https://doi.org/10.2310/7800.S05C13.

Kedia S, Ahuja V, Tandon R. Management of acute severe ulcerative colitis. World J Gastrointest Pathophysiol. 2014;5:579–88.

Márquez MF, Martínez ÁH, Duarte ÁR, CobiánRR. Current status of the treatment of fulminant colitis. Cir Esp. 2015;93:276–82.

Neal MD, Alverdy JC, Hall DE, Simmons RL, Zuckerbraun BS. Diverting loop ileostomy and colonic lavage: an alternative to total abdominal colectomy for the treatment of severe, complicated Clostridium difficile associated disease. Ann Surg. 2011;254:423–7.

Portela F, Lago P. Fulminant colitis. Best Pract Res Clin Gastroenterol. 2013;27:771–82.

Sartelli M, Coimbra R, Pagani L, Rasa K, editors. Infections in surgery prevention and management. Cham: Springer Nature Switzerland AG; 2021.

# Clostridium Infections

# 84

Giada Fasani, Angela Pieri, and Leonardo Pagani

**Learning Goals**
The aim of this chapter is to provide stronger knowledge on risk factors for the onset of *Clostridioides difficile* infection, especially in healthcare setting; to update the microbiological basis of toxin production and identification, and current methods of lab diagnosis; how to prevent or tackle the spread of the infection within facilities and how to treat it with old or newer drug treatment options, exploring also the current opportunity offered by non-pharmacological alternatives.

## 84.1 Introduction

*Clostridioides difficile* (CD) is an anaerobic, fastidious, spore-forming, toxigenic gram-positive bacillus, which colonizes the large intestine of humans, domestic, and wild mammals [1, 2].

First identified in 1935 as *Bacillus difficilis* in the fecal flora of healthy newborns, it remained unrecognized as a cause of human infection until 1977, when it was identified as the predominant bacterial cause of antibiotic-associated diarrhea and pseudomembranous colitis [3, 4].

Formerly known as *Clostridium difficile*, it was officially renamed in 2016 to highlight the taxonomic differences between this specie and other members of the *Clostridium* genus [4]; it remains the major cause of healthcare-associated diarrhea [5–7] and it has progressively become the most commonly identified cause of healthcare-associated infection in adults in the United States [8].

Furthermore, the rates of death are rising and *Clostridium difficile* has become both the leading cause of antibiotic-associated diarrhea in long-term care setting and a major community pathogen [5, 6, 8, 9]: the infection occurs also in populations that were previously considered to be at low risk, such as young or healthy persons living in the community, and peripartum women [9].

Because of the lack of resistance to colonization of the newborn and infant fecal flora, 60–70%

G. Fasani
Antimicrobial Stewardship Program, Bolzano Central Hospital, Bolzano, Italy

Division of Infectious Diseases, Department of Diagnostics and Public Health, University of Verona, Verona, Italy

A. Pieri
Division of Infectious Diseases, Bolzano Central Hospital, Bolzano, Italy

L. Pagani (✉)
Antimicrobial Stewardship Program, Bolzano Central Hospital, Bolzano, Italy

Division of Infectious Diseases, Bolzano Central Hospital, Bolzano, Italy
e-mail: lpagani.id@gmail.com

© The Author(s), under exclusive license to Springer Nature Switzerland AG 2023
F. Coccolini, F. Catena (eds.), *Textbook of Emergency General Surgery*,
https://doi.org/10.1007/978-3-031-22599-4_84

of healthy infants are asymptomatic carriers of *C. difficile* during the first year of life [2, 10].

The organism is spread via the oral-fecal route: potential reservoirs include asymptomatic carriers, infected patients, the contaminated environment, and animal intestinal tract (canine, feline, porcine, avian) [4].

To increase comparability between clinical settings, the use of available standardized case definitions is mandatory: *C. difficile* infections (CDI) are commonly divided into healthcare-associated and community-associated CDI [8].

### 84.1.1 Healthcare-Associated CDI (HCA-CDI)

HCA-CDI are characterized by symptom onset at least 48 hours after hospital admission [11].

Given the major impact of this infections, even institutions with limited resources should conduct regular surveillance [8].

In this setting, the transmission of the spores occurs primarily via the contaminated hands of health-care workers (HCWs); anyway, environmental contamination (e.g., beds, doors, baths, food utensils) and medical devices can also be involved [1].

### 84.1.2 Community-Associated (CA-) CDI

CA-CDI was first described in the 1980s in patients who received antibiotics in the outpatient setting [11].

Since then, many classifications have been proposed; widely accepted is the one suggested in 2007 by the Centers for Disease Control and Prevention (CDC): symptom onset in the community or within 48 h after admission to a healthcare institution provided that symptom onset was more than 12 weeks after the last discharge from a healthcare institution [1, 11].

The incidence has almost doubled in the last 20 years and in the United States approximately half of all cases can nowadays be considered community-acquired [11].

Although affected individuals are often asymptomatic and younger (also infants) [1, 11], the predominant ribotypes correspond with those isolated in hospital, suggesting a strong interconnection between the two settings [1].

As the awareness among physicians is low and laboratories infrequently examine stool samples from community patients to identify *C. difficile*, the disease often goes unrecognized and undiagnosed [5, 11].

### 84.1.3 Indeterminate and Unknown CDI

Cases that do not fit the above criteria (e.g., symptom onset in the community but patient discharged from the same or another healthcare institution within 12 weeks before symptom onset) can be defined as indeterminate. When the exposure setting cannot be determined because of lack of available data, the case is defined "unknown" [11].

### 84.1.4 Pediatric Setting

Around 70% of asymptomatic neonates may be colonized with toxin-producing *C. difficile* in the first months of life, perhaps due to the lack of receptors for *C. difficile* toxin in their immature intestine or due to their overall immature immune response [10].

The infants who are exclusively breast-fed show significantly less frequent colonization with *C. difficile* [10].

The disease is typically mild, and severe complications rarely occur in children [10].

## 84.2 Epidemiology

Until 2000s, *Clostridioides difficile* infections were described only in sporadic cases [3]; in the following 10 years, these infections have progressively become a global health challenge as a consequence of a dramatic worldwide increase in incidence and severity [1].

After the international peak recorded in 2010, CDI rates have declined remarkably in many European countries, while this positive trend has gone slower in the United States [8].

In the United States, an estimated 450,000 cases of *C. difficile* infection occurred in 2011, resulting in approximately 30,000 deaths [5, 8, 12]. The estimated burden of CDI decreased in the US between 2011 and 2017, probably as a result of improved infection control measures and concomitant overall decline of healthcare-associated infections [5].

About 345,000 cases occur outside the hospital, with almost half of them considered purely community-associated. Anyway, the most of these patients present close contacts with healthcare services (e.g., a visit in an outpatient healthcare setting) [5].

Epidemiological data are scarcer in Europe. The lack of a standardization of diagnostic procedures in hospitals, as well as the heterogeneity in the presence and the methodology of national surveillance, and the availability of molecular typing, hinders a more accurate overview of the burden of CDI [5].

In 2008, a study involving 34 European countries showed an overall incidence of 4.1 per 10,000 patient-days per hospital [5].

In 2012, the European Centre for Disease Prevention and Control (ECDC) reported that 48% of in-hospital gastrointestinal infections, and 7.7% of all healthcare-associated infections were due to CDI, concluding that CD is the eighth most frequent pathogen causing nosocomial infections [3].

Between 2016 and 2017, it was the sixth most frequent responsible for healthcare-associated infections, with an annual estimated number of cases of 189,256 [5].

In 2016, the EUCLID study (European, multicenter, prospective, biannual, point-prevalence study of CDI in hospitalized patients with diarrhea) reported that the CDI rate in Europe was 7.0 cases per 10,000 patient-days with wide differences among countries [3].

Due to the lack of clinical suspicion or suboptimal laboratory methods, about 23% of all positive CDI samples are not diagnosed. As a result, an estimated 40,000 inpatients are potentially undiagnosed per year [5].

CDI is a potentially severe complication among patients hospitalized also in Italian Internal Medicine wards [13]. A study conducted in nine hospitals of an Italian Local Health Authority between 2010 and 2015 showed an overall incidence of 3.7/10,000 patients-days: the majority were HCA-CDI (86.1%) and many patients presented both comorbidities (91.1%) and antibiotic exposure (76.2%) [14].

## 84.3 027 Ribotype

Outbreaks of infection characterized by major clinical severity, high relapse rate, and significant mortality have been described both in North America and in Europe in the last 15 years [1, 9, 10, 15].

The responsible is a hypervirulent strain of *C. difficile* identified in 2001. It is known as polymerase chain reaction (PCR)-ribotype 027 (North American pulsed-field gel electrophoresis type 1 (NAP1), or restriction endonuclease analysis group BI) [1–3, 15].

The increased virulence is thought to be associated with a single base pair deletion at position 117 of the *tcdC* gene [15]: it may lead to an increased and prolonged production of toxins (about 16 and 23 times for toxin A and B, respectively) [11, 15] and likely to the production of a binary toxin [15].

Initially reported in Canada, with the Quebec having been heavily affected [15, 16], it rapidly spread throughout North America and Europe [4, 5, 15] and became a major strain, responsible for almost half of CDI cases [3, 5].

In 2005, after the first important outbreaks in Europe [3], many countries developed surveillance studies about the rapid spread of this ribotype [15].

Clinical presentation is worrisome: it has been associated with increased disease severity, recurrences, poor response to metronidazole and fluoroquinolone therapy, and consequent significant higher death rate [1, 3].

A rise in the number of cases of fulminant colitis associated with multiple organ failure has also been demonstrated [1].

In the United States, it remains one of the most commonly identified strains especially involved in HCA-CDIs [8].

Even though its prevalence is decreasing in Europe [1, 5], the emergence of another virulent strain, named ribotype 078, has been reported first in the Netherlands [2, 5, 11], and then also in some other countries [15]. Often found in swine and cattle, it owns both severity pattern and virulence factors similar to the ones typical of ribotype 027 [5, 15].

## 84.4 Risk Factors

Although mostly related to the overuse and abuse of antibiotics [3], many other risk factors can be involved in infection onset and the major factors are host predisposing factors, exposure to spores, and colonic microbiome disruption [1].

### 84.4.1 Host Predisposing Factors

1. *Age*: patients aged 65 years and over present a five to tenfold increased risk of infection. They are also at risk of poor clinical outcome including severity and mortality [4].
2. *Comorbidities*: immunodeficiency (specifically malignant neoplasms, chemotherapy and transplantations), gastrointestinal diseases (inflammatory bowel diseases, malnutrition, obesity specifically with body mass index [BMI] ≥35), AIDS, diabetes mellitus, chronic kidney diseases, respiratory, and cardiovascular diseases and anemia [1, 4] are the most commonly associated comorbidities. The higher risk can be related not only with the concomitant illnesses themselves but also with the more frequent hospitalizations and antibiotic treatments [1].
3. *Gender*: females present a not clearly explained higher risk [1].

### 84.4.2 Exposure to Spores

The longer the hospital stay, the higher the risk [1]: after a month, up to 50% of patients in many hospital settings are colonized [4] and hospitalization history within 12 weeks is considered one of the main risk factors [5].

Because of persistent spore survival in the environment (it can last several months), toilets, clinic furnishings, phones, and medical devices (thermometers, stethoscopes) should be all considered as reservoirs [4].

Anyway, hands of healthcare personnel still represent the major risk factor for hospitalized people [4].

### 84.4.3 Colonic Microbiome Disruption

The main protective barrier against CDI is the normal intestinal microflora [4]: it ensures a direct inhibition of other pathogens through bacteriocins production, nutrient depletion, and host immune defenses stimulation [1]. Bacteroides and Firmicutes seem to play the major role in immunological responses against *C. difficile* [2, 4].

Gut microbiome diversity reduction or even its disruption is often a direct consequence of antibiotic therapy [1], even if relatively short: the treatment might dramatically reduce the amount of intestinal microbiota and a complete recovery may last several months [3, 4].

Although enteral nutrition is helpful in maintaining mucosal integrity, enterally-fed patients are more prone to develop CDI, probably as a consequence of a prolonged use of elemental diets responsible for the suppression of colonic fermentation that may contribute to normal gut flora disruption [1].

Finally, bile acids could also play a role: on the one side the primary bile acids, cholesterol derivatives produced and transformed in the liver are involved in spore germination; on the other side, secondary bile acids seem to inhibit this process. Although some recent studies have shown that there is a higher concentration of secondary bile acids in feces of healthy people and a higher concentration of primary bile in feces of patients with recurrent CDI, a full comprehension of the exact mechanism is still lacking [4].

### 84.4.4 Antibiotic Exposure

In 1974, Tedesco et al. published a prospective study of clindamycin-associated colitis, which was endemic in many hospitals, showing that 21% of patients treated with clindamycin developed diarrhea often associated with a severe intestinal damage [1, 4].

It is now well known that the risk for CDI development is six- to tenfold higher during antimicrobial therapy and in the subsequent month afterwards [1, 4]. The longer the treatment, the higher the risk: it strongly rises after 10 days [1]. However, the risk cannot be fully rule out even for short antibiotic courses, nor for single-dose surgical antibiotic prophylaxis [1, 3].

Although nearly all antibiotics have been associated with CDI, broad-spectrum antibiotics (specifically clindamycin, third-generation cephalosporins, penicillins, and fluoroquinolones) pose the greatest risk [1, 3, 4].

### 84.4.5 Other Medications

Exposure to gastric acid-suppressive medications, such as histamine-2 blockers and PPIs, may be a potential risk factor, specifically when antibiotics are administered concomitantly [1].

PPIs increase the pH of the stomach, which is barrier to ingested bacteria [3] but the explanation is not easy because acid gastric do not kill the spores. A possible explanation is that the vegetative forms play a more important pathogenic role than anticipated [17].

According to some studies, also nonsteroidal anti-inflammatory drugs (NSAIDs) may also be linked to the development of CDI [3].

### 84.4.6 Surgery

Colectomy, small-bowel, or gastric resection and lower-extremity amputation are associated with the highest risk of CDI. The risk is higher in case of emergency procedures [1], whereas gynecological and endocrine surgeries apparently present the lowest rates [1]; the role of appendectomy and bariatric surgery is still debated [1].

However, CDI development in surgical patients is more likely associated with common risk factors (e.g., antibiotic consumption and fragile patients) than with surgery itself [1].

### 84.4.7 Risk Factors for CA-CDI

While the potential role of environmental contamination (e.g., food and water) in the onset or transmission of *C. difficile* in the community setting is still debated [1], broad-spectrum antibiotic exposure [1, 11], emergency department visit [1], strict contacts with farms and livestock [11], comorbidities (cardiac disease, chronic kidney disease, IBD, hematologic malignancy, diabetes mellitus), and acid suppression medicaments [1] have been identified as the most common risk factors for acquisition of *C. difficile* outside the healthcare system [1, 11].

Finally, despite the presence of similar strains shared between humans and animals, transmission from animals has never been identified as a major transmission source to humans [10].

## 84.5 Clinical Features

Although the incubation period has never been precisely defined, it should be about 2–3 days or slightly longer [4].

Symptoms typically develop within the first 5–10 days after antibiotic exposure; however, they can present from the first day of antibiotic administration to 6 weeks after the end of the treatment [18].

CDI can present as a spectrum of symptoms: patients may even be asymptomatic, but the most typical feature is a mild, self-limiting diarrhea possibly associated with fever, abdominal pain, cramps, and abdominal distension [1].

Illness can also progress becoming more severe and presenting as a fulminant colitis or a toxic megacolon, which can lead to dehydration, bowel perforation, sepsis, or multi-organ failure [1, 4, 8], requiring prompt surgical intervention and intensive care unit admission [3].

The basis for this range of clinical manifestations is not fully understood, but it is likely related to host-pathogen interactions [1].

Most patients can spontaneously recover after 5–10 days of antibiotic therapy withdrawing [4].

Mortality rate directly due to CDI is estimated at 5%, whereas mortality associated with CDI complications reaches 15–25%, and up to 34% in intensive care units [4].

In the following paragraphs, we briefly describe the different possible scenarios.

### 84.5.1 Asymptomatic Patients

Asymptomatic colonization occurs when *C. difficile* is detected in the absence of symptoms of infection [1].

Among healthy adults, the prevalence ranges between 0% and 15% [1, 19]. The proportion is slightly higher (3–26%) in hospitalized patients [5]. As already explained, even 60–70% of infants can be colonized [4].

Although at higher risk of progressive disease [1, 5], only 25–30% of colonized patients will develop diarrhea [4].

Long-standing asymptomatic colonization with not toxinogenic strains could have a protective effect both for the presence of humoral immunity against toxins and for the nutrient competition [1, 5].

However, some mechanisms might trigger toxin production by a capable strain and the conversion of a non-toxigenic strain to a toxin producer by horizontal transfer might be also possible [1].

In any case, asymptomatic colonized individuals can still act as an infection reservoir, playing a role in spore shedding into the environment, responsible for secondary infection among patients [1, 3, 10].

### 84.5.2 Mild-to-Moderate CDI

Mild disease is defined as non-bloody, watery, self-limiting diarrhea possibly accompanied by abdominal pain, cramps, fever, and leukocytosis [1, 11].

Other non-specific signs and symptoms include nausea, malaise, hypoalbuminemia, and lower gastrointestinal tract bleeding. No systemic symptoms are usually present [11].

Profuse diarrhea, abdominal distension with consequent pain, fever, tachycardia, and oliguria are signs of progression to moderate or even severe disease [11].

If prolonged, the disease may result in altered electrolyte balance and dehydration [11].

Although this is the typical presentation of CA-CDI, approximately 40% require hospitalization: severity has usually been linked to hypervirulent ribotypes 027 and 078, both linked to poorer outcomes [11].

### 84.5.3 Severe CDI

Despite a wide variety of severity predictors has been described, international consensus for the definition of severe CDI is still lacking [1].

It is characterized by the presence of severe systemic symptoms and signs such as renal failure, hemodynamic instability with vasopressor requirement, and cardiopulmonary failure requiring mechanical ventilation [20, 21].

In 2014, the European Society for Clinical Microbiology and Infectious Diseases (ESCMID) defined "severe disease" as an episode of CDI with one or more specific signs and symptoms of severe colitis or a complicated course of disease, with significant systemic toxin effects and shock, resulting in need for ICU admission, colectomy, or death. White blood cells (WBCs) >15,000 cell/mm, hypoalbuminemia (<3 g/dL) and rise in serum creatinine level (≥133 μM/L or ≥1.5 times the premorbid level) can likely be present [2–4].

More recently, the guidelines of the Infectious Diseases Society of America (IDSA) used criteria based on expert opinion, defining a severe disease only by the presence of WBCs >15,000 cell/mm$^3$ or serum creatinine level >1.5 mg/day [3].

Another possible definition, known as ATLAS, combines five simple and commonly available clinical and laboratory variables: Age, antibiotic Treatment, Leucocyte count, serum Albumin, and Serum creatinine levels [1, 5].

Temperature (specifically, 38 °C or over) [1], bowel movements (specifically more than 10 per day), and severe abdominal pain [8] are also included as predictors in some definitions.

### 84.5.4 Fulminant CDI

The progression to fulminant *C. difficile* colitis is relatively infrequent (3–8% of all CDI), but it is well known to have a high mortality rate (35–80%) [1, 22].

Many scores to predict the probability to develop a fulminant CDI can be found in the literature but none is universally accepted [1].

Predictive clinical and laboratory features include age (>70 years), prior CDI, leukocytosis (>20,000–25,000/mm$^3$), hemodynamic instability with admission to intensive care unit [1, 4], serum lactate levels >3–5 mmol/L, or any evidence of severe organ failure [4, 23].

Mortality rate in this setting is high because of the possible development of hypotension or hypovolemic shock, ileus, toxic megacolon with colonic perforation, peritonitis, septic shock, and subsequent organ dysfunction [1, 3, 8].

Neither absence of diarrhea nor changes in mental status should be underestimated because the first can be a sign of progression and the second of significant toxemia [1].

Although characterized by high morbidity and mortality rates, the surgical timing is controversial because of the lack of clear factors to guide surgical decisions: a gray zone is present between the medically treatable and the surgery requiring cases [22].

### 84.5.5 Toxic Megacolon

Toxic megacolon is characterized by radiological signs of distension of the colon (> 6 cm in transversal width of colon) associated with the signs of systemic toxicity such as hemodynamic instability, marked elevated WBCs (>25,000/mm$^3$), hypoalbuminemia, and need of cardiorespiratory support [3]. These patients must immediately undergo evaluation for surgical intervention [3].

### 84.5.6 Cure

Initial cure is defined as disappearance of diarrhea for 2 consecutive days after completion of standard-of-care antibiotic therapy. Sustained (or global) cure is defined as initial clinical cure of the baseline episode of CDI and no recurrent infection through 12 weeks' follow-up [6].

## 84.6 Mechanism of Action

The ingested spores survive the acidic environment of the stomach and germinate into vegetative bacteria in the small intestine once exposed to bile acids [1, 3, 4].

The pathogen is not invasive; its virulence is mostly due to enzymes (collagenase, hyaluronidase, chondroitin-sulfatase) and toxins [3, 4].

Because the gut can act as a reservoir for *C. difficile*, it can both facilitate spread among patients and contribute to the high recurrence rates [1].

## 84.7 Toxins

Most disease-causing strains secrete two exotoxins, toxins A (an enterotoxin) and B (a cytotoxin), the primary virulence factors [1, 4, 24].

These toxins share a common molecular mechanism of action: once transported into the cytoplasm, they promote the inactivation of Rho GTPases through their irreversible glycosylation, leading to disorganization of the cytoskeleton, cell death, disruption of tight junctions, and neutrophil adhesion [1–4, 24].

The net effect of this severe inflammation and of the gut barrier integrity breakdown is a rapid fluid loss into the intestinal lumen, with onset of diarrhea as direct consequence [24]. In more severe cases, microulcerations covered with pseudomembranes (composed of destroyed intestinal cells, neutrophils, and fibrin) occur on the intestinal mucosal surface [4].

The respective roles and importance of toxins A and B remain contentious: although toxin A was thought to be the major virulence factor for many years, toxin B probably plays the most important role [1, 24].

All toxigenic strains contain TcdB, with or without the presence of TcdA [2]: TcdA+/TcdB− mutants are attenuated in virulence in comparison to the wild-type (TcdA+/TcdB+) strain, whereas TcdA−/TcdB+ mutants are fully virulent [24].

TcdB alone is associated with both severe localized intestinal and systemic organ damage, suggesting that this toxin might be both responsible for the onset of multiple organ dysfunction syndrome (MODS) and the primary factor inducing the host innate immune and inflammatory responses [24]. Moreover, toxins seem to be involved also in CDI extra-intestinal effects [1].

Many human and animal strains, including ribotype 027, produce a third toxin, known as binary toxin (CDT), encoded by the *cdtA* and *cdtB* genes [4, 24], whose specific role remains debated; however, it could be involved in adherence and colonization of *C. difficile* and it may also own an ADP-ribosyltransferase function, which leads to actin depolymerization [1, 2, 4, 24]. Thanks to two mutations in the toxin regulatory gene tcdC, the production of toxins A and B is markedly increased [4].

Finally, it has recently been demonstrated that human serum albumin acts as a "buffer system" by binding *C. difficile* toxins A and B in the blood vessels impairing their internalization into host cells; in severe CDI characterized by hypoalbuminemia, it cannot neutralize all *C. difficile* toxins, leading to severe toxemia [1, 22].

Considering the major role played by toxins, it is easy to guess why non-toxigenic *C. difficile* strains are non-pathogenic [1].

## 84.8 Recurrences

Recurrent CDI (rCDI) is defined as reappearance of symptoms within 8 weeks after the onset of a previous episode, provided that the symptoms from that episode have completely resolved and after exclusion of any other possible diagnostic hypothesis [1, 6]. As many as 10–30% of patients develop recurrence after a first CDI episode [1, 8].

For a patient with 1–2 previous episodes, the risk of further recurrences is 40–65% [1, 4, 9]: about half of the recurrent CDI cases are due to relapses of infection with the original strain caused by resident spores' germination, whereas the other half is caused by re-infection with different strains [1, 4].

Persisting dysbiosis often associated with impaired immune response to toxins on one side and new exposure to spores in high risk setting on the other are the main responsible for these recurrences [4, 6, 8].

Recurrent infections can be less severe than the first episode at onset [1], but they are often difficult to treat with consequent higher hospitalization-rate and costs, and more severe outcomes than the first episode [25].

Patients who can't stop antibiotic therapy for infections other than CDI are at higher risk of recurrences (mostly under fluoroquinolone treatment) [1]. Whenever possible, antibiotics strongly linked to CDI onset should be stopped and antibiotic treatment continued with agents less frequently involved, such as parenteral aminoglycosides, sulfonamides, macrolides, vancomycin, or tetracycline/tigecycline [1, 4].

The identification of patients at the greatest risk is the key for preventing recurrent infection: age (particularly older than 65 years), hospital exposure, comorbid conditions, severe underlying illnesses, concomitant receipt of antacid medications, hypoalbuminemia, impaired humoral immunity, poor quality of life, disease severity, and previous recurrent CDI are among major risk factors [1].

## 84.9 Diagnosis

CDI is defined by clinical signs and symptoms (specifically the presence of new-onset diarrhea) in combination with laboratory tests capable to identify free toxins or to demonstrate the presence of toxigenic *C. difficile* in a stool sample [1, 8]. They could be either a stool test positive for toxins or the detection of toxigenic *C. difficile*. Colonoscopic or histopathologic findings revealing pseudomembranous colitis are also considered affordable [8].

Since *C. difficile* can colonize the intestinal tract of healthy individuals, diagnostic testing for CDI should be performed only on diarrheic stools from symptomatic patients [1].

CDI should be suspected in patients with acute diarrhea (defined as a stool frequency of three or more loose stools per day, corresponding to Bristol stool chart types 5–7) with no obvious alternative explanation (such as laxative use), particularly in the setting of relevant risk factors [1, 3, 8].

For patients with ileus who may be unable to produce stool specimens, collection of perirectal swabs provides an acceptable alternative [1, 3].

The optimal approach for the diagnosis of CDI is still debated [3], and in the next paragraphs, we briefly describe the major available laboratory techniques.

### 84.9.1 Glutamate Dehydrogenase (GDH)

GDH is an enzyme produced by *C. difficile* in relatively larger amounts than toxins [1].

Enzyme immunoassay (EIA) and rapid tests such as LFA (15–30 min) present high sensitivity and specificity for its the detection [5].

A positive assay only documents the presence of *C. difficile* but does not discriminate between toxigenic and non-toxigenic strains (about 20% of the *C. difficile* population) [1, 4].

Therefore, a second test for toxin production is necessary for confirmation. GDH screening tests for C. *difficile* used in association with toxin A/B enzyme immunoassays (EIA) testing give an accurate test result quickly even if the sensitivity of such strategy is lower than NAATs [1].

### 84.9.2 Toxins

EIA for toxin A/B is fast (around 30 min to 4 h), easy-to-use, convenient, and inexpensive [1, 5].

It owns high specificity (95–100%), but it is not recommended alone due to its relatively low sensitivity (75–85%) [1, 4, 5].

Proper management in the pre-analytical phase is extremely important, as the toxin present in a stool sample is easily degraded at room temperature, and after about 2 h, it can be no longer detected in the acquired material. Once the stool sample is obtained, it should be stored at refrigerator temperature (+4 °C) and used for testing within 24 h [4].

### 84.9.3 Nucleic Acid Amplification Tests (NAATs)

Used since the early 1990s, nucleic acid amplification tests (NAAT) for *C. difficile* toxin genes, are characterized by excellent sensitivity and specificity, low complexity, and improved turnaround time. Therefore, they are considered the standard diagnostic test for CDI [1].

There are several commercially available NAATs such as a real-time PCR (RT-PCR) assay and loop-mediated isothermal amplification (LAMP) assay, both of which have an overall high analytical sensitivity (80–100%) and specificity (87–99%) [4].

Currently available NAAT assays are only qualitative (positive or negative) and cannot characterize the bacterial load and the viability of CD [5].

As a direct consequence of its high sensitivity, this test is unable to accurately distinguish between colonization and active disease or between alive and death bacteria, which may result in overdiagnosis and overtreatment, and in delaying recognition of other causes of diarrheal illness [1, 5].

Actually, PCR detects the presence of a toxin encoding gene, thus confirms the presence of *C. difficile* toxin-producing strain, but it does not necessarily mean that the strain produces any toxins at the moment [4].

Therefore, it should be performed only in patients with high suspicion for CDI and normally it is included in two-step algorithm [1, 8].

Anyway, some NAATs such as multiplex ones can simultaneously detect *C. difficile* strains and toxin encoding genes from stool samples [1].

Most NAAT assays detect only the toxin A/B encoding genes *tcdA* and/or *tcdB*, which are usually sufficient for the diagnosis. Some NAAT assays (e.g., Verigene, Xpert *C. difficile*) can also detect the binary toxin genes (*cdt*) and the deletion at nucleotide position 117 on the regulatory *tcdC* gene typical of ribotype 027 strains and of other related strains. This allows also a more stringent healthcare surveillance system [5].

The high cost and the already explained interpretation difficulties are the major limits of this technique [4].

### 84.9.4 Culture

Although long considered gold standard methods according to their sensitivity, toxigenic culture (TC) and cell cytotoxicity assays (CCA) are nowadays rarely performed as a routine diagnostic test as a consequence of their slow turnaround time (about 48–72 h), complexity, and lack of standardization [1, 4, 5].

The procedure, performed only by expert microbiologists, includes stool culture on a selective differential medium (e.g., cycloserine-cefoxitin-fructose agar, or CCFA) and then a specific assay to test the ability of the colonies to produce toxins [1].

### 84.9.5 Best Diagnostic Method: Algorithm

According to the fact that no single technique is suitable as a stand-alone test, diagnostic algorithms have become mandatory [1, 4, 5, 26].

Recently, both ESCMID and IDSA guidelines have recommended to use a two- or three wise-step algorithms [2, 3, 5, 8, 13].

Possible multistep algorithms are glutamate dehydrogenase [GDH] plus toxin; GDH plus toxin, arbitrated by nucleic acid amplification test [NAAT]; or NAAT plus toxin [8].

First of all, a screening test with high sensitivity and negative predictive value (NPV), e.g., NAAT or GDH tests, should be performed [1, 4].

If negative, it excludes CDI [4].

If positive, it should be followed by a more specific test with high positive predictive value (PPV) to confirm the diagnosis, e.g., ELISA detecting free toxins [3, 5].

If both positive, the diagnosis is confirmed [3–5].

In case of negativity of the second test, accurate clinical evaluation is mandatory because three scenarios are possible:

1. Real CDI infection with toxin levels below the threshold of detection
2. Carriage of a toxinogenic strain (without active toxin-production)
3. False-negative toxin A/B EIA result (uncommon) [3–5]

Samples with a negative GDH result but that are positive for toxin need to be retested, as this is an invalid result [4].

Before NAAT introduction in routine diagnostic facilities, GDH positive and toxins negative tests required additional analyses usually performed by culture and toxins research: they were associated with higher sensitivity but required several days. Now a three-step algorithm is often chosen: GDH plus ELISA for free toxins followed by NAAT in case of discordance [5] (Fig. 84.1).

Marked underdiagnosis is the direct consequence of suboptimal laboratory diagnostic [3], great heterogeneity in diagnostic practices between centers, lack of robust surveillance systems in all countries [5], and low clinical suspicion in community setting [3, 5].

To improve diagnostic efficacy, not only samples with a specific physician's request but at least all submitted unformed stool samples from patients 3 year- or older should be tested for CDI [26].

On the other side, repeating tests within 7 days after a first negative sample during the same diarrheal episode may be useful only in selected cases with ongoing clinical suspicion during an epidemic situation [1]; in all other cases, it gives no additive information being only a time and money waste [8].

Despite the lack of any evidence, in critically ill patients with hemodynamic instability and without a definitive diagnosis, it might be appropriate to repeat the tests within a short timeframe (e.g., 48 h) even in patients with atypical presentations [3].

Stool from asymptomatic patients may be tested only for epidemiological surveillance [8].

### 84.9.6 Other Diagnostic Methods

Only few and discordant data are present in the literature about fecal lactoferrin or other biologic markers [8].

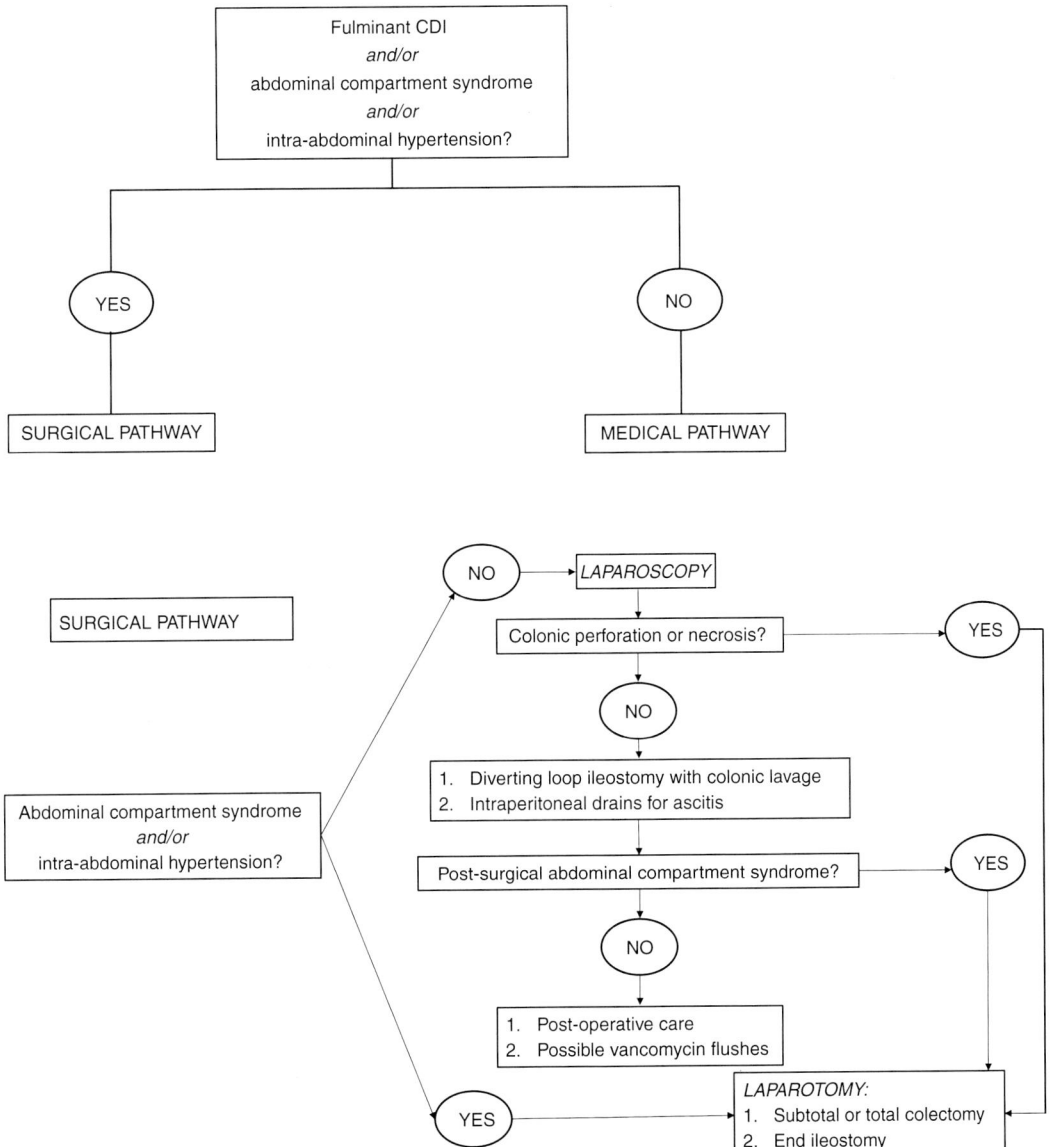

**Fig. 84.1** Three step- and two step-algorithms currently in use for diagnostic purposes

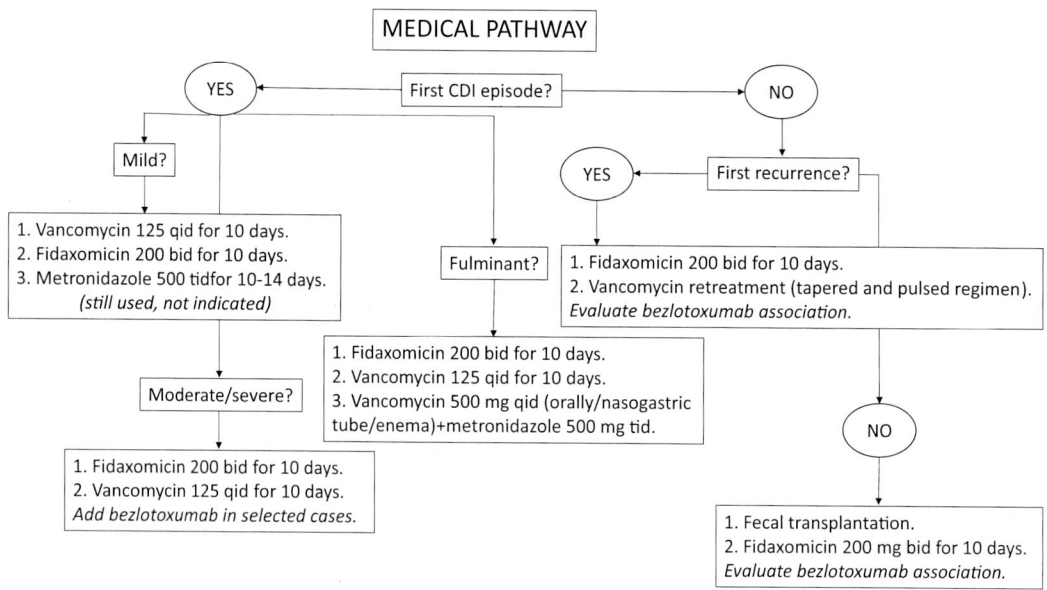

**Fig. 84.1** (continued)

## 84.9.7 Radiological Diagnostic Imaging

Computed tomography (CT) scan can both provide an early diagnosis and help assess disease severity [1].

Although considered the most common CT finding, colonic wall thickening is non-specific and can be found in other forms of colitis even if less pronounced [1, 3].

Other possible signs are dilatation, pericolonic fat stranding, "accordion sign" (high-attenuation oral contrast in the colonic lumen alternating with low-attenuation inflamed mucosa), "double-halo sign, target sign" (intravenous contrast displaying varying degrees of attenuation caused by submucosal inflammation and hyperemia), and ascites [1, 3, 27].

X-rays can reveal distended bowel loops, often with wall thickening [4], while ultrasound imaging is an especially good method of monitoring the width of colon [4] and is often used in critically ill patients who cannot be transported to the CT scan room [1]. It can evidence a thickened colonic wall with heterogeneous echogenicity as well as narrowing of the colonic lumen and hyperechoic lines covering the mucosa which are probably pseudomembranes. The presence of submucosal gaps may indicate extension of tissue damage into deeper structures and intraperitoneal free fluid is seen in more than 70% of cases [1].

## 84.9.8 Endoscopy

Even if useful for the diagnosis, flexible sigmoidoscopy should be used sparingly considering the potential risk of perforation [1]. It can be also helpful in ruling out other illnesses, especially when the stool tests are negative or clinical status worsens [3]. As a matter of fact, it is still the only method that allows the clear detection of pseudomembranes: they are elevated, white to yellow lesions, typically about 2 cm in diameter, irregularly distributed and separated by normal mucosa [4].

## 84.9.9 Laboratory Tests

High leukocytosis, elevated C-reactive protein, hypoalbuminemia, and signs of acute kidney injury are commonly found even if aspecific [4].

## 84.9.10 Diagnosis in Pediatric Setting

Because of the high prevalence of asymptomatic carriage of toxigenic *C. difficile* in infants, the more recent IDSA guidelines recommend against testing in newborns and infants <12 months with diarrhea [8, 10].

Tests should not be routinely performed in children with diarrhea who are 1–2 years of age unless other infectious or noninfectious causes have been excluded and is recommended only in case of prolonged or worsening diarrhea associated with risk factors (e.g., underlying inflammatory bowel disease or immunocompromising conditions) or relevant exposures in older children [8, 10].

## 84.10 Antibiotic Therapy

Since antibiotic therapy is the most important risk factor for the development of this disease, unnecessary antibiotic agents should be immediately discontinued: they may also decrease the clinical response and increase the risk of further recurrences [1, 3, 8, 9]. Whenever not feasible, the spectrum should be almost narrowed [3].

Empirical therapy for CDI should be avoided unless there is a strong suspicion or the results of the specific test are not available in a few hours [1, 3, 8].

In the following paragraphs, we briefly describe the different available antibiotic options.

### 84.10.1 Metronidazole

Although associated with possible side effects and treatment failures (especially in patients infected with the emergent 027/BI/NAP1 strain), oral metronidazole 500 mg three times per day for 10–14 days is often still used for treating an initial episode of mild-to-moderate CDI [1, 8].

Nausea, headache and taste aversion are common side effects [9] whereas peripheral neuropathy and irreversible neurotoxicity can be recorded in case of repeated or prolonged courses [1, 8]. Due to its potential toxicity for the fetus, metronidazole should be avoided in pregnant or breastfeeding women [4].

Both the difference in clinical cure rate for mild and moderate cases and the risk of recurrence are quite similar for patients treated with metronidazole, vancomycin or with the combination of the two drugs. Metronidazole has been proved to be inferior only in severe cases [1, 8].

Anyway, the most recent IDSA guideline, suggest choosing metronidazole only in case of an initial episode of non-severe CDI in settings where access to vancomycin or fidaxomicin is limited because, only in these cases, the higher availability and the far lower cost can represent a major advantage [1, 8].

Indeed, being efficiently absorbed, only small concentrations of this drug reach the lower gastrointestinal tract causing a pharmacodynamic disadvantage in a primarily mucosal or luminal infection: this can explain the limited effectiveness of the drug [6, 9].

### 84.10.2 Vancomycin

Because of its good concentration in the gut lumen, oral vancomycin owns superior pharmacokinetic properties compared to metronidazole and therefore it is the first-choice antibiotic in both mild-moderate and severe cases [1, 3, 28, 29].

It is also the best option for retreatment of patients with mild-moderate disease who do not respond to metronidazole [1].

The recommended dosage is 125 mg orally four times per day for 10 days [1, 8].

Above all in the ICU setting, doses of up to 500 mg four times a day orally or via enema in combination with intravenous metronidazole 500 mg three times a day have been successfully used with a reduction of the mortality rate [1, 3], although evidence is not strong [5]. It should be remarked that intravenous vancomycin has no effect on CDI, since the antibiotic is not excreted into the colon [1].

Whenever oral antibiotics cannot promptly reach the colon or if ileus is present, it may be administered per rectum every 6 h as retention enema via a large rectal tube or catheter [1, 5, 8].

In such cases, intravenous metronidazole can be administered together at the dosage of 500 mg every 8 h [8].

### 84.10.3 Fidaxomicin

Fidaxomicin (previously referred to as OPT-80), available since 2011, is a macrocyclic, bactericidal narrow spectrum-antibiotic, able to inhibit both toxin production and bacterial sporulation. Being minimally systemic absorbed and primarily directed against gram-positive pathogens, it is extremely specific with low impact on the normal gut microbiome [3, 4, 9].

The recommended dosage is 200 mg orally twice daily for 10 days [1, 8].

In vitro, it is more active than vancomycin, by a factor of approximately 8, against clinical isolates of *C. difficile*, including NAP1/BI/027 strains [9].

Both non-inferior to vancomycin for initial cure and even more effective in patients receiving concomitant antibiotics for other infections [1], fidaxomicin is also associated with a lower recurrence rate [1, 3].

Therefore, fidaxomicin is probably the best available choice for people considered at high risk for recurrence (e.g., elderly patients with multiple comorbidities who are receiving concomitant antibiotics) [1].

This drug has been already used among critically ill patients with efficacy comparable to that of general patients, even when crushed and administered via nasogastric tube [3].

Systemic side effects are uncommon [1, 9].

A significant limitation is still represented by the price [3] but a major benefit could be the elimination of additional costs for the treatment of further episodes [9].

### 84.10.4 Treatment

In 2014, the ESCMID guidelines indicated two drugs as cornerstone for CDI infection: metronidazole in non-severe and vancomycin in severe cases [4].

In the latter years, different studies outlined the vancomycin and fidaxomicin superiority over metronidazole. Therefore, in 2017, both IDSA and the Society for Healthcare Epidemiology of America (SHEA) updated their guidelines, pointing out that vancomycin and fidaxomicin should be the cornerstone of CDI treatment [3, 4, 6, 8].

In any case, clinical cure has never posed a real challenge: almost 80% of cases can be resolved both with metronidazole and vancomycin. Only in severe cases, the efficacy of metronidazole has proven limited [5].

A summary of the current treatment options is reported in Tables 84.1 and 84.2.

At this time, there are insufficient data to recommend extending the length of anti–*C. difficile* treatment beyond the indicated 10 days or restarting a drug empirically for patients who require a retreatment for another infection shortly after CDI treatment completion [5, 8] although some authors suggest extending the treatment up to 14 days whenever symptoms have not resolved [23].

### 84.10.5 Other Options

The usage of many other drugs, specifically tigecycline, rifaximin [1, 4, 6], fusidic acid, teicoplanin, and nitazoxanide has been described in the literature, but none can be currently recommended for general use and they can be considered only when standard therapeutic options have run out [1, 4].

### 84.10.6 Newer Antibiotics

1. *Surotomycin*: an orally administered, minimally absorbed semisynthetic narrow-spectrum cyclic peptide, formed by enzymatical cleavage of daptomycin able to disrupt the bacterial membrane by acting as a calcium-dependent cell membrane depolarizing agent. It has a fourfold greater in vitro potency than vancomycin with a minimal impact on intestinal microbiota [6].
2. *Cadazolid*: a bacterial protein synthesis inhibitor classified as an oxazolidinone antibiotic

**Table 84.1** Main CDI treatment options

| Drug | Indications | Dosage | Pros | Cons |
|---|---|---|---|---|
| Metronidazole | None. Anyway, still prescribed in initial mild to moderate CDI. | 500 mg tid for 10–14 days. | 1. Cheap. 2. Well-known. | 1. Higher probability of recurrences. 2. Peripheral neuropathy and irreversible neurotoxicity as possible side effects. 3. Forbidden in pregnant and breast-feeding women. |
| Vancomycin | First choice in both mild and severe CDI. | 125 mg qid for 10 days. | 1. Well-known. 2. More effective than metronidazole even in mild cases. | 1. Only orally available for CDI. 2. Less effective than fidaxomicin in reducing recurrences. |
| Fidaxomicin | FDA approved for CDI. First choice in both mild and severe CDI. First antibiotic choice in recurrences. | 200 mg bid for 10 days. | 1. Low impact on gut microbiome. 2. Almost as effective as vancomycin in mild to severe cases. 3. More effective than vancomycin in reducing recurrences. 4. Uncommon side effects. | 1. Expensive. 2. Newer than metronidazole and vancomycin; therefore less known. |
| Bezlotoxumab | Adjunctive treatment in patients at risk for rCDI. | 10 mg/kg iv once during antibiotic therapy. | Recurrence reduction. | 1. Diarrhea and nausea as common side effects. 2. Warning for patients with heart failure. 3. Expensive. |
| Fecal transplantation | Useful in case of multiple recurrences. | Several administration ways: colonoscopy/ retention enema, nasojejunal/nasoduodenal tube, capsules. | Recurrence reduction. | 1. Complicated selection of donors. 2. Laborious preparation. 3. Expensive. |

**Table 84.2** Recommended treatment regimens according to the severity of the disease

| Episode type | Indications |
|---|---|
| Mild | 1. Vancomycin 125 qid for 10 days. 2. Fidaxomicin 200 bid for 10 days. 3. Metronidazole 500 tid for 10–14 days (*still used, although no more indicated*) |
| Moderate to severe | 1. Fidaxomicin 200 bid for 10 days. 2. Vancomycin 125 qid for 10 days. *Add bezlotoxumab in selected cases.* |
| Fulminant | 1. Fidaxomicin 200 bid for 10 days. 2. Vancomycin 125 qid for 10 days. 3. Vancomycin 500 mg qid (orally/nasogastric tube/enema) + metronidazole 500 mg tid. |
| First recurrence | 1. Fidaxomicin 200 bid for 10 days. 2. Vancomycin retreatment (tapered and pulsed regimen)[a]. *Evaluate bezlotoxumab association.* |
| Multiple recurrences | 1. Fidaxomicin 200 mg bid for 10 days. 2. Fecal transplantation. *Evaluate bezlotoxumab association.* |

[a] 125 mg qid for 10 days, followed by – 125 mg tid for 1 week, then – 125 mg bid for 1 week, then – 125 mg q24h for 1 week, then – 125 mg q48h for 1 week, then – 125 mg once every third day for 1 week

although containing parts of the chemical structure of the fluoroquinolones [6].
3. *Ribaxamase*: a b-lactam cleaving enzyme, designed for oral administration concomitantly with iv b-lactam antibiotics, which acts via enzymatic degradation of excess b-lactam antibiotics in the small intestine. It could be able to reduce not only CDI incidence but also dysbiosis in gut microbiota therefore preventing recurrences [6].

### 84.10.7 Treatment of Recurrences

Metronidazole is not recommended as initial treatment of recurrent CDI as sustained response rates are lower than those with vancomycin [1, 5, 8].

Although both vancomycin and fidaxomicin are equally effective in resolving CDI symptoms, the latter is associated with a lower likelihood of CDI recurrence after a first episode [1, 5]: 15% with fidaxomicin versus 25% with vancomycin [4].

Fidaxomicin is also superior in lowering recurrent episodes in patients who experienced CDI recurrence a month after the end of treatment [4].

Antibiotic treatment for patients with more than one recurrence is complicated and still debated: fidaxomicin could be a good option as well as oral vancomycin administered with a tapered and pulsed regimen: anyway, the advantage of this scheme never been definitely proved [1, 5, 8]. A standard course of oral vancomycin followed by rifaximin is another possible option [1, 8]. Fecal transplantation (described below) seems to be the best solution.

## 84.11 Monoclonal Antibodies

Tough the level of circulating antibodies against toxin A and B has been correlated with protection against primary and recurrent *C. difficile* infection [25], the development of human monoclonal antibodies able to prevent toxins action could be another successfully strategy in both CDI management and recurrence prevention [1].

Already available, there are actoxumab against toxin A, and bezlotoxumab against toxin B [25].

Bezlotoxumab (MK-6072), a recombinant human IgG1/kappa isotype monoclonal antibody [8], binds to regions of toxin B that partially overlap with the putative receptor [6] therefore preventing the binding of the toxin to host cells [1, 6].

Data come from two double-blind, randomized, placebo-controlled, phase 3 trials, MODIFY I and MODIFY II, involving 2655 adults receiving oral standard-of-care antibiotics for primary or recurrent *C. difficile* infection: participants were randomized to receive also an infusion of bezlotoxumab (10 mg/kg of body weight), actoxumab plus bezlotoxumab (10 mg/kg each) or placebo; the administration of actoxumab alone (10 mg/kg) was interrupted after an interim analysis because of higher rates of death and serious adverse events with no clear explanation [25].

The primary end point was recurrent infection (new episode after initial clinical cure) within 12 weeks after infusion in the modified intention-to-treat population [25].

The rates of initial clinical cure were 80% with bezlotoxumab alone, 73% with actoxumab plus bezlotoxumab, and 80% with placebo; the rates of sustained cure (initial clinical cure without recurrent infection in 12 weeks) were 64%, 58%, and 54%, respectively [25].

Bezlotoxumab, responsible for the effect, was associated to a lower rate of recurrent infection than either placebo [1, 4, 5] and standard-of-care therapy [11, 25] and this effect was sustained throughout 12 weeks [25].

Actoxumab was not efficacious when given alone and provided no additional benefit when given with bezlotoxumab [11, 25].

The number of patients to treat in order to prevent a single episode of recurrent *C. difficile* infection is 10 but lower (about 6) among people aged 65 years or older and among people with previous *C. difficile* infection [25].

In 2016, the FDA approved bezlotoxumab for use as an adjunctive treatment in patients at risk for rCDI (including old age and/or use of antibiotics other than anti-CDI treatment) [1, 6] but open questions remain the exact definition of the target population and the cost-efficiency relationship [5].

Bezlotoxumab seems to be cost-effective in the following subgroups of patients: people aged 65 years and over, immunocompromised, patients with severe CDI, history of CDI in the previous 6 months [1, 5] or affected by ribotypes 027/078 [1, 5].

Its usage is limited by high cost and potential side effects: diarrhea and nausea are the most common but, although rare, an acute onset of acute heart-failure has been reported [4, 25].

## 84.12 Fecal Transplantation

The first description of fecal microbiota transplantation (FMT) comes from the traditional Chinese medicine: doctor Ge Hong (284–364 BC) applied human fecal suspension orally to patients with severe diarrhea or food poisoning. The first experiment in modern medicine was made by Eiseman in 1958: he used a fecal enema as therapy for pseudomembranous enterocolitis. Only in 1983, the procedure was officially described for the treatment of a patient affected by *C. difficile* [4].

FMT may be useful in all cases of multiple recurrences when antibiotic have failed [1, 3, 5, 8] and, with or without additional antibiotic treatment, it might also be a promising curative therapy for severe and complicated CDI [3, 6].

The procedure consists in infusion of intestinal microorganisms (in a suspension of healthy donor stool) into the gastrointestinal tract of the patient to restore gut microbiota and to normalize the bowel function [1, 3].

The donated stool is normally mixed with saline solution, homogenized, and filtrated to separate the solid parts obtaining fluid material [4].

Fecal transplant can be administrated via lower gastrointestinal tract procedures (colonoscopy, retention enema), or upper gastrointestinal tract procedures (nasojejunal/nasoduodenal tube) [1, 4]: the lower via seems to have a little superiority (95% vs 78%) [1, 5].

Administering consecutive courses of FMT following failure of first FMT may have in an incremental effect [1, 5].

Since antibiotics destroy the transplant, antibiotic withdrawal together with FMT probably have the highest rate of prevention of recurrent CDI [3, 4].

Several studies have already shown that frozen material is comparable to fresh stools: this allows to make the procedure easier, specifically for the donors [1, 5]. Stool samples can be stored at −80 °C and used during next 5–6 months. Some stool banks extend storing period for 2 years [4].

Another challenge is the use of galenics to deliver the transplant: oral capsules are as efficient as colonoscopy [1, 4, 5] and this strategy is commonly better tolerated because of its lower invasivity [1].

Being the selection of the donor very specific and complicated with significant variations among countries, an idea to simplify the procedure in the next future is to obtain artificial, not donor-related products [5].

A better understanding of the mechanism associated with success is mandatory: according to some recent studies, sterile filtrate from donor stool was sufficient to restore normal stool habits and eliminate symptoms. This suggests a potential role of bacterial cell wall components or DNA fragments, but bacteriophage could also be involved. This awareness could be the basis to favor more targeted approaches such as the manipulation of the gut microbiota implementing the safety particularly in high-risk patients [5].

Adverse events are very uncommon [1]: this procedure is highly safe also in fragile and immunocompromised patients, at least in the short-term, while long-term safety data still lack [3].

With the increased awareness of the native gut microbiome involvement in a lot of different areas (including metabolism, immunology, response to cancer therapy, lung-gut and brain-gut axis), there have been concerns about the long-term effect of transplanted stool [1, 5].

Anyway, the major possible risk associated with this procedure is the transfer of infectious pathogens to the recipient, in case of inappropriate donor screening [4].

Therefore, potential donors should be healthy, have daily formed bowel movement and be screened for bacterial, viral, and parasites infections [4].

Uncommon potential complications of FMT may be linked to delivery procedure (e.g., perforation with colonoscopy, aspiration pneumonia with upper GI administration) [4].

Although FMT has high success rates with long-term durability, few disadvantages still exist. In particular, the manipulation of feces and the classical enteral administration methods are laborious and tend to make the procedure rather unattractive for physicians and patients [1].

Widely accepted as treatment for further episodes, FMT should be compared with vancomycin (also pulsed or tapered) and to fidaxomicin (also extended pulsed) also as treatment for the first recurrence [5].

Several large "feces banks" have already been developed. In the Netherlands, treatment with FMT is organized at a national level by the "Netherlands Donor Feces Bank" at Leiden University Medical Center [4].

Beyond CDI, FMT could represent a promising strategy to another relevant issue, that are the MDR infections. By restoring the healthy gut microbiota, FMT could promote the decrease of antibiotic resistance gene expression in the gut of the patient [3].

## 84.13 Other Possible Therapies

### 84.13.1 Supportive Care

Supportive measures, including intravenous fluid resuscitation, albumin supplementation, and electrolyte replacement, should be provided to all patients with severe *C. difficile* infection [1].

Early detection of shock and aggressive management of underlying organ dysfunction are essential to improve the outcome in patients with fulminant colitis [1].

### 84.13.2 Probiotics

Considering the role of gut microbiome diversity disruption as a consequence of antibiotic treatment, the probiotic use aims to restore the normal gut flora capable to prevent *C. difficile* overgrowth [1, 10].

Limited evidence supports their use both for treatment and for prevention and the efficacy could also be both strain- and disease-specific [1]. The short-term use is probably safe in patients who are not immunocompromised or severely debilitated [1]. Probiotics are contraindicated in immunocompromised patients due to a rare but serious risk of gut translocation with consequent bacteremia, fungemia, and even sepsis [1, 10].

### 84.13.3 Intravenous Immunoglobulin

According to knowledge that the level of immune response to *C. difficile* colonization is the major determinant of the magnitude of clinical manifestations [1] and that asymptomatic carriers have high concentrations of antibodies directed against toxins, attempts with administration of passive immunization with intravenous immunoglobulins have been made with success in small case series [1, 4].

### 84.13.4 Antimotility Agents

The use of anti-peristaltic agents for the treatment of CDI should be discouraged. If anti-peristaltic agents are used to control persistent symptoms in patients with CDI, they must always be accompanied by medical therapy [1].

## 84.14 Surgical Management

Patients with severe and fulminant colitis who progress to systemic toxicity (organ failure, increased serum lactate and vasopressor requirement) need prompt surgical intervention and therefore deserve early surgical consultation [1, 8]. Surgical intervention should be performed before shock develops as a strategy to improve the outcome (source control) [1, 30].

A major problem is that surgical timing is controversial because of the lack of concrete decision-making factors: there are no reliable clinical and/or laboratory findings that can predict those patients who will respond to medical therapy and those who will need surgery [1, 22]. Indeed, some reports show that a short period of medical optimization can improve outcomes before colectomy [1]. Although optimal timing remains controversial, early intervention (within 48–72 h from the onset of systemic toxicity) is associated with a better outcome [3].

White blood cell, albumin, creatinine and body temperature are good markers which can help in rapid decision making because they can be evaluated objectively and bedside [22]. Many other factors (acute renal failure, mental status changes, or cardiopulmonary impairment) suggest the need of prompt surgical intervention, but patients are already strongly compromised at that point [1].

Resection of the entire colon should be considered to treat patients with fulminant colitis [1], colonic perforation, ischemia and when clinical conditions rapidly worsen despite correct antibiotic therapy [3].

If possible, a subtotal colectomy with preservation of the rectum can be considered [3, 8].

A conservative surgical approach associating loop ileostomy with intraoperative colonic lavage with warmed polyethylene glycol and antegrade vancomycin flushes every 6 hours for 10 days is a useful alternative to improve the outcome [1, 3, 5, 8, 31, 32].

Recent studies demonstrated no difference in in-hospital mortality for patients treated with the two different techniques [5].

> **Dos and Don'ts**
>
> **Dos**
> - Prescribe antibiotic courses only when necessary, after collection of adequate diagnostic samples; clearly indicate the reason to start antibiotics.
> - Take a time out to reassess the choice at 48–72 h, when microbiology comes back.
> - Place a definitive order of antibiotic prescription as shortest as possible.
> - Warrant any barrier precaution and optimized infection control and prevention measures.
>
> **Don'ts**
> - Avoid prolonged antibiotic courses, unless strictly mandatory (i.e., endocarditis or osteomyelitis).
> - Do not treat putative recurrence of *C. difficile* infection only on the basis of toxins results.
> - Do not go for newest treatment when simpler ones are very likely to still work.
> - Do not forget to put in place all the infection control procedures whenever indicated.

Figure 84.2 summarizes the medical or surgical pathway of CDI management, according to clinical course.

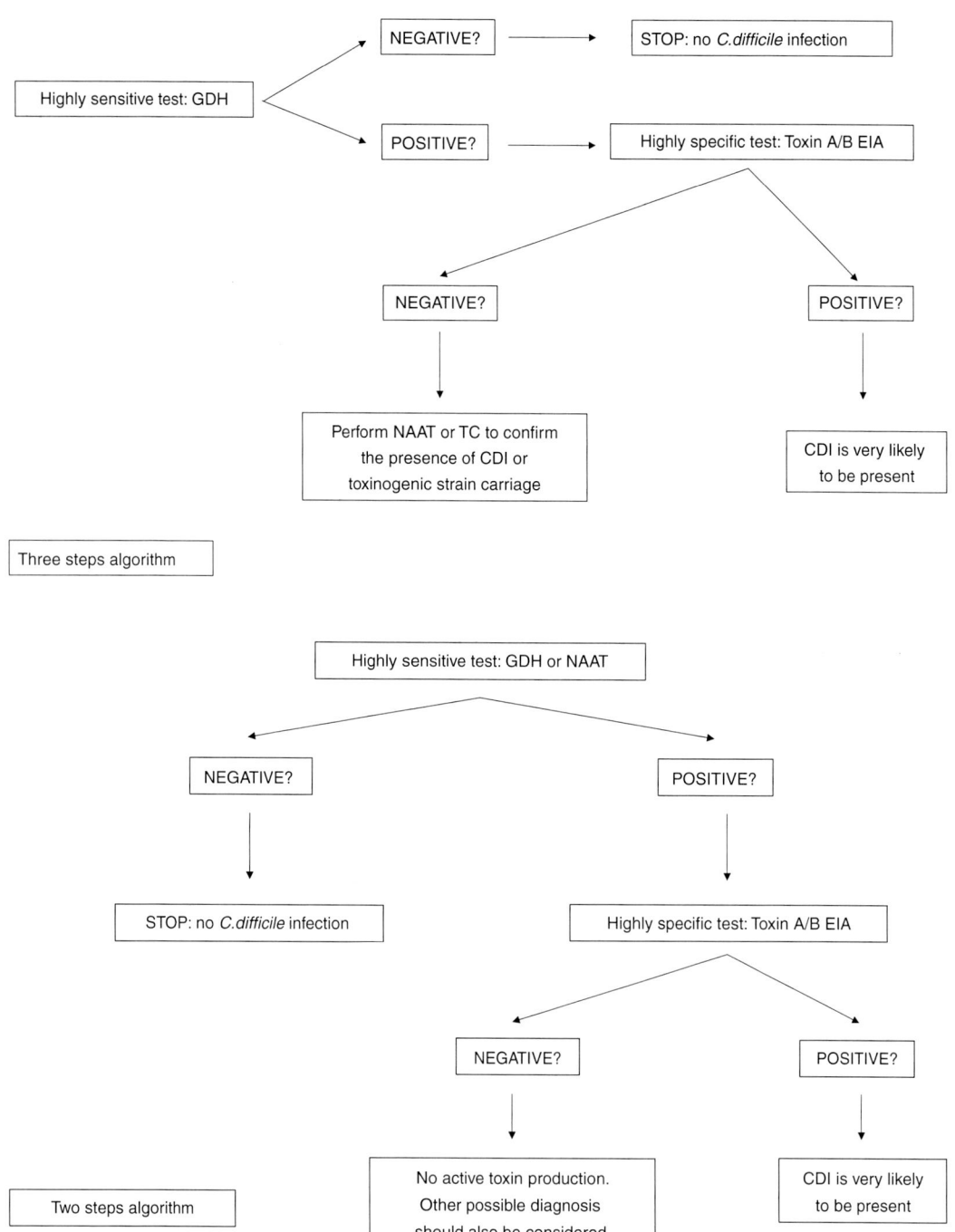

**Fig. 84.2** Medical or surgical pathway of CDI management, according to clinical course

## 84.15 Stewardship and Infection Control

Increased hospital length-of-stay, higher medical care costs, hospital re-admissions, and higher mortality rates are well-known direct consequences of CDI infection both in medical and surgical wards [1, 33].

Indeed, the rapid evolution of antibiotic resistance in *C. difficile* is a matter of concern for public health: multi-drug resistant (MDR) *C. difficile* strains are increasing (about 60% of the epidemic strains circulating in hospital settings show resistance to three or more antibiotics) [1].

Essential strategies to prevent transmission include antibiotic stewardship, contact precautions, hand hygiene, and barrier precautions (gloves and gowns), environmental cleaning. Still unclear and debated is the role of asymptomatic patients screening [1, 3].

## 84.15.1 Antibiotic Stewardship

Globally, up to 25% of antibiotic administration is not indicated [3].

Stewardship programs aim to help clinicians in limiting broad-spectrum antimicrobials prescription (e.g., cephalosporins, clindamycin, and quinolones) and in optimizing doses and duration of treatment [1, 3, 8].

Both persuasive (education and guidance) and restrictive (approval required, removal) strategies have shown to be effective [1].

## 84.15.2 Contact Precautions

*C. difficile* carriers should be promptly identified to be placed in contact (enteric) precautions in order to reduce contamination as spores can survive for months in the environment, despite regular use of environmental cleaning agents [1].

Patients should be isolated in private rooms with dedicated toilet facilities [1, 8] and priority should be accorded to those with stool incontinence when the number of rooms is limited [8].

If this possibility is over, patients may be cohorted in the same area, ensuring at the same time that they are not discordant carriers of other multidrug-resistant pathogens [8].

No indirect contact between patients (e.g., reading the same books/magazines, using the same phone) can be allowed anyway [4].

Contact (enteric) precautions should be maintained almost until the patient has diarrhea [10].

Despite the clearance of the organism from stool, residual contamination can persist in the environment and on the skin also after treatment completion [10]: therefore, it is better to maintain isolation measures for at least 48 h after symptom resolution [1, 8, 10].

Contact precautions should be prolonged until discharge if CDI rates remain high despite implementation of standard infection control measures against CDI [8].

Nearly half of the patients who respond to treatment with symptom relief continue to eliminate spores for up to 6 weeks, and some develop persistent colonization after clinical illness [10].

If there is a lag before the results are available, patients with suspected CDI infection should be placed on preemptive contact precautions [1, 8].

## 84.15.3 Hand Hygiene and Barrier Precautions (Gloves and Gowns)

Hand hygiene with soap and water is the cornerstone in *C. difficile* infection prevention [1, 3].

HCWs should perform accurate hand-hygiene before and after contact with a patient with CDI. They can use either soap and water or alcohol-based hand hygiene product [8].

The latter are highly effective against non-spore-forming organisms, but they do not damage *C. difficile* spores [1, 4, 10] whereas the mechanical hand washing with the use of running water and soap prevents the spores spread [4, 10].

Therefore, in cases of outbreaks or in hyperendemic settings, hand hygiene must be performed with soap and water. The same is valid in case of direct contact with feces or perineal region [3, 8].

Low HCWs' hand washing compliance and difficult access to sinks are major problems in infection control strategies [1].

Both health-care personnel and visitors must wear disposable gloves and gowns during care of a patient with CDI [1, 4, 8, 10].

To reduce the burden of spores on the skin, patients should wash hands regularly and bath daily [8, 10].

Whenever possible, disposable patient equipment should be used and then cleaned and disinfected with a sporicidal disinfectant if reusable [8].

## 84.15.4 Environmental Cleaning

Most disinfectants commonly used for environmental cleaning are not sporicidal and so the implementation of sodium hypochlorite solutions usage is warrant [1, 3, 4]. Spores can persist for even 5 months on the contaminated surfaces [34].

Daily to twice daily disinfection of high-touch surfaces (including bed rails) as well as terminal cleaning of rooms after patient discharge with chlorine-based products are probably the most effective interventions [1, 4, 10]. A sporicidal agent should be considered almost during endemic high rates or outbreaks, or if there is evidence of repeated cases of CDI in the same room [8, 10].

Physical wiping of surfaces can also mechanically remove spores [10].

The use of cleaning robots, such as UV light or hydrogen peroxide mist emitting devices, may have a role as adjunctive cleaning methods but they are still unable to take the place of manual cleaning [1, 10].

## 84.15.5 Screening of Asymptomatic Patients

Considering that colonization has never proved to be a direct independent precursor for CDI and that the role of asymptomatic patients in environmental contamination is controversial, screening and treatment of this population is not indicated yet [1, 4, 5, 8].

Knowing the importance of transmission trough patient and HCWs' hands and the role played by spores in the environment, limiting contamination of the hospital environment may play a crucial role in infection disease burden reduction [1, 3]. Studies show that about a quarter of all isolates from HCA-CDI are highly related to isolates from asymptomatic patients identified upon admission screening [5].

The challenge is to understand who to test: universal screening of every patient admitted or target screening of high-risk patients? [5].

Finally, the ESCMID study group for *C. difficile* (ESGCD) recently published a set of guidelines regarding measures for prevention:

1. To use personal protective equipment (gloves and gowns/disposable aprons)
2. To use contact precautions
3. To introduce daily environmental sporicidal disinfection and terminal disinfection of rooms of patients with CDI
4. To perform surveillance of CDI in combination with timely feedback of infection rates on both the hospital and ward level
5. To implement restriction protocols of antibiotic agents/classes
6. To implement protocols to reduce the duration of antibiotic therapy
7. To educate HCWs on prevention of CDI to enhance their knowledge and skills on prevention strategies [1]

## 84.15.6 Open Issues

Strong and uniform CDI definitions, standardized diagnostic algorithms, new and more objective tools to assess the response to treatment and a robust international surveillance system are strongly needed [5].

Ongoing epidemiological surveillance of cases of CDI with periodic characterization of the strains involved is also required to detect clustering of cases in time and space and to monitor the emergence of new, highly virulent clones [15].

> **Take-Home Messages**
> - *C. difficile* infection is a serious threat, especially in healthcare settings; antimicrobial misuse or abuse are the major drivers for the onset of new cases by

altering physiological gut microbiota and favoring the emergence of toxin-producing strains.
- The presence of risk factors should be clearly assessed in the presence of unexplained nosocomial diarrhea, or at referral of at-home recent antimicrobial course. Prompt diagnosis and treatment, either medical or surgical, or both, are essential to improve patients' outcome and to save lives.
- Healthcare professional should warrant optimized infection control and prevention measures and procedures to avoid the spread within hospitals and facilities.

## Questions and Answers

1. In which year was *Bacillus difficilis* identified in the fecal flora of healthy newborns, before being confirmed as human pathogen several years later?
   A. 1908
   B. **1935**
   C. 1969
   D. 1977
2. How high can the percentage of healthy infants be as asymptomatic carriers of *C. difficile* in the first year of life?
   A. Less than 5%
   B. Between 10% and 25%
   C. **60–70%**
   D. Over 90%
3. What is the name of the hypervirulent *C. difficile* PCR-ribotype that caused serious outbreaks in the last 15 years in many Western countries?
   A. X43
   B. **027**
   C. 21R
   D. 007
4. Which one among these couples of antimicrobials is much more associated with the risk of *C. difficile* infection?
   A. **Clindamycin and third generation cephalosporins**
   B. Penicillins and trimethoprim
   C. Fosfomycin and ofloxacin
   D. Daptomycin and linezolid
5. What is the name of the toxin associated with both severe localized intestinal and systemic organ damage?
   A. **TcdB**
   B. TcdA
   C. TBcd
   D. cdTA
6. What is the percentage of CA-CDI that may require hospitalization?
   A. Less than 5%
   B. Around 20%
   C. **40%**
   D. More than half of the cases
7. What is the most reliable lab procedure to diagnose *C. difficile* infection?
   A. NAAT
   B. Toxins
   C. **Diagnostic algorithms**
   D. Identification and culture
8. What are the two drugs of choice for the treatment of mild to moderate first-episode *C. difficile* infection?
   A. Moxifloxacin and piperacillin
   B. **Vancomycin and metronidazole**
   C. Fosfomycin and clindamycin
   D. Trimethoprim and fidaxomicin
9. Bezlotoxumab, a new treatment option, is a monoclonal antibody targeting:
   A. **Toxin B**
   B. Both toxin A and toxin B
   C. The bacterial cell wall
   D. The spores
10. What is the most promising alternative treatment for severe cases of CDI?
    A. Bezlotoxumab
    B. Herbal extracts
    C. **Fecal microbiota transplantation**
    D. Probiotics

# References

1. Sartelli M, Di Bella S, McFarland LV, et al. 2019 update of the WSES guidelines for management of *Clostridium difficile* infection in surgical patients. World J Emerg Surg. 2019;14:8. https://doi.org/10.1186/s13017-019-0228-3.
2. Burke KE, Lamont JT. *Clostridium difficile* infection: a worldwide disease. Gut Liver. 2014;8(1):1–6. https://doi.org/10.5009/gnl.2014.8.1.1.
3. Antonelli M, Martin-Loeches I, Dimopoulos G, Gasbarrini A, Vallecoccia MS. *Clostridioides difficile* (formerly *Clostridium difficile*) infection in the critically ill: an expert statement. Intensive Care Med. 2020;46(2):215–24. https://doi.org/10.1007/s00134-019-05873-x.
4. Czepiel J, Dróżdż M, Pituch H, Kuijper EJ, Perucki W, Mielimonka A, Goldman S, Wultańska D, Garlicki A, Biesiada G. *Clostridium difficile* infection: review. Eur J Clin Microbiol Infect Dis. 2019;38(7):1211–21. https://doi.org/10.1007/s10096-019-03539-6.
5. Kampouri E, Croxatto A, Prod'hom G, Guery B. *Clostridioides difficile* infection, still a long way to go. J Clin Med. 2021;10(3):389. https://doi.org/10.3390/jcm10030389.
6. Ooijevaar RE, van Beurden YH, Terveer EM, Goorhuis A, Bauer MP, Keller JJ, Mulder CJJ, Kuijper EJ. Update of treatment algorithms for *Clostridium difficile* infection. Clin Microbiol Infect. 2018;24(5):452–62. https://doi.org/10.1016/j.cmi.2017.12.022. Epub 2018 Jan 6.
7. Abt MC, McKenney PT, Pamer EG. *Clostridium difficile* colitis: pathogenesis and host defence. Nat Rev Microbiol. 2016;14(10):609–20. https://doi.org/10.1038/nrmicro.2016.108.
8. Clifford McDonald L, Gerding DN, Johnson S, Bakken JS, Carroll KC, Coffin SE, Dubberke ER, Garey KW, Gould CV, Kelly C, Loo V, Shaklee Sammons TJ, Sandora TJ, Wilcox MH. Clinical practice guidelines for *Clostridium difficile* infection in adults and children: 2017 update by the Infectious Diseases Society of America (IDSA) and Society for Healthcare Epidemiology of America (SHEA). Clin Infect Dis. 2018;66(7):e1–48. https://doi.org/10.1093/cid/cix1085.
9. Louie TJ, Miller MA, Mullane KM, Weiss K, Lentnek A, Golan Y, Gorbach S, Sears P, Shue YK. Fidaxomicin versus vancomycin for *Clostridium difficile* infection. N Engl J Med. 2011;364(5):422–31. https://doi.org/10.1056/NEJMoa0910812.
10. Dolla M, Marrab AR, Apisarnthanarakd A, Al-Maanie AS, Abbasf S, Rosenthalg VD. Prevention of *Clostridioides difficile* in hospitals: a position paper of the International Society for Infectious Diseases. Int J Infect Dis. 2021;102:188–95. https://doi.org/10.1016/j.ijid.2020.10.039.
11. Ofori E, Ramai D, Dhawan M, Mustafa F, Gasperino J, Reddy M. Community-acquired *Clostridium difficile*: epidemiology, ribotype, risk factors, hospital and intensive care unit outcomes, and current and emerging therapies. J Hosp Infect. 2018;99(4):436–42. https://doi.org/10.1016/j.jhin.2018.01.015.
12. Lessa FC, Mu Y, Bamberg WM, et al. Burden of *Clostridium difficile* infection in the United States. N Engl J Med. 2015;372:825–34.
13. Cioni G, Viale P, Frasson S, Cipollini F, Menichetti F, Petrosillo N, Brunati S, Spigaglia P, Vismara C, Bielli A, Barbanti F, Landini G, Panigada G, Gussoni G, Bonizzoni E, Gesu GP. Epidemiology and outcome of *Clostridium difficile* infections in patients hospitalized in internal medicine: findings from the nationwide FADOI-PRACTICE study. BMC Infect Dis. 2016;16(1):656. https://doi.org/10.1186/s12879-016-1961-9.
14. Roncarati G, Dallolio L, Leoni E, Panico M, Zanni A, Farruggia P. Surveillance of *Clostridium difficile* infections: results from a six-year retrospective study in nine hospitals of a North Italian local health authority. Int J Environ Res Public Health. 2017;14(1):61. https://doi.org/10.3390/ijerph14010061.
15. Kuijper EJ, Barbut F, Brazier JS, Kleinkauf N, Eckmanns T. Update of *Clostridium difficile* infection due to PCR Ribotype 027 in Europe, 2008. Euro Surveill. 2008;13(31):18942.
16. Pépin J, Valiquette L, Cossette B. Mortality attributable to nosocomial *Clostridium difficile*–associated disease during an epidemic caused by a hypervirulent strain in Quebec. CMAJ. 2005;173(9):1037–42. https://doi.org/10.1503/cmaj.050978.
17. Tleyjeh IM, Bin Abdulhak AA, Riaz M, Garbati MA, Al-Tannir M, Alasmari FA, AlGhamdi M, Rahman Khan A, Erwin PJ, Sutton AJ, Baddour LM. The association between histamine 2 receptor antagonist use and *Clostridium difficile* infection: a systematic review and meta-analysis. PLoS One. 2013;8(3):e56498. https://doi.org/10.1371/journal.pone.0056498.
18. Kim MJ, Kim BS, Kwon JW, Ahn SE, Lee SS, Park HC, Lee BH. Risk factors for the development of *Clostridium difficile* colitis in a surgical ward. J Korean Surg Soc. 2012;83:14–20.
19. Furuya-Kanamori L, Marquess J, Yakob L, et al. Asymptomatic *Clostridium difficile* colonization: epidemiology and clinical implications. BMC Infect Dis. 2015;15:516. https://doi.org/10.1186/s12879-015-1258-4.
20. Bagdasarian N, Rao K, Malani PN. Diagnosis and treatment of *Clostridium difficile* in adults: a systematic review. JAMA. 2015;313:398–408.
21. Kim PK, Zhao P, Teperman S. Evolving treatment strategies for severe *Clostridium difficile* colitis: defining the therapeutic window. In: Sartelli M, Bassetti M, Martin-Loeches I, editors. Abdominal sepsis. Hot topics in acute care surgery and trauma. Springer; 2018.
22. Asanoa S, Katsurab M. Determining the optimal surgical timing of fulminant *Clostridium difficile* colitis by using four objective factors and computed tomography findings: a case report. Int J Surg Case Rep. 2021;80:105633. https://doi.org/10.1016/j.ijscr.2021.02.019.

23. Zar FA, Bakkanagari SR, Moorthi KM, Davis MB. A comparison of vancomycin and metronidazole for the treatment of *Clostridium difficile*-associated diarrhea, stratified by disease severity. Clin Infect Dis. 2007;45:302–7.
24. Carter GP, Chakravorty A, Pham Nguyen TA, Mileto S, Schreiber F, et al. Defining the roles of TcdA and TcdB in localized gastrointestinal disease, systemic organ damage, and the host response during *Clostridium difficile* infections. mBIO. 2015;6(3):e00551.
25. Wilcox MH, Gerding DN, Poxton IR, Kelly C, Nathan R, Birch T, Cornely OA, Rahav G, Bouza E, Lee C, Jenkin G, Jensen W, Kim YS, Yoshida J, Gabryelski L, Pedley A, Eves K, Tipping R, Guris D, Kartsonis N, Dorr MB. Bezlotoxumab for prevention of recurrent *Clostridium difficile* infection. N Engl J Med. 2017;376(4):305–17. https://doi.org/10.1056/NEJMoa1602615.
26. Crobach MJT, Planche T, Eckert C, Barbut F, Terveer EM, Dekkers OM, Wilcox MH, Kuijper EJ. European Society of Clinical Microbiology and Infectious Diseases: update of the diagnostic guidance document for *Clostridium difficile* infection. Clin Microbiol Infect. 2016;22(4):S63–81. https://doi.org/10.1016/j.cmi.2016.03.010.
27. Lee DY, Chung EL, Guend H, Whelan RL, Wedderburn RV, Rose KM. Predictors of mortality after emergency colectomy for *Clostridium difficile* colitis: an analysis of ACS-NSQIP. Ann Surg. 2014;259:148–56.
28. Johnson S, Louie TJ, Gerding DN, et al. Polymer alternative for CDI treatment (PACT) investigators. vancomycin, metronidazole, or tolevamer for *Clostridium difficile* infection: results from two multinational, randomized, controlled trials. Clin Infect Dis. 2014;59:345–54.
29. Gough E, Shaikh H, Manges AR. Systematic review of intestinal microbiota transplantation (fecal bacteriotherapy) for recurrent *Clostridium difficile* infection. Clin Infect Dis. 2011;53:994–1002.
30. Clanton J, Fawley R, Haller N, Daley T, Porter J, Paranjape C, Bonilla H. Patience is a virtue: an argument for delayed surgical intervention in fulminant *Clostridium difficile* colitis. Am Surg. 2014;80:614–9.
31. Neal MD, Alverdy JC, Hall DE, Simmons RL, Zuckerbraun BS. Diverting loop ileostomy and colonic lavage: an alternative to total abdominal colectomy for the treatment of severe, complicated *Clostridium difficile* associated disease. Ann Surg. 2011;254:423–37.
32. Ferrada P, Callcut R, Zielinski MD, Bruns B, Yeh DD, Zakrison TL, et al. EAST Multi-Institutional Trials Committee. Loop ileostomy versus total colectomy as surgical treatment for *Clostridium difficile*-associated disease: an Eastern Association for the Surgery of Trauma multicenter trial. J Trauma Acute Care Surg. 2017;83:36–40.
33. Halabi WJ, Nguyen VQ, Carmichael JC, Pigazzi A, Stamos MJ, Mills S. *Clostridium difficile* colitis in the United States: a decade of trends, outcomes, risk factors for colectomy, and mortality after colectomy. J Am Coll Surg. 2013;217:802–12.
34. Fekety R, Kim KH, Brown D, Batts DH, Cudmore M, Silva J Jr. Epidemiology of antibiotic associated colitis; isolation of *Clostridium difficile* from the hospital environment. Am J Med. 1981;70(4):906–8.

# Bowel Parasitic Surgical Emergencies

# 85

Ibrahima Sall, Magatte Faye, and Ibrahima Diallo

## 85.1 Introduction

Bowel parasitic affections (BPA) are common in tropical areas and beyond the world. These affections may lead to acute abdomen requiring emergency surgery [1, 2].

BPA are gastrointestinal infectious diseases of poverty, poor sanitation, dirty water, and crowded living; in tropical warm temperature and humidity areas [3]. Nevertheless, considering populations migration, we must be aware of the worldwide dissemination in order to manage the disease if observed.

Bowel parasites have been known to infect humans since prehistoric times and they have evolved with humans throughout history [4]. Parasitism is the condition in which one organism (the parasite) neither harms its host; in some way lives at the expense of the host.

During our relatively short history on Earth, humans have acquired an amazing number of parasites, about 300 species of helminth worms and over 70 species of protozoans [5].

The major parasitic diseases infecting humans are listed in two categories: those caused by protozoans (single-celled organisms) and those caused by metazoans (multiple-celled organisms called helminths or worms). The most common helminths (metazoans) that inhabit the human gut are nematodes (Nemathelminthes, roundworms) and Platyhelminthes (flatworms) including cestodes (tapeworms), trematodes (flukes). The major protozoan that inhabits the human gut is *Entamoeba histolytica* (EH) (causing amoebiasis) [6].

Bowel parasitic surgical emergencies (BPSE) are represented by the acute abdomens requiring emergency surgery as the consequence of parasites involvement in the bowel. Even if the frequency has drastically decreased to less than 0.5% of acute abdomens in endemic areas, because of the large diffusion of medical treatment [1], we must be aware that the causing factors (poverty, poor sanitation, migration, internally displaced people or refugee's conflict camps …) can still challenge us. The natural history of these parasites (see in physiopathology) will show the different mechanisms of diseases, and the different lesions observed. So, the purpose of this chapter review has been centered on these parasites, causing bowel parasitic surgical emergencies.

I. Sall (✉) · M. Faye
Departement of General Surgery, Military Teaching Hospital, Hôpital Principal de Dakar, Dakar, Senegal

I. Diallo
Departement of Gastroenterology and Hepatology, Military Teaching Hospital, Hôpital Principal de Dakar, Dakar, Senegal

> **Learning Goals**
> - Understand the worldwide burden of bowel parasitic diseases.
> - Identify parasites found in the human gastrointestinal tract, and their parasitism characteristics.
> - Describe the physiopathology and the corresponding clinical syndrome of bowel parasitic surgical emergencies.
> - Master the therapeutic principles.

## 85.1.1 Epidemiology

In fact, one-fourth of the known human infectious diseases are caused by the helminth and protozoan groups [4].

Ascariasis still remains the most common intestinal parasite with 807–1221 million infections globally; and the most prevalent in East Asia, sub-Saharan Africa, and India. Whipworm (*Trichuris trichiura* [TT]) and hookworm (Ancylostoma) account for 604–795 and 576–740 million infections, respectively [7]. A study in South Africa confirmed that human infestation with Ascaris lumbricoides (AL) was responsible for 20% of acute admissions annually to the pediatric surgical wards of the Red Cross Children's Hospital in Cape Town in the 1980s. Of these admissions, 66% were in the bowel, 30% in the hepatobiliary tract, and 4% in the pancreas [8].

Amoebiasis is the second leading cause of death due to parasitic diseases (after malaria), killing about 40,000–100,000 people per year globally [9].

Despite the relative frequency described in low– and middle income countries (LMICs), intestinal or bowel parasitism is a global health concern because of migration and globalization. Intestinal parasites may be transmitted directly (hand-to-hand contact) or indirectly (contact with food or environmental surfaces). Regardless of route of transmission, the human hand, the skin contact with dirty water, and poor sanitation act as a common denominator in the transmission of intestinal parasites [4].

The natural cycle of parasitism can lead to bowel lesions and complications requiring surgery. BPSE may account to 5% of surgical acute abdomens in tropical regions [1].

## 85.1.2 Etiology

Parasites found in the human gastrointestinal tract can be largely categorized into two groups: metazoans (multicellular animals) and protozoans (single-celled organisms). Table 85.1 summarizes the most common bowel parasites and their characteristics leading to surgical complications [1, 10–14]. Biliopancreatic obstruction migration from the bowel via the ampulla is taken under consideration. The tropism of *Fasciola hepatica* (FH) involves essentially the liver, but we have decided to cite it because of its bowel crossing and rare inflammatory bowel lesions reported [11].

## 85.1.3 Physiopathology

The digestive tract is communicating directly with the external environment through food ingestion and soil defecation. So, the small and large bowels are a favorable environment for the parasitism cycle. The imbalance between parasitism, level of infestation, and immune system of the host is responsible of microscopic and macroscopic anomalies that may lead to surgical complications.

Bowel obstruction is the most frequent complications reported [1, 15, 16]. It may be a true obstruction, often correlated to ascariasis heavy worm infestation. It may be a paralytic ileus reported with strongyloidiasis. Pseudo-inflammatory tumors revealed by obstruction are also reported with amoebiasis, fascioliasis, schistosomiasis, and trichuriasis [1, 8, 9, 11, 12]. Bowel volvulus is reported in case of massive heavy worm infestation by *Ascaris lumbricoides* (AL) or *Trichuriasis trichiura* (TT). Intestinal invagination is another mechanism reported with TT, AL. Among surgical complications due to ascariasis, intestinal obstruction may be occurred in 74% [17].

**Table 85.1** Most common bowel parasite's characteristics leading to surgical complications

| Classification | Subclassification | Illness | Parasite | Bowel lesions |
|---|---|---|---|---|
| Metazoans | Nematodes (roundworms) Nemathelminthes | Ascariasis | Ascaris lumbricoides (AL) 10–30 cm length / 2–4 mm width Oral transmission | • Mucosal erosion<br>• Aggregated masses of worms<br>• Volvulus<br>• Invagination<br>• Appendicitis<br>• Biliopancreatic obstruction |
| | | Ankylostomiasis | Ankylostoma (hookworm) (AK) 7–13 mm / 0.3–0.6 mm Skin or oral transmission | • Mucosal inflammation and erosion<br>• Bleeding |
| | | Strongyloidiasis (Anguillulosis) | Strongyloides stercoralis (SS) 2–3 mm / 50 µm Skin transmission | • Duodenal obstruction<br>• Intestinal ileus<br>• Biliary obstruction |
| | | Trichuriasis (Trichocephalosis) | Trichuris Trichiura (TT) (whipworm) 3–5 cm / 1–2 mm Oral transmission | • Aggregated masses of worm<br>• Appendicitis<br>• Invagination |
| | | Enterobiasis (Oxyurosis) | Enterobius Vermicularis (EV) (pinworm) 1–3.8 mm (male) 9–13 mm (female) / 0.1–0.2 mm Oral transmission | • Appendicitis |
| | | Anisakiasis | Anisakis (AS) 3–10 cm / 1–3 mm Oral transmission (fish) | • Perforation |
| | Platyhelminthes (flatworms): Cestodes (tapeworms) | Taeniasis | Taenia saginata (beef) (TS) 4–12 m / 1–2 cm Taenia Solium (pork) 1–3 m / 1 mm Oral transmission | • Perforation<br>• Biliary obstruction |
| | Platyhelminthes (flatworms): Trematodes (flukes) | Fasciolasis | Fasciola Hepatica (FH) 15–30 mm / 10 mm Oral transmission | • Granuloma formation<br>• Inflammatory masses<br>• Biliary tract obstruction |
| | Platyhelminthes (flatworms): Trematodes (flukes) | Schistosomiasis | Schistozoma mansoni (SM) 15 à 25 mm / 8–12 mm Skin transmission | • Bowel wall inflammation<br>• Granuloma formation |
| Protozoans | | Amoebiasis | Entamoeba histolytica (EH) 12–40 µm Oral transmission | • Colon mucosal ulceration and necrosis<br>• Vessels thrombosis<br>• Amebomas (inflammatory masses)<br>• Perforation<br>• Rupture of liver abscesses |

Peritonitis is the result of intestinal perforation and contamination of the peritoneal cavity, often reported with amoebiasis, ascariasis, anisakiasis, and taeniasis. The crossing of a parasite through the intestinal wall is favored by a pre-existing impairment such as typhoid disease, tuberculosis, or malignant tumors [1]. Amoebiasis's acute pancolitis is less reported nowadays, but is a very serious complication [18]. Peritonitis may also be the result of bowel volvulus necrosis. Rupture of liver abscess due to amoebiasis, in the peritoneal cavity, is a frequent cause of peritonitis in endemic areas [1].

Appendicitis due to the migration of AL in the lumen of the vermiform appendix is still debatable since the symptoms of this migration can mimic appendicitis but rarely are the cause [19]. Surgical complications due to ascariasis's appendicular perforation may reach 7% of all surgical complications due to ascariasis [17]. Parasitic infections are reported to be greatly implicated in the pathophysiology of acute appendicitis. Enterobius vermicularis (EV) may be found in 10% of removed appendices [20]. The presence of parasites in the appendix may produce symptoms like acute appendicitis or be an incidental finding [21]. In endemic areas, almost 10% of appendicitis may be associated with parasites like TT, AL, and *Enterobius vermicularis* (EV) [22].

Biliary tract obstruction and Cholangitis are reported with Anisakis (AS), *Strongyloides stercoralis* (SS), *Taenia saginata* (TS), and FH [13, 23, 24]. The transpapillary crossing of parasites is favored mainly by surgical or endoscopic procedures on the Vater's ampulla. This parasite migration may also lead to pancreatitis, reported with AL SS, TS, and FH [13].

Acute gastrointestinal hemorrhage is extremely rare, but may lead to indicate surgery [25]. Mucosal and vessels erosions are responsible of the bleeding.

## 85.2 Diagnosis

Physicians and surgeons practicing in parasite's endemic areas should be aware of the potential surgical complications, in order to find good diagnosis and take the best strategies according to the bowel parasite in question.

### 85.2.1 Clinical Presentation

The clinical presentation is related to the physiopathologic characteristics. Signs, symptoms and physical findings are initially nonspecific. This clinical presentation may be considered according to five scenarios: the bowel obstruction syndrome (obstruction, volvulus, tumor), the peritonitis syndrome, the appendicitis syndrome, the biliopancreatic obstruction syndrome (jaundice, cholangitis or pancreatitis), and the gastrointestinal hemorrhage (bleeding) syndrome. These syndromes, related to acute abdomen, are not far different from their classic descriptions.

The clinical pattern is not specific and the etiological diagnosis is usually intraoperative [26], by visualization of the worm. The diagnosis of the parasite may be oriented by the endemic areas or its elimination by vomiting or in feces. The site of entry of the filariform larvae of SS is characterized by larva currens, a migrating pruritic (itchy) rash in which the subcutaneous parasites can move up to 5–10 cm/h. As the larvae pass through the lungs, Loeffler's syndrome (fever, wheezing, cough, shortness of breath) can be observed [12].

### 85.2.2 Tests

#### 85.2.2.1 Biology

Blood test may reveal anomalies related to the different complicated syndromes, but they are not specific of parasitism. Eosinophilia is common in bowel parasitism but do not specify the type of parasite. Anemia is also common with malnutrition, iron deficiency, and gastrointestinal bleeding induced by the parasitism.

Serum antibody detection is possible using immunofluorescence, immuno-hema-agglutination, the latex agglutination test, the gel diffusion precipitation test, immuno-electrophoresis, and ELISA [12]; but serology tests are expensive and not wide released.

Parasitology with fecal (stool) examination, to find the parasite or eggs, is the cornerstone of the parasite's identification (Figs. 85.1, 85.2, 85.3, 85.4, 85.5, and 85.6). Metazoans may be identified at macroscopic direct observation or

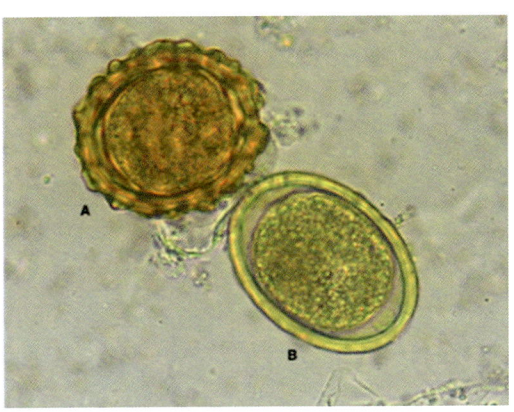

**Fig. 85.1** Eggs of Ascaris lumbricoïdes (A = typical; B = atypical). (With permission and courtesy of Pr. Seck MC. Laboratory of parasitology and mycology at Le Dantec Hospital of Dakar, in Senegal)

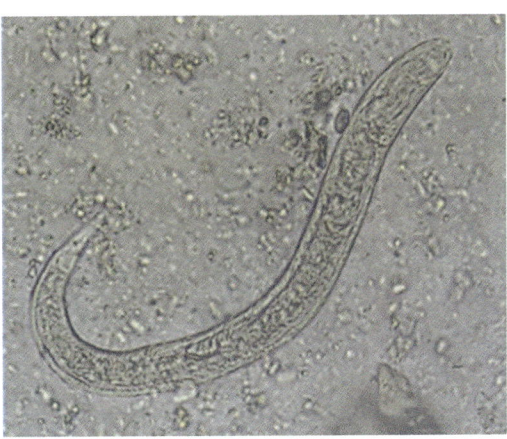

**Fig. 85.3** Larvae of Strongyloides stercoralis. (With permission and courtesy of Pr. Seck MC. Laboratory of parasitology and mycology at Le Dantec Hospital of Dakar, in Senegal)

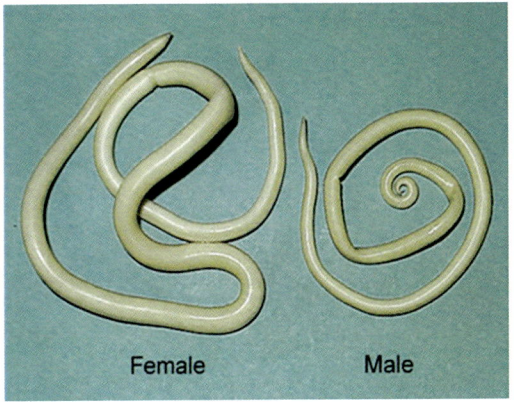

**Fig. 85.2** Ascaris lumbricoides. (With permission and courtesy of Pr. Seck MC. Laboratory of parasitology and mycology at Le Dantec Hospital of Dakar, in Senegal)

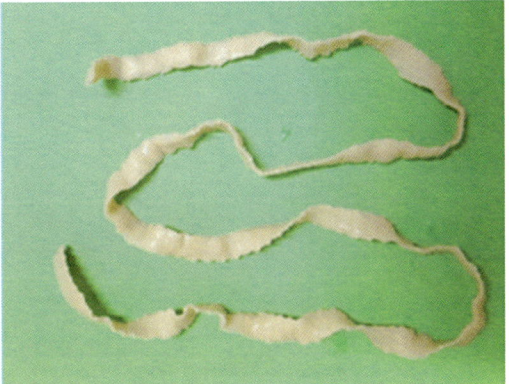

**Fig. 85.4** Taenia solium. (With permission and courtesy of Pr. Seck MC. Laboratory of parasitology and mycology at Le Dantec Hospital of Dakar, in Senegal)

microscopy. Protozoans are identified by microscopic exam.

Diagnosis of ascariasis is made through microscopy of nematode eggs (Fig. 85.1) in human feces or by finding of adult worms (Fig. 85.2). Diligent examination of stool specimens is needed to identify larvae of SS (Fig. 85.3). Patients with *Taenia saginata* and *Taenia solium* (Fig. 85.4) infections often recognize individual or short chains of motile proglottids in their stool. Definitive diagnosis of fascioliasis depends on the finding of FH eggs in the feces or in duodenal aspiration, serology, demonstration of adult flukes on liver biopsy, and surgical specimen. Stool examination demonstrates eggs or worm of SM (Fig. 85.5).

The finding of trophozoites of EH (Fig. 85.6) in the stool is consistent with invasive amoebiasis. If invasive amoebiasis is still suspected after negative stool examinations, serologic testing can be performed.

### 85.2.2.2 Imaging

Ultrasound (US) and computed tomography (CT) are useful for the diagnosis of acute abdomen. Imaging findings are not often specific but some lesions may have oriented the diagnosis [27]. Ultrasound abdominal examination may reveal intestinal or biliopancreatic ascariasis [8, 23]. In longitudinal US section, Ascaris is seen as a lin-

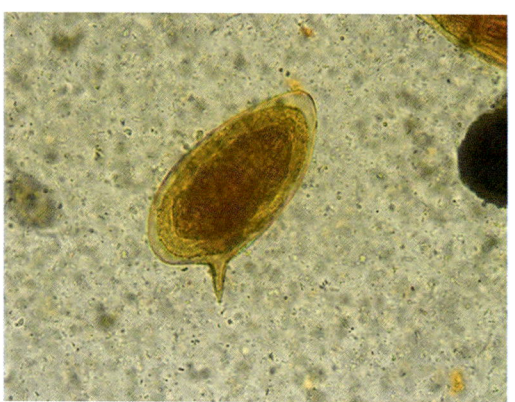

**Fig. 85.5** Egg of Schistosoma mansoni. (With permission and courtesy of Pr Seck MC. Laboratory of parasitology and mycology at Le Dantec Hospital of Dakar, in Senegal)

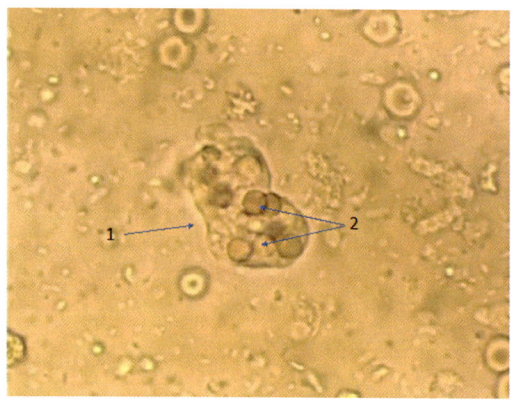

**Fig. 85.6** Entamoeba histolytica [vegetative form (20–40 μm) (1) containing red blood cells (2)]. (With permission and courtesy of Pr Seck MC. Laboratory of parasitology and mycology at Le Dantec Hospital of Dakar, in Senegal)

ear or curved, tubular echogenic image made of 3 thin, parallel, hyper-echogenic lines; without acoustic shadowing. This appearance is known as "triple line" sign. On transverse section, Ascaris appears like a round hyper-echogenic structure with hypo-echogenic center [23, 28–30]. US and cholangiography may identify flukes in the biliary tree [12, 23]. US and CT are the most useful imaging methods in the context of acute abdomen; magnetic resonance imaging (MRI) exceptionally may help [31].

### 85.2.2.3 Endoscopy

Endoscopy can directly show adult worms [30], but in the context of acute abdomen, it is prescription is limited. Histology diagnosis from endoscopic biopsies is especially useful when stool samples are negative. Histological examination of duodenal, jejuna biopsy, or appendicectomy specimens can demonstrate SS, EV, and TT adult worms embedded in the mucosa [29].

> **Differential Diagnosis**
> Differential diagnosis concerns the other acute abdomen causes. Considering the endemic areas, tests results, surgical findings, and histopathology lesions will lead to the diagnosis confirmation.

### 85.2.3 Final Diagnosis

The suspicion of diagnosis raises up with clinical syndrome, and/or endemic areas, and/or parasite elimination by vomiting or in feces, and/or imaging, and/or serology.

The final diagnosis in face of bowel obstruction syndrome is confirmed with:

- Surgery and parasitology for Ascariasis, Strongyloidiasis (Anguillulosis);
- Surgery, histopathology exam, and parasitology for Trichuriasis (Trichocephalosis), fascioliasis, and Amoebiasis;
- Histopathology exam and parasitology for Schistosomiasis.
- The final diagnosis in face of peritonitis syndrome is confirmed with:
- Surgery, histopathology exam and parasitology for Amoebiasis and Anisakiasis;
- Surgery and Parasitology for Ascariasis and Taeniasis.
- The final diagnosis in face of appendicitis syndrome is confirmed with:
- Surgery, histopathology exam and parasitology for Ascariasis, Enterobiasis, and Trichuriasis.

The final diagnosis in face of biliary obstruction (jaundice, cholangitis or pancreatitis) is confirmed with:

- Surgery and parasitology for Ascariasis, Strongyloidiasis, and Taeniasis;
- Surgery, histopathology exam and parasitology for fascioliasis.

The final diagnosis in face of gastrointestinal hemorrhage (bleeding) syndrome is confirmed with:

- Endoscopy, surgery and parasitology for Ascariasis and Ancylostomiasis.

## 85.3 Treatment

### 85.3.1 Medical Treatment

#### 85.3.1.1 Drugs

Three classes of drugs are used to treat majority of digestive parasites: 5-nitro-imidazoles (metronidazole, ornidazole, and tinidazole) for protozoa; benzimidazoles (albendazole, Triclabendazole, flubendazole, and mebendazole) for roundworms and praziquantel for tapeworms. Albendazole is also indicated for Taeniasis. Ivermectin henceforth is the therapeutic arsenal for strongyloidiasis, whose treatment was historically more delicated. These treatments are handling easy, usually quickly effective and well tolerated. Other molecules (antibiotics, nitazoxanide, fumagillin) recognize more confidential indications and are reserved for situations of failure and in cases of immunosuppression [28]. Medical drugs are always necessary to eradicate the parasitism.

#### 85.3.1.2 Endoscopy

Endoscopic exam has the possibility of diagnosing and treating biliary parasite migration, with or without sphincterotomy [24, 30].

### 85.3.2 Surgical Treatment

#### 85.3.2.1 Principles

Surgery is indicated to manage bowel complications but not to eradicate the parasitic disease. The principles of surgical treatment are to raise up bowel obstruction, to restore intestinal continuity, to realize appendectomy, to raise up biliopancreatic obstruction, and/or to assure hemostasis. Bowel resection may be necessary in case of perforation, bowel necrosis, or pseudo-inflammatory tumor. But without these complications we must consider medical conservative treatment [30, 32]. The choice between open and mini-invasive surgical techniques will depend on surgical expertise.

#### 85.3.2.2 Indications

In face of parasitic bowel obstruction diagnosis before laparotomy, most of the patients respond well to the non-operative management with a regimen that includes an adequate fluid and electrolyte replacement, a nasogastric suction tube, a specific antihelminthic therapy (piperazine or mebendazole administered via the nasogastric tube); glycerine + liquid paraffin emulsion enemas and antibiotics (in order to check the proliferation and translocation of the bowel flora exacerbated by the obstruction). The results of the non-operative therapeutic modality in well-selected patients are highly rewarding [17, 30, 33]. At the other extreme, with the patient who comes in with severe signs of peritoneal irritation, an aggressive resuscitation is required and emergency laparotomy for intestinal resection with anastomosis or stoma [32, 34, 35].

In face of parasitic bowel obstruction diagnosis at laparotomy, when no major alteration of the intestinal wall is observed, some authors have reported to manually express and advance the parasitic bundle toward the colon with maximal delicacy, in order to avoid disruption and perforation of the bowel wall; pouring saline solution over the bowel wall, for the purpose of lubrication, is helpful in the prevention of this serious mishap [17]. If successful advancement of the bundles of worms toward the colon is not achieved their extraction through enterotomy is also reported [1, 17]. But the risk of parasite migration causing anastomosis leakage is real.

Intestinal ileus reported with strongyloidiasis is a particular parasitic bowel obstruction syndrome. Surgery has no defined role in the treatment of strongyloidiasis. Most instances of abdominal exploratory surgery for intestinal SS infection could have been avoided if the obstruction had been treated with thiabendazole administered via a nasogastric tube [12].

In face of Peritonitis, the management comprises: resuscitation; infection source control (suture or diversion); antibiotherapy and fluid support. Removing of any infective source and damaged tissues, opening spaces and compartment, evacuating pus or others fluids, deriving (stoma) or resecting of any intestinal critical ischemic tracts (with anastomosis or stoma) are mandatory.

In face of appendicitis, appendectomy will not be the subject of discussion.

In face of biliopancreatic obstruction, parasite extraction is realized by choledocotomy [23, 24] or duodenotomy [1]. But endoscopic extraction, with or without sphincterotomy, must be the first choice.

In face of gastrointestinal hemorrhage (bleeding) indicating surgery, intestinal resection may be necessary [25].

### 85.3.3 Prognosis

Peritoneal rupture of a liver amoebiasis abscess is a major cause of peritonitis and is still associated with postoperative high mortality rate of 41%. Preoperative diagnosis could lead to nonoperative management that may be associated with better prognosis [1]. Prevention is the cornerstone to avoid parasitism and its complications. National prevention and control programs should be implemented in countries with high prevalence of infestation.

> **Dos and Don'ts**
> - Consider the epidemiology of bowel parasites in face of acute abdomen.
> - Consider surgery without any delay if indicated, especially in face of peritonitis and bowel obstruction.
> - Consider imaging and laboratory tests, if suitable, to improve diagnosis.
> - Do not forget medical treatment as mandatory for parasitism eradication.
> - Think about prevention for other family members.

> **Take-Home Messages**
> - The natural cycle of bowel parasitism can lead to bowel lesions and complications requiring surgery. Bowel parasitic surgical emergencies may account to 5% of surgical acute abdomens in tropical regions.
> - The final diagnosis is a combination of clinical syndrome, epidemiology, imaging and/or biology, surgical findings, histopathology, and parasitology in last but not least.
> - Surgery is indicated to manage bowel complications but not to eradicate the parasitic disease. Medical drugs are always necessary to eradicate the parasitism.
> - Preoperative diagnosis could lead to nonoperative management that may be associated with better prognosis.
> - Prevention is the cornerstone to avoid parasitism and its complications.

> **Multiple Choice Questions (*Correct Answer)**
> 1. Parasitism is the condition in which:
>    A. A parasite always harms its host.
>    B. A parasite never harms its host.
>    C. The parasite either harms its host or in some way lives at the expense of the host.*
>    D. One organism only lives at the expense of the host.
> 2. One fourth of the known human infectious diseases are caused:
>    A. Malaria.
>    B. HIV.
>    C. Influenza.
>    D. By the helminth and protozoan groups, in correlation with parasitism.*

3. The most common parasites that inhabit the human gut are:
   A. Protozoans.
   B. Metazoans.
   C. Protozoans and metazoans.
   D. The helminths group (metazoans: multiple-celled organisms) and Entamoeba histolytica (a protozoan: single-celled organism).*

4. Bowel parasitic surgical emergencies:
   A. Are represented by the acute abdomens requiring emergency surgery as the consequence of parasites involvement in the bowel.*
   B. Are represented by the incidental finding of parasites during surgery.
   C. Are represented by the natural history of parasitism.
   D. Are represented by the surgical treatment of parasites.

5. Bowel parasitic surgical emergencies:
   A. Are the consequences of poverty and poor sanitation.
   B. Are the consequences of amoebiasis, ascariasis, and taeniasis.
   C. Are the consequences of fascioliasis, schistosomiasis and trichuriasis.
   D. Are the consequences of the imbalance between parasitism, level of infestation and immune system of the host; that may lead to microscopic and macroscopic anomalies.*

6. Bowel parasitic surgical emergencies may be revealed by clinical syndrome scenarios:
   A. The bowel obstruction syndrome and the peritonitis syndrome.
   B. The bowel obstruction syndrome; the peritonitis syndrome; the appendicitis syndrome; the biliopancreatic obstruction syndrome and the gastrointestinal hemorrhage syndrome.*
   C. The peritonitis syndrome; the appendicitis syndrome.
   D. The bowel obstruction syndrome; the peritonitis syndrome; the appendicitis syndrome.

7. Bowel obstruction is mostly reported for:
   A. Ascariasis heavy worm infestation.*
   B. Strongyloidiasis.
   C. Amoebiasis.
   D. Fascioliasis, schistosomiasis and trichuriasis.

8. Peritonitis is the result of intestinal perforation and contamination of the peritoneal cavity, often reported with:
   A. Ascariasis heavy worm infestation.
   B. Appendicitis.
   C. Fascioliasis, schistosomiasis and trichuriasis.
   D. Amoebiasis, ascariasis, anisakiasis, taeniasis.*

9. Three classes of drugs are used to treat majority of digestive parasites:
   A. Metronidazole, ornidazole and tinidazole.
   B. 5-Nitro-imidazoles for protozoa, benzimidazoles for roundworms and praziquantel for tapeworms.*
   C. Albendazole, Triclabendazole, flubendazole.
   D. Antibiotics, nitazoxanide, fumagillin.

10. Bowel parasitic surgical emergencies require:
    A. Definitive surgery to eradicate parasitic disease.
    B. Always surgery to eradicate parasitic disease.
    C. Only medical drugs to eradicate the parasitism.
    D. Surgery to manage bowel complications and medical drugs to eradicate the parasitism.*

## References

1. Essomba A, ChichomMefire A, Fokou M, Ouassouo P, MassoMisse P, Esiene A, et al. Acute abdomens of parasitic origin: retrospective analysis of 135 cases. Ann Chir. 2006;131:194–7.
2. Malonga E, Mbock AM, Edzoa T, Niat G. Role of parasitosis in nontraumatic abdominal emergencies in a tropical milieu. Chirurgie. 1986;112:274–81.

3. Harhay MO, Horton J, Olliaro PL. Epidemiology and control of human gastrointestinal parasites in children. Expert Rev Anti-Infect Ther. 2010;8(2):219–34.
4. Alum A, Rubino JR, Ijaz MK. The global war against intestinal parasites—should we use a holistic approach? Int J Infect Dis. 2010;14:e732–8.
5. Ashford RW, Crewe W. The parasites of Homo sapiens. Liverpool: Liverpool School of Tropical Medicine; 1998.
6. Cummings R, Turco S. Parasitic infections. Essentials of glycobiology. 2nd ed. Harbor, NY: Cold Spring Harbor Laboratory Press; 2009.
7. Bethony J, Brooker S, Albonico M, Geiger SM, Loukas A, Diemert D, Hotez PJ. Soil transmitted helminth infections: ascariasis, trichuriasis, and hookworm. Lancet. 2006;367:1521–32.
8. Rode H, Cullis S, Millar A, et al. Abdominal complications of Ascaris lumbricoides in children. Pediatr Surg Int. 1990;5:397–401.
9. Stanley SL Jr. Amoebiasis. Lancet. 2003;22(361):1025–34.
10. Delarocque-Astagneau E, Hadengue A, Degott C, Vilgrain V, Erlinger S, Benhamou JP. Biliary obstruction resulting from Strongyloides stercoralis infection. Gut. 1994;35:705–6.
11. Makay O, Gurcu OB, Caliskan C, Nart D, Tuncyurek M, Korkut M. Ectopic fascioliasis mimicking a colon tumor. World J Gastroenterol. 2007;13(18):2633–5.
12. Mayer DA, Fried B. Aspects of human parasites in which surgical intervention may be important. Adv Parasitol. 2002;51:1–94.
13. Uysal E, Dokur M. The helminths causing surgical or endoscopic abdominal intervention: a review article. Iran J Parasitol. 2017;12(2):156–68.
14. Yasunaga H, Horiguchi H, Kuwabara K, Hashimoto H, Matsuda S. Clinical features of bowel anisakiasis in Japan. Am J Trop Med Hyg. 2010;83(1):104–5.
15. Baba AA, Ahmad SM, Sheikh KA. Intestinal ascariasis: the commonest cause of bowel obstruction in children at a tertiary care center in Kashmir. Pediatr Surg Int. 2009;25(12):1099–102.
16. Toure A, Soumaoro L, Toure F, Nabe D, Diakite S, Keita A. Abdominal surgical complications of intestinal parasites: a review of 13 cases from Conakry Ignace Deen National Hospital, Guinea. Int J Surg. 2013;30(4):1–5.
17. Ochoa B. Surgical complications of ascariasis. World J Surg. 1991;15:222–7.
18. Bikandou G, Kokolo J, Massengo R. Paracute amoebic colitis in the Brazzaville C.H.U. Med Afr Noire. 1992;39(1):48–52.
19. Wani I, Maqbool M, Amin A, Shah F, Keema A, Singh J, et al. Appendiceal ascariasis in children. Ann Saudi Med. 2010;30:63–6.
20. Helmy AH, Abou Shousha T, Magdi M, et al. Appendicitis; appendectomy and the value of endemic parasitic infestation. Egypt J Surg. 2000;19:87–91.
21. Julien C, Omouri A. Parasite in the appendix. N Engl J Med. 2020;383:e72.
22. Dorfman S, Cardozo J, Dorfman D, Del Villar A. The role of parasites in acute appendicitis of pediatric patients. Investig Clin. 2003;44:337–40.
23. Diémé EGPA, Ousmane Thiam O, Guèye ML, Sall I, Touré AO, Ogougbémy M, Cissé M, Dieng M. Ascariasis of the biliary tract: report of 2 cases at the General Surgery Department of Aristide Le Dantec Teaching Hospital and review of the literature. Batna J Med Sci. 2018;6:68–71.
24. Mbaye PS, Fall F, Collet-Burgel C, Sylla B, KlotzF. Angiocholite et pancréatite aiguës par enclavement d'un ascaris adulte dans la papille de Vater. Acta Endosc. 1999;29:495–8.
25. Dewi SD, Li SS. Acute lower gastrointestinal haemorrhage secondary to small bowel ascariasis. Malays J Med Sci. 2012;19(2):92–5.
26. Diouf HB, Vovor VM, Spay G, Toure P. Helminthiases chirurgicales, à propos de 103 observations. Médecine d'Afrique Noire. 1973;12:577–84.
27. Carnero PR, Mateo PH, Martín-Garre S, Pérez AG, Del Campo L. Unexpected hosts: imaging parasitic diseases. Insights Imaging. 2017;8:101–25.
28. Cinquetti G, Massoure MP, Rey P. Traitement des parasitoses digestives (amoebose exclue). EMC Gastroentérol. 2013;8(1):1–10. [Article 9-062-A-60]
29. Mohamed AE, Ghandour ZM, Al-Karawi M, Yasawy MI, Sammak B. Gastrointestinal parasite presentations and histological diagnosis from endoscopic biopsies and surgical specimens. Saudi Med J. 2000;21:629–34.
30. Ndiaye AR, Diallo I, Klotz F. Ascaridiose. EMC Pédiatr Maladies Infect. 2012;7(4):1–10. [Article 4-350-A-30]
31. Park M, Kim KW, Ha HK, Lee DH. Intestinal parasitic infection. Abdom Imaging. 2008;33:166–71.
32. Wasadikar PP, Kulkarni AB. Intestinal obstruction due to ascariasis. Br J Surg. 1997;84:410–2.
33. Gangopadhyay AN, Upadhyaya VD, Gupta DK, Sharma SP, Kumar V. Conservative treatment for round worm intestinal obstruction. Indian J Pediatr. 2007;74(12):1085–7.
34. Hesse AAJ, Nouri A, Hassan HS, Hashish AA. Parasitic infestations requiring surgical interventions. Semin Pediatr Surg. 2012;21:142–50.
35. Villamizar E, Mendez M, Bonilla E, Varon H, de Onatra S. Ascaris lumbricoides infestation as a cause of intestinal obstruction in children: experience with 87 cases. J Pediatr Surg. 1996;31:201–4.

## Further Reading

Essomba A, Chichom Mefire A, Fokou M, Ouassouo P, Masso Misse P, Esiene A, et al. Acute abdomens of parasitic origin: retrospective analysis of 135 cases. Ann Chir. 2006;131:194–7.

Hesse AAJ, Nouri A, Hassan HS, Hashish AA. Parasitic infestations requiring surgical interventions. Semin Pediatr Surg. 2012;21:142–50.

Mayer DA, Fried B. Aspects of human parasites in which surgical intervention may be important. Adv Parasitol. 2002;51:1–94.

Ochoa B. Surgical complications of ascariasis. World J Surg. 1991;15:222–7.

# Anorectal Emergencies

**86**

Antonio Tarasconi and Gennaro Perrone

**Learning Goals**
- Differential diagnosis of patients referring to emergency department (ED) with anorectal pain or bleeding as main complaint.
- Correct laboratory and imaging workup for every anorectal emergencies.
- Appropriate acute care management of anorectal emergencies, including non-operative management, endoscopy, angiography and surgery.

## 86.1 Introduction

The term "anorectal emergencies" comprises a wide variety of diseases that share the same presenting symptoms, that is, anorectal pain or bleeding. Most of the anorectal emergencies can be managed conservatively and do not require an inpatient management, but some of them could be life-threatening and need a prompt recognition and treatment. An incorrect recognition is frequent for anorectal diseases and it is well known that a delayed diagnosis is related to an adverse outcome [1]. Furthermore, the embarrassment related to the affected anatomical region delays the presentation of the patient in many cases, making a correct and timely diagnosis even more important. Lastly, anorectal diseases remain a common condition with relevant healthcare costs, such as impaired quality of life and work day loss. To help surgeons and emergency clinicians, we identified seven main topics that thoroughly cover this challenging subset of pathologies (anorectal abscess, perineal necrotizing fasciitis, complicated hemorrhoids, bleeding anorectal varices, complicated anorectal prolapse, retained anorectal bodies, and acute anal fissure) and performed a throughout revision of the available literature, to make evidence-based recommendation for their management.

### 86.1.1 Classification

Anorectal emergencies could be classified either according to the etiology (Table 86.1) or to the clinical presentation (Table 86.2). In clinical practice, this latter classification is probably more useful; in fact, making the correct initial diagnosis is crucial, but is probably the hardest task in these cases for multiple reasons: first, the clinical presentation of different anorectal emergencies is often overlapping and the acute and sometimes excruciating pain could preclude a thorough clinical examination; fur-

A. Tarasconi (✉) · G. Perrone
Emergency Surgery Department, Parma University Hospital, Parma, Italy
e-mail: gperrone@ao.pr.it

**Table 86.1** Etiological classification of anorectal emergencies

| Main diagnosis | Subtypes |
|---|---|
| 1 Anorectal abscesses | Intersphincteric<br>Perianal<br>Ischiorectal<br>Supralevator |
| 2 Perineal necrotizing fasciitis (Fournier's gangrene) | |
| 3 Complicated hemorrhoids | Bleeding<br>Thrombosed<br>strangulated |
| 4 Bleeding anorectal varices | |
| 5 Anorectal foreign bodies | Low-lying<br>High-lying<br>Drug concealment |
| 6 Complicate rectal prolapse | Irreducible<br>Strangulated |
| 7 Acute anal fissure | |

**Table 86.2** Classification according to clinical presentation

| Clinical presentation | Pathology |
|---|---|
| Anorectal pain/sepsis | Anorectal abscesses<br>Perineal necrotizing fasciitis (Fournier's gangrene)<br>Thrombosed/strangulated hemorrhoids<br>Complicated rectal prolapse<br>Anorectal foreign bodies<br>Anal fissure |
| Anorectal bleeding | Bleeding hemorrhoids<br>Bleeding anorectal varices<br>Complicated rectal prolapse<br>Anorectal foreign bodies<br>Acute anal fissure |

thermore, the embarrassment related to the affected anatomical region usually delays patients' presentation.

## 86.2 Anorectal Abscess

### 86.2.1 Epidemiology

Anorectal abscesses and fistulae are fairly common among the general population. It is almost impossible to accurately determine the incidence of anorectal abscesses, because they often drain spontaneously or are incised and drained in an outpatient setting or in a physician's office. Extrapolating from the fistula numbers, the incidence of anorectal abscess falls between 68,000 and 96,000 per annum in the United States; most patients are comprised between the ages of 20 and 60, with a mean age of 40. In adult patients, the male to female ratio is approximately 2:1 [2].

### 86.2.2 Etiology

Anorectal abscesses usually originate from an infection in the anal glands. Other rarer causes of anorectal abscesses are anorectal Crohn's disease, traumatic perforation of the anorectum (acuminated ingests, penetrating trauma, iatrogenic lesions), or infections spreading downwards from the pelvis (appendicitis, diverticulitis, or gynecologic sepsis) [2].

### 86.2.3 Pathophysiology

The opening of anal glands is located into the anal crypts and their ramifications extend into the submucosa and the internal anal sphincter; their anatomical structure allows the infection to extend from the anal lumen into the wall of the anal canal. Perforations of the anorectum create a communication between the rectal lumen and the surrounding tissue, thus allowing pathogens and rectal content to spread outside the rectum.

The infection may extend laterally to the perineal area (*perineal abscess*) or cephalad to the ischiorectal region (*ischiorectal abscess*) or along the rectal wall (*supralevator abscess*). Anorectal fistulae usually arise as consequence of an abscess and can be considered the chronic phase of an anorectal abscess.

### 86.2.4 Diagnosis

#### 86.2.4.1 Clinical Presentation

The clinical presentation is typically characterized by localized pain. Sing and symptoms may vary according to the anatomical location of the abscess: swelling, cellulites, and tenderness are typical of superficial abscesses, while deeper abscesses may present with fever, systemic toxicity, pain referred to the perineum, low back, and buttocks or with symptoms that mimic an intra-abdominal condition; discharge of pus could also be present and occasionally patients with anorectal abscesses will present with urinary retention. Furthermore, a draining fistula may be present.

### 86.2.4.2 Tests

Laboratory tests and radiological studies are not usually needed for the diagnosis of an anorectal abscess but can be useful in some special situations. The prescription of routine laboratory tests (complete blood count, serum creatinine, C-reactive protein, procalcitonin, lactates, and coagulation assessment) can give an insight on the general status of the patient and can help physicians understanding the severity of situation, especially in case of patients potentially candidates to emergency surgery or with signs of hemodynamic instability.

The use of imaging techniques could be helpful in all those cases with an atypical presentation, when the physical examination suggests a supralevator or horse-shoe abscess or whenever there is a suspicion of an ongoing perianal Crohn's disease or perineal gangrene. Magnetic resonance imaging (MRI) has high detection rates for anorectal abscesses [3], as well as endoscopic ultrasound (EUS), but both these imaging techniques have multiple downsides: MRI requires long acquisition time, while EUS necessitates of dedicated skills and its use is invariably precluded by the intense anal pain.

In this setting the use of contrast enhanced computed tomography (CT) scan, with its widespread availability and the short acquisition time, is suggested. CT scan also allows a complete study of the abdomen, to rule out intra-abdominal causes of the suppuration.

**Differential Diagnosis**
The differential diagnosis of anorectal abscesses is wide and comprehends all the possible causes of anal pain or swelling: hemorrhoids, anal fissures, sexually transmitted disease, proctitis, cancer, and Fournier's gangrene. The prompt distinction from this latter disease is of utmost importance, given the rapid evolution of the necrotizing fasciitis.

Usually a focused, detailed medical history and a complete physical examination, including anorectal examination, are sufficient to make the diagnosis. When the diagnosis remains unclear, an imaging investigation is suggested and the choice should be guided by patient's medical history and clinical presentation, local availability of resources and skills.

## 86.2.5 Treatment

### 86.2.5.1 Medical Treatment

Treatment of anorectal abscesses is mainly surgical and medical therapy has a supportive role. Antibiotics should be administered promptly in case of sepsis and should be continued after drainage in case of persistent sepsis/septic shock, cellulitis, or disturbances of the immune system. For a throughout discussion of the appropriate antibiotic regimens, we suggest to refer to the World Society of Emergency Surgery (WSES) guidelines for soft-tissue [4] and intra-abdominal infections [5].

Support therapy should also include proper analgesia.

Referring to interventional radiology, percutaneous drainage of anorectal abscesses is not recommended currently, given the high risk of persistence and recurrence.

### 86.2.5.2 Surgical Treatment

Surgical treatment should be prompt and include an ample incision to completely drain the abscess.

The approach depends on the anatomical location of the abscess and on the patient's condition: superficial abscesses in fit patients can be managed as outpatients, with office-based incision under local anesthesia; on the contrary, abscesses located deeper, with systemic toxicity or in unfit patients, should be drained in operating room under general or regional anesthesia, thus allowing for an accurate exploration of the involved tissue and a complete drainage of the collections. Drainage of large abscesses requires multiple counter incisions and the placement of soft drains encircling the remaining skin, to delay the healing and to allow the closure of the abscess progressing from the depth to the skin.

The role of wound packing is debated, and it is still unclear whether its use provides a benefit to the healing process, but it is well known that its use is associated with intense pain [6, 7]. Wound packing could play a role in case of continuous oozing of blood from the deeper areas that are not amenable of conventional hemostasis.

The search for an associated fistula is debated as well. There is evidence that suggests that the treatment of an associated fistula during the first operation could reduce the risk of recurrence, but it's burdened by an increased incidence of long-term continence disturbances [8, 9]. This increase is probably related to the edema and anatomical distortion caused by acute infection. The conclusion is that if an experienced surgeon could clearly identify an obvious fistula, its treatment during the first operation (either via fistulotomy or with the placement of a loose seton, according to the portion of sphincter involved) improves patient outcome. On the contrary, in case of unexperienced surgeon or unobvious fistula, it is not recommended to search for it, to avoid iatrogenic trauma.

### 86.2.6 Prognosis

Prognosis is usually good, with complete resolution of the abscess after adequate drainage. Obviously, the anatomical location and the presence of underlying diseases (e.g., Crohn's disease, malignancies) highly affect prognosis, healing time, and recurrence. It is important to keep in mind that high and voluminous abscesses may cause a systemic derangement with possible life-threatening consequences if not treated promptly. The most common sequela of anorectal abscess is a fistula, which may be the cause of a recurrent abscess. The reported incidence of fistulae following an abscess ranges from 26 to 37% [2].

## 86.3 Perineal Necrotizing Fasciitis (Fournier's Gangrene)

### 86.3.1 Epidemiology

A large population-based epidemiological study found an overall incidence of 1.6 cases per 100,000 males annually; males are predominantly affected, with a male to female ratio of 42:1, and the mean age is 50 [10]. Affected patients usually have comorbidities, with diabetes and obesity the most frequently associated pathologies. Furthermore, patients with an impaired host resistance from reduced cellular immunity (i.e., alcoholism, HIV, leukemia) have an increased risk of Fournier's gangrene [11].

### 86.3.2 Etiology

The etiology is infective and the most commonly accepted definition was proposed by Smith et al.: "an infective necrotizing fasciitis of the perineal, genital or perianal region" [12]. The infection is typically polymicrobial, with *Streptococcus*, *Staphylococcus*, and *Escherichia* commonly present, and three possible sites of origin are usually described: the perineal skin (24%), the colorectal region (21%), and the genitourinary tract (19%); an unknown origin still remains for about 36% of the cases [11].

### 86.3.3 Pathophysiology

The pathophysiology of the fasciitis starts with the presence of a localized infection that allows the entrance of normally commensal bacteria into the perineum: the subsequent inflammatory response results in an obliterative endarteritis, with vessels thrombosis and tissue ischemia. This reduction in blood flow promotes further anaerobic bacteria proliferation and fascial necrosis and digestion [13].

### 86.3.4 Diagnosis

#### 86.3.4.1 Clinical Presentation

Diagnosis is mainly clinical: a focused and detailed medical history and a complete physical examination including a careful inspection of the perineum) are usually enough to make the diagnosis. Fournier's gangrene is characterized by local signs and symptoms, like scrotal pain, swelling and erythema, and systemic features, such as fever, tachycardia, and other sign of sepsis. Examination may also reveal purulent discharge, crepitus, and patches of necrotic tissue with surrounding oedema. During physical examination, it is important to keep in mind that cutaneous manifestations tend to appear later in the disease process. Fournier's gangrene can rapidly progress to sepsis and multi organ failure and it is important to continuously monitor vital signs, to early detect an impending septic shock.

#### 86.3.4.2 Tests

Diagnosis can be guided by several risk scores, such as Laboratory Risk Indicator for Necrotising Fasciitis (LRINEC) [14], Fournier's gangrene Severity Index (FGSI) [15], and its simplified version (SFGSI) [16]. These scores seem to be reliable tools in diagnosing and prognosing the Fournier's gangrene.

Complete blood count, the dosage of serum creatinine and electrolytes, C-reactive protein, procalcitonin, and arterial hemogas analysis allow the assessment of the patient's status, identifying signs of systemic infection or sepsis.

Imaging tests are suggested in stable patients, but should not delay a timely surgical treatment. Plain radiographs, US, CT scan, and MRI may demonstrate air in the soft tissue planes as well as help determine the extent of the disease [17]. CT has high sensitivity (90%) and specificity (93.3%) for diagnosis necrotizing soft tissue infections, and may also reveal the underlying cause [18]. On the other hand, US can be promptly performed at the patient's bedside, can evaluate the scrotal contents, and does not require radiation nor intravenous contrast. For these reasons, US can be suggested whenever a CT scan is not available or not feasible.

> **Differential Diagnosis**
> Differential diagnosis includes all the causes of perineal pain and of sepsis. Usually clinical findings (excruciating pain, cutaneous necrosis, crepitus) are enough to make a correct diagnosis, but in doubtful cases imaging techniques could be requested.

### 86.3.5 Treatment

#### 86.3.5.1 Medical Treatment

The tendency to spread widely and extremely quickly makes Fournier's gangrene a time sensitive disease: a prompt recognition and treatment are of utmost importance. The cornerstones of treatment are antibiotic therapy, hemodynamic resuscitation and emergent surgical therapy.

Antibiotic therapy must be prompt and aggressive and it is recommended to start an empiric antimicrobial therapy including gram-positive, gram-negative, aerobic, and anaerobic organisms, as soon as the diagnosis of Fournier's gangrene is considered. The use of an anti-methicillin-resistant *Staphylococcus aureus* (MRSA) agent should be based on local epidemiology. Aside from antibiotics, medical therapy is supportive and aimed to treat the signs of sepsis and septic shock.

#### 86.3.5.2 Surgical Treatment

Surgical treatment of Fournier's gangrene is mandatory and should be performed as soon as possible. The aim of surgery is to drain fluid collection and perform a complete debridement of necrotic tissue. Subsequent surgical revisions should be planned based on the patient conditions (ideally every 12–24 h) and should be continued until the patient is free of necrotic tissue.

Surgical approach should be aggressive, multidisciplinary, and tailored on patients' conditions. The decision to perform a diverting ostomy or suprapubic cystostomy should be guided by the degree of fecal contamination of the wound and by the possible urethral disruption or stricture [19, 20]. Orchiectomy or other genitalia disfiguring surgery should be performed only if strictly necessary.

### 86.3.6 Prognosis

Prognosis is poor if not treated promptly. Mortality rates varies widely among different studies, ranging from 7.5% to 88% [10]. Mortality rates improve with an aggressive and prompt surgical approach [21, 22], but morbidity and long-term sequelae are frequent.

When disfiguring surgery and sexual dysfunction may not be avoided, the subsequent complex reconstructive surgery should be planned by a dedicated and multidisciplinary team. Patient's psychological burden should not be overlooked and should be addressed by the managing team.

## 86.4 Complicated Hemorrhoid (Thrombosed, Strangulated, or Bleeding)

### 86.4.1 Epidemiology

The exact prevalence of hemorrhoids is not known, because most of the times patients use self-medications, but this disease is very common as it is estimated that up to 75% of American citizens will suffer of hemorrhoids at some time in their lives [23]. Hemorrhoids are more frequent in elderly adults and in pregnant women.

### 86.4.2 Etiology

Increased intra-abdominal pressure, with the compromission of the venous drainage of hemorrhoid plexus, and prolonged straining are known predisposing factors for the development of hemorrhoids. Foods and lifestyle habits, such as low fiber diet, low water intake, spicy foods, and alcohol intake, are also related to hemorrhoids development.

### 86.4.3 Pathophysiology

Hemorrhoids are symptomatic enlargements or prolapse of anal cushions. Anal cushions are normally present in the anal mucosa and are formed by connective tissue, smooth muscle and a dense vascular plexus that creates a communication between portal and systemic circulation. The alteration of the venous drainage of the hemorrhoidal plexus, mainly due to increased intra-abdominal pressure, leads to the engorgement and enlargement of the plexus itself. This increased volume, when associated to the mechanical action of prolonged straining, promotes the protrusion of hemorrhoids through the anal canal. Recent studies also suggest that tissue inflammation and hyperperfusion of the hemorrhoidal plexus could play a role in the pathogenesis of hemorrhoids [24]. The protrusion is a risk factor for thrombosed hemorrhoids. Enlarged and engorged veins are also at increased risk of bleeding, usually due to the traumatic action of hard stools. Furthermore, hemorrhoids could become strangulated, either for torsion of a single hemorrhoid on its vascular axis or for the protrusion of the plexus through the anal canal.

### 86.4.4 Diagnosis

#### 86.4.4.1 Clinical Presentation
The usual presentation of patients with complicated hemorrhoids is either acute anal pain (also called hemorrhoidal crisis) or anorectal bleeding. The blood is typically bright red and coated on the surface of stools or found during cleansing. Diagnosis is clinical, based on patient's medical history and complete physical examination (comprehensive of digital rectal examination and anoscopy, when feasible). Vital signs and hemodynamic parameters should be checked repeatedly in patients presenting with anorectal bleeding.

Physical examination could identify a painless rectal bleeding or the presence of prolapsed anal tissue, usually with signs of thrombosis, painful at digital pressure and not easily reducible.

#### 86.4.4.2 Tests

There is no evidence in literature on the role of lab tests in case of hemorrhoidal crisis; imaging and laboratory tests should be performed in case of doubtful diagnosis, to exclude other causes of acute anal pain (e.g., anorectal abscesses, Fournier's gangrene, and anal fissures). However, patients referring for anorectal bleeding should be investigated to exclude other causes of bleeding, to define the severity of bleeding and to correctly stratify the risk for every patient. Blood tests should include a complete blood count, serum electrolytes, creatinine, liver function and a coagulation assessment. Blood type and cross-match should also be ordered at the time of initial assessment for patients with signs of severe bleeding.

Imaging investigation (CT scan, MRI or endo-anal ultrasound) are suggested only if there is suspicion of concomitant anorectal diseases (e.g., sepsis/abscess, inflammatory bowel disease, neoplasm).

> **Differential Diagnosis**
>
> Thrombosed, strangulated, and prolapsed hemorrhoids should be differentiated from rectal prolapse, and differential diagnosis is usually made on the base of clinical examination: rectal prolapse involves a concentric, complete protrusion, whereas prolapsed hemorrhoids are a radial bulging and prolapse of discrete anal cushions.
>
> Regarding bleeding hemorrhoids (Fig. 86.1), it is extremely important not to blindly attribute painless rectal bleeding to hemorrhoids, because it may be a sign of other diseases. Endoscopic evaluation of the entire colon is necessary if patient's personal and family history and physical examination raise concerns for inflammatory bowel disease or cancer (anemia, atypical bleeding or no obvious source of bleeding, alteration of bowel habits, preceding weight loss, personal and family history of colorectal cancer or inflammatory bowel disease). Furthermore, bleeding hemorrhoids must be differentiated from bleeding anorectal varices because treatment differs importantly (see Sect. 86.5).

### 86.4.5 Treatment

#### 86.4.5.1 Medical Treatment

Non-operative management is always recommended as first-line therapy for patients with complicated hemorrhoids. Medical management includes dietary and lifestyle changes (i.e., increased fiber and water intake together with adequate bathroom habits) [25, 26], the use of Flavonoids [27] and, in case of thrombosed or strangulated hemorrhoids, the use of topical muscle relaxant [28]. Available literature does not allow to make any recommendation regarding the role of nonsteroidal anti-inflammatory drugs

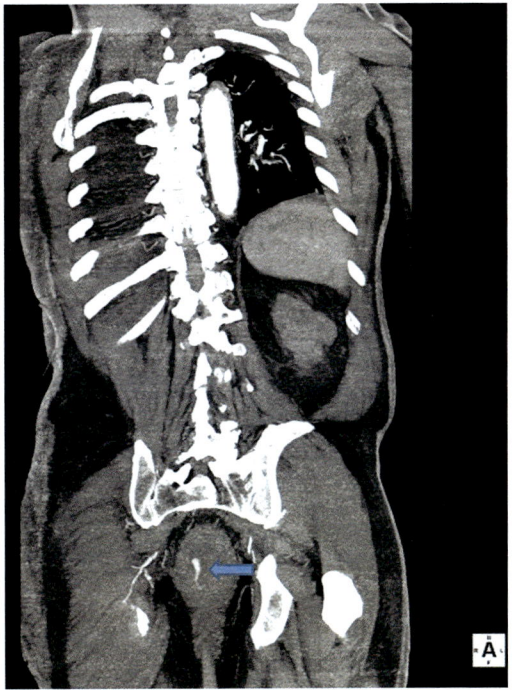

**Fig. 86.1** CT scan of active hemorrhoidal bleeding (arrow)

(NSAIDs), topical steroids, other topical agents, or injection of local anesthetics for complicated hemorrhoids.

Patients with severe bleeding requires prompt resuscitation and should be treated according to the principle for management of hemorrhagic shock.

Office-based procedures (e.g., rubber band ligation, injection sclerotherapy, infrared coagulation, cryotherapy, radiofrequency ablation, and laser therapy) are often used in an elective setting and there is growing evidence that angiography and angioembolization could play a role for the treatment of hemorrhoids, but the available literature on the use of these procedure is heterogeneous and of low quality and does not allow to make any recommendation for complicated hemorrhoids.

### 86.4.5.2 Surgical Treatment

Regarding thrombosed hemorrhoids, the studies comparing non-operative management and surgery led to contrasting results: some evidence suggest that conservative treatment could be associated with shorter patient stay and less anal sphincter damage [29], while other studies suggest that surgery may be superior to conservative management resulting in more rapid symptom resolution, lower incidence of recurrence, and longer remission intervals [30].

Incision of thrombosed hemorrhoids with clot removal is still a popular procedure, but should be abandoned because of subsequent persistent bleeding and significantly higher recurrence rates [31].

The evidence about stapled hemorrhoidectomy is scarce and, also given the potential for life-threatening complications of this procedure in the elective setting [32], its application in emergency setting should be carefully evaluated.

Based on the paucity of available studies and on the small numbers of patients included, it seems that hemorrhoidectomy can be beneficial in selected patients and the decision between non-operative management and early surgical excision (within 72 h from the onset of symptoms) should be based on physician's expertise and patient's preference, remembering the increased risk of sphincter damage related to emergency surgery and the increased risk of recurrence related to conservative management. There is growing evidence that angioembolization (Figs. 86.2 and 86.3) could have a role in the management of hemorrhoidal bleeding, but the evidences are still scarce.

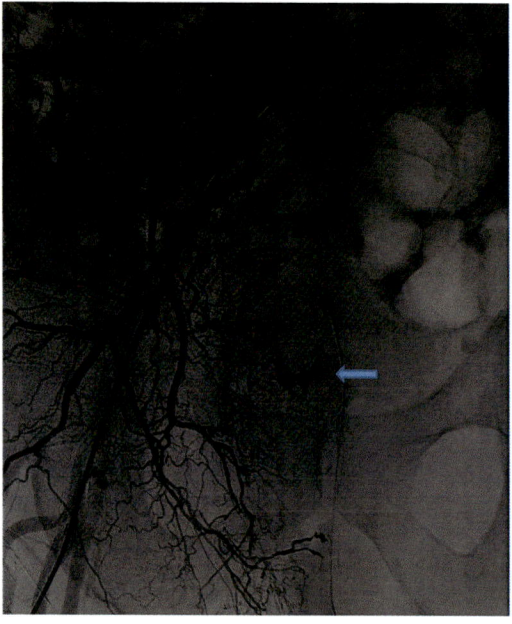

**Fig. 86.2** Active bleeding(arrow) from right hemorrhoidal artery during angiography

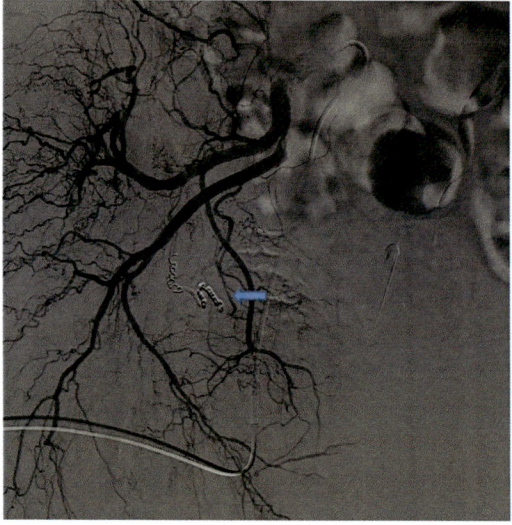

**Fig. 86.3** Bleeding interrupted after angioembolization (arrow) of the right hemorrhoidal artery

This literature review could not identify any data regarding the role of surgery for bleeding hemorrhoids, so no recommendations could be made in this setting.

### 86.4.6 Prognosis

For thrombosed and strangulated hemorrhoids prognosis is usually good, with resolution of symptoms usually after 10–15 days of non-operative management. Recurrence rate is high and definitive surgery should be carefully discussed with patients.

Bleeding from hemorrhoids is usually self-limiting, but on some cases, bleeding can be severe and life threatening, thus requiring prompt and aggressive management.

## 86.5 Bleeding Anorectal Varices

### 86.5.1 Epidemiology

Anorectal varices are isolated, dilated, submucosal veins, not contiguous with the anal columns and/or pectinate line, extending cranially into the rectum. They are associated with portal hypertension and can occur in up to 89% of patients with a portal pressure above 10 mm Hg. Despite the high prevalence of rectal varices, clinically significant bleeding is rare and occurs in less than 5% of patients [33].

### 86.5.2 Etiology

The underlying etiology can vary widely, including every cause of portal hypertension: cirrhosis, splenic vein obstruction, pancreatitis, mesenteric vein obstruction, cavernous malformation of the portal vein, and other congenital vascular anomalies, congestive heart failure.

### 86.5.3 Pathophysiology

Anorectal varices are portalsystemic collaterals which develop in response to portal hypertension. Esophageal and gastric varices, portal hypertensive gastropathy, and caput medusae are caused by the same pathogenic mechanism.

### 86.5.4 Diagnosis

#### 86.5.4.1 Clinical Presentation

The collection of throughout medical history is crucial: in fact, the presence of anorectal bleeding in patients with a history of long-standing or uncontrolled portal hypertension should raise the suspicion of bleeding anorectal varices. Typical presentation is a significant rectal bleeding not accompanied by rectal or anal pain, but possibly associated with other sign and symptoms of prolonged portal hypertension. A complete physical examination, including a digital rectal examination, allows to rule out other causes of lower gastrointestinal (GI) bleeding. These bleeding can be fatal and it is important to frequently check vital signs, to early identify an impending hemorrhagic shock.

#### 86.5.4.2 Tests

Laboratory tests are aimed to define the entity of bleeding, to stratify patient's risk and to evaluate liver function. Blood test should include a complete blood count, serum electrolytes, blood urea nitrogen, creatinine, liver function and coagulation assessment. Blood grouping and crossmatch for packed red blood cells should also be requested for patients with severe bleeding.

Endoscopy (anoproctoscopy or flexible sigmoidoscopy) is the first diagnostic tool, as it can also have a therapeutic role [34].

Imaging is supplementary and could be useful in case of doubtful diagnosis after endoscopy. Endoscopic ultrasound (EUS), with the implementation of Color Doppler evaluation, can detect deep rectal varices even in patients with a negative routine endoscopy, showing precisely the anatomy of the rectal venous plexus and the hemodynamics of varices. In all those cases where EUS is not feasible or not conclusive, contrast enhanced CT scan is the next step. CT scan has an overall sensitivity for acute hemorrhage up to 92% and can identify other findings to suggest a cause or site of origin for the bleeding, even in cases where a site of active extravasation is not identified [35].

> **Differential Diagnosis**
> Differential diagnosis can be difficult, especially when bleeding is massive thus preventing a correct examination and visualization of the rectum. The differential diagnosis includes all the pathologies that can present with painless anorectal bleeding, mainly neoplasm and bleeding hemorrhoids.

## 86.5.5 Treatment

### 86.5.5.1 Medical Treatment

The goal of medical treatment is to reduce portal hypertension and variceal blood flow, while preventing systemic hypotension and hemorrhagic shock. The early involvement of the hepatology specialist is suggested and allows optimal control of comorbid conditions.

A prompt resuscitation and correction of coagulopathy are mandatory. Targets for resuscitation are Hb level of at least >7 g/dL (4.5 mmol/L) and mean arterial pressure > 65 mm Hg, but avoiding fluid overload. The presence of massive bleeding should prompt the activation of a dedicated transfusional protocol. A helpful maneuver to gain time in case of massive bleeding is the endorectal placement of a compression tube (i.e., Sengstaken-Blakemore tube or a Linton-Nachlas balloon compression tube) [36].

The use of vasopressin, somatostatin, and terlipressin, in adjunct to vasoactive drugs, could lower portal pressure and offer the endoscopist a clearer field [37]. Propranolol and carvedilol can reduce portal pressure gradient by 20% in about 50–75% of patients, respectively, but hypotension is a contraindication to the use of beta-blockers [38].

Anti-fibrinolytic therapy could be helpful in patients with persistent bleeding and impaired clot integrity [39].

A short course of prophylactic antibiotic therapy provides clear benefits in terms of survival and decrease the risk of spontaneous bacterial peritonitis [40].

However, after all these measures are put in place, rebleeding is almost universal if another modality of treatment is not instituted. Definitive treatment is made via a step-by-step approach, starting with local endoscopic procedures (variceal band ligation, sclerotherapy or EUS-guided glue injection) and moving up to radiological (embolization, balloon-occluded retrograde transvenous obliteration, transjugular intrahepatic portosystemic shunt) and then surgical procedures.

### 86.5.5.2 Surgical Treatment

Surgery is the last step when all the other procedures failed.

Surgical methods include simple suture ligation, inferior mesenteric vein occlusion and portocaval shunt surgery, but most of these patients have poor general condition and will not tolerate an invasive approach. Direct suture ligation is technically challenging and often not successful, especially in cases of massive bleeding. For these reasons this procedure is not routinely advised and is reserved for patients who are unfit for any other procedures and when no other treatment is available. Stapled anopexy provided encouraging results in few case-reports, but it is hardly feasible in case of massive bleeding.

## 86.5.6 Prognosis

Prognosis is generally poor, with a 2-month mortality rate up to 80%, usually related to hepatic failure rather than to the hemorrhage itself [41]. Another study demonstrated that a favorable prognosis may not be expected even when initial hemostasis is achieved, with cumulative survival rates of 64 and 33% at 6 and 12 months, respectively [42].

In the light of the above it could be supposed that bleeding from anorectal varices may occur in patients with liver cirrhosis at the final stage of progression.

## 86.6 Complicated Rectal Prolapse (Irreducible or Strangulated)

### 86.6.1 Epidemiology

A complete rectal prolapse is defined as the protrusion of all layers of the rectal wall through the anal canal, and should be distinguished from a mucosal prolapse.

According to a Finnish epidemiological study, the annual incidence of rectal prolapse is 2.5 per 100,000 population. Rectal prolapse affects mainly female patients (male to female ratio 1:10) over 50 years old (median age 69 years) [43].

### 86.6.2 Etiology

Patients with rectal prolapse usually present a weak pelvic floor and a mobile rectum. Long-standing constipation and straining over many years, due to evacuation disorders, are believed to be key factors for the development of rectal prolapse.

### 86.6.3 Pathophysiology

Straining and pudendal neuropathy, caused by aging or obstetric injury, cause a pathologic relaxation of the pelvic floor and worsen pudendal nerve damage; this neural damage in turn leads to weakness of the internal and external anal sphincters. The combination of these mechanisms facilitates protrusion of the rectal wall through the anus [44]. Furthermore, the ligamentous attachments of the rectum and presacral fascia could become attenuated by the continuous downward pushing and often a redundant sigmoid colon is present.

The prolapsed bowel quickly increases its volume, due to the bowel edema caused by the reduced venous and lymphatic outflow. The dimensional increase of the prolapse could preclude the return of the bowel to its normal intra-abdominal position. A rectal prolapse is defined incarcerated when it became no longer reducible but no signs of ischemic damage are present; when ischemic damage arises, due either to impaired arterial supply or to blocked venous outflow, the prolapse is defined strangulated.

### 86.6.4 Diagnosis

#### 86.6.4.1 Clinical Presentation

Diagnosis is clinical and is based on patient's medical history and symptoms and on clinical examination. The most common complaint is a protrusion of the rectum through the anus associated to lower abdominal pain; passage of mucus and blood is frequent. Patients usually complain of chronic constipation or incontinence.

#### 86.6.4.2 Tests

The prescription of laboratory or imaging tests should be guided by the physical examination and patient's general status. Laboratory tests, including complete blood count, serum creatinine, inflammatory markers (e.g., C-reactive protein, procalcitonin and lactates) and coagulation assessment are useful to assess the status of the patient and to exclude the presence of underlying sepsis. In stable patients with complicated rectal prolapse, a contrast enhanced abdomen pelvic CT scan should be performed to investigate potential associated conditions (e.g., colorectal cancer, bowel obstruction, signs of perforation, and peritonitis, prolapse of other pelvic organs). In patients with complicated rectal prolapse and persistently unstable after proper resuscitation, an appropriate and timely management should not be delayed to perform imaging investigations.

> **Differential Diagnosis**
> Differential diagnosis with prolapsed hemorrhoids is not always easy but a rectal prolapse involves a concentric, complete protrusion, whereas prolapsed hemorrhoids are a radial bulging and prolapse of discrete anal cushions.

## 86.6.5 Treatment

### 86.6.5.1 Medical Treatment

Not infrequently, incarcerated rectal prolapse could became reducible after appropriate maneuvers, aimed to reduce the edema of prolapsed bowel. In fact, in patients with incarcerated rectal prolapse without signs of ischemia or perforation, an attempt of non-operative management is the first-line therapy, because it allows to plan an elective definitive surgery in optimal patient's conditions. Conversely, non-operative management is not indicated when signs of gangrene or perforation are present and in a hemodynamically unstable patient.

Non-operative management comprehends:

- Submucosal adrenaline injections;
- Topical application of granulated sugar or of hypertonic solutions of sugar [45];
- Submucosal infiltration of hyaluronidase [46];
- Elastic compression wrap [47].

All these maneuvers should be performed with the patient in Trendelenburg position and after administration of analgesia or under mild sedation and anesthesia.

### 86.6.5.2 Surgical Treatment

Definitive treatment of rectal prolapse is surgical and, traditionally, consists of either transabdominal or perineal approaches, each with their own advantages and disadvantages. While choosing an approach for an individual patient, important factors that should be taken into account are: surgeon skills and expertise, severity of symptoms, patient's fitness and preferences, presence of peritonitis/ischemia/perforation, concomitant colorectal cancer, patient's hemodynamic status. Up to now, there is no high-quality evidence regarding the best surgical approach in an emergency setting. Perineal procedures require a specific set of skills and expertise and are associated with higher recurrence rates, but could be performed under spinal anesthesia and presents lower operative morbidity and mortality, making them a feasible option for elderly or medically unfit patients. Transabdominal approaches have the benefit of entering the abdominal cavity and are required in case of associated peritonitis or other intra-abdominal complications. Hartmann's procedure could be an option, especially in case of patients with previous rectal incontinence or in case of damage control surgery. Moreover, most of the transabdominal procedures could be safely performed by emergency general surgeons. Lastly, when a colorectal or coloanal anastomosis is performed, the creation of a diverting loop colostomy or ileostomy should be considered in presence of risk factors for anastomotic leakage.

## 86.6.6 Prognosis

Prognosis is strictly related to the general status of the patient. Patients without signs of ischemia/sepsis/perforation and successfully treated with non-operative management have good prognosis, despite being at high risk of recurrence. Conversely, patients with bowel perforation and septic shock with hemodynamic instability have a reserved prognosis with high risk of death. In between these two extremes we found all the spectrum of patients with complicated rectal prolapse.

## 86.7 Retained Anorectal Foreign Bodies

### 86.7.1 Epidemiology

Anorectal foreign bodies are commonly seen in most large hospitals but precise epidemiological data are not available. There is a great prevalence of male patients, with a male to female ratio of 37:1 [48]. Most patients are in their forties, and anorectal foreign bodies are very uncommon in children and are usually the result of assault or child abuse.

### 86.7.2 Etiology

Erotic stimulation is the most common cause of retained anorectal foreign body; other reported causes are assault, accidental or iatrogenic events, ingestion, psychiatric diseases, drug trafficking, and self-treatment of fecal impaction.

A multitude of different objects can be found retained into the rectum and this variety leads to different clinical presentations, degrees of damage to local tissues and management implications.

### 86.7.3 Pathophysiology

The pathophysiology of anorectal foreign bodies is usually traumatic and related to the kinetics of insertion or from sharp edges. Patients' efforts to remove the foreign body may cause additional damage. The structures interested are the anal sphincters and the colorectal walls. The determination of site of injury is important for management and it could be divided into two main categories: intra-peritoneal or extra-peritoneal.

Other rarer pathophysiological processes are toxic effects related to the insertion/concealment of drugs and occur when the package disrupts and the active ingredient is adsorbed by the rectal mucosa.

### 86.7.4 Diagnosis

#### 86.7.4.1 Clinical Presentation

Common complaints include rectal or abdominal pain, constipation or incontinence, and bright red blood per rectum. In case of rectal or colonic perforation tachycardia, fever, signs of sepsis, and of peritonism may be present. It is important to remember that hospital presentation is usually delayed and preceded by effort to remove the foreign body at home. Reported time from insertion to hospital presentation ranges from 2 to 7 days, but delays up to 6 months have been reported [48]. This delay is due to embarrassment and for the same reasons a high percentage of patients initially conceal the presence of the foreign body.

In the light of the above, a great degree of suspect is necessary and a careful physical examination is mandatory. Digital rectal examination could be dangerous due to the presence of sharp objects and should be performed carefully and possibly after the acquisition of an abdomen X-ray.

All findings must be accurately reported, including presence of abrasions or bruising of the perianal area and the status of the anal sphincters, to investigate a possible sexual assault.

#### 86.7.4.2 Tests

When medical history and physical examination exclude the presence of a bowel perforation or anal sphincter damage, routine laboratory exams are necessary only in those cases requiring extraction under spinal or general anesthesia.

On the other hand, in case of suspected bowel perforation it is suggested to assess patient's status with the request of complete blood count, serum creatinine, electrolytes, liver function, and inflammatory markers (e.g., C-reactive protein, procalcitonin and lactates). Coagulation assessment is also required in case of surgical treatment. Furthermore, serum toxicology is mandatory in cases of use or concealment of illicit drugs.

Regarding imaging, lateral and anteroposterior plain X-ray of the chest, abdomen and pelvis could identify the foreign body, determine its position, shape, and size and detect the possible presence of pneumoperitoneum. A contrast enhanced CT scan is helpful in locating non-radiopaque objects, in case of suspected bowel perforation or abscess or in the diagnosis of bowel obstruction. The advantages of CT scan are a short acquisition time, a precise localization of the foreign body, the detection of its related complications and an accurate study of the pelvic extraperitoneal region. Imaging investigation should not delay a prompt surgical intervention in case of patients with retained anorectal foreign bodies and signs of hemodynamical instability persisting after proper resuscitation.

MRI is usually not included into the diagnostic workup, due to the possible presence of magnetic foreign bodies.

> **Differential Diagnosis**
> Differential diagnosis includes all the causes of anorectal pain and bleeding, as well as colorectal perforation. Correct diagnosis is usually made with the collection of an accurate medical history and a complete physical examination. In doubtful cases, thoracic and abdominal plain X-ray and contrast enhanced CT scan could help making the diagnosis.

## 86.7.5 Treatment

### 86.7.5.1 Medical Treatment

Appropriate treatment differs according to patient's condition, object's location, shape and number. First, patients with signs of bowel perforation/peritonitis should be managed surgically with a trans-abdominal approach. Patients without signs of perforation could undergo an attempt of trans-anal extraction. Low-lying objects have greater rates of success of bedside trans-anal extraction. These patients, in case of failure of bedside extraction, could be taken to the operating theater to try trans-anal extraction after pudendal nerve block, spinal anesthesia, intravenous conscious sedation or general anesthesia. Patients with high-lying, non-palpable objects, should undergo an attempt of endoscopic extraction as first-line therapy, under adequate analgesia. Sharp or fragile objects (e.g., light bulbs) must be handled with care, to avoid iatrogenic trauma and an upfront surgical approach may be considered. These indications do not applies to specific subset of patients, the "body packers" [49]. In case a drug pack is encountered inside the rectum, every maneuver that can cause the disruption of the drug package should be avoided to protect the patient from the life-threatening complications of drug overdose. For this reason, endoscopic retrieval is contraindicated by different authors and specialist societies. Furthermore, a complete radiological survey of the GI tract is required, as many of these drug packs are swallowed rather than inserted retrograde.

### 86.7.5.2 Surgical Treatment

Surgical approach is suggested in case of bowel perforation or in case of failure of trans-anal extraction. In patients with perforation and hemodynamic instability, an emergent laparotomy and a damage control surgery approach are recommended. In case of perforation and hemodynamic stability, surgical approach could be laparoscopic or laparotomic according to individual patient's condition and local expertise. Primary suture of the perforation is feasible only in case of small and recent perforation with limited peritoneal contamination, if the colonic tissues appear healthy and well vascularized and an approximation of perforation edges could be performed without tension. When primary suture is not feasible, the decision between resection with primary anastomosis, with or without a diverting stoma, and Hartmann's procedure should be based on patient's clinical conditions and the presence of risk factor for anastomotic leakage (e.g., chronic steroidal therapy, requirement of vasopressors, pre-existing comorbid conditions).

For patients without bowel perforation and failure of trans-anal extraction a step-up approach is suggested, starting with downward milking, then up to intraoperative assisted colonoscopy and proceeding to colotomy only when milking/transanal extraction fails.

## 86.7.6 Prognosis

Prognosis is strictly related to the degree of damage of sphincters and colorectal walls. Objects who are amenable of trans-anal extraction and did not cause any traumatic damage have a very benign prognosis. At the other extreme we found patients with bowel perforation and septic shock with hemodynamic instability, who have a reserved prognosis with high risk of death. In between these two extremes we found all the spectrum of patients with retained foreign anorectal bodies.

## 86.8 Acute Anal Fissure

### 86.8.1 Epidemiology

Anal fissure is a longitudinal tear within the anal canal that can be extended from the dentate line to the anal verge. Fissures are defined chronic when persisting beyond 6 weeks. They are very common and occur in young patients without any difference among sex [50]. A precise determination of their incidence is difficult, because most of the times patients do not refer to the hospital or are managed on an office-base setting.

Approximately 90% of anal fissures are located posteriorly in the midline, while anterior fissures occur in 10% of women and 1% of men. Fewer than 1% of fissures are located laterally or are multiple in number and should raise the suspect of a different underlying disease (Crohn's disease, sexually transmitted diseases, anal cancer, or tuberculosis) [51].

### 86.8.2 Etiology

The exact etiology of anal fissure is still unknown. The two most accredited theories at present are traumatic and ischemic.

### 86.8.3 Pathophysiology

The pathophysiology may be different for anterior, posterior, and lateral fissures. For posterior fissures, the passage of bulky and hard stools creates a mechanical trauma to the anal canal, creating pain and a tear in the mucosa and resulting in intense pain during defecation. Anal pain creates a deleterious feedback loop: firstly it creates fear of defecation and stool retention, that became harder and cause more trauma during the passage through the anal canal; on the other hand, anal pain increases the basal tone of internal anal sphincter, reducing blood flow and a relative ischemia of the posterior commissure. Ischemia is believed to be involved in fistula formation according to some experimental evidences: post-mortem studies demonstrated how the posterior commissure is poorly perfused in 85% of patients, while study of anal manometry in patients with chronic anal fissures demonstrated hypertonia of the internal sphincter and fewer relaxations.

Regarding anterior anal fissures, there are some studies that suggest occult external sphincter injury and impaired external sphincter function, when compared with posterior fissure patients.

Lateral fissures are extremely rare and are usually correlated with other underlying pathologies.

### 86.8.4 Diagnosis

#### 86.8.4.1 Clinical Presentation
Typical presentation of acute anal fissures is characterized by anal pain during and after defecation, spasm, and bleeding. At clinical examination, acute anal fissures appear as a linear tear in the anoderm, with well-demarcated edges, while chronic fissures are usually characterized by a distal sentinel tag, a proximal hypertrophied anal papilla, raised edges, and exposed internal sphincter muscle fibers.

#### 86.8.4.2 Tests
Laboratory tests and imaging are not necessary in case of typical fissures. For lateral and atypical fissures, when concomitant diseases are suspected, laboratory tests, imaging, and endoscopy should be based on the supposed associated disease.

> **Differential Diagnosis**
> Differential diagnosis comprehends all the causes of anal pain/bleeding, but usually the diagnosis is straight forward and based on the findings of the physical examination.

## 86.8.5 Treatment

### 86.8.5.1 Medical Treatment

Acute anal fissures should be managed with a combination of dietary and lifestyle modification and medical therapy. The goals of this approach are:

- Achieve sphincter relaxation, thus reducing pain, increasing blood flow and facilitating the healing process. The so called "chemical sphincterotomy" can be obtained with warm sitz baths, local application of calcium channel blockers (CCBs, like Diltiazem or Nifedipine), local application of Nitrates (Nitroglycerin) and Botulinum injection. CCBs and nitrates also induce an increase in local blood flow. A recent meta-analysis suggested a superiority of CCBs over nitrates in terms of increased healing rate and lower side effects (nitrates could cause headache and hypotension) [52].
- Minimize anal trauma, with the use of stool softeners (increased intake of oral fluids, high-fiber diet or fiber supplement, bulk forming laxatives).
- Treat pain, to reduce sphincter hypertonus; Lidocaine is the most commonly prescribed topical anesthetic, while administration of pain killers (e.g., paracetamol or ibuprofen) and/or perianal infiltration of anesthetics is indicated for patients with severe acute pain.

Manual anal dilatation is no longer suggested, due to the high risk of incontinence [53]. Conversely, less traumatic, precise, measurable, and reproducible techniques of anal dilatation (i.e., balloon dilatation and staged dilatation) could be taken into account before surgical treatment of chronic anal fissure [54].

### 86.8.5.2 Surgical Treatment

Surgery is suggested only in the chronic phase, after the failure of 6–8 weeks of medical therapy. For chronic fissures, lateral internal sphincterotomy is the preferred technique with a lower recurrence rate, a higher patient satisfaction and a healing rate of over 90% [55].

## 86.8.6 Prognosis

Prognosis is good, as most of acute anal fissures will resolve only with medical therapy. Dietary and lifestyle changes are recommended to reduce the recurrence rate. If the fissure does not heal within 6–8 weeks, it becomes chronic and should be treated accordingly.

> **Dos and Don'ts**
> - Always collect an accurate and focused medical history.
> - Carefully perform a complete physical examination.
> - Be respectful and empathic with the patients, remembering that the involved anatomic area is deeply intimate.
> - Never underestimate an anorectal bleeding.

> **Take-Home Messages**
> - Anorectal bleeding should never be overlooked, as it could be life-threatening and could be the first sign of a colorectal malignancy or inflammatory bowel disease.
> - Timely diagnosis and management of anorectal sepsis save lives.
> - Given the overlapping signs and symptoms of most of the anorectal emergencies, accurate collection of patient's medical history and a complete physical examination are mandatory to correctly start the diagnostic workup.
> - Early involve an acute care surgeon in the management of patients with anorectal emergencies.
> - The anatomical conformation and the specific function of the area require utmost attention to preserve the sphincterial complex.

## Multiple Answer Questions

1. In case of anorectal abscess with no obvious fistula at surgical exploration, what is the correct action?
   A. Accurately probe or use hydrogen peroxide to search for a possible fistula.
   B. Avoid probing to prevent iatrogenic trauma.
   C. Early surgical re-exploration to identify a possible fistula.
   D. None of the above.

   **Correct Answer: B**

2. Which is the cornerstone of Fournier's gangrene management?
   A. Resuscitation and hemodynamic support, timely surgical treatment, appropriate antibiotic therapy.
   B. Early surgical treatment, but after acquisition of contrast enhanced CT scan.
   C. Medical therapy with antibiotics, hemodynamic support and pain control.
   D. Surgical treatment and hyperbaric therapy.

   **Correct Answer: A**

3. Is it important to differentiate bleeding hemorrhoids from bleeding anorectal varices?
   A. No, treatment does not differ.
   B. Yes, treatment is completely different.
   C. No, they are just two names for the same disease.
   D. Yes, it is important for proper patient classification, but treatment does not differ.

   **Correct Answer: B**

4. When is it indicated to perform a full colonoscopy for bleeding hemorrhoids?
   A. Always, every patient with lower gastrointestinal bleeding should undergo a full colonoscopy.
   B. Never.
   C. In presence of risk factors for colorectal cancer or inflammatory bowel disease (anemia, atypical bleeding, alteration of bowel habits, preceding weight loss, suggestive personal and family history).
   D. In case of recurrent bleeding.

   **Correct Answer: C**

5. Is surgical approach indicated in case of acute anal fissures?
   A. Yes, lateral internal sphincterotomy is the correct surgical approach.
   B. Yes, posterior internal sphincterotomy is the correct surgical approach.
   C. No, surgical approach is reserved to chronic anal fissures.
   D. Surgical treatment of acute anal fissures is based on surgeon's expertise and patient's preference.

   **Correct Answer: C**

6. Medical treatment of thrombosed or strangulated hemorrhoids is based on:
   A. Flavonoids.
   B. Topical muscle relaxants.
   C. Dietary and lifestyle changes.
   D. All of the above.

   **Correct Answer: D**

7. Which is the appropriate surgical approach to a strangulated rectal prolapse?
   A. Perineal.
   B. Transabdominal.
   C. Laparoscopic, when dedicated skills are available.
   D. Surgical approach should be decided based on patient's characteristics, presence of bowel perforation/peritonitis and surgeon's expertise.

   **Correct Answer: D**

8. Which subset of patients with retained anorectal foreign body requires great attention and a differentiated management?
   A. Patients carrying drug packages, because casing disruption could cause a fatal drug overdose.
   B. Patients with high-lying objects.
   C. Patients with low-lying objects.
   D. Childs and elderly patients.

**Correct Answer: A**

9. What is the role of surgery in case of thrombosed hemorrhoids?
   A. Surgery is never indicated.
   B. Surgery is the first-line therapy.
   C. Surgery is indicated is symptoms persist after 72 h of non-operative management.
   D. Early surgical approach (within 72 h from the onset of symptoms) could be indicated in selected patients, based on physician's expertise and patient's preference.

**Correct Answer: D**

10. Which of the following is correct regarding Fournier's gangrene?
    A. Surgery is the last chance after failure of non-operative management.
    B. It is a benign disease and the appropriate treatment should be guided by a correct imaging study.
    C. Medical treatment is only supportive and immediate and aggressive surgery is mandatory.
    D. Time elapsed before surgery does not affect morbidity and mortality.

**Correct Answer: C**

## References

1. Goldstein ET. Outcomes of anorectal disease in a health maintenance organization setting. The need for colorectal surgeons. Dis Colon Rect. 1996;39(11):1193–8.
2. Abcarian H. Anorectal infection: abscess-fistula. Clin Colon Rectal Surg. 2011;24(1):14–21.
3. Garcia-Granero A, et al. Management of cryptoglandular supralevator abscesses in the magnetic resonance imaging era: a case series. Int J Color Dis. 2014;29(12):1557–64.
4. Sartelli M, et al. 2018 Wses/Sis-E consensus conference: recommendations for the management of skin and soft-tissue infections. World J Emerg Surg. 2018;13:58.
5. Sartelli M, et al. The management of intra-abdominal infections from a global perspective: 2017 Wses guidelines for management of intra-abdominal infections. World J Emerg Surg. 2017;12(1):29.
6. Smith SR, et al. Internal dressings for healing perianal abscess cavities. Cochrane Database Syst Rev. 2016;8:Cd011193.
7. Pearce L, et al. Multicentre observational study of outcomes after drainage of acute perianal abscess. Br J Surg. 2016;103(8):1063–8.
8. Schouten, W.R. And T.J. Van Vroonhoven, Treatment of anorectal abscess with or without primary fistulectomy. Results of a prospective randomized trial Dis Colon Rect. 1991. 34(1): P. 60–63.
9. Malik, A.I., R.L. Nelson, And S. Tou, Incision and drainage of perianal abscess with or without treatment of anal fistula. Cochrane Database Syst Rev, 2010. 22(7): Cd006827.
10. Sorensen, M.D. And J.N. Krieger Fournier''s gangrene: epidemiology and outcomes in the general us population. Urol Int, 2016. 97(3): P. 249–259.
11. Eke N. Fournier's gangrene: a review of 1726 cases. Br J Surg. 2000;87(6):718–28.
12. Smith, G.L., C.B. Bunker, And M.D. Dinneen, Fournier's Gangrene. Br J Urol, 1998. 81(3): P. 347–355.
13. Singh A, et al. Fournier's gangrene. A clinical review. Androl. 2016;88(3)
14. Wong CH, et al. The Lrinec (laboratory risk indicator for necrotizing fasciitis) score: a tool for distinguishing necrotizing fasciitis from other soft tissue infections. Crit Care Med. 2004;32(7):1535–41.
15. Laor E, et al. Outcome prediction in patients with Fournier's gangrene. J Urol. 1995;154(1):89–92.
16. Lin TY, et al. Validation and simplification of Fournier's gangrene severity index. Int J Urol. 2014;21(7):696–701.
17. Rajan, D.K. And K.A. Scharer Radiology of Fournier's gangrene. AJR Am J Roentgenol, 1998. 170(1): P. 163–168.
18. Martinez M, et al. The role of computed tomography in the diagnosis of necrotizing soft tissue infections. World J Surg. 2018;42(1):82–7.
19. Ozturk, E., Y. Sonmez, And T. Yilmazlar, What are the indications for a stoma in Fournier's gangrene?*. Color Dis, 2011. 13(9): P. 1044–1047.
20. Yanar H, et al. Fournier's gangrene: risk factors and strategies for management. World J Surg. 2006;30(9):1750–4.
21. Sorensen MD, et al. Fournier's gangrene: management and mortality predictors in a population based study. J Urol. 2009;182(6):2742–7.
22. Corman, J.M., J.A. Moody, And W.J. Aronson, Fournier's gangrene in a modern surgical setting:

23. Lohsiriwat V. Treatment of hemorrhoids: a coloproctologist's view. World J Gastroenterol. 2015;21(31):9245–52.
24. Lohsiriwat V. Approach to hemorrhoids. Curr Gastroenterol Rep. 2013;15(7):332.
25. Alonso-Coello P, et al. Fiber for the treatment of hemorrhoids complications: a systematic review and meta-analysis. Am J Gastroenterol. 2006;101(1):181–8.
26. Alonso-Coello P, et al. Laxatives for the treatment of hemorrhoids. Cochrane Database Syst Rev. 2005;4:Cd004649.
27. Alonso-Coello P, et al. Meta-analysis of flavonoids for the treatment of haemorrhoids. Br J Surg. 2006;93(8):909–20.
28. Tjandra JJ, et al. Rectogesic (glyceryl trinitrate 0.2%) ointment relieves symptoms of haemorrhoids associated with high resting anal canal pressures. Color Dis. 2007;9(5):457–63.
29. Allan A, et al. Prospective randomised study of urgent haemorrhoidectomy compared with non-operative treatment in the management of prolapsed thrombosed internal haemorrhoids. Color Dis. 2006;8(1):41–5.
30. Chan, K.K. And J.D. Arthur External haemorrhoidal thrombosis: evidence for current management. Tech Coloproctol, 2013. 17(1): P. 21–25.
31. Čavčić J, et al. Comparison of topically applied 0.2% glyceryl trinitrate ointment, incision and excision in the treatment of perianal thrombosis. Dig Liver Dis. 2001;33(4):335–40.
32. Guy, R.J. And F. Seow-Choen Septic complications after treatment of haemorrhoids. Br J Surg, 2003. 90(2): P. 147–156.
33. Maslekar S, et al. Systematic review of anorectal varices. Color Dis. 2013;15(12):E702–10.
34. Misra SP, et al. Colonic changes in patients with cirrhosis and in patients with extrahepatic portal vein obstruction. Endoscopy. 2005;37(5):454–9.
35. Raman SP, Horton KM, Fishman EK. Mdct and Ct angiography evaluation of rectal bleeding: the role of volume visualization. AJR Am J Roentgenol. 2013;201(3):589–97.
36. Kim, K.S., G.J. Suh, And W.Y. Kwon, Successful bridging hemostasis using a Sengstaken-Blakemore tube in massive rectal variceal bleeding Korean J Crit Care Med, 2014. 29(3).
37. Biecker E. Portal hypertension and gastrointestinal bleeding: diagnosis, prevention and management. World J Gastroenterol. 2013;19(31):5035–50.
38. Rodrigues SG, Mendoza YP, Bosch J. Beta-blockers in cirrhosis: evidence-based indications and limitations. Jhep Rep. 2020;2(1):100063.
39. O'leary JG, et al. Aga clinical practice update: coagulation in cirrhosis. Gastroenterology. 2019;157(1):34–43 E1.
40. Chavez-Tapia NC, et al. Meta-analysis: antibiotic prophylaxis for cirrhotic patients with upper gastrointestinal bleeding - an updated Cochrane review. Aliment Pharmacol Ther. 2011;34(5):509–18.
41. Bittinger M, et al. Bleeding from rectal varices in patients with liver cirrhosis - an ominous event. Gastrointest Endosc. 2004;59(5)
42. Yoshino K, et al. Therapeutic strategy for patients with bleeding rectal varices complicating liver cirrhosis. Hepatol Res. 2014;44(11):1088–94.
43. Kairaluoma, M.V. And I.H. Kellokumpu, Epidemiologic aspects of complete rectal prolapse. Scand J Surg, 2005. 94(3): P. 207–210.
44. Felt-Bersma, R.J., E.S. Tiersma, And M.A. Cuesta, Rectal prolapse, rectal intussusception, rectocele, solitary rectal ulcer syndrome, and enterocele. Gastroenterol Clin N Am, 2008. 37(3): P. 645–668, Ix.
45. Shapiro, R., E.H. Chin, And R.M. Steinhagen, Reduction of an incarcerated, prolapsed ileostomy with the assistance of sugar as a desiccant. Tech Coloproctol, 2010. 14(3): P. 269–271.
46. Chaudhuri A. Hyaluronidase in the reduction of incarcerated rectal prolapse: a novel use. Int J Color Dis. 1999;14(4–5):264.
47. Sarpel, U., B.P. Jacob, And R.M. Steinhagen, Reduction of a large incarcerated rectal prolapse by use of an elastic compression wrap. Dis Colon Rectum, 2005. 48(6): P. 1320–1322.
48. Kurer MA, et al. Colorectal foreign bodies: a systematic review. Color Dis. 2010;12(9):851–61.
49. Cappelletti, S., D. Piacentino, And C. Ciallella, Commentary on confounding definitions and descriptions of body packing. Abdom Imaging, 2015. 40(8): P. 3365–3366.
50. Jamshidi R. Anorectal complaints: hemorrhoids, fissures, abscesses, fistulae. Clin Colon Rectal Surg. 2018;31(2):117–20.
51. Zaghiyan, K.N. And P. Fleshner, Anal fissure Clin Colon Rectal Surg, 2011. 24(1): P. 22–30.
52. Nelson RL, et al. A systematic review and meta-analysis of the treatment of anal fissure. Tech Coloproctol. 2017;21(8):605–25.
53. Nielsen MB, et al. Risk of sphincter damage and anal incontinence after anal dilatation for fissure-in-ano. An endosonographic study. Dis Colon Rectum. 1993;36(7):677–80.
54. Pinsk, I., et al., The long-term effect of standardized anal dilatation for chronic anal fissure on anal continence. Ann Coloproctol, 2021 37(2):115-119.
55. Karamanlis E, et al. Prospective clinical trial comparing sphincterotomy, nitroglycerin ointment and xylocaine/lactulose combination for the treatment of anal fissure. Tech Coloproctol. 2010;14(Suppl 1):S21–3.

## Further Reading

Tarasconi A, et al. Anorectal emergencies: WSES-AAST guidelines. World J Emerg Surg. 2021;16(1):48.

# Gynaecological Surgical Emergencies

**87**

Robert Tchounzou, André Gaetan Simo Wambo, and Alain Chichom-Mefire

### Learning Goals
- List the five most common causes of gynaecological surgical emergencies across the world.
- Propose an approach to the management of pelvic pain in the female patient of reproductive age.
- Identify and solve immediately life-threatening gynaecological surgical emergencies.
- Provide an accurate and timely diagnosis in stable patients relying on clinical examination and simple tools such as emergency room ultrasound.
- Discuss the place of laparoscopy in the management of gynaecological surgical emergencies.
- Understand the need for protection of reproductive function in the course of management of all gynaecological surgical emergencies.

## 87.1 Introduction

Gynaecological surgical emergencies are frequent life-threatening conditions and are major contributors to morbidity and mortality worldwide [1]. Although the challenges of their diagnosis and management are not the same in various settings, their causes seem to have frozen over decades.

Whatever the setting of practice, the main objectives are almost always the same: identifying and resolving without delay immediately life-threatening situations, and in stable patients, providing an accurate diagnosis within a relatively short period of time to guarantee appropriate and timely management, permanently keeping in mind the need for preserving patient's procreation capabilities as this is often a major concern in reproductive ages in all settings. Health care providers located in low- and middle-income countries (LMICs) face a special challenge related to the need for ensuring equitable access to surgical care in frail health systems often characterized by limited technical background and the absence of minimal universal health coverage. They consequently need to be permanently inventive in defining strategies that will ensure provision of minimum standard care in the emergency settings with little equipment. When it comes to gynaecological emergencies, very often, it's NOT about what you have but how you use the little that you have. This chapter intends among other objectives

R. Tchounzou · A. G. S. Wambo
Department of Obstetric/Gynaecology, Faculty of Health Sciences, University of Buea,
Buea, Cameroon

A. Chichom-Mefire (✉)
Department of Surgery, Faculty of Health Sciences, University of Buea, Buea, Cameroon

to discuss some tips often used by providers facing such special challenges.

Often manifesting with abdomino-pelvic pain and/or non-menstrual vaginal bleeding [2–5], gynaecological surgical emergencies are usually centred on four major issues often overlapping in their clinical expression: ectopic pregnancies, acute complications of adnexal masses, pelvic inflammatory disease (PID; and its main complication: tubo-ovarian abscess [TOA]) and vulvo-vaginal trauma including genital mutilations [6, 7]. There is one additional problem which is a major burden in many low- and middle-income countries (LMICs) and worth discussing: complications of unsafe abortions. The discussion in this chapter will be centred on these frequent causes of gynaecological emergencies. However, while attending to a patient with pelvic pain, one should keep in mind the possibility of the involvement of a digestive or urologic component as they could be often misleading [8].

Over decades, routine practice has established the fact that combination of a careful clinical assessment and pelvic ultrasound permits the proper assessment and accurate diagnosis of a wide range of gynaecological surgical emergencies [8, 9]. Ultrasound is now often available even in the most remote areas, especially since the advent and expansion of portable ultrasound devices. If judiciously associated with some basic biological work-up also available nearly everywhere such as pregnancy test, inflammatory markers like erythrocyte sedimentation rate (ESR) and C-reactive protein (CRP), the diagnostic capabilities are almost completely covered. The possibility of obtaining additional information such as beta-human chorionic gonadotropin (β-HCG) levels and calcitonin levels could be a decisive advantage in some specific situations. **Sophisticated imaging tools and biological work-up are not required to efficiently face most gynaecological surgical emergencies!**

The overall philosophy of the management of gynaecological emergencies is now guided by two major concepts:

- The advent and massive development of minimally invasive surgical approaches.
- The increasing need to preserve pelvic organs and their contributions to reproductive function, with particular emphasis on Fallopian tubes and ovaries.

Their operative management is now largely dominated by the constant progress and the large diffusion of minimally approaches which, in a few decades, have overtaken centuries of routine gynaecological practice. They can now be used for the management of almost all related situations with very few exceptions [10, 11], and their scope keeps extending. They also represent the best option for the possibility of preserving procreation capabilities [10]. One specific aspect of this philosophy of gynaecological surgery is Natural Orifice Transluminal Endoscopic Surgery (NOTES) in Gynaecological in which the vagina could be used to access abdominal cavity and solve a wide range of clinical issues in gynaecology and general surgery leaving the patient with no scar [11, 12]. The implementation and diffusion of these approaches which have proven to be economically beneficial in various aspects should be considered a priority in countries lagging behind.

This chapter aims at reviewing timely diagnostic and management tips of most common gynaecological surgical emergencies form different angles and visions of clinical practice. We have chosen to exclude children and adolescent younger than reproductive age from this discussion.

## 87.2 Ectopic Pregnancy

### 87.2.1 Introduction

This happens when a fertilized egg is wrongly implanted outside of the uterine endometrial cavity. It is considered the most common gynaecological emergency as it could affect up to 2% of pregnancies worldwide [12, 13]. It MUST be considered whenever a female patient of reproductive age presents to the emergency department with a pelvic pain, especially when associated with an unusual pattern of bleeding [14]. Suspicion must

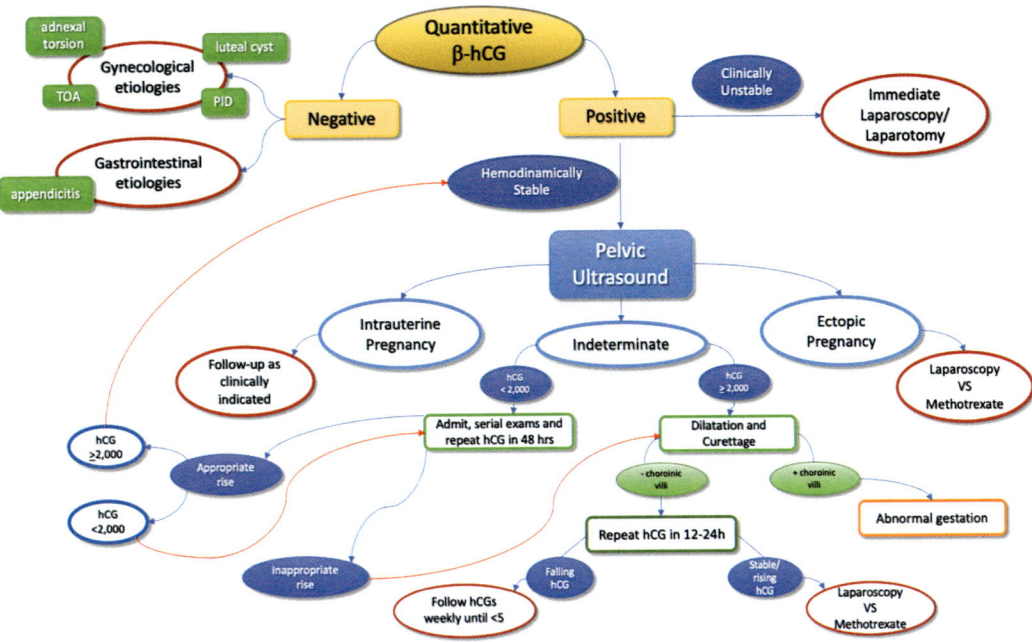

**Fig. 87.1** Ectopic pregnancies diagnostic and therapeutic algorithm

be even greater in patients with current or past pelvic inflammatory disease (PID), past history of pelvic surgery including tubal ligation and history of abortion [15, 16]. The localization of the egg in this often life-threatening condition is extremely variable, from the very common and dangerous location in the Fallopian tube to the abdominal cavity. The advent of in vitro fertilization (IVF) seems to have favoured the arousal of more unusual localizations such as the myometrium or the scar of a segmental caesarean section [17, 18]. It has even been suggested that the absence of a uterus does not exclude the possibility of an ectopic pregnancy [19]. Sometimes, identifying the location seems really difficult in what is sometimes temporarily referred to as 'pregnancy of unknown location' [20].

Easy to handle when suspected and confirmed on time, it becomes immediately life-threatening when ruptured, especially when localized in the Fallopian tubes. Major disparities have been reported in the clinical presentations of ectopic pregnancies with unacceptable proportions presenting as the often-deadly ruptured form in numerous LMICs [21–23]. Under such conditions, ectopic pregnancy must be considered in every woman diagnosed with 'acute abdomen', especially when it is associated with signs of anaemia.

Figure 87.1 reports the suggested flowcharts for ectopic pregnancies management.

## 87.2.2 Diagnosis

It seems possible to diagnose ectopic pregnancy on clinical grounds alone in over 85% of cases, especially when it has ruptured [22]. A simple positive pregnancy test combined to suggestive clinical criteria strongly supports the diagnosis and guide a decision in the absence of imaging facilities or training. Ultrasound would confirm the absence of an embryo in the uterine cavity and often visualize the ectopic embryo, especially in the Fallopian tube. Using a vaginal probe makes it even more sensitive [14]. A baseline value of β-HCG should be obtained whenever possible as its trends in serial measurements might serve in diagnosis and follow-up of a non-surgical treatment [20].

### 87.2.3 Management

Most authorities still agree on the fact that all patients diagnosed with ectopic pregnancy (EP) must be admitted until considered safe [20]. Currently, three treatment options can be offered to the patient diagnosed with ectopic pregnancy: expectant management, conservative medical management with a single injection of methotrexate and surgical (operative) management.

A single intramuscular dose of methotrexate, which could be repeated once if the fall in β-HCG levels is not satisfactory, has been established for decades as a valid treatment option in early, non-complicated EP [16, 20, 24]. This is a grade A recommendation [24]. Patients undergoing this treatment option MUST display a drop of β-HCG levels indicating resolution of trophoblastic activity within 48 hours or be prepared to be moved to surgical treatment [25].

The concept of 'expectant management' arouse from the suggestion that spontaneous resolution is a possible natural course of EP. Several clinical trials have been conducted to compare this option to methotrexate injection. Recently, in meta-analysis and systematic review, Colombo et al. failed to demonstrate any significant differences between expectant management and medical treatment with methotrexate in terms of resolution of the EP and avoidance of surgery [26]. Consequently, caution is highly recommended when making a decision on which conservative option should be applied while waiting for results of more decisive randomized trials.

Obviously, conservative management should not even be envisaged in the absence of repeated ultrasound and serial β-HCG follow-up facilities.

Surgical management is generally indicated in ruptured EP and when conservative management is contraindicated. As indicated earlier, the salvation of Fallopian tube should always be envisaged as long as it does not seem to increase the risk of a future EP on the same tube. Ruptured ectopic pregnancy is considered an immediately life-threatening condition because of the associated, often massive haemoperitoneum and should be handled immediately. Timely diagnosis and management could result in 100% survival rate even in austere environments [27]. In almost all situations, this treatment can be performed through a laparoscopic approach now available in most countries at least in urban centres [16]. Situations of massive haemoperitoneum have not been considered a contraindication to laparoscopic approach for over two decades now [28].

Even in 2021, there is nothing wrong in managing EP, complicated or not, with a laparotomy, sometimes explorative in suspicious cases backed by a strong beam of clinical arguments and in the absence of the most basic imaging facilities such as ultrasound. If wrong, in such situations the surgeon will likely still discover another surgically correctable condition.

The future of the management of ectopic pregnancy might significantly depend on the possibility of more precocious and precise diagnosis based on novel 'metabolomics' profiling using new biological markers [29].

> **Dos and Don'ts**
> **Dos:**
> - Ask about the last menstrual period.
> - Always admit the patient with a suspicion of ectopic pregnancy, especially in places where they cannot be traced.
> - Request a β-HCG from the time of suspicion as it will serve for diagnosis and follow-up. If not possible, a simple pregnancy test can help.
> - Use laparoscopic approach whenever possible.
> - Preserve the ovaries and the tubes whenever possible.
>
> **Don'ts:**
> - Request sophisticated investigations such as computed tomography (CT) scan or extensive biological work-up, except in really confusing situations.
> - Apply expectant management until further evidence of its efficacy is provided.
> - Apply conservative management if you do not have access to follow-up facilities (β-HCG measurements and ultrasound).
> - Systematically perform salpingectomy for tubal ectopic pregnancies.

## 87.3 Adnexal Torsion

### 87.3.1 Introduction

This occurs following the rotation of one ovary on its vascular pedicle causing in a stepwise manner oedema, haemorrhagic infarction and necrosis of all adnexal structures if not timely and properly diagnosed and surgically treated. As adnexal torsion is relatively frequent in very young females, the preservation of adnexal structures and chances of procreation are at stake [30].

### 87.3.2 Diagnosis

Its diagnosis is challenging because of the extremely polymorphic and often misleading clinical presentation. In its acute form, it could combine pelvic pain, vomiting, fever, urinary symptoms and sometimes elevated white cell count, mimicking not only a number of other gynaecological conditions, but also digestive or urologic involvements such as pyelonephritis, appendicitis or urolithiasis [30, 31]. It also can take a more sluggish sub-acute, intermittent or even chronic form, mimicking a malignancy, especially in older patients [4]. Though it frequently involves a healthy ovary [4], it most often complicates a pre-existing adnexal mass of which the most common is any form of ovarian cyst. For all these reasons, diagnosis of adnexal torsion is not easy and it can easily be missed or confused with something else, turning in many situations in a discovery of surgical exploration often initiated for another indication.

In the absence of clear-cut, decisive clinical criteria as is often the case in up to half of patients [4], pelvic ultrasound plays a key role in guiding the diagnosis, especially if Doppler mode is available. If performed by a trained staff, it could detect adnexal torsion in the form of a pelvic mass in over 95% of cases [31]. However, the Doppler ultrasound cannot be used to guide clinical decision because it cannot be relied on to rule out torsion and ischaemia as vascular supply could be preserved due to the double origin of blood supply to the ovary. In such doubtful situations, CT scan or magnetic resonance imaging (MRI) could be discriminatory though they should not be proposed as first line [30, 32].

### 87.3.3 Management

All the diagnostic uncertainties explain why suspicion of adnexal torsion if often considered enough justification for surgical exploration. Laparoscopic approach represents the best option for an extensive exploration of the pelvis, including digestive and urologic differential diagnosis. The only limit to this approach seems to be the size of the mass at the origin of the torsion [31]. All surgical gestures including detorsion or untwisting, oophorectomy and adnexectomy are possible under laparoscopic approach, but the surgical management of adnexal torsion is now dominated by the attempt to preserve the ovary and tube at all cost despite the controversial suspicion of risk of sequelae such as post-operative adhesions and even tubal occlusion [33, 34]. Some suggest that the ovary be preserved regardless of its appearance except if it falls apart as the result of complete necrosis [4].

**Dos and Don'ts**

**Dos:**
- Perform bi-manual palpation during clinical assessment for a pelvic mass.
- Always request a pelvic ultrasound. Whenever possible, this should be performed by a trained staff that can use the Doppler mode.
- In the presence of a painful adnexal mass, surgical exploration is an acceptable option.
- Use laparoscopic approach whenever possible.

**Don'ts:**
- Remove ovary except if certain of its complete and irreversible necrosis.

## 87.4 PID and Tubo-Ovarian Abscess

### 87.4.1 Introduction

pelvic inflammatory disease (PID) and tubo-ovarian abscess (TOA) represent two stages of the same entity affecting females of reproductive age. PID is a relatively benign disease if timely identified and addressed and the main concern about it is usually the possible sequelae and their impact on procreation potential and risk of EP [35, 36]. The real challenge of PID is to be able to timely capture evolution towards TOA and take appropriate action.

### 87.4.2 Diagnosis

Often manifesting in patients who display a temporary reduction of the effectiveness of the barrier function of the cervix including carriers of an intrauterine device, its clinical presentation ranges from the severe acute pelvic pain warranting admission to much milder pictures [35–38]. Examination might reveal moderate signs of localized peritonitis. Imaging work-up does NOT contribute directly to the diagnosis of uncomplicated PID. However, obtaining a baseline value of ESR and CRP could help monitor evolution and guide decision. Whenever possible, an **ENDOCERVICAL** bacteriological sample obtained through speculum examination should be collected. **A sample obtained from the vagina or exocervix would be misleading!**

It is suggested that TOA is actually present in 15% of patients at the time they are diagnosed with PID [39]. This entity is much more dangerous and could be life-threatening in the event of rupture and development of sepsis [40]. Though its clinical presentation if highly variable, TOA should be suspected in every woman of reproductive age who displays the combination of fever, diarrhoea and leucocytosis, especially (but not only) if diagnosed with a PID [41]. Ultrasound must be requested and could contribute to identify the adnexal inflammatory mass and even guide decision as per the need for an invasive treatment [42]. Patients carrying an intrauterine device seem to develop much larger TOA on ultrasound though it does not result in an increase need for surgery [38]. Serial measurements of absolute values of CRP and ESR when available would also indicate failure of conservative management and sometimes guide decision of the need for an invasive action [43, 44].

### 87.4.3 Management

The effort for bacteriological documentation of the infection should not delay the start of empiric antibiotic therapy guided by the general biology of PID which is dominated by *Chlamydia trachomatis*, *Neisseria gonorrhoeae*, *Streptococcus spp*, some anaerobes and gram-negative bacteria. *Mycoplasma genitalium* also seems to play an increasing role [37, 45]. The choice of antibiotics is of critical importance as antimicrobial resistance is developing as a worldwide community concern [46]. Current guidelines consider the combination of ceftriaxone-doxycycline-metronidazole as a good starting line of treatment. Intravenous administration should be preferred whenever possible at least for the first days. Fluoroquinolones combined to metronidazole could supplement for patients with allergy issues or contra-indications [45].

Antibiotic therapy based on the same regimen is still considered the first line treatment for TOA [38, 47]. It is estimated that this regimen will fail in 25% of patients who will require a more invasive treatment [39]. The decision to shift to a surgical treatment is generally guided by clinical assessment combined with ultrasound (large abscess, complex cystic image) and biological markers mentioned earlier [43]. Serum calcitonin levels also seem to play a role [39]. When surgical decision has been taken, it is highly suggested that imaging-guided drainage is superior to laparoscopic or open drainage as it ensues in significantly better results in terms of success of drainage, complication rate and duration of hospital stay [43, 47].

Recently, an objective score combining age at admission, leucocytosis on admission, ultrasonographic measurement of TOA and bilaterality of the collection has been used in predicting antibiotic treatment failure in patients with TOA but still needs to be validated [48].

> **Dos and Don'ts**
>
> **Dos:**
> - Obtain baseline CRP and ESR values whenever possible.
> - Start empirical antibiotics targeting relevant germs as soon as possible.
> - Use ultrasound-guided drainage rather than surgery for TOA whenever possible.
>
> **Don'ts:**
> - Take a sample in the vagina or exocervix for bacteriological diagnosis.
> - Wait for results of bacteriological analysis before starting antibiotics.
> - Use a single antibiotic for the treatment of PID.
> - Apply a surgical option until clear signs of failure of antibiotic treatment.

## 87.5 Female Non-obstetric Genital Injuries

Female genitalia could get injured in three different ways: general traumatic mechanism, sexual activity (consensual and non-consensual) and ritual genital mutilations. Isolated genital injuries rarely result into death and thus tend to be minimized [49]. They represent only about 0.2% of cases in a national trauma data bank [50]. They, however, require specific attention because of their potential to generate disturbing consequences such as genital fistulas, chronic discomfort, dyspareunia and fertility problems [49]. Initial management in the emergency setting sometimes play a key role in avoiding these complications and providing emotional and mental support. Examination of a female displaying an injury to the genitalia should whenever possible be performed in a spirit of forensic analysis and history of injury is often misleading, especially when provided by someone else than the victim.

Non-sexual injury to female genitalia occurs following a wide variety of mechanism including blunt trauma, crush injury, burns of all types, impalement and straddle injury, falls, cow horn, sports injury and intentional injury using a variety of objects and often combined with sexual violence [51–53]. Though they most often involve anatomical structures of the vulva and vagina, possibilities of involvement of the anus, urethra, bony pelvis and even internal organs must be kept in mind during assessment in the emergency department [49].

Sexual violence remains a major worldwide concern, disproportionally affecting particularly vulnerable females such as adolescents and young adults [52, 54]. Examination of victims must be performed in the forensic spirit with the idea of collecting evidence to help action of justice, including information on the perpetrators who are often closed family members [52]. One should keep in mind that this examination cannot be limited to genitalia and anus as injuries to other body parts are often discovered, especially when the perpetrator used a weapon [52, 54, 55].

An increasing number of females are received in the emergency department for injuries sustained during consensual sex. Male-to-female disproportion and the practice of 'dry sex' seem to be major risk factors. Examination often discovers rupture of posterior fornix and vaginal lacerations generally requiring minor, but mandatory surgical repair [53, 56].

Female genital mutilation is still performed in many areas in the world, especially in Africa and middle-East [57, 58]. It could still be observed in western countries in immigrants [58]. According to WHO, it affects around 200 million women [59]. Lesions observed range from clitoridectomy to the extremely devastating infibulation [57, 59]. The major concern in the emergency department is the risk of bleeding which could be deadly and the need to prepare for the possible future reversal of the mutilation through plastic surgery.

Generally, surgical intervention is not always required following genital injury. This is particularly true for victims of sexual assault [50]. Whatever the treatment option selected, it is important to remember antibiotic prophylaxis and anti-tetanic prophylaxis in open, penetrating injuries involving the vagina and vulva, especially when a foreign object is involved [53].

## 87.6 Unsafe Abortions

Complications of unsafe abortions are still a tragedy in some areas and major contributors to maternal death and disability. Half of abortions in the world are conducted under conditions which are considered unsafe [60], especially in countries where abortion is still illegal. It is now generally admitted that restriction of access to abortion is the main explanation to the high burden of unsafe abortions. When performed in a clandestine setting, abortion frequently involves violent methods such as use of sharp curettage and insertion of objects in the genital tract [61]. Additionally, the illegal environment is incompatible with early consultation when complications develop, often interpreted as signs of success of the procedure. Consequently, patients tend to remain 'clandestine' until late in the course of developing these complications. Those requiring emergency surgery include retained product of conception often associated to bleeding of various severity, septic complications often requiring urgent surgical intervention for source control, injuries to the genital tract and sometimes to internal organs [62].

---

MCQs
1. Which of the following investigations is/are indispensable for the diagnosis of ectopic pregnancy?
    A. Ultrasound.
    B. β-HCG.
    C. Pelvic CT scan.
    D. All of the above.
    E. **None of the above.**
2. According to WHO, how many women are affected by female genital mutilations every year?
    A. 1 million.
    B. 5 million.
    C. 10 million.
    D. 100 million.
    E. **200 million.**
3. What proportion of patients with a PID actually have a TOA at the time of reception in the emergency department?
    A. 10%.
    B. **15%.**
    C. 20%.
    D. 25%.
    E. 30%.
4. Which of the following would be useful to decision making in cases of suspicion of adnexal torsion?
    A. Doppler ultrasound.
    B. CT scan.
    C. MRI.
    D. **All of the above.**
    E. None of the above.
5. In a case of ruptured ectopic pregnancy with minimal haemoperitoneum, which of the following options should be preferred?
    A. Single injection of Methotrexate.
    B. Expectant management.
    C. **Laparoscopy.**
    D. Laparotomy.
    E. All of the above.
6. Which of the following is often associated with an increased risk of ectopic pregnancy? (Select all that apply).
    A. **History of PID and TOA.**
    B. History of diffuse peritonitis.
    C. **History of previous ectopic pregnancy.**
    D. History of adhesive bowel obstruction.
    E. All of the above.
7. What proportion of patients with TOA will eventually require drainage?
    A. 10%
    B. 15%

C. **25%**
D. 50%
E. 100%.

8. Which of the following antibiotics could be included in combinations for empirical treatment in PID? (Select all that apply).
   A. Ampicillin.
   B. **Metronidazole.**
   C. **Doxycycline.**
   D. **Ceftriaxone.**
   E. **Ofloxacin.**

9. Which of the following approaches to gynaecological surgical emergency interventions leaves the patient with no scar?
   A. Laparotomy.
   B. Laparoscopy.
   C. Robotic surgery.
   D. Da Vinci.
   E. **NOTES.**

10. The following anatomical parts of female genitalia are often injured following coital injuries in the context of consensual sex, mandating surgical repair:
    A. Labia majora.
    B. Clitoris.
    C. **Posterior fornix.**
    D. **Vaginal walls.**
    E. Cervix.

# References

1. Fawole A, Awonuga D. Gynaecological emergencies in the tropics: recent advances in management. Ann Ib Postgrad Med. 2007;5(1):12–20. https://doi.org/10.4314/aipm.v5i1.63539. PMID: 25161432; PMCID: PMC4110985
2. Dewey K, Wittrock C. Acute pelvic pain. Emerg Med Clin North Am. 2019;37(2):207–18. https://doi.org/10.1016/j.emc.2019.01.012.
3. Abam DS. Overview of gynaecological emergencies [internet]. Contemporary Gynecologic Practice. IntechOpen; 2015 [cited 2021 May 13]. https://www.intechopen.com/books/contemporary-gynecologic-practice/overview-of-gynaecological-emergencies.
4. Adnexal Torsion in Adolescents: ACOG Committee opinion no, 783. Obstet Gynecol. 2019;134(2):e56–63. https://doi.org/10.1097/AOG.0000000000003373.
5. Pokharel HP, Dahal P, Rai R, Budhathoki S. Surgical emergencies in obstetrics and gynaecology in a tertiary care hospital. JNMA J Nepal Med Assoc. 2013;52(189):213–6.
6. Burnett LS. Gynecologic causes of the acute abdomen. Surg Clin North Am. 1988;68(2):385–98. https://doi.org/10.1016/s0039-6109(16)44484-1.
7. McWilliams GD, Hill MJ, Dietrich CS 3rd. Gynecologic emergencies. Surg Clin North Am. 2008;88(2):265–83., vi. https://doi.org/10.1016/j.suc.2007.12.007.
8. Pages-Bouic E, Millet I, Curros-Doyon F, Faget C, Fontaine M, Taourel P. Acute pelvic pain in females in septic and aseptic contexts. Diagn Interv Imaging. 2015;96(10):985–95. https://doi.org/10.1016/j.diii.2015.07.003. Epub 2015 Oct 3
9. Ignacio EA, Hill MC. Ultrasound of the acute female pelvis. Ultrasound Q. 2003;19(2):86–98; quiz 108–10. https://doi.org/10.1097/00013644-200306000-00004.
10. Promecene PA. Laparoscopy in gynecologic emergencies. Semin Laparosc Surg. 2002;9(1):64–75.
11. Jallad K, Walters MD. Natural orifice transluminal endoscopic surgery (NOTES) in gynecology. Clin Obstet Gynecol. 2017;60(2):324–9. https://doi.org/10.1097/GRF.0000000000000280.
12. Li CB, Hua KQ. Transvaginal natural orifice transluminal endoscopic surgery (vNOTES) in gynecologic surgeries: a systematic review. Asian J Surg. 2020;43(1):44–51. https://doi.org/10.1016/j.asjsur.2019.07.014. Epub 2019 Aug 20
13. Jacob L, Kalder M, Kostev K. Risk factors for ectopic pregnancy in Germany: a retrospective study of 100,197 patients. Ger Med Sci. 2017;15:Doc19. https://doi.org/10.3205/000260. PMID: 29308062; PMCID: PMC5738501
14. Lee R, Dupuis C, Chen B, Smith A, Kim YH. Diagnosing ectopic pregnancy in the emergency setting. Ultrasonography. 2018;37(1):78–87. https://doi.org/10.14366/usg.17044. Epub 2017 Aug 19. PMID: 29061036; PMCID: PMC5769947
15. Shaikh NB, Shaikh S, Shaikh F. A clinical study of ectopic pregnancy. J Ayub Med Coll Abbottabad. 2014;26(2):178–81.
16. Oron G, Tulandi T. A pragmatic and evidence-based management of ectopic pregnancy. J Minim Invasive Gynecol. 2013;20(4):446–54. https://doi.org/10.1016/j.jmig.2013.02.004. Epub 2013 Apr 12
17. Boukhanni L, Ait Benkaddour Y, Bassir A, Aboulfalah A, Asmouki H, Soummani A. A rare localization of ectopic pregnancy: intramyometrial pregnancy in twin pregnancy following IVF. Case Rep Obstet Gynecol. 2014;2014:893935. https://doi.org/10.1155/2014/893935. Epub 2014 Mar 18. PMID: 24744925; PMCID: PMC3976907
18. Pędraszewski P, Wlaźlak E, Panek W, Surkont G. Cesarean scar pregnancy - a new challenge for

19. Ilea C, Stoian I, Carauleanu D, Socolov D. A case of ectopic tubal pregnancy eight years after a hysterectomy presenting as a diagnostic challenge. Am J Case Rep. 2019 Oct;31(20):1596–600. https://doi.org/10.12659/AJCR.918894. PMID: 31666499; PMCID: PMC6849500
20. Hendriks E, Rosenberg R, Prine L. Ectopic pregnancy: diagnosis and management. Am Fam Physician. 2020;101(10):599–606.
21. Cornelius AC, Onyegbule A, Onyema UET, Duke OA. A five year review of ectopic pregnancy at Federal Medical Centre, Owerri, South East, Nigeria. Niger J Med. 2014;23(3):207–12.
22. Akaba GO, Agida TE, Onafowokan O. Ectopic pregnancy in Nigeria's federal capital territory: a six year review. Niger J Med. 2012;21(2):241–5.
23. Pradhan P, Thapamagar SB, Maskey S. A profile of ectopic pregnancy at Nepal medical college teaching hospital. Nepal Med Coll J. 2006;8(4):238–42.
24. Marret H, Fauconnier A, Dubernard G, Misme H, Lagarce L, Lesavre M, Fernandez H, Mimoun C, Tourette C, Curinier S, Rabishong B, Agostini A. Overview and guidelines of off-label use of methotrexate in ectopic pregnancy: report by CNGOF. Eur J Obstet Gynecol Reprod Biol. 2016;205:105–9. https://doi.org/10.1016/j.ejogrb.2016.07.489. Epub 2016 Aug 3
25. Condous G. Ectopic pregnancy: challenging accepted management strategies. Aust N Z J Obstet Gynaecol. 2009;49(4):346–51. https://doi.org/10.1111/j.1479-828X.2009.01032.x.
26. Colombo GE, Leonardi M, Armour M, Di Somma H, Dinh T, da Silva CF, Wong L, Armour S, Condous G. Efficacy and safety of expectant management in the treatment of tubal ectopic pregnancy: a systematic review and meta-analysis. Hum Reprod Open. 2020;2020(4):hoaa044. https://doi.org/10.1093/hropen/hoaa044. PMID: 33134560; PMCID: PMC7585644
27. Ngwenya S. Challenges in the surgical management of ectopic pregnancy in a low-resource setting: Mpilo central hospital, Bulawayo, Zimbabwe. Trop Doct. 2017;47(4):316–20. https://doi.org/10.1177/0049475517700810. Epub 2017 Mar 26
28. Rizzuto MI, Oliver R, Odejinmi F. Laparoscopic management of ectopic pregnancy in the presence of a significant haemoperitoneum. Arch Gynecol Obstet. 2008;277(5):433–6. https://doi.org/10.1007/s00404-007-0473-7. Epub 2007 Sep 29
29. Turkoglu O, Citil A, Katar C, Mert I, Kumar P, Yilmaz A, Uygur DS, Erkaya S, Graham SF, Bahado-Singh RO. Metabolomic identification of novel diagnostic biomarkers in ectopic pregnancy. Metabolomics. 2019;15(11):143. https://doi.org/10.1007/s11306-019-1607-1.
30. Robertson JJ, Long B, Koyfman A. Emergency medicine myths: ectopic pregnancy evaluation, risk factors, and presentation. J Emerg Med. 2017;53(6):819–28. https://doi.org/10.1016/j.jemermed.2017.08.074. Epub 2017 Oct 27
31. Lo LM, Chang SD, Horng SG, Yang TY, Lee CL, Liang CC. Laparoscopy versus laparotomy for surgical intervention of ovarian torsion. J Obstet Gynaecol Res. 2008;34(6):1020–5. https://doi.org/10.1111/j.1447-0756.2008.00806.x.
32. Ssi-Yan-Kai G, Rivain AL, Trichot C, Morcelet MC, Prevot S, Deffieux X, De Laveaucoupet J. What every radiologist should know about adnexal torsion. Emerg Radiol. 2018;25(1):51–9. https://doi.org/10.1007/s10140-017-1549-8. Epub 2017 Sep 7
33. Mandelbaum RS, Smith MB, Violette CJ, Matsuzaki S, Matsushima K, Klar M, Roman LD, Paulson RJ, Matsuo K. Conservative surgery for ovarian torsion in young women: perioperative complications and national trends. BJOG. 2020;127(8):957–65. https://doi.org/10.1111/1471-0528.16179. Epub 2020 Mar 9. PMID: 32086987; PMCID: PMC7772940
34. Fujishita A, Araki H, Yoshida S, Hamaguchi D, Nakayama D, Tsuda N, Khan KN. Outcome of conservative laparoscopic surgery for adnexal torsion through one-stage or two-stage operation. J Obstet Gynaecol Res. 2015;41(3):411–7. https://doi.org/10.1111/jog.12534. Epub 2014 Nov 3
35. Chappell CA, Wiesenfeld HC. Pathogenesis, diagnosis, and management of severe pelvic inflammatory disease and tuboovarian abscess. Clin Obstet Gynecol. 2012;55(4):893–903. https://doi.org/10.1097/GRF.0b013e3182714681.
36. Lareau SM, Beigi RH. Pelvic inflammatory disease and tubo-ovarian abscess. Infect Dis Clin N Am. 2008;22(4):693–708. https://doi.org/10.1016/j.idc.2008.05.008.
37. Cazanave C, de Barbeyrac B. Les infections génitales hautes : diagnostic microbiologique. RPC infections génitales hautes CNGOF et SPILF [Pelvic inflammatory diseases: Microbiologic diagnosis - CNGOF and SPILF Pelvic Inflammatory Diseases Guidelines]. Gynecol Obstet Fertil Senol. 2019;47(5):409–17. French. https://doi.org/10.1016/j.gofs.2019.03.007. Epub 2019 Mar 13
38. Kapustian V, Namazov A, Yaakov O, Volodarsky M, Anteby EY, Gemer O. Is intrauterine device a risk factor for failure of conservative management in patients with tubo-ovarian abscess? An observational retrospective study. Arch Gynecol Obstet. 2018;297(5):1201–4. https://doi.org/10.1007/s00404-018-4690-z. Epub 2018 Feb 24
39. Sordia-Hernández LH, Serrano Castro LG, Sordia-Piñeyro MO, Morales Martinez A, Sepulveda Orozco MC, Guerrero-Gonzalez G. Comparative study of the clinical features of patients with a tubo-ovarian abscess and patients with severe pelvic inflammatory disease.

Int J Gynaecol Obstet. 2016;132(1):17–9. https://doi.org/10.1016/j.ijgo.2015.06.038. Epub 2015 Sep 19
40. Kinay T, Unlubilgin E, Cirik DA, Kayikcioglu F, Akgul MA, Dolen I. The value of ultrasonographic tubo-ovarian abscess morphology in predicting whether patients will require surgical treatment. Int J Gynaecol Obstet. 2016;135(1):77–81. https://doi.org/10.1016/j.ijgo.2016.04.006. Epub 2016 Jun 17
41. Inal ZO, Inal HA, Gorkem U. Experience of Tubo-ovarian abscess: a retrospective clinical analysis of 318 patients in a single tertiary Center in Middle Turkey. Surg Infect. 2018;19(1):54–60. https://doi.org/10.1089/sur.2017.215. Epub 2017 Nov 17
42. Ribak R, Schonman R, Sharvit M, Schreiber H, Raviv O, Klein Z. Can the need for invasive intervention in Tubo-ovarian abscess be predicted? The implication of C-reactive protein measurements. J Minim Invasive Gynecol. 2020;27(2):541–7. https://doi.org/10.1016/j.jmig.2019.04.027. Epub 2019 Aug 31
43. Verdon R. Prise en charge thérapeutique des infections génitales hautes non compliquées. RPC infections génitales hautes CNGOF et SPILF [Treatment of uncomplicated pelvic inflammatory disease: CNGOF and SPILF Pelvic Inflammatory Diseases Guidelines]. Gynecol Obstet Fertil Senol. 2019;47(5):418–30. French. https://doi.org/10.1016/j.gofs.2019.03.008. Epub 2019 Mar 13
44. Sartelli M, Labricciosa FM, Barbadoro P, Pagani L, Ansaloni L, Brink AJ, Carlet J, et al. The Global Alliance for Infections in Surgery: defining a model for antimicrobial stewardship-results from an international cross-sectional survey. World J Emerg Surg. 2017;12:34. https://doi.org/10.1186/s13017-017-0145-2. eCollection 2017. PubMed PMID: 28775763; PubMed Central PMCID: PMC5540347
45. Karaca K, Ozkaya E, Kurek Eken M, Uygun I, Kopuk SY, Alpay M. Serum procalcitonin levels together with clinical features and inflammatory markers in women with tubo-ovarian abscess for discriminating requirements for surgery for full recovery. J Obstet Gynaecol. 2018;38(6):818–21. https://doi.org/10.1080/01443615.2017.1405927. Epub 2018 Mar 9
46. Kairys N, Roepke C. Tubo-Ovarian Abscess. 2020 Jun 27. In: StatPearls [Internet]. Treasure Island, FL: StatPearls Publishing; 2021.
47. Goje O, Markwei M, Kollikonda S, Chavan M, Soper DE. Outcomes of minimally invasive management of Tubo-ovarian abscess: a systematic review. J Minim Invasive Gynecol. 2021;28(3):556–64. https://doi.org/10.1016/j.jmig.2020.09.014. Epub 2020 Sep 28
48. Fouks Y, Cohen A, Shapira U, Solomon N, Almog B, Levin I. Surgical intervention in patients with Tubo-ovarian abscess: clinical predictors and a simple risk score. J Minim Invasive Gynecol. 2019;26(3):535–43. https://doi.org/10.1016/j.jmig.2018.06.013. Epub 2018 Aug 11
49. Lopez HN, Focseneanu MA, Merritt DF. Genital injuries acute evaluation and management. Best Pract Res Clin Obstet Gynaecol. 2018;48:28–39. https://doi.org/10.1016/j.bpobgyn.2017.09.009. Epub 2017 Sep 28
50. Gambhir S, Grigorian A, Schubl S, Barrios C, Bernal N, Joe V, Gabriel V, Nahmias J. Analysis of non-obstetric vaginal and vulvar trauma: risk factors for operative intervention. Updat Surg. 2019;71(4):735–40. https://doi.org/10.1007/s13304-019-00679-4. Epub 2019 Sep 19
51. Merritt DF. Genital trauma in children and adolescents. Clin Obstet Gynecol. 2008;51(2):237–48. https://doi.org/10.1097/GRF.0b013e31816d223c.
52. Santos JC, Neves A, Rodrigues M, Ferrão P. Victims of sexual offences: medicolegal examinations in emergency settings. J Clin Forensic Med. 2006;13(6–8):300–3. https://doi.org/10.1016/j.jcfm.2006.06.003. Epub 2006 Aug 23
53. Habek D, Kulas T. Nonobstetrics vulvovaginal injuries: mechanism and outcome. Arch Gynecol Obstet. 2007;275(2):93–7. https://doi.org/10.1007/s00404-006-0228-x. Epub 2006 Aug 22
54. Riggs N, Houry D, Long G, Markovchick V, Feldhaus KM. Analysis of 1,076 cases of sexual assault. Ann Emerg Med. 2000;35(4):358–62. https://doi.org/10.1016/s0196-0644(00)70054-0.
55. Grossin C, Sibille I, Lorin de la Grandmaison G, Banasr A, Brion F, Durigon M. Analysis of 418 cases of sexual assault. Forensic Sci Int. 2003;131(2–3):125–30. https://doi.org/10.1016/s0379-0738(02)00427-9.
56. Tchounzou R, Chichom-Mefire A. Retrospective analysis of clinical features, treatment and outcome of coital injuries of the female genital tract consecutive to consensual sexual intercourse in the Limbe Regional Hospital. Sex Med. 2015;3(4):256–60. https://doi.org/10.1002/sm2.94. PMID: 26797059; PMCID: PMC4721037
57. Carcopino X, Shojai R, Boubli L. Les mutilations génitales féminines: généralités, complications et prise en charge obstétricale [Female genital mutilation: generalities, complications and management during obstetrical period]. J Gynecol Obstet Biol Reprod (Paris). 2004;33(5):378–83. French. https://doi.org/10.1016/s0368-2315(04)96544-1.
58. Farage MA, Miller KW, Tzeghai GE, Azuka CE, Sobel JD, Ledger WJ. Female genital cutting: confronting cultural challenges and health complications across the lifespan. Womens Health (Lond). 2015;11(1):79–94. https://doi.org/10.2217/whe.14.63.
59. Puppo V. Female genital mutilation and cutting: an anatomical review and alternative rites. Clin Anat. 2017;30(1):81–8. https://doi.org/10.1002/ca.22763. Epub 2016 Sep 6
60. Cameron S. Recent advances in improving the effectiveness and reducing the complications of abortion. F1000Res. 2018;7:F1000 Faculty Rev-1881. https://doi.org/10.12688/f1000research.15441.1. PMID: 30631424; PMCID: PMC6281004
61. Ratovoson R, Kunkel A, Rakotovao JP, Pourette D, Mattern C, Andriamiadana J, Harimanana A, Piola P. Frequency, risk factors, and complications

of induced abortion in ten districts of Madagascar: results from a cross-sectional household survey. BMC Womens Health. 2020;20(1):96. https://doi.org/10.1186/s12905-020-00962-2. PMID: 32375746; PMCID: PMC7203894

62. Ekanem EI, Etuk SJ, Ekabua JE, Iklaki C. Clinical presentation and complications in patients with unsafe abortions in University of Calabar Teaching Hospital, Calabar, Nigeria Niger. J Med. 2009;18(4):370–4. https://doi.org/10.4314/njm.v18i4.51245.

# Nontraumatic Urologic Emergencies

Dyvon Walker, Rodrigo Donalisio da Silva, and Fernando J. Kim

## 88.1 Introduction

**Learning Goals**
Nontraumatic urologic emergencies can involve any part of the genitourinary system, including kidneys, ureters, bladder, urethra, penis, scrotum, and perineal area. Expeditious diagnosis and treatment of these conditions are imperative to maintain normal function and prevent progression to more deleterious or lethal outcomes such as sepsis or organ loss.

**Table 88.1** Urologic emergencies

| Non traumatic | Traumatic |
|---|---|
| Hematuria | Renal trauma |
| Penile emergencies | Ureteral injury |
| Priapism | Bladder trauma |
| Paraphimosis | Urethral injury |
| Testicular torsion | Testicular trauma |
| Fournier's gangrene | |
| Obstructing nephrolithiasis | |
| Acute urinary retention (AUR) | |

## 88.2 Penile Emergencies (Table 88.1)

### 88.2.1 Priapism

**Epidemiology**—Priapism is a completely rigid, painful erection without sexual stimulation lasting greater than 4 h.

Priapism may occur at all ages. The incidence rate of priapism in the general population is low (0.5–0.9 cases per 100,000 person-years) [1]. In patients with sickle cell disease (SCD), the prevalence of priapism is up to 3.6% in patients <18 years of age [2] increasing up to 42% in patients ≥18 years of age [3].

### 88.2.2 Classification and Pathophysiology

Priapism is categorized into **ischemic, stuttering, and nonischemic types**; *Ischemic ("low-flow") priapism* requires emergent treatment as there is minimal to no vascular perfusion into the corpora cavernosa, which could lead to permanent erectile dysfunction (ED) if left untreated. In one study, erectile function was preserved in 92% of patients if ischemic priapism was reversed in less than 24 h, compared to 22% preservation in patients with priapism lasting greater than 7 days [2].

With a lifetime probability of developing priapism of 29–42%, individuals with sickle cell disease (SCD) are among those highest at risk [4]. Also at risk are individuals with neuro-

D. Walker · R. D. da Silva · F. J. Kim (✉)
Division of Urology, Department of Surgery, Denver Health Medical Center and University of Colorado, Denver, CO, USA
e-mail: dyvon.walker@cuanschutz.edu;
rodrigo.donalisiodasilva@dhha.org

logic conditions affecting the spinal cord, and rarely, those with white blood cell disorders such as leukemia. Additionally, medications such as trazodone, those for erectile dysfunction (ED), and intracavernosal injections, among others, put individuals at increased risk of developing ischemic priapism, with a prevalence of up to 35% [5].

*Stuttering priapism* causes recurrent unwanted, persistent, and painful erection with intervening periods of detumescence. This priapism often requires multiple visits to an emergency medical center for management. These episodes are often self-limiting and terminate within 3 h. Each episode carries a risk of fibrotic injury to the corpora cavernosa if the priapism continues and is not reduced promptly. The prevalence of stuttering priapism is greater in patients with sickle cell disease owing to hyperviscosity, increased adhesiveness of the blood to the vascular endothelium, and disrupted vascular homeostasis [6].

*Nonischemic (arterial, high-flow) priapism* usually is due to pelvic trauma. Often, penile arteriography is diagnostic and when the arteriocavernous fistula is identified by the interventional radiologists, the fistula can be effectively treated by embolization.

## 88.2.3 Diagnosis

Diagnostically, apart from physical examination and basic laboratory analysis, it is important to differentiate between ischemic and nonischemic priapism (which is usually caused by trauma). This can be done by obtaining a penile blood gas aspirated from the corpus cavernosum. An ischemic penile blood gas usually reveals a partial pressure of oxygen ($PO_2$) < 30 mm Hg, a partial pressure of carbon dioxide ($PCO_2$) > 60 mm Hg, and a pH < 7.25 [7].

The nonischemic (arterial, high-flow) priapism penile aspirate is consistent with normal arterial blood gas values (pH, 7.4; $PO_2$, >90 mm Hg; $PCO_2$, <40 mm Hg).

## 88.2.4 Treatment (Medical)

### 88.2.4.1 Ischemic (Low Flow) Priapism

Hydration and analgesia are the first steps for the treatment of priapism, as they can, along with supplemental oxygen, lead to detumescence in SCD patients in an acute sickle crisis. Subsequently, the goal of treatment is to empty the cavernosal spaces of blood and clots, and thus, needle aspiration should be employed with subsequent intracavernosal injection of phenylephrine (100–200 mg every 5–10 minutes with a max of 1000 mg) [7]. If these measures fail, then surgical intervention via a shunt between the corpora spongiosa and cavernosum may be warranted. If this approach fails, surgical treatment is advised for a corpora-urethral shunt.

### 88.2.4.2 Stuttering Priapism

Most widely used treatments are hormonal (e.g., androgen receptor antagonists, gonadotropin-releasing hormone agonists, and 5-alpha reductase inhibitors). The strategy of treatment is to prevent recurrences.

### 88.2.4.3 Nonischemic (Arterial, High-Flow) Priapism

Penile arteriography will determine the arteriocavernous fistula and embolization can effectively treat the priapism.

## 88.2.5 Prognosis

Overall, the treatment of priapism is effective and ultimately can lead to placement of penile implantation in cases of erectile dysfunction post the acute treatment.

## 88.3 Penile Ring Entrapment

Penile rings are rings usually made of metal or silicone that are used to sustain erection during sexual intercourse to enhance pleasure. The rings exert their effect by reducing the outflow of blood from cavernosal tissue, but when left on for extended periods of time, can lead to penile ring entrapment (PRE) causing tissue necrosis, gangrene, and potential for penile amputation [8].

The primary goal of management is to restore blood supply to the penis, and according to various case studies, treatment methods include sliding, cutting, and surgical intervention, with post-treatment cystoscopy to assess for urethral damage. Sliding involves the use of lubricants to attempt to slide the ring off followed by compression of the edematous tissue, and is the safest option to preserve underlying tissue [8]. If the sliding method is unsuccessful, then cutting is the next approach. In our experience, an electric axel driver, or a diamond-tipped Midas Drill and Dremel tool, is effective and offers a safe and expeditious treatment. When the cutting method is used, however, it is important to protect underlying tissue from thermal and mechanical damage.

### 88.3.1 Paraphimosis

Paraphimosis is the entrapment of foreskin behind the penile glans, causing constriction of venous return from the glans. Immediate treatment is warranted as tissue ischemia and necrosis can occur if left untreated.

A history of phimosis, or constriction of the prepuce distal to the glans preventing retraction, is the most common cause of paraphimosis. Additionally, a significant cause of paraphimosis is iatrogenic, during urethral catheterization of an uncircumcised patient; therefore, it is of utmost importance to replace the foreskin after inserting a urethral catheter in an uncircumcised male [9]. In the evaluation of a patient with paraphimosis, the findings include constrictive tissue preventing reduction of the foreskin over the penis, penile swelling, and penile pain.

Apart from pain medication, the first step of treatment is attempting manual reduction by manually compressing the edematous foreskin. If initial attempts are unsuccessful, needle puncture into the edematous portion to remove blood may allow sufficient decompression to allow for reduction. If manual reduction remains unsuccessful, then surgical intervention via a dorsal slit procedure or circumcision is warranted. Additionally, surgical intervention is recommended in patients who have a history of significant paraphimosis, given the significant risk of recurrence [9].

### 88.3.2 Prognosis

The treatment of constrictive penile ring and paraphimosis is effective and does not cause any permanent damage to the organ when treated expeditiously.

> **Dos and Don'ts**
> **Dos:**
> - Pain management can be achieved effectively with regional block of the penis for all conditions described for penile issues.
> - When removing penile ring, protect the underlying penile skin so the drill does not perforate the penile skin.
>
> **Don'ts:**
> - Do not use local anesthetic with Epinephrine.

## 88.4 Nontraumatic Scrotal Emergencies

### 88.4.1 Testicular Torsion

#### 88.4.1.1 Epidemiology
Testicular torsion has a bimodal age distribution, with the first peak occurring at ages 1–2 and the second, higher peak occurring in adolescence [10].

#### 88.4.1.2 Etiology
Testicular torsion occurs when twisting of the spermatic cord causes lack of blood flow to the

testis from the testicular artery and lack of venous drainage, leading to edema and the potential for ischemia and necrosis.

### 88.4.1.3 Pathophysiology
Individuals with the highest predisposition to developing testicular torsion are those in whom the tunica vaginalis is abnormally fixed proximally on the cord, otherwise known as a "bell-clapper deformity," which is present in up to 12% of the male population [11].

## 88.4.2 Diagnosis

### 88.4.2.1 Clinical Presentation
Patients will present with acute onset, one-sided testicular pain with scrotal edema and absent or reduced cremasteric reflex. The testicle may even be oriented horizontally because of twisting of the spermatic cord.

### 88.4.2.2 Imaging
The diagnosis of testicular torsion can be supported by a scrotal color Doppler ultrasonography that will demonstrate lack of vascular flow to the affected testis.

The history is pivotal to make the diagnosis and to understand the testis ischemia time so we can predict salvageability of the organ.

> **Differential Diagnosis**
> Since testicular torsion is an emergency, it is important to differentiate it from other common causes of acute scrotum such as epididymitis.
>
> Patients with epididymitis will present with gradual onset pain over days to weeks, will have an intact cremasteric reflex, and will usually have pyuria and leukocytosis on urinalysis.

### 88.4.2.3 Treatment (Surgical)
When testicular torsion is suspected, manual detorsion should be attempted at the bedside to relieve symptoms. For definitive treatment, the patient should be emergently taken to the operating room to undergo scrotal exploration, detorsion of the testicle, and bilateral orchiopexy. Depending on the amount of time from onset of pain to treatment, the patient may require orchiectomy of the affected testicle [2, 12].

### 88.4.2.4 Prognosis
The viability of the testis is inversely related to the duration of the torsion. If detorsion occurs within 4 h after onset of pain, the salvage rate is 96%, which drops to 10% after 24 h.

> **Dos and Don'ts**
> **Dos:**
> - Make the diagnosis expeditiously as soon as the patient arrives in the Emergency Department and call the urologist on call asap.
>
> **Don'ts:**
> - Do not attempt manual detorsion more than once.

## 88.5 Fournier Gangrene

### 88.5.1 Epidemiology

Fournier gangrene has a strong predilection for males as opposed to females with a 10 to 1 ratio. The incidence in males 1.6 per 100,000 cases. Fournier gangrene is seen most commonly in men ages 50 to 79, with an incidence of 3.3 per 100,000 cases. These frequencies appear in all patients both in the US and worldwide [13].

Individuals that are immunocompromised, have a history of poorly controlled diabetes or alcohol use disorder, or have a history of instrumentation, are at significantly increased risk of developing Fournier gangrene. Additionally, increased mortality rates are associated with patients who have diabetes, heart disease, renal failure, or kidney disease [14].

## 88.5.2 Etiology

Fournier gangrene is a type of necrotizing fasciitis (NF) or gangrene usually affecting the perineum and/or external genitalia rapidly spreading to contiguous fascia at a rate up to 1 in. per hour [15].

It was named after French venereologist Jean-Alfred Fournier in 1883. Infection typically arise when polymicrobial commensal organisms are introduced from the gastrointestinal, genitourinary systems or skin into an immunosuppressed host.

## 88.5.3 Pathophysiology

Often group A hemolytic streptococcus and *Staphylococcus aureus*, alone or in synergism initiate infection. Anaerobic bacteria may be present, usually in combination with aerobic gram-negative organisms and proliferate in a hypoxic environment. Due to lower oxidation-reduction potential, gases such as hydrogen, nitrogen, hydrogen sulfide and methane, are produced which may accumulate in soft tissue spaces [16].

## 88.5.4 Diagnosis and Clinical Presentation

The hallmark of Fournier presentation is palpable crepitus, which is sufficient for diagnosis. Additionally, patients typically present with a swollen, erythematous, and tender scrotum, inguinal area, or perineum, often with dark purple or black discoloration of the skin [17]. Patients will often report systemic symptoms such as fever, chills, nausea, vomiting, urinary retention, and malaise.

## 88.5.5 Tests

Evaluation of Fournier gangrene involves a combination of both blood work and imaging.

Blood work in Fournier gangrene should include complete blood count (CBC) with differential and comprehensive metabolic panel (CMP). The CBC will often show elevated white blood count (WBC) with the potential for a left shift. The CMP may show any electrolyte abnormalities such as hyponatremia or metabolic acidosis, as well as any concurrent renal failure. Blood cultures and lactate can help to evaluate for associated bacteremia and sepsis. Arterial blood gas may be obtained to assess for acid/base status. Wound cultures are necessary to guide antibiotic treatment.

The most specific form of imaging in the diagnosis of Fournier gangrene is computed tomography (CT) imaging. CT imaging findings include fascial thickening, subcutaneous air, and fluid collections such as an abscess [18].

If a periurethral source is suspected, a retrograde urethrogram should be performed. If a perirectal source is suspected, proctoscopy may expose the source [10].

> **Differential Diagnosis**
> The differential diagnosis for Fournier gangrene includes testicular torsion, epididymitis, cellulitis, abdominal wall cellulitis, perianal/periurethral abscess, gangrenous balanitis, gangrenous vulvitis, inguinal lymphogranulomatosis, syphilis, chancre, tissue edema, herpes simplex, vasculitis, toxic shock syndrome, toxic epidermal necrolysis, and Stevens-Johnson syndrome [19].

## 88.5.6 Treatment

Fournier gangrene is a life-threatening true urological emergency. The treatment encompasses both surgical and medical resuscitation due to the severe septic state of the patient [11].

**Medical** intervention revolves around the initiation of empiric broad-spectrum antibiotics while awaiting culture sensitivities. Antibiotic therapy has historically involved triple therapy in covering for the previously mentioned gram-positive, gram-negative, and aerobic organisms that are associated with Fournier gangrene. The combination of a third-generation cephalosporin or aminoglycoside, in addition to penicillin and metronidazole, is classically used as triple therapy antibiotic coverage. Current antibiotic regimens include the use of carbapenems or piperacillin-tazobactam. In addition to antibiotic therapy, fluid resuscitation is of great importance as patients may present with hypotension. Diabetic patients suffering from Fournier gangrene will need correction of any blood glucose abnormalities.

**Surgical** intervention is based on wide resection of necrotic, gangrenous tissue. The time of presentation to surgical intervention has had associations with improved prognosis. Surgical debridement is based on the separation of the skin and subcutaneous tissue with debridement halting when the skin and subcutaneous tissue can no longer be easily separated and viability of tissue demonstrate good blood flow. Often, more than one surgical debridement and reconstruction of the affected areas is necessary.

### 88.5.7 Prognosis

The prognosis of Fournier gangrene is multifactorial.

Researchers attempted to create a scoring system to predict the clinical outcome for Fournier gangrene patients. Some of the factors included int the scoring systems included temperature, heart rate, respiratory rate, serum potassium and sodium, creatinine, bicarbonate levels, hematocrit, and white blood count [20]. Electrolyte abnormalities that are associated with a worse prognosis include elevated calcium and low magnesium levels [20].

A patient's age, as well as the extent of tissue involvement, also determines the prognosis. Patient prognosis declines with advancing age. The larger the degree of tissue involvement is similarly associated with a worse prognosis.

As previously mentioned, the time of onset of the disease to surgical treatment is key; patients who present earlier often having better outcomes. Diabetic patients with a HbA1c greater than 7 have also been found to have a worse prognosis [21].

With an average mortality rate of 20%, Fournier gangrene requires immediate treatment and emergent surgical debridement. Evidence suggests that the highest mortality rates are due to sepsis and multiple organ failure, followed by respiratory, renal, cardiovascular, and lastly, hepatic mortality [14]. Medical treatment includes fluid resuscitation as well as broad spectrum antibiotics. The most important treatment, however, is surgical debridement to extensively resect all infected tissue, followed by frequent dressing changes and re-debridement if necessary.

> **Dos and Don'ts**
> **Dos:**
> - Early diagnosis and imaging request (CT scan of abdomen and pelvis) to identify air present between the skin/subcutaneous tissue and fascia.
> - Early start of fluid resuscitation, as well as broad spectrum antibiotics.
> - Perform surgical debridement in the operating room as often as needed.
> - Establish interprofessional team strategies for improving care coordination and communication to advance Fournier gangrene and improve outcomes.
>
> **Don'ts:**
> - Delay in treatment can cause death.

## 88.6 Obstructing Nephrolithiasis

### 88.6.1 Epidemiology

According to the National Health and Nutrition Examination Survey, the prevalence of kidney stone disease has doubled from 1994 to 2010 [22].

Kidney stone disease typically presents between the ages of 20 and 60 and is more prevalent in hot climates. It affects about 10% of people over their lifetime, incidence increasing with age; 50% will have a recurrence within 5–10 years and 75% within 20 years. Developed countries have seen rapid increases over the last 30 years, especially in women in whom incidence is now almost equal to that of men [23].

## 88.6.2 Etiology

There is an association with stone formation in individuals who have diabetes, inflammatory bowel disease, hyperparathyroidism, sarcoidosis, cystinuria, gout, and recurrent urinary tract infections [24].

The most common type of stone is the Calcium Oxalate stones. The stone growth starts with the formation of crystals in supersaturated urine which then adhere to the urothelium, thus creating the nidus for subsequent stone growth. The biological processes that anchor crystals to the urothelium are incompletely understood. Then the stone could obstruct the urinary system causing pain and often infections. There are other types of stones that will not be described here since we will be discussing the acute treatment of infected stones obstructing the urinary system.

## 88.6.3 Pathophysiology

Obstructing infected kidney stones refer to stones that form because of urinary tract infections with urease-producing bacteria, secondarily infected stones of any composition, or stones obstructing the urinary tract leading to pyelonephritis.

Obstructive pyelonephritis is a urologic emergency as it can result in sepsis and even death.

## 88.6.4 Diagnosis

### 88.6.4.1 Clinical Presentation
Clinical symptoms include: Flank pain, abdominal pain, fevers, chills, dysuria, hematuria, urgency, frequency. The patient may have a urologic history of urinary tract infection, pyelonephritis, and urolithiasis.

On physical examination patient may present with signs and symptoms of infection, fever, malaise, hypothermia, costovertebral angle tenderness, and abdominal/suprapubic tenderness.

### 88.6.4.2 Laboratory Tests
Urinalysis and urine culture, ± Blood cultures (if presenting acutely with fever/concern for sepsis).

Radiology-Noncontrast CT urogram (gold standard), KUB, and/or renal US (best used for follow-up).

> **Differential Diagnosis**
> The other conditions that could mimic this condition will depend on the side of the obstruction. On the right side, consider pelvic inflammatory disease, appendicitis, gastrointestinal diseases, and on the left side, diverticular disease, testicular torsion in males.

### 88.6.4.3 Medical Treatment
Intravenous fluid resuscitation and broad-spectrum antibiotics.

### 88.6.4.4 Surgical Treatment
Immediate drainage of the affected urinary system. The placement of ureteral stent is preferred method but the placement of percutaneous nephrostomy tube should be considered depending on the size of the stone and/or issues with risk of perforation of the ureter in cases of impacted ureteral stones.

## 88.6.5 Prognosis

When proper drainage of the urinary system is re-established and appropriate broad-spectrum antibiotics is given patients may experience improvement of the clinical symptoms.

> **Dos and Don'ts**
> **Dos:**
> - Establish drainage of urinary system either via ureteral stent placement or percutaneous tube placement ipsilateral to the obstructed side.
>
> **Don'ts:**
> - Do not delay treatment.

## 88.7 Acute Urinary Retention (AUR)

Acute urinary retention (AUR) is a common urological emergency associated with inability to empty the bladder to completion.

### 88.7.1 Epidemiology

The incidence of AUR has been estimated as 3.0–6.8 cases per 1000 person-years in the general male population [25]. AUR is more prevalent in men because of longer urethra and presence of the prostate. By the eighth decade of life, the incidence of AUR in men increases fivefold to tenfold from rates in middle age, with an estimated 10% of men in their 70s, and 33% of men in their 80s experiencing AUR at some point [26].

This contrasts to an earlier study from the Hospital Episode Statistics database in England, which showed decreasing trend for primary AUR by 7% between 1998 and 2003 [27].

Maybe the resurgence of AUR is due to increased life expectancy leading to more hospitalizations of the elderly population [28].

### 88.7.2 Etiology

Acute urinary retention (AUR) presents as a sudden inability to voluntarily void and can be caused by obstruction or a dysfunctional bladder. Obstructive etiologies are more common in men and are typically secondary to benign prostatic hyperplasia (BPH), which is the most common cause of AUR [29]. Other obstructive etiologies include urethral stricture and bladder neck contracture, which can occur from previous urologic surgery, prior catheterization, or urinary tract/sexually transmitted infections. When the etiology of AUR is due to a dysfunctional bladder, it is usually caused by medication side effects and occurs more commonly in women. Common etiologic medications include anticholinergics, opioids, and after general anesthesia.

Neurologic conditions such as spinal cord injury, multiple sclerosis, or Parkinson disease can also cause AUR, and in patients who are presenting with hematuria, the presence of clots can cause obstruction leading to AUR.

### 88.7.3 Classification

There is no classification of AUR that is used clinically.

### 88.7.4 Pathophysiology

The exact etiology of AUR is unclear and is thought to be multifactorial. It is postulated that a combination of mechanical (BPH, urethral stricture, clot retention) or dynamic obstruction (increased alpha-adrenergic activity, prostatic inflammation), bladder over-distension (immobility, constipation, drugs inhibiting bladder contractility, high alcohol intake), and neuropathic mechanisms (diabetes mellitus, multiple sclerosis) are attributable for AUR [30].

### 88.7.5 Diagnosis and Clinical Presentation

Along with reporting inability to spontaneously void, most patients experiencing AUR will complain of suprapubic or lower abdominal pain. In older men, history of BPH is common. Patients with a neurologic etiology (multiple sclerosis, trauma, Diabetes Mellitus) or those who have chronic urinary retention may not be sensitive to the pain associated with retention but may instead present with overflow incontinence. Bedside ultrasound of the bladder can rapidly identify and quantify bladder volume [31].

### 88.7.6 Clinical Presentation

It is important to obtain a detailed history of trauma to the spine, pelvis and genital area. Also, other neurological problems may cause AUR, that is, diabetes mellitus and multiple sclerosis, as well as medications that decrease emptying of the bladder.

### 88.7.7 Tests

Uroflowmetry and post void residuals (PVR) volume should be obtained.

Uroflow is a study to determine the flow rate of your urine during voiding.

PVR is the amount of urine retained in the bladder after a voluntary void measured by ultrasonography.

> **Differential Diagnosis**
> The different causes of AUR include acute prostatitis, male and female pelvic malignances, female organ vaginal prolapse, vulvovaginitis, sexually transmitted disease, fecal impaction, and existing or newly diagnosed neurologic disease (multiple sclerosis, Parkinson's disease, diabetic neuropathy, and stroke).

### 88.7.8 Treatment

#### 88.7.8.1 Medical Treatment

In cases where an enlarged prostate is the etiology of AUR, the two main classes of medications used are alpha blockers and 5-alpha reductase inhibitors. Alpha blockers have been shown to reduce rates of catheter reinsertion after a trial without catheter [29]. Due to their hormone-mediated mechanism of action, 5-alpha reductase inhibitors are unlikely to improve AUR in the short-term, but are beneficial in preventing ongoing prostate hypertrophy and future episodes of retention [32].

#### 88.7.8.2 Surgical Treatment

Placement of either indwelling Foley catheter with or without assistance of cystoscopy or supra-pubic catheter placement. Often, in male patients the urethra dilatation may be needed to place the indwelling Foley catheter. Ultimately, treatment of underlying causes should be performed after the acute episode [33].

### 88.7.9 Prognosis

It will be dependent on the underlying cause of obstruction and/or functional causes of bladder emptying.

> **Dos and Don'ts**
> **Dos:**
> - Perform bladder ultrasonography when placing a suprapubic catheter to prevent bowel injury, especially in patients that had prior abdominal surgery.
>
> **Don't:**
> - Do not delay treatment to prevent bladder injury and acute deterioration of renal function.

> **Take-Home Messages**
> Apart from flank and/or abdominal pain on the side of the stone, patients often experience nausea, vomiting, dysuria, hematuria, frequency, and radiation of pain to the groin. In cases with an infected stone, which requires immediate urologic intervention, patients will also exhibit systemic symptoms such as fever and chills. Urinalysis will often be positive for nitrites, leukocyte esterase, bacteria, or white blood cells, and patients will likely have a positive urine culture.

Ureteral stent placement to divert urine around the obstructing stone should be the first step in treatment, especially in the setting of infected stones. Once the patient is stable, definitive stone treatment via ureteroscopy with laser lithotripsy and stone extraction may be warranted. CT imaging remains the gold standard for diagnosis of nephrolithiasis or urolithiasis because it visualizes almost all stone types, evaluates for the presence of hydronephrosis, and has sensitivities and specificities greater than 95% [34].

### Multiple Choice Questions

1. Fournier gangrene:
   A. **Must be operated as soon as possible.**
   B. Can be treated with antibiotics only.
   C. Can be treated with hyperbaric oxygen only.
   D. It is a skin infection.
2. Testicular torsion.
   A. Can be treated conservatively.
   B. **It is a surgical emergency.**
   C. It is a bilateral disease.
   D. It is always associated with inguinal hernia.
3. Flank pain.
   A. It is caused always by acute appendicitis.
   B. It is caused only by biliary colic.
   C. **Can be related to renal colic.**
   D. It is never related to stone disease.

## References

1. Eland IA, et al. Incidence of priapism in the general population. Urology. 2001;57(5):970–2.
2. Manjunath AS, Hofer MD. Urologic emergencies. Med Clin North Am. 2018;102(2):373–85. https://doi.org/10.1016/j.mcna.2017.10.013.
3. Adeyoju AB, et al. Priapism in sickle-cell disease; incidence, risk factors and complications - an international multicentre study. BJU Int. 2002;90(9):898–902.
4. Emond AM, Holman R, Hayes RJ, Serjeant GR. Priapism and impotence in homozygous sickle cell disease. Arch Intern Med. 1980;140(11):1434–7.
5. Wein AJ, Kavoussi LR, Campbell MF. Campbell-Walsh urology. 11th ed. Elsevier; 2015.
6. Keoghane SR, Sullivan ME, Miller MA. The aetiology, pathogenesis and management of priapism. BJU Int. 2002;90:149–54.
7. Burnett AL, Bivalacqua TJ. Priapism: current principles and practice. Urol Clin North Am. 2007;34(4):631–42, viii. https://doi.org/10.1016/j.ucl.2007.08.006.
8. Dawood O, Tabibi S, Fiuk J, Patel N, El-Zawahry A. Penile ring entrapment - a true urologic emergency: grading, approach, and management. Urol Ann. 2020;12(1):15–8. https://doi.org/10.4103/UA.UA_16_19.
9. Bragg BN, Kong EL, Leslie SW. Paraphimosis. Treasure Island, FL: StatPearls; 2021.
10. Samm BJ, Dmochowski RR. Urologic emergencies. Conditions affecting the kidney, ureter, bladder, prostate, and urethra. Postgrad Med. 1996;100(4):177–80, 83-4. https://doi.org/10.3810/pgm.1996.10.100.
11. Gatti JM, Patrick MJ. Current management of the acute scrotum. Semin Pediatr Surg. 2007;16(1):58–63. https://doi.org/10.1053/j.sempedsurg.2006.10.008.
12. Kessler CS, Bauml J. Non-traumatic urologic emergencies in men: a clinical review. West J Emerg Med. 2009;10(4):281–7.
13. Sorensen MD, Krieger JN. Fournier's gangrene: epidemiology and outcomes in the general US population. Urol Int. 2016;97(3):249–59.
14. El-Qushayri AE, Khalaf KM, Dahy A, Mahmoud AR, Benmelouka AY, Ghozy S, et al. Fournier's gangrene mortality: a 17-year systematic review and meta-analysis. Int J Infect Dis. 2020;92:218–25. https://doi.org/10.1016/j.ijid.2019.12.030.
15. Sarani B, Strong M, Pascual J, Schwab CW. Necrotizing fasciitis: current concepts and review of the literature. J Am Coll Surg. 2009;208(2):279–88.
16. Akilov O, Pompeo A, Sehrt D, Bowlin P, Molina WR, Kim FJ. Early scrotal approximation after hemiscrotectomy in patients with Fournier's gangrene prevents scrotal reconstruction with skin graft. Can Urol Assoc J. 2013;7(7-8):E481–5.
17. Paty R, Smith AD. Gangrene and Fournier's gangrene. Urol Clin North Am. 1992;19(1):149–62.
18. Mallikarjuna MN, Vijayakumar A, Patil VS, Shivswamy BS. Fournier's gangrene: current practices. ISRN Surg. 2012;2012:942437.
19. Chernyadyev SA, Ufimtseva MA, Vishnevskaya IF, Bochkarev YM, Ushakov AA, Beresneva TA, Galimzyanov FV, Khodakov VV. Fournier's gangrene: literature review and clinical cases. Urol Int 2018;101(1):91-97.]
20. Laor E, Palmer LS, Tolia BM, Reid RE, Winter HI. Outcome prediction in patients with Fourniers gangrene. J Urol 1995 Jul;154(1):89-92.

21. Sen H, Bayrak O, Erturhan S, Borazan E, Koc MN. Is hemoglobin A1c level effective in predicting the prognosis of Fournier gangrene? Urol Ann. 2016;8(3):343–7.
22. Scales CD Jr, Smith AC, Hanley JM, Saigal CS. Urologic Diseases in America P. Prevalence of kidney stones in the United States. Eur Urol. 2012;62(1):160–5. https://doi.org/10.1016/j.eururo.2012.03.052.
23. Dawson CH, Tomson CRV. Kidney stone disease: pathophysiology, investigation and medical treatment. Clin Med (Lond). 2012;12(5):467–71. https://doi.org/10.7861/clinmedicine.12-5-467.
24. Lorenz EC, Lieske JC, Vrtiska TJ, Krambeck AE, Li X, Bergstralh EJ, et al. Clinical characteristics of potential kidney donors with asymptomatic kidney stones. Nephrol Dial Transplant. 2011;26(8):2695–700. https://doi.org/10.1093/ndt/gfq769.
25. Fong YK, Milani S, Djavan B. Natural history and clinical predictors of clinical progression in benign prostatic hyperplasia. Curr Opin Urol. 2005;15(1):35–8. https://doi.org/10.1097/00042307-200501000-00009.
26. Jacobsen SJ, Jacobson DJ, Girman CJ, Roberts RO, Rhodes T, Guess HA, et al. Natural history of prostatism: risk factors for acute urinary retention. J Urol. 1997;158(2):481–7. https://doi.org/10.1016/s0022-5347(01)64508-7.
27. Cathcart P, van der Meulen J, Armitage J, Emberton M. Incidence of primary and recurrent acute urinary retention between 1998 and 2003 in England. J Urol. 2006;176:200–4; discussion 4
28. Armitage JN, Sibanda N, Cathcart PJ, Emberton M, van der Meulen JH. Mortality in men admitted to hospital with acute urinary retention: database analysis. Br Med J. 2007;335:1199–202.
29. Emberton M, Anson K. Acute urinary retention in men: an age old problem. BMJ. 1999;318(7188):921–5. https://doi.org/10.1136/bmj.318.7188.921.
30. Yoon PD, Chalasani V, Woo HH. Systematic review and meta-analysis on management of acute urinary retention. Prostate Cancer Prostatic Dis. 2015;18(4):297–302.
31. Thomas K, Chow K, Kirby RS. Acute urinary retention: a review of the aetiology and management. Prostate Cancer Prostatic Dis. 2004;7:32–7.
32. Fisher E, Subramonian K, Omar MI. The role of alpha blockers prior to removal of urethral catheter for acute urinary retention in men. Cochrane Database Syst Rev. 2014;(6):CD006744. https://doi.org/10.1002/14651858.CD006744.pub3.
33. Hallett JM, Stewart GD, McNeill SA. The management of acute urinary retention: treating the curse of the aging male. Curr Bladder Dysfunct Rep. 2013;8:242–9.
34. White WM, Zite NB, Gash J, Waters WB, Thompson W, Klein FA. Low-dose computed tomography for the evaluation of flank pain in the pregnant population. J Endourol. 2007;21(11):1255–60. https://doi.org/10.1089/end.2007.0017.

# Non-Obstetric Abdominal Surgical Emergencies in Pregnancy and Puerperium

## 89

Goran Augustin

**Learning Goals**

**Acute Appendicitis**
- To understand the etiopathogenesis of acute appendicitis during pregnancy and its relation to clinical presentation.
- To understand the differences in accuracy of different imaging modalities in pregnancy in diagnosing acute appendicitis and their proper use in pregnancy.
- To know abdominal wall access techniques to reach the appendix during pregnancy and potential specific complications related to pregnancy.
- To understand the relationship of duration of complicated acute appendicitis or its postoperative complications on obstetric outcomes.

**Acute Biliary Disease**
- To understand the etiopathogenesis of acute cholecystitis during pregnancy and its relation to clinical presentation.
- To understand the potential causes of increased laboratory findings of the liver and pancreatic enzymes during pregnancy, with and without acute cholecystitis.
- To understand which imaging modalities are the most accurate for the specific underlying cause of surgical biliary disease.
- To know differential diagnoses of acute cholecystitis during pregnancy, related and unrelated to pregnancy.
- To know abdominal wall access techniques to reach the gallbladder during pregnancy and potential specific complications related to pregnancy.
- To understand the relationship of severe or complicated acute cholecystitis or its postoperative complications on obstetric outcomes.

**Acute Pancreatitis**
- To know the share of most common causes of acute pancreatitis during pregnancy.
- To understand the order of imaging modalities for the diagnosis and follow-up of acute pancreatitis during pregnancy.
- To understand the indications for medical and surgical treatment of acute pancreatitis during pregnancy.

G. Augustin (✉)
Department of Surgery, University Hospital Centre Zagreb, School of Medicine University of Zagreb, Zagreb, Croatia

**Symptomatic Abdominal Wall Hernias**
- To understand the most common causes for the development or progression of abdominal wall hernias during pregnancy.
- To know potential differential diagnoses of abdominal wall hernias during pregnancy, especially for umbilical and groin hernias.
- To understand the options and indications for both conservative and operative therapy of abdominal wall hernias during pregnancy.

**Intestinal Obstruction**
- To know the incidence of the causes of intestinal obstruction during pregnancy, different from the general population.
- To understand which imaging modalities are necessary for the diagnosis, partly depending on the potential cause.
- To know the indications for conservative and surgical therapy of different causes of intestinal obstruction.
- To understand surgical treatment options and related obstetric management.

**Maternal Abdominal Trauma**
- To understand different types of the pathophysiology of maternal abdominal trauma in pregnancy depending on the injured organ(s).
- To understand the specificities of prehospital care and resuscitation of the injured pregnant patients.
- To understand the indications for the use of different diagnostic imaging modalities depending on the type of abdominal trauma in pregnancy.
- To understand the indications of nonoperative management and principles of surgical treatment sometimes combined with obstetric management.
- To know maternal and fetal prognosis depending on the type and severity of abdominal trauma, and specific organs injured.

## 89.1 Background

### 89.1.1 Epidemiology

The rate of AA during pregnancy in the most recent four population-based studies is 1/1000–1/4167 pregnancies [1]. Complications of gallstones represent the second most common non-gynecologic condition requiring surgery in pregnancy. The incidence of acute cholecystitis during pregnancy is 1/1000–1/10,000 pregnancies [2], and 40% of pregnant patients with symptomatic cholelithiasis require cholecystectomy during pregnancy [3, 4]. 1/1200 pregnancies are complicated by CBD stones [5]. Acute pancreatitis incidence varies more significantly than in the general population (4.8–24.2/100,000 [6]), ranging from 1/1000 to 1/12,000 pregnancies, and rarely progresses to the necrotizing form [7, 8].

An inguinal hernia in pregnancy has a reported incidence of 1/1000–1/3000 with 75% occurring in multiparas [9]. The incidence of incarcerated/strangulated groin hernias in pregnancy is unknown but is at least 10 times lower. Intestinal obstruction incidence varies from 1/1500 to 1/66,431 [10]: major causes of intestinal obstruction in pregnant women include adhesions (mostly postoperative), volvulus, and intussusceptions [10]. Maternal abdominal trauma injuries resulting in an emergency department visit occur in 3–7% of pregnancies [11]. Most reports claim 0.3–0.4% of pregnant women require hospital admission because of trauma, some even 0.9% [12].

### 89.1.2 Etiology

Constipation is a risk factor for AA [13].

The presence of sludge in the first trimester of pregnancy correlated with a higher risk of developing gallstones. Multiparity is a risk factor due to hormonal changes that directly influence gallstone formation [14]. Diabetes mellitus is a risk factor for gallstones. As the prevalence of overweight and obesity in young women increases [15], pregnancy-associated gallbladder disease may become a greater problem.

Nearly 70% of cases are secondary to biliary stones or sludge, followed by hyperlipidemia and alcohol abuse in approximately 20% of cases, respectively [16]. AP appears to be more prevalent with the advanced gestational stage, occurring most commonly in the third trimester [17].

The risk factors (family history, collagen diseases, smoking, renal failure, chronic lung disease, diabetes mellitus, steroid use, malignancy, malnutrition, cirrhosis, ascites, obesity) for abdominal wall hernias are the same as for the general population plus the increase of intra-abdominal pressure due to an enlarging gravid uterus. Pregnancy carries a 1.72-fold increased risk for a hernia.

Intra-abdominal adhesions are associated with 60–77% of intestinal obstruction in pregnancy [10]. Intestinal volvulus is responsible for 25% of bowel obstructions in pregnant women but only 3–5% in nonpregnant patients [10].

Blunt abdominal trauma has similar mechanisms despite its cause. Most commonly it is due to a MVA, domestic violence, and falls. Only the affected area and the magnitude of force could be different. There is a remarkable increase in uterine pressure during impact. The maximum pressure on the uterus during MVA even with belted patients was approximately 10 times that observed during labor [18]. Seatbelts could reduce injuries by 51% [19], lap belts by 35%, and diagonal belts by 60–80% [20].

### 89.1.3 Pathophysiology

Because AA is an inflammatory process, the inverse relationship between pregnancy and AA could suggest that a Th1-mediated inflammatory response is partly responsible [21]. Increased pelvic vascularity and displacement or kinking (especially if partly fixed) of the appendix by the growing uterus may hasten obstruction or strangulation, and increased local lymphatic drainage together with interference with omental migration due to the enlarged uterus may favor the systemic spread of the inflammatory process.

Pregnancy is associated with an increased percentage of colic acid, increased cholesterol secretion, increased bile acid pool size, decreased enterohepatic circulation, and decreased percentage of chenodeoxycholic acid [22]. The progesterone-induced smooth muscle relaxation of the gallbladder reduces gallbladder emptying and promotes stasis of the bile [23]. Progesterone also reduces bile acid secretion and increases the risk of cholelithiasis and acute cholecystitis [24]. There is a decrease in the gallbladder emptying rate and an increase in fasting and residual gallbladder volumes after emptying in the second and third trimesters [25]. Estrogen increases the risk for the formation of cholesterol gallstones by promoting the hepatic secretion of biliary cholesterol that induces an increase in cholesterol saturation of the bile [26]. Also, high levels of estrogen significantly enhance the activity of 3-hydroxy-3-methylglutaryl coenzyme A (HMG-CoA) reductase, the rate-limiting enzyme in hepatic cholesterol biosynthesis, even under high dietary cholesterol loads [26].

The trimester distribution of acute pancreatitis is consistent with (1) a potential lithogenic effect of estrogen during pregnancy [27], (2) a physiological type of insulin resistance in the second and third trimesters of pregnancy [28], (3) a progressive physiologic increase in both serum cholesterol and triglyceride concentrations, with peak levels reached at term, in response to elevated estrogen levels, (4) possible compression effect of the uterus on a biliary tree, pancreatic vessels and pancreas itself, and (5) significant rise in intra-abdominal pressure due to prolonged second stage of labor [29]. Pregnancy promotes biliary lithiasis and biliary sludge with increased frequency of biliary AP.

The hormone relaxin relaxes abdominal wall musculature to make more intra-abdominal space for the growing uterus. Despite this effect, there is a slight increase in intra-abdominal pressure during pregnancy which induces and promotes abdominal wall hernias.

It is not proven that pregnancy contributes to the development of intussusception. Most patients without the lead point are in the second or third trimester [30]. The long-standing obstipation, common in pregnancy, as well as the direct pressure exerted by the gravid uterus upon the rectum in the direction of the sacrum, tends to produce this entity without the leading point.

Mechanisms of MVA and domestic violence are the same as in the general population. Falls accounted for more than half of classifiable reported maternal injuries during pregnancy, and about 3% of all mothers reported at least one fall during pregnancy. Falls may be a more common mechanism of injury during pregnancy, particularly in the second and third trimesters, because of (1) weight gain, (2) the shift of the center of gravity to accommodate the expanding uterus, and (3) increased joint mobility [31].

Penetrating trauma mostly includes injury of enlarged uterus and fetus, with a significantly lower incidence of displaced maternal internal organs.

## 89.2 Diagnosis

### 89.2.1 Acute Appendicitis

#### 89.2.1.1 Clinical Presentation

*Constant abdominal pain* is the most common symptom [32], and pain in the RLQ, present in 67–84% of patients, is the most reliable symptom [32]. Classical pain migration is present in 50–70% [33, 34]. After the third month of pregnancy, the pain could slightly change the location and migrate progressively upward and laterally. A growing pregnant uterus could displace a mobile cecum with the appendix but not the completely/partly fixed cecum or (retrocecal) appendix. The appendix returns to its normal position by postpartum day 10. *Nausea* is nearly always present, and vomiting in 70–87% of patients [35]. It can be present in normal pregnancy and suspicion should be raised if new-onset nausea is present. *Anorexia* is common in early pregnancy, but new-onset anorexia should raise suspicion of AA. *An atypical clinical picture* commonly presents with RUQ pain (12%), uterine contractions, dysuria (20%), and diarrhea [36, 37]. With obstetric complications, such as *miscarriage* [38] or *preterm labor* [39, 40], a careful examination should always exclude AA which could cause these obstetric complications.

There is not a single, reliable sign that can aid in the diagnosis of AA in pregnancy. *Abdominal tenderness* in the RLQ on direct palpation is always present [36]. *Rebound tenderness* is present in 55–93% [36], and *abdominal muscle rigidity* in 50–65% [41]. These two signs are more likely to be present during the first trimester. In the second and the third trimester, as the abdominal wall distends, the anterior abdominal wall is distanced from the inflamed appendix losing the ability to elicit guarding and rigidity [42]. *Rovsing's sign* is variable, in 18–60% of patients [43]. *The psoas sign* is observed less frequently during pregnancy (5–50% [44]) when compared with nonpregnant patients with AA [45]. *Obturator sign* is positive in 21% of patients [46]. *Rectal or pelvic tenderness* may occur in early pregnancy but is unusual in late pregnancy as the appendix is dislodged from its pelvic location and shielded with the enlarged uterus [42]. Around 36% of patients with proven AA had positive *Alders' sign* [46], without a comparison between trimesters. *Bryan's sign* is abdominal pain produced by shifting the gravid uterus to the right, by some the most reliable sign [47]. Less than 50% of pregnant patients with AA have a low-grade fever [35]. In one series 72% of patients who had AA (with or without perforation) had temperatures of less than 37.5 °C [48]. Also, pregnant patients with a low-grade fever have leukocytosis, a fact that further complicates definitive diagnosis [35].

#### 89.2.1.2 Tests

*Leukocytosis* is not diagnostic due to the physiologic rise in some pregnant patients in the second and third trimesters reaching 20,000/mm$^3$ in early labor [49]. The degree of leukocytosis is an indicator of perforation and is rarely present if the values are below 16,000 mm$^3$ [46]. If WBC values during previous normal pregnancy were within normal limits, then RLQ pain with elevated WBC should be taken seriously. *Neutrophil granulocytosis with the left shift* is a diagnostic of acute infection. A *C-reactive protein* (CRP) value >40 mg/L should raise suspicion, especially if the pain lasts more than 12 h [50]. All patients with perforation had elevated CRP (mean 55 mg/L) [34].

*Alvarado Score* has a positive predictive value of 60% with a score of 5–7 and 100% with a score of ≥9. The sensitivity and specificity of AS

7 are around 80%. *Modified AS for pregnant patients* [51] has similar accuracy.

Transabdominal ultrasound is the initial imaging modality of choice for suspected AA in pregnancy [52]. Sonographic criteria are the same as in the nonpregnant population for the diagnosis of AA [36]. The positive predictive value is almost 100%. For women in the late second trimester or third trimester, it is recommended that the patient is placed in the left posterior oblique or left lateral decubitus position, which allows displacement of an enlarged uterus and use of the graded-compression technique without difficulty [53]. Also, to identify underlying pathology it can identify cervical incompetence [54] important for obstetric complications. Doppler sonography can produce high intensities and should be used judiciously, keeping the exposure time and acoustic output to the lowest level possible [55]. Transvaginal Doppler sonography is used for defining adnexal torsion or vascularized tumors. Some recommend transvaginal sonography as the first US diagnostic tool for female patients with low abdominal pain [56]. The European Society of Urogenital Radiology [57] and the American College of Radiology [58] recommend performing MRI after the indeterminate US. The MRI criteria for AA are the same as for US. The MRI criteria that exclude AA are (1) appendiceal diameter < 6 mm or (2) appendiceal diameter of 6–7 mm with no evidence of periappendicitis. The second MRI scenario warrants close clinical follow-up. Abdominal CT is used if MRI is not available. The CT criteria for AA are the same as for US. A low-dose (<2.5 mGy) protocol is sufficient to confirm or rule out AA in 83% [59]. The diagnosis of the remaining case can be performed by standard-dose CT.

**Differential Diagnosis**

Differential diagnosis is more extensive (Table 89.1) than in nonpregnant patients because of:

- Less reliable history and physical examination.
- Higher incidence of some pathologic conditions that mimic AA.

**Table 89.1** Differential diagnosis of acute appendicitis during pregnancy and puerperium

| Non-obstetric/nongynecologic conditions | Gynecologic/obstetric conditions |
|---|---|
| Gastroenteritis | Ruptured/hemorrhagic ovarian cyst |
| Urinary tract infections | Adnexal torsion |
| Pyelonephritis | Salpingitis |
| Nephrolithiasis | Tubo-ovarian abscess |
| Acute cholecystitis | Threatened abortion |
| Acute pancreatitis | Placental abruption |
| (incarcerated) hernia | Chorioamnionitis |
| Bowel obstruction | Pelvic inflammatory disease |
| Cecal carcinoma | Degenerative fibroid |
| Mesenteric adenitis | Ectopic pregnancy |
| Spontaneous rectus hematoma | Preeclampsia |
| Pulmonary embolism | Round ligament syndrome/pain |
| Right lower lobe pneumonia | Varicose veins in the parametria |
| Meckel's diverticulitis | Preterm labor |
| Sickle cell disease | Pelvic endometriosis |
| Stump appendicitis | Metritis |
| Inflammatory bowel disease | Ovarian vein syndrome |

### 89.2.2 Acute Biliary Disease

#### 89.2.2.1 Clinical Presentation

Symptoms of gallstone disease during pregnancy are the same as in nonpregnant patients [60]. Increasing severity of colicky pain, fever, or chills (rigors) usually implies an underlying complication, that is, cholecystitis, AP, or cholangitis. If persistent jaundice is present, common bile duct (CBD) stones should be suspected. *Direct abdominal tenderness* in the upper right quadrant is most common. Due to somewhat distant locations of the enlarging uterus and gallbladder, there is no significant blunting of symptoms and signs. *Murphy's sign* (cessation of inspiration during palpation of the inflamed gallbladder) may be elicited less frequently in pregnant patients and indicates acute cholecystitis [61]. *Abdominal muscle rigidity* is present with gallbladder perforation and biliary peritonitis, but abdominal wall laxity in late pregnancy might mask the classical signs of peritonitis [42]. *Fever* and *tachycardia* are variably present and not sensitive signs.

The clinical presentation of CBD stones is the same as in the nonpregnant population. Classic symptoms include abdominal pain, jaundice, nausea, vomiting, and itching.

#### 89.2.2.2 Tests

Only granulocytosis (left shift) indicates a bacterial infection. C-reactive protein (CRP) is elevated and bacterial infection is expected with values >40 mg/L. Serum bilirubin and transaminases may be elevated, as in nonpregnant women. Serum alkaline phosphatase is less helpful because estrogen causes its elevation (levels may double during normal pregnancy). Serum amylase levels are elevated transiently in up to 33%.

The accuracy of transabdominal ultrasound for gallbladder disease in pregnancy is 95–98% [62]. If gallstones are the only pathologic finding, then the state is defined as biliary colic. For the diagnosis of acute cholecystitis, further findings should be present: (1) gallbladder calculi, (2) wall thickening (>3 mm), (3) pericholecystic fluid, (4) sonographic Murphy's sign (focal tenderness under the ultrasound transducer positioned over the gallbladder). Another finding that should be ruled out is common bile duct obstruction because confirmation or suspicion changes the therapeutic approach.

MRCP is indicated if dilatation of intrahepatic and extrahepatic ducts is present on abdominal ultrasound. It can also differentiate between CBD stones and external compression due to Mirizzi syndrome. The pancreas is frequently obscured by overlying bowel gas during ultrasound evaluation, and MRCP better evaluates the pancreas for edema, the pancreatic duct for obstruction in the setting of biliary AP, and the peripancreatic tissues for inflammation.

> **Differential Diagnosis**
> Many diseases present with pain in the upper right abdominal quadrant. However, with adequate history taking and clinical examination, most of them could be excluded. The list of the most common differential diagnoses is presented in Table 89.2.

> Several entities should be included in the differential diagnosis of CBD stones and cholangitis. Most of them could be easily excluded after an abdominal ultrasound or MRCP. The two most common are intrahepatic cholestasis of pregnancy and acute fatty liver of pregnancy (AFLP).

### 89.2.3 Acute Pancreatitis

#### 89.2.3.1 Clinical Presentation

The predominant symptom is upper abdominal pain which is usually midepigastric and could radiate to the back in about 40% of the cases. Pain is commonly accompanied by midepigastric tenderness, nausea, and vomiting [63]. Fever may be present [63]. Some cases may have persistent vomiting, abdominal distension, and tenderness in the whole abdomen. The duration of symptoms may vary from 1 day up to 3 weeks. In severe cases, sinus tachycardia, hyperventilation, and the smell of acetone of the breath are also present. If accompanied by fever, unstable respiratory and circulatory function, shock, and gastrointestinal bleeding, these are strong indications for severe AP.

**Table 89.2** Differential diagnosis of right upper quadrant pain in pregnancy

| Jaundice[a] | No jaundice |
|---|---|
| CBD stones | Diaphragmatic myocardial infarction |
| Hepatitis | Acute appendicitis |
| Intrahepatic cholestasis | Pancreatitis |
| Preeclampsia-eclampsia | Symptomatic/perforated peptic ulcer |
| HELLP syndrome | Pyelonephritis/nephrolithiasis |
| Acute fatty liver in pregnancy | Radiculopathy |
| Hepatic malignancy | Herpes zoster (shingles) |
| Cholangitis | Perihepatitis (Fitz-Hugh-Curtis sy.) |
| Hepatic vascular engorgement | Rib fracture/costal margin pain |
| Hepatic hematoma | Pleural effusion |
| | Pneumonia |
| | Colon cancer (hepatic flexure) |

[a] Jaundice in these conditions is not obligatory

Sometimes the cause of the AP can be found during emergent operation for acute abdomen. Intraperitoneal fluid can be milky and lipemic. Similarly, if the emergent CS is indicated placenta can appear to be covered with milky fluid which contributes to the diagnosis of hyperlipidemic AP.

#### 89.2.3.2 Tests

The diagnosis relies on at least a threefold elevation of serum amylase and lipase levels. [64]. HTG-induced AP is triggered when TG levels exceed 1000 mg/dL (10 mmol/L) unless accompanied by lactescent (milky coloration) serum [65], found in 45% of patients [65]. PHPT is diagnosed when total serum calcium concentration is greater than 10.1 mg/dL (2.52 mmol/L) during the second or 8.8 mg/dL (2.2 mmol/L) during the third trimester with elevated or normal intact PTH level [66]. Maternal serum calcium falls by about 10% in pregnancy, therefore when evaluating calcium, it may be prudent to draw ionized calcium. An elevated GGT level can help us to evaluate the history of alcohol use.

Transabdominal ultrasound (US) is the initial imaging technique of choice to confirm the AP and to estimate fetal growth and development (length of the femur) and fetal vitality by measuring indirect parameters, such as oligohydramnios.

MRCP has high sensitivity and specificity for choledocholithiasis and other common forms of bile duct pathology. MRCP also obviates the need for intraoperative cholangiography. The third advantage is the ability to evaluate the entire pancreas and abdomen for AP and fluid collections [67] and can define pancreatic pseudocysts.

> **Differential Diagnosis**
> Hyperamylasemia has been reported to occur with perforated peptic ulcer, perforated appendicitis, intestinal obstruction, mesenteric infarction, pulmonary embolism, pneumonia, myocardial infarction, lymphoma, hyperemesis gravidarum [68], and several tubo-ovarian pathologies, including ruptured ectopic pregnancy, salpingitis, pelvic inflammatory disease, ovarian papillary serous cystadenocarcinoma, ovarian adenosquamous carcinoma, ovarian endometrioid carcinoma, mucinous tumors, and surface papillary carcinoma [69].
> Hyperlipidemia has been reported to appear in the event of cholecystitis, esophagitis, peptic ulcer disease, enteritis, peritonitis, and bowel obstruction and infarction [70].

### 89.2.4 Symptomatic Abdominal Wall Hernias

#### 89.2.4.1 Clinical Presentation

Diagnosis is made by the presence of a reducible or nonreducible lump, which demonstrates an expansile cough impulse and the exclusion of other causes of a lump. Palpation of hernia content can differentiate a solid structure (greater omentum or uterine fibroid) from the intestine (gas sounds on pressure). Assessment of the region is made by applying the Valsalva maneuver.

If incarceration occurs, there is severe abdominal pain with nausea and sometimes vomiting. If the bowel is incarcerated, then severe vomiting sometimes with the absence of stool and flatus is present. Fever develops if perforation due to distension or strangulation occurs. In such cases, redness of the overlying skin can be found due to the spread of infection through the abdominal wall.

#### 89.2.4.2 Tests

Transabdominal ultrasound confirms the diagnosis of hernia and defines the contents of the hernia sac. For groin hernia color Doppler US is recommended due to many other potential diagnoses which are mostly treated nonoperatively.

> **Differential Diagnosis**
> There are many causes of a groin swelling/mass, while in other hernia positions the list of other possible etiologies is smaller.

## 89.2.5 Intestinal Obstruction

### 89.2.5.1 Clinical Presentation

Intestinal obstruction presents a large scale of severity of obstructive symptoms and signs which depend upon (1) location of the obstruction, (2) the degree of obstruction, (3) the rate of progression of obstruction, (4) intestinal perforation, and (5) underlying malignancy. The symptomatology is the same as in the nonpregnant population. All colicky pain in pregnancy is not necessarily uterine in origin and that premature labor can complicate intestinal obstruction and vice versa [71].

**Plain Abdominal X-Rays**

Plain abdominal radiograph findings depend on the degree of intestinal obstruction. With complete obstruction, air-liquid levels are present. Potentially misleadingly normal findings are present with retrograde intussusception after RYGB.

### 89.2.5.2 Transabdominal Ultrasound

The classic features include "target," "doughnut," or "crescent-in-doughnut" signs on a transverse view and the "pseudokidney" sign in the longitudinal view or multiple concentric rings of intussusceptum. CT shows similar findings, and currently, MRI is more frequently used and shows the same findings as CT.

> **Differential Diagnosis**
> The most common differential diagnoses are constipation, irritable bowel syndrome, postpartum acute intestinal pseudo-obstruction, hyperemesis gravidarum, acute pancreatitis.

## 89.2.6 Maternal Abdominal Trauma

### 89.2.6.1 Blunt Abdominal Trauma

Blunt abdominal trauma always presents with abdominal pain of variable intensity and location. Minor injuries are never accompanied by signs of peritonism. If intra-abdominal bleeding is present, abdominal pain is progressively worse, sometimes with signs of peritonism or Kehr's sign. With massive bleeding hemodynamic shock and instability are present. The seat belt sign indicates more severe intra-abdominal injury.

### 89.2.6.2 Penetrating Abdominal Trauma

The gravid uterus works as a maternal shield, protecting more vital maternal structures from injury. As a result, the incidence of visceral injuries in pregnant women with penetrating abdominal trauma is 16–38% [72], significantly lower than that in the general population, where it is 80–90% with anterior abdominal gunshot wounds and may exceed 95% with evidence of peritoneal penetration [73]. Clinical presentation depends on the type of injury, the number of wounds, degree of every organ injured. An entrance and exit wounds predict the bullet path and possible intra-abdominal injuries, but high-velocity projectiles are often unpredictable, and multiple wounds can exist concomitantly. If the uterus is damaged, continued or intermittent vaginal bleeding can be found [74].

### 89.2.6.3 Fetomaternal Hemorrhage

FMH or transplacental hemorrhage is a physiological event of the transplacental passage of low fetal blood volume (fetal cells) into the maternal circulation and thus remains clinically insignificant and undetected. *Severe* FMH is defined as a fetal blood loss >30 ml [75]. Symptoms can be neonatal anemia, followed by decreased or absent fetal movement as well as stillbirth. Also, fetal hydrops, pathological CTG pattern, and intrauterine growth restriction are potential signs [75].

### 89.2.6.4 Amniotic Fluid Embolism

The most common presentation of all-cause AFE is cardiac arrest. It typically presents with sudden onset of hypoxia, hypotension with shock, altered mental status, and disseminated intravascular coagulation. Other common signs and symptoms are seizures, evidence of fetal distress, and maternal constitutional symptoms (fever, nausea, and headache). At the scene of a car crash, the condition is far worse than expected from the injuries sustained, with cardiorespiratory collapse.

## 89.2.6.5 Laboratory Findings

Decreased *hemoglobin* and *hematocrit* levels could be due to physiologic anemia of pregnancy, but decreasing levels are signs of intra-abdominal bleeding. Serum βHCG levels should be obtained for all females of reproductive age who were exposed to trauma because in 5.4–8% of patients an undiagnosed pregnancy is found [76]. With the *Kleihauer-Betke test*, fetal red blood cells containing fetal hemoglobin are identified by erythrosine staining. Using the *Rosette test* a sample of maternal blood is incubated with Rho(D) immune globulin, which will bind to any fetal Rh-positive red blood cells if present. Upon the addition of enzyme-treated cDE indicator cells, the presence of Rh-positive fetal blood causes rosetting, which can be seen by light microscopy. *Flow cytometry* using monoclonal antibodies directed against HbF has some important advantages over the Kleihauer-Betke test in the quantitation of FMH: (1) cytometric methods can accurately distinguish adult F-cells from fetal RBCs; (2) flow cytometry rapidly analyzes a greater number of cells ($\geq 50,000$), improving quantitative accuracy; [3] as flow cytometry is automated, it has greater reproducibility [77] *Base deficit* $\leq -6$ and *increased pulse rate* indicates that there is a markedly enhanced risk for intra-abdominal bleeding.

There is no specific routine diagnostic test to confirm amniotic fluid embolism. The diagnosis is largely a clinical one and essentially a diagnosis of exclusion. In pregnant trauma patients, other causes of collapse should be ruled.

## 89.2.6.6 Plain Abdominal X-Rays

A plain abdominal X-ray confirms maternal skeletal trauma or maternal pneumoperitoneum from the rupture of the hollow viscus. The most common fractures include pelvic ring fractures and diastasis of the pubic symphysis.

## 89.2.6.7 Transabdominal Ultrasound

Focused abdominal sonography for trauma (FAST) is an important method of evaluating patients with blunt abdominal trauma. Sensitivities for the detection of free fluid with this method range 42–100% [78], while in pregnancy around 83% [79]. One explanation for the marked number of false-negative results is that FAST is performed early in the resuscitation process, at a time when hemoperitoneum may not have accumulated to a detectable amount. A marked number of false-negative results (27.5%) is observed in patients with bowel and mesenteric injuries [78].

## 89.2.6.8 Abdominal CT

Abdominal CT is used in polytrauma patients or when US is nondiagnostic. Except for the diagnosis of injury of a specific organ and its severity, placental abruption can be detected.

> **Differential Diagnosis**
> With abdominal trauma, either blunt or penetrating differential diagnosis is very narrow. The only difficulty is to determine the organ(s) injured and the severity of the injury of a specific organ.

## 89.3 Treatment

### 89.3.1 Acute Appendicitis

#### 89.3.1.1 Medical Treatment

Currently, conservative management is not recommended, although it is more common than expected, ranging from 5.8 to 9% [80]. Abdominal MRI findings [81] should dictate the type of therapy [82]. Still, there is no consensus on the route, type, and duration of antibiotic therapy. Another indication is (1) bridge therapy or (2) definitive therapy in remote or inaccessible areas. The shortcomings include a 25% failure rate even with uncomplicated AA in the first and second trimester [82]; an increased incidence of recurrent AA during the same pregnancy and the unknown impact of prolonged antibiotic therapy followed by surgery due to treatment failure on the fetus. If the patient is in active labor and delivery is imminent, the operation may be delayed for a short time (until the placenta is delivered), but immediate appendectomy is advised if prolonged labor is anticipated [83].

#### 89.3.1.2 Surgical Treatment

Surgical treatment is recommended. It can be performed by open or laparoscopic approach. The operation should be completed with (1) minimal or no uterine manipulation, (2) good hemostasis, and (3) and prevention of cooling and drying of the uterine surfaces, which increases the risk of postoperative uterine contractions [84]. The most experienced abdominal surgeon available should perform the procedure to shorten the operative time, anesthesia time [85], and immobilization time, and reduce potential intra- and postoperative complications.

Standard position McBurney incision is recommended with an open approach. It can be performed (1) throughout the pregnancy regardless of the gestational age, (2) with the direct access to the suppurative process without spreading it in clean areas, (3) with minimization or elimination of uterine manipulation, and (4) with gridiron incision with extremely low risk for acute disruption or late postoperative hernia.

Lower midline laparotomy is used when an acute abdomen with diffuse peritoneal irritation is present for three main reasons [41]: (1) dealing with unexpected surgical findings, (2) completion of "difficult" appendectomy started through other incisions or laparoscopy, and (3) CS performed through the same incision if necessary.

Laparoscopic appendectomy has many advantages. Laparoscopy expands the ability to explore the abdomen with less uterine manipulation [86]. Further, it increases the ability to locate and treat dislocated appendix and results in relatively small incisions compared with the OA or helps in detecting other unexpected causes of acute abdomen [87]. Reduced cecal manipulation during LA with less cecal trauma causes earlier restoration of large bowel function and earlier passage of the first flatus and first postoperative stool. With an open (Hasson) technique for the first trocar placement, there is almost no possibility of injury to intra-abdominal organs. In addition to the general advantage of smaller incisions, less postoperative pain, and earlier return to normal activity, lower rates of abdominal wall dehiscence or herniation during labor are another potential benefit. *Laparoscopic appendectomy may be performed safely in pregnant patients with suspicion of appendicitis. Laparoscopic appendectomy can be performed safely in any trimester and is considered by many to be the standard of care for gravid patients with suspected appendicitis* (SAGES clinical practice guideline (2009 and 2011)).

#### 89.3.1.3 Prognosis

A 66% perforation rate has been reported when the operation is delayed by more than 24 h compared with 0% when surgical management is initiated less than 24 h after the presentation [88]. The timing of intervention varies by trimester: 90% of patients in the first trimester undergo the operation within 24 h of the onset of symptoms, whereas in the third trimester, up to 64% of the patients have symptoms for more than 48 h before operation [89]. Diagnostic and therapeutic delay of more than 48 h is especially seen during labor and the early puerperium [90, 91]. Perforation can also result in an increased risk of generalized peritonitis because the omentum cannot isolate the infection [92].

Today, overall, maternal mortality is <1% [5, 34, 93], or even 0% even with perforated AA [94]. It is rare in the first trimester and increases with advancing gestational age due to the prolonged period between admission and operation in the third trimester [92].

When the appendix is not perforated (simple AA), fetal mortality is 0–5% [95]; while perforation raises fetal mortality to 10–36% [5, 35, 36, 93, 95]. Women undergoing appendectomy in the third trimester have a 1.6 times greater risk of preterm birth than those in the first or second trimesters, and a 3.4 times greater likelihood of birth at gestational ages <33 weeks [96].

### 89.3.2 Acute Biliary Disease

#### 89.3.2.1 Medical Treatment

Biliary colic could be treated nonoperatively but with the risk of recurrent attacks. Traditional indication for medical therapy is to delay the cholecystectomy until the second trimester when the spontaneous abortion rate after cholecystectomy is the lowest (12% in the first trimester and 5.6% in the second trimester) [97]. Delay of surgery until the second trimester may lead to further complications of gallstone disease such as acute cholecystitis and biliary AP, risk of maternal malnutrition, and reduction in fetal growth rate caused by lack of maternal oral intake leading to higher spontaneous abortion rates and preterm labor (PTL) [60].

The only indication for conservative therapy of acute cholecystitis is the advanced third trimester of pregnancy. Women who had a cholecystectomy in the third trimester had a longer hospital length of stay, a higher cost of the cholecystectomy admission episode, and increased 30-day nonobstetric readmissions compared with women undergoing an operation in the 3 months postpartum [98]. Preterm delivery rates are two- to three-fold higher with cholecystectomy performed during the third trimester compared to the operation performed up to 3 months postpartum [98].

ERCP for CBD in pregnancy tends to be safe for both the mother and the fetus, but the procedure should be largely restricted to therapeutic indications with additional intraprocedural safety measures [99]. is a potential risk of electrocautery to the fetus. The complications in pregnancy consist mainly of post-ERCP AP (6–16%) [100], PTL, and post-sphincterotomy bleeding [99]. There is no difference in rates of perforation, infection, and bleeding of ERCPs performed in pregnant women and nonpregnant women [101]. Laparoscopic cholecystectomy and ERCP during pregnancy are safe. ERCP for the treatment of CBD stones and acute cholangitis in pregnancy is preferred to the surgical approach [22, 99].

#### 89.3.2.2 Surgical Treatment

Maternal and fetal outcomes are similar after laparoscopic (LC) and open cholecystectomy (OC) [102]. LC carries a decreased risk of spontaneous abortion in the first trimester and PTL in the third trimester. There is an almost significantly lower incidence of premature contractions with LC compared to OC [102]. *Laparoscopic cholecystectomy is the treatment of choice in a pregnant patient with gallbladder disease, regardless of the trimester* (SAGES Guidelines 2007 [103]).

OC is performed in a standard fashion as in the general population. LC is performed also with the standard position of the trocars. Open, Hasson approach is recommended, although during the first 20 weeks Veress needle can be used. The third trimester poses certain difficulties mainly regarding the diminished working space available owing to the enlarging uterus, the risk of injuring the uterus, and the perceived risk for excessive manipulation of the gravid uterus leading to PTL. The most serious complication of the uterine injury includes that of fetal loss owing to pneumoamnion resulting from inadvertent injury during Veress needle insertion for pneumoperitoneum [104]. A near-term gravid uterus makes an LC technically impossible, and near-term pregnancy is the only absolute indication for OC [105]. Median laparotomy is reserved for the patients with an indication for CS along with cholecystectomy.

#### 89.3.2.3 Prognosis

Maternal mortality is nil and morbidity is similar to the nonpregnant population concerning all surgical procedures. Cesarean section rate in conservatively treated patients is significantly higher (35%) than in the patients who received cholecystectomy [100]. Preterm labor is currently <5%. Fetal mortality and morbidity are around zero for both laparoscopic and open cholecystectomy. Prognosis after CBD surgery during pregnancy is excellent, with no fetal morbidity or mortality [106].

### 89.3.3 Acute Pancreatitis

#### 89.3.3.1 Medical Treatment

Treatment should include the treatment of the AP itself, and specific treatment/elimination of the cause of AP. The initial management of AP during pregnancy is similar to management in nonpregnant patients: fluid restoration, oxygen, analgesics, antiemetics, and monitoring of vital signs. Parenteral nutrition is considered to be safe and necessary in pregnancy [27], to maintain normal fetal development. Continuous renal replacement therapy and hemoperfusion are reserved for severe AP. Lipid-lowering medications, insulin and heparin, and finally plasmapheresis is used for hypertriglyceridemic AP.

### 89.3.3.2 Surgical Treatment

Surgical treatment includes operative intervention for the AP itself and management of associated local (biliary tract disease, pancreatic tumor) or distant (PHPT, HTG, etc.) causes of the AP during an attack or once the acute inflammation subsides.

Surgery for necrotizing AP should be delayed as long as possible [16] and can be also performed during the CS through median laparotomy. Therefore, the indications for surgery are [16]: (1) pancreatic necrosis and infection (3–4 weeks after the onset of symptoms), (2) large intra-abdominal exudates, and (3) maternal or fetal deterioration.

The decompression and percutaneous drainage help to avoid or delay surgery in most patients with SAP [16]. For patients with pancreatic abscess, drainage is recommended [107].

Therapeutic delivery is indicated to cure the pregnancy (hormone)-induced AP of any cause, resistant to conservative, and/or surgical treatment of AP.

### 89.3.3.3 Prognosis

Maternal mortality is <1% [27], with several studies without maternal deaths [16]. Non-gallstone AP had worse maternal and fetal outcomes than simple gallstone AP. Recent perinatal mortality rate is 0.57–4.7% [16, 27, 106], and 19% of preterm labor [16].

## 89.3.4 Symptomatic Abdominal Wall Hernia

### 89.3.4.1 Medical Treatment

Pregnant patients presenting with asymptomatic reducible groin or umbilical hernias during pregnancy can safely be managed nonoperatively until postpartum. Growing uterus blocks hernia orifices and incarceration during pregnancy is extremely rare.

### 89.3.4.2 Surgical Treatment

Pregnant hernioplasty is performed when the hernia is painful, irreducible, or incarcerated. With large hernia, skin necrosis or skin defect is also an indication for the operation. If CS is indicated the simultaneous repair of umbilical or groin hernia can be performed. A groin hernia is exposed through an extended skin incision of Pfannenstiel incision, while umbilical hernia can be repaired through Pfannenstiel incision (internal hernia repair) or separate incision (external hernia repair). Simultaneous repair during CS is mandatory if the gravid uterus is in the hernia sac because there is no possibility of vaginal delivery.

Elective umbilical and epigastric hernia repair should, if possible, be postponed until after pregnancy and preferably until after the last pregnancy in women of childbearing age. If hernia repair cannot be postponed until after the last pregnancy, a sutured repair is suggested for umbilical and epigastric hernias in women of childbearing age. A mesh repair could be performed after the last pregnancy [108].

### 89.3.4.3 Prognosis

Mortality is nil, but there are no data about surgical site infections, postherniorrhaphy pain, or recurrence rate. Simultaneous repair of umbilical or groin hernia with CS does not carry an increased recurrence rate.

## 89.3.5 Intestinal Obstruction

### 89.3.5.1 Medical Treatment

The usual measures employed to deal with adhesive bowel obstruction such as blind nasogastric tube insertion have no place in RYGB patients as they can lead to bowel perforation at the gastrojejunostomy and false sense of decompression while the biliopancreatic limb can remain obstructed.

### 89.3.5.2 Surgical Treatment

Almost all patients are explored by laparotomy, but recently, laparoscopy is more frequently used to minimize abdominal wall trauma and shorten postoperative hospital stay [109]. Principles for manual repositioning and bowel resection are the same as in the general population.

For sigmoid volvulus, in the first trimester, a nonoperative procedure using colonoscopic detorsion and rectal tube decompression is recommended until the second trimester when sigmoid colectomy is performed for recurrent cases [110]. In the advanced third trimester, if sufficient intestinal exposure cannot be obtained due to the enlarged uterus, a CS must be carried out [111]. Right hemicolectomy is the treatment of choice for cecal volvulus in pregnancy.

### 89.3.5.3 Prognosis

For intestinal intussusception, maternal prognosis, both after resection for ischemic bowel or without bowel resection is excellent [109, 112]. Higher rates of spontaneous abortion and preterm labor are present [112], especially if perforation with peritonitis occurs.

For colonic volvulus, maternal mortality has been reported to be 5% if the bowel is viable but rises to over 50% if perforation has occurred. Most maternal and fetal deaths occurred when a delay in presentation and surgical intervention was >48 h.

## 89.3.6 Maternal Abdominal Trauma

### 89.3.6.1 Prehospital Treatment

The initial key to the survival of both mother and fetus is prehospital management. Oxygen supplementation by nasal cannula or face mask should be routine. Pregnancy is considered a triage criterion for transport to a trauma center by the *American College of Surgeons Committee on Trauma*. Whenever possible, transportation should be to a center that can provide obstetrical care, as long-term monitoring is usually required. There are 9 well-known indicators for the transfer of patients to level I trauma centers).

Avoidance of supine hypotension syndrome (uterocaval compression) should be a paramount part of all initial resuscitative measures in pregnant trauma patients. Placing the patient on a backboard with a 15° angle to the left should be employed in all patients beyond 20 weeks of gestation. Significantly decreased cardiac output of up to 60% due to uterocaval compression leads to prolonged resuscitation with increased acidosis and vasopressor requirements [113]. Below 24 weeks *manual left lateral displacement* might be sufficient. There is the 1-handed and 2-handed technique [114]. In gestations of >24 weeks, a 30° lateral tilt is recommended. Although this reduces the efficacy of CPR compared to the supine position, in the pregnant patient, the slightly reduced efficacy of chest compressions is outweighed by improved cardiac preload and overall cardiac output [113]. Placement of a hard backboard in the supine position might not be tolerable for third-trimester gravida. The increased work of breathing due to increased diaphragmatic splinting might lead to respiratory failure. In this circumstance, transport in a 30° reversed Trendelenburg position seems acceptable [115].

### 89.3.6.2 Observation

The optimal length of time necessary to monitor women in hospitals with minor or no obvious injuries following an MVA is 24 h in most cases, without any adverse impact on complication rates [116]. After a visit, careful evaluation following repeated abdominal trauma and costly routine hospitalization for 24 h or more appears to be dispensable as in single-event cases [117]. Patients without premature uterine contractions or abdominal tenderness and with normal findings in the clinical evaluation, in the screening ultrasound, and the continuous 4 h nonstress test may safely be sent home along with instructions for a proper follow-up in the outpatient clinic.

### 89.3.6.3 Interventional Radiology

Hemorrhage into the pelvis (zone 3 of the retroperitoneum) is difficult to control operatively and is usually managed with interventional embolization if there is no indication for the operative fixation of the pelvic fracture which, apart from bone stabilization, also stabilizes retroperitoneal hematoma. The radiation dose required for the interventional radiologic procedure(s), however, can be prohibitive.

### 89.3.7 Surgical Treatment Blunt Trauma

An absolute indication for surgical management is maternal hemodynamic instability. Depending on the organ injured the proper procedure is performed as in the general population.

#### 89.3.7.1 Surgical Treatment Penetrating Trauma

Most stab wounds without maternal hard signs, such as hypotension, evisceration, hemorrhage, or peritonitis, can be managed nonoperatively. If the patient is hemodynamically stable, every wound should be explored in local anesthesia.

Proposed criteria for nonoperative management of gunshot wounds are:

- A fetus is dead,
- Entrance wound is below the level of the fundus,
- The bullet is radiographically shown to be in the uterus,
- Maternal evaluation is reassuring,
- Hematuria or rectorrhagia must be absent.

Exploration of the maternal abdomen due to maternal abdominal gunshot wound does not mandate CS. Indications for associated emergency CS are [118]:

- Surgical,
- Pregnant uterus mechanically limits exploration or surgical repair,
- Fetal,
- Hemorrhage,
- Interference with the fetal-maternal exchange,
- Infection.

### 89.3.8 Obstetric Treatment

Management of obstetric complications and fetal trauma is out of the scope of this textbook. Obstetric complications include traumatic placental abruption, placental tear, traumatic uterine rupture, amniotic fluid embolism, and preterm labor.

Perimortem CS should only be considered in the emergency department when [119]:

- Uterine size exceeds the umbilicus or gestation >24 weeks,
- Evidence of fetal heart activity (Doppler or M-mode ultrasound),
- Unsuccessful maternal CPR <4–5 min (up to 15 min if fetal vital signs persist).

If the fetus is dead or previable and the uterine damage is not extensive, the uterus may be sutured and a vaginal delivery allowed [120]. If the fetus is alive and viable, and the uterine damage is not extensive, uterine wound repair and CS is indicated to explore potentially correctable fetal injuries. Extensive uterine damage or uncontrollable hemorrhage is an indication for CS and hysterectomy if the uterus is severely damaged or bleeding uncontrollable.

### 89.3.9 Prognosis Blunt Abdominal Trauma

Trauma is the most common cause of maternal mortality with an incidence of 46.3% [121]. Head injury is the most common cause of maternal death, followed closely by hemorrhagic shock [122]. Maternal hemorrhagic shock carries a maternal mortality rate of 66.6% [123].

#### 89.3.9.1 Prognosis Penetrating Abdominal Trauma

Maternal survival from stab wounds is ≈100% while maternal mortality rate from gunshot wounds is from 3.9 to 10.5% [123] with many cases as a result of additional head trauma.

## Dos and Don'ts

**Acute Appendicitis**
- Always use abdominal ultrasound in the diagnostic work-up.
- Do not use an abdominal CT scan for the diagnosis after the unequivocal abdominal ultrasound if MR is available.
- Do not delay appendectomy if complicated acute appendicitis is anticipated.

**Acute Biliary Disease**
- Treat biliary colic conservatively.
- Do not treat conservatively acute cholecystitis during the first and second trimester of pregnancy.
- Start conservative treatment of acute cholecystitis during the advanced third trimester to avoid high conversion rate to open surgery and second abdominal wall incision if Cesarean section is indicated.

**Acute Pancreatitis**
- An adequate volume of intravenous fluid should be administered promptly.
- Use parenteral nutrition to maintain optimal maternal nutrition and normal fetal development.
- Use plasmapheresis if lipid-lowering agents are not successful.

**Symptomatic Abdominal Wall Hernia**
- Examine the patient to exclude bowel incarceration or strangulation in the abdominal wall hernia.
- Start conservative treatment if there are no signs of bowel obstruction.
- Operate the patient at least 6 weeks after delivery.

**Intestinal Obstruction**
- Include parenteral nutrition in conservatively treated patients.
- Immediately operate on cecal volvulus.
- Perform colonoscopy for sigmoid volvulus.

**Maternal Abdominal Trauma**
- Always give oxygen to a pregnant patient with abdominal trauma.
- Initially treat the hemodynamically stable patient conservatively.
- Do not resuscitate patient in advanced pregnancy in the supine position.

## Take-Home Messages

**Acute Appendicitis**
- Conservatively treated AA before pregnancy has a significantly higher incidence of AA during pregnancy.
- Graded compression transabdominal ultrasound is the preferred initial imaging method for suspected acute appendicitis during pregnancy.
- MRI in pregnant patients with suspected appendicitis, if this resource is available, is recommended after the inconclusive transabdominal ultrasound.
- Acute appendicitis should not be treated non-operatively during pregnancy until further high-level evidence is available.
- Laparoscopic appendectomy during pregnancy is safe in terms of risk of fetal loss and preterm delivery and it is preferable to open surgery as associated with a shorter length of hospital stay and lower incidence of surgical site infection.

**Acute Biliary Disease**
- Conservative treatment of acute cholecystitis during pregnancy carries a high risk of recurrence during the same pregnancy.
- Early (laparoscopic) cholecystectomy minimizes the risk of obstetric complications, especially small for gestational age.
- Both conservative and operative treatment of acute cholecystitis are permitted during the advanced third trimester.

- Common bile duct stones should be treated with minimal dose ERCP followed by laparoscopic cholecystectomy with maternal pelvic shielding.

**Acute Pancreatitis**
- Incidence of the causes of acute pancreatitis during pregnancy is different from those in the general population, with hyperlipidemic acute pancreatitis being one of the leading causes.
- MRCP helps in the early diagnosis and treatment of biliary acute pancreatitis.
- An adequate volume of intravenous fluid should be administered promptly to correct the volume deficit and maintain a basal fluid requirement.
- Parenteral nutrition is considered to be safe and should be given to maintain normal fetal development.
- A therapeutic Cesarean section is an option after all treatments options are unsuccessful, especially in hyperlipidemic pancreatitis.
- Acute pancreatitis during pregnancy still carries a high risk of miscarriage, preterm labor, or spontaneous abortion.

**Symptomatic Abdominal Wall Hernia**
- Incarcerated or strangulated abdominal wall hernia during pregnancy is extremely rare because growing gravid uterus blocks hernia orifices.
- Clinical examination is highly accurate in defining incarcerated or strangulated abdominal wall hernia during pregnancy.
- Pregnant patients presenting with asymptomatic reducible groin or umbilical hernias during pregnancy can safely be managed nonoperatively until postpartum.
- Surgical treatment in pregnancy is reserved for incarcerated and strangulated abdominal wall hernia.

- Any umbilical or groin hernia can be repaired during Cesarean section for obstetric indications.

**Intestinal Obstruction**
- Plain abdominal X-rays are often diagnostic.
- Volvulus of the sigmoid colon can be easily diagnosed on plain abdominal Y-rays enabling colonoscopic detorsion if indicated.
- For sigmoid volvulus, in the first trimester, a nonoperative procedure using colonoscopic detorsion and rectal tube decompression is recommended.
- From the second trimester, colonoscopic detorsion is rarely successful, and sigmoid colectomy is indicated.
- Sigmoid colectomy is indicated for recurrent cases.
- In the advanced third trimester, if sufficient intestinal exposure cannot be obtained due to the enlarged uterus, a CS must be carried out.
- Right hemicolectomy is the treatment of choice for cecal volvulus in pregnancy.

**Maternal Abdominal Trauma**
- Uterine blood flow may decrease by up to 30% before the mother demonstrates clinical signs of shock.
- Minor abdominal trauma does not preclude the possibility of placental abruption.
- Continuous electronic fetal monitoring is more sensitive in detecting placental abruption than ultrasonography, intermittent monitoring, Kleihauer–Betke test, or physical examination.
- The optimal duration of maternal hospital monitoring with minor or no obvious injuries following an MVA is 24 h.

## Multiple Choice Questions

1. When a pregnant patient presents with sigmoid volvulus, colonoscopic decompression is indicated in
   A. **First trimester.**
   B. Second trimester.
   C. Third trimester.
   D. All trimesters.
2. Pregnant patient with minor abdominal trauma can be safely sent home after.
   A. Normal clinical examination + laboratory findings.
   B. A + normal transabdominal ultrasound.
   C. **Up to 24 h of normal cardiotocography**
   D. At least 48 h of normal cardiotocography.
3. Which hernias are not repaired simultaneously with Cesarean section?
   A. Unilateral groin hernia.
   B. Bilateral groin hernia.
   C. **Umbilical hernia.**
   D. Perineal hernia.

## References

1. Zingone F, Sultan AA, Humes DJ, West J. Risk of acute appendicitis in and around pregnancy: a population-based cohort study from England. Ann Surg. 2015;261:332–7.
2. Morrell DG, Mullins JR, Harrison P. Laparoscopic cholecystectomy during pregnancy in symptomatic patients. Surgery. 1992;112:856–9.
3. Graham G, Baxi L, Tharakan T. Laparoscopic cholecystectomy during pregnancy: a case series and review of the literature. Obstet Gynecol Surv. 1998;53:566–74.
4. Wishner JD, Zolfaghari D, Wohlgemuth S, et al. Laparoscopic cholecystectomy in pregnancy. A report of 6 cases and review of the literature. Surg Endosc. 1996;10:314–8.
5. McKay AJ, O'Neill J, Imrie C. Pancreatitis, pregnancy and gallstones. BJOG. 1980;87:47–50.
6. Go VL, Everhart J. Pancreatitis. In: Everhart JE, editor. Digestive diseases in the United States: epidemiology and impact. Washington, DC: US Government Printing Office NIH Publication no. 94-1447; 1994. p. 693.
7. Ramin KD, Ramin SM, Richey SD, Cunningham F. Acute pancreatitis in pregnancy. Am J Obstet Gynecol. 1995;173:187–91.
8. Robertson KW, Stewart IS, Imrie C. Severe acute pancreatitis and pregnancy. Pancreatology. 2006;6:309–15.
9. Carilli S. Hernia repair during cesarean section. Int J Clin Med. 2015;6:1–6.
10. Perdue PW, Johnson HW Jr, Stafford PW. Intestinal obstruction complicating pregnancy. Am J Surg. 1992;164(4):384–8. http://ac.els-cdn.com/S0002961005809109/1-s2.0-S0002961005809109-main.pdf?_tid=7e435fc0-1677-11e4-bb93-00000aab0f01&acdnat=1406566500_b0d064d2c33a9a108694e5d1e390be37
11. Barraco RD, Chiu WC, Clancy T, et al. Practice management guidelines for the diagnosis and management of injury in the pregnant patient: the EAST practice management guidelines work group. J Trauma. 2010;69:211–4.
12. Shah KH, Simons RK, Holbrook T, Fortlage D, Winchell RJ, Hoyt DB. Trauma in pregnancy: maternal and fetal outcomes. J Trauma. 1998;45(1):83–6. http://www.ncbi.nlm.nih.gov/pubmed/9680017
13. Maes U. A surgical consideration of appendicitis in pregnancy. Am J Obstet Gynecol. 1934;27:214–24.
14. Bolukbas FF, Bolukbas C, Horoz M, et al. Risk factors associated with gallstone and biliary sludge formation during pregnancy. J Gastroenterol Hepatol. 2006;21:1150–3.
15. Mokdad AH, Ford ES, Bowman B, et al. Prevalence of obesity, diabetes, and obesity-related health risk factors, 2001. JAMA. 2003;289:76–9.
16. Hernandez A, Petrov MS, Brooks D, et al. Acute pancreatitis in pregnancy: a 10-year single center experience. J Gastrointest Surg. 2007;11:1623–7.
17. Rakshit A, Dey R, De M, Biswas RR, Biswas S. Pancreatitis in pregnancy – a scenario in a tertiary care Centre. Al Ameen J Med Sci. 2010;3:332–6.
18. Smith RN, Crosby W. Unpublished observations on labor in the baboon.
19. Lister RD, Milsom B. Car seat belts: an analysis of the injuries sustained by car occupants. Practitioner. 1963;191:332–40.
20. Lindgren S, Warg E. Seat belts and accident prevention. Practitioner. 1962;188:467–73.
21. Confavreux C, Hutchingson M, Hours M, et al. Rate of pregnancy-related relapses in multiple sclerosis. N Engl J Med. 1998;339:285–91.
22. Sungler P, Heinerman PM, Steiner H, et al. Laparoscopic cholecystectomy and interventional endoscopy for gallstone complications during pregnancy. Surg Endosc. 2000;14:267–71.
23. Davis M, Ryan J. Influence of progesterone on Guinea pig gallbladder motility in vitro. Dig Dis Sci. 1986;31:513–8.
24. Behar J. Clinical aspects of gallbladder motor function and dysfunction. Curr Gastroenterol Rep. 1999;1:91–4.

25. Braverman DZ, Johnson ML, Kern F. Effects of pregnancy and contraceptive steroids on gallbladder function. New Engl J Med. 1980;302:362–4.
26. Wang HH, Afdhal NH, Wang DQ-H. Overexpression of estrogen receptor alpha increases hepatic cholesterogenesis, leading to biliary hypersecretion in mice. J Lipid Res. 2006;47(4):778–86. http://www.ncbi.nlm.nih.gov/pubmed/16380638
27. Eddy JJ, Gideonsen MD, Song J, et al. Pancreatitis in pregnancy. Obstet Gynecol. 2008;112:1075–81.
28. Kautzky-Willer A, Prager R, Waldhausl W, et al. Pronounced insulin resistance and inadequate beta-cell secretion characterize lean gestational diabetes during and after pregnancy. Diabetes Care. 1997;20:1717–23.
29. Ross G. Pancreatitis following pregnancy. BMJ. 1955;1:349–50.
30. Penney D, Ganapathy R, Jonas-Obichere M, El-Refeay H. Intussusception: a rare cause of abdominal pain in pregnancy. Ultrasound Obstet Gynecol. 2006;28(5):723–5.
31. Cunningham FG, Leveno KJ, Bloom SL, Spong CY, Dashe JS, Hoffman BL, et al. Williams obstetrics 24th edition [Internet]. 2014. http://www.ncbi.nlm.nih.gov/pubmed/15003161%5Cn, http://cid.oxfordjournals.org/lookup/doi/10.1093/cid/cir991%5Cn, http://www.scielo.cl/pdf/udecada/v15n26/art06.pdf%5Cn, http://www.scopus.com/inward/record.url?eid=2-s2.0-84861150233&partnerID=tZOtx3y1
32. Unal A, Sayharman SE, Ozel L, et al. Acute abdomen in pregnancy requiring surgical management: a 20-case series. Eur J Obstet Gynecol Reprod Biol. 2011;159:87–90.
33. King RM, Anderson G. Appendicitis and pregnancy. Calif Med. 1962;97:158–62.
34. Andersen B, Nielsen T. Appendicitis in pregnancy: diagnosis, management and complications. Acta Obstet Gynecol Scand. 1999;78:758–62.
35. Zhang Y, Zhao YY, Qiao J, Ye R. Diagnosis of appendicitis during pregnancy and perinatal outcome in the late pregnancy. Chin Med J. 2009;122:521–4.
36. Onder A, Kapan M, Arikanoglu Z, et al. Acute appendicits in pregnancy: evaluation of 129 patients during 20 years. J Curr Surg. 2012;2:4–10.
37. Mourad J, Elliott JP, Erickson L, Lisboa L. Appendicitis in pregnancy: new information that contradicts long-held clinical beliefs. Am J Obstet Gynecol. 2000;182:1027–9.
38. Heaton G. Some peculiarities of appendicitis in the female sex, with special reference to appendicitis occuring during pregnancy. BMJ. 1905;1(2305):463–5.
39. Auguste T, Murphy B, Oyelese Y. Appendicitis in pregnancy masquerading as recurrent preterm labor. Int J Gynaecol Obstet. 2002;76:181–2.
40. Dasari P, Maurya D. The consequences of missing appendicitis during pregnancy. BMJ Case Rep. 2011;2011:bcr.05.2011.4185.
41. Cunningham FG, McCubbin J. Appendicitis complicating pregnancy. Obstet Gynecol. 1975;45:415–20.
42. DeVore G. Acute abdominal pain in the pregnant patient due to pancreatitis, acute appendicitis, cholecystitis, or peptic ulcer disease. Clin Perinatol. 1980;7:349–69.
43. Hinshaw J. The acute abdomen complication pregnancy. J Oklahoma Med Assoc. 1963;56:4–7.
44. Bailey LE, Finley J, RK; Miller, SF; Jones L. Acute appendicitis during pregnancy. Am Surg. 1986;52:218–21.
45. El Ghali MA, Kaabia O, Ben MZ, Jgham M, Tej A, Sghayer A, et al. Acute appendicitis complicating pregnancy: a 33 case series, diagnosis and management, features, maternal and neonatal outcomes. Pan Afr Med J. 2018;30:212.
46. Chen CF, Yen SJ, Tan K, et al. Acute appendicitis during pregnancy. J Med Sci. 1999;19:256–62.
47. Kurtz GR, Davis RS, Sproul J. Acute appendicitis in pregnancy and labor, a report of 41 cases. Obstet Gynecol. 1964;23:528–32.
48. Masters K, Levine BA, Gaskill HV, Sirinek K. Diagnosing appendicitis during pregnancy. Am J Surg. 1984;148:768–71.
49. Amos JD, Schorr SJ, Norman P, et al. Laparoscopic surgery during pregnancy. Am J Surg. 1996;171:435–7.
50. Hoshino T, Ihara Y, Suzuki T. Appendicitis during pregnancy. Int J Gynaecol Obstet. 2000;69:271–3.
51. Saddique M, Oqbal P, Ghazi A. Appendicitis in pregnancy; does modified Alvarado score have a predictive value. Pak J Surg. 2009;25:25–8.
52. Rosen MP, Ding A, Blake M, et al. ACR appropriateness criteria right lower quadrant pain-suspected appendicitis. J Am Coll Radiol. 2011;8:749–55.
53. Lim HK, Bae SH, Seo G. Diagnosis of acute appendicitis in pregnant women: value of sonography. Am J Roentgenol. 1992;159:539–42.
54. Negrete LM, Spalluto LB. Don't be short-sighted: cervical incompetence in a pregnant patient with acute appendicitis. Clin Imaging. 2018;51:35–7.
55. Abramowicz JS, Kossoff G, Marsal K, et al. Safety Statement, 2000 (reconfirmed 2003). International Society of Ultrasound in obstetrics and gynecology (ISUOG). Ultrasound Obstet Gynecol. 2003(21):100.
56. Bramante R, Radomski M, Nelson M, Raio C. Appendicitis diagnosed by emergency physician performed point-of-care transvaginal ultrasound: case series. West J Emerg Med. 2013;14:415–8.
57. Masselli G, Derchi L, McHugo J, Rockall A, Vock P, Weston M, et al. Acute abdominal and pelvic pain in pregnancy: ESUR recommendations. Eur Radiol. 2013;23:3485–500.
58. Garcia EM, Camacho MA, Karolyi DR, Kim DH, Cash BD, Chang KJ, et al. ACR Appropriateness Criteria® right lower quadrant pain-suspected appendicitis. J Am Coll Radiol. 2018;15:S373–87.

59. Poletti PA, Botsikas D, Becker M, Picarra M, Rutschmann OT, Buchs NC, et al. Suspicion of appendicitis in pregnant women: emergency evaluation by sonography and low-dose CT with oral contrast. Eur Radiol. 2019;29:345–52.
60. Davis A, Katz VL, Cox R. Gallbladder disease in pregnancy. J Reprod Med Obstet Gynecol. 1995;40:759–62. http://ovidsp.ovid.com/ovidweb.cgi?T=JS&PAGE=reference&D=emed3&NEWS=N&AN=1995346225
61. Augustin G, Majerovic M. Non-obstetrical acute abdomen during pregnancy. Europ J Obstet Gynecol Reprod Biol. 2007;131:4–12.
62. Rambal S, Manhas K, Sharma S, Gupta S. Ultrasound evaluation of gallbladder disease in pregnancy. JK Sci. 2001;3:78–83.
63. Kennedy A. Assessment of acute abdominal pain in the pregnant patient. Semin Ultrasound CT MR. 2000;21:64–77.
64. Sreelatha S, Nataraj V. Acute pancreatitis in pregnancy. Indian J Clin Pr. 2012;23:231–2.
65. Fortson MR, Freedman SN, Webster P 3rd. Clinical assessment of hyperlipidemic pancreatitis. Am J Gastroenterol. 1995;90:2134–9.
66. Kokrdova Z. Pregnancy and primary hyperparathyroidism. J Obstet Gynaecol. 2010;30:57–9.
67. Oto A, Ernst R, Ghulmiyyah L, et al. The role of MR cholangiopancreatography in the evaluation of pregnant patients with acute pancreaticobiliary disease. Br J Radiol. 2009;82:279–85.
68. Pacheco R, Nishioka Sde A, de Oliveira L. Validity of serum amylase and lipase in the differential diagnosis between acute/acutized chronic pancreatitis and other causes of acute abdominal pain. Arq Gastroenterol. 2003;40:233–8.
69. Norwood SH, Torma MJ, Fontenelle L. Hyperamylasemia due to poorly differentiated adenosquamous carcinoma of the ovary. Arch Surg. 1981;116:225–6.
70. Vissers R, Abu-Laban R, McHugh D. Amylase and lipase in the emergency department evaluation of acute pancreatitis. J Emerg Med. 1999;17:1027–37.
71. Hudson C. Ileostomy in pregnancy. Proc R Soc Med. 1972;65:281–3.
72. Buchsbaum H. Penetrating injury of the abdomen. In: Buchsbaum H, editor. Trauma in pregnancy. 1st ed. Philadelphia, PA: WB Saunders; 1979. p. 82–142.
73. Moore EE, Moore JB, Van Duzer-Moore S, Thompson J. Mandatory laparotomy for gunshot wounds penetrating the abdomen. Am J Surg. 1980;140:847–51.
74. Geggie N. Gunshot wound of the pregnant uterus with survival of the fetus. CMAJ. 1961;84:489–91.
75. Wylie BJ, D'Alton ME. Fetomaternal hemorrhage. Obstet Gynecol. 2010;115(5):1039–51.
76. Bochicchio GV, Napolitano LM, Haan J, Champion H, Scalea T. Incidental pregnancy in trauma patients. J Am Coll Surg. 2001;192(5):566–9.
77. Kim Y, Makar R. Detection of fetomaternal hemorrhage. Am J Hematol. 2012;
78. Richards JR, Ormsby EL, Romo MV, Gillen M, a, McGahan JP. Blunt abdominal injury in the pregnant patient: detection with US. Radiology. 2004;233(2):463–70.
79. Goodwin H, Holmes JF, Wisner DH. Abdominal ultrasound examination in pregnant blunt trauma patients. J Trauma. 2001;50(4):689–93; discussion 694. http://www.ncbi.nlm.nih.gov/entrez/query.fcgi?cmd=Retrieve&db=PubMed&dopt=Citation&list_uids=11303166
80. Cheng HT, Wang YC, Lo H, et al. Laparoscopic appendectomy versus open appendectomy in pregnancy: a population-based analysis of maternal outcome. Surg Endosc. 2015;29:1394–9.
81. Amitai MM, Katorza E, Guranda L, Apter S, Portnoy O, Inbar Y, et al. Role of emergency magnetic resonance imaging in the workup of suspected appendicitis in pregnant women. Isr Med Assoc J. 2016;18:600–4.
82. Joo JI, Park HC, Kim MJ, Lee BH. Outcomes of antibiotic therapy for uncomplicated appendicitis in pregnancy. Am J Med. 2017;130:1467–9.
83. Black W. Acute appendicitis in pregnancy. BMJ. 1960;1:1938–41.
84. McGory ML, Zingmond DS, Tillou A, et al. Negative appendectomy in pregnant women is associated with a substantial risk of fetal loss. J Am Coll Surg. 2007;205:534–40.
85. Hiersch L, Yogev Y, Ashwal E, et al. The impact of pregnancy on the accuracy and delay in diagnosis of acute appendicitis. J Matern Fetal Neonatal Med. 2014;27:1357–60.
86. Bennett TL, Estes N. Laparoscopic cholecystectomy in the second trimester of pregnancy: a case report. J Reprod Med. 1993;38:833–4.
87. Sadot E, Telem DA, Arora M, et al. Laparoscopy: a safe approach to appendicitis during pregnancy. Surg Endosc. 2010;24:383–9.
88. Tamir IL, Bongard FS, Klein S. Acute appendicitis in the pregnant patient. Am J Surg. 1990;160:571–6.
89. Basaran A, Basaran M. Diagnosis of acute appendicitis during pregnancy - a systematic review. Obstet Gynecol Surv. 2009;64:481–8.
90. Kuvacic I, Skrablin S, Zupancic B, Lovric H. Appendicitis in the early puerperium: case report. Gynaecol Perinatol Gynaecol Perinatol. 2003;12:130–2.
91. Irvine SW, Devereaux RS, Wang H. Postpartum appendicitis manifesting as umbilical purulence. Am J Emerg Med. 2010;28(262):e1–3.
92. Tracey M, Fletcher H. Appendicitis in pregnancy. Am Surg. 2000;66:555–60.
93. Al-Mulhim A. Acute appendicitis in pregnancy. A review of 52 cases. Int Surg. 1996;81:295–7.
94. Corneille MG, Gallup TM, Bening T, et al. The use of laparoscopic surgery in pregnancy: evaluation of safety and efficacy. Am J Surg. 2010;200:363–7.

95. Ueberrueck T, Koch A, Meyer L, et al. Ninety-four appendectomies for suspected acute appendicitis during pregnancy. World J Surg. 2004;28: 508–11.
96. Buitrago G, Arevalo K, Moyano JS, Caycedo R, Gaitan H. Appendectomy in third trimester of pregnancy and birth outcomes: a propensity score analysis of a 6-year cohort study using administrative claims data. World J Surg. 2020;44:12–20.
97. Curet MJ, Allen D, Josloff RK, Pitcher DE, Curet LB, Miscall BG, et al. Laparoscopy during pregnancy. Arch Surg. 1996;131(5):546–50.
98. Fong ZV, Pitt HA, Strasberg SM, Molina RL, Perez NP, Kelleher CM, et al. Cholecystectomy during the third trimester of pregnancy: proceed or delay? J Am Coll Surg. 2019;228:494–502.e1.
99. Tham TC, Vandervoort J, Wong R, et al. Safety of ERCP during pregnancy. Am J Gastroenterol. 2003;98:308–11.
100. Othman MO, Stone E, Hashimi M, et al. Conservative management of cholelithiasis and its complications in pregnancy is associated with recurrent symptoms and more emergency department visits. Gastrointest Endosc. 2012;76:564–9.
101. Inamdar S, Berzin TM, Sejpal DV, Pleskow DK, Chuttani R, Sawhney MS, et al. Pregnancy is a risk factor for pancreatitis after endoscopic retrograde cholangiopancreatography in a National Cohort Study. Clin Gastroenterol Hepatol. 2016;14:107–14.
102. Barone JE, Bears S, Chen S, et al. Outcome study of cholecystectomy during pregnancy. Am J Surg. 1999;177:232–6.
103. https://www.sages.org/publications/guidelines/guidelines-for-diagnosis-treatment-and-use-of-laparoscopy-for-surgical-problems-during-pregnancy/.
104. Friedman JD, Ramsey PS, Ramin K, et al. Pnuemoamnion and pregnancy loss after second trimester laparoscopic surgery. Obstet Gynecol. 2002;99:512–3.
105. Ogura JM, Francois KE, Perlow JH, Elliott J. Complications associated with peripherally inserted central catheter use during pregnancy. Am J Obstet Gynecol. 2003;188:1223–5.
106. Date RS, Kaushal M, Ramesh A. A review of the management of gallstone disease and its complications in pregnancy. Am J Surg. 2008;196:599–608.
107. Wada K, Takada T, Hirata K, et al. Treatment strategy for acute pancreatitis. J Hepatobiliary Pancreat Sci. 2010;17:79–86.
108. Dave SP, Reis ED, Hossain A, Taub PJ, Kerstein MD, Hollier LH. Splenic artery aneurysm in the 1990s. Ann Vasc Surg. 2000;14(3):223–9.
109. Harma M, Harma MI, Karadeniz G, et al. Idiopathic ileoileal invagination two days after cesarean section. J Obstet Gynaecol Res. 2011;37:160–2.
110. Alshawi J. Recurrent sigmoid volvulus in pregnancy: report of a case and review of the literature. Dis Colon Rectum. 2005;48:1811–3.
111. Allen JR, Helling TS, Langenfeld M. Intraabdominal surgery during pregnancy. Am J Surg. 1989;158(6):567–9. 1988;43:123–31
112. Bosman WM, Veger HT, Hedeman Joosten PP, Ritchie E. Ileocaecal intussusception due to submucosal lipoma in a pregnant woman. BMJ Case Rep. 2014;2014:bcr2013203110.
113. GAD R, Willis BA. Resuscitation in late pregnancy. Anaesthesia. 1988;43(5):347–9.
114. Vanden Hoek TL, Morrison LJ, Shuster M, Donnino M, Sinz E, Lavonas EJ, et al. Part 12: cardiac arrest in special situations: 2010 American Heart Association guidelines for cardiopulmonary resuscitation and emergency cardiovascular care. Circulation. 2010;122(18 Suppl 3):S829–61.
115. Lavery JP, Staten-McCormick M. Management of moderate to severe trauma in pregnancy. Obs Gynecol Clin North Am. 1995;22:69–90.
116. Vivian-Taylor J, Roberts CL, Chen JS, Ford J. Motor vehicle accidents during pregnancy: a population-based study. BJOG. 2012;119:499–503.
117. Rogers FB, Rozycki GS, Osler T, et al. A multi-institutional study of factors associated with fetal death in injured pregnant patients. Arch Surg. 1999;134:1274–7.
118. Buchsbaum HJ, Caruso P. Gunshot wound of the pregnant uterus. Case report of fetal injury, deglutition of missile, and survival. Obstet Gynecol. 1969;33:673–6.
119. ACOG Educational Bulletin. Obstetric aspects of trauma management. Number 251, September 1998. Int J Gynaecol Obs. 1999;64:87–94.
120. Kobak AJ, Hurwitz C. Gunshot wounds of the pregnant uterus: review of the literature and two case reports. Obstet Gynecol. 1954;4:383–91.
121. Fildes J, Reed L, Jones N, et al. Trauma: the leading cause of maternal death. J Trauma. 1992;32:643–5.
122. Pearlman MD, Tintinalli JE, Lorenz R. Blunt trauma during pregnancy. New Engl J Med. 1990;323:1609–13.
123. Srinarmwong C. Trauma during pregnancy: a review of 38 cases. Thai J Surg. 2007;28:138–42.

# Enterovesical and Enterogenital Fistulae

## 90

Krishanth Naidu and Francesco Piscioneri

## 90.1 Introduction

> **Learning Goals**
> - Understand that EVF and EGF are uncommon but occur as a consequence of both benign and malignant processes.
> - The aetiology of a fistula can be determined from the patient's history.
> - Acknowledge that the diagnosis and treatment of EVF and EGF are challenging and therefore consider interprofessional assessment and planning.
> - Sepsis must be controlled prior to attempting definitive surgery.
> - Inflammatory bowel disease (IBD) related EVF and EGF should have their disease medically optimized prior to surgery.

K. Naidu
Department of Colorectal Surgery—Concord Hospital, University of Sydney,
Sydney, NSW, Australia

F. Piscioneri (✉)
Department of General Surgery—Canberra Hospital,
Australian National University,
Canberra, ACT, Australia
e-mail: frank@arkpacific.com

### 90.1.1 History and Classification

A fistula is defined as an abnormal communication between two epithelialized surfaces [1–5]. With fistula nomenclature, it is pertinent that the organ of origin is stated first [5]. However, at times, this is not easily discernible. Reassuringly, in clinical practice, the most commonly encountered fistulae are of bowel origin [3, 6]. The earliest known observation of an EVF was described by Rufus of Ephesus, a Greek physician in the second Century AD [3]. In relation to inciting events, the pendulum has swung from diseases of the past such as typhoid and tuberculosis to diverticulitis and malignancy [3]. Though the use of the term *bowel* traditionally implies the small bowel, it is interchangeably used to refer to both small and large bowel [1]. It is best to use appropriate prefixes to ensure both specificity and clarity in the description as it has diagnostic and treatment implications (e.g. *jejuno-, ileo- and colo*) [7].

EVF is classified according to the bowel segment involved [4, 8]. Table 90.1 defines the various EVF and their incidences.

### 90.1.2 Aetiology

EVF and EGF are usually the result of an underlying pathology involving the gastrointestinal or genitourinary tract and take between months and

**Table 90.1** Classification of EVF

| | |
|---|---|
| Colovesicle (CVF) | 70% |
| Rectovesicle & rectourethral | 11% |
| Ileovesicle | 16% |
| Appendicovesicle | 7% |

**Table 90.2** Summary of fistulae aetiologies

| |
|---|
| Congenital disorders |
| Acquired disorders |
| Trauma |
| Operative |
| Obstetric |
| Traumatic |
| Infection/sepsis |
| Inflammatory bowel disease |
| Radiation |
| Carcinoma |

years to form [5, 9]. The true incidence is difficult to ascertain [5].

The common causes are:

1. Diverticulitis:
   - ~60% of EVF.
   - Sigmoid colon is the most common organ of origin.
   - Only 2% of patients with the diverticular disease develop EVF.
2. Malignancy:
   - ~20% of EVF.
   - Colorectal cancer accounts for ~1% of EVF [2, 10].
   - Primary bladder cancer rarely culminates in a fistula, possibly owing to the relatively early detection [5].
3. Inflammatory bowel disease:
   - Crohn's disease (~2%) is implicated owing to the transmural inflammation inherent in the disease process.
4. Chemoradiation
   - Presents after a relatively long dormant period.
5. Iatrogenic
   - Obstetric: ~0.5% of all vaginal deliveries with an increased incidence in the developing countries [11, 12]. Chronic rectovaginal fistulae, as a consequence of birth trauma, are a huge personal burden in developing countries. The highly specialized treatment, often requiring multiple operations and tissue transfers, and need for dedicated centres, is the rate-limiting step with quality care in these patients.
   - Gynaecology: Hysterectomy, pelvic organ prolapse repair ± mesh.
   - Colorectal operations: ~3–10% following low anterior resections, haemorrhoidectomy.
6. Foreign bodies.
7. Trauma.
8. Inflammation/infection.
   - Anorectal cryptoglandular disease
   - Bartholin gland abscess.
   - Human immunodeficiency virus (HIV).
   - Lymphogranuloma venereum.
   - Tuberculosis.

Further to formation, non-closure of fistulae is a significant issue. The mnemonic *FRIEND* can be applied to potential reasons for non-healing [13].

*F*—Foreign bodies.
*R*—Radiation treatment.
*I*—Inflammation/infection.
*E*—Epithelized tract.
*N*—Neoplasm.
*D*—Distal obstruction.

Table 90.2 provides a non-exhaustive list of aetiologies.

## 90.1.3 Epidemiology

EVF has a male preponderance (i.e. 3:1), owing to the intimacy between the sigmoid colon and the bladder. This is dissimilar to the female anatomy, where the bladder and colon interface is separated by the uterus, except in post-hysterectomy patients [1, 9, 14].

Spontaneous fistula closure rates are reported in as many as ½ of patients with diverticulitis [3].

In both the developing and developed world, the female incidence of iatrogenic induced fistulae, such as CVxF, ureterovaginal and vesicovaginal are more common than CVF [3, 9, 15, 16]. Those with CVF tend to be older with a history of

**Table 90.3** Norwegian women diagnosed with a gynaecological fistula during 2008–2014 (n = 1627) [4, 9, 31]

| Colovaginal (CVxF) | 43% |
|---|---|
| Enterovaginal | 8% |
| Enterouterine | 4% |
| Rectovaginal | 5% |

hysterectomy. Uterine atrophy has been postulated as contributory to the process of fistula formation. Though EGF occurs in both sexes, the true incidence in males is difficult to define owing to the rarity with its encounter.

Urogenital fistulae related to the rectum tend to be observed in the postoperative setting, (e.g. prostatectomy) or as a consequence of infection or tissue destruction. Table 90.3 provides a summary of gynaecological fistulas.

As CVF and CVxF are the most common fistulae seen in clinical practice, the contents of this chapter will apply to them unless it is otherwise indicated.

## 90.1.4 Pathophysiology

Fistulae may be either congenital or acquired. Congenital EVF is extremely rare and often associated with an imperforate anus [3].

Table 90.2 provides a list of acquired causes of EVF.

### 90.1.4.1 Inflammatory

Inflammatory processes account for approximately 60% of EVF, with diverticulitis causative in up to 70% of situations. The fistulae in this situation are almost always colonic in origin [3, 8]. Risk factors for such a process include localized perforation with an associated abscess or phlegmonous diverticulitis.

Inflammatory bowel disease accounts for approximately 10% of EVF, owing to its characteristic transmural inflammation and resultant organ intimacy and erosion. Crohn's disease tends to result in ileovesicle fistulae most commonly, with some centres describing a 10% formation rate in those with regional ileitis. It is worth noting that most patients are under 40 years of age with the median onset of fistula symptoms being 10 years from Crohn's diagnosis [17].

Less-common inflammatory causes of fistulae include Meckel diverticulum, appendicitis and genitourinary infections (e.g. actinomycosis).

### 90.1.4.2 Malignant

Malignant processes are the second most common cause of fistulae as seen in up to 20% cases [10]. Reassuringly, owing to earlier diagnosis and treatment, the incidence is decreasing. Given how commonly rectal and distal colonic carcinoma is encountered, rectovesicle fistulae and CVF are infrequently seen. Invasion of adjacent organs and structures results as a consequence of space obliteration with growth and inflammation, culminating in an epithelialized tract. Occasionally, genitourinary malignancies are causative. As EVF goes, in the pelvis, fistulizing into the prostate is uncommon owing to the strength of Denonvilliers fascia. Interestingly, this barrier is penetrable by infection as the rectum and prostate share a common vascular and lymphatic system [18]. The presence of an empty prostatic capsule and an obstruction to urinary flow contribute to the manifestation and persistence of a prostatorectal fistula [18].

### 90.1.4.3 Iatrogenic

Surgical procedures, primary or adjunctive to chemo-radiotherapy and post-procedural infections are possible iatrogenic causes. Surgeries for both benign and malignant conditions have been implicated (i.e. laparoscopic inguinal hernia repair, rectal polyp excisions, anterior resections, prostatectomies) [3, 19]. Unrecognized viscous injury is an uncommon cause of CVF and EVF.

Radiotherapy treatment encompasses a field that can implicate the bowel and other adjacent organs and thus lead to fistula formation. Radiotherapy-related complications are considered to smoulder for years prior to manifesting as a fistula. The incidence of radiation-induced rectovaginal fistulae is approximately 1% [20].

Cytotoxic and immune-based therapy related fistula formation is rare but has been reported [21].

#### 90.1.4.4 Trauma

Penetrating abdominal or pelvic trauma and foreign bodies, such as a gunshot, swallowed bones, bezoars and gallstones may cause gastrointestinal (GI) fistulae [22].

## 90.2 Diagnosis

### 90.2.1 Clinical Presentation

There are no pathognomic features for EVF or EGF. The severity, presenting symptoms and signs vary considerably but can be understood if one acknowledges the concept below:

1. Origin (Viscera).
2. Destination (Viscera).
3. Duration.
4. Disease process.
5. Complications.

Urogenital symptoms such as suprapubic pain, flank pain, dysuria, frequency, tainted/malodorous urine, haematuria, pneumaturia and vaginal discharge are suspicious of an EVF/EGF. *Gouverneur's syndrome*, characterized by a constellation of suprapubic pain, urinary frequency, dysuria and tenesmus has been ascribed to diagnosing EVF [23]. However, none of these are diagnostic of fistula disease.

Pneumaturia tends to occur in patients with diverticulitis or Crohn's disease rather than those with a malignant aetiology [3]. Faecaluria is seen in up to 40% of those with an EVF [24]. Interestingly, the reverse passage of urine via the colon/rectum is rarely seen [24].

Clinicians ought to be cognizant of the variety in presentation severity—chronic urinary tract infections, fulminant urosepsis and shock. In EVF, patients frequently report not only extended duration of antibiotics but multiple courses, particularly in men, should lead to questions. With EGF, fungal vaginal infections superimposed with excoriated mucosal surfaces can be seen as a consequence of the effluent.

In those with IBD and complicated diverticular disease, further to abdominal pain, a palpable mass is occasionally noted in up to 30% of patients [24].

History of known diseases causing fistulae should concern treating clinicians, particularly with symptoms and signs such as weight loss, change in bowel habits, per rectal bleeding and fever.

### 90.2.2 Tests

EVF is neither an easy nor straightforward disease to evaluate and manage. Flow Chart 90.1 provides a summary to guide the process and is based on the fundamentals of good surgical practice.

The process begins with confirming the diagnosis followed by characterizing the anatomy (site, size and complexity) of the fistula. It is important to clarify the underlying pathology. This then allows the ability to consolidate and plan the management and follow-up.

Laboratory, imaging and procedural diagnostic studies are considered, usually in combination to provide guidance toward a diagnosis.

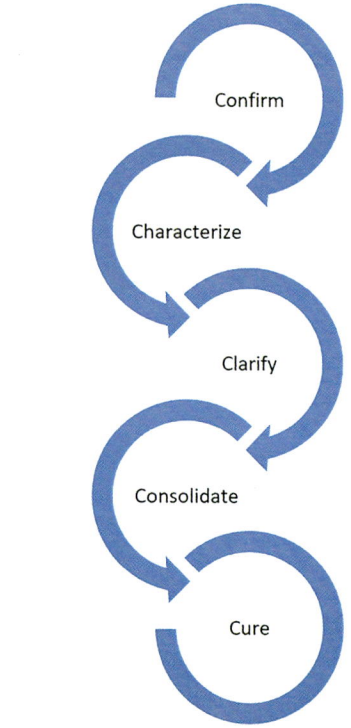

**Flow Chart 90.1** Approach to a fistula

- **Laboratory**
  - Urinalysis is usually undertaken as a point of care investigation. It can portray indices of infection such as white blood cells, nitrites, protein and glucose content. Historically, *cellulose* test has been used [3, 25]. The sample can also be sent for culture and microscopy, with *Escherichia coli* the most commonly identified organism. As alluded to before, clinicians ought to have a high index of suspicion of the prospect of EVF in situations with recurrent positive cultures.
  - A full blood panel consisting of a complete blood cell count, blood urea nitrogen, renal profile, electrolytes and C-reactive protein should be considered. Anaemia and leucocytosis may be found in cases of malignancy and unremedied sepsis respectively. For the most part, the blood panel is undisturbed.
  - The value of undertaking blood cultures via peripheral or central access cannot be stressed enough in septic and shocked situations.
- **Imaging**
  Several imaging modalities are available to achieve the goal of establishing the diagnosis and clarifying the anatomy and pathology.
  - Computed tomography (CT).
    This modality is considered the most sensitive as EVF detection, thus advocating a CT of the abdomen and pelvis as part of the primary work-up. The value of CT is seen with the identification and delineation of air, fluid and complex structures (e.g. abscess and masses). 3-D reconstruction abilities allow clarity and characterization of anatomy. Its use is superior to magnetic resonance imaging owing to the resource cost and time to acquisition of images. Though the value of oral contrast is debated, rectal contrast CT scans are highly regarded in situations where a fistula is thought to originate from the distal colon or rectum. Bladder contrast CT scans have been used with variable outcomes.
  - Magnetic resonance imaging (MRI).
    T1 and T2 weighted images allow the identification of inflammatory changes in fat planes and fluid collections respectively. In combination, fistula tracts and their underlying pathology can be mapped owing to superior soft tissue delineation. The practical application of MRI in EVF is limited owing to the image quality acquisition, lower costs and increased availability of CT scans.
  - Fistulogram/contrast enterography.
    Is routinely done in conjunction with a CT or MRI.
  - Barium enema.
    The use of this now somewhat historical fluoroscopy-based procedure has dwindled owing to its ability to reveal EVF unreliably.
  - Cystography.
  - *Herald* and *beehive* signs have been described with bladder fistulae [26, 27]. The former represents a perivesicular abscess. A crescentic defect is seen on the superior aspect of the bladder in an oblique view.
  - Ultrasonography (US).
    As with cystography, US is rarely used for primary EVF imaging.
- **Diagnostic Procedures**
  - Cystoscopy/vaginoscopy/hysteroscopy.
    The instrumentation of these hollow structures is helpful in diagnostic evaluation. Apart from suggesting the presence of a fistula, the direct inspection of the mucosa allows the evaluation of malignancy (e.g. biopsy).
    With EVF, a herald patch (mucosal inflammation, oedema and pseudo-polyp formation) or cobble stoning may be seen in the bladder with gas and discharge seen in up to 90% of patients [26, 27]. A beehive sign describes the vesicular end of an EVF with its constellation of densely packed homogenous openings.
  - Endoscopy.
    Colonoscopy is valuable in determining the aetiology of the fistula and thus forms an integral part of EVF investigation, particularly if malignancy or IBD is considered as this consolidates information for surgical planning [27].
  - Laparoscopy/laparotomy and examination under anaesthesia.
    Though considered invasive, these procedures are useful particularly in women, owing to the complex anatomy that may not be well represented in the above radiologic methods. In some instances, these exploratory procedures allow not only diagnosis but therapy.

- Poppy seed test [25].

    This is a novel diagnostic tool that consists of approximately 1 g of poppy seeds ingested with a liquid medium. The urine is judiciously checked over the next 2 days for excreted seeds.

    This tool yielded a 100% detection rate for fistulae when compared to CT scans. However, it is limited by its inability to characterize a fistula.

> **Differential Diagnosis**
> - Urinary tract infection.
> - Appendicitis.
> - Abdominal trauma—blunt and penetrating.
> - Peptic ulcer disease.
> - Colorectal malignancy.
> - Inflammatory bowel disease.
> - Aortic injury.

## 90.3 Treatment

Treatment of fistulae encompasses management of the entire disease spectrum, i.e. the fistula itself and the underlying pathology if it is treatable. It is worth emphasizing, especially with a situation as elaborate as fistulae, good clinical practice is a marriage of the least aggressive treatment modality with the best success rate and consideration of resources.

### 90.3.1 Medical Treatment

In patients harbouring urinary tract infections and diverticulitis, medical treatment of their symptoms should be undertaken. Similarly, in patients with IBD, the aim is to maximize medical treatment of the underlying disease with promising long-term remission. Zhang and colleagues reported 1/3 of patients with Crohn's disease achieved long-term remission of EVF over a mean of 4.7 years with antibiotics, steroids, and a combination of immunomodulators [28].

Patients with malignant bladder invasions can be treated with an in-dwelling or percutaneous drainage system.

Endoscopic and other novel interventional remediation methods have been proposed (i.e. sealants, glues and clips) but these are not currently recommended due to limited and conflicting data in relation to their outcomes.

Medical management is the only treatment of choice for those who are nonsurgical candidates.

The role and value of maintaining a well-nourished individual through the stages of investigations and diagnosis cannot be stressed enough. Nutrition can be administered parenterally or enterally, with parenteral hyperalimentation considered in those with proximal fistulae. Enteral nutrition is best suited for low to moderate volume distal enteric fistulae. H2 blockers should also be used to reduce gastric acid output. Often overlooked is the importance of skin protection, particularly with cutaneous termination of the fistulae tracts. The above is best achieved through a multi-disciplinary model.

### 90.3.2 Surgical Treatment

Historically, fistula surgery was a staged process. Nowadays, not only are single-stage procedures (good health, well-organized fistulae and the absence of systemic infection) considered almost routine, but laparoscopic approaches are advocated. In saying that, from small and limited series, the conversion rates in laparoscopic surgery are as high as 30% [29].

The principle of surgery with fistulae is to excise the diseased segment of the bowel and fistula with the restoration of enteric continuity. The extent of resection is dependent on the underlying aetiology (i.e. limited excision in diverticular processes and IBD). It is rare to excise the involved bladder or vagina as primary closure with an absorbable suture is usually sufficient.

In situations where a densely adherent abdomen is found and fistula suspected with an unknown aetiology, consideration should be made for a frozen section prior to radical resections.

In some instances, a diverting stoma and drainage of intra-abdominal sepsis are all that should be contemplated in the immediate period. A permanent stoma should be considered in situations of aggressive malignancy and reduced fitness for extensive surgery. The latter offers a long-term strategy to mitigate sepsis with the maintenance of quality of life.

### 90.3.3 Prognosis

With a reported mortality and complication rate of 3.5 and 27%, respectively, the invasive management of fistulae has consequences [30]. Furthermore, recurrences are seen in up to 5% patients [30]. Apart from the traditional general surgical complications (i.e. fever, deep vein thrombosis (DVT), and wound breakdown), specific issues such as anastomotic disruptions, bladder leaks, abdominal abscesses and obstruction may occur. Most of these issues are largely preventable with postoperative adjuncts and enhanced recovery pathways with multidisciplinary input.

The outcome is generally excellent in patients with non-radiation or non-malignant aetiology. Where there is malignant involvement of adjacent viscera, a less favourable outlook is seen owing to an aggressive biological process.

> **Dos and Don'ts**
> - **Do** control sepsis before embarking on definitive surgery.
> - **Do** consult with other relevant subspecialties (e.g. urology) before embarking on surgery in complex cases.
> - **Do not** undertake surgical intervention prior to complete planning.
> - **Do not** underestimate the value of a suitably nourished and optimized patient.
> - **Do not** perform a primary anastomosis for acute obstruction unless in a specialist centre with experience in these cases.
> - **Do not** operate on inflammatory bowel disease until medically controlled.

> **Take-Home Messages**
> - Confirm, characterize, clarify, consolidate and cure.
> - Optimize the patient.
> - Define and treat the underlying disease process.
> - Multidisciplinary management is key.

> **Multiple Choice Question**
> 1. The most common organism found in the urine of colovesical fistulae are
>    A. Predominantly anaerobic.
>    B. Staphylococcal family.
>    C. Enteroviruses.
>    D. Mixed enteric organisms.
>    **Answer: D**
> 2. Malignancies can lead to fistula formation. The most common arises in
>    A. Sigmoid colon.
>    B. Bladder.
>    C. Uterus.
>    D. Transverse colon.
>    **Answer: A**
> 3. In long-standing colo-vesical fistula, the most common **abdominal** finding is
>    A. Generalized peritonitis.
>    B. Direct tenderness over the bladder.
>    C. Pain centred mainly over the left iliac fossa.
>    D. Often there are minimal or no abdominal signs.
>    **Answer: D**
> 4. What is the most common cause of colovesicle fistula?
>    A. Malignancy
>    B. Inflammatory bowel disease.
>    C. Diverticular disease.
>    D. Pelvic radiation.
>    **Answer: C**
> 5. How common is fistula formation in acute diverticulitis?
>    A. 1–2%
>    B. 5%

    C. 20%
    D. 50%.
    
    **Answer: C**

6. Which is the most common fistula in acute diverticulitis?
    A. Colouterine.
    B. Colovesicle.
    C. Coloenteric.
    D. Colovaginal.
    
    **Answer: B**

7. What prevents fistulae closure?
    A. Distal obstruction.
    B. Larger body mass index (BMI).
    C. Long tract.
    D. Older patients.
    
    **Answer: A**

8. Which is the most **sensitive** in fistula investigation?
    A. US.
    B. CT.
    C. Barium enema.
    D. Fistulogram.
    
    **Answer: B**

9. Which EVF aetiology has the **least** predictable course?
    A. Malignancy
    B. Inflammatory bowel disease.
    C. Diverticular disease.
    D. Radiation.
    
    **Answer: D**

10. What is the most common complication following EVF surgery?
    A. Recurrence of fistula.
    B. Wound infection.
    C. DVT.
    D. Anastomotic disruption.
    
    **Answer: B**

# References

1. Pugh JI. On the pathology and behaviour of acquired non-traumatic vesico-intestinal fistula. Br J Surg. 1964;51:644–57.
2. Farooqi N, Tuma F. Intestinal fistula. Treasure Island, FL: StatPearls; 2021.
3. Basler JAE. Enterovesical Fistula: WebMD; 2020 [updated 24th Dec 2020]. https://emedicine.medscape.com/article/442000-overview
4. Golabek T, Szymanska A, Szopinski T, Bukowczan J, Furmanek M, Powroznik J, et al. Enterovesical fistulae: aetiology, imaging, and management. Gastroenterol Res Pract. 2013;2013:617967.
5. Shaydakov ME, Pastorino A, Tuma F. Enterovesical Fistula. Treasure Island, FL: StatPearls; 2021.
6. Scozzari G, Arezzo A, Morino M. Enterovesical fistulas: diagnosis and management. Tech Coloproctol. 2010;14(4):293–300.
7. Tuma F, McKeown DG, Al-Wahab Z. Rectovaginal fistula. Treasure Island, FL: StatPearls; 2021.
8. Keady CHD, Joyce M. When the bowel meets the bladder: optimal management of colorectal pathology with urological involvement. World J Gastrointest Surg. 2020;12(5):208–25.
9. Sardinha TC, Yebara SM, Wexner SD. Surgical therapy: mutual and combined aspects—enterourinary fistula. In: Davila GW, Ghoniem GM, Wexner SD, editors. Pelvic floor dysfunction. Philadelphia, PA: Springer; 2006.
10. Balsara KP, Dubash C. Complicated sigmoid diverticulosis. Indian J Gastroenterol. 1998;17(2):46–7.
11. ER R. Rectovaginal fistula. In: Beck D. SS, Wexner S, editor. Fundamentals of anorectal surgery. 3rd ed. Philadelphia, PA: Springer; 2019.
12. Champagne BJ, McGee MF. Rectovaginal fistula. Surg Clin North Am, Table of Contents. 2010;90(1):69–82.
13. Schecter WP, Hirshberg A, Chang DS, Harris HW, Napolitano LM, Wexner SD, et al. Enteric fistulas: principles of management. J Am Coll Surg. 2009;209(4):484–91.
14. Karamchandani MC, West CF Jr. Vesicoenteric fistulas. Am J Surg. 1984;147(5):681–3.
15. De Ridder D. An update on surgery for vesicovaginal and urethrovaginal fistulae. Curr Opin Urol. 2011;21(4):297–300.
16. Lawes DEJ. Rectovaginal and rectourethral fistula. In: Zbar AP, Wexner SD, editors. Coloproctology. 1st ed. Springer; 2010. p. 169–84.
17. Charua-Guindic L, Jimenez-Bobadilla B, Reveles-Gonzalez A, Avendano-Espinosa O, Charua-Levy E. Incidence, diagnosis and treatment of colovesical fistula. Cir Cir. 2007;75(5):343–9.
18. Graber P. Prostatorectal fistulas. In: Marti MC, Givel J-C, editors. Surgery of anorectal diseases. Berlin: Springer; 1990.
19. Gray MR, Curtis JM, Elkington JS. Colovesical fistula after laparoscopic inguinal hernia repair. Br J Surg. 1994;81(8):1213–4.
20. Levenback C, Gershenson DM, McGehee R, Eifel PJ, Morris M, Burke TW. Enterovesical fistula following radiotherapy for gynecologic cancer. Gynecol Oncol. 1994;52(3):296–300.
21. Ansari MS, Nabi G, Singh I, Hemal AK, Pandey G. Colovesical fistula an unusual complication of

cytotoxic therapy in a case of non-Hodgkin's lymphoma. Int Urol Nephrol. 2001;33(2):373–4.
22. Crispen PL, Kansas BT, Pieri PG, Fisher C, Gaughan JP, Pathak AS, et al. Immediate postoperative complications of combined penetrating rectal and bladder injuries. J Trauma. 2007;62(2):325–9.
23. Driver CP, Anderson DN, Findlay K, Keenan RA, Davidson AI. Vesico-colic fistulae in the Grampian region: presentation, assessment, management and outcome. J R Coll Surg Edinb. 1997;42(3):182–5.
24. Pontari MA, McMillen MA, Garvey RH, Ballantyne GH. Diagnosis and treatment of enterovesical fistulae. Am Surg. 1992;58(4):258–63.
25. Kwon EO, Armenakas NA, Scharf SC, Panagopoulos G, Fracchia JA. The poppy seed test for colovesical fistula: big bang, little bucks! J Urol. 2008;179(4):1425–7.
26. Kaisary AV, Grant RW. "Beehive on the bladder": an indication of colovesical disease. Br J Urol. 1984;56(1):35–7.
27. Lavery IC. Colonic fistulas. Surg Clin North Am. 1996;76(5):1183–90.
28. Fiocchi C. Closing fistulas in Crohn's disease—should the accent be on maintenance or safety? N Engl J Med. 2004;350(9):934–6.
29. Nevo Y, Shapiro R, Froylich D, Meron-Eldar S, Zippel D, Nissan A, et al. Over 1-year followup of laparoscopic treatment of enterovesical fistula. JSLS. 2019;23(1)
30. Woods RJ, Lavery IC, Fazio VW, Jagelman DG, Weakley FL. Internal fistulas in diverticular disease. Dis Colon Rectum. 1988;31(8):591–6.
31. Borseth KF, Acharya G, Kiserud T, Trovik J. Incidence of gynecological fistula and its surgical treatment: a national registry-based study. Acta Obstet Gynecol Scand. 2019;98(9):1120–6.

## Further Reading

Beck D, Steele S, Wexner S, editors. Fundamentals of anorectal surgery. 3rd ed. Philadelphia, PA: Springer International Publishing; 2019.
Clark S. Colorectal surgery: a companion to specialist surgical practice. 6th ed. St. Louis, MO: Elsevier; 2018.
Strickland M, Burnstein M, Cohen Z, et al. Colovesical fistula 2019 June 24. UpToDate (Internet) 2021.
Townsend C, Beauchamp RD, Evers BM, et al. Sabiston textbook of surgery-the biological basis of modern surgical practice. 20th ed. Philadelphia, PA: Elsevier; 2016.

# Enterocutaneous and Enteroatmospheric Fistulae

**91**

Ashleigh Phillips, Eu Jhin Loh, and Francesco Amico

## 91.1 Introduction

> **Learning Goals**
> - Implications of anatomy of enterocutaneous and enteroatmospheric fistulae.
> - Optimal timing for the management of enterocutaneous and enteroatmospheric fistulae.
> - FRIEND and SNAP acronyms.

### 91.1.1 Definitions

An enterocutaneous fistula is an abnormal opening between a part of the gastrointestinal tract and the skin. They are distinct from stomas as they arise pathologically, rather than being created to serve a purpose. An enteroatmospheric fistula (EAF) is a particular type of enterocutaneous fistula (ECF), which has its opening into an abdominal wound, which has been left open, rather than onto the skin. Strictly speaking, an ECF or EAF is an opening between the small bowel and the skin; however, the terms have entered the medical lexicon as general terms for fistulae arising from any gastrointestinal organ. Fistulae can be further named for the organ from which they arise (e.g. colocutaneous, gastrocutaneous).

The formation of ECFs and EAFs complicates numerous surgical procedures and inflammatory conditions. They are uncommon complications; however, they are associated with significant morbidity for the patients who suffer from them. They present a significant challenge to all clinicians who care for these patients and their successful management relies on a highly skilled multidisciplinary team.

### 91.1.2 Epidemiology

There is a highly variable incidence of ECF and EAF across the numerous aetiologies. It has been described as 1.1% following emergency general surgical procedures on the gastrointestinal tract [1]. If considering different parts of the enteric tract, small bowel resections are the procedure most frequently resulting in fistulizing disease followed by colorectal resections, with an incidence of 2.8 and 1.3% respectively [1]. In terms of conditions, Crohn's disease is a prevalent cause of ECF. Approximately 0.3% of people living with Crohn's disease will have an ECF at any one time, and ECF represents approximately 9% of fistulizing Crohn's disease [2, 3].

Mortality resulting from ECFs varies from 6 to 33%. This large variation is predominantly due to the heterogeneous nature of the fistulae [4]. The high variability between types of fistulae and patients with fistulae makes it difficult to accurately state the mortality rate of ECFs. Most deaths from enterocutaneous fistula are from sepsis associated with the fistula or fistula repair surgery [5]. Such operations are in fact burdened with frequent complications and long sequelae. These often-malnourished patients often struggle to overcome the fistula, establish adequate anabolic metabolism and achieve a full recovery.

ECFs are responsible for a significant burden of disease on communities and health systems. This burden is manifested in lengthy hospital admissions, reduced quality of life and the intensive usage of resources. A study on trauma laparotomy patients compared intensive care unit length of stay in individuals with and without EFCs. This study demonstrated that patients with an ECF had an average 22-day longer length of stay than patients without ECF. In the same cohort, the hospital length of stay was found to be 66 days longer for the patient with ECFs than for matched controls without fistula. ECFs and EAFs are associated with significantly increased hospital care costs. It has been shown that costs related to the index hospital admission were on average around USD$36,000 higher for patients who developed ECF [6]. Lengthy admissions, intensive investigation and therapies, prolonged periods of rehabilitation and multiple invasive interventions all contribute to the significant impact that ECFs and EAFs have on the quality of life.

## 91.1.3 Aetiology

The aetiology of enterocutaneous fistulae is diverse and often multifactorial. An understanding of the cause of a particular ECF or EAF is key in planning its subsequent management. ECF and EAFs can be classified as iatrogenic or spontaneous based on their aetiology. Furthermore, patient factors contribute to the development and persistence of ECFs.

The pathophysiology of enterocutaneous fistula first begins with an insult, which allows for there to be a communication between the gut and the skin. Constant flow of fluid causes a tract to form with gradual epithelialization of this tract. Once the tract is fully epithelialized, there is a much higher chance of the fistula persisting [4]. From a molecular standpoint, these fistulae are formed via epithelial to mesenchymal transition. This process is driven by both transforming growth factor $\beta$ (TGF$\beta$) and interleukin-13 (IL-13). A recent study of Crohn's disease associated fistulae has shown IL-13 to be upregulated in cells lining the fistula tracts, which then induces the expression of molecules responsible for invasive cell growth and epithelial to mesenchymal transition. This finding has led the way for further research into IL-13 inhibition for the treatment of these fistulae [7].

### 91.1.3.1 Aetiology—Iatrogenic ECFs and EAFs

Iatrogenic ECFs are the most common type of fistula [8, 9]. They occur following major abdominal surgery, often for traumatic injury or overwhelming abdominal sepsis. Small and large bowel resections are commonly implicated because approximately 75% of enterocutaneous fistulae arise from the anastomotic breakdown [10]. Another common cause is missed enterotomies (either traumatic or iatrogenic). Lastly, ECFs can be caused by erosion into the gastrointestinal tract from prosthesis such as abdominal mesh.

EAFs are a particularly difficult form of iatrogenic fistula to manage. They often occur in conjunction with an abdomen that is left open following the index laparotomy. When a laparostomy is present, the incidence of EAFs increases proportionally with time to definitive fascial closure. Also, in this circumstance, EAF is more likely to develop when anastomoses are present, particularly when exposed to the atmosphere. EAF can develop rapidly, sometimes within 8 days of the initial laparotomy [11].

Some specific operative factors are worth mentioning owing to an increased risk of developing an ECF or EAF, when present. Namely, operations performed in an emergency setting, operations for traumatic injury and operations involving a primary anastomosis following bowel resections are all associated with an increased risk of developing ECF postoperatively. In one series of 278 patients with ECF, approximately 70% were resulting from emergency operations [12]. Other factors including the presence of concurrent sepsis, multiple anastomoses, implantation of foreign material and missed enterotomies increase the risk of ECF [1, 9, 11, 13, 14].

Multiple factors correlate with iatrogenic ECFs and are implicated in their persistence once an ECF is established. The acronym FRIEND can facilitate memorizing the main ones and is described as follow [4]:

- Foreign body.
- Radiation.
- Inflammation and infection.
- Epithelialization.
- Neoplasia.
- Distal obstruction.

### 91.1.3.2 Aetiology—Spontaneous ECFs

The most common cause of spontaneous ECFs is Crohn's disease. Fistulizing Crohn's disease commonly manifests as anorectal fistulae; however, ECFs and EAFs can represent up to 9% of fistulizing Crohn's disease [2, 3, 15]. An EAF or ECF may develop in the wound of an operation performed as a complication of Crohn's disease, but an ECF may also develop on virgin abdominal skin, not in conjunction with any surgical intervention. Fistulizing Crohn's is associated with the transmural inflammation, a key characteristic of Crohn's disease. An epithelial defect arises from the ongoing inflammation and is extended through the lamina propria and muscularis mucosa layers of the bowel. As this defect deepens, there is infiltration of inflammatory cells and cytokines, which enable the fistula tract to form and extend to the skins surface. Once there is a formed tract, intestinal epithelial cells migrate along the tract, lining it and allowing it to persist [16].

Patient-specific risk factors play a role in the establishment of a spontaneous ECF or EAF. Modifiable risk factors, including smoking and malnutrition, can tentatively be addressed preoperatively to reduce the likelihood of ECF formation. Non-modifiable risk factors include immunosuppression, concurrent infection at surgery and inflammatory bowel disease.

### 91.1.4 Classification

The classification of an enterocutaneous fistula is a key element in planning further management because this will guide the management strategy. Fistulae have a very diverse clinical picture and will require a personalized approach. Adequate classification also provides prognostic information useful to predict the likely course of the fistula. Additionally, to the aetiology-based classification presented above, another useful classification criterion is the output. Finally, an anatomical classification is possible once the fistula has been fully investigated.

The output of ECFs and EAFs offers a functional way to classify fistulae into three groups: low-output fistulae producing <200 mL/day, moderate output producing 200–500 mL/day and high-output fistulae producing more than 500 mL of effluent daily. The output of an enterocutaneous fistula is a crucial consideration as it correlates with its likely natural history. In fact, a low-output fistula is much more likely to resolve with conservative measures than a high-output fistula, because ongoing fluid passage contributes to epithelialization and persistent inflammatory infiltration of the fistula tract. Moreover, the fistula output defines the likely nutritional requirements of patients, because of the loss of digestive enzymes, nutrient-rich chyme and relative defunctioning of the distal bowel.

Once clarified, the anatomy of the fistula also offers an opportunity to classify different types of

ECFs and EAFs. The fistula anatomy sometimes correlates with the characteristics of the effluent; however, advanced imaging is required to precisely delineate which enteric segment is involved. Anatomically, four types of ECFs and EAFs have been described [14]:

- Type I fistulae arising from upper gastrointestinal organs including the oesophagus, stomach, duodenum and the biliary tree.
- Type II fistulae arising from the small bowel distal to the ligament of Treitz.
- Type III fistulae arising from the large bowel, including the rectum.
- Type IV fistulae are all enteroatmospheric fistulae, regardless of the organ of origin.

An anatomical classification of the fistula is important as it often defines the likely losses and guides any appropriate fluid and nutrients replacement strategy. In fact, based on which gastrointestinal organ is involved different electrolytes and nutrients are lost. This directly correlates with the need for replacement when formulating any required supporting therapy. But also, varying acidity of the effluent implies different techniques required to manage the wound relating to the potential for different enteric products to degrade the skin. Another obvious implication is also the ability for the fistula to heal. These are some of the factors correlating with how favourable the spontaneous closure of different types of EAF and ECFs might be (Table 91.1) [17].

**Table 91.1** Factors predicting favourable or unfavourable closure

| Factor | Favourable | Unfavourable |
|---|---|---|
| Organ of origin | Oesophageal Duodenal stump Pancreatic, biliary Jejunal Colonic | Gastric Lateral duodenal Ligament of Treitz Ileal |
| Aetiology | Postoperative (anastomotic leakage) Appendicitis Diverticulitis | Malignancy Inflammatory bowel disease |
| Output | Low (<200–500 mL/day) | High (>500 mL/day) |
| Nutritional status | Well-nourished Transferrin >200 mg/dL | Malnourished Transferrin <200 mg/dL |
| Sepsis | Absent | Present |
| State of bowel | Intestinal continuity Absence of obstruction | Diseased adjacent bowel Distal obstruction Large abscess Bowel discontinuity Previous irradiation |
| Fistula characteristics | Tract >2 cm Defect <1 cm | Tract <1 cm Defect >1 cm |

## 91.2 Diagnosis

Diagnosing the presence of an ECF or EAF is often simple, the patient has a typical history accompanied by the presence of enteric contents outpouring from a skin opening or found in the wound. The diagnostic challenge for ECFs then comes in the characterization of the fistula, which often requires extensive investigation including advanced imaging. The clinical features of ECFs will be described, followed by an approach to the investigation and characterization of the fistula.

### 91.2.1 Clinical Presentation

#### 91.2.1.1 History
Patients who develop an ECF or EAF typically have a history of an inciting event. Many patients will have had significant abdominal surgery, while others may have had a flare of Crohn's disease. Carefully considering other aetiologies of fistulae is important. Following this index event, many patients follow a troubled postoperative course, which is often accompanied by a combination of failure to normal recovery, wound breakdown and recurrent abdominal sepsis. Following this, the ECF or EAF will declare itself, with the obvious leak of enteric contents.

In the early stages of an enterocutaneous fistula, abdominal sepsis is often a key feature of the presentation. Enquiring about and treating the abdominal sepsis is an important step toward managing these patients. Abdominal sepsis can present in myriad ways but commonly features increasing abdominal pain and symptoms of dysfunction of the gut, with the possibility of this representing a prodromic sign of ECF and EAF.

### 91.2.1.2 Examination

There are two distinct parts of the clinical examination—first directly examining the fistula and its local complications, second general examination of the patient for the systemic complications of the fistula.

Examination of the fistula is not always immediately clear. The telltale sign of the presence of a fistula is the presence of enteric contents in the wound. The wound should be carefully examined for local areas of dehiscence, exudate, erythema and induration. A fistula tract may or may not be evident. Findings should be carefully recorded, and the use of clinical photographs (with appropriate consent) can be a valuable tool to monitor serial wound changes. The surrounding skin should be examined for signs of localized irritation from the presence of enteric fluid. If there is doubt about the presence of a fistula on the examination, an inert dye such as methylene blue can be added to food or enteric feeding solutions. A fistula is confirmed when this dye is expressed into the wound. Cautious local wound exploration is also an option worth considering.

ECFs and EAFs can be associated with significant morbidity because of the systemic complications they can lead to. The careful clinician must watch for signs of sepsis, especially if complicated by multi-organ dysfunction. Closely monitoring the patient's nutritional and fluid volume status is of paramount importance for patients at risk of ECF and EAFs. Additionally to standard physical examination, the nutritional status of the patient can be examined in several ways including their general level of functioning and serially monitoring the patient's weight.

## 91.2.2 Tests

Investigations serve several purposes once an enterocutaneous fistula is clinically suspected. Firstly, they are of assistance in identifying any associated pathology in the abdomen but also, confirm the diagnosis and define the anatomy of an ECF. Investigations play an important role in monitoring the consequences of ECFs and EAFs. In the long term, if adequate imaging is taken, investigations play an important role in surgical planning for definitive closure, as needed.

### 91.2.2.1 Identifying Associated Abdominal Pathology

An ECF or EAF rarely exists in isolation, and it is important to investigate an underlying pathology. In the acute and postacute phase both at the onset of the disease and further into its management, this is achieved largely through monitoring inflammatory markers in the blood (such as white cell count and c-reactive protein) and cross-sectional imaging. The most frequently used imaging modality used in this phase is computed tomography (CT) performed with intravenous contrast to enhance image quality. This provides detailed information about the presence of any associated complications, for example, abscesses and collections found intraperitoneally or within the thickness of the abdominal wall. Other complications such as bowel obstruction and resulting dilated bowel are also accurately detected by contrast-enhanced CT. In the acute phase, CT is usually not able to precisely define the anatomy of an ECF, with the fistula tract sometimes not yet established, if the disease is of recent onset.

### 91.2.2.2 Defining the Anatomy of an ECF

Cross-sectional imaging is the mainstay of imaging to define the anatomy of an ECF or EAF. CT is a valuable tool as it is readily available and rapidly provides quality images [18]. While CT is often undertaken in the acute phase while the diagnosis is being established, imaging to define the anatomy of a fistula is best deferred 7–10 days after the complete resolution of sepsis. CT is not always indicative of the source of an enterocutaneous fistula; however, it can provide valuable information about distal obstruction, which need to be addressed aiming for fistula closure [8]. Further information can be gained by using contrast within the lumen of the digestive tract, either orally, rectally, or through the fistula tract itself.

Fluoroscopy is another tool that can provide information on the anatomy of an ECF or EAF [8, 18], useful to define intestinal continuity. Depending on the location of the fistula, contrast can be introduced orally, with a nasogastric tube, or rectally. Fistulogram can also be performed with contrast media being instilled directly into the fistula opening. Depending on the calibre of the opening, it can be cannulated with a fine nasogastric feeding tube, larger nasogastric tube, or Foley catheter. It can often be useful for the surgical team to be present and assist with cannulation of the fistula tract, especially if multiple tracts are present to maximize gathering information required for surgical planning.

Magnetic resonance imaging has emerged as an important tool in the workup of ECFs or EAFs as it became more widely available [9]. It is a very useful technique owing to its superior soft tissue differentiation when compared to CT. One of the reasons MRI is not useful in the acute phase is its prolonged image acquisition time. In the acute phase, it can be difficult to minimize respiratory and peristalsis artefact which can significantly degrade the quality of images obtained [18]. Like CT and fluoroscopy, utility of MRI can be enhanced with the use of contrast media. Intravenous gadolinium contrast can help to define the hypervascularity of active inflammation around the fistula. Oral contrast enterography can also provide important detail about the lumen of the bowel.

### 91.2.2.3 Investigations for the Sequelae of ECF and EAF

Judicious use of investigations can reveal and monitor the major consequences of ECFs and EAFs—namely sepsis and malnutrition. Clinicians should always be suspicious of septic complications in these patients, both acutely and in the chronic phase. Derangement of inflammatory markers is an early clue that septic complications may be developing. If there is a suspicion of septic complications, a systematic approach should be used including taking samples for microscopy, culture and sensitivity. It is important to culture samples from the blood, vascular access devices, if any, and urine. Wounds may also be swabbed; however, results should be interpreted with caution and any resulting treatment might benefit from the input of a specialized microbiology input. Also, if an abscess is identified and drained a fluid sample should be sent for culture.

Careful monitoring of the patients' nutritional status is an ongoing challenge and nutritional requirements will change throughout the disease course. Overreliance on a single measure can be misleading and several blood markers should be used to provide a complete picture. Useful markers include blood-based proteins such as albumin, prealbumin and transferrin. In addition, close monitoring of electrolytes, urea and creatinine can guide the adequacy of fluid provision. Many patients with enterocutaneous fistula receive at least partial parenteral nutrition, if not total parenteral nutrition. Monitoring of parenteral nutrition also entails close monitoring of liver function, serum electrolytes and trace minerals to allow the parenteral nutrition formula to be titrated to the requirement.

### 91.2.2.4 Investigations to Plan Definitive Closure of ECFs and EAFs

Choosing the right time to surgically intervene in an ECF or EAF is critical to maximizing the chance of success. If the patient is not acutely systemically unwell, tolerating dressings and the nutritional regimen, some centres will wait for up to 12 months before planning definitive closure [9, 19]. Before proceeding with closure, it is important to aim for the patient to be as free from infection as possible and nutritionally replete. Transferrin can be a useful marker of protein sufficiency as it has a shorter half-life than albumin

(5–8 days vs 23–26 days). This allows it to be a timely measure of the current nutritional status. Repeated cross-sectional imaging close to the time of surgery can determine any change in the fistula characteristics and guide the surgical approach.

> **Differential Diagnosis**
> The diagnosis of ECFs or EAFs is often clear; however, a few important differentials should be considered. The main differential is surgical site infection. A superficial surgical site infection can present with a significant exudate from the wound; however, no fistula tract will be identified either clinically or radiologically. Deep surgical site infections with intra-abdominal collection may have formed a sinus tract draining to the skin. This can be considered with contrast-based investigations showing no communication between the sinus and the lumen of the gut.

## 91.3 Treatment

### 91.3.1 Principles of Treatment

There are two key phases of treatment for an ECF: the acute phase followed by the subacute and chronic phases. Management of the enterocutaneous fistula and its local and systemic complications should proceed in a stepwise fashion to maximize the chances of spontaneous closure. The approach to enterocutaneous fistula management is summarized by the SNAP mnemonic [20]:

- S—skin protection and sepsis control.
- N—nutrition optimization.
- A—define fistula anatomy.
- P—plan for definitive closure.

Acutely, the major concerns are skin and sepsis control and optimization of nutrition. It is important to note from this stepwise approach that planning for definitive management of the fistula is the last step. Neither ECFs nor EAFs need urgent closure and this should not be attempted. There is evidence to show that mortality and morbidity are increased if surgical intervention is attempted between 10 and 45 days after the development of a fistula [8, 21]. Additionally, a large proportion of fistulae will close spontaneously with conservative measures. Generally speaking, a sufficient trial period of conservative measures should be observed, and after this, fistulae which persist are unlikely to close spontaneously and should be worked up for surgical treatment.

Enterocutaneous fistulae are highly complex conditions, which are associated with significant morbidity for patients. For this reason, the early involvement of a well-coordinated multidisciplinary team is important. Medical specialists which will need to be involved include intensivists, in the acute phase if a systemic compromise is present, skilled radiologists and surgeons with experience in managing these patients. The medical team needs significant input from nursing and allied health colleagues. Patients with ECFs and EAFs require very intensive nursing due to the complexity of the dressings and the need to provide supplemental nutrition. Additionally, the involvement of social workers and mental health professionals can aid patients and families in adjusting to life with a fistula and help to prevent or minimize comorbid mental illness resulting from the fistula.

### 91.3.2 Medical Treatment

#### 91.3.2.1 Wound Management

Fastidious attention to detail in the management of fistula wounds is imperative to their successful management. There are several goals when considering a plan to manage these wounds. These goals include minimizing skin loss, managing wound pain, containing and quantifying effluent, promoting closure of the fistula and minimizing the social impact on the patient from odours and obtrusive dressings. No two fistulae are alike, and each patient will require a tailored approach to dressings and devices. A patient with more than one fistula will require a specific approach for each fistula. Early involvement of specialist wound care and stomal therapy nurses is invaluable.

A dressing strategy should protect the peri fistular skin. In fact, skin breakdown can impair spontaneous closure and is also a source of infection. The deleterious effects of effluent can be due to several factors including the volume of fluid on the skin, the introduction of enteric bacteria to threatened skin and perhaps most importantly, the corrosive effects of enteric fluid. The origin of enteric fluid varies its corrosive nature, it may be acidic or alkaline and often contains digestive enzymes, which indiscriminately break down the skin's surface.

A key factor in devising a strategy to manage a wound with an enterocutaneous fistula is the output of the fistula. As output increases, so too does the complexity of the dressing required to manage it. A low-output fistula may be able to be managed with a simple absorptive dressing. The dressing should be able to draw effluent away from the skin's surface to prevent enzymatic degradation or maceration from fluid exposure.

Moderate and high-output fistulae often need to be managed with pouches or ostomy devices. Pouches allow effluent to be taken away from the perifistular skin and facilitate measurement of effluent without the cumbersome need to weigh dressings. Pouch devices also reduce the frequency of dressing changes, thereby reducing local trauma to the skin. Many pouches have been designed to be impenetrable or resistant to odours [22], which can contribute to improving patients' quality of life significantly.

In addition to pouches, many other tools can be employed to protect the skin. These can include skin wafers, adhesive powders and stomal pastes. These can improve the longevity of pouch application and reduce the frequency of dressings. These adjunctive tools also facilitate the application of a pouch to uneven skin or around skin folds.

Negative pressure wound therapy dressings can be useful for managing perifistular wounds, particularly in the setting of EAFs. Direct application onto the fistula is often complicated by tube blockages, loss of vacuum and need for frequent changes. The dressing sponge can also retain fluid and leave it in contact with the skin or wound preventing healing. Creating islands within the dressing foam around the fistula and managing the fistula separately can be a useful approach. There is no evidence to show that negative pressure wound therapy speeds spontaneous closure of the fistula or improves rates of spontaneous closure.

#### 91.3.2.2 Treating Sepsis

Once sepsis has been recognized, time is of the essence and rapid intervention is mandatory. Broad spectrum, intravenous antibiotics should be commenced within 1 h of recognizing sepsis [23] and immediately after samples are taken for culture. The antibiotic regimen should cover-gram-positive, gram-negative and anaerobic organisms, as well as reaching therapeutic concentrations in the target tissue. When choosing an antibiotic regimen, local patterns of antibiotic resistance should be considered, particularly if there are high rates of colonization with multi-resistant organisms in the local community or high rates of nosocomial infection within the institution. Many appropriate empiric regimens exist, all of which are combinations of two or more agents. These can include piperacillin and tazobactam, ampicillin, gentamicin and metronidazole or ceftriaxone and metronidazole. Patients with severe penicillin allergy can be managed with gentamicin and clindamycin [24].

Aside from antibiotic therapy, patients need aggressive supportive care and early referral to intensive care in the setting of deterioration. Supportive measures include adequate fluid resuscitation, supplemental oxygen and close fluid balance monitoring.

If investigations identify an intra-abdominal collection, local source control can be performed in addition to the above measures. Patients should be referred to interventional radiology if a collection is amenable to percutaneous drainage. CT or ultrasound-guided drainage is a safe procedure, which is often done with only local anaesthesia [9].

### 91.3.2.3 Measures to Reduce Fistula Output

Reducing fistula output can reduce the complexity of dressings, reduce nutritional requirements and increase the likelihood of spontaneous closure. Several strategies exist to achieve this. In the early stages, a period of complete bowel rest with total parenteral nutrition may be sufficient to reduce output enough for the fistula to close. Oral and enteral feeding can be associated with increased fistula output. If there is a significant increase, replacing some or all the oral feeds with either elemental enteral feeding or parenteral nutrition can be trialled.

Pharmacological measures are used to reduce the secretory functions of the gut and promote bulking of enteric fluid. Medications can be used to reduce gastric acid secretion—namely proton pump inhibitors and histamine H2-receptor antagonists. This has the additional benefit of reducing the corrosive effects of acidic fistula effluent in a proximal fistula. Antidiarrheal drugs such as loperamide and codeine can reduce the fluid content of the effluent and reduce output. In very high output fistulae (>1 L/day), particularly those associated with the biliary tract, somatostatin analogues such as octreotide can be used to reduce secretions. Downregulation of receptors can reduce the efficacy of octreotide over time; however, it can be a valuable tool to bring fistula output down to a manageable level.

### 91.3.2.4 Optimizing Nutritional Status

Patients with ECFs and EAFs can have significant differences in their nutritional requirements when compared to the normal adult population. Optimizing nutrition in conjunction with a dietitian can promote the healing of a wound associated with a fistula as well as improving the chances of spontaneous closure. Loss of effluent can lead to the loss of important kilojoules, protein, micronutrients and fluid. Patients with higher output fistulae tend to have higher nutritional requirements. Adequate kilojoule and protein intake are especially important to promote healing. Kilojoule requirements can be up to 1.5 times greater than normal. Protein requirements vary according to fistula output but can be 1.5 times normal for a low-output fistula and up to 2.5 times greater for a high-output fistula. Vitamin C requirement can be as much as 5–10 times normal.

Nutrition can be provided orally, enterally through feeding tubes or parenterally. Ideally, as much of the diet should be given orally as can be tolerated. Despite this, oral feeding can be associated with greatly increased fistula output and reducing the volume of oral feeds can be of assistance in reducing fistula output. Enteral nutrition can be used to supplement or replace oral intake however does also have limitations in increasing fistula output, this can be circumvented by using an elemental formula for enteral feeding. Sometimes partial or total parenteral nutrition may be needed. This should be for as short a period as possible; however, it may need to continue until after the definitive surgical closure of the fistula. Novel approaches are being developed for distal refeeding of fistula effluent [25]. This can improve nutritional absorption from the gut as well as improve intestinal continuity. It relies on well-defined proximal and distal limbs of the fistula, an appropriate refeeding device and well-trained nursing staff.

### 91.3.2.5 Fibrin Sealant and Glue Closure of the Fistula

Fibrin sealant and Histoacryl glue have both been investigated as potential options for the closure of recalcitrant fistulae [2]. They have the clear advantage of being able to be performed bedside without the need for anaesthesia. This is achieved by injecting 3 mL of sealant via a flexible cannular passing through the outer fistula orifice to the intestinal lumen. As soon as the sealant comes in contact with living tissue, it polymerizes, generating a film with high tensile resistance [26].

Careful patient selection is needed to improve the chances of success and most patients will require multiple treatments to achieve closure. This approach generally works best for low-output fistulae with a long, narrow fistula tract. There must be no evidence of distal obstruction or active inflammatory disease before attempting fibrin sealant or glue injection, as this will preclude fistula closure.

### 91.3.2.6 Novel Methods in Wound Management and Surgical Control of ECFs and EAFs

Deep fistulae are often more challenging to manage and increase the risk of sepsis, peritonitis and catabolic syndrome [27]. Therefore, when possible, they should be converted to a superficial fistula. Several novel methods have been developed with the aim of stabilizing a deep fistula by isolating the fistula from the surrounding tissue while protecting the skin and granulation tissue from irritation or caustic fluid. These methods include the utilization of a 12 mm silastic stoma stud (Kapitex Healthcare Ltd., Wetherby, West Yorkshire, UK) to stent the cutaneous component of the fistula [28]. Another method called the Wound Crown technique involves collecting the fistula drainage in an ostomy appliance attached to a collapsible fistula isolation device [29].

Another solution to wound isolation involves the use of a vacuum-assisted wound closure system. The negative pressure of the vacuum enables the wound to be drained effectively and promotes the migration of tissue healing factors [30, 31]. This method remains controversial primarily due to some reports of increased association in the formation of new fistulae and mortality [31]. However, these results lack robust data with poor outcomes being multi-factorial and relating to multi-organ failure, intestinal anastomosis and abdominal sepsis contributing to increased mortality [32].

In the setting of a frozen or hostile abdomen, a Foley or Malecot catheter could be used in conjunction with vacuum-assisted closure to promote granulation tissue formation over the bowel and allow for subsequent skin grafting [33]. Another method describes a parachuting technique to suturing the rectus abdominis muscle over the fistula opening to facilitate safe fascial closure and mitigate high-output fistulae [34]. The advantages of this method are that it provides a tension-free closure of the fistula without compromising tissue viability or necessitating bowel resection. Patients could also return to early enteral nutrition and mobilization.

### 91.3.3 Surgical Treatment

Most fistulae that have not closed by 2 months are unlikely to close spontaneously. Despite this, most experts suggest waiting at least 3–6 months before attempting surgical closure of a fistula and some suggest delaying for up to 12 months. The main reason for this delay is the obliterative peritonitis, which develops in the context of intra-abdominal sepsis and enterocutaneous fistula. Intervening too early increases the risk of iatrogenic injury and fistula recurrence. Delaying allows time for these dense adhesions to soften somewhat. Other benefits of delaying include allowing time for nutritional optimization and allowing the skin and subcutaneous tissues time to heal and scar following the initial insult.

The surgical challenge of these cases should not be understated. These are highly challenging cases, which must be approached patiently and meticulously. Sometimes the case is performed by two teams in sequence, firstly the general surgical team which addresses the entry to the abdomen and resection of the fistula followed by an abdominal wall or plastic surgical team which addresses the abdominal wall closure with advanced techniques if needed. The patient should be nutritionally replete.

The main goal of the operation is complete resection of the affected segment of bowel and primary anastomosis of the bowel. Attempts have been made at wedge resections and oversewing the fistula tract; however, these have had unacceptably high rates of fistula recurrence. The challenge of the operation comes in gaining entry to the abdomen without causing an iatrogenic enterotomy.

A midline laparotomy is made, often through the existing scar and dissected down to the peritoneum. This will often need to be made longer than the original wound to allow for adequate access to the fistula and affected segment of the bowel.

Adhesiolysis can be tedious and must be performed slowly and carefully until the section of bowel involved in the fistula can be defined. Following this, the bowel is resected and anastomosed. If the distal obstruction cannot be excluded based on preoperative imaging, it may be necessary to release the entire small bowel to ensure continuity and avoid downstream obstructions.

Once the implicated segment of bowel has been resected and anastomosis performed, the final challenge is closure of the abdominal wall. The abdominal wall should be mobilized laterally so that it is free from adhesions posteriorly. Ideally, the abdominal wall is closed primarily with tension-free closure between good quality native tissues. If this is not possible, component separation techniques may need to be employed. If the defect is so large that even component separation techniques are inadequate a musculoskeletal flap represents an option to reconstruct the abdominal wall. The use of non-absorbable synthetic meshes should be avoided if appropriate and when possible owing to their propensity to causing infections and increasing the risk of refistulization.

Postoperatively, the patient should be closely monitored. Providing early enteral feeds has been shown to improve outcomes [35]. Diet can be gradually reintroduced. While this is in progress, enteral or parenteral nutrition should be gradually weaned and cycled. Provision of continuous parenteral or enteral nutrition can suppress appetite and slow the establishment of a normal oral diet. Involvement of acute pain service for management of postoperative analgesia is recommended as standard of care. The wound should be carefully cared for and examined for complications such as surgical site infection or a dreaded fistula recurrence.

> **Dos and Don'ts**
> - Do not rush into operative management of enterocutaneous and enteroatmospheric fistulae.
> - Do understand the anatomy of the fistula and correlate it with optimal management of the effluent for the best management strategy and outcome.

> **Take-Home Messages**
> - Best management of enterocutaneous and enteroatmospheric fistulae requires team approach and senior input.
> - Prehabilitation is key to good surgical outcomes.
> - Investigation of patients with the fistulizing disease requires multimodal imaging at different stages of this condition following the onset of disease.

> **Multiple Choice Questions**
> 1. Many enterocutaneous fistulae arise because of iatrogenic injury. The most frequent event underlying fistula formation is:
>    A. Repair of unintentional enterotomies.
>    B. Erosion of foreign body implants.
>    C. Insufficient abdominal washout.
>    **D. Anastomotic breakdown.**
> 2. The three most useful classification tools for enterocutaneous fistula are:
>    A. Anatomical, pathological and biological.
>    B. Aetiology, output and pathological.
>    **C. Anatomical, aetiology and output.**
>    D. Output, pathological and physiological.
> 3. Mitchell, 45 M, is in the Intensive Care Unit, day 10 post trauma laparotomy with ileal resection and primary anastomosis. Initially, he was improving well; however, he has deteriorated over the last few days. He now has persistent abdominal pain, elevated C-reactive protein and fevers. What is the key finding on examination which would make you concerned for an enterocutaneous fistula?
>    A. Abdominal distension.
>    **B. Presence of chyme in the wound.**
>    C. Abdominal percussion tenderness.
>    D. Skin dehiscence.

4. You now wish to investigate Mitchell further to confirm your suspicion of enterocutaneous fistula formation, you will start with a CT today. What is the primary role of performing a CT abdomen and pelvis with IV and oral contrast in the acute setting?
   A. Planning fistula repair.
   B. Defining fistula anatomy.
   C. **Excluding other intra-abdominal pathology.**
   D. Deciding whether to proceed with a barium enema.
5. Providing adequate nutrition presents a significant challenge in the management of enterocutaneous fistula. Which of the following blood markers provides the most up to date information on the patient's nutritional status?
   A. Albumin.
   B. Ferritin.
   C. Insulin.
   D. **Transferrin.**
6. MRI is an important modality for investigating enterocutaneous fistula. It is particularly useful in planning definitive surgical closure of the fistula. This is because of its.'
   A. Avoidance of ionizing radiation.
   B. **Superior soft tissue differentiation.**
   C. Ability to investigate for associated pathology.
   D. Usefulness in the acute phase of enterocutaneous fistula.
7. Which of the following is the first priority in managing an enterocutaneous fistula wound?
   A. Nutrition.
   B. Define anatomy.
   C. **Skin and sepsis management.**
   D. Planning definitive closure.
8. Many novel approaches to managing enterocutaneous fistula have been developed. One of the key aims for these novel approaches is to convert a deep fistula to a superficial one. The benefits of this include.
   A. **Mitigating the risk of sepsis, peritonitis and catabolic syndrome.**
   B. Reducing the need for enteral nutrition.
   C. Reducing fistula output.
   D. Aiding in the definitive closure of the fistula.
9. Patients with an enterocutaneous fistula are often in a catabolic state and can have greatly increased nutritional requirements. Compared with a healthy individual, how much more protein will a patient with a high- output fistula require?
   A. 1.2 times greater
   B. 1.5 times greater
   C. **2.5 times greater**
   D. 3.5 times greater.
10. When conservative measures fail, a definitive closure of enterocutaneous fistula should be performed. This can be a highly challenging operation. Which of the following is NOT a way to mitigate the challenges of this operation?
    A. Involving a specialist surgical team to perform advanced abdominal closure.
    B. **Avoid performing total adhesiolysis of the small bowel.**
    C. Wait for at least 3–6 months for obliterative peritonitis to reduce.
    D. Extending the incision beyond the initial surgical scar.

**Conflict of Interest and Sources of Funding** None declared.

# References

1. Hatchimonji JS, Passman J, Kaufman EJ, Sharoky CE, Ma LW, Scantling D, et al. Enterocutaneous fistula after emergency general surgery: mortality, read-

1. mission, and financial burden. J Trauma Acute Care Surg. 2020;89(1):167–72.
2. Nielsen OH, Rogler G, Hahnloser D, Thomsen OO. Diagnosis and management of fistulizing Crohn's disease. Nat Clin Pract Gastroenterol Hepatol. 2009;6(2):92–106.
3. Schwartz DA, Tagarro I, Carmen Diez M, Sandborn WJ. Prevalence of fistulizing Crohn's disease in the United States: estimate from a systematic literature review attempt and population-based database analysis. Inflamm Bowel Dis. 2019;25(11):1773–9.
4. Cowan KB, Cassaro S. Enterocutaneous fistula. 2020 10 Aug 2020 [cited 17/04/2021]. In: StatPearls [Internet]. Treasure Island, FL: StatPearls Publishing; 2021.
5. Hollington P, Mawdsley J, Lim W, Gabe SM, Forbes A, Windsor AJ. An 11-year experience of enterocutaneous fistula. Br J Surg. 2004;91(12):1646–51.
6. Brooks NE, Idrees JJ, Steinhagen E, Giglia M, Stein SL. The impact of enteric fistulas on US hospital systems. Am J Surg. 2021;221(1):26–9.
7. Scharl M, Frei S, Pesch T, Kellermeier S, Arikkat J, Frei P, et al. Interleukin-13 and transforming growth factor β synergise in the pathogenesis of human intestinal fistulae. Gut. 2013;62(1):63–72.
8. Stein SL. Enterocutaneous and enteroatmospheric fistulas. In: Bulger EM, Lamont JT, Soybel DI, Chen W, editor. UpToDate: 2021.
9. Tuma F, Crespi Z, Wolff CJ, Daniel DT, Nassar AK. Enterocutaneous fistula: a simplified clinical approach. Cureus. 2020;12(4):e7789.
10. Berry SM, Fischer JE. Classification and pathophysiology of enterocutaneous fistulas. Surg Clin North Am. 1996;76(5):1009–18.
11. Martin N, Sarani B. Management of the open abdomen in adults. In: K C, editor, Tet W. Post. Waltham, MA. UpToDate2021.
12. Quinn M, Falconer S, McKee RF. Management of Enterocutaneous Fistula: outcomes in 276 patients. World J Surg. 2017;41(10):2502–11.
13. Teixeira PGRMD, Inaba KMSMD, DuBose JMD, Salim AMD, Brown CMD, Rhee PMD, et al. Enterocutaneous fistula complicating trauma laparotomy: a major resource burden. Am Surg. 2009;75(1):30–2.
14. Gribovskaja-Rupp I, Melton GB. Enterocutaneous fistula: proven strategies and updates. Clin Colon Rectal Surg. 2016;29(2):130–7.
15. Michelassi F, Stella M, Balestracci T, Giuliante F, Marogna P, Block GE. Incidence, diagnosis, and treatment of enteric and colorectal fistulae in patients with Crohn's disease. Ann Surg. 1993;218(5):660–6.
16. Scharl M, Rogler G. Pathophysiology of fistula formation in Crohn's disease. World J Gastrointest Pathophysiol. 2014;5(3):205–12.
17. Evenson AR, Fischer JE. Current management of enterocutaneous fistula. J Gastrointest Surg. 2006;10(3):455–64.
18. Tonolini M, Magistrelli P. Enterocutaneous fistulas: a primer for radiologists with emphasis on CT and MRI. Insights Imaging. 2017;8(6):537–48.
19. Osborn C, Fischer JE. How I do it: gastrointestinal cutaneous fistulas. J Gastrointest Surg. 2009;13(11):2068–73.
20. Kaushal M, Carlson GL. Management of enterocutaneous fistulas. Clin Colon Rectal Surg. 2004;17(2):79–88.
21. Fazio VW, Coutsoftides T, Steiger E. Factors influencing the outcome of treatment of small bowel cutaneous fistula. World J Surg. 1983;7(4):481–8.
22. Hoedema R, Suryadevara S. Enterostomal therapy and wound care of the enterocutaneous fistula patient. Clin Colon Rectal Surg. 2010;23(03):161–8.
23. Epstein JC, Anderson ID. Abdominal sepsis and abdominal compartment syndrome. In: Paterson-Brown SMMMSFFFCSF, Paterson HMBMMDF, editors. Core topics in general and emergency surgery, Elsevier, Amsterdam. 2019. p. 281–94.
24. Complete e. Empirical therapy for sepsis and septic shock from a biliary or gastrointestinal tract source. 2021.
25. Communications R. New Zealand surgeon's work to change patients' lives. Surg News. 2020;22(1):10–2.
26. Committee AT, Bhat YM, Banerjee S, Barth BA, Chauhan SS, Gottlieb KT, et al. Tissue adhesives: cyanoacrylate glue and fibrin sealant. Gastrointest Endosc. 2013;78(2):209–15.
27. Lee SH. Surgical management of enterocutaneous fistula. Korean J Radiol. 2012;13(Suppl 1):S17–20.
28. Alexander RJ, Nash GF. Enterocutaneous fistula stent. Ann R Coll Surg Engl. 2009;91:619–20.
29. Heineman JT, Garcia LJ, Obst MA, Chong HS, Langin JG, Humpal R, et al. Collapsible enteroatmospheric fistula isolation device: a novel, simple solution to a complex problem. J Am Coll Surg. 2015;221(2):e7–14.
30. Subramaniam MH, Liscum KR, Hirshberg A. The floating stoma: a new technique for controlling exposed fistulae in abdominal trauma. J Trauma. 2002;53(2):386–8.
31. Rao M, Burke D, Finan PJ, Sagar PM. The use of vacuum-assisted closure of abdominal wounds: a word of caution. Color Dis. 2007;9(3):266–8.
32. Fischer JE. A cautionary note: the use of vacuum-assisted closure systems in the treatment of gastrointestinal cutaneous fistula may be associated with higher mortality from subsequent fistula development. Am J Surg. 2008;196(1):1–2.
33. Layton B, Dubose J, Nichols S, Connaughton J, Jones T, Pratt J. Pacifying the open abdomen with concomitant intestinal fistula: a novel approach. Am J Surg. 2010;199(4):e48–50.
34. de Weerd L, Kjæve J, Nergård S. The parachute design as a new extraperitoneal method of closing a recalcitrant high-output enterocutaneous fistula: report of a case. Surg Today. 2012;42(7):681–5.
35. Badrasawi M, Shahar S, Sagap I. Nutritional management in enterocutaneous fistula. What is the evidence? Malays J Med Sci. 2015;22(4):6–16.

## Further Reading

Kumpf VJ, de Aguilar-Nascimento JE, Diaz-Pizarro Graf JI, Hall AM, McKeever L, Steiger E, Winkler MF, Compher CW. ASPEN-FELANPE clinical guidelines. J Parenter Enter Nutr. 2017;41:104–12. https://doi.org/10.1177/0148607116680792.

https://www.nice.org.uk/guidance/ipg507/evidence/overview-pdf-497308861

# Complication of Bariatric Surgery

## 92

Doron Kopelman and Uri Kaplan

## 92.1 Introduction

According to the World Health Organization (WHO) report, obesity rates have almost tripled in the last four decades [1]. Obesity has become a significant public health concern and is associated with increased risk to develop chronic diseases such as hypertension, diabetes mellitus, hyperlipidemia, and obstructive sleep apnea. It is also associated with increased morbidity and mortality.

Bariatric surgical procedures have been shown to be the best treatment option for achieving sustained weight loss and improvement in obesity-related comorbidities [2, 3]. In the last 20 years, with the introduction of laparoscopy to bariatric surgery, it has become increasingly popular with short lengths of hospital stay. Nowadays, most bariatric cases are performed in centers of excellence by trained bariatric surgeons as part of multidisciplinary teams. These factors improve significantly the outcome of bariatric surgery.

The introduction of the tourist medical industry along with outpatient cases has led to a short postoperative hospital stay. Patients with postoperative complications arrive to local emergency rooms or clinics where the physician may have limited knowledge in the field of bariatric surgery. The aim of this chapter is to review the most common bariatric procedures, outline the common complications postbariatric procedures, and provide diagnostic tools and treatment options for patients who present to the emergency department.

**Learning Goals**
- At the end of this chapter, you'll be able to describe and define the anatomical changes after common bariatric procedures.
- At the end of this chapter, you'll be able to assess patients with a bariatric surgery complication who arrive to the emergency department.
- At the end of this chapter, you'll be able to identify the common bariatric surgery complications who present to the emergency department and choose the correct initial treatment.

### 92.1.1 Epidemiology

Obesity has become a global epidemic and is a major public health challenge of the twenty-first century. According to the WHO, in 2016, 39% of

D. Kopelman (✉)
Emek Medical Center and the Technion—Israel Institute of Technology, Afula, Israel
e-mail: kopelman_d@clalit.org.il

U. Kaplan
General Surgery B, Emek Medical Center, Afula, Israel

adults (more than 1.9 billion) in the world were overweight (defined as body mass index (BMI) $\geq 25$ kg/m$^2$) and 13% (over 650 million) were obese defined as BMI $\geq 30$ kg/m$^2$) [1]. In 2014, the global prevalence of morbid obesity (BMI $\geq 40$ or BMI $\geq 35$ with at least one obesity related comorbidity) was 0.64% in men and 1.6% in women [4]. There are disparities in the prevalence of obesity across countries. This trend continues within the country among sex, age, ethnic group, and socioeconomic status [5].

The morbidity of commonly performed bariatric procedure is between 5 and 10%. In 5% of them, the complications will happen at home [6]. With that being said, the rate of emergency department (ED) visits of bariatric patients is much higher. The frequency of ED visits within 30 days of surgery is around 11% with readmission rate of 4.4–5.5%. Around 50% of those visits and readmissions occur in hospitals other than the one where the bariatric procedure was performed [7, 8].

## 92.1.2 Etiology

Obesity is a multifactorial disease. It involves social, psychological, and endocrine processes. The complex adipostatic system in our body maintains a constant weight despite energy fluctuations [9]. There are several key organs that balance body energy. The hypothalamus is an important control center. The gastrointestinal tract produces several hormones including ghrelin, glucagon-like peptide-1, and leptin. These hormones exert positive and negative feedback on the hypothalamus promoting hunger or satiety sensation. Psychological and social factors also affect obesity as eating is considered by many as a pleasurable and social activity.

The fact that dieting induces the body to adapt to physiological starvation could be the explanation for the low successful results in the long term [10]. Bariatric surgery success stems from the alteration of physiological processes that maintain weight homeostasis.

Bariatric procedures are classified as either restrictive, reducing the volume of food patients can digest, malabsorptive, reducing the absorption of food at the mucosal level, or both. However, it is reasonable to associate the beneficial influence of surgery on the body adipose system as the key factor for bariatric surgery success [11].

### 92.1.2.1 Types of Bariatric Surgery

The clinical practice guidelines for bariatric surgery are well established [12, 13]. The fifth International Federation for the Surgery of obesity and metabolic disorders (IFSO) global registry report, which was published in 2019, contains data from over 60 countries on over 833,000 operations [14]. The four most common operations worldwide are sleeve gastrectomy (SG) (58.6%), Roux-en-Y gastric bypass (RYGB) (31.2%), Omega anastomosis gastric bypass/Mini gastric bypass (OAGB/MGB) (4.1%) and adjustable gastric band (AGB) (3.7%). Globally, over the last 11 years, there is a trend toward a reduction in gastric banding and RYGB while there is a rise in SG and OAGB/MGB procedures. Nowadays, almost all bariatric procedures are performed laparoscopically (99.1%) [14]. Currently, there is no evidence regarding which operation suits each patient and this is the main reason for many operative options.

### 92.1.2.2 Sleeve Gastrectomy (SG)

The operation was developed as the first stage for duodenal switch operation; however, due to comparable outcomes, it became a stand-alone procedure. Most of the stomach (approximately 70–80%) is excised. The greater curvature of the stomach is denuded from its blood supply from the angle of His to a point 4–6 cm proximal to the pylorus. A bougie, between 34 and 42 French, is inserted along the lesser curvature and using a linear stapler the fundus body and part of the antrum of the stomach is excised, creating a tubular sleeve-like pouch. The excised part of the stomach is removed (Fig. 92.1I). The procedure is safe (mortality rate of 0.1–0.2%) with low complication rate [15, 16].

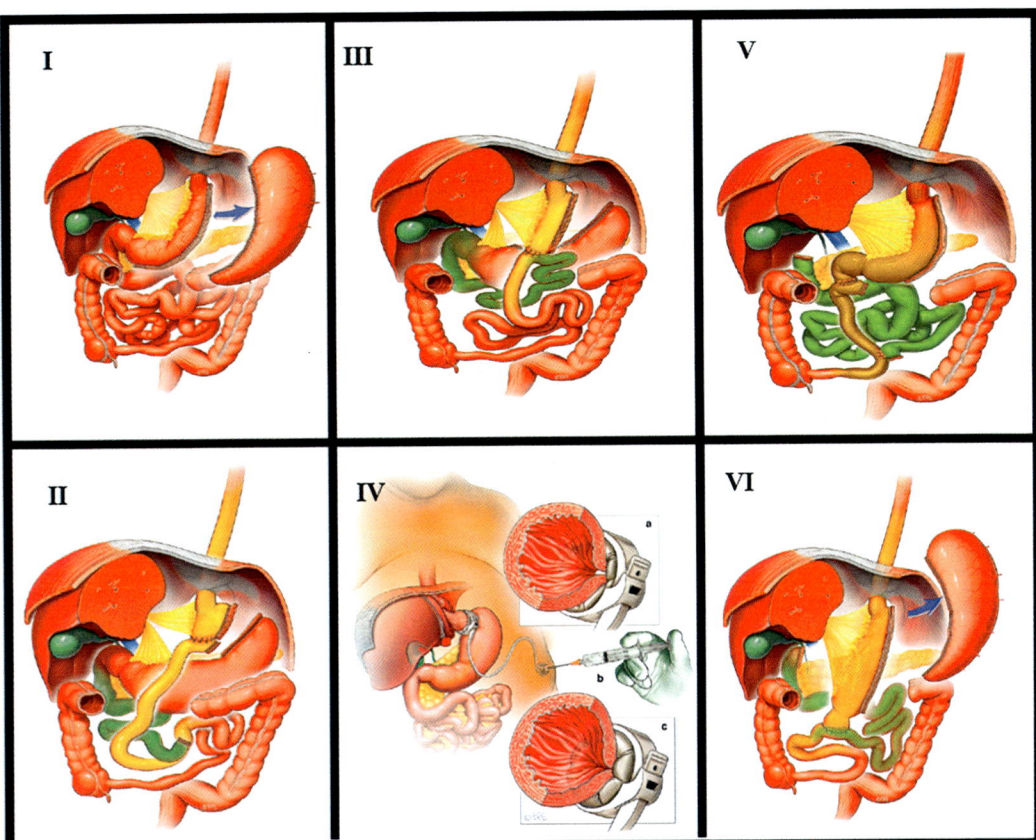

**Fig. 92.1** Common bariatric surgeries: *I*—Sleeve gastrectomy, *II*—Roux-en-Y gastric bypass, *III*—Omega anastomosis gastric bypass/mini gastric bypass, *IV*—Adjustable gastric banding (**a**–deflated band, **b**–subcutaneous port, **c**–inflated band), *V*—Duodenal switch, *VI*—Single anastomosis duodenoileal anastomosis with sleeve gastrectomy (SADI-S). Reprinted with permission from Ramos AC, Carraso HJ, Bastos EL. (2021). Bariatric Procedures: Anatomical and Physiological Changes. Bhaskar AG, Kantharia N, Baig S, Priya P, Lakdawala M, Sancheti MS (Eds). Management of Nutritional and Metabolic Complications of Bariatric Surgery. (pp. 41–50). Springer Nature

### 92.1.2.3 Roux-En-Y Gastric Bypass (RYGB)

The operation is considered the gold standard of bariatric surgery. The procedure involves the creation of a small proximal gastric pouch of approximately 30 mL. The pouch is separated from the rest of the stomach which is left in situ. The small bowel is divided 50–150 cm distal to the duodenojejunal (DJ) flexure. The distal limb of small bowel is anastomosed to the gastric pouch in an antecolic or retrocolic fashion and is called the roux limb. The proximal part, termed biliopancreatic limb (BP limb), is anastomosed 100–150 cm distal to the gastrojejunostomy anastomosis (Fig. 92.1II). The proximal anastomosis is termed gastrojejunostomy (GJ) and the distal anastomosis is called jejunojejunostomy (JJ). Any mesenteric defects are closed. The procedure is safe with slightly higher morbidity and mortality compared to SG with no statistical significance [15, 16].

### 92.1.2.4 Omega Anastomosis Gastric Bypass/Mini Gastric Bypass (OAGB/MGB)

OAGB/MGB is a recent modification of the RYGB. The procedure is easier to perform. It begins with the creation of a long and narrow, sleeve like, proximal gastric pouch, which ends at the area of the gastric incisura. The rest of the stomach is left in situ. The small bowel, approximately 200 cm from the DJ flexure, is anastomosed in an antecolic loop fashion to the gastric pouch (Fig. 92.1III). The procedure is safe with comparable results to the RYGB [17].

#### 92.1.2.5 Adjustable Gastric Banding (AGB)

The band is an inflatable silicone ring connected by a tube to a subcutaneous injection port. The band is located around the angle of His creating a small gastric pouch of around 30 mL. The band lies in the 2-to-8 o'clock position and is usually secured with gastrogastric sutures overlying the fundus to the proximal pouch. Insertion or aspiration of fluid from the band, via the subcutaneous port, adjusts the degree of constriction (Fig. 92.1IV). The procedure is safe with low complication rate [18].

#### 92.1.2.6 Other Bariatric Procedures

Duodenal switch (DS) involves the creation of gastric sleeve followed by the division of the duodenum in its first part. The Ileum is divided 250 cm proximal to the ileocolic valve and is anastomosed to the duodenum in a Roux-en-Y fashion (Fig. 92.1V). Single anastomosis duodenoileostomy (SADI) is similar to DS in terms of the gastric sleeve and duodenum division. However, the ileum is anastomosed to the duodenum in a loop fashion 250–300 cm from ileocolic valve (Fig. 92.1VI). Both procedures are mainly malabsorptive with acceptable safety [19].

### 92.1.3 Classification

The classification of complication postbariatric surgery can be classified according to the type of surgery or initial presentation. Most patients will be evaluated by general surgeons not necessarily experienced in bariatric surgery. For that reason, we chose to use the initial presentation classification. In general, the three main complaints to the emergency department will be bleeding, obstruction, or sepsis. The classification is summarized in Table 92.1.

### 92.1.4 Pathophysiology

Complications postsurgical procedures can be classified to nonsurgical, mainly related to general anesthesia and immobilization and surgical, specific to the procedure itself.

#### 92.1.4.1 Nonsurgical Complications

The nonsurgical complications are similar to other operative procedures and include cardiorespiratory complications, nutritional deficiencies, which are more common in malabsorptive procedures, and cholelithiasis.

Table 92.1 Complication of common bariatric surgeries

| Procedure | Bleeding | Obstruction | Sepsis |
|---|---|---|---|
| Adjustable gastric banding | • Esophagitis | • Band overtight<br>• Band slippage<br>• Band erosion<br>• Port site hernia | • Port/band infection<br>• Esophageal perforation<br>• Gastric perforation |
| Sleeve gastrectomy | • Hemorrhage (intraluminal or intraperitoneal) | • Stricture<br>• Twist<br>• Port site hernia | • Staple line leak |
| Roux-en-Y gastric bypass/omega anastomosis gastric bypass/min gastric bypass | • Hemorrhage (intraluminal or intraperitoneal)<br>• Marginal ulcers | • Internal hernia<br>• Intussusception<br>• Stricture<br>• Port site hernia | • Anastomotic leak<br>• Staple line leak |
| General | • Cardiopulmonary complications (including PE, MI)<br>• Nutritional deficiencies<br>• Cholelithiasis | | |

Cardiorespiratory complications are usually presented with chest pain or discomfort, shortness of breath, and tachycardia. Analysis of death within 30-days of surgery found that cardiac causes account for 28% of death cases and pulmonary embolism for 17% [20]. Bariatric patients are predisposing to thromboembolic events due to numerous factors, including obesity itself, immobility, hypoventilation syndrome, and venous stasis disease. The rate of either deep vein thrombosis or pulmonary embolism up to 30 days postbariatric surgery is 2.2%, with a death rate of 0.03% [21]. Patients with chest pain and SOB should have immediate 12-lead ECG, measurement of myocardial enzymes, and chest X-ray. While massive pulmonary embolism is usually fatal, a low threshold for CT angiogram can contribute to rapid diagnosis.

Nutritional deficiencies are common postbariatric procedures. The most common is anemia due to iron, B12, or folic acid deficiency, abnormalities in bone metabolism and other vitamins and minerals deficiency. Thiamine (B1) deficiency can occur within 8–15 weeks postsurgery and is related to inadequate repletion and persistent vomiting. Acute presentation, such as Wernicke's encephalopathy, can present with nutritional polyneuropathy, ophthalmoparesis, ataxia, and confusion. Early initiation of supplemental therapy can prevent permanent deficits and recovery typically occurs within 3–6 month [22].

Cholelithiasis formation is common after bariatric surgery due to rapid weight loss. The incidence of gallstones formation ranges from 10 to 38%. During rapid weight loss, cholesterol travels from adipose tissue to bile forming high saturation index. This, in turn, encourages the formation of cholesterol crystals that eventually form stones. The progression of asymptomatic cholelithiasis to symptomatic ones is less than 5% and the rate of cholecystectomy after RYGB is 6.8% [23]. Choledocholithiasis is infrequent post-RYGB, with the rate of 0.2–5.3% of cases with cholelithiasis [23]. As in any patient who presents with right upper quadrant abdominal pain, the biliary disease could be the cause for the ED visit.

### 92.1.4.2 Surgical Complications

Surgical complications can be subdivided by the time from surgery (early, within weeks of the primary surgery, or late) or type of surgery. We chose to divide complications according to initial presentation to the emergency department and type of surgery.

### Bleeding

#### General

Although massive bleeding postbariatric surgery is usually diagnosed during the perioperative hospitalization, patient can present with hemorrhagic shock and even exsanguination. The main reasons for bleeding are from staple lines, mesenteric or omental vessels, short gastric vessels, and other iatrogenic injuries. In early postoperative period, port site bleeding should be included in the differential diagnosis. The incidence of postoperative bleeding ranges from 0.5% to 4% [24]. The rate of reoperation due to bleeding ranges from 0.8% to 2.5% of all postoperative bleeding post bariatric surgery [25]. Bleeding can be intraperitoneal or intraluminal. The clinical symptoms are tachycardia, oliguria, decreased consciousness, and decreased hemoglobin (Hb) level. Gastrointestinal (GI) bleeding can also present with vomiting of blood, hematochezia, or melena. Intraperitoneal bleeding presents as abdominal discomfort or abdominal pain, abdominal swelling, and even as peritonitis.

#### Sleeve Gastrectomy

The most common cause of bleeding in patients post-SG is related to the gastric staple line. Erosion at the staple line can cause intraperitoneal or intraluminal bleeding. Bleeding will occur in 0–20% of cases with reoperation in 1.4% of major bleeding [26]. The presentation is usually in the early post-surgery phase. Hematemesis or melena is the common presentation.

#### Roux-En-Y Gastric Bypass and Omega Anastomosis Gastric Bypass/Mini Gastric Bypass

As in SG, the early bleeding post-RYGB or OAGB/MGB results are mainly due to the staple lines. The rate of bleeding post-RYGB is 1–4%. The most common site for bleeding is gastric remnant staple line (40%) followed by GJ (30%) and JJ (30%). Major bleeding in OAGB/MGB occurs in 0.2–28.6% of cases with 0.3–0.58% of these cases necessitate intervention including reoperation [26]. GJ bleeding will present as hematemesis or melena. Remnant stomach and JJ bleeding will usually present as melena. The main cause for late bleeding in patients post RYGB and OAGB/MGB is a bleeding marginal ulcer (MU). MU is an ulcer that develops at the GJ anastomosis, usually at the jejunal side, with multifactorial etiology. The incidence of MU is 0.6–16%, of whom 9.27% will require surgical intervention [27]. Symptoms include heartburn, epigastric pain nausea, and vomiting. Risk factors include nonsteroidal anti-inflammatory medications (NSAIDs) or corticosteroids treatment, nicotine use, and *Helicobacter Pylori* infection.

## Obstruction

### General

Bariatric surgery patients, like any other general surgery patients, can suffer from post-surgery intraabdominal adhesions. The rate of intestinal obstruction due to adhesions in bariatric patients is 13.7% [28]. Bariatric patients are prone to develop incisional hernia due to their excess weight and comorbidities. The rate of port site hernia postbariatric surgery has been reported to be as high as 37% [29]. The rate of symptomatic or incarcerated port site hernia is not well documented and for that reason is unknown. Symptoms include nausea, vomiting, and usually focal abdominal pain around one or more of the surgical scars. Palpating the thick abdominal wall may interfere with early accurate diagnosis.

### Sleeve Gastrectomy

The main reason for obstruction post SG is stricture, usually at the incisura angularis (Fig. 92.2). The common causes for obstruction in the early phase after SG are food intolerance and tissue edema. Twisting or kinking of the gastric sleeve are the main reasons for obstruction after SG. They account for 1.4% of SG surgeries and the average interval for diagnosis is 37 days [30].

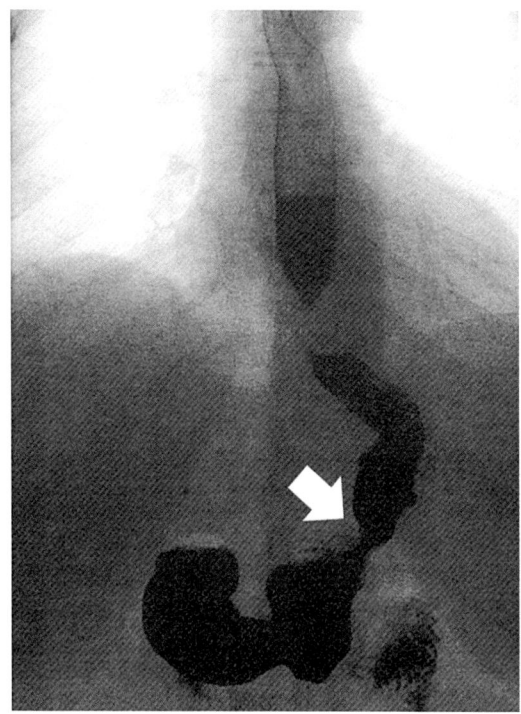

**Fig. 92.2** Upper Gastrointestinal contrast swallow test showing narrowing of the sleeve (white arrow)

### Roux-En-Y Gastric Bypass

Internal hernia (IH) is the most common and dreadful cause of small bowel obstruction after RYGB. It can occur at any time postsurgery but mainly has a late presentation. The incidence ranges from 1% to 5.8%. IH that is not treated surgically have a mortality rate of over 50% [31]. Post Roux-en-Y reconstruction small bowel can pass through new anatomic spaces. This passage can cause twisting, obstruction, and even incarceration of small bowel. Nowadays, most RYGB is performed in an antecolic approach which means there are two anatomic spaces: between the two mesenteries of the small bowel at the area of the JJ anastomosis and between the mesentery of the roux limb and the meso of the transverse colon and the retroperitoneum. The latter is also called Peterson's hernia. In retrocolic approach, a third space is the defect in the mesentery of the transverse colon (Fig. 92.3). The most common site for IH is the JJ mesenteric defect. Patients have intermittent obstruction and usually do not vomit. The episodic abdominal pain usually delays the diagnosis and imaging may also be

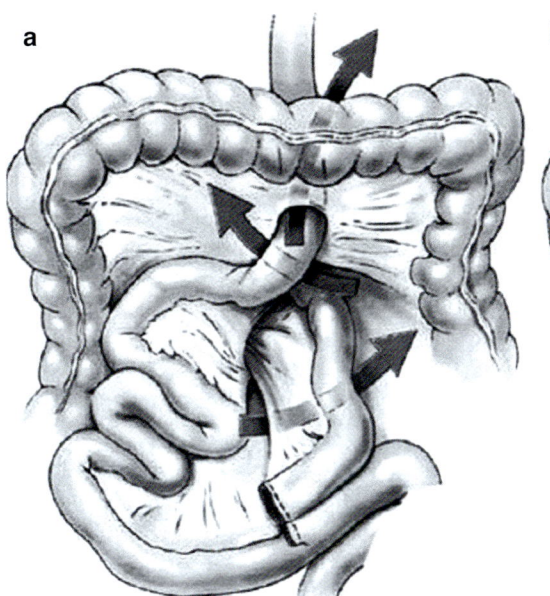 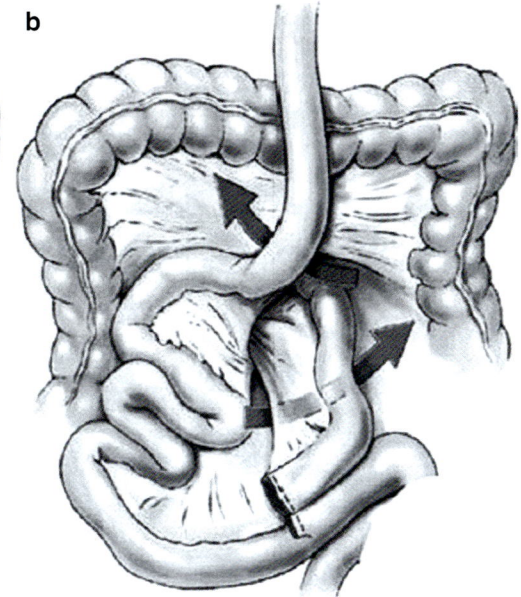

**Fig. 92.3** Mesenteric defects in Roux-en-Y gastric bypass: (**a**) Retrocolic approach creating three defects. (**b**) Antecolic approach creating two defects. Reprinted from Palermo M, Acquafresca PA, Serra E. (2020). Closing the Mesentery Defects. Ettinger J, Azaro E, Weiner R, Higa KD, Neto MG, Teixeira AF, Jawad M (Eds). Gastric Bypass Bariatric and metabolic Surgery Perspectives. (pp. 181–185). Springer Nature

negative. Patients with a suspected diagnosis of internal hernia and negative imaging may need to undergo diagnostic laparoscopy.

Strictures in the GJ anastomosis or JJ anastomosis are the main cause of early obstruction. The causes for GJ stricture are tension and/or ischemia at the anastomosis. The same goes for JJ anastomosis. Blood clots at the JJ can obstruct the anastomosis. Unlike the GJ anastomosis stenosis, which can present more slowly (up to weeks), JJ anastomosis stenosis has a more acute presentation and is more difficult to diagnose, due to the altered anatomy. They present with epigastric pain or discomfort due to gastric remnant distension and even as peritonitis due to gastric remnant perforation.

Other causes for small bowel obstruction include retrograde intussusception at the JJ anastomosis site, adhesions, and incarcerated port site hernia.

### Omega Anastomosis Gastric Bypass/Mini Gastric Bypass

In OAGB/MGB, there is only one anatomic space that can cause IH. The space, which resembles Peterson hernia in RYGB, is between the mesentery of the small bowel loop, the mesentery of the transverse colon, and the retroperitoneum. OAGB/MGB has a lower rate of internal hernia compared to the RYGB [17]. The rate of GJ stricture is low and was reported as high as 0.2% in revisional OAGB/MGB [32].

### Adjustable Gastric Banding

AGB is designed to partially cause obstruction in the cardia of the stomach. As such, patient can present with symptoms that resemble obstruction. With that being said the rate of early obstruction is very low. Late obstruction can be caused by band slippage or overtightening of the band. The mean rate of slippage is 4.93% [33]. Band slippage can involve prolapse of the posterior pouch, anterior pouch, or concentric. Ischemia of the gastric wall is the worst complication of band slippage. It should be considered if symptoms do not respond to percutaneous decompression.

Band erosion into the lumen mean reported rate is 1.46% (0.23–32.65%) [34]. Most cases do not mandate emergency treatment unless the presenting symptom is peritonitis or infection. Most cases will be asymptomatic; however, others can present as loss of restriction, bleeding, port infection, or dysphagia. Proximal migration can cause obstruction of the gastroesophageal junction (GEJ).

## Systemic Inflammatory Response Syndrome (SIRS)/Sepsis

The most common cause for sepsis post-bariatric surgery is gastrointestinal leak. Although early recognition is difficult in morbidly obese patients, prompt diagnosis is crucial and can minimize the risk of developing chronic fistula or progression to septic shock. The etiology of leaks can be divided into technical issues and patients' related issues. The most common presentation is tachycardia, fever, and abdominal pain. The patient will be described as ill-appearing.

Sleeve gastrectomy leak is the most dreadful complication of SG. The rate of gastric leak is 1–3% in primary cases and more than 10% in revision procedures [35]. The most common site is near the GEJ. The main two reasons are ischemia and distal obstruction due to stenosis, twist, or kink at the incisura angularis. Leak should be categorized according to their occurrence time postsurgery; acute—less than 7 days, early—within 1–6 weeks, late—within 6–12 weeks, and chronic—more than 12 weeks [36].

## Roux-En-Y Gastric Bypass and Omega Anastomosis Gastric Bypass/Mini Gastric Bypass

Small bowel leaks post-RYGB and OAGB/MGB are usually diagnosed earlier, within 3 days of surgery. The rate of leak post-RYGB ranged from 0.1 to 5.8% [26]; however, this rate is gradually decreasing and today is around 0.3% [37]. The most common sites for leaks are at the GJ anastomosis. Other sites include gastric remnant staple line, JJ anastomosis, and along the small bowel due to iatrogenic injuries. The rates of leaks post-OAGB/MGB is 0.8–1.6% in primary cases and 4.08% in revisional procedures [26].

Perforated marginal ulcer is another cause for bariatric patients to present with sepsis. The rate of perforated marginal ulcer post-RYGB is 0.83% [38]. The etiology and outcome of this event is not well understood.

## Adjustable Gastric Banding

Esophageal or gastric perforation can present to the emergency department 48 h postsurgery. This complication is rare but should be considered. Infected band due to erosion or port site infection can lead to intra-abdominal abscess and sepsis.

## Abdominal Pain/Discomfort

Abdominal pain is a common complaint for patients postbariatric procedure. Abdominal pain was presented in 21.6% of the bariatric patients who presented to the ED. In 33.4% of these patients, no explanation for the pain was found [39]. The pathologic features that contribute to the pain are divided into surgical, nonsurgical, and psychological or behavioral. These patients usually undergo numerous tests including imaging, endoscopy, and even surgery.

## 92.2 Diagnosis

Most bariatric patients will present with complaints of abdominal pain. Emergency department physician needs to complete the diagnosis based on the patients chief complaint and the procedure they have had. Other abdominal pathologies such as pancreatitis, appendicitis, diverticulitis, nephrolithiasis, and hepatitis should be included in the differential diagnosis.

### 92.2.1 Clinical Presentation

Any patient who arrives to the ED should initially be assessed and stabilized according to ABCs (airway, breathing, and circulation). Initial treatment based on ABCs warrants a special consideration for the obese patient.

#### 92.2.1.1 Airway

Patients may present with inadequate oxygenation due to problems with airway. It is essential to be prepared for difficult airway management due to their habitus and difficulties in landmarks identification. Preparing an adequate airway management strategy is of paramount importance. Placing the patient in ramped position and adequate preoxygenation is always imperative and apneic oxygenation, using high flow nasal cannula, should be considered [40].

### 92.2.1.2 Breathing
Tachypnea can present as an indicator for pulmonary or cardiac disease; however, it may be an indicator for a systemic acidotic process. Obese patients have reduced functional residual capacity and as a result suffer from limited oxygen reserve [40]. Calculation of tidal volume during mechanical ventilation should be based on ideal body weight and not actual weight.

### 92.2.1.3 Circulation
Tachycardia in obese patients should be taken seriously as it can serve as a clue for underlying pathology [41]. It can indicate hypovolemia due to dehydration or bleeding and it can also be the presenting symptom of pulmonary embolus or anastomotic leak. Hypotension is usually a sign of hypovolemia, due to bleeding, dehydration, or sepsis. Resuscitation should be initiated with IV crystalloid solution in case of hypovolemia or packed red blood cell transfusion in case of active GI bleeding.

### 92.2.1.4 History
Abdominal pain is the most common principal diagnosis associated with ED visits followed by metabolic disorders and infection [8], whereas abdominal pain, nausea/vomiting, and dehydration are the main symptoms associated with ED visits. A focused history can help narrow the differential diagnosis. Initial assessment should be in the search for evidence of obstruction, GI bleeding, or infection/sepsis. A meticulous question regarding the nature of the pain can assist the diagnosis. Epigastric pain can indicate GEJ or GJ anastomosis pathology whereas dull or nonspecific pain could indicate small bowel pathology. Hematemesis, melena, or hematochezia are obvious sign of GI bleeding but can be seen in GI perforation as well. Particular importance should be given to the bariatric procedure itself. Type and time since surgery could give clues regarding the diagnosis. Surgical report is the preferable method; however, surgery that was performed in foreign country or long interval time since surgery could make it difficult to know which procedure the patient had. Medical history including underlying comorbidities, which can alter the initial treatment, as well as current medication and recent medication withhold should be sought.

### 92.2.1.5 Physical Examination
Abdominal examination could be misleading in the obese patient. The wide distance between the skin and abdominal wall muscles can make it harder to identify signs of peritonitis. Signs of wound infection or localized pain should be sought. Focal tenderness, guarding, and rebound will be difficult to elicit. A benign abdominal examination should not give a false assumption that abdominal pathology is not present.

## 92.2.2 Tests

### 92.2.2.1 Laboratory Tests
Initial tests should include complete blood cell count, renal and liver function, lipase, blood gases, and CRP. In case of suspected cardiac ischemia troponin level should be obtained. Elevated liver enzymes could be seen in gallbladder and bile ducts diseases or obstruction of the biliopancreatic limb along with elevated lipase. Lactic acidosis can be found in bowel ischemia or sepsis. Blood cultures should be taken in any patients with suspected sepsis or fever. Type and crossed blood products should be prepared in bleeding patients.

### 92.2.2.2 Imaging Studies

**X-Ray**
During the early postoperative period, chest X-ray can help in the diagnosis of patients with dyspnea. Atelectasis, pleural effusion, and pneumonia can easily be seen. Free air under the dia-

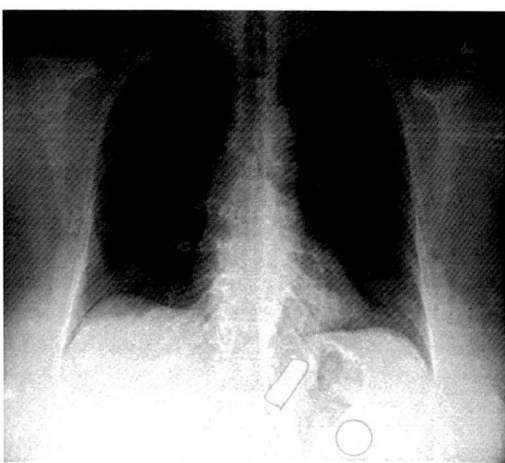

**Fig. 92.4** X-ray study showing a normally positioned gastric band at approximately 45° to the spine. The band and port are outlined in gray line

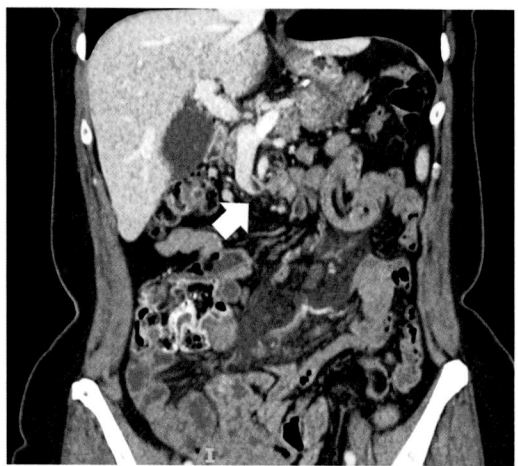

**Fig. 92.5** CT scan image shows superior mesenteric vein beaking sign. Internal hernia was diagnosed in this post-RYGB patient during a diagnostic laparoscopy

phragm, in case of bowel perforation, can be seen in patients with severe abdominal pain who are unstable. Plain X-ray can determine the position of a gastric band. The correct position should be in 1–2 to 7–8 position as seen in Fig. 92.4. Other positions of the band may indicate slippage of the band.

## Upper Gastrointestinal Contrast Swallow Test

Upper gastrointestinal contrast swallow test is used to diagnose obstruction due to band slippage or prolapse. It can be helpful in the diagnosis of stenosis at the GJ anastomosis or in the gastric tube after SG. Contrast swallow study may help in the diagnosis of leaks at the area of anastomosis or along staple lines; however, the low sensitivity (22–75%) and the high availability of computed tomography in the ED made its use scarce.

### 92.2.2.3 Computed Tomography (CT)

CT is the main diagnostic tool in the assessment of bariatric patient at the ED and should be considered in the early assessment of patients with signs of obstruction or sepsis. In clinically stable patients with suspected bariatric surgery complication, CT of the abdomen and pelvis with intravenous and small amount of oral contrast has higher sensitivity and specificity than contrast swallow study in identifying leak along with the ability to identify abscess, internal hernia, and other pathologies [42]. The addition of the chest to the study can help in ruling out PE or other pulmonary complications. CT detects leaks in the GJ anastomosis or in SG in 60–80% of the cases [43].

CT has a major role in the diagnosis of internal hernia (IH), which is one of the most difficult pathologies to identify. There are several signs of internal hernia in CT exam including swirled mesentery, small bowel obstruction (SBO) hurricane eye, and, superior mesenteric vein (SMV) beaking, as seen in Fig. 92.5. The overall accuracy and sensitivity for the diagnosis of IH were mesenteric swirl and SBO; however, SMV beaking with SBO had the highest specificity [44]. In case of clinical suspicion, a negative CT study does not rule out the diagnosis and surgery should be considered.

### 92.2.2.4 Endoscopy

Endoscopy is the modality of choice in the diagnosis and treatment of bleeding complications. It can diagnose MU and treat active bleeding. Band erosion is easily diagnosed during endoscopy and, in certain conditions, can be treated by endoscopy. Stricture, leaks, and fistula can also be diagnosed and treated [45]. Most cases of GI bleeding necessitate early endoscopic intervention. Endoscopy is the modality of choice in the diagnosis of band erosion. The decision regarding the use of endoscopy during the diagnosis and treatment of other complications mandates a consultation between the surgeon and the gastroenterologist.

### 92.2.2.5 Ultrasound (US)

The use of US in the bariatric patient is questionable due to their habitus. However, patients with suspected gallbladder disease may benefit from a US exam.

> **Differential Diagnosis**
> The differential diagnosis should be assessed according to the presenting symptoms and type of procedure the patient had (Table 92.1).

## 92.3 Treatment

### 92.3.1 Medical Treatment

Initial treatment should start with a rapid assessment of hemodynamic stability. Most patients will require IV crystalloid fluids. Anti-emetic and PPI medications should be considered. Urgent surgical consults should be ordered in unstable patients post- bariatric surgery. The decision regarding explorative laparotomy vs. laparoscopy will be decided based on surgeon's experience and preference.

Table 92.1 summarizes the treatment for common bariatric surgery complications.

#### 92.3.1.1 Bleeding

The treatment of patients, who present with GI bleeding, should include the initiation of IV PPI medication and preparation of type and crossed blood products. Anti-dote for anticoagulation treatment should be considered based on hemodynamic status and type of procedure planned. Upper endoscopy for diagnosis and treatment should be ordered in patients with intraluminal bleeding. Esophagitis or gastritis can be treated conservatively. Most MU will be treated with PPI, sucralfate, and treating causative factors. The most common indication for surgical solution includes perforation, bleeding, gastrogastric fistula, and refractory disease.

#### 92.3.1.2 Obstruction

Patients with obstructive symptoms are usually dehydrated. The initial treatment should include IV fluids, electrolyte supplementations, and urinary output monitoring. Endoscopy is used for the final diagnosis and treatment in case of stenosis after SG or at the GJ anastomosis. Dilatation is performed with gradual pneumatic balloon dilatation. Multiple sessions are usually required. IH is treated surgically. Any patient with suspected IH should have immediate surgical consultation.

Slipped or overinflated gastric band can be treated by deflation of the band. Band deflation should be performed under strict aseptic conditions by any general surgeon. Port site can be difficult to palpate but usually the patient knows the exact place. A noncoring needle, Huber needle, is preferably used; however, any needle can be used. The port should be held firmly between the thumb and index finger of the nondominant hand and the needle should be inserted at the dome of the port until it touches the metallic base of the port. After complete aspiration of the fluid, immediate resolution of symptoms should be noted. Patient with complete resolution should be sent to his bariatric surgeon. If symptoms do not resolve, surgical exploration is warranted.

#### 92.3.1.3 Systemic Inflammatory Response Syndrome (SIRS)/ Sepsis

The treatment of staple line leak is challenging. After blood cultures, broad-spectrum IV antibiotics, covering gram-negative, anaerobic, and gram-positive in case of wound complication, should be initiated. Patients who are ill-appearing or hemodynamic unstable should have an emergent surgical consult. While "contained cause" (e.g., abscess, contained leak) can be treated conservatively, patients with signs of peritonitis warrant prompt surgical intervention. Initial treatment of leaks includes no oral intake (NPO),

IV fluids, PPI, and parenteral nutrition. Percutaneous drainage of collection should be made by interventional radiology (IR). Surgical consultation, as well as contacting the bariatric surgeon is warranted. Other treatment options include stenting, double pig tail drain inserted endoscopically, glue and surgical washout and drainage. In proximal leaks after SG, conservative treatment should last at least 12 weeks before reoperation is considered [36].

### 92.3.2 Surgical Treatment

Patients with a bariatric surgery complication and signs of peritonitis or unstable patients should have emergent surgical consultation for prompt surgical intervention. The decision on laparoscopic or open intervention is decided based on surgeon experience. If the patient is stable, transfer to an experienced bariatric center is recommended due to the availability of surgical experience and supporting multidisciplinary team.

Surgical intervention for bleeding MU who failed endoscopic treatment can include suture of the ulcer with absorbable sutures under endoscopic surveillance, longitudinal enterotomy with suture of the ulcer bed followed by transverse closure of the enterotomy or redo of the GJ anastomosis. The recurrence rate of MU after surgical intervention is 24% after 12 months [27]. The treatment for perforated MU includes primary suture or omental Graham patch with or without gastrostomy to the remnant stomach. Redo of the GJ anastomosis is another surgical option.

Acute SG leak can be treated with surgical irrigation and drainage of the staple line. Resuture is an option if the patient is no longer than postoperative day 3 and the tissue is not friable. Surgical treatment, post failed conservative treatment, can include total gastrectomy with Roux-en-Y esophagojejunostomy or Roux-en-Y fistulojejunostomy.

Obstruction at the JJ warrants surgical treatment. CT scan can help in identifying the precise location—at the BP limb, Roux limb, or both. It can also identify whether the cause is blood clot or not. In the case of blood clot, enterotomy with clot removal is an option, whereas JJ anastomosis stenosis warrants redo the stenotic part or resection of the JJ with the reconstruction of a new JJ anastomosis.

The treatment for IH is emergent surgical exploration. In most cases, the bowel in Peterson's hernia traverse from left to right and in the case of mesenteric hernia at the area of JJ anastomosis from right to left. Running the small bowel from the ileocecal valve to the DJ flexure can help with orientation during surgery. During surgery, after returning the bowel to its anatomic place, the mesenteric defects are closed with non-absorbable sutures.

Acute band slippage that does not respond to percutaneous band deflation is an indication for urgent surgical intervention. Laparoscopic band removal is usually the treatment of choice. After lysis of adhesions, the band is unclipped or cut and removed. Special attention should be made to divide the band capsule in order to relieve the obstruction symptoms. Percutaneous removal of the port and connecting tube end the procedure. Band erosion is usually not treated operatively unless the presenting symptoms are peritonitis or infection. Band erosion above 50% of its circumference can be treated endoscopically. Subcutaneous removal of the port before the procedure is mandatory. In case of peritonitis or infection, the treatment of choice is laparoscopic removal of the eroded band, repair of gastric the wall and drainage.

### 92.3.3 Prognosis

Bariatric procedures are considered safe. The mortality rate ranges from 0.03% to 0.2% and is constantly decreasing in the last 20 years. The 30 days serious adverse events rate is less than 6%. Rate of early reoperation and readmission is 0.5–3% and 2.8–4.8% for SG, respectively, and 0.7–5% and 4.7–6.5% for RYGB [46]. Long-term studies found that the rate of reoperations or reinterventions ranges from 5% to 22.1% [46].

## Dos and Don'ts

- Early assessment of vital signs in order to decide hemodynamic stability.
- Meticulous medical history, including obesity related comorbidities, could enlighten the cause for ED referral.
- Accurate surgical history and especially the precise bariatric procedure are of utmost importance in order to anticipate the related surgical complications.
- Don't let normal abdominal examination fool you.
- Normal CT scan does not rule out internal hernia.
- Assess nutritional deficiencies in post-bariatric surgery patients who present with gait or neurological abnormalities.

## Take-Home Messages

- Bariatric surgery is a safe procedure
- Tachycardia in postbariatric surgery patients is an alarming sign.
- Normal abdominal exam does not rule out an abdominal catastrophe.
- Know the anatomy of bariatric procedures.
- For bariatric patient with nonspecific abdominal pain, CT scan should be used to rule out internal hernia or other related complications.

**Algorithm 92.1: Emergency Department Assessment and Treatment for Patient with Bariatric Surgery Complications**

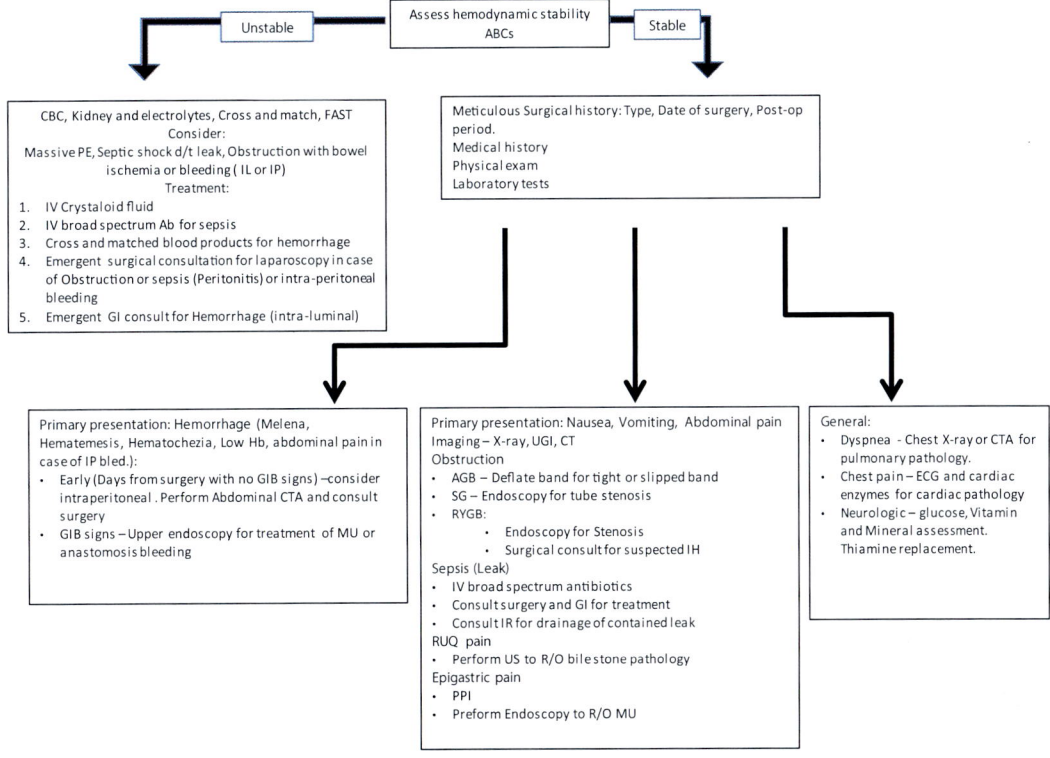

*ABC* airway, breathing, circulation, *CBC* complete blood count, *FAST* focal assessment sonography for trauma, *IL* intraluminal, *IP* intraperitoneal, *Hb* hemoglobin, *GIB* gastrointestinal bleeding, *CTA* computed tomography angiogram, *MU* marginal ulcer, *UGI* upper gastrointestinal contrast study, *US* ultrasound, *PPI* proton pump inhibitors, *ECG* electrocardiogram, *AGB* adjustable gastric banding, *SG* sleeve gastrectomy, *RYGB* Roux-en-Y gastric bypass

**Chapter's Questions**

1. A 55 y/o male with a history of hypertension, diabetes mellitus, and hypercholesteremia had laparoscopic Roux-en-Y gastric bypass 2 weeks ago, present to the ED with chest pain and shortness of breath started 20 min ago. The patient is diaphoretic with the vital sign of 100/60, 65 b/m and saturation of 95%. What is the next step in assessment of the patient?
   A. Order laboratory tests.
   B. Order abdominal CT.
   C. **Perform ECG to R/O cardiac pathology.**
   D. Order consult for emergency endoscopy.

2. A 45 y/o female had laparoscopic adjustable gastric banding 4 months ago. Present to the ED with symptoms of nausea and vomiting started 4 h ago. She had a normal postoperative period. What is the best next step in the assessment of the patient?
   A. **Abdominal X-ray.**
   B. Abdominal CT.
   C. Endoscopy.
   D. Consult surgery for diagnostic laparoscopy.

3. A 47 y/o male had laparoscopic Rouxen-Y 2 years ago. Present with a history of 4 months of intermittent periumbilical abdominal pain. Abdomen is soft and not tender. Laboratory tests are normal. She had an upper endoscopy last month that was normal. Abdominal US was negative for bile stones and CT of the abdomen is normal. This is her third ED referral. What is the best treatment option for him?
   A. D/C home with pain medication prescription.
   B. Consult psychiatry.
   C. **Consult bariatric surgeon for diagnostic laparoscopy.**
   D. Offer laparoscopic cholecystectomy.

4. A patient 35 y/o arrive to ED 10 days post-RYGB with 2 days of shortness in breath. Vital sign: tachycardia of 110 b/m and dyspnea of 20 b/m. Abdominal exam is normal. Lab is normal. What would be the best next test?
   A. Upper GI contrast study.
   B. D/C home.
   C. **CTA of chest.**
   D. Upper endoscopy.

5. A patient 42 y/o arrive to the ED 4 days postlaparoscopic sleeve gastrectomy with symptoms of nausea, vomiting, and fever of 38.5° in the last 24 h. Abdominal exam is normal except for mild LUQ pain. WBC—12 K. Electrolytes, liver panel, and amylase are normal. Chest X-ray is normal and upper GI contrast study is normal. What is the best next diagnostic study?
   A. Abdominal US.
   B. Upper endoscopy.
   C. **Abdominal CT.**
   D. Diagnostic laparoscopy.

6. What CT finding has the best specificity for the diagnosis of internal hernia?
   A. Swirled mesentery and small bowel obstruction.
   B. **Superior mesenteric vein beaking and small bowel obstruction.**
   C. Hurricane eye and swirled mesentery.
   D. Hurricane eye and small bowel obstruction.

7. A patient 35 y/o woman arrives to ED with a complaint of fatigue and epigastric pain. She had laparoscopic Rouxen-Y 2 years ago. She mentions black stool in the last 2 days. Her abdomen is soft with mild epigastric pain. Her hemoglobin level is 10 g/dL. What would be the best next diagnostic test?
   A. Abdominal X-ray.
   B. Abdominal US.
   C. Upper GI contrast study.
   D. **Upper endoscopy.**

8. A 35 y/o male arrives to the emergency ED with severe abdominal pain that started 2 h ago. He had laparoscopic adjustable gastric banding 1 day ago. His abdomen is tender with signs of peritonitis. WBC—15 K. Chest X-ray shows small amount of free air. What is the best next treatment option?
   A. **Perform emergent diagnostic laparoscopy.**
   B. Order emergent upper endoscopy.
   C. Admit for further evaluation.
   D. Order CT scan.
9. A 55 y/o male arrives to the ED with his family due to multiple falls in the last days. He suffers from nausea and vomiting for the last 2 months. He had omega anastomosis gastric bypass/mini gastric bypass 4 months ago. Abdominal exam is normal. Glucose level is normal. What is the best next treatment?
   A. CT abdomen.
   B. **Give IV thiamine (B1).**
   C. Upper endoscopy.
   D. IV broad-spectrum antibiotics.
10. A 25 y/o male arrives to ED with 2 days history of abdominal pain that started in the epigastrium and now shifted to RLQ. His abdomen is soft except for mild tenderness in RLQ. He had a laparoscopic Roux-en-Y gastric bypass 1 year ago. WBC-13 K, the rest of laboratory tests is normal. What is the best next diagnostic test?
    A. **Lower abdomen US.**
    B. CT chest-abdomen.
    C. Pain medication and d/c home.
    D. US of upper abdomen.

# References

1. World Health Organiztion. Obesity and overweight fact sheet. 2020. http://www.who.int/news-room/fact-sheets/detail/obesity-and-overweight. Accessed 13 March 2021.
2. Buchwald H, Avidor Y, Braunwald E, et al. Bariatric surgery: a systematic review and meta-analysis. JAMA. 2004;292(14):1724–37.
3. Colquitt JL, Pickett K, Loveman E, Frampton GK. Surgery for weight loss in adults. Cochrane Database Syst Rev. 2014;8:CD003641.
4. Meisinger C, Ezzati M, Di Cesare M. Trends in adult body-mass index in 200 countries from 1975 to 2014: a pooled analysis of 1698 population-based measurement studies with 19.2 million participants. Lancet. 2016;387(10026):1377–96.
5. McLaren L. Socioeconomic status and obesity. Epidemiol Rev. 2007;29(1):29–48.
6. Bradley JF III, Ross SW, Christmas AB, et al. Complications of bariatric surgery: the acute care surgeon's experience. Am J Surg. 2015;210(3):456–61.
7. Telem DA, Yang J, Altieri M, et al. Rates and risk factors for unplanned emergency department utilization and hospital readmission following bariatric surgery. Ann Surg. 2016;263(5):956–60.
8. Mora-Pinzon MC, Henkel D, Miller RE, et al. Emergency department visits and readmissions within 1 year of bariatric surgery: a statewide analysis using hospital discharge records. Surgery. 2017;162(5):1155–62.
9. Tadross JA, Le Roux CW. The mechanisms of weight loss after bariatric surgery. Int J Obes. 2009;33(1):S28–32.
10. Fildes A, Charlton J, Rudisill C, Littlejohns P, Prevost AT, Gulliford MC. Probability of an obese person attaining normal body weight: cohort study using electronic health records. Am J Public Health. 2015;105(9):e54–9.
11. Miras AD, Le Roux CW. Mechanisms underlying weight loss after bariatric surgery. Nat Rev Gastroenterol Hepatol. 2013;10(10):575.
12. Mechanick JI, Youdim A, Jones DB, et al. Clinical practice guidelines for the perioperative nutritional, metabolic, and nonsurgical support of the bariatric surgery patient2013 update: cosponsored by American Association of Clinical Endocrinologists, The Obesity Society, and American Society for Metabolic & Bariatric Surgery. Endocr Pract. 2013;19(2):337–72.
13. Di Lorenzo N, Antoniou SA, Batterham RL, et al. Clinical practice guidelines of the European Association for Endoscopic Surgery (EAES) on bariatric surgery: update 2020 endorsed by IFSO-EC, EASO and ESPCOP. Surg Endosc. 2020;34(6):2332–58.
14. Ramos A, Kow L, Brown W, et al. 5th IFSO global registry report. Int Fed Surg Obes Metab Disord. 2019;29(3):782–95.
15. Kumar SB, Hamilton BC, Wood SG, Rogers SJ, Carter JT, Lin MY. Is laparoscopic sleeve gastrectomy safer than laparoscopic gastric bypass? A comparison of 30-day complications using the MBSAQIP data registry. Surg Obes Relat Dis. 2018;14(3):264–9.
16. Peterli R, Wölnerhanssen BK, Peters T, et al. Effect of laparoscopic sleeve gastrectomy vs laparoscopic Roux-en-Y gastric bypass on weight loss in patients with morbid obesity: the SM-BOSS randomized clinical trial. JAMA. 2018;319(3):255–65.

17. Magouliotis DE, Tasiopoulou VS, Tzovaras G. One anastomosis gastric bypass versus Roux-en-Y gastric bypass for morbid obesity: an updated meta-analysis. Obes Surg. 2019;29(9):2721–30.
18. O'Brien PE, Hindle A, Brennan L, et al. Long-term outcomes after bariatric surgery: a systematic review and meta-analysis of weight loss at 10 or more years for all bariatric procedures and a single-centre review of 20-year outcomes after adjustable gastric banding. Obes Surg. 2019;29(1):3–14.
19. Moon RC, Kirkpatrick V, Gaskins L, Teixeira AF, Jawad MA. Safety and effectiveness of single-versus double-anastomosis duodenal switch at a single institution. Surg Obes Relat Dis. 2019;15(2):245–52.
20. Smith MD, Patterson E, Wahed AS, et al. Thirty-day mortality after bariatric surgery: independently adjudicated causes of death in the longitudinal assessment of bariatric surgery. Obes Surg. 2011;21(11):1687–92.
21. Stein PD, Matta F. Pulmonary embolism and deep venous thrombosis following bariatric surgery. Obes Surg. 2013;23(5):663–8.
22. Becker DA, Balcer LJ, Galetta SL. The neurological complications of nutritional deficiency following bariatric surgery. J Obes. 2012;2012:608534.
23. Leyva-Alvizo A, Arredondo-Saldaña G, Leal-Isla-Flores V, et al. Systematic review of management of gallbladder disease in patients undergoing minimally invasive bariatric surgery. Surg Obes Relat Dis. 2020;16(1):158–64.
24. Kitahama S, Smith MD, Rosencrantz DR, Patterson EJ. Is bariatric surgery safe in patients who refuse blood transfusion? Surg Obes Relat Dis. 2013;9(3):390–4.
25. Augustin T, Aminian A, Romero-Talamás H, Rogula T, Schauer PR, Brethauer SA. Reoperative surgery for management of early complications after gastric bypass. Obes Surg. 2016;26(2):345–9.
26. Silecchia G, Iossa A. Complications of staple line and anastomoses following laparoscopic bariatric surgery. Ann Gastroenterol. 2018;31(1):56.
27. Pyke O, Yang J, Cohn T, et al. Marginal ulcer continues to be a major source of morbidity over time following gastric bypass. Surg Endosc. 2019;33(10):3451–6.
28. Husain S, Ahmed AR, Johnson J, Boss T, O'Malley W. Small-bowel obstruction after laparoscopic Roux-en-Y gastric bypass: etiology, diagnosis, and management. Arch Surg. 2007;142(10):988–93.
29. Karampinis I, Lion E, Hetjens S, et al. Trocar site HERnias after bariatric laparoscopic surgery (HERBALS): a prospective cohort study. Obes Surg. 2020;1–7.
30. Rebibo L, Hakim S, Dhahri A, Yzet T, Delcenserie R, Regimbeau J-M. Gastric stenosis after laparoscopic sleeve gastrectomy: diagnosis and management. Obes Surg. 2016;26(5):995–1001.
31. Martin LC, Merkle EM, Thompson WM. Review of internal hernias: radiographic and clinical findings. Am J Roentgenol. 2006;186(3):703–17.
32. Kermansaravi M, Shahmiri SS, DavarpanahJazi AH, et al. One anastomosis/mini-gastric bypass (OAGB/MGB) as revisional surgery following primary restrictive bariatric procedures: a systematic review and meta-analysis. Obes Surg. 2020:1–14.
33. Singhal R, Bryant C, Kitchen M, et al. Band slippage and erosion after laparoscopic gastric banding: a meta-analysis. Surg Endosc. 2010;24(12):2980–6.
34. Egberts K, Brown WA, O'Brien PE. Systematic review of erosion after laparoscopic adjustable gastric banding. Obes Surg. 2011;21(8):1272–9.
35. Abou Rached A, Basile M, El Masri H. Gastric leaks post sleeve gastrectomy: review of its prevention and management. World J Gastroenterol WJG. 2014;20(38):13904.
36. Rosenthal RJ, Panel ISGE. International sleeve gastrectomy expert panel consensus statement: best practice guidelines based on experience of> 12,000 cases. Surg Obes Relat Dis. 2012;8(1):8–19.
37. Vidarsson B, Sundbom M, Edholm D. Incidence and treatment of small bowel leak after Roux-en-Y gastric bypass: a cohort study from the Scandinavian obesity surgery registry. Surg Obes Relat Dis. 2020;16(8):1005–10.
38. Altieri MS, Pryor A, Yang J, et al. The natural history of perforated marginal ulcers after gastric bypass surgery. Surg Endosc. 2018;32(3):1215–22.
39. Pierik AS, Coblijn UK, de Raaff CAL, van Veen RN, van Tets WF, van Wagensveld BA. Unexplained abdominal pain in morbidly obese patients after bariatric surgery. Surg Obes Relat Dis. 2017;13(10):1743–51.
40. Aceto P, Perilli V, Modesti C, Ciocchetti P, Vitale F, Sollazzi L. Airway management in obese patients. Surg Obes Relat Dis. 2013;9(5):809–15.
41. Kassir R, Debs T, Blanc P, et al. Complications of bariatric surgery: presentation and emergency management. Int J Surg. 2016;27:77–81.
42. Kim J, Azagury D, Eisenberg D, DeMaria E, Campos GM. ASMBS position statement on prevention, detection, and treatment of gastrointestinal leak after gastric bypass and sleeve gastrectomy, including the roles of imaging, surgical exploration, and nonoperative management. Surg Obes Relat Dis. 2015;11(4):739–48.
43. Lim R, Beekley A, Johnson DC, Davis KA. Early and late complications of bariatric operation. Trauma Surg Acute Care Open. 2018;3(1):e000219.
44. Dilauro M, McInnes MDF, Schieda N, et al. Internal hernia after laparoscopic Roux-en-Y gastric bypass: optimal CT signs for diagnosis and clinical decision making. Radiology. 2017;282(3):752–60.
45. Joo MK. Endoscopic approach for major complications of bariatric surgery. Clin Endosc. 2017;50(1):31.
46. Arterburn DE, Telem DA, Kushner RF, Courcoulas AP. Benefits and risks of bariatric surgery in adults: a review. JAMA. 2020;324(9):879–87.

## Further Reading

Colquitt JL, et al. Surgery for weight loss in adults. Cochrane Database Syst Rev. 2014:8.

Mechanick JI, et al. Clinical practice guidelines for the perioperative nutritional, metabolic, and nonsurgical support of the bariatric surgery patient2013 update: cosponsored by American Association of Clinical Endocrinologists, The Obesity Society, and American Society for Metabolic & Bariatric Surgery. Endocr Pract. 2013;19(2):337–72.

Di Lorenzo N, et al. Clinical practice guidelines of the European Association for Endoscopic Surgery (EAES) on bariatric surgery: update 2020 endorsed by IFSO-EC, EASO and ESPCOP. Surg Endosc. 2020;34(6):2332–58.

Magouliotis DE, Tasiopoulou VS, Tzovaras G. One anastomosis gastric bypass versus Roux-en-Y gastric bypass for morbid obesity: an updated meta-analysis. Obes Surg. 2019;29(9):2721–30.

Kim J, et al. ASMBS position statement on prevention, detection, and treatment of gastrointestinal leak after gastric bypass and sleeve gastrectomy, including the roles of imaging, surgical exploration, and nonoperative management. Surg Obes Relat Dis. 2015;11(4):739–48.

Arterburn DE, et al. Benefits and risks of bariatric surgery in adults: a review. JAMA. 2020;324(9):879–87.

# 93

# Intra-Abdominal Hypertension and Abdominal Compartment Syndrome

Tyler Lamb, Andrew W. Kirkpatrick, and Derek J. Roberts

**Learning Goals**
- Understand the pathophysiology, presentation, and diagnosis of intra-abdominal hypertension (IAH) and abdominal compartment syndrome (ACS).
- Describe the medical, interventional, and surgical management of IAH/ACS.
- Understand evidence-informed approaches to open abdominal management, temporary abdominal closure, and fascia-to-fascia closure of the open abdomen after decompressive laparotomy.

## 93.1 Introduction

Intra-abdominal hypertension (IAH) is commonly encountered in critically ill or injured patients, has repeatedly been reported to be an independent risk factor for in-hospital mortality, and may progress to development of abdominal compartment syndrome (ACS) [1, 2]. ACS may result in cardiac, respiratory, renal, hepatic, and neurologic dysfunction or failure. Despite this, surveys suggest that as few as 60% of physicians working in intensive care units (ICUs) are aware of relevant IAH and ACS definitions and clinical practice guidelines, and as many as 18% never measure intra-abdominal pressure (IAP) in critically ill patients [3]. This chapter reviews the classification, epidemiology, pathophysiology, presentation, diagnosis, and medical, interventional, and surgical management of IAH/ACS. We also highlight the consensus definitions, recommendations, and suggestions published in the most recent clinical practice guideline by the WSACS—The Abdominal Compartment Society.

T. Lamb
Division of General Surgery, Department of Surgery, University of Ottawa, Ottawa, ON, Canada

The Ottawa Hospital, Civic Campus, Ottawa, ON, Canada
e-mail: tlamb@toh.ca

A. W. Kirkpatrick
Departments of Surgery and Critical Care Medicine and the Regional Trauma Program, University of Calgary, Calgary, AB, Canada

Foothills Medical Centre, Calgary, AB, Canada
e-mail: andrew.kirkpatrick@albertahealthservices.ca

D. J. Roberts (✉)
The Ottawa Hospital, Civic Campus, Ottawa, ON, Canada

Division of Vascular and Endovascular Surgery, Department of Surgery, School of Epidemiology and Public Health, University of Ottawa, Ottawa, ON, Canada

Clinical Epidemiology Program, The Ottawa Hospital Trauma Program and the Ottawa Hospital Research Institute, Ottawa, ON, Canada

The O'Brien Institute for Public Health, University of Calgary, Calgary, AB, Canada

### 93.1.1 History of IAH and ACS

Clinical research investigating IAH/ACS dates back to the nineteenth century, when an inverse relationship was observed between rectal IAP and urine output [2, 4, 5]. From the late nineteenth century through the twentieth century, numerous experimental and clinical observations were subsequently made regarding the various systemic effects of increased IAP. This translated to surgical recommendations such as performing repair of omphaloceles in two stages and opting for delayed abdominal closure to prevent "acute tension pneumoperitoneum" in some cases [2, 5, 6]. Finally, the term "intra-abdominal compartment syndrome" was first used to describe a series of patients with decreased urine output, increased respiratory pressure, and significant abdominal distention following massive fluid resuscitation during and after surgical repair of ruptured abdominal aortic aneurysms (AAAs) [2, 5, 7].

The establishment of the World Society of the Abdominal Compartment Syndrome (WSACS) in 2004, which has since been renamed the WSACS—The Abdominal Compartment Society (WSACS), was a major milestone in the history of the study of IAH and ACS. This group sought to "promote research, foster education, and improve the survival of patients with IAH and ACS" at a time where there was substantial heterogeneity regarding definitions of IAH and ACS, and in classifying the degree of severity of IAH, in the literature [2, 8]. Updated WSACS—The Abdominal Compartment Society IAH/ACS consensus definitions and clinical practice guidelines were published in 2013 [1, 8].

### 93.1.2 Normal IAP

The normal reference range for IAP, representing the "steady-state pressure concealed within the abdominal cavity," is approximately 5–7 mm Hg in healthy adults, compared to approximately 10 mm Hg in critically ill adults and 4–10 mm Hg in critically ill children [1, 2, 8]. Clinical practice guidelines recommend measuring IAP via the bladder with a maximal instillation volume of 25 mL of sterile saline in the supine position at end expiration, and expressing it in mm Hg [1, 9]. Despite this, as many patients benefit from having their head of bed (HOB) elevated to reduce risk of ventilator-associated pneumonia, updated clinical practice guidelines should examine whether IAP may be best measured with the head at 30° [10, 11]. IAP is generally constant across the abdominal cavity when supine because the intra-abdominal contents are non-compressive and fluid in density [9]. However, IAP may increase with diaphragmatic contraction during inspiration and decrease with relaxation of the diaphragm during expiration [1, 9, 12].

Body mass index (BMI) and abdominal diameter are important predictors of increased IAP. As BMI and abdominal diameter increase, IAP rises [13, 14]. Previous studies have suggested IAP ranges between 7 and 14 mm Hg in obese patients. Further, the IAP range for overweight (BMI 25.0–29.9 kg/m$^2$) patients is 6.3–11.2 mm Hg, obese (BMI 30.0–39.9 kg/m$^2$) patients is 7.4–13.7 mm Hg, and morbidly obese (BMI ≥ 40.0 kg/m$^2$) patients is 8.4–16.2 mm Hg [14]. However, it must be noted that attribution of elevated IAP to BMI should only been done when pathologic causes for IAH have been ruled out. Moreover, an IAP above 15 mm Hg is rare even among healthy obese patients [13].

### 93.1.3 IAH and ACS

A complete list of relevant definitions related to IAH/ACS and related concepts has been published in the 2013 WSACS—The Abdominal Compartment Society IAH/ACS consensus definitions and clinical practice guidelines [1]. IAH is defined as a sustained or repeated IAP ≥12 and 10 mm Hg among adults and children, respectively [1, 8]. In adults, IAH is further classified into four grades based on severity of sustained or repeated elevations in IAP: Grade I (12–15 mm Hg), Grade II (16–20 mm Hg), Grade III (21–25 mm Hg), and Grade IV (>25 mm Hg) [1, 8]. Abdominal perfusion pressure (APP) can be calculated by subtracting the IAP from the mean arterial pressure (MAP) [APP = MAP–IAP], and has been reported to be an important and accurate measure of perfusion and resuscitation [1, 2, 15]. In terms of predicting survival, it may be superior to IAP, MAP, urine output, arterial pH, lactate, and base deficit among adult surgical critical care patients [2, 15]. Despite this, APP remains uncommonly measured or used in clinical practice.

In adults, ACS is defined as a sustained IAP above 20 mm Hg and new or progressive organ dysfunction or failure attributed to elevated IAP [1, 8]. When the evidence of organ dysfunction is clinically readily apparent, such as with hypotension or hemodynamic instability, increased peak airway pressures, and oliguria, this is referred to as overt ACS [1, 16]. In children, the threshold IAP used to define ACS in the setting of new or progressive organ dysfunction is 10 mm Hg [1]. Importantly, close attention should be paid to new organ dysfunction regardless of these thresholds, as IAH can produce such effects at lower IAPs as well [2].

IAH and ACS can be primary, secondary, recurrent (sometimes termed tertiary), or quaternary [1, 17]. Abdominopelvic injury or disease (e.g., acute pancreatitis or a ruptured AAA) is the cause of primary IAH/ACS, and surgical or interventional therapies are commonly required for treatment [1, 17]. Secondary IAH/ACS arises from causes outside the abdomen or pelvis, such as vascular injury to an extremity, or which involve capillary leak syndrome and peripheral vasoplegia, such as sepsis or burns [1, 17]. Recurrent (or tertiary) IAH/ACS represents IAH/ACS that redevelops despite treatment of IAH/ACS [1]. Finally, quaternary IAH is a unique type of IAH without other complications that frequently occur in the setting of abdominal wall reconstruction, and may potentially be managed conservatively [18, 19].

### 93.1.4 Epidemiology

The incidence of IAH ranges from 21% to 58% and ACS from 1% to 12% among mixed populations of critically ill adults in the ICU [20–23]. The wide range reported for these estimates is likely secondary to differences in patient characteristics, diagnostic criteria, and methods of IAP measurement. A meta-analysis that included 1669 adult ICU patients and utilized WSACS—The Abdominal Compartment Society definitions of IAH/ACS reported a 27.7% prevalence of IAH and 2.7% prevalence of ACS upon admission to the ICU [23].

As the above estimates apply to ICU patients in general, they may underestimate the incidence among those at higher risk for IAH/ACS [21, 24–30]. Historically, the prevalence of IAH and ACS was reported to be as high as 53% and 12% among trauma and emergency general patients, respectively [21]. However, with advances in trauma resuscitation strategies that emphasize rapid hemorrhage control and use of blood products instead of large amounts of crystalloid fluids, the incidence of post-injury ACS has markedly declined [31, 32]. Patients with extensive burns have reported risks of IAH and ACS of 34% and 17–20%, respectively [29, 30]. The risk of IAH/ACS increases in burn patients with total body surface area burns >50%, inhalational injury, and excessive fluid and crystalloid resuscitation, regardless of abdominal involvement of burns [2, 28–30]. Those who have a particularly high risk of IAH/ACS are those with severe acute pancreatitis (where the incidence of IAH ranges between 30 and 93% and ACS approaches 50%) [2, 25–27]. Finally, patients with ruptured AAAs, particularly those who are managed with endovascular abdominal aortic aneurysm repair, have been reported to have an incidence of ACS of approximately 8% [33].

### 93.1.5 Pathophysiology

Bowel ischemia is an important driver of the pathophysiology of IAH and ACS, ultimately leading to a cyclical and self-perpetuating process [2, 34–37]. Following fluid resuscitation after development of a shock state, pro-inflammatory cytokines are released as part of the ischemia–reperfusion pathway [34–39]. If the primary insult is intra-peritoneal (e.g., hemorrhage, sepsis resulting from leakage from a hollow viscus), this drives a peritoneal inflammatory response, but a systemic inflammatory response is common among those with IAH/ACS regardless of the primary insult [34–38]. These cytokines result in bowel injury by increasing permeability of the mesenteric capillaries and bowel wall, permitting release of bacteria and endotoxins into circulation, leading to neutrophil priming, systemic inflammation, and extravasation of fluid into the bowel wall and mesentery [34–41].

As a result of this increased permeability and extravasation, subsequent fluid resuscitation leads to third-spacing of liters of fluid within the bowel and mesentery [34, 42]. As the edema increases, so does IAP, causing reduced lymphatic drainage out of the abdomen due to lymphatic obstruction, again further increasing IAP [34, 38]. Increased IAP also results in a reduction in capillary blood flow at the level of the bowel mucosa, eventually causing ischemia and necrosis [38]. In a cyclical fashion, the result of the ongoing bowel ischemia is increased bowel wall permeability and release of pro-inflammatory cytokines and toxic media into systemic circulation, which further worsens bowel wall edema and IAP in a repetitive fashion [38]. This self-perpetuating process has been described as a two-hit phenomenon, wherein the initial bowel injury is the "first hit" [2].

Bowel injury results in release of pro-inflammatory ascites, which is associated with adverse outcomes and the systemic propagation of toxic biomediators [43]. Visceral injury, peritoneal irritation, and intra-abdominal contamination are triggers for release of interleukin-6 (IL-6), IL-8, tumor necrosis factor-α (TNF-α), and IL-1β [44]. Uptake of these cytokines via the lymphatic system, and their subsequent release into the systemic circulation, leads to a systemic inflammatory response [45]. Consequently, clinical studies continue to investigate whether removal or dilution of inflammatory ascites to prevent their uptake into the lymphatic and circulatory systems may blunt the systemic inflammatory response and improve patient outcomes [39, 43].

### 93.1.6 Systemic Effects of IAH/ACS

The systemic effects of IAH/ACS are detailed below, by organ system, and in Table 93.1.

**Table 93.1** Systemic effects of abdominal compartment syndrome. Table reproduced from Roberts DJ, De Waele JJ, Kirkpatrick AW, Malbrain MLNG. Intra-abdominal hypertension and the abdominal compartment syndrome. In: O'Donnell JM, Nácul FE, editors. Surgical Intensive Care Medicine. Cham: Springer International Publishing; 2016. p. 621–44

| Central nervous system | Cardiovascular | Respiratory |
|---|---|---|
| *Supradiaphragmatic effects* | | |
| ↑ Intra-cranial pressure | *Cardiac* | *Pressures* |
| ↓ Cerebral perfusion pressure | ↓ Cardiac venous return and preload | ↑ Intra-thoracic pressure |
| ↑ Blood-brain barrier disruption | ↑ Central venous pressure | ↑ Pleural pressure |
| | ↑ Pulmonary artery pressure | ↑ Auto positive end expiratory pressure |
| | ↑ Pulmonary artery occlusion pressure | ↑ Peak airway pressure |
| | ↓ Ventricular compliance | ↑ Plateau airway pressure |
| | ↓ Ventricular contractility | *Compliance* |
| | ↓ Ventricular regional wall motion | ↓ Static chest wall compliance |
| | =/↓ Right ventricular end diastolic volume | ↓ Static respiratory system compliance |
| | =/↓ Global end diastolic blood volume index | = Static lung compliance |
| | =/↓ Heart rate | ↓ Dynamic compliance |
| | ↓ Cardiac output | Lung capillary leak syndrome |
| | *Systemic arterial* | ↑ Alveolar edema and extravascular lung water |

**Table 93.1** (continued)

| Central nervous system | Cardiovascular | | Respiratory | |
|---|---|---|---|---|
| | ↑ Systemic vascular resistance and afterload | | ↓ Lung volumes (simulating restrictive disease) | |
| | ↓ Mean arterial pressure | | ↑ Compressive atelectasis | |
| | | | *Ventilation and gas exchange* | |
| | | | ↑ Dead-space ventilation | |
| | | | ↑ Intra-pulmonary shunting | |
| | | | Hypercarbia | |
| | | | ↓ $PaO_2$ and $PaO_2/FiO_2$ ratio | |
| | | | ↑ Activated lung neutrophils | |
| | | | ↑ Pulmonary inflammatory cell infiltration | |
| Gastrointestinal | Renal | Hepatic | Abdominal wall | Endocrine |
| *Subdiaphragmatic effects* | | | | |
| *Mesenteric blood flow* | *Renal blood flow* | *Hepatic blood flow* | ↓ Rectus sheath blood flow | ↓ Adrenal blood flow |
| ↓ Abdominal perfusion pressure | ↓ Renal perfusion pressure | ↓ Hepatic arterial flow | ↓ Compliance | |
| ↓ Celiac artery flow | ↓ Renal blood flow | ↓ Portal venous flow | ↑ Wound complication | |
| ↓ Superior mesenteric artery flow | ↑ Renal vein compression | ↑ Portocollateral flow | | |
| ↓ Bowel mucosal flow | ↑ Renal vascular resistance | *Hepatic function* | | |
| ↑ Mesenteric vein compression | *Renal function* | ↓ Lactate clearance | | |
| *Bowel function* | ↓ Filtration gradient | ↓ CYP450 enzyme activity | | |
| ↓ Intra-mucosal pH | ↓ Urine output | ↓ Indocyanine green clearance | | |
| ↑ Intestinal permeability | ↓ Tubular function | | | |
| ↑ Bacterial translocation | ↓ GFR | | | |
| ↑ Risk of multiple organ dysfunction | ↑ Angiotensin II | | | |
| ↓ Successful enteral feeding | ↑ Antidiuretic hormone | | | |
| | ↑ Ureteral compression | | | |

*GFR* glomerular filtration rate, *CYP450* cytochrome P450

## 93.1.7 Neurological

Elevated IAP is associated with increased intracranial pressure (ICP) and decreased cerebral perfusion pressure [46]. There are two proposed mechanisms for these changes: (1) rising jugular venous pressure as a result of increased intrathoracic pressure reduces cerebral venous drainage, and (2) impediments in cerebrospinal fluid drainage from the superior sagittal sinus and lumbar venous plexus [46, 47]. Interestingly, disruption of the blood–brain barrier has been observed with more than 4 h of IAH and the disruption was reversed by decreasing IAP by abdominal decompression [47, 48].

## 93.1.8 Cardiovascular

IAH/ACS decreases cardiac output and MAP through several mechanisms [49]. First, increased IAP compresses the intra-abdominal inferior vena cava (IVC), which decreases venous return to the heart [2, 34, 49]. IVC compression begins at an IAP of 15 mm Hg and compression of the renal and mesenteric veins occurs above 20 mm Hg [2, 49, 50]. Compression of intra-abdominal arterioles also increases systemic vascular resistance and afterload [50]. Finally, increased IAP induces indirect compression of the heart, lungs, and intra-thoracic vasculature [34, 49, 50]. Collectively, the above results in impaired cardiac contractility and compliance, increased pulmonary vascular resistance, and decreased preload and increased afterload [2, 49, 50].

### 93.1.9 Respiratory

Approximately half of IAP can be transmitted to the thoracic cavity [2, 34, 49, 51]. In addition to the increased pulmonary vascular resistance noted above, this causes a reduction in chest wall compliance and increased airway pressures [2, 34, 49, 51]. Coupled with compressive atelectasis and increased alveolar dead-space, this results in decreased lung volumes, which increases ventilation–perfusion mismatch and leads to progressive hypoxemia due to respiratory failure [2, 34, 49, 51].

### 93.1.10 Renal

Early in IAH, increased IAP causes renal vein compression [52]. As IAH worsens and ACS develops, renin–angiotensin system activation, renal vascular resistance, and renal dysfunction increase [52]. Patients often develop oliguria at an IAP of 15 mm Hg and progress to anuria beyond 30 mm Hg of IAP [52]. Overall, IAH results in reduced blood flow to nephrons, decreased glomerular filtration, and diminished urine output [2, 52].

### 93.1.11 Gastrointestinal

In porcine models, reductions in blood flow through the mesenteric and hepatic arteries have been reported to be as high as 73% and 55%, respectively, at an IAP of 20 mm Hg [53]. Worsening bowel ischemia subsequently often leads to increased bowel wall permeability, bacterial translocation, and sepsis and/or septic shock [54]. Animal models illustrate dramatic effects of even modest IAH. With only 6 h of IAH at 25 mm Hg, an 80% reduction in mucosal blood flow, an exponential increase in mucosal permeability, and erosion and necrosis of jejunal villi have been observed [38]. These changes may facilitate both bacterial and pro-inflammatory mediator translocation across the bowel wall and into systemic circulation [55]. Further, while gut ischemia may be the most "occult" sequalae of IAH, it may potentially be the most critical as the gut houses the human microbiome, which has profound effects on health and critical illness, and of which we are only in the infancy of understanding [56].

## 93.2 Diagnosis

### 93.2.1 When Should IAP Be Measured?

IAP is recommended to be measured in any critically ill or injured patient with any known risk factor for IAH or ACS [1]. Table 93.2 presents evidence-informed risk factors for IAH and ACS reported by a systematic review and meta-analysis of 2500 ICU patients by Holodinsky, Roberts, and colleagues [57]. These authors reported that large volume crystalloid resuscitation, respiratory dysfunction or failure [acute respiratory distress syndrome, need for mechanical ventilation, positive end-expiratory pressure (PEEP) >10 cm $H_2O$], shock, and hypotension were the most significant risk factors for IAH/ACS [57]. In injured and postoperative patients, significant risk factors for IAH/ACS included worsening base deficit, while those for IAH/ACS in general ICU patients included obesity, sepsis, abdominal surgery, and ileus [57]. Transfusion of multiple units of packed red blood cells (pRBCs), as well as a greater ratio of crystalloid to pRBCs administered, were also reported as potential risk

**Table 93.2** Significant risk factors for intra-abdominal hypertension and abdominal compartment syndrome among critically ill patients [57]

| Risk factor | Population | Odds ratio (95% confidence interval) |
|---|---|---|
| *Intra-abdominal hypertension* | | |
| Obesity | Mixed ICU patients | 5.10 (1.92–13.58) |
| Age (1-year increase) | Mixed ICU patients | 2.75 (1.01–3.09) |
| Sepsis | Mixed ICU patients | 2.38 (1.34–4.23) |
| Abdominal surgery | Mixed ICU patients | 1.93 (1.30–2.85) |
| Laparotomy | Trauma patients | 5.72 (1.50–21.43) |
| Pancreatitis | Mechanically ventilated mixed ICU patients | 4.73 (1.96–11.41) |
| Hepatic failure or cirrhosis | Mechanically ventilated mixed ICU patients | 2.07 (2.07–28.81) |
| Hepatic dysfunction | Mixed ICU patients | 2.25 (1.10–4.58) |
| Gastrointestinal bleeding | Mechanically ventilated mixed ICU patients | 3.37 (1.43–7.94) |
| Ileus | Mixed ICU patients | 2.05 (1.40–2.98) |
| APACHE II score (one-point increase) | Pancreatitis patients | 1.65 (1.13–2.41)[a] |
| Base deficit | Trauma patients | 1.15 (1.01–1.33) |
| Acidosis | Mixed ICU patients | 1.93 (1.12–3.45) |
| Vasopressor use | Mechanically ventilated mixed ICU patients | 2.33 (1.02–5.35) |
| Shock | Mixed ICU patients | 4.68 (1.93–6.44) |
| Hypotension | Mixed ICU patients | 2.12 (1.05–4.50) |
| CVP (1 mm hg increase) | Mixed ICU patients | 1.30 (1.10–1.60) |
| PEEP >10 cm $H_2O$ | Mechanically ventilated mixed ICU patients | 2.41 (1.57–3.70) |
| Respiratory failure $PaO_2/FiO_2 < 300$) | Mechanically ventilated mixed ICU patients | 1.87 (1.22–2.87) |
| ARDS | Mixed ICU patients | 3.61 (1.60–9.06) |
| Mechanical ventilation | Mixed ICU patients | 6.78 (1.94–59.03) |
| Pre-ICU crystalloid | Trauma patients | 1.40 (1.00–1.96) |
| Fluid balance | Mixed ICU patients | 5.22 (2.03–7.45) |
| Fluid collections | Pancreatitis patients | 2.021 (1.30–3.13)[a] |
| Fluid resuscitation (>3.5 L crystalloid or colloid) | Mixed ICU patients | 2.17 (1.30–3.63) |
| *Abdominal compartment syndrome* | | |
| OR within 75 min of ED admission | Trauma patients | 102.70 (9.65 to 999.99) |
| APACHE II score > 20.3 | Severe acute pancreatitis | 1.14 (1.01–1.29) |
| Glasgow-Imrie score > 9.1 | Severe acute pancreatitis | 1.22 (1.00–1.49) |
| Temperature ≤ 34 °C | Trauma patients | 22.90 (1.39–378.25) |
| Hemoglobin ≤ 80 g/L | Trauma patients | 252.20 (9.89–999.99) |
| Hemoglobin ≤8 0 g/L (primary ACS) | Trauma patients | 206.10 (7.41–999.99) |
| Base deficit ≥ 12 | Trauma patients | 3.50 (1.37–839.50) |
| Urine output ≤ 150 mL/24 h | Trauma patients | 64.10 (5.48–749.68) |
| Serum creatinine > 217.7 μmol/L | Severe acute pancreatitis | 1.12 (1.02–1.22)[a] |
| Systolic blood pressure < 86 mm hg in ED | Trauma patients | 4.90 (1.78–13.99) |
| $GAP_{CO2}$ ≥ 16 | Trauma patients | >999.99 (22.10–999.99) |
| $GAP_{CO2}$ ≥ 16 (primary ACS) | Trauma patients | 54.30 (2.15–999.99) |
| Cardiac index < 2.6 L/min/m² | Trauma patients | 12.50 (1.02–153.64) |
| Crystalloid ≥ 3 L in ED | Trauma patients | 23.00 (6.38–83.10) |
| Crystalloid ≥3 L in ED (primary ACS) | Trauma patients | 69.80 (10.21–477.70) |

(continued)

**Table 93.2** (continued)

| Risk factor | Population | Odds ratio (95% confidence interval) |
|---|---|---|
| Crystalloid ≥3 L in ED (secondary ACS) | Trauma patients | 15.80 (1.74–143.85) |
| Crystalloid ≥ 7.5 L | Trauma patients | 166.20 (4.76–999.99) |
| Crystalloid ≥ 7.5 L (secondary ACS) | Trauma patients | 38.70 (3.19–469.55) |
| Pre-hospital crystalloid | Extremity injury patients | 1.99 (1.07–3.73) |
| ED crystalloid | Extremity injury patients | 1.85 (1.08–3.15) |
| pRBC ≥3 units in ED | Trauma patients | 5.60 (1.03–30.83) |
| Crystalloid to pRBC ratio | Trauma patients | 2.30 (1.40–3.80) |
| Crystalloid (L) to pRBC (units) ratio > 1.5:1 | Trauma patients | 3.60 (1.30–9.70) |

*APACHE II* acute physiology and chronic health evaluation II, *CVP* central venous pressure, *PEEP* positive end-expiratory pressure, *ARDS* acute respiratory distress syndrome, *OR* operating room, *ED* emergency department, *ACS* abdominal compartment syndrome, $GAP_{CO2}$ gastric mucosal $CO_2$ minus end tidal $CO_2$, *pRBC* packed red blood cells
[a] Unadjusted

factors for IAH/ACS [57]. Finally, higher APACHE-II and Glasgow-Imrie scores and creatinine levels were important risk factors in patients with acute pancreatitis [57].

### 93.2.2 How Should IAP Be Measured?

Appropriate IAP measurement is essential for the diagnosis of IAH and ACS. IAP should be measured at end expiration via the bladder following instillation of no more than 25 mL of sterile saline (higher volumes may falsely elevate the measurements) [1, 9]. The patient should be supine and there should be no contraction of the abdominal wall musculature. Measurements in awake patients should be interpreted cautiously because pain, muscle contraction, and forceful respiration may render obtained values inaccurate [1, 9]. The transducer should be zeroed at the level of the midaxillary line. While measurement via the bladder is most often recommended due to simplicity and low costs, IAP can also be measured directly with intra-peritoneal devices or indirectly via the stomach, uterus, rectum, or IVC [1, 9]. Measurement of IAP via the bladder is illustrated in Fig. 93.1.

IAP varies with patient position and increases with greater degrees of HOB elevation [11, 13, 58]. At 30° elevation, the IAP is approximately 4 mm Hg higher, and at 45° it is approximately 9 mm Hg higher [13]. The effects of this positioning are important because many ICU patients are positioned with the HOB at 30° to reduce risk of ventilator-associated pneumonia [10, 13].

### 93.2.3 Clinical Signs

Use of clinical findings for diagnosis of IAH/ACS is associated with low sensitivities and specificities of 56–61% and 81–87%, respectively [57, 59]. Clinical signs may include abdominal distention, elevated peak inspiratory/airway pressures, elevated central venous pressure (CVP), oliguria or anuria, and hypotension [2, 34]. While computed tomography (CT) may be useful for determining the etiology of primary IAH, it is not recommended for diagnosis of IAH/ACS [1]. CT findings of IAH/ACS are primarily related to the sequelae of increased IAP, and may include compression of the IVC and solid organs, bowel wall thickening, elevation of the diaphragm, and bilateral inguinal herniation [60, 61]. "Round belly sign" may also be seen on CT in patients with IAH/ACS. This sign occurs when the ratio of the anteroposterior to transverse abdominal diameters (excluding subcutaneous fat and measured at level where the left renal vein crosses the aorta) exceeds 0.8 [60, 61].

# 93 Intra-Abdominal Hypertension and Abdominal Compartment Syndrome

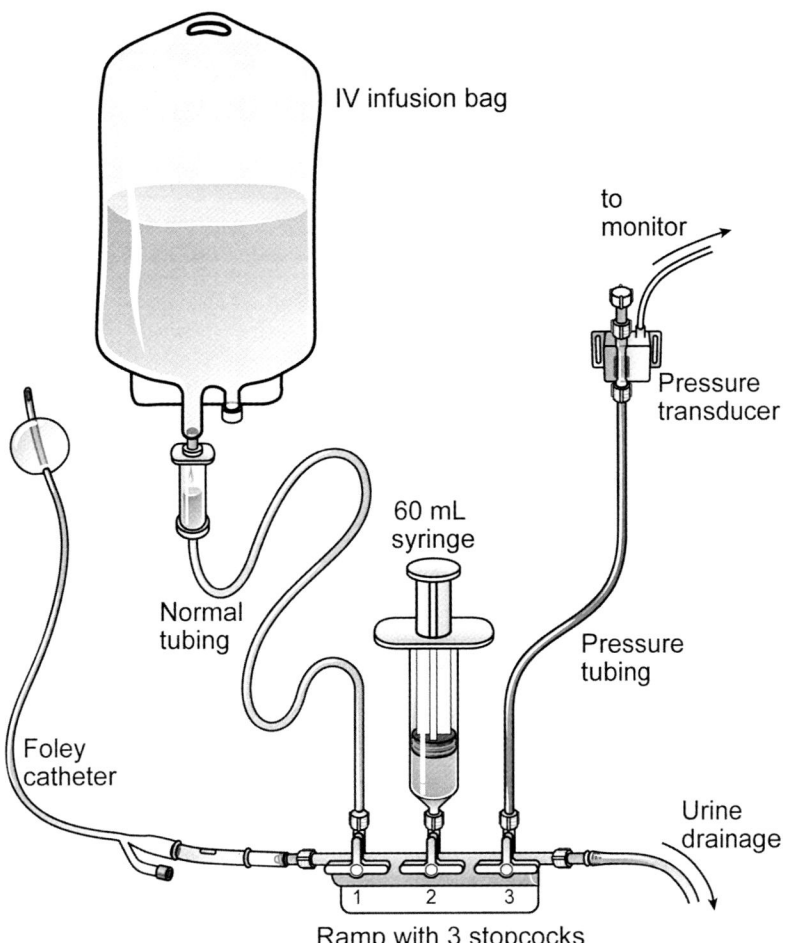

**Fig. 93.1** Intra-abdominal pressure measurement via the bladder. Following Foley catheter insertion, a ramp with three three-way stopcocks is connected between the Foley and the tubing for urine drainage. Connected to the stopcocks, moving from the one closest to the Foley, are infusion tubing with a bag of normal saline, a 60 mL syringe, and a pressure transducer with rigid transducer tubing. After flushing the system and ensuring appropriate supine positioning and zeroing at the level of the midaxillary line at the iliac crest, the stopcocks are switched to "off," allowing urine to flow into the drainage bag. To measure the IAP, the urine drainage tube is clamped distal to the ramp/stopcocks and the transducer stopcock is switched "on" to the transducer and "off" to the urine drainage tube. The first stopcock is switched to "on" to the saline infusion tubing and the second stopcock is switched to "on" to the infusion bag and syringe. 25 mL of saline is aspirated into the syringe and the first stopcock is switched to "off" to the infusion bag and on to the patient. The 25 mL is then instilled into the bladder via the Foley catheter. Once the first and second stopcocks are switched to "on" to the patient and "off" to the infusion bag and syringe, the bladder pressure can be measured by the transducer. Figure reproduced from supplementary material in Kirkpatrick AW, Roberts DJ, De Waele J, Jaeschke R, Malbrain MLNG, De Keulenaer B, et al. Intra-abdominal hypertension and the abdominal compartment syndrome: updated consensus definitions and clinical practice guidelines from the World Society of the Abdominal Compartment Syndrome. Intensive Care Med. 2013 Jul;39 (7):1190–206

## 93.3 Treatment

In 2013, WSACS—The Abdominal Compartment Society published consensus statements (Table 93.3) and IAH/ACS management algorithms (Figs. 93.2 and 93.3). These were developed through a systematic review of the literature and grading of the "quality" of evidence using the Grading of Recommendations, Assessment, Development, and Evaluation (GRADE) guide-

**Table 93.3** 2013 WSACS consensus management statements. Table reproduced from Kirkpatrick AW, Roberts DJ, De Waele J, Jaeschke R, Malbrain MLNG, De Keulenaer B, et al. Intra-abdominal hypertension and the abdominal compartment syndrome: updated consensus definitions and clinical practice guidelines from the World Society of the Abdominal Compartment Syndrome. Intensive Care Med. 2013 Jul;39 (7):1190–206

*Recommendations*
1. We recommend measuring IAP when any known risk for IAH/ACS is present in a critically ill or injured patient [GRADE 1C]
2. Studies should adopt the trans-bladder technique as the standard IAP measurement technique [not GRADED]
3. We recommend use of protocolized monitoring and management of IAP versus not [GRADE 1C]
4. We recommend efforts and/or protocols to avoid sustained IAH as compared to inattention to IAP among critically ill or injured patients [GRADE 1C]
5. We recommend decompressive laparotomy in cases of overt ACS compared to strategies that do not use decompressive laparotomy in critically ill adults with ACS [GRADE 1D]
6. We recommend that among ICU patients with open abdominal wounds, conscious and/or protocolized efforts be made to obtain an early or at least same-hospital-stay abdominal fascial closure [GRADE 1D]
7. We recommend that among critically ill/injured patients with open abdominal wounds, strategies utilizing negative pressure wound therapy be used versus not [GRADE 1C]

*Suggestions*
1. We suggest that clinicians ensure that critically ill or injured patients receive optimal pain and anxiety relief [GRADE 2D]
2. We suggest brief trials of neuromuscular blockade as a temporizing measure in the treatment of IAH/ACS [GRADE 2D]
3. We suggest that the potential contribution of body position to elevated IAP be considered among patients with, or at risk of, IAH or ACS [GRADE 2D]
4. We suggest liberal use of enteral decompression with nasogastric or rectal tubes when the stomach or colon are dilated in the presence of IAH/ACS [GRADE 1D]
5. We suggest that neostigmine be used for the treatment of established colonic ileus not responding to other simple measures and associated with IAH [GRADE 2D]
6. We suggest using a protocol to try and avoid a positive cumulative fluid balance in the critically ill or injured patient with, or at risk of, IAH/ACS after the acute resuscitation has been completed and the inciting issues have been addressed [GRADE 2C]
7. We suggest use of an enhanced ratio of plasma/packed red blood cells for resuscitation of massive hemorrhage versus low or no attention to plasma/packed red blood cell ratios [GRADE 2D]
8. We suggest use of PCD to remove fluid (in the setting of obvious intraperitoneal fluid) in those with IAH/ACS when this is technically possible compared to doing nothing [GRADE 2C]. We also suggest using PCD to remove fluid (in the setting of obvious intraperitoneal fluid) in those with IAH/ACS when this is technically possible compared to immediate decompressive laparotomy as this may alleviate the need for decompressive laparotomy [GRADE 2D]
9. We suggest that patients undergoing laparotomy for trauma suffering from physiologic exhaustion be treated with the prophylactic use of the open abdomen versus intraoperative abdominal fascial closure and expectant IAP management [GRADE 2D]
10. We suggest not to routinely utilize the open abdomen for patients with severe intraperitoneal contamination undergoing emergency laparotomy for intra-abdominal sepsis unless IAH is a specific concern [GRADE 2B]
11. We suggest that bioprosthetic meshes should not be routinely used in the early closure of the open abdomen compared to alternative strategies [GRADE 2D]

*No recommendations*
1. We could make no recommendation regarding use of abdominal perfusion pressure in the resuscitation or management of the critically ill or injured
2. We could make no recommendation regarding use of diuretics to mobilize fluids in hemodynamically stable patients with IAH after the acute resuscitation has been completed and the inciting issues have been addressed
3. We could make no recommendation regarding the use of renal replacement therapies to mobilize fluid in hemodynamically stable patients with IAH after the acute resuscitation has been completed and the inciting issues have been addressed
4. We could make no recommendation regarding the administration of albumin versus not, to mobilize fluid in hemodynamically stable patients with IAH after acute resuscitation has been completed and the inciting issues have been addressed
5. We could make no recommendation regarding the prophylactic use of the open abdomen in non-trauma acute care surgery patients with physiologic exhaustion versus intraoperative abdominal fascial closure and expectant IAP management
6. We could make no recommendation regarding use of an acute component separation technique versus not to facilitate abdominal fascial closure

*ACS* abdominal compartment syndrome, *IAP* intra-abdominal pressure, *IAH* intra-abdominal hypertension, *PCD* percutaneous catheter drainage

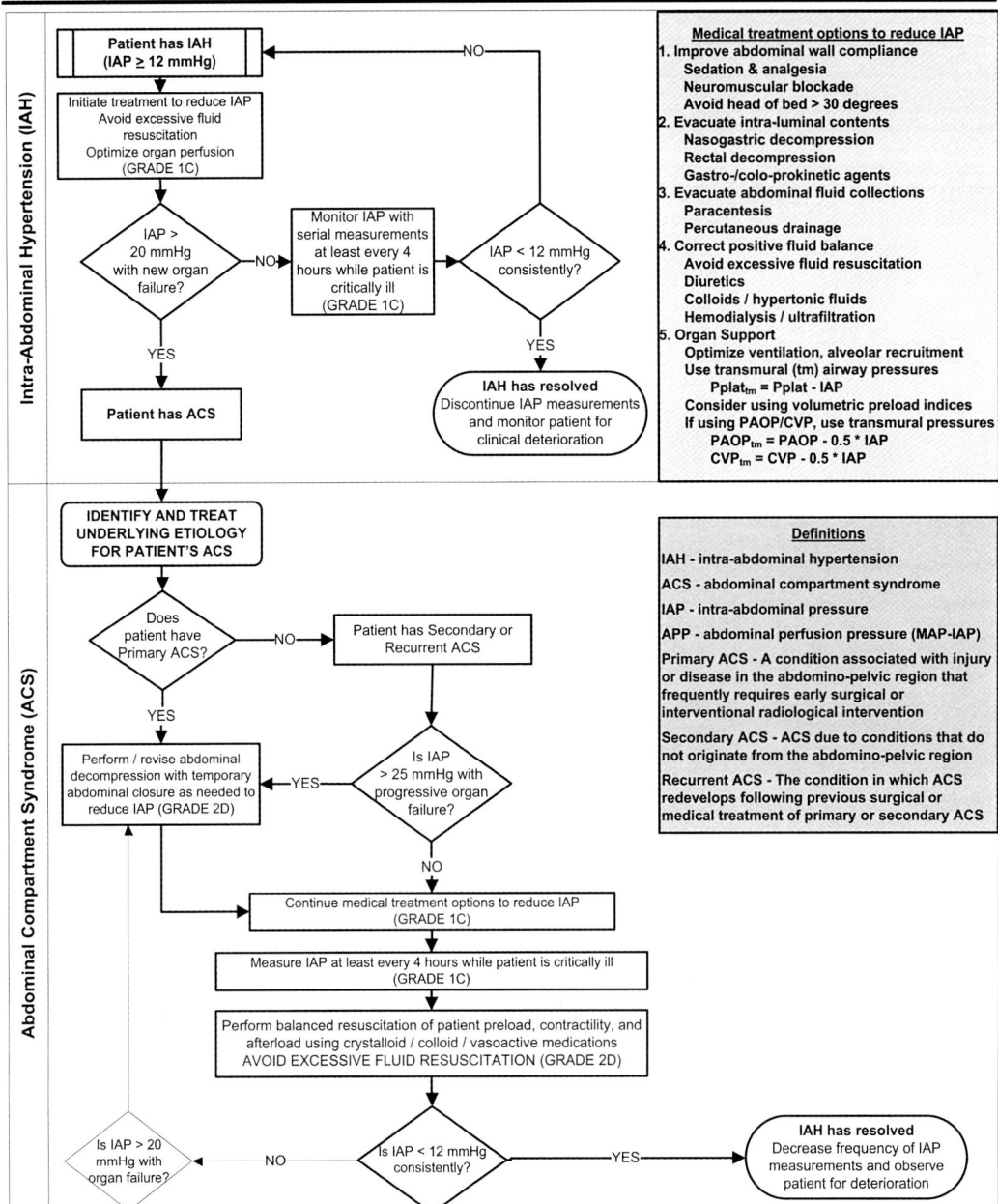

**Fig. 93.2** WSACS 2013 intra-abdominal hypertension/abdominal compartment syndrome management algorithm. Figure reproduced from Kirkpatrick AW, Roberts DJ, De Waele J, Jaeschke R, Malbrain MLNG, De Keulenaer B, et al. Intra-abdominal hypertension and the abdominal compartment syndrome: updated consensus definitions and clinical practice guidelines from the World Society of the Abdominal Compartment Syndrome. Intensive Care Med. 2013 Jul;39 (7):1190–206

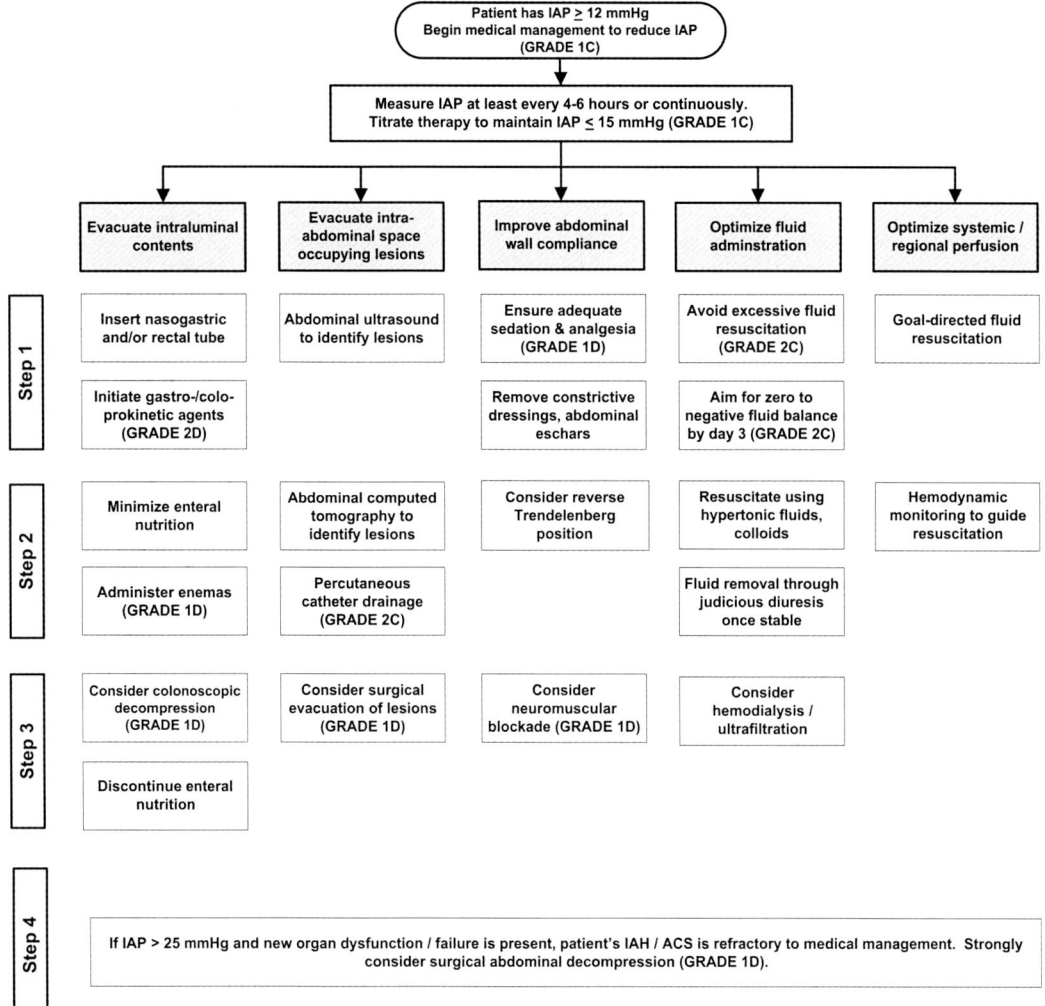

**Fig. 93.3** WSACS 2013 intra-abdominal hypertension medical management algorithm. Figure reproduced from Kirkpatrick AW, Roberts DJ, De Waele J, Jaeschke R, Malbrain MLNG, De Keulenaer B, et al. Intra-abdominal hypertension and the abdominal compartment syndrome: updated consensus definitions and clinical practice guidelines from the World Society of the Abdominal Compartment Syndrome. Intensive Care Med. 2013 Jul;39 (7):1190–206

lines [1]. This section presents medical, interventional, and surgical management options for adults and children with IAH/ACS [1].

### 93.3.1 Medical Management

Medical management of IAH/ACS aims to increase abdominal wall compliance, reduce overall fluid balance, and evacuate gastrointestinal contents [1]. The compliance of the abdomen refers to the change in volume for a given change in IAP and is a measure of ease of abdominal expansion [1, 8]. Abdominal compliance may be increased at least temporarily (e.g., in patients with ACS who are being transferred to the operating room for decompressive laparotomy) by administering neuromuscular blocking agents [62]. These agents have been reported to decrease IAP by as much as 4 mm Hg in as little as 15 min [62]. Further, while sedation and analgesia are often recommended to reduce pain and anxiety (and therefore abdominal muscular tone) there is a paucity of evidence to support that sedation improves IAP in patients with IAH/ACS. Interestingly, fentanyl may actually increase IAP during laparoscopy due to its effect on expiratory activity [63]. Decompression of the gastrointestinal tract with nasogastric or rectal tubes is commonly used in patients with IAH/ACS, especially if there is evidence of stomach, small bowel, or colon dilation [1]. Such dilation has been linked to IAH/ACS in porcine models and in cases of humans undergoing endoscopy [64]. By decreasing the intra-abdominal volume occupied by enteric contents, IAP is decreased, particularly when abdominal wall compliance is reduced. Correction of positive fluid balance and avoidance of excessive fluid resuscitation is of critical importance in preventing and managing IAH/ACS. In support of this, in a retrospective study of trauma patients, ACS incidence decreased from 7.4% to 0% over a 5-year period as total crystalloid administration decreased from 12.8 L to 6.6 L [65]. Although diuretics, hemodialysis, and several other modalities may also decrease overall fluid balance, evidence supporting their use in patients with or at risk of IAH/ACS is lacking [1].

### 93.3.2 Interventional Management

Percutaneous drainage of intra-abdominal fluid collections in patients with IAH/ACS may decrease IAP and avoid need for decompressive laparotomy in some situations [1, 66]. The largest accessible collections should be targeted. In one retrospective cohort study, percutaneous drainage was as effective as decompressive laparotomy at reducing IAP in patients with accessible intra-abdominal fluid collections [67]. It has also been reported to potentially obviate the need for operative intervention in as many as 81% of patients, and may reduce mortality, complications, and ICU admissions among patients with severe acute pancreatitis [67, 68]. However, to date no randomized controlled trial has been performed to estimate the outcomes of percutaneous drainage in patients with IAH/ACS.

Prospective studies have investigated other interventions, including instillation of hyperosmolar fluids into the peritoneum among individuals with intra-abdominal sepsis or an open abdomen, termed direct peritoneal resuscitation (DPR) [69]. DPR has been reported to potentially decrease abdominal fascial closure rates [69]. There is also evidence that DPR, through arteriolar dilation, can reduce cellular hypoxia and organ ischemia, particularly in the bowel [70, 71]. In animal models, it also mitigates the overall inflammatory response when compared to intravenous fluids alone [71–73].

### 93.3.3 Surgical Management

Surgical intervention has a role to play across the continuum of care for patients with or at risk of IAH/ACS. Surgical care for patients with or at risk of IAH/ACS can be divided into several stages, including prevention of IAH/ACS, surgical decompression, temporary abdominal closure (TAC), open abdominal management in the ICU, prevention of wound complications, and staged abdominal reconstruction.

### 93.3.4 Prevention of IAH/ACS

Surgical decision making has an important role to play in IAH/ACS prevention. Specifically, surgeons should consider leaving the abdomen open in patients undergoing laparotomy who have received a large volume of fluids for resuscitation and have significant visceral edema or develop severe IAH or signs of ACS with attempted closure [74, 75]. Evidence of persistent hypothermia, acidemia, and coagulopathy should also prompt surgeons to consider leaving the abdomen open [1]. However, valid evidence to support use of the open abdomen in trauma, emergency general surgery, or other surgical patients with metabolic derangements or physiological impairment is lacking.

### 93.3.5 Surgical Decompression

ACS that does not respond to medical management and/or percutaneous drainage is recommended to be managed with decompressive midline laparotomy [1, 76]. If decompressive laparotomy in the operating room cannot be facilitated expeditiously, it can be performed at the bedside in the ICU [2]. A recent systematic review investigated the effect of decompressive laparotomy for patients with ACS [77]. Following decompressive laparotomy, there were significant reductions in IAP (−18.2 mm Hg), heart rate (−12.2 beats per minute), CVP (−4.6 mm Hg), and peak inspiratory pressure (−10.1 mm Hg) [77]. Cardiac index, ratio of partial pressure of arterial oxygen and fraction of inspired oxygen (P/F ratio), and urine output were also significantly increased following laparotomy [77]. Of note, while organ dysfunction may improve, IAH itself may persist after decompression [77]. Mortality in patients undergoing decompressive laparotomy approaches 50%, most commonly due to organ dysfunction [77]. Although rare, close attention should be paid to the potential development of reperfusion syndrome after decompressive laparotomy due to acidemic blood from the mesenteric vasculature being released into blood, resulting in acidemia and hemodynamic instability [2, 76].

Several minimally invasive fasciotomies have also been suggested as alternatives to decompressive laparotomy [2, 66]. These include bilateral subcutaneous anterior rectus sheath fasciotomies, midline subcutaneous fasciotomies, and subcutaneous or open linea alba fasciotomies [2, 66]. Further research is required to elucidate whether these fasciotomies can be recommended over decompressive laparotomy, which remains the current recommendation for treatment of ACS that fails to respond to medical or interventional therapies [1].

### 93.3.6 TAC

TAC of the open abdomen is frequently accomplished with a commercially available negative pressure wound therapy device (e.g., ABThera™ Open Abdomen Negative Pressure Therapy System [Kinetic Concepts Inc., San Antonio, TX, USA]) or a Barker's vacuum pack (Figs. 93.4 and 93.5) [78–83]. Animal studies have shown that negative pressure wound therapy for TAC may be more effective in removing peritoneal fluid than alternate TAC devices and may remove proinflammatory mediators present in peritoneal fluid [84]. A prospective cohort study of patients who underwent TAC after laparotomy for trauma or emergency general surgery also reported improved mortality and fascial closure rates with the ABThera™ versus the Barker's vacuum pack [79, 85]. However, these findings have been contested in other studies, which have failed to demonstrate mortality benefits with commercial negative pressure wound therapy devices [86]. A single-center randomized controlled trial published by Kirkpatrick, Roberts, and colleagues allocated patients with intra-abdominal trauma or sepsis to the ABThera™ or the Barker's vacuum pack [87]. In this study, peritoneal drainage was

## ABThera™ Open Abdomen NPT System

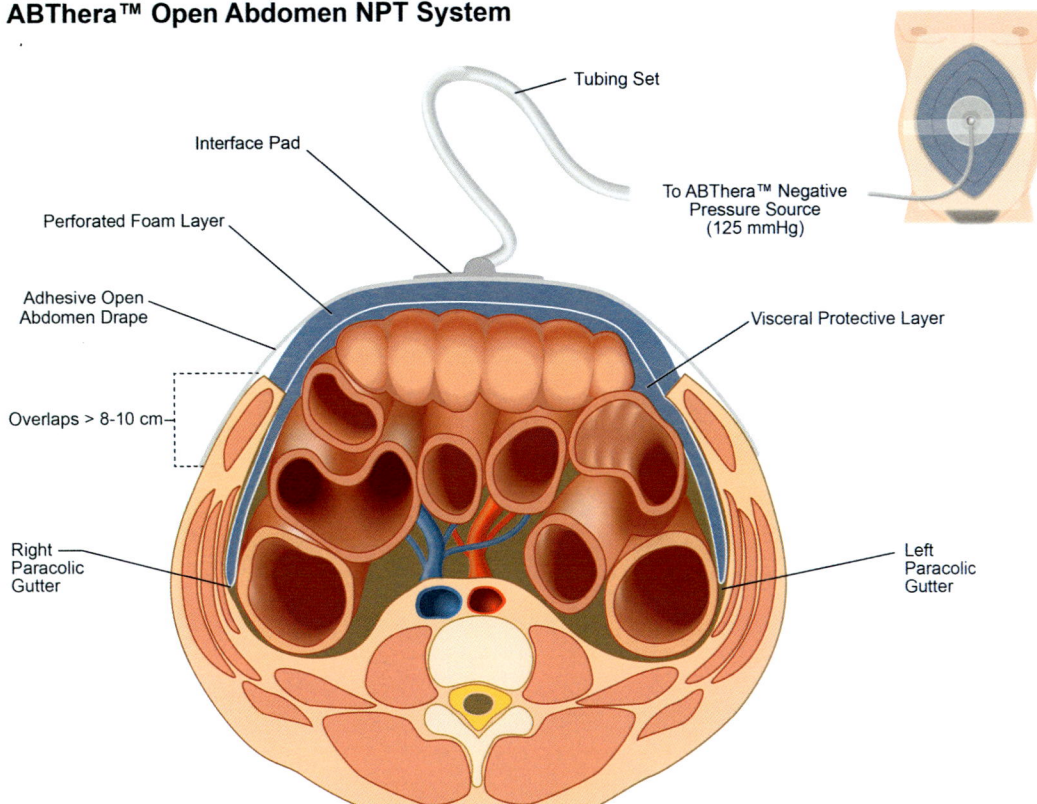

**Fig. 93.4** Schematic of the ABThera™ open abdomen negative pressure therapy system [Kinetic Concepts Inc., San Antonio, TX, USA]). Figure reproduced from Roberts DJ, De Waele JJ, Kirkpatrick AW, Malbrain MLNG. Intra-abdominal hypertension and the abdominal compartment syndrome. In: O'Donnell JM, Nácul FE, editors. Surgical Intensive Care Medicine. Cham: Springer International Publishing; 2016. p. 621–44

surprisingly lower in the ABThera™ arm. Further, there were no significant differences in the peritoneal or plasma concentrations of pro-inflammatory cytokines [87]. However, there was a significant improvement in 90-day mortality in the ABThera™ group, which may have been due to a type I error [87].

In patients with an open abdominal wound who are managed with negative pressure wound therapy, ACS may develop in rare but unique circumstances [2, 88]. These devices may increase drainage of peritoneal fluid, which helps to offset IAP increases [88]. However, when they are placed onto patients with limited intra-peritoneal fluid, predominantly visceral edema, substantial intra-abdominal packing, or retroperitoneal bleeding or hematoma, IAH or ACS may develop because the reduced compliance of the abdominal wall during negative pressure wound therapy is not offset by an associated increase in intra-peritoneal fluid drainage. Table 93.4 provides a summary of various TAC methods [2, 74, 78, 79, 81–83, 88].

### 93.3.7 Wound Management and Complications

Management of open abdominal wounds is complex and requires appropriate expertise to minimize complications. The original Bjork classification was modified in 2013 by the WSACS—The Abdominal Compartment Society to further standardize classification of open abdominal wounds [1, 89]. There exist four classifications, with subclassifications within each:

## Barker's Vacuum Pack

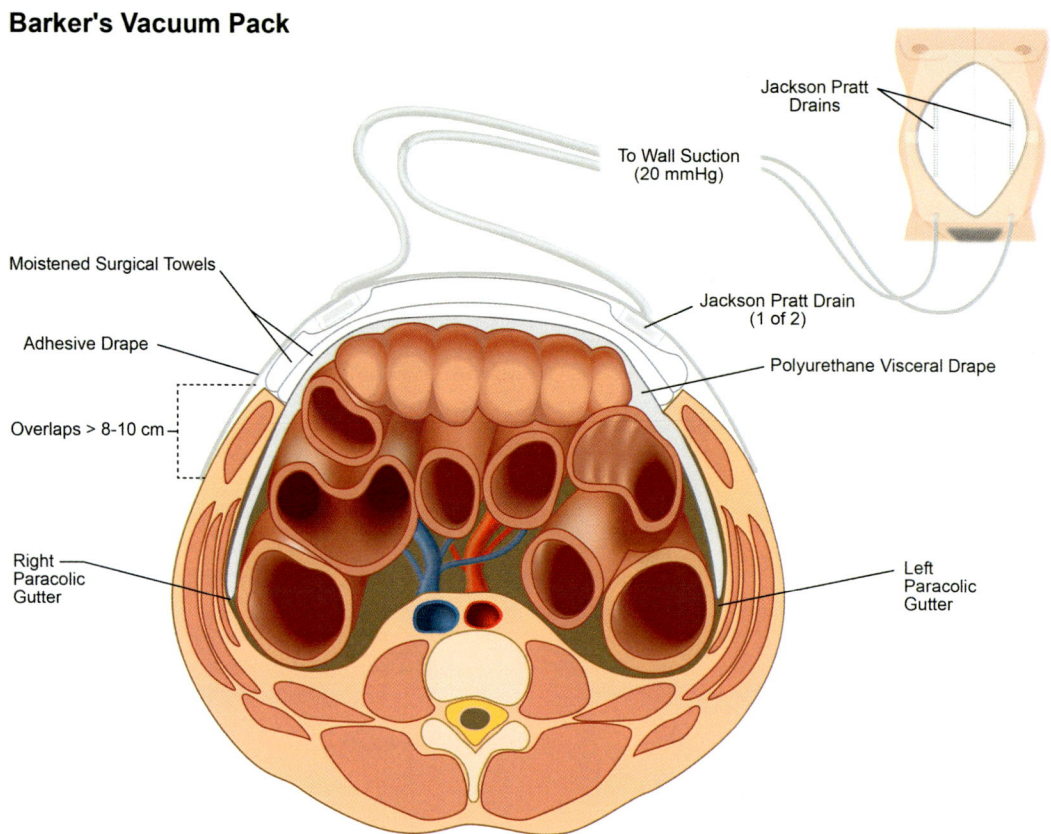

**Fig. 93.5** Schematic of the Barker's vacuum pack. Figure reproduced from Roberts DJ, De Waele JJ, Kirkpatrick AW, Malbrain MLNG. Intra-abdominal hypertension and the abdominal compartment syndrome. In: O'Donnell JM, Nácul FE, editors. Surgical Intensive Care Medicine. Cham: Springer International Publishing; 2016. p. 621–44

(1) No fixation, (2) developing fixation, (3) frozen abdomen, and (4) established enteroatmospheric fistula and frozen abdomen [1, 89]. Classes 1 and 2 are further subdivided as (A) clean, (B) contaminated, or (C) enteric leak, while class 3 is subdivided as (A) clean or (B) contaminated [1, 89].

Enteroatmospheric fistula is perhaps the most feared complication of open abdominal management. The incidence of enteroatmospheric fistula formation is approximately 5% in trauma patients [90, 91]. Risk factors for development of these fistulae in the open abdomen include receipt of greater than 10 L of fluid resuscitation (or 5–10 L by 48 h), large bowel resection, and an increasing number of abdominal re-explorations (likely reflecting increasing degrees of enteric trauma induced by repeated small bowel manipulation) [81, 90, 91]. The length of time that the abdomen is left open may also increase the risk of fistula formation, suggesting that closing the abdomen as soon as possible after it is opened should be a surgical priority [92].

Deep soft tissue infections, intra-abdominal sepsis, and complex ventral herniae are also important complications of open abdominal management [81, 91]. Upwards of 25% of patients with an open abdomen will experience at least one complication, and there is a dramatic increase in this risk after the abdomen has been left open for more than 8 days (from 12% to 52%) [91]. As patients with an open abdomen have high metabolic needs and suffer from significant insensible losses of fluids, enteral feeding is recommended

**Table 93.4** Temporary abdominal closure methods and devices [2, 74, 78, 79, 81–83, 88]. Table reproduced from Roberts DJ, De Waele JJ, Kirkpatrick AW, Malbrain MLNG. Intra-abdominal hypertension and the abdominal compartment syndrome. In: O'Donnell JM, Nácul FE, editors. Surgical Intensive Care Medicine. Cham: Springer International Publishing; 2016. p. 621–44

| Type | Description | Advantages | Disadvantages | Prognostic estimates[a] | | | |
|---|---|---|---|---|---|---|---|
| | | | | 1° Fascial closure | Mortality | Fistula | Abscess |
| *Skin approximation* | | | | | | | |
| Towel clips[b] | The abdominal skin is closed using towel clips placed 2–3 cm apart along the length of the skin incision | Low cost, may be applied rapidly, Universally available | High risk of recurrent IAH/ACS, towel clips may interfere with angiography and diagnostic imaging, does not prevent fascial retraction or adhesion formation | 43% | 39% | NA | NA |
| Suture[b] | The abdominal skin is closed by placing a running suture (typically nylon) along the length of the skin incision | Low cost, may be applied rapidly, universally available | High risk of IAH/ACS, does not prevent fascial retraction or adhesion formation | | | | |
| *Silo* | | | | | | | |
| Bogotá bag | A sterile X-ray cassette or 3 L Urological irrigation bag is sutured between the skin or fascial edges | Low cost, universally available, prevents desiccation, ability to visualize the bowel postoperatively | Does not prevent fascial retraction or adhesion formation, may damage skin or fascia, does not remove or control peritoneal fluid | 28–29% | 30–41% | 0–8% | 6–12% |
| *Mesh/sheet* | | | | | | | |
| Synthetic absorbable | An absorbable sheet [e.g., Polyglycolic acid (Dexon) or polyglactin 910 (Vicryl)] is sutured between the fascial edges | Does not need to be removed, may be plicated, pleated, or reduced in size to achieve progressive fascial closure | Does not prevent adhesion formation | 36% | 30% | 8% | 9% |
| Synthetic non-absorbable | A non-absorbable sheet [e.g., Polyprolene (Marlex), polypropylene (Prolene) or expanded polytetrafluoroethylene (Gortex)] is sutured between the fascial edges | May be plicated, pleated, or reduced in size to achieve progressive fascial closure | Must be removed before definitive abdominal closure, does not prevent adhesion formation, a high rate of fistula formation has been reported with use of polypropylene | | | | |

(continued)

Table 93.4 (continued)

| Type | Description | Advantages | Disadvantages | Prognostic estimates[a] | | | |
|---|---|---|---|---|---|---|---|
| | | | | 1° Fascial closure | Mortality | Fistula | Abscess |
| Biologic | A biologic material [e.g., Human acellular dermal matrix (Alloderm)] is sutured between the fascial edges | Does not need to be removed during abdominal closure | Expensive, does not prevent adhesion formation, a high rate of abdominal wall laxity has been reported during medium-term follow-up | NA | NA | NA | NA |
| *Artificial burr* | | | | | | | |
| Wittmann patch[b] | Two opposing Velcro sheets are sutured to the fascial edges, which overlap in the middle, allowing for progressive fascial reapproximation | Has been associated with a high primary fascial closure rate in prognostic studies | Sutures may potentially increase risk for ischemia/necrosis of the fascial edges, does not control peritoneal fluid (unless combined with negative pressure wound therapy) | 78–90% | 16–17% | 2–3% | 2–3% |
| *Negative pressure wound therapy[c]* | | | | | | | |
| Barker's vacuum pack | The abdominal viscera is covered with a perforated, nonadherent plastic sheet, which is tucked under the parietal peritoneum and into the pericolic gutters. This drape is covered with surgical towels and two closed suction, surgical drains (the towels may be omitted if there is concern about the viability of the bowel). After a transparent adhesive drape is placed over the wound to create an airtight seal, the drains are connected to wall suction | Low cost, may be applied rapidly, universally available, controls peritoneal fluid, prevents visceral adhesion to the peritoneum, may maintain constant negative pressure on the laparotomy wound without damaging the fascia | May not provide as effective or uniform negative pressure to the laparotomy wound or peritoneum (particularly in the pericolic gutters) when compared to the VAC or ABThera™ | 52% | 27% | 6% | 4% |
| VAC RENASYS-F/AB abdominal dressing (Smith and Nephew, Inc., Canada and USA) or KCI VAC (San Antonio, TX, USA) | The abdominal viscera is covered with a nonadherent, perforated plastic drape and a piece of black polyurethane foam is placed between the Laparotomy wound edges. After a transparent adhesive drape is placed over the wound and surrounding skin, this airtight seal is pierced by a suction drainage system and connected to a suction pump and fluid collection system | May be applied rapidly, controls Peritoneal fluid, prevents visceral adhesion to the peritoneum, maintains constant negative pressure on the laparotomy wound without damaging the fascia | Relatively more expensive, concern regarding a higher rate of abdominal fistulae and recurrent ACS | 60% | 18% | 3% | 3% |

| | | | | | | |
|---|---|---|---|---|---|---|
| ABThera™ Open abdomen NPT system (San Antonio, TX, USA) | The abdominal viscera is covered by a protective layer Comprised of 6 radiating foam extensions enveloped in a sheet with small fenestrations. A superficial perforated foam layer is then placed over top of the protective layer. An adhesive open abdomen drape is then placed atop the wound and adjacent skin and an interface pad with a tubing system is applied and connected to a negative pressure source | May be applied rapidly, effectively drains fluid throughout the peritoneum in theory, prevents visceral adhesion to the peritoneum, maintains constant negative pressure on the laparotomy wound without damaging the fascia | Relatively more expensive, concern regarding a higher rate of abdominal fistulae and recurrent ACS | NA | NA | NA |

*KCI* Kinetic Concepts, Inc., *NA* not available, *NPT* negative pressure therapy, *RCT* randomized controlled trial, *VAC* vacuum-assisted closure
[a] Estimates derived from systematic reviews of largely unweighted, uncontrolled cohort studies that included heterogeneous populations of surgical patients, many of whom would not have had ACS at the time of the index laparotomy
[b] Presently, these methods are likely uncommonly used for patient management in the intensive care unit post-decompressive laparotomy [78]
[c] The WSACS—The Abdominal Compartment Society recommends strategies that employ negative pressure wound therapy for TAC [1]

in patients without discontinuity of the gastrointestinal tract [83]. Enteral tube feeding is associated with improved fascial closure rates, reduced complications, and increased survival, though the ideal site for delivery of feeds (e.g., stomach, duodenum, or jejunum) remains to be elucidated [2, 93].

### 93.3.8 Abdominal Reconstruction

Ideally, patients with TAC return to the operating room as soon as safe and possible for attempted fascial closure. When such closure is not possible, patients should undergo staged abdominal reconstruction, which is generally feasible in patients with wounds without fixation or those developing fixation that lack contamination (classes 1 and 2A, as discussed above) [94]. Numerous methods of staged abdominal reconstruction exist, including vacuum-assisted closure, vacuum-assisted mesh-mediated fascial traction, the Wittmann patch, dynamic retention with sutures or commercial devices, the Abdominal Re-Approximation Anchor (ABRA®) abdominal wall closure device (CJ Medical), and progressive closure with plication or pleating of a synthetic patch between the edges of the fascia [80, 94–100]. The underlying principles of staged abdominal reconstruction include preventing fixity of the abdominal viscera for the underlying peritoneal peritoneum, minimization of bowel manipulation (to prevent fistula formation), prevention of lateralization of the abdominal wall by maintaining tension toward the midline, and progressively closing the fascia between dressing changes [1, 94, 101]. Despite all efforts, some patients cannot be primarily closed on the index hospitalization. Abdominal closure should therefore be planned after a convalescence period in which the patient regains their health and cardiovascular fitness, BMI is reduced, and CT evaluation of the abdominal wall assesses the anatomy to allow re-approximation of the rectus muscles with or without advanced techniques such as anterior component or transversus abdominis releases.

### 93.3.9 Prognosis

IAH and ACS are associated with considerable morbidity and mortality. A higher risk of multi-organ dysfunction in general ICU patients has been reported in patients with IAH than those without it after adjusting for differences in case-mix [17, 21]. Further, there is an up to 24% increase in mortality associated with IAH in ICU patients and a near-50% mortality among those patients undergoing laparotomy for ACS [23, 102, 103]. Therefore, preventing IAH and reducing IAP may potentially reduce morbidity and mortality. However, no randomized controlled trial has yet been conducted to substantiate this.

## 93.4 Conclusions

IAH is commonly encountered during critical care, but the majority of individuals working in the ICU may be unaware of the relevant clinical guidelines. IAH is graded based on the severity of sustained or repeated intra-abdominal pressure elevations, while ACS is defined by an intra-abdominal pressure > 20 mm Hg with organ dysfunction attributable to IAH. IAH/ACS can have broad and severe effects on nearly all organ systems, and ACS is associated with considerable mortality. IAH should be measured in any at-risk, critically ill patient, with treatment initiated promptly. Medical management should focus on increasing abdominal wall compliance, avoiding over-resuscitation (especially with crystalloid fluids), reducing overall fluid balance, and evacuating gastrointestinal contents, while interventional or surgical intervention is recommended for treatment of ACS. A number of methods exist for TAC and staged abdominal reconstruction following decompressive laparotomy, and efforts should be made to close the abdomen as soon as is feasible.

The understanding and management of IAH/ACS is an evolving area of research. To date, no randomized controlled trial has reported that measurement of IAP and treatment of IAH improves patient-important outcomes in critically ill or injured patients. Moving forward, further studies are required to investigate whether multifaceted strategies of measuring and treating IAH are associated with improved patient-important outcomes in critically ill or injured patients. Lack of clinical trial evidence to support such strategies may explain why some clinicians do not routinely measure IAP. This type of evidence may therefore improve guideline adherence and further understanding of optimal management strategies for IAH/ACS.

> **Dos and Don'ts**
> - *Do* avoid excessive fluid resuscitation in critically ill or injured patients where possible.
> - *Do* focus on improving abdominal wall compliance and evacuating intra- and extraluminal contents in patients with IAH.
> - *Do* proceed with decompressive laparotomy in patients who develop overt ACS when other interventions have failed.
> - *Do not* perform primary fascial closure when signs of ACS develop during closure.
> - *Do* close the abdomen after opening it as soon as is feasible.

> **Take-Home Messages**
> - IAP should be measured in any critically ill or injured patient with any known risk factor for IAH or ACS.
> - IAP should be measured at end expiration via the bladder following instillation of no more than 25 mL of sterile saline with the patient supine and an absence of contraction of the abdominal wall musculature.
> - In adult patients, IAH is graded as Grade I (12–15 mm Hg), Grade II (16–20 mm Hg), Grade III (21–25 mm Hg), and Grade IV (>25 mm Hg), while ACS is defined as IAP ≥20 mm Hg with new organ dysfunction.
> - Medical management of IAH involves improving abdominal wall compliance, correction of positive fluid balance, and evacuation of gastrointestinal contents, while overt ACS should be managed with emergent decompressive laparotomy in the operating room or ICU.
> - Following decompressive laparotomy, TAC should be facilitated with a negative pressure wound therapy device.

**Suggested Reading**
- WSACS Consensus Definitions and Clinical Guidelines [1].
- The Open Abdomen in Trauma and Non-Trauma Patients: The World Society of Emergency Surgery Guidelines [75].
- Eastern Association of Trauma: Open Abdomen in Trauma and Emergency General Surgery, Management of: Part 1 [83].
- Eastern Association of Trauma: Open Abdomen Management, A Review: Part 2 [104].

> **Review Questions**
> 1. In healthy adults, the normal IAP is expected to be:
>    A. 1–4 mm Hg.
>    B. **5–7 mm Hg.**
>    C. 7–14 mm Hg.
>    D. 15–20 mm Hg.
> 2. Which of the following is not predictive of increased IAP?
>    A. BMI.
>    B. Abdominal diameter.
>    C. **Supine positioning, compared to HOB elevation.**
>    D. Critical illness.
> 3. ACS is:
>    A. Diagnosed in all patients with IAP over 25 mm Hg.

B. A diagnosis best made using imaging studies (e.g., CT scan).
   C. Treated by opening the abdomen via laparotomy and leaving the abdomen open as long as possible.
   D. **Diagnosed based on a sustained IAP above 20 mmHg and new or progressive organ dysfunction or failure.**
4. IAP should be measured:
   A. **In any critically ill or injured patient with any known risk factor for IAH or ACS.**
   B. Via the rectum after instillation of 25 mL of water via the rectal tube.
   C. With the HOB elevated to 30°, to reduce risk of pneumonia.
   D. Only in patients undergoing emergency laparotomy.
5. Medical management of IAH/ACS includes all of the following, except:
   A. Decompression of the gastrointestinal tract with nasogastric or rectal tubes.
   B. **Preferential use of fentanyl, as it has been shown to reduce IAP.**
   C. Correction of highly positive fluid balance.
   D. Administering neuromuscular blocking agents as a bridge to surgical intervention.
6. A 63-year-old-man is admitted to the ICU with severe acute pancreatitis. He is intubated and sedated, has nasogastric and rectal tubes in situ, and recently had a large intra-abdominal fluid collection drained percutaneously. IAP measured via the bladder is 29 mm Hg and he is increasingly distended with minimal urine output. His oxygen requirements are increasing, he is now tachycardic at 125 beats per minute, and is newly requiring vasopressor support with two agents. The best treatment at this time is:
   A. Increased sedation to try to relax the abdominal wall further.
   B. Urgent CT and drainage of any other intra-abdominal collections.
   C. **Urgent decompressive laparotomy.**
   D. Intravenous furosemide to diurese the patient and decrease his fluid balance.
7. Following decompressive laparotomy for a 48-year-old woman with overt ACS, which of the following TAC methods is recommended?
   A. **A negative pressure wound therapy device.**
   B. Closure of the skin only with sutures or towel clips.
   C. Definitive fascial closure regardless of signs of ACS during attempted closure.
   D. Up-front component separation in all patients at the index laparotomy to facilitate eventual fascial closure.
8. Definitive fascial closure following decompressive laparotomy should be attempted:
   A. **As soon as safe and possible.**
   B. Only after interval management with a planned ventral hernia for 4–6 weeks.
   C. Only once the abdominal viscera develop fixation.
   D. In a staged fashion as long as the wound is class 3 or 4 (frozen abdomen or established enteroatmospheric fistula and frozen abdomen).
9. Which of the following is not a risk factor for development of enteroatmospheric fistula?
   A. Receipt of greater than 10 L of fluid resuscitation.

B. Large bowel resection.
C. Increased length of time that the abdomen is left open.
D. **Early re-exploration to attempt abdominal closure.**

10. Which of the following patients are at high risk of IAH/ACS?
    A. A patient with extensive burns to the thorax and upper/lower extremities, but sparing the abdomen.
    B. A patient admitted to the ICU following repair of a ruptured AAA.
    C. A patient with severe acute pancreatitis.
    D. **All of the above.**

## References

1. Kirkpatrick AW, Roberts DJ, De Waele J, Jaeschke R, Malbrain MLNG, De Keulenaer B, et al. Intra-abdominal hypertension and the abdominal compartment syndrome: updated consensus definitions and clinical practice guidelines from the world Society of the Abdominal Compartment Syndrome. Intensive Care Med. 2013;39(7):1190–206.
2. Roberts DJ, De Waele JJ, Kirkpatrick AW, Malbrain MLNG. Intra-abdominal hypertension and the abdominal compartment syndrome. In: O'Donnell JM, Nácul FE, editors. Surgical intensive care medicine. Cham: Springer International Publishing; 2016. p. 621–44.
3. Wise R, Rodseth R, Blaser A, Roberts D, De Waele J, Kirkpatrick A, et al. Awareness and knowledge of intra-abdominal hypertension and abdominal compartment syndrome: results of a repeat, international, cross-sectional survey. Anaesthesiol Intensive Ther. 2019;51(3):186–99.
4. Emerson H. Intra-abdominal pressures. Arch Intern Med. 1911;VII(6):754–84.
5. Schein M, Ivatury R. Intra-abdominal hypertension and the abdominal compartment syndrome. BJS. 1998;85(8):1027–8.
6. Baggot M. Abdominal blow-out: a concept. Curr Res Anesth Analg. 1951;30(5):295–9.
7. Fietsam RJ, Villalba M, Glover JL, Clark K. Intra-abdominal compartment syndrome as a complication of ruptured abdominal aortic aneurysm repair. Am Surg. 1989;55(6):396–402.
8. Malbrain MLNG, Cheatham ML, Kirkpatrick A, Sugrue M, Parr M, De Waele J, et al. Results from the international conference of experts on intra-abdominal hypertension and abdominal compartment syndrome. I Definitions. Intensive Care Med. 2006;32(11):1722–32.
9. Malbrain MLNG. Different techniques to measure intra-abdominal pressure (IAP): time for a critical reappraisal. Intensive Care Med. 2004;30(3):357–71.
10. Collard HR, Saint S, Matthay MA. Prevention of ventilator-associated pneumonia: an evidence-based systematic review. Ann Intern Med. 2003;138(6):494–501.
11. Cheatham ML, De Waele JJ, De Laet I, De Keulenaer B, Widder S, Kirkpatrick AW, et al. The impact of body position on intra-abdominal pressure measurement: a multicenter analysis. Crit Care Med. 2009;37(7):2187–90.
12. Ball CG, Kirkpatrick AW. "Progression towards the minimum": the importance of standardizing the priming volume during the indirect measurement of intra-abdominal pressures. Crit Care. 2006;10(4):153.
13. De Keulenaer BL, De Waele JJ, Powell B, Malbrain MLNG. What is normal intra-abdominal pressure and how is it affected by positioning, body mass and positive end-expiratory pressure? Intensive Care Med. 2009;35(6):969–76.
14. Sugerman H, Windsor A, Bessos M, Wolfe L. Intra-abdominal pressure, sagittal abdominal diameter and obesity comorbidity. J Intern Med. 1997;241(1):71–9.
15. Cheatham ML, White MW, Sagraves SG, Johnson JL, Block EF. Abdominal perfusion pressure: a superior parameter in the assessment of intra-abdominal hypertension. J Trauma. 2000;49(4):621–7.
16. Ball CG, Kirkpatrick AW, McBeth P. The secondary abdominal compartment syndrome: not just another post-traumatic complication. Can J Surg. 2008;51(5):399–405.
17. Reintam A, Parm P, Kitus R, Kern H, Starkopf J. Primary and secondary intra-abdominal hypertension—Different impact on ICU outcome. Intensive Care Med. 2008;34(9):1624–31.
18. Kirkpatrick AW, Nickerson D, Roberts DJ, Rosen MJ, McBeth PB, Petro CC, et al. Intra-abdominal hypertension and abdominal compartment syndrome after abdominal wall reconstruction: quaternary syndromes? Scand J Surg. 2017;106(2):97–106.
19. Petro CC, Raigani S, Fayezizadeh M, Rowbottom JR, Klick JC, Prabhu AS, et al. Permissible intraabdominal hypertension following complex abdominal wall reconstruction. Plast Reconstr Surg. 2015;136(4):868–81.
20. Reintam Blaser A, Regli A, De Keulenaer B, Kimball EJ, Starkopf L, Davis WA, et al. Incidence, risk factors, and outcomes of intra-abdominal

hypertension in critically ill patients: a prospective multicenter study (IROI study). Crit Care Med. 2019;47(4):535–42.
21. Vidal MG, Ruiz Weisser J, Gonzalez F, Toro MA, Loudet C, Balasini C, et al. Incidence and clinical effects of intra-abdominal hypertension in critically ill patients. Crit Care Med. 2008;36(6):1823–31.
22. Malbrain MLNG, Chiumello D, Pelosi P, Bihari D, Innes R, Ranieri VM, et al. Incidence and prognosis of intraabdominal hypertension in a mixed population of critically ill patients: a multiple-center epidemiological study. Crit Care Med. 2005;33(2):315–22.
23. Malbrain MLNG, Chiumello D, Cesana BM, Reintam Blaser A, Starkopf J, Sugrue M, et al. A systematic review and individual patient data meta-analysis on intra-abdominal hypertension in critically ill patients: the wake-up project. World initiative on abdominal hypertension epidemiology, a unifying project (WAKE-up!). Minerva Anestesiol. 2014;80(3):293–306.
24. Chen X, Gestring ML, Rosengart MR, Billiar TR, Peitzman AB, Sperry JL, et al. Speed is not everything: identifying patients who may benefit from helicopter transport despite faster ground transport. J Trauma Acute Care Surg. 2018;84(4):549–57.
25. Ke L, Ni H-B, Sun J-K, Tong Z-H, Li W-Q, Li N, et al. Risk factors and outcome of intra-abdominal hypertension in patients with severe acute pancreatitis. World J Surg. 2012;36(1):171–8.
26. Chen H, Li F, Sun J-B, Jia J-G. Abdominal compartment syndrome in patients with severe acute pancreatitis in early stage. World J Gastroenterol. 2008;14(22):3541–8.
27. Keskinen P, Leppaniemi A, Pettila V, Piilonen A, Kemppainen E, Hynninen M. Intra-abdominal pressure in severe acute pancreatitis. World J Emerg Surg. 2007;2:2.
28. Hobson KG, Young KM, Ciraulo A, Palmieri TL, Greenhalgh DG. Release of abdominal compartment syndrome improves survival in patients with burn injury. J Trauma. 2002;53(6):1124–9.
29. Ivy ME, Atweh NA, Palmer J, Possenti PP, Pineau M, D'Aiuto M. Intra-abdominal hypertension and abdominal compartment syndrome in burn patients. J Trauma. 2000;49(3):387–91.
30. Oda J, Yamashita K, Inoue T, Harunari N, Ode Y, Mega K, et al. Resuscitation fluid volume and abdominal compartment syndrome in patients with major burns. Burns. 2006;32(2):151–4.
31. Roberts DJ, Ball CG, Feliciano DV, Moore EE, Ivatury RR, Lucas CE, et al. History of the innovation of damage control for management of trauma patients: 1902-2016. Ann Surg. 2017;265(5):1034–44.
32. Balogh ZJ, Lumsdaine W, Moore EE, Moore FA. Postinjury abdominal compartment syndrome: from recognition to prevention. Lancet. 2014;384(9952):1466–75.
33. Karkos CD, Menexes GC, Patelis N, Kalogirou TE, Giagtzidis IT, Harkin DW. A systematic review and meta-analysis of abdominal compartment syndrome after endovascular repair of ruptured abdominal aortic aneurysms. J Vasc Surg. 2014;59(3):829–42.
34. Carr JA. Abdominal compartment syndrome: a decade of progress. J Am Coll Surg. 2013;216(1):135–46.
35. Malbrain MLNG, De laet I. It's all in the gut: introducing the concept of acute bowel injury and acute intestinal distress syndrome. Crit Care Med. 2009;37:365–6.
36. Malbrain MLNG, Vidts W, Ravyts M, De Laet I, De Waele J. Acute intestinal distress syndrome: the importance of intra-abdominal pressure. Minerva Anestesiol. 2008;74(11):657–73.
37. Al-Mufarrej F, Abell LM, Chawla LS. Understanding intra-abdominal hypertension: from the bench to the bedside. J Intensive Care Med. 2012;27(3):145–60.
38. Cheng J, Wei Z, Liu X, Li X, Yuan Z, Zheng J, et al. The role of intestinal mucosa injury induced by intra-abdominal hypertension in the development of abdominal compartment syndrome and multiple organ dysfunction syndrome. Crit Care. 2013;17(6):R283.
39. Emr B, Sadowsky D, Azhar N, Gatto LA, An G, Nieman GF, et al. Removal of inflammatory ascites is associated with dynamic modification of local and systemic inflammation along with prevention of acute lung injury: in vivo and in silico studies. Shock. 2014;41(4):317–23.
40. Shah SK, Jimenez F, Walker PA, Aroom KR, Xue H, Feeley TD, et al. A novel mechanism for neutrophil priming in trauma: potential role of peritoneal fluid. Surgery. 2010;148(2):263–70.
41. Shah SK, Jimenez F, Walker PA, Xue H, Feeley TD, Uray KS, et al. Peritoneal fluid: a potential mechanism of systemic neutrophil priming in experimental intra-abdominal sepsis. Am J Surg. 2012;203(2):211–6.
42. Miller PR, Thompson JT, Faler BJ, Meredith JW, Chang MC. Late fascial closure in lieu of ventral hernia: the next step in open abdomen management. J Trauma. 2002;53(5):843–9.
43. Clements TW, Tolonen M, Ball CG, Kirkpatrick AW. Secondary peritonitis and intra-abdominal sepsis: an increasingly global disease in search of better systemic therapies. Scand J Surg. 2021;1457496920984078
44. Yamamoto T, Umegae S, Matsumoto K, Saniabadi AR. Peritoneal cytokines as early markers of peritonitis following surgery for colorectal carcinoma: a prospective study. Cytokine. 2011;53(2):239–42.
45. Cavriani G, Domingos HV, Soares AL, Trezena AG, Ligeiro-Oliveira AP, Oliveira-Filho RM, et al. Lymphatic system as a path underlying the spread of lung and gut injury after intestinal ischemia/reperfusion in rats. Shock. 2005;23(4):330–6.
46. Bloomfield GL, Ridings PC, Blocher CR, Marmarou A, Sugerman HJ. A proposed relation-

46. ship between increased intra-abdominal, intrathoracic, and intracranial pressure. Crit Care Med. 1997;25(3):496–503.
47. Youssef AM, Hamidian Jahromi A, Vijay CG, Granger DN, Alexander JS. Intra-abdominal hypertension causes reversible blood-brain barrier disruption. J Trauma Acute Care Surg. 2012;72(1):183–8.
48. Joseph DK, Dutton RP, Aarabi B, Scalea TM. Decompressive laparotomy to treat intractable intracranial hypertension after traumatic brain injury. J Trauma. 2004;57(4):685–7.
49. Ivatury R. Abdominal compartment syndrome. CRC Press; 2006.
50. Ridings PC, Bloomfield GL, Blocher CR, Sugerman HJ. Cardiopulmonary effects of raised intra-abdominal pressure before and after intravascular volume expansion. J Trauma. 1995;39(6):1071–5.
51. Mutoh T, Lamm WJ, Embree LJ, Hildebrandt J, Albert RK. Volume infusion produces abdominal distension, lung compression, and chest wall stiffening in pigs. J Appl Physiol. 1992;72(2):575–82.
52. Mohmand H, Goldfarb S. Renal dysfunction associated with intra-abdominal hypertension and the abdominal compartment syndrome. J Am Soc Nephrol. 2011;22(4):615–21.
53. Diebel LN, Dulchavsky SA, Wilson RF. Effect of increased intra-abdominal pressure on mesenteric arterial and intestinal mucosal blood flow. J Trauma. 1992;33(1):45–9.
54. Diebel LN, Dulchavsky SA, Brown WJ. Splanchnic ischemia and bacterial translocation in the abdominal compartment syndrome. J Trauma. 1997;43(5):852–5.
55. Kirkpatrick AW, Roberts DJ, De Waele J, Laupland K. Is intra-abdominal hypertension a missing factor that drives multiple organ dysfunction syndrome? Crit Care. 2014;18(2):124.
56. Kirkpatrick AW, Hamilton DR, McKee JL, MacDonald B, Pelosi P, Ball CG, et al. Do we have the guts to go? The abdominal compartment, intra-abdominal hypertension, the human microbiome and exploration class space missions. Can J Surg. 2020;63(6):E581–93.
57. Holodinsky JK, Roberts DJ, Ball CG, Blaser AR, Starkopf J, Zygun DA, et al. Risk factors for intra-abdominal hypertension and abdominal compartment syndrome among adult intensive care unit patients: a systematic review and meta-analysis. Crit Care. 2013;17(5):R249.
58. Yi M, Leng Y, Bai Y, Yao G, Zhu X. The evaluation of the effect of body positioning on intra-abdominal pressure measurement and the effect of intra-abdominal pressure at different body positioning on organ function and prognosis in critically ill patients. J Crit Care. 2012;27(2):222.e1–6.
59. Kirkpatrick AW, Brenneman FD, McLean RF, Rapanos T, Boulanger BR. Is clinical examination an accurate indicator of raised intra-abdominal pressure in critically injured patients? Can J Surg. 2000;43(3):207–11.
60. Al-Bahrani AZ, Abid GH, Sahgal E, O'shea S, Lee S, Ammori BJ. A prospective evaluation of CT features predictive of intra-abdominal hypertension and abdominal compartment syndrome in critically ill surgical patients. Clin Radiol. 2007;62(7):676–82.
61. Sugrue G, Malbrain MLNG, Pereira B, Wise R, Sugrue M. Modern imaging techniques in intra-abdominal hypertension and abdominal compartment syndrome: a bench to bedside overview. Anaesthesiol Intensive Ther. 2018;50(3):234–42.
62. De Laet I, Hoste E, Verholen E, De Waele JJ. The effect of neuromuscular blockers in patients with intra-abdominal hypertension. Intensive Care Med. 2007;33(10):1811–4.
63. Drummond GB, Duncan MK. Abdominal pressure during laparoscopy: effects of fentanyl. Br J Anaesth. 2002;88(3):384–8.
64. Souadka A, Mohsine R, Ifrine L, Belkouchi A, El Malki HO. Acute abdominal compartment syndrome complicating a colonoscopic perforation: a case report. J Med Case Rep. 2012;6:51.
65. Joseph B, Zangbar B, Pandit V, Vercruysse G, Aziz H, Kulvatunyou N, et al. The conjoint effect of reduced crystalloid administration and decreased damage-control laparotomy use in the development of abdominal compartment syndrome. J Trauma Acute Care Surg. 2014;76(2):457–61.
66. Ouellet J-F, Leppaniemi A, Ball CG, Cheatham ML, D'Amours S, Kirkpatrick AW. Alternatives to formal abdominal decompression. Am Surg. 2011;77(Suppl 1):S51–7.
67. Cheatham ML, Safcsak K. Percutaneous catheter decompression in the treatment of elevated intraabdominal pressure. Chest. 2011;140(6):1428–35.
68. Peng T, Dong L-M, Zhao X, Xiong J-X, Zhou F, Tao J, et al. Minimally invasive percutaneous catheter drainage versus open laparotomy with temporary closure for treatment of abdominal compartment syndrome in patients with early-stage severe acute pancreatitis. J Huazhong Univ Sci Technol. 2016;36(1):99–105.
69. Coccolini F, Gubbiotti F, Ceresoli M, Tartaglia D, Fugazzola P, Ansaloni L, et al. Open abdomen and fluid instillation in the septic abdomen: results from the IROA study. World J Surg. 2020;44(12):4032–40.
70. Zakaria ER, Garrison RN, Spain DA, Matheson PJ, Harris PD, Richardson JD. Intraperitoneal resuscitation improves intestinal blood flow following hemorrhagic shock. Ann Surg. 2003;237(5):703–4.
71. Weaver JL, Smith JW. Direct peritoneal resuscitation: a review. Int J Surg. 2016;33(Pt B):237–41.
72. Weaver JL, Matheson PJ, Matheson A, Graham VS, Downard C, Garrison RN, et al. Direct peritoneal resuscitation reduces inflammation in the kidney after acute brain death. Am J Physiol Renal Physiol. 2018;315(2):F406–12.
73. Smith JW, Ghazi CA, Cain BC, Hurt RT, Garrison RN, Matheson PJ. Direct peritoneal resuscitation

improves inflammation, liver blood flow, and pulmonary edema in a rat model of acute brain death. J Am Coll Surg. 2014;219(1):79–87.
74. Godat L, Kobayashi L, Costantini T, Coimbra R. Abdominal damage control surgery and reconstruction: world society of emergency surgery position paper. World J Emerg Surg. 2013;8(1):53.
75. Coccolini F, Roberts D, Ansaloni L, Ivatury R, Gamberini E, Kluger Y, et al. The open abdomen in trauma and non-trauma patients: WSES guidelines. World J Emerg Surg. 2018;13:7.
76. Anand RJ, Ivatury RR. Surgical management of intra-abdominal hypertension and abdominal compartment syndrome. Am Surg. 2011;77(Suppl 1):S42–5.
77. Van Damme L, De Waele JJ. Effect of decompressive laparotomy on organ function in patients with abdominal compartment syndrome: a systematic review and meta-analysis. Crit Care. 2018;22(1):179.
78. Boele van Hensbroek P, Wind J, Dijkgraaf MGW, Busch ORC, Goslings JC. Temporary closure of the open abdomen: a systematic review on delayed primary fascial closure in patients with an open abdomen. World J Surg. 2009;33(2):199–207.
79. Barker DE, Green JM, Maxwell RA, Smith PW, Mejia VA, Dart BW, et al. Experience with vacuum-pack temporary abdominal wound closure in 258 trauma and general and vascular surgical patients. J Am Coll Surg. 2007;204(5):783–4.
80. De Waele JJ, Leppäniemi AK. Temporary abdominal closure techniques. Am Surg. 2011;77(Suppl 1):S46–50.
81. Demetriades D, Salim A. Management of the open abdomen. Surg Clin North Am. 2014;94(1):131–53.
82. Quyn AJ, Johnston C, Hall D, Chambers A, Arapova N, Ogston S, et al. The open abdomen and temporary abdominal closure systems: historical evolution and systematic review. Color Dis. 2012;14(8):e429–38.
83. Diaz JJJ, Cullinane DC, Dutton WD, Jerome R, Bagdonas R, Bilaniuk JW, et al. The management of the open abdomen in trauma and emergency general surgery: part 1 - damage control. J Trauma. 2010;68(6):1425–38.
84. Kubiak BD, Albert SP, Gatto LA, Snyder KP, Maier KG, Vieau CJ, et al. Peritoneal negative pressure therapy prevents multiple organ injury in a chronic porcine sepsis and ischemia/reperfusion model. Shock. 2010;34(5):525–34.
85. Cheatham ML, Demetriades D, Fabian TC, Kaplan MJ, Miles WS, Schreiber MA, et al. Prospective study examining clinical outcomes associated with a negative pressure wound therapy system and Barker's vacuum packing technique. World J Surg. 2013;37(9):2018–30.
86. Carlson GL, Patrick H, Amin AI, McPherson G, MacLennan G, Afolabi E, et al. Management of the open abdomen: a national study of clinical outcome and safety of negative pressure wound therapy. Ann Surg. 2013;257(6):1154–9.
87. Kirkpatrick AW, Roberts DJ, Faris PD, Ball CG, Kubes P, Tiruta C, et al. Active negative pressure peritoneal therapy after abbreviated laparotomy: the intraperitoneal vacuum randomized controlled trial. Ann Surg. 2015;262(1):38–46.
88. Roberts DJ, Zygun DA, Grendar J, Ball CG, Robertson HL, Ouellet J-F, et al. Negative-pressure wound therapy for critically ill adults with open abdominal wounds: a systematic review. J Trauma Acute Care Surg. 2012;73(3):629–39.
89. Björck M, Bruhin A, Cheatham M, Hinck D, Kaplan M, Manca G, et al. Classification - important step to improve management of patients with an open abdomen. World J Surg. 2009;33(6):1154–7.
90. Bradley MJ, Dubose JJ, Scalea TM, Holcomb JB, Shrestha B, Okoye O, et al. Independent predictors of enteric fistula and abdominal sepsis after damage control laparotomy: results from the prospective AAST open abdomen registry. JAMA Surg. 2013;148(10):947–54.
91. Miller RS, Morris JAJ, Diaz JJJ, Herring MB, May AK. Complications after 344 damage-control open celiotomies. J Trauma. 2005;59(6):1364–5.
92. Coccolini F, Ceresoli M, Kluger Y, Kirkpatrick A, Montori G, Salvetti F, et al. Open abdomen and entero-atmospheric fistulae: An interim analysis from the international register of open abdomen (IROA). Injury. 2019;50(1):160–6.
93. Burlew CC, Moore EE, Cuschieri J, Jurkovich GJ, Codner P, Nirula R, et al. Who should we feed? Western trauma association multi-institutional study of enteral nutrition in the open abdomen after injury. J Trauma Acute Care Surg. 2012;73(6):1380–8.
94. Björck M, D'Amours SK, Hamilton AER. Closure of the open abdomen. Am Surg. 2011;77(Suppl 1):S58–61.
95. Acosta S, Bjarnason T, Petersson U, Pålsson B, Wanhainen A, Svensson M, et al. Multicentre prospective study of fascial closure rate after open abdomen with vacuum and mesh-mediated fascial traction. Br J Surg. 2011;98(5):735–43.
96. Acosta S, Björck M, Wanhainen A. Negative-pressure wound therapy for prevention and treatment of surgical-site infections after vascular surgery. Br J Surg. 2017;104(2):e75–84.
97. Wittmann DH, Aprahamian C, Bergstein JM, Edmiston CE, Frantzides CT, Quebbeman EJ, et al. A burr-like device to facilitate temporary abdominal closure in planned multiple laparotomies. Eur J Surg. 1993;159(2):75–9.
98. Miller PR, Meredith JW, Johnson JC, Chang MC. Prospective evaluation of vacuum-assisted fascial closure after open abdomen: planned ventral hernia rate is substantially reduced. Ann Surg. 2004;239(5):606–8.
99. Haddock C, Konkin DE, Blair NP. Management of the open abdomen with the abdominal Reapproximation anchor dynamic fascial closure system. Am J Surg. 2013;205(5):528–33; discussion 533

100. Bjarnason T, Montgomery A, Ekberg O, Acosta S, Svensson M, Wanhainen A, et al. One-year follow-up after open abdomen therapy with vacuum-assisted wound closure and mesh-mediated fascial traction. World J Surg. 2013;37(9):2031–8.
101. Ball CG. Damage control resuscitation: history, theory and technique. Can J Surg. 2014;57(1):55–60.
102. De Waele JJ, Hoste EA, Malbrain ML. Decompressive laparotomy for abdominal compartment syndrome—a critical analysis. Crit Care. 2006;10(2):R51.
103. Smit M, Koopman B, Dieperink W, Hulscher JBF, Hofker HS, van Meurs M, et al. Intra-abdominal hypertension and abdominal compartment syndrome in patients admitted to the ICU. Ann Intensive Care. 2020;10(1):130.
104. Diaz JJJ, Dutton WD, Ott MM, Cullinane DC, Alouidor R, Armen SB, et al. Review of the management of the open abdomen: part 2 - management of the open abdomen. J Trauma. 2011;71(2):502–12.

# Open Abdomen Management

Pradeep Navsaria, Deidre McPherson, Sorin Edu, and Andrew Nicol

**Learning Goals**
- Indications for open abdomen—when to leave the abdomen open?
- Techniques of TAC—which method of OA should I use?
- Managing the OA—how do I maintain a good OA dressing?
- Complications of OA—how do I prevent and manage complications of an OA?

## 94.1 Introduction

Open abdomen (OA) care has expanded rapidly over the last four decades. The OA is associated with significant morbidity and high mortality. OA management poses a formidable challenge to the surgeon and wound care practitioners. The benefits of managing patients with OAs include prevention of intra-abdominal hypertension (IAH) and abdominal compartment syndrome (ACS), and allow for ease of re-entry for planned relook laparotomies and early identification of intra-abdominal complications such as bleeding anastomotic breakdown and fistulae. Despite these benefits, the application and maintenance of an OA presents numerous technical management challenges especially once the development of sepsis and fistulae occurs. Furthermore, prolonged maintenance of an OA may also result in fixation of the abdominal contents and lateralization of the aponeurosis with reduced chances of re-approximation of the fascia resulting in large complex ventral hernias. With increasing adoption of the OA there is an increased demand for temporary abdominal closure (TAC) methods (laparostomy) to protect the exposed viscera. Several techniques of TAC have been described but their safety and effectiveness remain under considerable debate and scrutiny. Negative pressure wound therapy (NPWT) has revolutionized TAC methods and features as a dominant adjunct for TAC when managing the OA.

## 94.2 Aetiology

The acute care surgeon is frequently confronted with hypotensive patients either with catastrophic *traumatic intra-abdominal bleeding* or severe *intra-abdominal sepsis*.

P. Navsaria (✉) · D. McPherson · S. Edu · A. Nicol
Trauma Center, Groote Schuur Hospital, University of Cape Town, Cape Town, South Africa
e-mail: pradeep.navsaria@uct.ac.za; andrew.nicol@uct.ac.za

### 94.2.1 Traumatic Intra-Abdominal Bleeding

When presented with a shocked, hypotensive patient following abdominal trauma, *damage control resuscitation* (DCR) must be initiated in the prehospital period, emergency front-room and the operating theatre. The five pillars of DCR include *rewarming* the patient, correction of *acidosis*, *permissive* hypotension, *restricting* clear 'fluid' administration and applying *haemostatic* resuscitation protocols. In addition, damage control surgery (DCS) entails an abbreviated laparotomy aimed at arresting the bleeding and preventing intestinal spillage in an attempt to halt the vicious cycle of acidosis, hypothermia and coagulopathy. Following DCS, the abdomen is left open with application of a temporary dressing to allow for rapid and easy re-entry and prevention of IAH and ACS. Damage control surgery combined with DCR improves 30-day survival [1].

### 94.2.2 Intra-Abdominal Sepsis

Recent evidence suggests that leaving the abdominal cavity open together with negative pressure suction therapy has the potential to mitigate biomediator spillage from the abdominal cavity into the systemic circulation in presence of severe abdominal sepsis [2]. It has been suggested that this modus operandi allows for the early identification and increased drainage of any residual sepsis, control of the persistent source of infection, more effective removal of biomediator-rich peritoneal fluid, effective avoidance of IAH and to safely allow for delayed gastrointestinal anastomoses [3]. Despite the absence of compelling evidence of efficacy, use of the OA after laparotomy for sepsis is increasingly being recommended [4–6]. This includes consensus recommendations from recognized societies such as the World Society of the Abdominal Compartment Syndrome and the World Society of Emergency Surgery who have stated that despite lack of high-quality data, OA use might be an important option in the treatment of severe peritonitis [6], a position reaffirmed in 2018, although the lack of evidence was again emphasized [7]. Thus, although unexplained, significantly improved survival with more efficient OA management using safer temporary abdominal closure devices does seem to warrant continued studies, especially as there appears to be much clinical adoption without sound scientific evidence to base this upon. Therefore, a multi-centre multi-national prospective randomized trial addressing this question in those requiring source control laparotomies for severe complicated intra-abdominal sepsis has recently launched globally [3]. Although intensive care services are critically limited globally, employing the OA is logistically possible even in rudimentary critical care settings [8]. Thus, if this technique truly abrogates systemic sepsis and post-peritonitis multiple organ failure, then this may be a truly impactful surgical strategy. The surgical community is therefore hopeful that this.

collaboration answers two critical questions in the management of secondary peritonitis/IAS, as well as lays a collaborative framework to continue to definitely answer critical questions for some of the world's most vulnerable patients [9].

Having noted the above, there is no doubt that the surviving sepsis campaign (SSC) guidelines have improved mortality in patients with severe sepsis. The recently revised guidelines have combined the 3-h and 6-h bundles into a single 'hour-1- bundle' with the explicit intention of initiating immediate resuscitation and management by measuring lactate levels, obtaining blood cultures, administering broad spectrum antibiotics, rapid infusion of crystalloid at 30 mL/kg for hypotension or lactate levels >4 mmol/L, and application of vasopressors to maintain mean arterial pressure greater than 65 mmHg [10]. This is closely followed by a laparotomy for septic source-control with or without surgical damage control principles.

Fig. 94.1 summarizes the approach to patients who are hypotensive secondary to abdominal bleeding (traumatic haemorrhagic shock) and abdominal sepsis (septic shock).

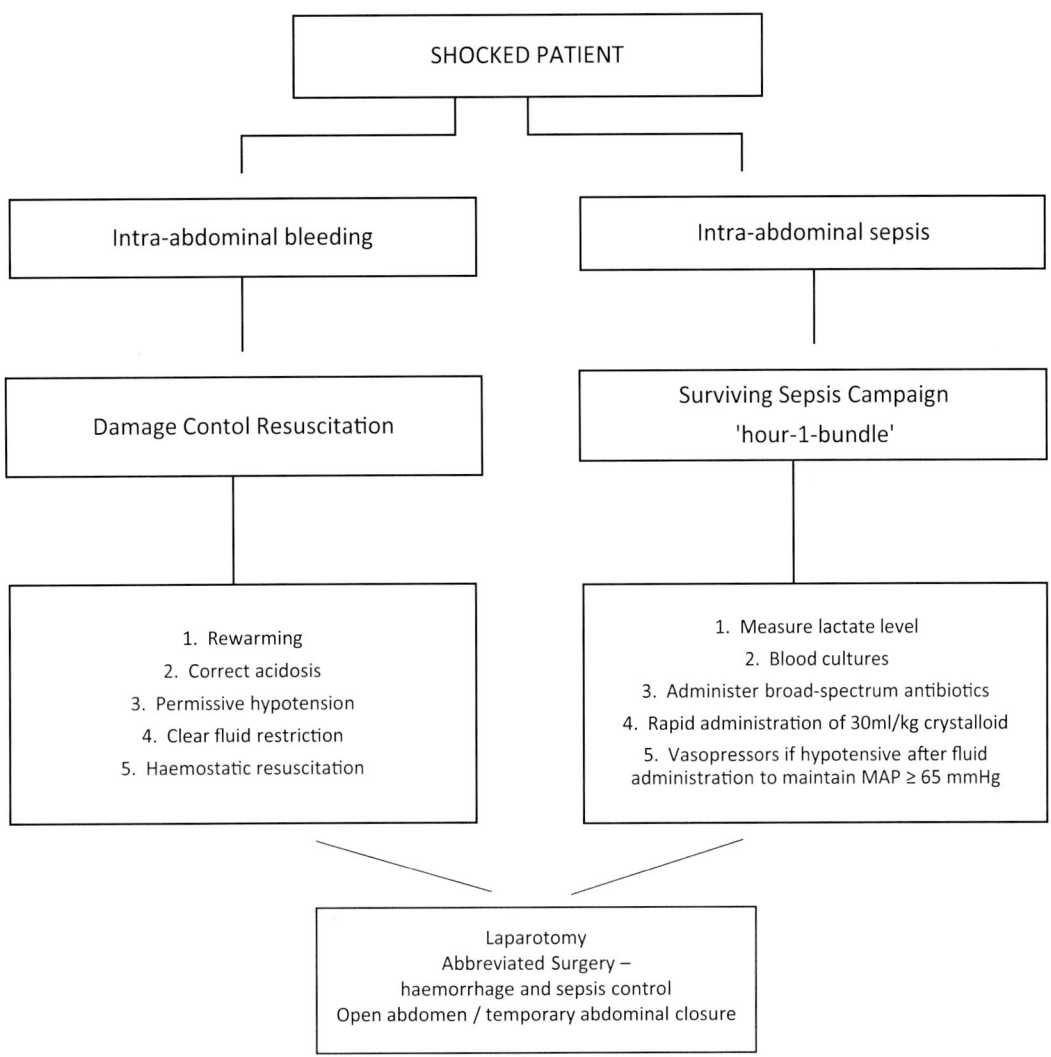

**Fig. 94.1** Management algorithm for the acutely shocked patient

## 94.2.3 Indications for OA: Trauma

- Damage control surgery in the presence of persistent hypotension, acidosis, hypothermia, coagulopathy and aggressive resuscitation.
- Risk factors for abdominal compartment syndrome: DCS, planned relooks, intra-abdominal packing.
- Established abdominal compartment syndrome.

## 94.2.4 Indications for OA: Non-Trauma

- Peritonitis: severe sepsis/septic shock requiring abbreviated laparotomy.
- Planned relook for intestinal ischaemia.
- Vascular emergencies: ruptured abdominal aortic aneurysm, occlusive and non-occlusive mesenteric ischaemia.
- Abdominal compartment syndrome associated with pancreatitis.

Table 94.1 Björck open abdomen classification (2016) [16]

| Grade | Description |
|---|---|
| 1A | Clean OA without adherence bowel and abdominal wall or fixity |
| 1B | Contaminated OA without adherence or fixity |
| 1C | Enteric leak, no fixation |
| 2A | Clean OA developing adherence or fixity |
| 2B | Contaminated OA developing adherence or fixity |
| 2C | Enteric leak, developing fixation |
| 3A | Clean, frozen abdomen |
| 3B | Contaminated frozen abdomen |
| 4 | Enteroatmospheric fistula, frozen abdomen |

A classification of the OA has been proposed to allow for improved reporting of OA status, standardization of clinical guidelines for improving OA management and to facilitate comparisons between studies and heterogenous patient populations [11]. This classification system will facilitate communication, clarify OA management and potentially improve patient care (Table 94.1).

## 94.3 Diagnosis

The term 'open abdomen' refers to an abdominal wall defect created by intentionally leaving an abdominal incision open that exposes abdominal viscera at the completion of intra-abdominal surgery or by opening or reopening the abdomen because of concern for abdominal compartment syndrome, ongoing intra-abdominal bleeding or intra-abdominal sepsis. The OA is managed with temporary abdominal closure using one of several techniques, followed by interval abdominal closure, preferably by bringing the edges of the abdominal fascia together primarily (primary closure) or, if this is not feasible, using a functional closure or simple coverage.

## 94.4 Treatment

### 94.4.1 Temporary Abdominal Closure Techniques

The ideal TAC dressing should be inexpensive and cost-effective, simple, easy and rapidly performed, allow for easy re-entry, keep the patient dry, allow for dressing change at the bedside, be able to both quantitate (how much?) and qualitate (blood, intestinal content, bile, urine) fluid loss, maintain sterility, material used should be biologically inert, preserve integrity of the abdominal wall and support a high definitive fascial closure rate, have a low fistula rate and prevent the abdominal compartment syndrome.

A variety of techniques of (TAC) have been described [12–20]. They are similar in surgical principles and allow for sequential re-entry into the abdomen. However, each method uses different materials and is a slight variation of the other. The authors employ the *modified sandwich-vacuum pack* [21]. This technique is an adaptation of three previously described techniques of TAC: the 'sandwich technique' (Schein et al. 1986) [12], the Barker 'vacuum-pack' (Brock et al. 1995) [13] and the 'Bogota Bag' by Torres and Borraez [22] (Fig. 94.2). In the original sandwich technique of TAC, a polypropylene mesh (Marlex) was *sutured* to the surrounding fascia and the wound covered by an adhesive polyurethane drape wound dressing with interposition suction tubes for drainage. The sutureless vacuum-pack described by Brock et al. consists of the placement of a *fenestrated* polyethylene sheet between the abdominal viscera and the anterior parietal peritoneum, the placement of a *sterile surgical towel* over the polyethylene sheet with two closed suction drains over the towel and the placement of an adhesive drape over the entire wound with continuous suction applied to the drains. The use of opened plastic bags, such as the type used for intravenous fluid or urological irrigation has been reported and sporadically acknowledged as a practice used extensively with success in hospitals in Columbia, South America [14]. The modified sandwich-vacuum pack differs in that a sterile surgical towel and Marlex mesh is not used, and no material is sutured to the rectus sheath. The technique, however, employs the insertion of interrupted tension-free sutures to the sheath to prevent retraction of the rectus sheath.

Unlike the previous methods described, we utilize NGTs as drainage and suction tubes and bring them out through the plastic adhesive drape

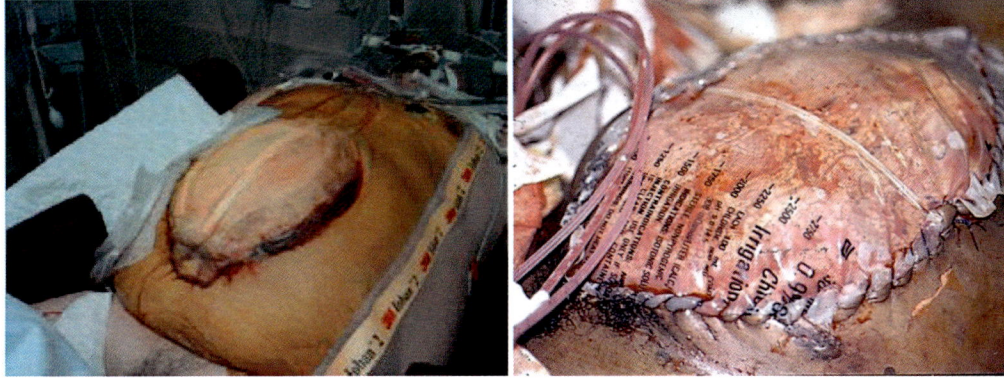

**Fig. 94.2** 'Sandwich technique', 'vacuum pack' and 'Bogota Bag' temporary abdominal closure. 'Sandwich technique' (Schein et al. [12]). Vacuum-pack (Brock et al. [13]). 'Bogota Bag' closure (Borraez et al. [14]). Reproduced with permission from Madbak FG and Lawless RA. Historical Perspective in Madbak FG, Dangleben DA, editors. Options in the Management of the Open Abdomen. Springer New York Heidelberg Dordrecht London; 2015. p 1–8.doi 10.1007/978-1-4939-1827-0.

through a drainage bag. The modified sandwich-vacuum pack technique utilizes an opened 3-L urological irrigation bag (Fig. 94.3). At the end of the laparotomy (a) the opened plastic bag is placed within the peritoneal cavity between the viscera and the parietal peritoneum of the anterior abdominal wall (b). The edges of the irrigation bag are placed at least 5 cm from the fascia edges. The rectus-sheath is then loosely approximated with tension-free interrupted 1-Nylon sutures (c). Two large-bore nasogastric tubes (NGTs) are placed into the middle of the wound, one into each apex, between the opened plastic irrigation bag and Nylon sutures (d). The surrounding skin is cleaned and dried. Old Fashioned Balsam Spray (Sangene Products cc, Newlands, South Africa) is applied to the surrounding skin and every effort is made to prevent any soiling of the skin. Any stomas and/or drain sites are covered with an appropriate pouching system. An Opsite™ (Smith & Nephew Medical Ltd., England) adhesive polyurethane drape is applied to the entire wound, with the two NGTs being brought through the centre of the drape through a small hole (e; f). A drainage bag is applied onto the adhesive drape over the site where the NGTs exit and the NGTs are brought out through the bottom of the drainage bag and a seal secured around the exit with 25 mm Elastoplast® fabric roll plaster (Smith & Nephew Ltd., Pinetown, South Africa) (h). The two NGTs are connected via a Y-connector to a wall pressure suction unit with a vacuum source of 80–100 mmHg (i). This forms the completed vacuum seal (j). The finished closure is secure, firm, airtight and dry. The fistula, definitive facial closure and mortality rates associated with this technique are 5, 53% and 45%, respectively. The advantages of the

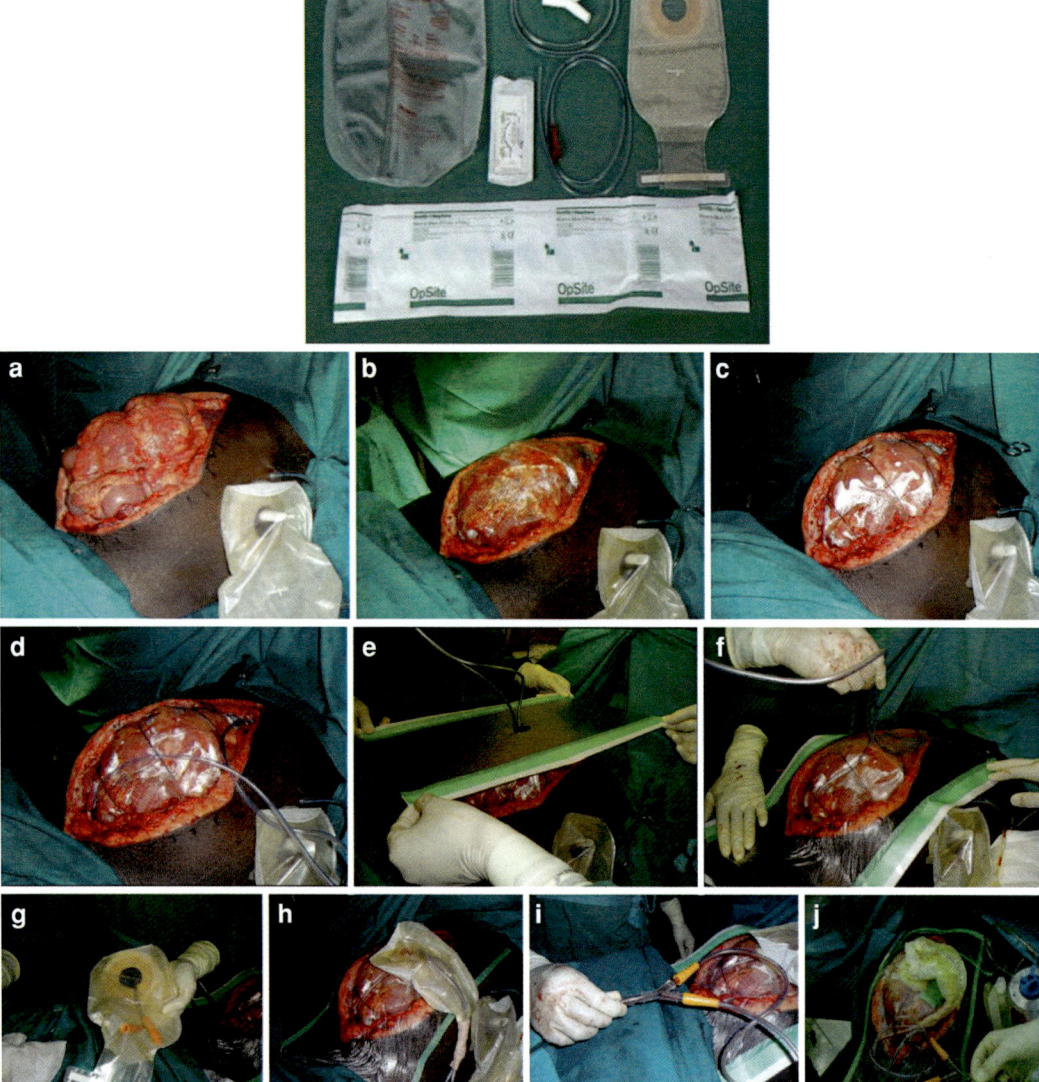

**Fig. 94.3** Temporary abdominal closure using readily available items found in any operating room[21]

technique described above are the ease in execution, low cost and readily available components required to establish a TAC dressing. The disadvantage, however, is the low fascial closure rate.

The two most commonly used commercially available negative-pressure TAC dressings systems are the ABThera™ System (KCI, USA, Inc., San Antonio, TX) and the RENASYS-AB™ Abdominal Dressing and RENASYS EZ pump (Smith & Nephew; St Petersburg, FL, USA). Both these commercially available products utilize an inert plastic covering as an organ protection layer, polyurethane foam dressing and a vacuum device to apply measured constant suction. The authors are most familiar with the latter system and the system is described here

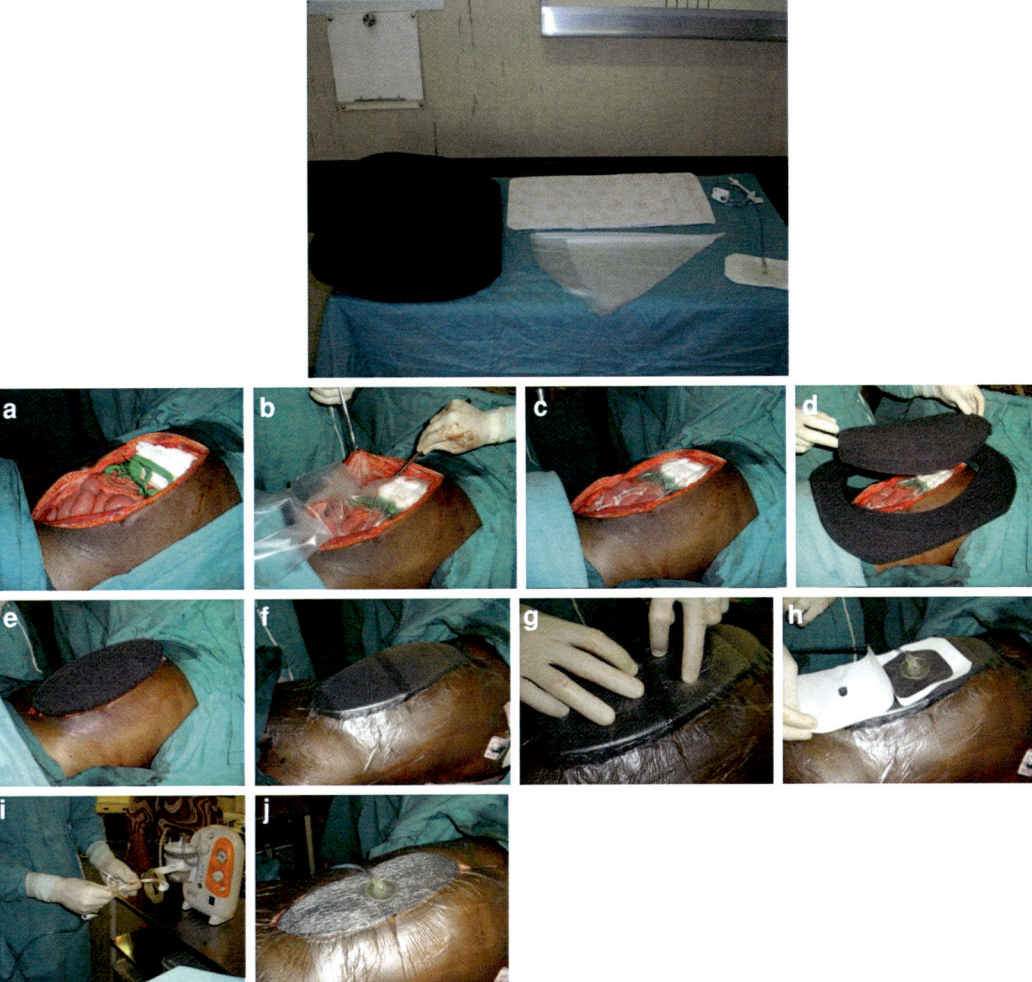

**Fig. 94.4** A commercial temporary abdominal closure dressing (RENASYS EZ™ pump, Smith & Nephew; St Petersburg, FL, USA)[23]

(Fig. 94.4) [23]. A fenestrated nonadherent film is placed directly over the exposed viscera but under the rectus sheath (a, b, c). Polyurethane foam is then reduced along pre-cut perforations to the appropriate size and placed on top of the film within the open abdomen (d, e). A transparent film then covers the foam (f) and the surrounding peri-wound skin before a suction port is connected to the NPWT pump (g, h). Negative pressure is delivered at a continuous −80 mm Hg (i, j). The primary fascial closure, fistula and mortality rates for the Abthera™ and Renasys™ devices are 90% and 65%, 3% and 5%, and 26% and 20%, respectively.

## 94.4.2 Complications

Significant complications are associated with the OA: enteroatmospheric fistulae, loss of abdominal domain with failure to achieve definitive fascial closure with resultant ventral hernias and intra-abdominal sepsis. These are difficult to manage, prolong intensive care and overall hospital stays with accompanying increased overall hospital costs.

### 94.4.2.1 Enteroatmospheric Fistula

Enteroatmospheric fistula is a serious, dreaded and challenging complication of the OA

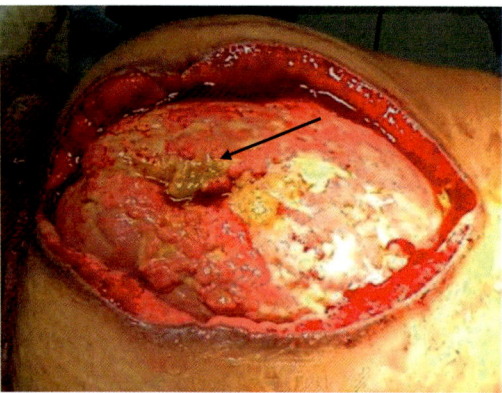

**Fig. 94.5** Enteroatmospheric fistula in an open abdomen (Grade 4 open abdomen)

(Fig. 94.5). Enteroatmospheric fistula can be associated with the primary aetiology of the OA. The high rates of fistula formation have been more often described in patients with an OA due to peritonitis; the type of materials used and there is also a concern of fistula formation especially regards the use of NPWT. The rate of enteroatmospheric fistula ranges from 0 to 55% in septic peritonitis patients with an overall fistula rate of 12%. In these septic patients, the highest rate is seen after mesh placement (17%), while NPWT with fascial traction shows the lowest fistula rate (6%) and NPWT without fascial traction has a fistula rate of 15%. The most commonly cited objection to the use of NPWT TAC is a perceived increase in fistula formation. The rate of fistula formation in the trauma population is about 3% (range 0–7%) [23]. It is possible that these relatively low levels of fistula formation are observed in this specific population of open abdomen patients [24] and that higher incidence of de novo fistula formation may occur in 'high risk' subsets of patients, i.e., those with more advanced grade of open abdomen (grade 3 or 4), sepsis, or in wounds where a bowel anastomosis following bowel surgery is present or where there is a delay or failure to achieve fascial closure. In fact, where concern has been expressed by several commentators [25–27] the patients described tend to be 'high risk.' The potential link between NPWT and fistula formation has been disputed by others [28] including in a systematic review [29]. Interestingly, their data showed that large-bowel resection, large-volume resuscitation, and an increasing number of re-explorations were statistically significant predictors for development of a fistula within an open abdomen after trauma. Another recent review of the available techniques for open abdomen management found a higher incidence of EAF occurring in septic open abdomen compared with nonseptic open abdomen (12.1 vs. 3.7% respectively) [30]. In addition, this review did not show any evidence of a relationship between use of negative-pressure wound therapy (NPWT) and fistula formation. More evidence is needed to determine whether use of NPWT on grade 3 or 4 open abdomen is effective and whether an increased risk of fistulization is indeed observed as a result of therapy in this subpopulation.

Patients with EAF must be managed according to standard fistula management guidelines paying attention to nutrition (oral, parenteral or both), strict fluid and electrolyte management, control of sepsis, fistula effluent control and protection of the wound and surrounding skin. The authors' approach is one of two techniques: laparostomy drainage (for moderate-to-high output fistula) (Fig. 94.6) and fistula isolation with NPWT (Fig. 94.7). The latter method is easy and quick to apply, consisting of a non-adherent protective dressing placed to protect the wound bed, with a hole cut for the enteric opening. The VAC sponge is accurately tailored to fit the wound and to match the fistula opening and is placed over the foam layer. An adherent polyurethane drape is eventually placed over the sponge and a hole is cut in this drape directly over the fistula, to allow placement of the appliance of an ostomy bag for collecting the fistula effluent. A number of refinements to this technique are described in the literature, all attempting to obtain a better sealing of fistula area from the rest of the wound [26–28]. We place a non-adherent liner to the wound with hole cut in it over the fistula. The VAC sponge is sized according to the wound and hole made over

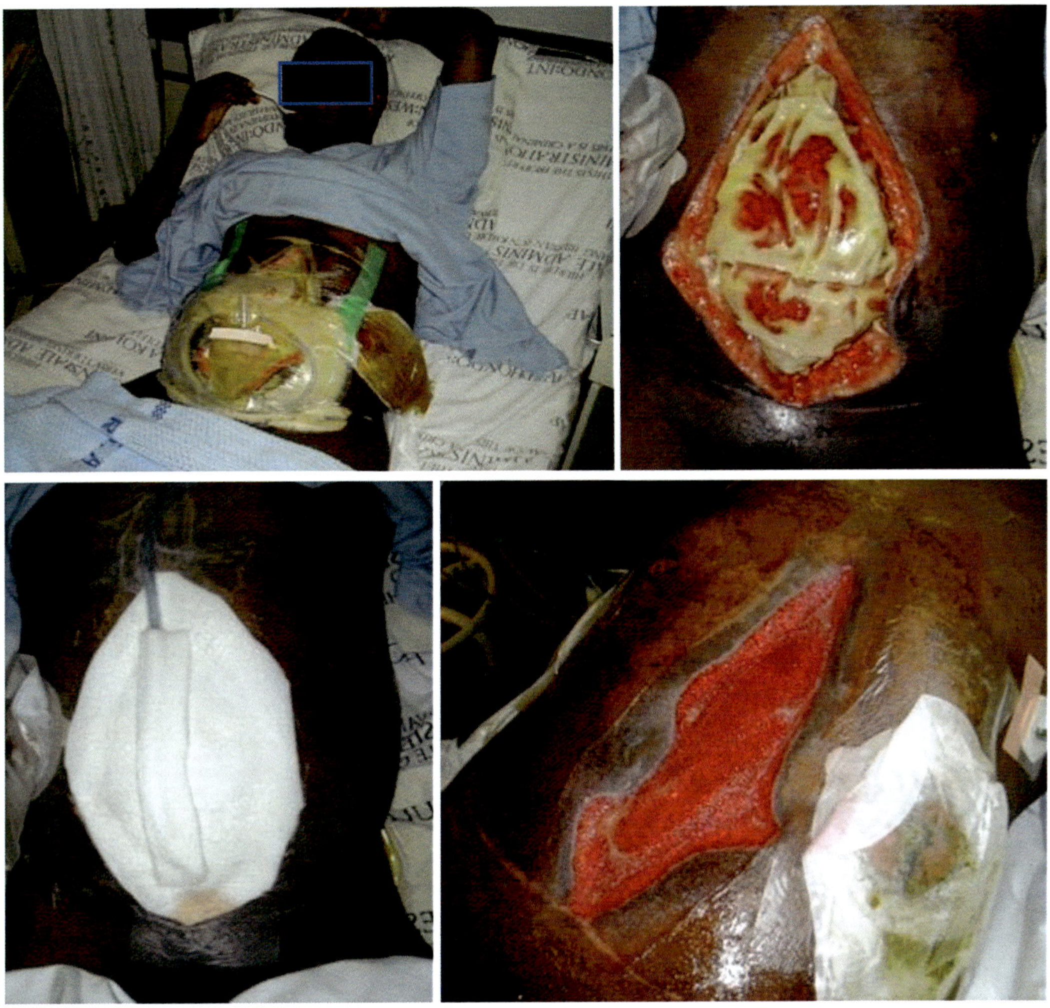

**Fig. 94.6** Patient with high-output EAF and laparostomy bag, spontaneous closure with standard medical management and foam NPWT resulting in healthy granulation tissue ready for split-skin grafting

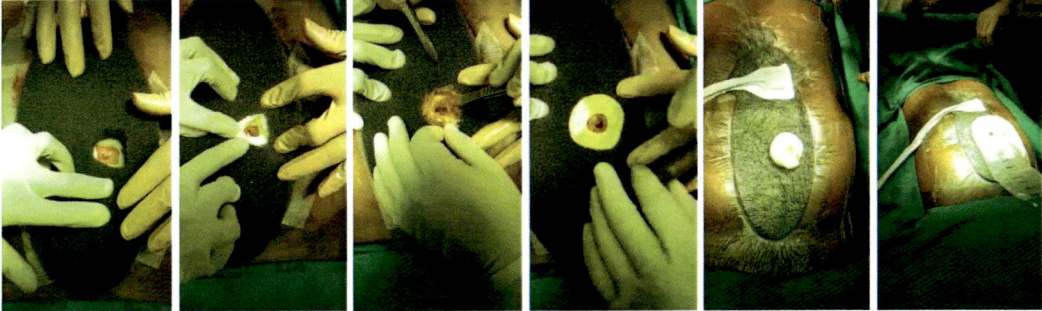

**Fig. 94.7** Fistula isolation within a vacuum dressing

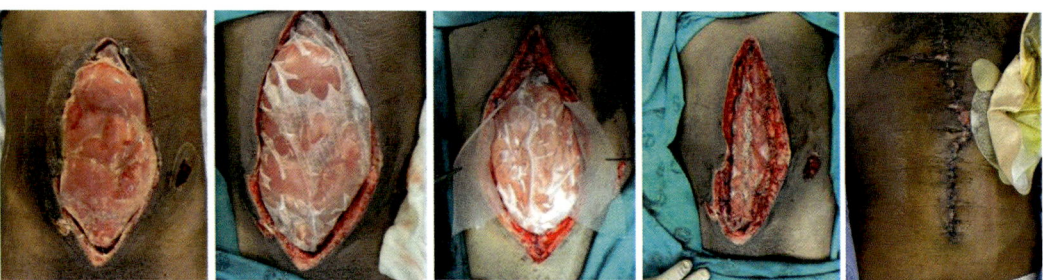

**Fig. 94.8** Vacuum-assisted mesh-mediated (VAMM) closure after 11 days and 3 dressing changes

the fistula. A funnel with rolled vaseline guaze is placed in the vac sponge and is topped and topped with two stoma rings. One is placed on the sponge and the second moulded into the funnel. Stoma paste is generously applied to allow for adherence to the sponge and vaseline gauze. Adherent polyurethane drapes and negative pressure is applied and a seal confirmed. An aperture is made over the stoma rings and a stoma bag applied. This isolation technique combined with NPWT allows for adequate wound management, re-epithelialization and eventual abdominal wall skin graft with conversion of the EAF into an enterostomy. Abdominal wall reconstruction and fistula excision are postponed at least 6 months. At this time, the evidence base for management recommendations for EAF is limited, suggesting that interventions should mainly be based on practical considerations such as resources and clinician skill. A proposed algorithm has been previously suggested [31].

### 94.4.2.2 Delayed Fascial Closure

Patients undergoing OA management are at risk of developing a 'frozen abdomen' and lower rates of definitive fascial closure. Every effort should be exerted to achieve primary fascial closure during the index admission and as soon as ongoing resuscitation has ceased, no further surgical re-exploration is needed and the patient can physiologically tolerate it without concerns of developing IAH/ACS. In many patients early definitive fascial closure may not be possible due to persistent bowel oedema or ongoing intra-abdominal sepsis. Early definitive fascial approximation and abdominal closure reduce mortality, complications and length of stay associated with the OA. Early fascial closure occurring within 4–7 days from the index operation is achieved more often following DCS for trauma than patients with abdominal sepsis. In the presence of a Grade 1A/2A open abdomen and failure to achieve early closure, the authors' approach is to employ the vacuum-assisted mesh-mediated (VAMM) facial traction technique as described by Petersson et al. [32] (Fig. 94.8). The intra-abdominal visceral protection layer of the NPWT system is inserted and tucked as far laterally to prevent adhesion formation between the intra-abdominal contents and the abdominal wall. The mesh is divided into two halves and sutured with a 2–0 running polypropylene suture to the fascial edges in an in-lay position on each side. The two mesh halves are thereafter pulled together under tension and sutured in the midline. The mesh-mediated tension on the abdominal wall prevents retraction of the lateral muscles, facilitating closure. The subcutaneous polyurethane foam is then placed between the abdominal wall edges, whereafter occlusive self-adhesive polyethylene films are applied to seal the wound. The tubing set is then applied, and the therapy unit of the NPWT system is set to −100 mmHg with continuous pressure. Every 72–96 h, the abdominal dressing is changed. The tubing set, occlusive self-adhesive polyethylene films and subcutaneous polyurethane foams are removed, and the mesh halves are opened in the midline. The intra-abdominal visceral protection layer is removed. When the abdominal cavity has been carefully inspected and loose adhesions are divided, a new intra-abdominal visceral protection layer is placed, and the mesh halves are re-sutured under tension in the midline. It is important to try to reduce the diastasis at each dressing change. When the fascial edges can be aligned in the midline, the mesh is removed by cutting the running suture holding the mesh in the in-lay position and the incision is then closed by a running absorbable suture.

The authors also occasionally use TopClosure ™ (Tension Relief System– TRS, IVT Medical Ltd., Israel) which is an innovative new technology created for skin stretching and secure wound closure, is a simple yet creative and effective manner of treating diverse and complex skin wounds such as post traumatic, surgical, acute and chronic skin wounds, which do not respond to conventional wound care (Fig. 94.9). The TopClosure® TRS is applied to secure wound closure in Grade 3A OA. Tension on the scar can be reduced or totally eliminated, thus avoiding dehiscence improving the quality and the aesthetics of the scar. When tension is too high to allow immediate primary closure of wound edges, skin is dressed and complete closure is deferred to a later stage. Mechanical creep is utilized gradually in a few days process. In this way the TopClosure® TRS prevents ischaemia and tearing of tissues caused in the process of wound closure by tension sutures. Additionally, the TopClosure® TRS can be applied simultaneously with regulated negative pressure treatment, to promote the healing process for chronic wound.

In the presence of a Grade 3A OA with large defects not amenable to VAMM or TRS closure, the authors persist with foam and NPWT to allow for healthy granulation to develop in the wound bed with subsequent split-skin grafting. Skin clips or sutures are strictly avoided to fix the skin graft to prevent iatrogenic EAF development. Instead, a foam dressing with negative pressure is applied to fix the graft. The ventral incisional hernias that develop are tackled at no less than 6 months later.

### 94.4.2.3 Incisional Ventral Hernias

Ventral hernias that develop as result of failure to achieve fascial closure following open abdomen management at the index admission differ from incisional hernias at the site of a previous surgical abdominal incisions. While the latter usually has all the hernia components of a defect, sac and content, ventral hernias following an open abdomen almost NEVER have as sac and the defects are generally large (Fig. 94.10). The authors' approach to these complex hernias is a simple

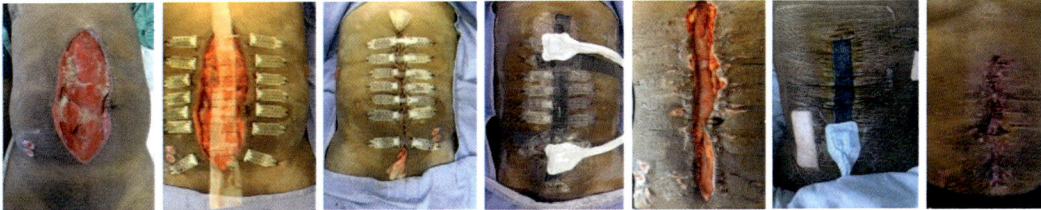

**Fig. 94.9** TopClosure™ tension relief system wound closure after 13 days

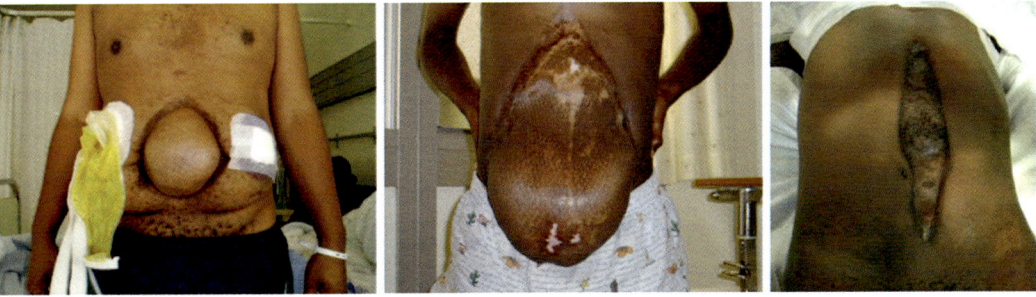

**Fig. 94.10** Complex incisional ventral hernias of varying sized abdominal wall defects

and uncomplicated one. Repair of these hernias are only considered once the patient's condition is completely stabilized and not before 6 months following hospital discharge. Patients are deemed ready for repair, once the healed skin graft can be clinically easily separated from the underlying bowel ('positive pinch test') or after a year, whatever comes first (Fig. 94.11). In the presence of stomas, loop colostomies are reversed, and hernia repair scheduled three months later. In the presence of end-stomas, mucus-fistulas or Hartmann's type stomas, the bowel prep is administered prior to the repair. Under general anaesthesia the skin graft is excised, the skin and subcutaneous tissue undermined and healthy sheath exposed. A lateral releasing incision is performed which consists only of elevation of the external oblique off the internal oblique. Following this, a tension-free fascial repair is done if feasible. The repair is reinforced with a onlay mesh (ProGrip™, Covidien, Medtronic, South Africa) (Fig. 94.12). Failure to achieve facial closure, a retrorectus composite mesh (Symbotex™, Covidien, Medtronic, South Africa) is used to repair the defect (Fig. 94.13).

An algorithm for the management of the OA is presented in Fig. 94.14.

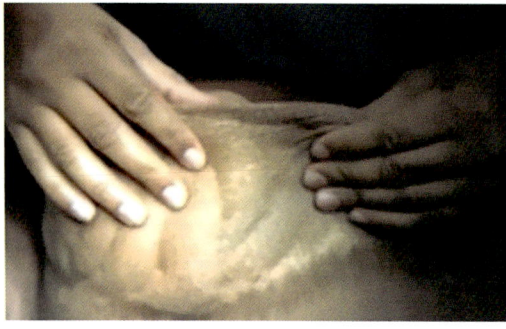

**Fig. 94.11** Clinical examination revealing healed graft 'separation' from underlying bowel suggestingreadiness for incisional hernia repair—'positive pinch test'

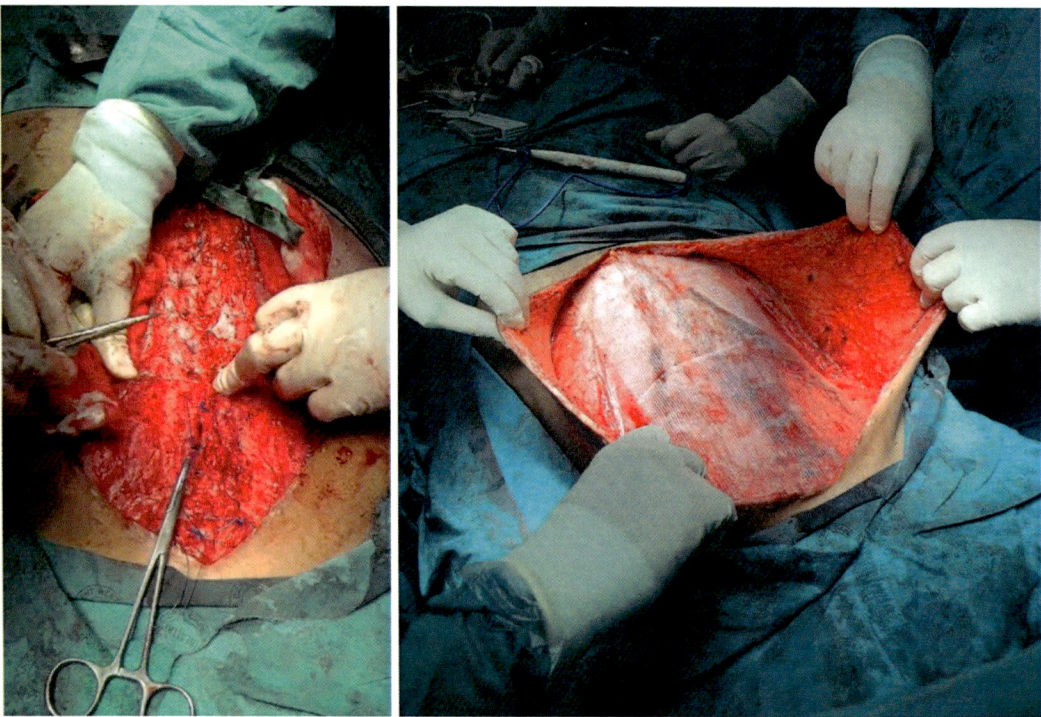

**Fig. 94.12** Incisional ventral hernia with tension-free fascial closure following component lateral release and reinforcement with an onlay mesh

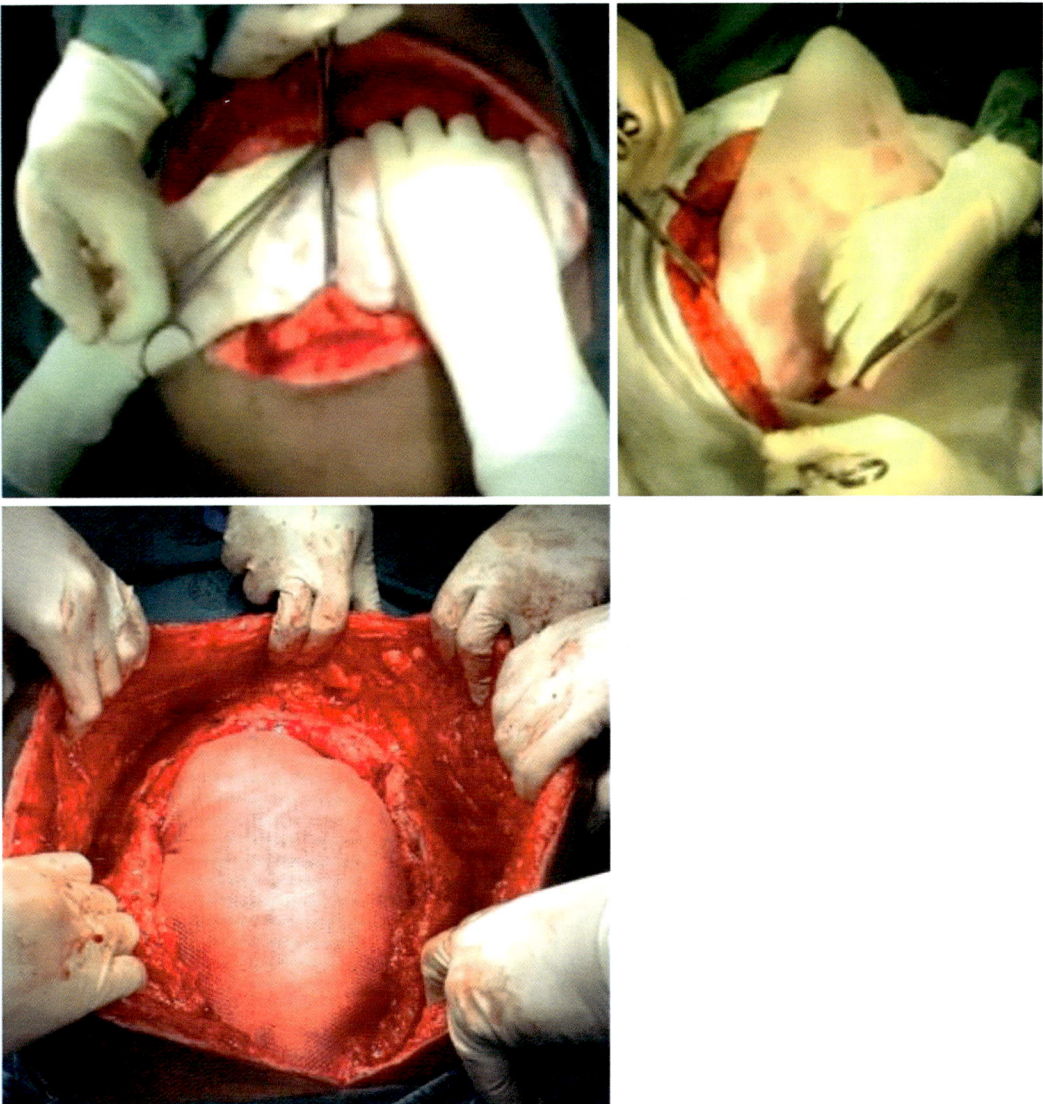

**Fig. 94.13** Incisional ventral hernia defect following component lateral release with retrorectus composite mesh closure

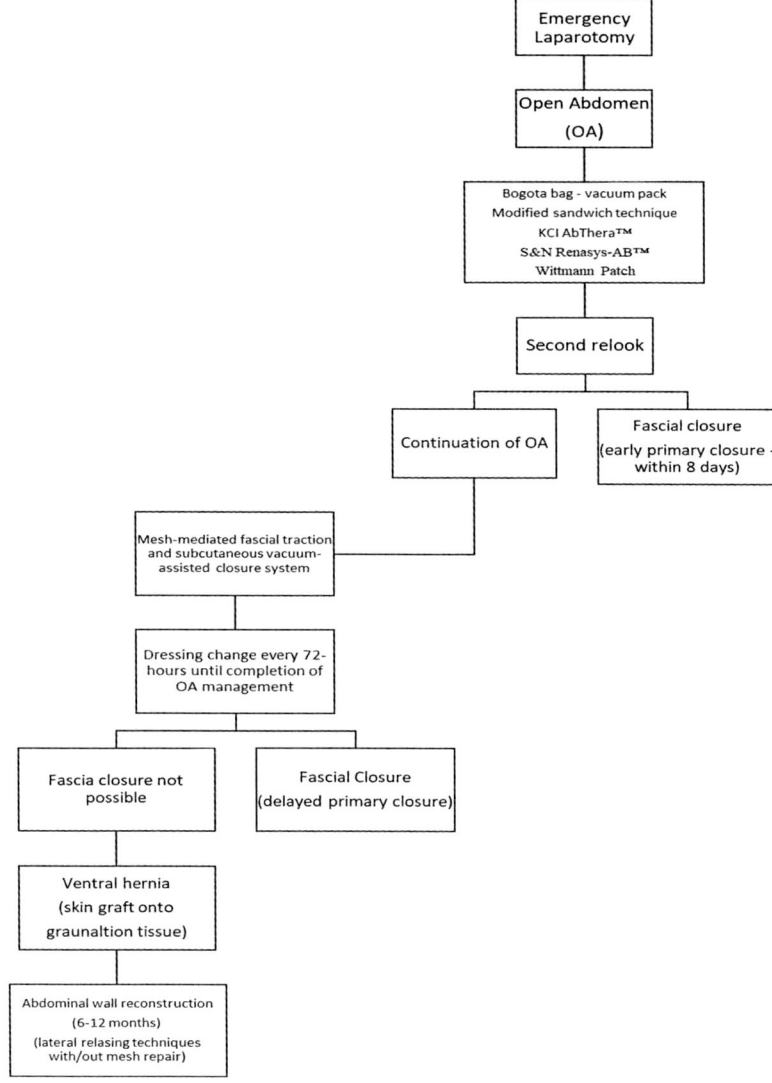

**Fig. 94.14** Management algorithm for the open abdomen. Modified with permission from Coccolini F, Biffl W, Catena F, Ceresoli M, Chiara O, Cimbanassi S et al. The open abdomen, indications, management and definitive closure. World J Emerg Surg. 2015;0:32. doi: 10.1186/s13017-015-0026-5 [33] and Willms A, Güsgen C, Schaaf S, Bieler D, von Websky M, Schwab R. Management of the open abdomen using vacuum-assisted wound closure and mesh-mediated fascial traction. Langenbecks Arch Surg. 2015 Jan;400(1):91–9. https://doi.org/10.1007/s00423-014-1240-4 [34]

### Dos and Don'ts
#### Dos
- Measure intra-abdominal pressure routinely.
- Leave the abdomen open following damage control surgery.
- ALWAYS use negative pressure.
- Attempt fascial closure within 7 days of index operation.
- Attempt mesh-mediated fascial closure when primary closure not feasible.
- ONLY use closed suction drains in an OA.
- Colostomies must be placed as lateral as possible with an OA.

#### Don'ts
- NEVER close the abdomen under tension.
- NEVER use skin staples to fix skin grafts on OA granulation bed.
- NEVER forget fluid homeostasis and nutritional support.

### Take-Home Messages
- DONOT close the abdomen under tension following laparotomy.
- DONOT close the abdomen following damage control surgery.
- Attempt to close the abdomen within 4–7 days of the index procedure.
- Always use negative pressure wound therapy.

AN ALIVE PATIENT WITH A LARGE VENTRAL HERNIA IS A BETTER OUTCOME THAN A DEAD PATIENT WITH A CLOSED ABDOMEN

### Multiple Choice Questions
1. All of the following are indications for an open abdomen except:
   A. Planned relook laparotomy.
   B. Abdominal compartment syndrome.
   C. **Patient undergoing isolated traumatic splenectomy with a lactate of 2.**
   D. Liver packing for haemorrhage control.
2. The following statement regarding negative pressure wound therapy in the management of the open abdomen is false:
   A. Increases fascial closure rates.
   B. **Increases risk of enteroatmospheric fistulas.**
   C. Ameliorates abdominal sepsis by removing peritoneal fluid-rich in biomediators.
   D. Nursing wound care burden is reduced.
3. The risk of enteroatmospheric fistula in an open abdomen is higher in the following except:
   A. Intra-abdominal sepsis.
   B. The use of mesh as temporary abdominal wall closure.
   C. **Negative pressure wound therapy.**
4. Early fascial closure is achieved more commonly under the following conditions except:
   A. Trauma patients (bleeding).
   B. 1A/2A open abdomen
   C. **Acute care surgery patients (sepsis).**
   D. Negative pressure wound therapy.
5. Mesh-mediated vacuum closure should be attempted in:
   A. **1A/2A open abdomen**
   B. Presence of fistula.
   C. Frozen abdomen.
   D. Ongoing sepsis.

6. Ventral incisional hernias as result of open abdomen management are similar to surgical site incisional hernias except:
   A. They both have a defect.
   B. **They both have a peritoneal sac.**
   C. They both have contents.
   D. OA defects tend to be larger.
7. Ventral hernias with residual defects despite component separation should have composite mesh placed:
   A. Onlay.
   B. **Retrorectus.**
   C. Between the recti.
   D. Avoided.
8. A 65-year-old man is involved in a motor vehicle collision. In the emergency room, he develops respiratory distress, goes into respiratory failure and is intubated. A chest radiograph reveals the liver to be in the right chest cavity. He is rushed to the operating room for repair of the ruptured diaphragm. Which of the following factors would not be an indication for leaving the abdomen open?
   A. **An operation lasting less the 120 min.**
   B. Bowel perforation with extensive spillage of intestinal content into peritoneal and pleural cavities.
   C. The inability to close.
   D. Severe intra-abdominal haemorrhage.

## References

1. Kaafarani HM, Velmahos GC. Damage control resuscitation in trauma. Scand J Surg. 2014;103:81–8. https://doi.org/10.1177/1457496914524388.
2. Clements TW, Tolonen M, Ball CG, Kirkpatrick AW. Secondary peritonitis and intra-abdominal sepsis: an increasingly global disease in search of better systemic therapies [published online ahead of print, 2021 Jan 7]. Scand J Surg. 2021;110(2):139–49. https://doi.org/10.1177/1457496920984078.
3. Kirkpatrick AW, Coccolini F, Ansaloni L, Roberts DJ, Tolonen M, McKee JL, et al. Closed or open after source control laparotomy for severe complicated intra-abdominal sepsis (the COOL trial): study protocol for a randomized controlled trial. World J Emerg Surg. 2018;13:26. Published 2018 Jun 22. https://doi.org/10.1186/s13017-018-0183-4.
4. Sartelli M, Viale P, Catena F, Ansaloni L, Moore E, Malangoniet M, et al. WSES guidelines for management of intra-abdominal infections. World J Emerg Surg. 2013;8:3. https://doi.org/10.1186/1749-7922-8-3.
5. De Waele JJ. Abdominal sepsis. Curr Infect Dis Rep. 2016;18:23. https://doi.org/10.1007/s11908-016-0531-z.
6. Sartelli M, Abu-Zidan FM, Ansaloni L, Bala M, Beltrán MA, Biffl WL, et al. The role of the open abdomen procedure in managing severe abdominal sepsis: WSES position paper. World J Emerg Surg. 2015;10:35. https://doi.org/10.1186/s13017-015-0032-7.
7. Coccolini F, Roberts D, Ansaloni L, Ivatury R, Gamberini E, Kluger Y, et al. The open abdomen in trauma and non-trauma patients: WSES guidelines. World J Emerg Surg. 2018;13:7. https://doi.org/10.1186/s13017-018-0167-4.
8. Scriba MF, Laing GL, Bruce JL, Clarke DL. Repeat laparotomy in a developing world tertiary level surgical service. Am J Surg. 2015;210:755–8. https://doi.org/10.1016/j.amjsurg.2015.03.024.
9. Doig CJ, Page SA, McKee JL, Moore EE, Abu-Zidan FM, Carroll R, et al. Ethical considerations in conducting surgical research in severe complicated intra-abdominal sepsis. World J Emerg Surg. 2019;14:39. https://doi.org/10.1186/s13017-019-0259-9. Erratum in: World J Emerg Surg 2019;14:47
10. Levy MM, Evans LE, Rhodes A. The surviving sepsis campaign bundle: 2018 update. Intensive Care Med. 2018;44:925–8. https://doi.org/10.1007/s00134-018-5085-0.
11. Björck M, Kirkpatrick AW, Cheatham M, Kaplan M, Leppäniemi A, De Waele JJ. Amended classification of the open abdomen. Scand J Surg. 2016;105:5–10. https://doi.org/10.1177/1457496916631853.
12. Schein M, Saadia R, Jamieson JR, Decker GAG. The 'sandwich technique' in the management of the open abdomen. Br J Surg. 1986;73:369–70. https://doi.org/10.1002/bjs.1800730514.
13. Brock WB, Barker DE, Burns RP. Temporary closure of open abdominal wounds: the vacuum pack. Am Surg. 1995;61:30–5.
14. Fernandez L, Norwood S, Roettger R, Wilkins HE III. Temporary intravenous bag silo closure in severe abdominal trauma. J Trauma. 1996;40:258–60. https://doi.org/10.1097/00005373-199602000-00014.
15. Sherck J, Seiver A, Shatney C, Oakes D, Cobb L. Covering the 'open abdomen': a better technique. Am Surg. 1998;64:854–7.
16. Ghimenton F, Thompson SR, Muckart DJJ, Burrows R. Abdominal content containment: practicalities and outcome. Br J Surg. 2000;87:106–9. https://doi.org/10.1046/j.1365-2168.2000.01337.x.

17. Nagy KK, Fildes JJ, Mahr C, Roberts RR, Krosner SM, Joseph KT, et al. Experience with three prosthetic materials in temporary abdominal wall closure. Am Surg. 1996;62:331–5.
18. Aprahamian C, Wittmann DH, Bergstein JM, Quebbeman EJ. Temporary abdominal closure (TAC) for planned relaparotomy (etappenlavage) in trauma. J Trauma. 1990;30:719–23. https://doi.org/10.1097/00005373-199006000-00011.
19. Howdieshell TR, Yeh KA, Hawkins ML, Cue JI. Temporary abdominal wall closure in trauma patients: indications, technique, and results. World J Surg. 1995;19:154–8. https://doi.org/10.1007/BF00317004.
20. Barker DE, Kaufman HJ, Smith LA, Ciraulo DI, Richart CL, Burns RP. Vacuum pack technique of temporary abdominal wall closure: a 7-year experience with 112 patients. J Trauma. 2000;48:201–6. https://doi.org/10.1097/00005373-200002000-00001.
21. Navsaria PH, Bunting M, Omoshoro-Jones J, Nicol AJ, Kahn D. Temporary closure of open abdominal wounds by the modified sandwich-vacuum pack technique. Br J Surg. 2003;90:718–22. https://doi.org/10.1002/bjs.4101.
22. Madbak FG, Lawless RA. Historical perspective. In: Madbak FG, Dangleben DA, editors. Options in the management of the open abdomen. New York/Heidelberg/Dordrecht/London: Springer; 2015. p. 1–8. https://doi.org/10.1007/978-1-4939-1827-0.
23. Navsaria P, Nicol A, Hudson D, Cockwill J, Smith J. Negative pressure wound therapy management of the "open abdomen" following trauma: a prospective study and systematic review. World J Emerg Surg. 2013;8(1):4. https://doi.org/10.1186/1749-7922-8-4.
24. Mentula P, Hienonen P, Kemppainen E, Puolakkainen P, Leppäniemi A. Surgical decompression for abdominal compartment syndrome in severe acute pancreatitis. Arch Surg (Chicago, IL, 1960). 2010;145:764–9. https://doi.org/10.1001/archsurg.2010.132.
25. Trevelyan SL, Carlson GL. Is TNP in the open abdomen safe and effective? J Wound Care. 2009;18:24–5. https://doi.org/10.12968/jowc.2009.18.1.32139.
26. Rao M, Burke D, Finan PJ, Sagar PM. The use of vacuum-assisted closure of abdominal wounds: a word of caution. Colorectal Dis. 2007;9:266–8. https://doi.org/10.1111/j.1463-1318.2006.01154.x.
27. Fischer JE. A cautionary note: the use of vacuum-assisted closure systems in the treatment of gastrointestinal cutaneous fistula may be associated with higher mortality from subsequent fistula development. Am J Surg. 2008;196:1–2. https://doi.org/10.1016/j.amjsurg.2008.01.001.
28. Shaikh IA, Ballard-Wilson A, Yalamarthi S, Amin AI. Use of topical negative pressure in assisted abdominal closure does not lead to high incidence of enteric fistulae. Colorectal Dis. 2010;12:931–4. https://doi.org/10.1111/j.1463-1318.2009.01929.x.
29. Stevens P. Vacuum-assisted closure of laparostomy wounds: a critical review of the literature. Int Wound J. 2009;6:259–66. https://doi.org/10.1111/j.1742-481X.2009.00614.x.
30. Bruhin A, Ferreira F, Chariker M, Smith J, Runkel N. Systematic review and evidence based recommendations for the use of negative pressure wound therapy in the open abdomen. Int J Surg. 2014;12:1105–14. https://doi.org/10.1016/j.ijsu.2014.08.396.
31. Di Saverio S, Tarasconi A, Inaba K, Navsaria P, Coccolini F, Costa Navarro D, et al. Open abdomen with concomitant enteroatmospheric fistula: attempt to rationalize the approach to a surgical nightmare and proposal of a clinical algorithm. J Am Coll Surg. 2015;220:e23–33. https://doi.org/10.1016/j.jamcollsurg.2014.11.020.
32. Petersson P, Petersson U. Dynamic fascial closure with vacuum-assisted wound closure and mesh-mediated fascial traction (VAWCM) treatment of the open abdomen-an updated systematic review. Front Surg. 2020;7:577104. Published 2020 Nov 5. https://doi.org/10.3389/fsurg.2020.577104.
33. Coccolini F, Biffl W, Catena F, Ceresoli M, Chiara O, Cimbanassi S, et al. The open abdomen, indications, management and definitive closure. World J Emerg Surg. 2015;10:32. https://doi.org/10.1186/s13017-015-0026-5.
34. Willms A, Güsgen C, Schaaf S, Bieler D, von Websky M, Schwab R. Management of the open abdomen using vacuum-assisted wound closure and mesh-mediated fascial traction. Langenbeck's Arch Surg. 2015;400(1):91–9. https://doi.org/10.1007/s00423-014-1240-4.

## Further Reading

Chen Y, Ye J, Song W, Chen J, Yuan Y, Ren J. Comparison of outcomes between early fascial closure and delayed abdominal closure in patients with open abdomen: a systematic review and meta-analysis. Gastroenterol Res Pract. 2014:784056. https://doi.org/10.1155/2014/784056.

Cirocchi R, Birindelli A, Biffl WL, Mutafchiysk V, Popivanov G, Chiara O, et al. What is the effectiveness of the negative pressure wound therapy (NPWT) in patients treated with open abdomen technique? A systematic review and meta-analysis. J Trauma Acute Care Surg. 2016;81:575–84. https://doi.org/10.1097/TA.0000000000001126.

Cristaudo A, Jennings S, Gunnarsson R, DeCosta A. Complications and mortality associated with temporary abdominal closure techniques: a systematic review and meta-analysis. Am Surg. 2017;83:191–216.

Quyn AJ, Johnston C, Hall D, Chambers A, Arapova N, Ogston S, et al. The open abdomen and temporary abdominal closure systems—historical evolution and systematic review. Color Dis. 2012;14:e429–38. https://doi.org/10.1111/j.1463-1318.2012.03045.x.

# Liver Trauma

## 95

Federico Coccolini, Camilla Cremonini, and Massimo Chiarugi

> **Learning Goals**
> - Know that the hemodynamic status is the determining factor in planning the decisional algorithm and management of liver trauma.
> - Remember that patients treated non-operatively require a strict follow-up with physical, laboratory, and radiological examinations in order to detect any change in the clinical status.
> - Know the role of interventional radiology as NOM extension.
> - Choose the optimal surgical strategy in case of operative treatment keeping in mind two main goals: hemorrhage and bile leak control.

## 95.1 Introduction

### 95.1.1 Epidemiology

The liver is the most frequently injured organ of the abdominal cavity, both in blunt and penetrating traumas. Its size and location make this organ highly susceptible to traumatic injuries: the liver is, in fact, the largest abdominal organ and occupies a large portion of the right thoraco-abdominal area. Liver injuries occur approximately in around 3–5% of all trauma admission and most injuries (80%) do not require surgical intervention, being amenable to non-operative management (NOM) [1].

Diagnosis and treatment, both non-operative and operative, has evolved and continues to evolve thanks to advanced technologies. Innovative techniques, such as interventional endovascular procedures and multimodal approaches (Endo-Vascular resuscitation and Trauma Management [EVTM]) [2], allow a wide range of options in trauma management that have increased the rate of patients successfully treated non-operatively even in case of severe injuries [3, 4]. Nowadays, in high-level trauma centers with rapidly available resources, NOM associated with the advancing techniques above mentioned can be considered as a feasible option even in transient responder patients [5]. However, some of the most severe liver injuries require an operative treatment and some of these lesions, such as retro-hepatic venous lesions as well as those of the portal triad, still represent a challenge for the surgeon and are related to high mortality rates.

---

F. Coccolini (✉) · C. Cremonini · M. Chiarugi
General Emergency and Trauma Surgery Department, Pisa University Hospital, Pisa, Italy
e-mail: massimo.chiarugi@unipi.it

## 95.1.2 Etiology: Mechanism of Injury

Blunt trauma (i.e., road traffic accidents or fall from height) is the leading cause of abdominal and more specifically liver traumas in European countries, whereas penetrating trauma (PT: stab wounds [SWs] and gunshot wounds [GSWs]) is a more common mechanism of injury in the USA and South Africa [6]. The liver parenchyma is fragile and the vessels inside are thin-walled with high-flow blood, so major injuries to the liver are usually associated with high blood loss. Blunt trauma may cause a hepatic injury with different mechanisms. First, deceleration forces can cause a tear in the parenchyma at the site of fixation points (i.e., ligaments) as the liver continues to move after impact. This can lead to severe lacerations of retro-hepatic inferior vena cava or hepatic veins. Second, the liver can be injured after direct blow to the abdomen, with laceration or hematoma of the parenchyma.

Penetrating trauma causes damage by direct transection of any structure encountered on its trajectory, (vein, artery, or biliary tree) and can be divided into two categories:

1. Low-energy PT: stab wound (SW) or low-velocity gunshot wounds (GSWs) such as handgun (<340 m/s).
2. High-energy PT: high-velocity GSW (>340 m/s) such as shotgun, rifles, or combat guns.

## 95.2 Classification

A uniform widespread classification works as a common language that can be used to communicate and to compare outcomes and efficacy of management techniques across different centers. In fact, classification of trauma injuries has always been essential to stratify and consequently treat trauma patients. Since its introduction in 1989 [7], the AAST-OIS (American Association of Surgery of Trauma—Organ Injury Scale) classification and its revisions [8], based on anatomical aspects and describing the

**Table 95.1** AAST-OIS liver injury scale (2018 revision)

| Grade | Injury type | Injury description |
|---|---|---|
| I | Hematoma | Subcapsular, <10% surface area |
|  | Laceration | Capsular tear; <1 cm parenchymal depth |
| II | Hematoma | Subcapsular, 10–50% surface area: Intraparenchymal <10 cm in diameter |
|  | Laceration | Capsular tear 1–3 parenchymal depth, <10 cm in length |
| III | Hematoma | Subcapsular, >50% surface area or expanding; ruptured subcapsular or parenchymal hematoma; intraparenchymal hematoma >10 cm |
|  | Laceration | >3 cm parenchymal depth |
| IV | Laceration | Parenchymal disruption involving 25–75% of hepatic lobe |
| V | Laceration | Parenchymal disruption involving >75% of hepatic lobe |
|  | Vascular | Juxta-hepatic venous injuries; i.e., retro-hepatic vena cava/central major hepatic veins |

Note: Advance one grade for multiple injuries up to grade III
Adapted from: R. A. Kozar et al., "Organ injury scaling 2018 update: Spleen, liver, and kidney," J. Trauma Acute Care Surg., vol. 85, no. 6, pp. 1119–1122, Dec. 2018

site and the extent of damage, have fulfilled this purpose proving itself to be a useful and effective tool in the decision-making process [9, 10]. Table 95.1 shows the AAST-OIS classification for liver injury ranging from Grade I to Grade V and describing both hematoma and laceration characteristics. In the last decades, NOM protocols integrated with endovascular procedures such as angioembolization (AE) were successfully applied in patients with anatomically severe lesions but stable hemodynamic parameters [11, 12]. This shows how physiology and anatomy are both keystones driving the trauma management choices and strategies. Accordingly, the World Society of Emergency Surgery (WSES) proposed a classification system anchored not only on the anatomical aspect of organ injuries but also on the physiological status of the patient [13, 14].

Hepatic injuries can be divided into three degrees according to the WSES classification

**Table 95.2** Liver trauma classification

|  | WSES grade | AAST | Hemodynamic |
|---|---|---|---|
| Minor | WSES grade I | I–II | Stable |
| Moderate | WSES grade II | III | Stable |
| Severe | WSES grade III | IV–V | Stable |
|  | WSES grade IV | Any | Unstable |

*WSES* World Society of Emergency Surgery, *AAST* American Association for the Surgery of Trauma
Adapted from: F. Coccolini et al., "Liver trauma: WSES 2020 guidelines," World J Emerg Surg. 2020 Mar 30;15(1):24

that considers the AAST-OIS classification (Table 95.1) and the hemodynamic status (Table 95.2) [13]:

- Minor (WSES class I).
- Moderate (WSES class II).
- Severe (WSES class III and IV).

## 95.3 Diagnosis of Liver Trauma

Diagnosis and subsequent management of a liver injury should follow at the beginning the Advanced Trauma Life Support (ATLS) principles that remain the foundation of trauma care. Early efforts should be focused on identifying and treating life-threatening lesions that may take precedence over possible internal injuries. However, severe liver injuries may be the cause of a hemorrhagic shock and need to be at least suspected during the primary survey.

When managing a trauma patient, the *hemodynamic status* plays a key role and drives the decision on what diagnostic study should be done. A proper trauma resuscitation, shifted in the last two decades to an early transfusion of blood in a 1:1 ratio trying to avoid the deadly triad of hypothermia, acidosis, and coagulopathy [5], may allow to stabilize the patient and gain some time for the assessment. Serum lactate and base deficit are sensitive diagnostic markers of grade of hemorrhagic shock and can be used to monitor the response to resuscitation [15].

The Extended Focused Assessment with Sonography for Trauma (E-FAST) occurs early during the primary survey and, although less reliable in detecting liver injury (especially in case of low-grade lesions), has high sensitivity in effectively and rapidly detecting intra-abdominal free fluid [14]. Sensitivity and specificity reported in the literature are around 80–85% and >95%, respectively [16]. A lower sensitivity has been reported in case of penetrating trauma [17]. Ultrasounds may also be unreliable if the hemoperitoneum is less than 300 cc or may be impaired by other factors including morbid obesity of the patient or extensive subcutaneous emphysema. A negative FAST exam does not exclude a liver injury. However, a positive FAST exam is a valuable information that needs to be combined with the physiological asset of the patient in deciding whether to perform an exploratory laparotomy or not.

*Computed tomography* (CT) scan with intravenous contrast is the gold standard for all hemodynamically stable trauma patients with a sensitivity and specificity that reach 95–100% [14]. In selected centers, under the strict supervision of the trauma team and with ongoing resuscitation, CT scan may be used also in transient responder patients or even in unstable patient in very selected situations/cases [18].

CT scan, other than detecting and defining the severity and the extent of the liver injury, helps in differentiating patients with active bleeding (active contrast extravasation, Fig. 95.1) from those with contained vascular injuries, and it also helps in driving subsequent procedures such as angiography (AG) and/or angioembolization.

Diagnostic peritoneal lavage (DPL) or aspiration (DPA) should be considered as diagnostic tools in low-resources setting or where FAST and CT are not available. It finds a role also in case of hemodynamically unstable patients with a negative or questionable positive FAST exam. Moreover, DPL may help in understanding free fluid composition allowing to detect eventual biomarkers (i.e., bilirubin) wherever advanced diagnostic techniques are not available.

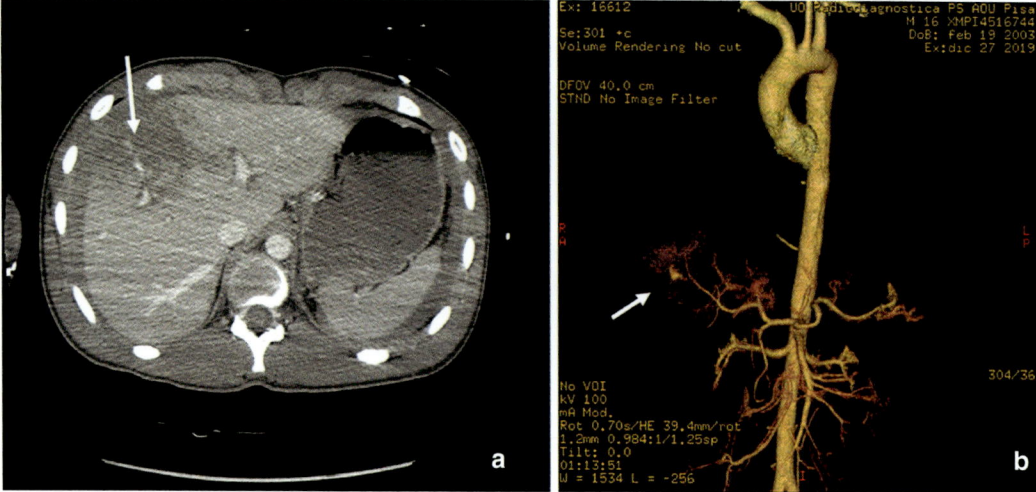

**Fig. 95.1** (**a**) CT scan image of a Grade IV (AAST) liver injury with active contrast extravasation (arrow). (**b**) CT scan vascular reconstruction of hepatic artery with evidence of the blush (arrow)

## 95.4 Management Strategies

As said above, the choice between NOM and operative management (OM) is mainly driven by the hemodynamic status of the patient rather than the severity of organ injury alone. Table 95.3 shows a summary of the indications of NOM and operative management (OM) in case of abdominal trauma, either blunt or penetrating, while Figs. 95.2 and 95.3 represent two algorithms for the management of hepatic injuries proposed by the World Society of Emergency Surgery (WSES) guidelines of liver trauma [14].

**Table 95.3** General management strategies

| Non-operative management (NOM) | Operative management (OM) |
|---|---|
| Hemodynamic stability | Hemodynamic instability with positive FAST (focused assessment with sonography for trauma) |
| Absence of other lesions requiring OM | Evisceration |
| | Impalement |
| | Peritonitis on abdominal examination |
| | CT scan evidence of intra-abdominal injury requiring surgery (i.e., hollow viscus injury) |
| | Failed NOM/embolization or persistent bleeding |

Very delicate scenario: Unevaluable patients (i.e., intoxicated, concomitant neurotrauma)

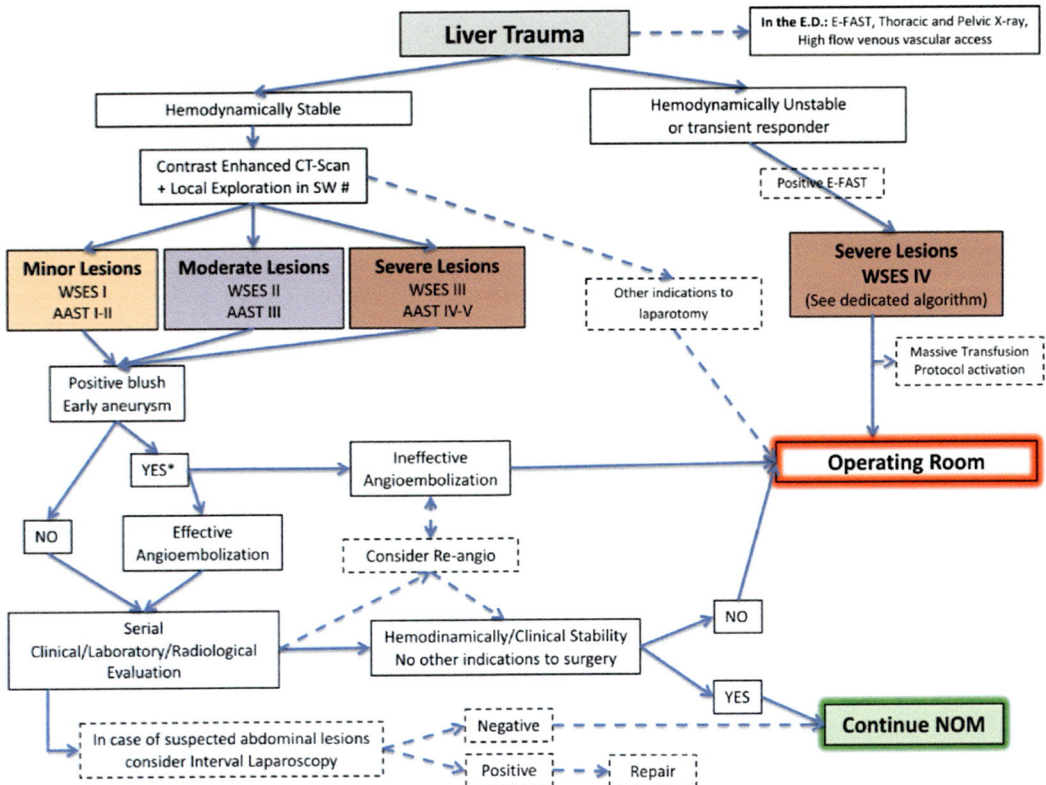

**Fig. 95.2** Liver trauma management algorithm. *SW* stab wound. # Wound exploration near the inferior costal margin should be avoided if not strictly necessary. * Angioembolization should be always considered for adults, only in selected patients and in selected centers for pediatrics. (With permission, from: F. Coccolini et al., "Liver trauma: WSES 2020 guidelines," World J Emerg Surg. 2020 Mar 30;15(1):24)

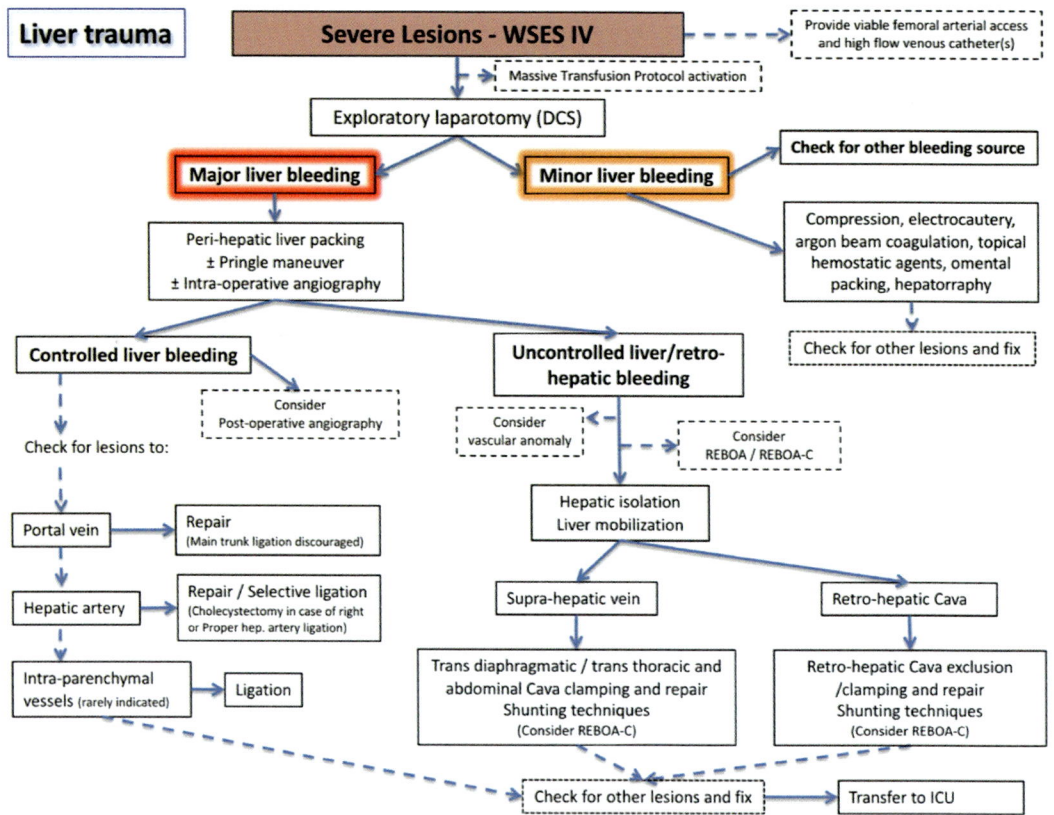

**Fig. 95.3** Hemodynamically unstable liver trauma management algorithm. *DCS* damage control surgery, *ICU* intensive care unit, *REBOA-C* resuscitative endovascular balloon occlusion of the aorta-cava. With permission, from: F. Coccolini et al., "Liver trauma: WSES 2020 guidelines," World J Emerg Surg. 2020 Mar 30;15(1):24)

## 95.5 Non-Operative Management (NOM) of Liver Injury

Non-operative management (NOM) has gained more and more consent over the past decades and is now considered the standard of care for traumatic patients who are hemodynamically stable and do not present other lesions requiring surgery (i.e., hollow viscous injury [HVI] documented at the CT scan) [14]. This line of treatment should be followed regardless of the grade of the liver injury [11]. Different studies showed high success rates, good outcomes, and low incidence of complications in stable trauma patients with severe liver injuries treated with NOM [3, 4]. Presence of a large subcapsular hematoma or a large volume of hemoperitoneum is not a strict indication for OM. Bleeding from hepatic parenchyma is usually of low pressure (being most commonly due to venous laceration, especially in blunt trauma) and frequently it stops spontaneously. The rationale for treating these patients with non-operative strategies lies in trying to avoid a non-therapeutic laparotomy and the consequent high rate of morbidity (reported to be between 20 and 40% [19]).

Moreover, in recent years, NOM indications are still expanding showing good results in terms of outcomes even in transient responder patients, reserving surgery for those who present in extremis or become hemodynamically unstable despite resuscitation [20]. This concept should be considered in selected settings where crucial resources related to trauma management such as massive transfusion protocol activation, trained surgeons, operating room, interventional radiology, continuous monitoring in emergency room (ER) and intensive care unit (ICU), etc. are all rapidly and 24/7 available [14].

In case of liver injuries treated with NOM, no standardized monitoring protocols exist; patients should be monitored with serial clinical examinations, and laboratory and eventually radiological exams, in order to detect any change in the clinical status. Level of hemoglobin, hematocrit, and transaminase are some of the laboratory exams that need to be monitored. Increasing level of transaminases may indicate a progressive intrahepatic parenchymal ischemia and may suggest the necessity to proceed with hepatic resection [21]. Moderate (WSES II–AAST III) and severe (WSES III–AAST IV–V) lesions may require intensive care unit admission, even in case of isolated liver injury.

As part of NOM, angiography with or without angioembolization (AG/AE) is the first-line intervention in case of hemodynamically stable patient with an active contrast extravasation documented at the CT scan (Fig. 95.4). AG/AE may be also indicated in case of other vascular injuries detected at CT scan like pseudoaneurysm (PSA) or arterio-venous fistula. There is no agreement in the literature regarding actual factor predicting NOM failure. Some studies showed how age, high Injury Severity Score (ISS), high grade of liver injury, associated intra-abdominal injuries, high necessity of blood transfusion, and high quantity of intra-abdominal free fluid may be related to higher risk of NOM failure [22–24]. Nevertheless, NOM seems less likely to fail in liver injuries than in splenic or kidney injuries [25].

It is important to note that in hemodynamically stable children the presence of active blush on CT scan is not an absolute indication for AG/AE [26].

### 95.5.1 NOM in Penetrating Trauma

NOM can be considered also in selected patients with liver injuries due to penetrating trauma (PT). High-energy GSW are less amenable to NOM since they usually cause extensive damage to the tissues; NOM success rates reported are around 10%, with OM required in 90% of cases [27, 28]. SWs and low-velocity GSWs are more likely to be successfully treated with NOM: 50% of the SWs to the anterior abdomen, 85% of the SWs to the back, and around 25% of the GSWs to the abdomen may be safely managed with NOM

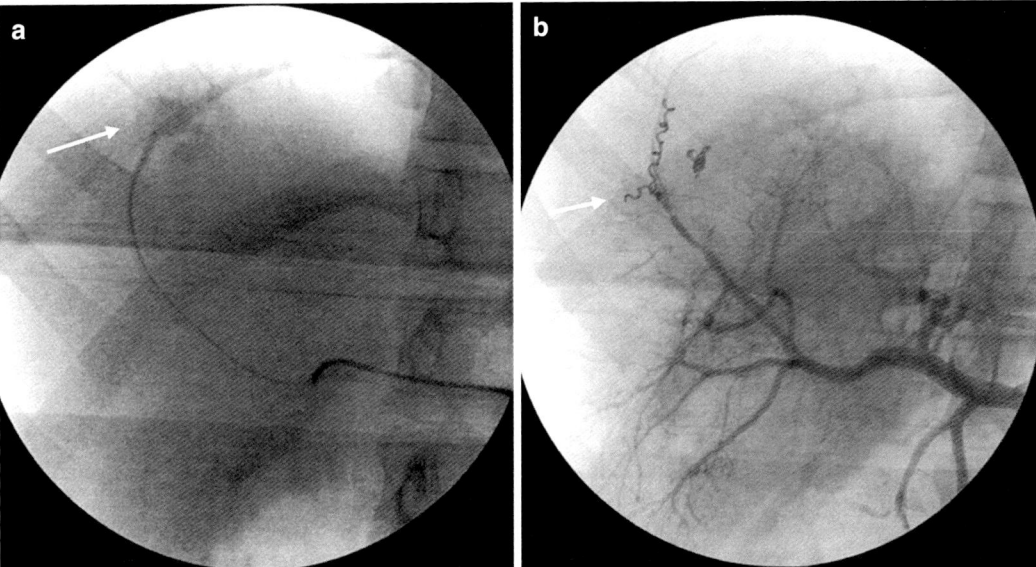

**Fig. 95.4** (a) Angiographic evidence of an arterial active contrast (arrow) from right hepatic artery. (b) Angioembolization of right hepatic artery with coils (arrow)

[14]. These rates of success were also confirmed by studies performed only on liver injuries after GSWs [12, 29, 30].

In case of PT patients managed with NOM, it is even more mandatory to strictly follow the evolution of the clinical status to detect any change. Serial clinical, laboratory, and radiological examinations are fundamental.

One of the main risks of NOM in general, and especially in PT, is missing intra-abdominal injuries, mainly hollow viscous perforation (HVI) and diaphragm laceration [31]. In stable and asymptomatic patients, these injuries can be suspected considering the trajectory of the bullet or of the stab tract. In this and other cases (see below: 5.3 Role of Laparoscopy), interval laparoscopy (IL) plays a key role.

### 95.5.2 Concomitant Neurotrauma

Hemodynamically stable patients with liver injury may present with concomitant neurotrauma (i.e., spinal cord or head trauma). In these cases, abdominal examination may be unreliable, and these patients may not present signs of peritonitis due to associated intra-abdominal injuries (i.e., HVI). Specific attention should be paid in managing these cases. In blunt trauma and no other indications to surgery, NOM should be considered as first-line strategy. In penetrating liver injuries, the gold standard is still debated and it seems that OM may be considered safer [14, 30, 32].

Moreover, patients with concomitant neurotrauma need high perfusion pressure to the brain to avoid secondary damage (following hypotension and hypoperfusion). In these patients, there are specific hemodynamic parameters that need to be met [14]:

1. Systolic blood pressure > 110 mmHg.
2. Central perfusion pressure of 60–70 mmHg in case of moderate head or spinal cord trauma.
3. Central perfusion pressure > 80 mmHg in case of severe head or spinal cord trauma.

### 95.5.3 Role of Laparoscopy

Alongside the shifting of trauma injuries management from OM to NOM when applicable, laparoscopy and more specifically interval laparoscopy (IL; exploratory laparoscopy without any associated surgical procedure) has been proven itself as an effective tool in several scenarios preventing unnecessary laparotomy in 34% of cases [33, 34]. It is of course indicated only in stable patients and should not be attempted in case of hemodynamic instability.

Interval laparoscopy should be considered as an "extension" of NOM in order to confirm/exclude injuries requiring surgery in all those patients where intra-abdominal injuries are suspected but not detected [14].

These are some of the scenarios where IL may play a role:

- In penetrating trauma, when peritoneal violation is in doubt or the trajectory is long and tangential or if the wound tract is hard to determine on CT scan, IL has been used to diagnose it as well as possible associated intra-abdominal lesions.
- In penetrating thoraco-abdominal trauma, due to the specific risks of injuries of this region (i.e., liver injury associated with a diaphragmatic lesion).
- In case of unreliable clinical examinations (due to intoxication or concomitant neurotrauma) associated with suspicious signs at the CT scan (i.e., localized bowel-wall thickening and free peritoneal fluid in the absence of a solid organ injury).
- More specifically in case of liver injury, IL is an important tool that may help evaluate the evolution of an injury with slow recovery or persistent abnormalities at the CT scan. It also may work as a bridge strategy to plan a step-up treatment (subsequent laparoscopic/laparotomic intervention). Finally, in case of intraoperative diagnosis of a liver injury that requires surgical repair, a laparoscopic repair may be attempted in hemodynamically stable patients [35].

## 95.6 Operative Management (OM)

OM should be the treatment of choice for hemodynamically unstable and non-responder patients (WSES IV), other than the general indications above mentioned [14].

Trauma laparotomy should be performed always through a midline incision from the xiphoid to the pubis with full surgical preparation of chest, abdomen, and groins, to rapidly access all cavities and to identify ongoing bleeding. Once any major bleeding is controlled or temporarily compressed with laparotomic pads, the remainder of the abdominal cavity should be inspected for bowel or other solid organ injuries. In the general sequence of repairing, simultaneous intraoperative intensive resuscitation with early administration of blood products aiming to maintain good organ perfusion and to contrast all trauma-induced physiological derangements is crucial [5, 14].

During laparotomy for liver injury, main goals are control of the hemorrhage and of the bile leak, and to stabilize the patient; thus damage control resuscitation should be initiated as soon as possible.

In case of *minor liver injury* or incidental lesion, compression with packs or finger compression of the wound may be sufficient to stop the bleed since many of these lesions do not require surgical fixation. In case of minor bleeding, this might be controlled with several hemostasis control tools, including electrocautery, bipolar devices, argon, or topical hemostatic agents [16, 36].

In case of *major hemorrhage* (Fig. 95.5), some fundamental passages may be applied in the following sequence (see below for more detailed descriptions):

- Taking down falciform ligament.
- Compress the liver manually by assistant and/or place surgical pads around the liver to compress it (liver packing) while doing palpatory evaluation of liver surface to rapidly understand lesion extent.

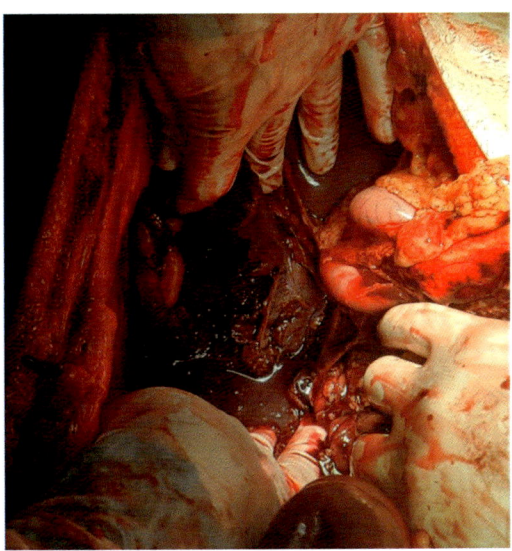

**Fig. 95.5** High-grade liver injury

- Pringle maneuver in the case of persistent bleeding.
- Consider retro-hepatic veins or cava vein lesions in case of persistent bleeding after correctly performed liver packing and Pringle maneuver or in the case of dark blood coming from behind the liver.

1. **Manual compression and liver packing**: In unstable patients with complex injuries not amenable to rapid definitive repair, consider packing and damage control surgery (DCS) that may be effective in stabilizing the patient. Packing technique is important: packs should be placed around the liver (above, below, and laterally), reproducing its anatomy to compress the parenchyma (Fig. 95.6a). Intact hepatic ligaments increase the chance of tamponade hence they do not need to be divided [37], especially in case of a hematoma of the ligament itself. This finding may indicate a vena cava or hepatic vein injury and taking down the ligament may lead to rapid exsanguination. Falciform ligament, however, should be divided as its section helps in more effective packing and in reducing the risk of traction and laceration on the parenchyma due to surgical pads' placement during packing.

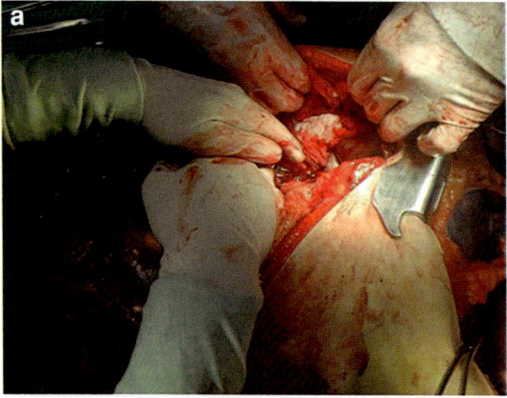

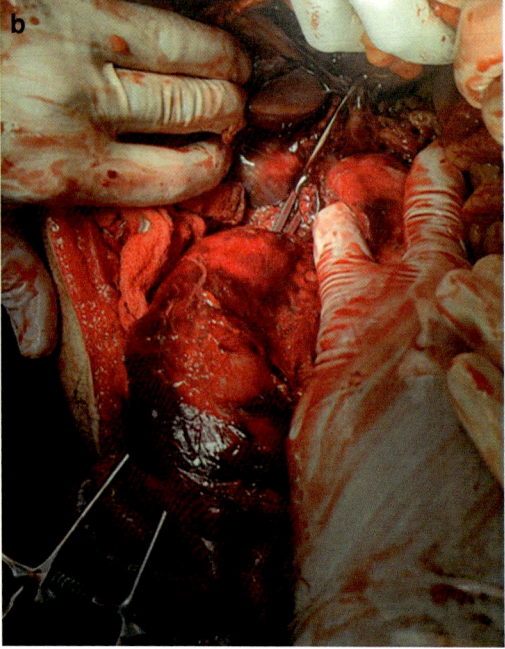

**Fig. 95.6** (**a**) Peri-hepatic packing with laparotomic packs. (**b**) Pringle maneuver

Hepatic packing is often useful in blunt venous injury, whereas is less effective in providing hemostasis in case of penetrating injury or arterial bleeding [32]. If the packing does not control the bleeding, next step is to perform Pringle maneuver. If the result is insufficient, progressively procced with unpacking and search the cause of bleeding whenever it is clear that it does not come from behind the liver as stated before. If the packing is successful, complete abdominal cavity exploration and perform a laparostomy. Then the patient should be rapidly taken to the next phase of management (usually ICU for optimal resuscitation and/or to the CT scan if not done before): intra- or post-operative AG/AE may be considered as an adjunctive procedure since it seems to improve patient survival [38]. Hepatic packing can be removed as soon as the patient is stabilized with subsequent abdominal wall early closure.

2. **Hepatic vessels flow temporary interruption (Pringle maneuver)**: In case of massive bleeding, a Pringle maneuver should be considered as an early step to achieve vascular control (reducing arterial and portal vein blood inflow to the liver; Fig. 95.6b). The maneuver should be kept in place for less than 30 min for each clamping period, thus reducing complications related to normothermic-ischemia time [32, 37]. If the Pringle maneuver fails and the bleeding continues, there are two options to consider: an aberrant hepatic artery or a retro-hepatic vena cava/hepatic vein laceration [14].

3. **Ligation of the vessels in the wound**: If the source of bleeding is localized, an attempt to repair it should be done. Bleeding from liver lacerations may be controlled by clipping or ligating (with a direct suture technique) any bleeders inside the wound [32].

4. **Hepatic debridement or finger fracture**: In deeper lacerations, a blunt dissection of the liver parenchyma between fingers ("finger fracture") allows for careful extension into the laceration and identification of bleeding vessel that can be legated with clips or direct suture. The opportunity of performing finger fracture however must be cautiously evaluated: the major risk is to extend the lesion without any effective hemostatic procedures or to create additional lesions. Endovascular procedures in fact may allow for effectively stopping the bleed without the necessity to enlarge the liver lesions in most of the cases.

5. **Balloon tamponade**: In case of through and through penetrating injuries, considering their great depth and length, it may be impossible to directly visualize the bleeding

source. Hence, inserting a "balloon" into the tract may achieve hemostasis. The balloon may be represented by a Foley catheter or by a Penrose drain tied at both ends and inflated with fluid [32, 37]. If successful, the balloon is left in the abdomen and removed 24–48 h later at a second laparotomy. It is important to dose the intra-balloon pressure in order to not disrupt perilesional parenchyma with excessive balloon distension. If the bleeding does not stop, consider dissection down to the injured liver segment ("tractotomy," a rarely used technique) or DCS followed by AG/AE [32].

6. **Hepatic vessels repair**: In case of hepatic artery or portal vein injuries, a first attempt of direct repair should be made. If not effective or not possible, consider hepatic artery ligation or selective ligation. In case of ligation of the right branch or common trunk of hepatic artery, perform or plan (in DCS procedures) a shortcoming subsequent cholecystectomy to avoid gallbladder necrosis [39]. Portal vein injuries should be repaired. Ligation of a portal vein main branch should be considered only in patients with an intact hepatic artery, because of the high risk of hepatic necrosis and bowel edema [14]. In these cases, high suspicion of necessity for subsequent segmental liver resection should be maintained [39].

7. **Complete vascular exclusion**: Different techniques of vascular exclusion have been described but they are rarely adopted because of the high mortality rates related [14]. Total vascular exclusion can be achieved by clamping the supra-hepatic and infra-hepatic inferior vena cava (Heaney maneuver) in addition to the Pringle maneuver and by an eventual infra-diaphragmatic aortic clamping. Otherwise, an atrio-caval shunting may be attempted by placing a chest tube through the right atrium into the infra-hepatic inferior vena cava. This shunt may allow to bypass the retro-hepatic vena cava and its laceration. These techniques are generally poorly tolerated by unstable patients with major bleeding [14].

### 95.6.1 Specific Considerations

1. *Suspected retro-hepatic cava or hepatic vein injuries*: Two strategies may be adopted: tamponade with hepatic packing or direct repair. These lacerations represent a challenge even for the skilled trauma surgeon.
2. *Major hepatic resections* should be avoided at first and only considered in subsequent operations.
   Some authors suggest hepatic resection in case of [32, 37]:
   - Extensive devitalized hepatic tissue.
   - Major bile leak from main intrahepatic duct laceration with no alternative mini-invasive treatments.
   - Persistent bleeding from destructive injuries.
   
   In case of need, a non-anatomic resection is preferred as safer and easier [14]. In patients with large areas of devitalized liver tissue, experienced surgeons may be involved in the management pathway.
3. *Resuscitative endovascular balloon occlusion of the aorta* (REBOA) may be used as a temporary bleeding control maneuver and as bridge to other more definitive procedures of hemorrhage control in hemodynamically unstable patients [14]. A concomitant use of resuscitative endovascular balloon occlusion of the vena cava (REBOVC) inflated at the level of retro-hepatic vena cava may achieve the goal of proximal and distal vascular control of a venous injury [14].
4. *Post-operative AG/AE* plays a role in different scenarios [14, 16]:
   - Persistent arterial bleeding despite emergency laparotomy and hemostasis attempts.
   - After hepatic packing as an adjunctive procedure [38].
   - After initial operative hemostasis, in stable or stabilized patients with contrast blush at completion CT scan.
   - After a successful post-operative AG/AE procedure in the event of a re-bleeding detected at CT scan in hemodynamically stable patient.

5. *Hepatic transplantation*: In case of massive crush injuries or devitalized hepatic parenchyma, hepatic transplantation has been successfully described [39]. This can be considered as an alternative for very few patients, with overall excellent chance of survival and minimal concomitant injury, especially other intra-abdominal or neurologic injuries [32].

## 95.7 Complications

Minor liver injuries usually heal without complications; grade III and IV injuries treated with NOM are more likely to develop some complication, with 12–14% rates [32]. Post-operative complications in patients with severe injuries have been reported in about 50% of cases [37]. Most frequent complications after liver trauma are:

1. Vascular complications: re-bleeding or secondary hemorrhage (i.e., subcapsular hematoma) either after operative treatment or AG/AE, pseudoaneurysm (PSA), and arterio-venous fistula.
2. Biliary complications: bile leak, biloma, biliary peritonitis, biliary fistula with bilemia, and hemobilia.
3. Hepatic necrosis and abscesses.
4. Abdominal compartment syndrome.

A *bile leak* is the most common complication and occurs more frequently after operative management [32]. It may present with abnormal liver function tests, abdominal pain, and distention or even fever if infected. Percutaneous drainage is a viable strategy of treatment in case of symptomatic or infected bilomas as well as intrahepatic abscesses [32]. If this first line of treatment fails, an endoscopic retrograde cholangio-pancreatography (ERCP) with biliary stenting may represent an effective tool. This technique may be also used in case of *bilio-venous fistula* (usually associated with bilemia) [40]. In case of *bile peritonitis*, laparotomy is indicated. Another valid alternative is represented by combined laparoscopic drainage/irrigation and endoscopic bile duct stenting [41, 42].

*Hemobilia*, defined as blood in biliary system, may occur in case of an arterio-biliary fistula (usually due to a PSA). It presents with pain, jaundice, anemia, or even hematemesis or melena. The treatment usually consists in an AE of the PSA [14, 32].

*Abscesses* are rare, especially after NOM, and are usually associated with high-grade injuries. CT scan guided percutaneous drainage, same as in biliary collections, is the treatment of choice, showing high success rate and low morbidity [14].

*Necrosis* of a liver segment may occur after AE or following the trauma itself. The patients may present with elevation of liver transaminases, coagulopathy, abdominal pain, feeding intolerance, respiratory compromise, renal failure, and sepsis [32]. After definitive diagnosis at the CT scan, surgical management may be indicated. Hepatic necrosis requiring surgical debridement is much less common in patients managed non-operatively [32].

*Re-bleeding* or secondary hemorrhage is another frequent complication after liver trauma, and is more commonly reported after NOM. Bleeding can be defined early if occurs within 24 h and tends to occur more often within the first 3 days of injury [14, 43]. AG/AE is usually the treatment of choice, hence the bleeding often presents without severe hemodynamic compromise. AG/AE should be considered also in case of hepatic artery pseudoaneurysm or subcapsular hematoma in order to prevent rupture [14, 32].

## 95.8 Thrombo-Prophylaxis, Feeding, and Mobilization

Bed rest and prolonged in-hospital observation are no longer required. Hospital length of stay should be based on the clinical status of the patient. Mechanical prophylaxis has been shown to be safe and early mobilization should be considered in all stable trauma patients, unless some contraindications exist [44].

Several studies showed that early (<24–48 h) thromboembolic prophylaxis in trauma patients with solid organ injuries is safe: administration of low molecular weight heparin (LMWH) should be started as soon as possible [45, 46]. In patients under anticoagulant therapy, it is important to evaluate the possible need of reversal therapy balancing the risk of bleeding with the risk of thromboembolic complications.

It is also recommended to start as soon as possible the enteral feeding, in the absence of contraindications.

## 95.9 Follow-Up

Currently, follow-up CT scans are generally indicated only for those patients who develop signs or symptoms suggestive of hepatic abnormality or present a change in the clinical status: persistent abdominal pain, fever, jaundice, or drop in the hemoglobin level.

After discharge, mandatory imaging follow-up for liver injury is not advocated. The majority of hepatic injuries seem to be resolved at the CT scan imaging in 4 months [32]. Patients may return safely to normal physical activity 3–4 months after trauma [14].

### Dos and Don'ts
- Always consider NOM in hemodynamically stable patients and in transient responders if treated in a level I trauma center.
- Do not base the management decision on the anatomical severity of the injury.
- Consider AG/AE as a precious adjunct in NOM or even after DCS and perihepatic packing.
- Do not perform major resection or complex procedures during index intervention: aim to rapidly treat the lesion with the simplest technique available when possible.

### Take-Home Messages
- The majority of liver injuries can be successfully treated non-operatively, with the eventual adjunct of angiography/angioembolization.
- NOM is the gold standard in stable patients with hepatic trauma regardless of the severity of the injury.
- Interventional radiology plays a key role not only as a NOM extension but also in managing eventual complications; NOM with AG/AE plays a role in transient responder patients in selected centers.
- Interval laparoscopy may be considered as an extension of NOM to evaluate suspected injuries or in a planned step-up treatment.
- In case of operative treatment, surgery has two main goals: hemorrhage and bile leak control.

### Multiple Choice Questions
1. In hemodynamically stable patients, the most valuable investigation to study liver injuries is:
   A. E-FAST exam.
   B. **CT scan with intravenous contrast.**
   C. Chest X-ray.
   D. Diagnostic peritoneal lavage.
2. Which classification system considers both the anatomical aspect of the injury and the hemodynamic status of the patient?
   A. The AAST classification.
   B. Both the AAST-OIS classification and the WSES classification.
   C. **The WSES classification.**
   D. Neither of them.

3. The main factor leading to the choice between operative and non-operative management (NOM) is:
   A. The anatomical aspect of the injury.
   B. The severity of the AAST grade.
   C. **The hemodynamic status of the patient.**
   D. The mechanism of injury: blunt or penetrating.
4. Severe liver injuries (i.e., large subcapsular hematomas with parenchymal disruption):
   A. Represent absolute indications to operative management.
   B. **May be managed with NOM in case of patient's hemodynamic stability and absence of associated injuries requiring surgery.**
   C. May be managed with NOM regardless of the hemodynamic stability.
   D. Need to be treated with angiography/angioembolization (AG/AE).
5. Angiography/angioembolization finds a role as NOM "extension" and is indicated:
   A. In case of hemodynamic stability and presence of contrast blush at the CT scan.
   B. In case of hemodynamic stability and presence of vascular injury (i.e., PSA or arterio-venous fistula) detected at the CT scan.
   C. **A and B.**
   D. In all severe cases (AAST grades III, IV, and V) regardless of the hemodynamic status of the patient.
6. Interval laparoscopy:
   A. Plays no role in case of liver trauma.
   B. Is a useful tool only in case of penetrating trauma.
   C. **May help in the evaluation of a slow-healing liver injury with persistent laboratoristic alterations or abnormal clinical examinations.**
   D. Cannot be considered a "NOM-extension" being a surgical procedure.
7. Operative management is indicated in case of:
   A. Hemodynamic instability.
   B. CT scan evidence of intra-abdominal injury requiring surgery (i.e., hollow viscous injury).
   C. NOM failure with persistent bleeding.
   D. **All of the above mentioned.**
8. In case of major hemorrhage from a liver injury, during laparotomy, which strategy can be followed:
   A. Hepatic packing.
   B. Pringle maneuver.
   C. Attempt to repair the vascular lesion.
   D. **All of the above mentioned.**
9. In order to achieve hemorrhage and bile leak control during laparotomy for traumatic liver injury:
   A. **Hepatic debridement and direct repair or ligation of vessels are strategies that may be attempted.**
   B. Always try to perform major hepatic resections.
   C. Liberally ligate the portal vein.
   D. Never try to repair a hepatic artery injury.
10. Select the correct sentence:
    A. AG/AE finds no role or indication after hepatic packing (performed during a damage control surgery) or persistent arterial bleeding despite laparotomy.
    B. **Resuscitative endovascular balloon occlusion of the aorta (REBOA) may be used as a temporary bleeding control maneuver and as bridge to other more definitive procedures of hemorrhage control in hemodynamically unstable patients.**
    C. Major hepatic resections are recommended in every trauma scenario where hemorrhage control from a liver injury is unsuccessful.
    D. In case of NOM, monitoring of clinical status, parameters, and blood test of the patients is not recommended.

11. Hemobilia (defined as blood in the biliary system):
    A. May happen as a complication after liver trauma and it is usually due to a post-traumatic PSA.
    B. May present with pain, jaundice, hematemesis, or unexplained anemia.
    C. Can be treated with angioembolization, with good results.
    D. **All of the above.**

# References

1. Richardson JD, et al. Evolution in the management of hepatic trauma: A 25-year perspective. Ann Surg. 2000;232(3):324–30. https://doi.org/10.1097/00000658-200009000-00004.
2. Hörer TM, et al. Endovascular Resuscitation and Trauma Management (EVTM)-Practical Aspects and Implementation. Shock. 2021;56(1S):37–41.
3. Zago TM, Tavares Pereira BM, Araujo Calderan TR, Godinho M, Nascimento B, Fraga GP. Nonoperative management for patients with grade IV blunt hepatic trauma. World J Emerg Surg. 2012;7(S1) https://doi.org/10.1186/1749-7922-7-s1-s8.
4. Van Der Wilden GM, et al. Successful nonoperative management of the most severe blunt liver injuries: A multicenter study of the Research Consortium of New England Centers for Trauma. Arch Surg. 2012;147(5):423–8. https://doi.org/10.1001/archsurg.2012.147.
5. Shrestha B, et al. Damage-control resuscitation increases successful nonoperative management rates and survival after severe blunt liver injury. J Trauma Acute Care Surg. 2015;78(2):336–41. https://doi.org/10.1097/TA.0000000000000514.
6. Badger SA, Barclay R, Campbell P, Mole DJ, Diamond T. Management of liver trauma. World J Surg. 2009;33(12):2522–37. https://doi.org/10.1007/s00268-009-0215-z.
7. Moore EE, et al. Organ injury scaling: Spleen, liver, and kidney. J Trauma Inj Infect Crit Care. 1989;29(12):1664–6. https://doi.org/10.1097/00005373-198912000-00013.
8. Kozar RA, et al. Organ injury scaling 2018 update: Spleen, liver, and kidney. J Trauma Acute Care Surg. 2018;85(6):1119–22. https://doi.org/10.1097/TA.0000000000002058.
9. Tinkoff G, et al. American Association for the Surgery of Trauma Organ Injury Scale I: Spleen, Liver, and Kidney, Validation Based on the National Trauma Data Bank. J Am Coll Surg. 2008;207(5):646–55. https://doi.org/10.1016/j.jamcollsurg.2008.06.342.
10. Croce MA, et al. AAST organ injury scale: correlation of CT-graded liver injuries and operative findings. J Trauma Inj Infect Crit Care. 1991;31(6):806–12. https://doi.org/10.1097/00005373-199106000-00011.
11. G. C. Velmahos et al., "High success with nonoperative management of blunt hepatic trauma the liver is a sturdy organ," 2003.
12. Schellenberg M, Benjamin E, Piccinini A, Inaba K, Demetriades D. Gunshot wounds to the liver: No longer a mandatory operation. J Trauma Acute Care Surg. 2019;87(2):350–5. https://doi.org/10.1097/TA.0000000000002356.
13. Coccolini F, et al. WSES classification and guidelines for liver trauma. World J Emerg Surg. 2016;11(1):50. https://doi.org/10.1186/s13017-016-0105-2.
14. Coccolini F, et al. Liver trauma: WSES 2020 guidelines. World J Emerg Surg. 2020;15(1):35. https://doi.org/10.1186/s13017-020-00302-7.
15. Rossaint R, et al. Management of bleeding following major trauma: an updated European guideline. Crit Care. 2010;14(2):R52. https://doi.org/10.1186/cc8943.
16. Coccolini F, et al. Liver trauma: WSES position paper. World J Emerg Surg. 2015;10(1):39. https://doi.org/10.1186/s13017-015-0030-9.
17. Soffer D, et al. A prospective evaluation of ultrasonography for the diagnosis of penetrating torso injury. J Trauma Inj Infect Crit Care. 2004;56(5):953–9. https://doi.org/10.1097/01.TA.0000127806.39852.4E.
18. Ordoñez CA, Parra M, Holguín A, Garcia C, Guzmán-Rodríguez M, Padilla N, Caicedo Y, Orlas C, Garcia, A, Rodríguez-Holguín F, Serna J. Whole-body computed tomography is safe, effective and efficient in the severely injured hemodynamically unstable trauma patient. Colombia Médica. 2020;51(4):e-4054362. https://doi.org/10.25100/cm.v51i4.4362.
19. Shih HC, Wen YS, Ko TJ, Wu JK, Su CH, Lee CH. Noninvasive evaluation of blunt abdominal trauma: Prospective study using diagnostic algorithms to minimize nontherapeutic laparotomy. World J Surg. 1999;23(3):265–70. https://doi.org/10.1007/PL00013178.
20. Brooks A, Reilly J-J, Hope C, Navarro A, Naess PA, Gaarder C. Evolution of non-operative management of liver trauma. Trauma Surg Acute Care Open. 2020;5(1):e000551. https://doi.org/10.1136/tsaco-2020-000551.
21. Letoublon C, et al. Management of blunt hepatic trauma. J Visc Surg. 2016;153(4):33–43. https://doi.org/10.1016/j.jviscsurg.2016.07.005.
22. Boese CK, Hackl M, Müller LP, Ruchholtz S, Frink M, Lechler P. Nonoperative management of blunt hepatic trauma: A systematic review. J Trauma Acute Care Surg. 2015;79(4):654–60. https://doi.org/10.1097/TA.0000000000000814.
23. Hommes M, Navsaria PH, Schipper IB, Krige JEJ, Kahn D, Nicol AJ. Management of blunt liver trauma in 134 severely injured patients. Injury. 2015;46(5):837–42. https://doi.org/10.1016/j.injury.2014.11.019.

24. Yanar H, Ertekin C, Taviloglu K, Kabay B, Bakkaloglu H, Guloglu R. Nonoperative treatment of multiple intra-abdominal solid organ injury after blunt abdominal trauma. J Trauma Inj Infect Crit Care. 2008;64(4):943–8. https://doi.org/10.1097/TA.0b013e3180342023.
25. Velmahos GC, et al. Nonoperative treatment of blunt injury to solid abdominal organs: A prospective study. Arch Surg. 2003;138(8):844–51. https://doi.org/10.1001/archsurg.138.8.844.
26. Wisner DH, et al. Management of children with solid organ injuries after blunt torso trauma. J Trauma Acute Care Surg. 2015;79(2):206–14. https://doi.org/10.1097/TA.0000000000000731.
27. Lamb CM, Garner JP. Selective non-operative management of civilian gunshot wounds to the abdomen: A systematic review of the evidence. Injury. 2014;45(4):659–66. https://doi.org/10.1016/j.injury.2013.07.008.
28. Biffl WL, Leppaniemi A. Management guidelines for penetrating abdominal trauma. World J Surg. 2015;39(6):1373–80. https://doi.org/10.1007/s00268-014-2793-7.
29. Demetriades D, et al. Gunshot injuries to the liver: The role of selective nonoperative management. J Am Coll Surg. 1999;188(4):343–8. https://doi.org/10.1016/S1072-7515(98)00315-9.
30. Navsaria P, Nicol A, Krige J, Edu S, Chowdhury S. Selective nonoperative management of liver gunshot injuries. Eur J Trauma Emerg Surg. 2019;45(3):323–8. https://doi.org/10.1007/s00068-018-0913-z.
31. Demetriades D, et al. Selective nonoperative management of penetrating abdominal solid organ injuries. Ann Surg. 2006;244(4):620–8. https://doi.org/10.1097/01.sla.0000237743.22633.01.
32. Bruns BR, Kozar RA. Liver and biliary trauma. In: Moore E, Feliciano DV, Mattox KL, editors. Trauma. 8th ed. New York: McGraw-Hill Education; 2017. p. 551–74.
33. Ortega AE, Tang E, Froes ET, Asensio JA, Katkhouda N, Demetriades D. Laparoscopic evaluation of penetrating thoracoabdominal traumatic injuries. Surg Endosc. 1996;10(1):19–22. https://doi.org/10.1007/s004649910003.
34. O'Malley E, Boyle E, O'Callaghan A, Coffey JC, Walsh SR. Role of laparoscopy in penetrating abdominal trauma: A systematic review. World J Surg. 2013;37(1):113–22. https://doi.org/10.1007/s00268-012-1790-y.
35. Fabiani P, et al. Diagnostic and therapeutic laparoscopy for stab wounds of the anterior abdomen. J Laparoendosc Adv Surg Tech Part A. 2003;13(5):309–12. https://doi.org/10.1089/109264203769681682.
36. Kozar RA, et al. Western trauma association/critical decisions in trauma: Operative management of adult blunt hepatic trauma. J Trauma Inj Infect Crit Care. 2011;71(1):1–5. https://doi.org/10.1097/TA.0b013e318220b192.
37. Inaba K, Vogt KN. Liver trauma. In: Demetriades D, Inaba K, Velmahos GC, editors. Atlas of surgical techniques in trauma. New York: Cambridge University Press; 2015. p. 198–208.
38. Matsushima K, et al. Adjunctive use of hepatic angioembolization following hemorrhage control laparotomy. J Trauma Acute Care Surg. 2020;88(5):636–43. https://doi.org/10.1097/TA.0000000000002591.
39. Peitzman AB, Marsh JW. Advanced operative techniques in the management of complex liver injury. J Trauma Acute Care Surg. 2012;73(3):765–70. https://doi.org/10.1097/TA.0b013e318265cef5.
40. Harrell DJ, Vitale GC, Larson GM. Selective role for endoscopic retrograde cholangiopancreatography in abdominal trauma. Surg Endosc. 1998;12(5):400–4. https://doi.org/10.1007/s004649900690.
41. Carrillo EH, Reed DN, Gordon L, Spain DA, Richardson JD. Delayed laparoscopy facilitates the management of biliary peritonitis in patients with complex liver injuries. Surg Endosc. 2001;15(3):319–22. https://doi.org/10.1007/s004640000300.
42. Carrillo EH, et al. Interventional techniques are useful adjuncts in nonoperative management of hepatic injuries. J Trauma Inj Infect Crit Care. 1999;46(4):619–24. https://doi.org/10.1097/00005373-199904000-00010.
43. Kozar RA, et al. Risk factors for hepatic morbidity following nonoperative management: Multicenter study. Arch Surg. 2006;141(5):451–9. https://doi.org/10.1001/archsurg.141.5.451.
44. London JA, Parry L, Galante J, Battistella F. Safety of Early Mobilization of Patients With Blunt Solid Organ Injuries. Arch Surg. 2008;143(10):972–6.
45. Rostas JW, et al. The safety of low molecular-weight heparin after blunt liver and spleen injuries. Am J Surg. 2015;210(1):31–4. https://doi.org/10.1016/j.amjsurg.2014.08.023.
46. Murphy PB, et al. Very early initiation of chemical venous thromboembolism prophylaxis after blunt solid organ injury is safe. Can J Surg. 2016;59(2):118–22. https://doi.org/10.1503/cjs.010815.

## Further Reading

Coccolini F, et al. Liver trauma: WSES 2020 guidelines. World J Emerg Surg. 2020;15(1):35. https://doi.org/10.1186/s13017-020-00302-7.

Hörer TM, et al. Endovascular resuscitation and trauma management (EVTM)-practical aspects and implementation. Shock. 2021;56(1S):37–41.

Inaba K, Vogt KN. Liver trauma. In: Demetriades D, Inaba K, Velmahos GC, editors. Atlas of surgical techniques in trauma. New York: Cambridge University Press; 2015. p. 198–208.

Letoublon C, et al. Management of blunt hepatic trauma. J Visc Surg. 2016;153(4):33–43. https://doi.org/10.1016/j.jviscsurg.2016.07.005.

# Splenic Trauma

## 96

Tian Wei Cheng Brian Anthony, Carlo Vallicelli, and Fausto Catena

## 96.1 Introduction

> **Learning Goals**
> - To understand the AAST and WSES classification of splenic injury.
> - To be able to recognize patients suitable for nonoperative management [NOM] and understand the nuances of NOM.
> - To have a good grasp on the latest evidence regarding angioembolization and its role in NOM.
> - To understand the indications for splenectomy.

## 96.2 Epidemiology

There is currently no consensus on the overall incidence of splenic injury. According to a European study, the incidence of blunt splenic injury is low, but it accounts for significant mortality [1]. Studies from the United States show that the overall mortality of blunt splenic injury varies from an average of 8.2 to 13% from 1981 to 2000 [2]. In a Taiwanese study, the incidence of blunt splenic injury was also not common (8.33 per million/year), with injured patient numbers being consistent every year [3].

## 96.3 Etiology

The spleen is typically injured when there is trauma involving the lower left chest or the upper left abdomen [4, 5], primarily because of its juxtaposition in the left upper abdomen to the 9th, 10th, and 11th ribs.

The three mechanisms of injury:

- Penetrating trauma, e.g. abdominal gunshot wounds.
- Blunt trauma, e.g. a punch or kick to the abdomen.
- Indirect trauma, e.g. a tear in the splenic capsule during colonoscopy or traction on the splenocolic ligament.

Most mechanisms of injuries are similar between children and adults. These include motor vehicle crashes and pedestrian accidents. Conversely, certain mechanisms of injury such as motorcycle accidents, sports injuries, gunshots or stab-related injuries, and assaults are more frequent in adults [6].

---

T. W. C. B. Anthony (✉)
Department of General Surgery, Singapore General Hospital, Singapore, Singapore
e-mail: brian.anthony.tian.w.c@singhealth.com.sg

C. Vallicelli · F. Catena
Department of General, Acute Care and Trauma Surgery, Bufalini Hospital, Cesena, Italy
e-mail: carlo.vallicelli@auslromagna.it;
fausto.catena@auslromagna.it

## 96.4 Classification

The traditional classification system is the AAST system (Table 96.1) which takes the anatomical insult as the main consideration in injury grading. However, this does not take into account the overall clinical status of the patient.

The World Society of Emergency Surgery (WSES) has recently published an updated classification, that factors the clinical picture into the management algorithm [7]. The WSES classification is as follows (Table 96.2):

- Minor (WSES class I) includes hemodynamically stable AAST grade I–II blunt and penetrating lesions.
- Moderate (WSES classes II) includes hemodynamically stable AAST grade III blunt and penetrating lesions.
- Moderate (WSES classes III) includes hemodynamically stable AAST grade IV–V blunt and penetrating lesions.
- Severe (WSES class IV) includes hemodynamically unstable AAST grade I–V blunt and penetrating lesions.

**Table 96.1** AAST classification of splenic trauma

| Grade | Injury description | |
|---|---|---|
| I | Hematoma | Subcapsular, <10% surface area |
|   | Laceration | Capsular tear, <1 cm parenchymal depth |
| II | Hematoma | Subcapsular, <10–50% surface area |
|   |   | Intraparenchymal, <5 cm diameter |
|   | Laceration | 1–3 cm parenchymal depth not involving a parenchymal vessel |
| III | Hematoma | Subcapsular, >50% surface area or expanding |
|   |   | Ruptured subcapsular or parenchymal hematoma |
|   |   | Intraparenchymal hematoma >5 cm |
|   | Laceration | >3 cm parenchymal depth or involving trabecular vessels |
| IV | Laceration | Laceration of segmental or hilar vessels producing major devascularization (>25% of spleen) |
| V | Laceration | Completely shatters spleen |
|   | Vascular | Hilar vascular injury which devascularized spleen |

**Table 96.2** WSES classification of splenic trauma

|  | WSESclass | Mechanism of injury | AAST | Hemodynamic status[a,b] | CT scan | First-Line treatment in adults | First-Line treatment in pediatric |
|---|---|---|---|---|---|---|---|
| Minor | WSES I | Blunt/penetrating | I–II | Stable | Yes + local exploration in SW[d] | NOM[c] + serial clinical/radiological evaluation Consider angiography/angioembolization | NOM[c] + serial clinical/radiological evaluation Consider angiography/angioembolization |
| Moderate | WSES II | Blunt/penetrating | III | Stable | | | |
| | WSES III | Blunt/penetrating | IV–V | Stable | | NOM[c] All angiography/angioembolization + serial clinical/laboratory/radiological evaluation | |
| Severe | WSES IV | Blunt/penetrating | I–V | Unstable | No | OM | OM |

*SW* stab wound, *GSW* gunshot wound

[a] *Hemodynamic instability in adults* is considered the condition in which the patient has an admission systolic blood pressure <90 mmHg with evidence of skin vasoconstriction (cool, clammy, decreased capillary refill) and an altered level of consciousness, or a blood pressure >90 mmHg but requiring bolus infusions/transfusions and/or vasopressor drugs and/or admission base excess (BE) > −5 mmol/L and/or shock index >1 and/or transfusion requirement of at least 4–6 units of packed red blood cells within the first 24 h. Conversely, transient responders are those patients who show an initial response to fluid resuscitation, and thereafter still have signs of ongoing loss and perfusion deficits.

[b] *Hemodynamic stability in pediatric patients* is considered as having a systolic blood pressure of 90 mmHg plus twice the child's age in years (the lower limit is inferior to 70 mmHg plus twice the child's age in years, or inferior to 50 mmHg in some studies). Stabilized or acceptable hemodynamic status is considered in children with a positive response to fluid resuscitation: 3 blouses of 20 mL/kg of crystalloid replacement should be administered before blood replacement; positive response can be indicated by the heart rate reduction, the sensorium clearing. the return of peripheral pluses and normal skin color, an increase in blood pressure and urinary output, and an increase in warmth of extremity. Clinical judgement is fundamental in evaluating children

[c] NOM should only be attempted in centers capable of a precise diagnosis of the severity of spleen injuries and capable of intensive management (close clinical observation and hemodynamic monitoring in a high dependency/intensive care, including serial clinical examination and laboratory assay, with immediate access to diagnostics, interventional radiology, and surgery and immediately available access to blood and blood products or alternatively in the presence of a rapid centralization system in those patients amenable to be transferred

[d] Wound exploration near the inferior costal margin should be avoided if not strictly necessary because of the high risk to damage the intercostal vessels

## 96.5 Diagnosis

### 96.5.1 Clinical Presentation

Patients will present with a history of trauma, abdominal pain, and varying stages of shock.

### 96.5.2 Diagnostic Imaging

1. Extended focused assessment sonography for trauma (E-FAST) has replaced diagnostic peritoneal lavage (DPL) in the management of abdominal trauma [8–10]. Studies have shown a sensitivity of up to 91% and a specificity of up to 96% for a small fluid amount [11, 12]. The E-FAST can detect the presence of free fluid and can also provide an ultrasonographic image of the spleen itself. Moreover, the E-FAST is readily available at the bedside, thus increasing its utility and applicability.

2. Contrast tomography (CT) scan is considered the gold standard in trauma with a sensitivity and specificity for splenic injuries near to 96–100% [9, 13, 14]. However, hilar injuries may be underestimated [9]. The main considerations prior to using the CT scanner, are that the

scanner must be rapidly available and must be performed only in hemodynamically stable patients or in those responding to fluid resuscitation [15, 16]. The CT scan is particularly useful as it can help delineate the anatomy of the injured spleen, which helps in the AAST grading of the injury. The delayed phase can also further differentiate patients with active bleeding from those with contained vascular injuries [17].

The identification of an active contrast extravasation is a classic sign of active hemorrhage [18]. Contrast blush occurs in about 17% of cases and has been demonstrated to be an important predictor of failure of NOM (>60% of patients with blush failed NOM). However, the absence of a blush on the CT scan in high-grade splenic injuries does not definitively exclude active bleeding and should not preclude angioembolization [13, 19, 20].

## 96.6 Management

### 96.6.1 Nonoperative Management (NOM) for Blunt Splenic Trauma

For hemodynamically stable patients, with the absence of other abdominal organ injuries that require surgery, these patients should undergo a trial of NOM regardless of injury grade [13, 21–24]. The caveat is that the hospital must have the capability for intensive monitoring, facilities and expertise for angioembolization, the ready access to available operating theatres, and immediate access to blood products. The presence of a CT scanner is paramount, as a baseline CT scan with intravenous contrast is necessary to define the anatomical splenic injury and to identify associated injuries.

The success rate of NOM in such circumstances is approximately 90% [25]. The advantages of NOM include reduced hospital costs, avoidance of nontherapeutic laparotomies, lower rates of blood transfusions, lower mortality, and the prevention of overwhelming post-splenectomy infection [OPSI] [23, 26, 27]. Routine laparotomy in hemodynamically stable patients with blunt splenic injury is not indicated [28, 29].

Risk factors for NOM failure include age > 55 years old, high ISS, and moderate to severe splenic injuries [15, 37, 40]. Other relative risk factors for NOM failure include age > 55 years old alone, large hemoperitoneum alone, hypotension before resuscitation, GCS < 12, low hematocrit level upon admission, associated abdominal injuries, blush at CT scan, anticoagulation drugs, HIV disease, drug addiction, cirrhosis, and need for blood transfusions [13, 17, 18, 25, 30–40].

An exception however exists for patients with WSES classes II–III spleen injuries with associated severe traumatic brain injury. In these patients, NOM could be considered only if absolutely efficient and rapid rescue therapy is available; otherwise, splenectomy should be performed.

### 96.6.2 Nonoperative Management (NOM) for Penetrating Trauma

Laparotomy has been the gold standard in penetrating abdominal trauma [e.g., gunshot and stab wounds]. Overall, the rate of negative laparotomy ranges between 9% and 14% [41, 42] in these cases. However, if the patient is found to have concomitant pancreatic, diaphragmatic, colic, and splenic injuries, they tend to have a significantly increased mortality rate [43]. The associated pancreatic injuries also frequently require spleno-pancreatectomy [43]. Although there is a trend toward adopting NOM for gunshot and stab injuries [44, 45], the decision for NOM in penetrating trauma should be still decided on a case-by-case basis.

### 96.6.3 Role of Angiography and Angioembolization [AG/AE] in NOM

The main indications for AG/AE are [46–48]:

1. WSES I and II patients who have vascular injuries detected via CT scan (contrast blush, pseudo-aneurysms, and arteriovenous fistula). Hemodynamically stable patients with WSES class I and II lesions without blush should not

undergo routine AG/AE but may be considered for prophylactic proximal embolization in presence of risk factors for NOM failure.
2. WSES III patients who are hemodynamically stable regardless of the presence of CT blush.
3. Patients who are stable with signs of persistent hemorrhage regardless of the absence of CT blush once extra-splenic source of bleeding has been excluded.

Some considerations during AG/AE:

1. In presence of a single vascular abnormality (contrast blush, pseudo-aneurysms and arteriovenous fistula) in minor and moderate injuries, it is unclear whether proximal or distal embolization should be adopted [49]. Both methods were found to be similar with regard to the incidence of major infarctions, infections, and major rebleeding [50].
2. In presence of multiple splenic vascular abnormalities or in presence of a severe lesion, proximal or combined AG/AE should be used, after confirming the presence of a permissive pancreatic vascular anatomy. Or in the absence of blush during angiography, if a blush was previously seen at CT scan, proximal angioembolization could be considered.
3. In performing AG/AE, coils should be preferred to temporary agents.
4. Conversely, when AG/AE is not rapidly available or in event of rapid hemodynamic deterioration, surgery should be considered.

The reported success rate of NOM with AG/AE ranges from 86 to 100% [46–48, 51–58]. AG/AE reduces the odds of splenectomy, with better results, the earlier the AG/AE was performed [58, 59]. Meta-analyses have shown a significant improvement in NOM success following introduction of AG/AE protocols (OR 0.26, 95% CI 0.13–0.53, $p < 0.002$) [37, 60–62].

Between 2.3 and 47% CT detected, contrast blushes could not be confirmed during angiography [63, 64]. Moreover an analysis on 143 patients with blush at CT scan suggested that an angiographic procedure without embolization increases twofold the risk of rebleeding and NOM failure [64].

The use of routine prophylactic AG/AE in high-grade splenic injuries is controversial [19, 46, 48, 54, 65–68]. NOM failure rates both with and without prophylactic AG/AE for high-grade injuries are 0–42% vs. 23–67%, respectively [19, 46, 48, 54, 65, 66]. Controversies exist regarding which kind of lesions should be considered as "high-grade" (AAST III–V or IV–V grade) and should undergo routine AG/AE [19, 46, 67, 68]. It has been reported that NOM could fail in up to 3% of grade III lesions without blush, with no AG/AE [19]. Considering the AG/AE-related morbidity of 47% (versus 10% related to NOM without AG/AE) [68], patients with grade III lesions without blush should not undergo routine AG/AE.

AG/AE major morbidity rates range from 3.7 to 28.5% including rebleeding, splenic infarction, splenic abscesses, acute renal insufficiency, pseudocysts, and puncture-related complications [19, 46, 48, 69–76]. The rates for minor morbidities range from 23 to 61% and include fever, pleural effusion, and coil migration [48, 69, 75, 76]. Comparatively, patients undergoing OM still reported significantly higher complication rates as compared to those who had AG/AE [68, 70, 71, 74].

AG/AE does not seem to totally compromise the splenic function, and, even in presence of an elevated leukocyte and platelet counts, no significant differences in immunoglobulin titers were found between splenic artery AG/AE patients and controls [66]. The spleen due to its intense vascularization, can maintain the necessary bloodflow to continue its immunological function.

### 96.6.4 Operative Management (OM)

The main indications of OM include:

1. Patients with hemodynamic instability or with associated lesions like peritonitis or bowel evisceration requiring surgical exploration. The severity of splenic injury seems to be related to the incidence of hollow viscus injury (1.9, 2.4, 4.9, and 11.6% in minor, moderate, major, and massive injuries, respectively) [77].
2. OM should be performed in moderate and severe lesions even in stable patients, in cen-

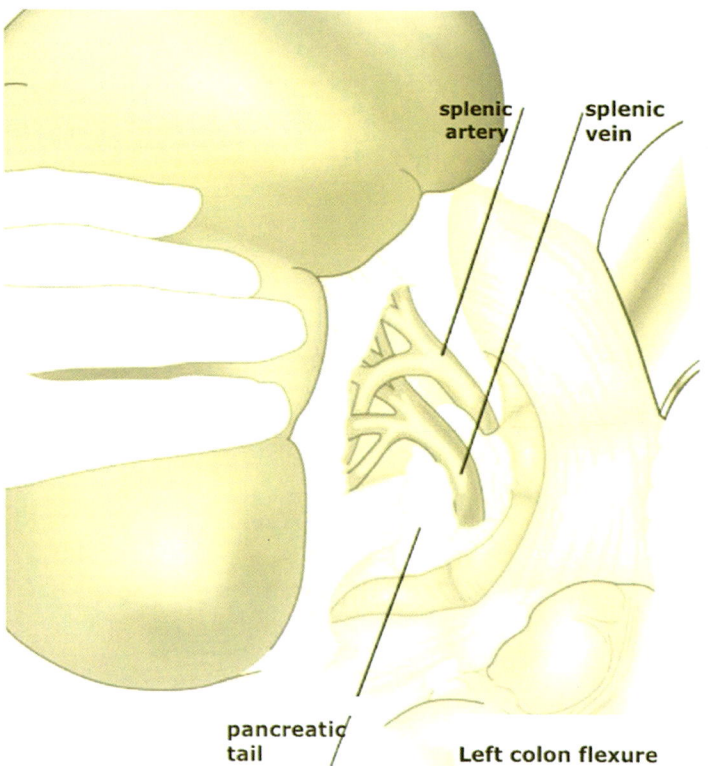

**Fig. 96.1** Open splenectomy

ters where intensive monitoring cannot be performed and/or when AG/AE is not rapidly available [78, 79].

3. When NOM with AG/AE fails and patient remains hemodynamically unstable or shows a significant drop in hematocrit levels or continuous transfusion is required, OM is also indicated.

During OM, salvage of a part of the spleen is controversial [80, 81]. The use of splenic autologous transplantation—leaving pieces of spleen inside the abdomen—to avoid infective risk from splenectomy has not been shown to reduce morbidity or mortality [82]. Overall mortality of splenectomy in trauma is approximately 2%, and the incidence of postoperative bleeding after splenectomy ranges from 1.6 to 3%, but with mortality near to 20% [83]. Laparoscopic splenectomy in bleeding trauma patients is not recommended, and open splenectomy is mandatory [84, 85] (Fig. 96.1).

WSES spleen trauma management algorithm for adult patients is reported in Fig. 96.2.

### 96.6.5 Thromboprophylaxis in Splenic Trauma

Trauma patients are at high risk of venous thromboembolism (VTE). The transition to a hypercoagulation state occurs within 48 h from injury [86–88]. For patients who survive beyond the first 24 h, pulmonary embolism (PE) is the third leading cause of death. Even with chemical prophylaxis, deep venous thrombosis (DVT) can be detected in 15% of patients. If this progresses to PE, the mortality is about 50% [86, 87].

DVT prophylaxis is paramount in trauma patients. Mechanical prophylaxis is very safe and should be considered in all patients without absolute contraindication to its use.

Regarding chemical prophylaxis, it is best to consider using LMWH-based prophylactic anticoagulation. Splenic trauma without ongoing bleeding is not an absolute contraindication to this. If anything, prophylactic anticoagulation should be started as soon as possible from trauma [120]. Bellal et al. [89] found no difference in hemorrhagic complication and NOM failure rate in patients with

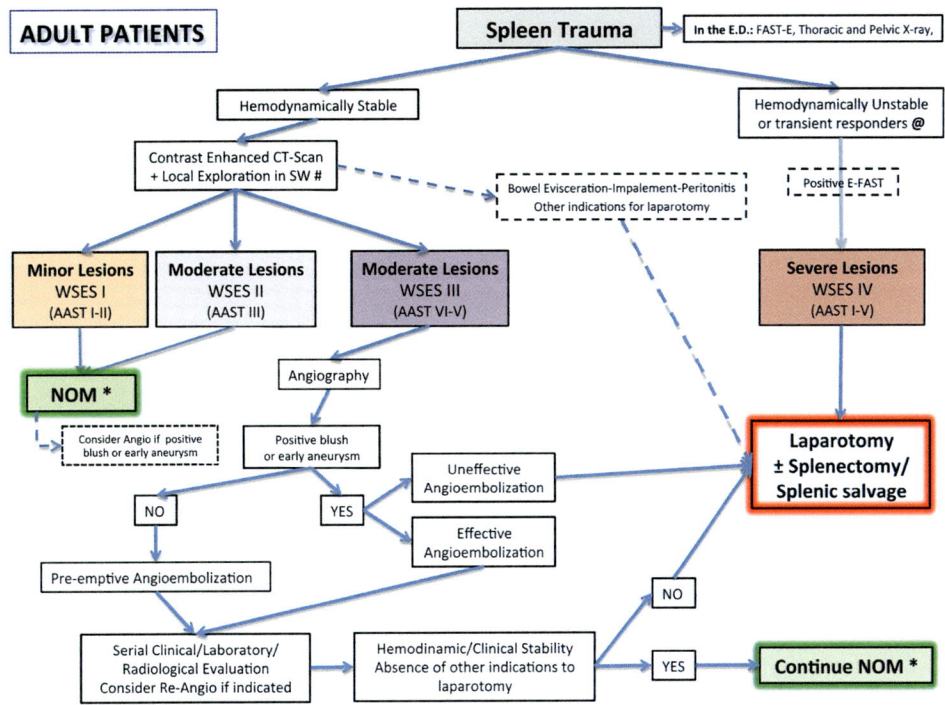

**Fig. 96.2** WSES spleen trauma management algorithm for adult patients

early (< 48 h), intermediate (48–72 h), and late (> 72 h) VTE prophylaxis. Rostas et al. [86] show that VTE rates were over fourfold greater when LMWH was administered after 72 h from admission. Pertaining to oral anticoagulants, the risk-benefit balance of reversal should be individualized. Failing to resume anticoagulation in a timely fashion is associated with poor outcomes [90].

## 96.7 Prognosis: Short- and Long-Term Follow-up for NOM

Complete bed rest for the first 48-72hours, is the cornerstone of NOM treatment for patients with moderate and severe splenic traumatic lesions [16]. 19% of splenic-delayed ruptures happen within the first 48 h, with the majority of delayed ruptures occuring most frequently between 4 to 10 days after the trauma. Patients can present for a delayed splenectomy after discharge, anytime between 3 and 146 days after injury, and the rate of readmission for splenectomy was 1.4% [91] with approximately 2% of patients requiring late intervention [92].

Savage et al. [92] found an average of healing time of 12.5 days for patients with grades I–II splenic injury, with a complete healing after 50 days. Conversely patients with grades III–V injuries required 37.2 and 75 days respectively. In 2–2.5 months, regardless of the severity of the splenic injury, 84% of patients had complete healing [92]. Crawford et al. suggested that an early discharge is safe because late failure occurs infrequently [39, 93]. Nonetheless, the mortality of delayed rupturse range from 5 to 15% compared with 1% mortality in cases of acute rupture [31, 94]. In any case, patients who have undergone NOM should be counseled to not remain alone or in isolated places for the first weeks after the discharge, and they should be warned about the red flag symptoms to watch out for.

Repeated CT scans during the admission should be considered in patients with moderate or severe lesions, or those with decreasing hematocrit, or patients who were found to have vascular anomalies or underlying splenic pathologies or coagulopathies, and in neurologically impaired patients. However, there is no consensus regarding the timing and type of imaging (CT vs. US) [16, 31, 95–

98]. More than 50% of patients demonstrated healing at an interval follow-up CT scan after 6 weeks, and subsequent further scans seemed to have no additional clinical utility [99]. However, routine post-discharge follow-up abdominal CT is not necessary in low-grade (AAST grade I or II) injuries [96].

Activity restriction may be suggested for 4–6 weeks in minor injuries and up to 2–4 months in moderate and severe injuries [92, 98, 100, 101]. Complete healing of almost all grades is observed 3 months after injury. The role of radiological follow-up before returning to normal activity remains controversial overall.

## 96.8 Pediatric Splenic Trauma (<15 Years Old)

The spleen is the most commonly injured solid organ in pediatric blunt trauma (25–30%) [6, 102]. The Eastern Association for the Surgery of Trauma (EAST) recommends NOM in blunt splenic trauma in all hemodynamically stable children irrespective of the AAST injury grade [103, 104].

NOM seems to be more effective in children [105] and is associated with reduced costs and lengths of hospital stay, less need for blood transfusions, vaccinations, and antibiotic therapy, as well as higher immunity and reduced rate of infections [106–110]. Even though it is not clear why NOM outcomes are superior in children compared with adults, this phenomenon may be related to certain unique pediatric characteristics (e.g., thicker splenic capsule, higher proportion of myoepithelial cells, more efficient contraction, and retraction of the splenic arterioles [111–116]).

WSES spleen trauma management algorithm for pediatric patients is reported in Fig. 96.3.

### 96.8.1 Diagnostic Procedures

*Contrast-enhanced computer tomography (CT)* is the gold standard for the evaluation of blunt abdominal trauma [6, 8]. However, patients

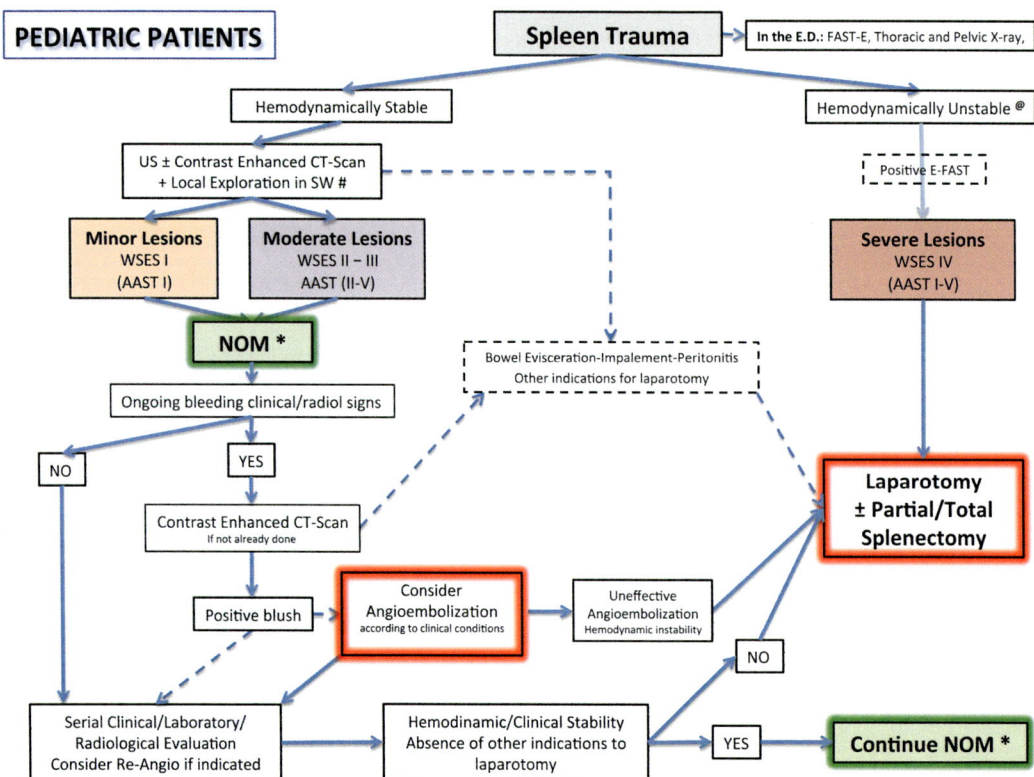

**Fig. 96.3** WSES spleen trauma management algorithm for pediatric patients

should be hemodynamically stable as well as cooperative or sedated. Of note, surgeons should interpret CT findings cautiously before opting for OM because more than 50% of children present with grade III–IV lesions [6].

*FAST (Focused Assessment with Sonography for Trauma)*: The role of FAST for the diagnosis of spleen injury in children is still unclear. The sensitivity of this imaging modality in children ranges from 50 to 92% [117–119]. The specificity of this exam is also quite low, and, therefore, in a hemodynamically stable patient, a positive FAST examination should be followed by an urgent CT. Bedside FAST may have utility in hemodynamically unstable patients to rapidly identify or rule out intraperitoneal hemorrhage when patients cannot undergo CT.

### 96.8.2 Nonoperative Management in Splenic Injury

NOM is recommended as first-line treatment for hemodynamically stable pediatric patients with blunt splenic trauma [105]. Patients with moderate-severe blunt and all penetrating splenic injuries should be considered for transfer to dedicated pediatric trauma centers after stabilization.

NOM of splenic injuries in children should be considered only in an environment that has the capability for patient continuous monitoring, angiography, trained surgeons, an immediately available OR, and immediate access to blood and blood products or alternatively in the presence of a rapid centralization system in those patients amenable to be transferred [120, 121]. NOM should be attempted even in the setting of concomitant head trauma, unless the patient is unstable due to intra-abdominal bleeding.

In particular, for blunt splenic injuries with hemodynamic stability and absence of other internal injuries requiring surgery, these patients should undergo an initial attempt of NOM irrespective of injury grade. The presence of contrast blush at CT scan is not an absolute indication for splenectomy or AG/AE in children. Intensive care unit admission in isolated splenic injury may be required only for moderate and severe lesions [122].

However, no sufficient data validating NOM for penetrating spleen injury in children exist. However, reports on successful nonoperative management of isolated penetrating spleen injuries in hemodynamically stable pediatric patients do exist [123–125].

NOM failure rates for pediatric splenic trauma have been shown to range from 2 to 5% [126, 127]. Of note, there is evidence suggesting that the rate of NOM failure peaks at 4 h and then declines over 36 h from admission [126]. Overall, the majority (72.5%) of NOM failures seem to occur during the first week after trauma, with 50% of them happening within the first 3–5 days [128].

### 96.8.3 The Role of Angiography/Angioembolization (AG/AE)

The vast majority of pediatric patients do not require AG/AE for CT blush or moderate to severe injuries [129–131].

However, there are several potential considerations:

1. AG/AE may be considered if the patient has signs of persistent hemorrhage not amenable to NOM, once extra-splenic source of bleeding has been excluded.
2. AG/AE may be considered for the treatment of post-traumatic splenic pseudo-aneurysms prior to patient discharge.
3. Patients of more than 15 years old, or children of less than 13–15 years old that are more vulnerable to OPSI, should be managed according to adults AG/AE-protocols [132, 133].

The role of embolization in the management of pediatric splenic pseudo-aneurysms is also unclear. Of note, PSAs often undergo spontaneous thrombosis and could resolve without any interventions [97, 108, 131].

Mortality and major complications are rarely reported following AG/AE [131, 132, 134, 135]. Nevertheless, a post-embolization syndrome (PES), consisting of abdominal pain, nausea, ileus, and fever, seems to occur in 90% of children undergoing AG/AE. This syndrome is usually self-limited and tends to resolve spontaneously in 6–9 days [136]. In addition, pleural effusion (9%), pneumonia (9%), and coil migration (4.5%) can also be seen after splenic embolization [132]. Overall, AG/AE seems to preserve splenic function without lasting complications, but most children do not need this intervention [130].

### 96.8.4 Operative Management in Blunt and Penetrating Injuries

Patients should undergo OM in cases of hemodynamic instability, failure of conservative treatment, severe coexisting injuries necessitating intervention, and peritonitis, bowel evisceration, and impalement [122, 137–140].

Splenic preservation (at least partial) should be attempted whenever possible. Partial (subtotal) splenectomy or splenorrhaphy are safe and viable alternatives to total splenectomy and can be performed even in high-grade injuries [139, 141–143]. 1% of pediatric patients who undergo immediate OM are readmitted for intestinal obstruction within a year [140].

### 96.8.5 Splenic Trauma Associated with Head Injuries

Head injury is an important cause of morbidity and mortality in trauma patients of all ages (50–60%) and can also result in altered mental status, which can complicate the process of clinical evaluation [144]. Especially in the setting of concurrent head injury, blood pressure and heart rate are poor markers of hemorrhagic shock in pediatric patients [122]. Nevertheless, an analysis of the National Pediatric Trauma Registry suggested that the association of altered mental status from head injury with spleen injuries should not impact the decision for observational management in pediatric patients (< 19 years old) [144].

### 96.8.6 Short- and Long-Term Follow-Up in Splenic Trauma (Blunt and Penetrating)

In hemodynamic stable children without a drop in hemoglobin levels for 24 h, bed rest should be suggested. Initial APSA guidelines [106] recommended bed rest for a number of days equal to the grade of injury plus 1 day [106]. However, recent studies suggest a shorter bed rest of one night in solitary grade I–II splenic trauma and two nights for patients with more severe injuries (grade ≥ III) and stable hemoglobin level [145]. Longer admissions should be considered in patients with lower hemoglobin levels on admission, higher injury grade, suspected other abdominal injuries (as pancreatic or small bowel injuries), blush on the CT scan, bicycle handlebar injuries, and recurrent bleeding or patients at risk for missed injuries [122].

US (DUS, CEUS) follow-up seems reasonable to minimize the risk of life-threatening hemorrhage and associated complications in children [146].

After NOM in moderate and severe injuries, the reprise of normal activity could be considered safe after at least 6 weeks. The APSA guidelines [106] recommended 2–5 months of "light" activity before restart with normal activities and recommended 3 week–3 months of limited activity at home. In fact, the risks of delayed splenic rupture and post-traumatic pseudocysts seem to be increase within the first 3 weeks (incidence 0.2 and 0.3%, respectively) [106, 147]. Canadian guidelines suggested a discharge at home after reprise and good toleration of oral intake, able mobilization, and analgesia with oral medications; without a need for any imaging prior to discharge [148]. They reported a restriction of activities of no more than 6–8 weeks [148].

## 96.9 Infection Prophylaxis in Asplenic and Hyposplenic Adult and Pediatric Patients

Patients should receive immunization against encapsulated bacteriae (*Streptococcus pneumoniae*, *Haemophilus influenzae*, and *Neisseria meningitidis*) [149, 150]. Vaccination programs should be started no sooner than 14 days after splenectomy or splenic total vascular exclusion. In fact, before 14 days, the antibody response is suboptimal [149, 151]; after that interval, the earlier the better. In asplenic/hyposplenic patients discharged before 15 days, where the risk to miss the vaccination is deemed high, the first vaccines should be given before discharge [151, 152]. The Center for Disease Control in 2016 proposed these last updated recommendations [153].

Most episodes of severe infections occur within the first 2 years after splenectomy, and for this reason, some authors recommended at least 2 years of prophylactic antibiotics after splenectomy. However, the duration of antibiotic prophylaxis is controversial.

Ideally, the vaccinations against *S. pneumoniae*, *H. influenzae* type B, and *N. meningitidis* should be given at least 2 weeks before splenectomy [6]. Patients should be informed that immunization can only reduce the incidence of OPSI (vaccines so far available do not allow an exhaustive coverage for *S. pneumoniae*—23 of 90 serotypes are included, nor for *N. meningitidis*—5 of 6 serotypes).

Annual immunization against seasonal flu is recommended for all patients over 6 months of age [154, 155]. Malaria prophylaxis is strongly recommended for travelers. Antibiotic therapy should be strongly considered in the event of any sudden onset of unexplained fever, malaise, chills, or other constitutional symptoms, especially when medical review is not readily accessible.

OPSI is a medical emergency. The risks of OPSI and associated death are highest in the first year after splenectomy, at least among young children, but remain elevated for more than 10 years and probably for life. The incidence of OPSI is 0.5–2%; the mortality rate is from 30 to 70%, and most death occurs within the first 24 h. Only prompt diagnosis and immediate treatment can reduce mortality [6, 150, 151, 154]. Asplenic/hyposplenic children younger than 5 years old have a greater overall risk of OPSI with an increased death compared with adults [149, 155]. The risk is more than 30% in neonates [6]. Evidence exists regarding the possible maintainence of function by the embolized spleen (hyposplenic patients); however, it is reasonable to consider it as less effective and proceed with vaccination as well [130, 156].

Asplenic/hyposplenic patients should be given an antibiotic supply in the event of any sudden onset of unexplained fever, malaise, chills, or other constitutional symptoms, especially when medical review is not readily accessible. The recommended options for emergency standby in adults include the following: (a) amoxicillin, 3 g starting dose followed by 1 g, every 8 h; (b) levofloxacin 500 mg every 24 h or moxifloxacin 400 mg every 24 h (for beta-lactam allergic patients). The recommended emergency standby treatment in children is amoxicillin 50 mg/Kg in three divided daily doses. For beta-lactam allergic patients, an alternative should be proposed by a specialist (fluoroquinolones are generally contraindicated in children, but due to the possible severity of OPSI, they might still be considered).

---

### Dos and Dont's

**Dos**

1. All hemodynamically stable patients with blunt splenic trauma should be managed nonoperatively, with angio-embolization applied when indicated.
2. All unstable patients with splenic trauma should be managed operatively.
3. Stable patients with severe injuries should be considered for operative management, if angioembolization and monitoring facilities are inadequate.

**Don'ts**

1. Do not operate on pediatric patients with splenic trauma unless absolutely indicated, e.g., concomitant injuries requiring surgery.

## MCQ

1. NOM for splenic trauma:
   A. Is always possible.
   B. **Is possible only for stable patients.**
   C. Is performed with splenectomy.
   D. Is not possible.
2. NOM for splenic trauma:
   A. Is performed in all hospitals (HUB and SPOKE).
   B. **Is performed in HUB trauma centers.**
   C. Is performed if surgical services are not available.
   D. Is performed without interventional radiology.
3. NOM for splenic trauma:
   A. Is performed always with splenic artery embolization.
   B. **Can be performed with bed rest and close observation alone.**
   C. Is performed always with splenic artery distal embolization.
   D. Is performed always with embolization.

### Take-Home Messages

- Nonoperative management is the first line of management for stable patients with blunt splenic trauma.
- If unstable, or if monitoring facilities are inadequate, surgical management is the first line option.
- For stable penetrating traumas, each case should be evaluated individually to decide if surgery or conservative management would be most ideal.

## References

1. Brady RRW, Bandari M, Kerssens JJ, Paterson-Brown S, Parks RW. Splenic trauma in Scotland: demographics and outcomes. World J Surg. 2007;31(11):2111–6.
2. Hartnett KL, Winchell RJ, Clark DE. Management of adult splenic injury: a 20-year perspective. Am Surg. 2003;69(7):608–11.
3. Soo KM, Lin TY, Chen CW, Lin YK, Kuo LC, Wang JY, Lee WC, Lin HL. More becomes less: management strategy has definitely changed over the past decade of splenic injury—a nationwide population-based study. Biomed Res Int. 2015;2015:124969. https://doi.org/10.1155/2015/124969. Epub 2015 Jan 5
4. Zarzaur BL, Rozycki GS. An update on nonoperative management of the spleen in adults. Trauma Surg Acute Care Open. 2017;2(1):e000075.
5. Yang K, Li Y, Wang C, Xiang B, Chen S, Ji Y. Clinical features and outcomes of blunt splenic injury in children: a retrospective study in a single institution in China. Medicine (Baltimore). 2017;96(51):e9419.
6. Lynn KN, Werder GM, Callaghan RM, Sullivan AN, Jafri ZH, Bloom DA. Pediatric blunt splenic trauma: a comprehensive review. Pediatr Radiol. 2009;39:904–16.
7. Coccolini F, Montori G, Catena F, et al. Splenic trauma: WSES classification and guidelines for adult and pediatric patients. World J Emerg Surg. 2017;12:40.
8. American College of Surgeon's Commitee on Trauma. Advanced Trauma Life Support® (ATLS®) student manual. 9th ed. Chicago, IL: American College of Surgeon; 2012.
9. Carr JA, Roiter C, Alzuhaili A. Correlation of operative and pathological injury grade with computed tomographic grade in the failed nonoperative management of blunt splenic trauma. Eur J Trauma Emerg Surg. 2012;38:433–8.
10. Kirkpatrick AW, Sirois M, Laupland KB, Liu D, Rowan K, Ball CG, et al. Hand-held thoracic sonography for detecting post-traumatic pneumothoraces: the extended focused assessment with sonography for trauma (EFAST). J Trauma. 2004;57:288–95.
11. Doody O, Lyburn D, Geoghegan T, Govender P, Monk PM, Torreggiani WC. Blunt trauma to the spleen: ultrasonographic findings. Clin Radiol. 2005;60:968–76.
12. El-Matbouly M, Jabbour G, El-Menyar A, Peralta R, Abdelrahman H, Zarour A, et al. Blunt splenic trauma: assessment, management and outcomes. Surgeon. 2016;14:52–8.
13. Bee TK, Croce MA, Miller PR, Pritchard FE, Fabian TC. Failures of splenic nonoperative management: is the glass half empty or half full? J Trauma. 2001;50:230–6.
14. Clark R, Hird K, Misur P, Ramsay D, Mendelson R. CT grading scales for splenic injury: why can't we agree? J Med Imaging Radiat Oncol. 2011;55:163–9.
15. Becker CD, Mentha G, Terrier F. Blunt abdominal trauma in adults: role of CT in the diagnosis and management of visceral injuries. Part 1: liver and spleen. Eur Radiol. 1998;8:553–62.
16. Shapiro MJ, Krausz C, Durham RM, Mazuski JE. Overuse of splenic scoring and computed tomographic scans. J Trauma. 1999;47:651–8.
17. Anderson SW, Varghese JC, Lucey BC, P a B, Hirsch EF, J a S. Blunt splenic trauma: delayed-phase CT for differentiation of active hemorrhage from

contained vascular injury in patients. Radiology. 2007;243:88–95.
18. Jeffrey RB, Olcott EW. Imaging of blunt hepatic trauma. Radiol Clin N Am. 1991;29:1299–310.
19. Bhullar IS, Frykberg ER, Tepas JJ, Siragusa D, Loper T, Kerwin AJ. At first blush: absence of computed tomography contrast extravasation in grade IV or V adult blunt splenic trauma should not preclude angioembolization. J Trauma Acute Care Surg. 2013;74:105–11; discussion 111-2
20. Hassan R, Aziz AA, Ralib ARM, Saat A. Computed tomography of blunt spleen injury: a pictorial review. Malaysian J Med Sci. 2011;18:60–7.
21. Juyia RF, Kerr HA. Return to play after liver and spleen trauma. Sports Health. 2014;6:239–45.
22. Fernandes TM, Dorigatti AE, Pereira BMT, Cruvinel Neto J, Zago TM, Fraga GP. Nonoperative management of splenic injury grade IV is safe using rigid protocol. Rev Col Bras Cir. 2013;40:323–9.
23. Stassen NA, Bhullar I, Cheng JD, Crandall ML, Friese RS, Guillamondegui OD, et al. Selective nonoperative management of blunt splenic injury: an eastern Association for the Surgery of trauma practice management guideline. J Trauma Acute Care Surg. 2012;73:S294–300.
24. Velmahos GC, Toutouzas KG, Radin R, Chan L, Demetriades D. Nonoperative treatment of blunt injury to solid abdominal organs: a prospective study. Arch Surg. 2003;138:844–51.
25. Smith J, Armen S, Cook CH, Martin LC. Blunt splenic injuries: have we watched long enough? J Trauma. 2008;64:656–63; discussion 663-5
26. Hafiz S, Desale S, Sava J. The impact of solid organ injury management on the US health care system. J Trauma Acute Care Surg. 2014;77:310–4.
27. Gaspar B, Negoi I, Paun S, Hostiuc S, Ganescu R, Beuran M. Selective nonoperative management of abdominal injuries in polytrauma patients: a protocol only for experienced trauma centers. Maedica. 2014;9:168–72.
28. Moore FA, Davis JW, Moore EE, Cocanour CS, West MA, McIntyre RC. Western trauma association (WTA) critical decisions in trauma: management of adult blunt splenic trauma. J Trauma. 2008;65:1007–11.
29. Rowell SE, Biffl WL, Brasel K, Moore EE, Albrecht RA, DeMoya M, et al. Western trauma association critical decisions in trauma: management of adult blunt splenic trauma-2016 updates. J Trauma Acute Care Surg. 2017;82:787–93.
30. Nix JA, Costanza M, Daley BJ, Powell MA, Enderson BL. Outcome of the current management of splenic injuries. J Trauma. 2001;50:835–42.
31. Peitzman AB, Heil B, Rivera L, Federle M, Harbrecht BG, Clancy K, et al. Blunt splenic injury in adults: multi-institutional study of the Eastern Association for the surgery of trauma. J Trauma Inj Infect Crit Care. 2000;49:177–89.
32. Malhotra AK, Latifi R, Fabian TC, Ivatury RR, Dhage S, Bee TK, et al. Multiplicity of solid organ injury: influence on management and outcomes after blunt abdominal trauma. J Trauma. 2003;54:925–9.
33. Velmahos GC, Zacharias N, Emhoff TA, Feeney JM, Hurst JM, Crookes BA, et al. Management of the most severely injured spleen: a multicenter study of the research consortium of New England centers for trauma (ReCONECT). Arch Surg. 2010;145:456–60.
34. Jeremitsky E, Kao A, Carlton C, Rodriguez A, Ong A. Does splenic embolization and grade of splenic injury impact nonoperative management in patients sustaining blunt splenic trauma? Am Surg. 2011;77:215–20.
35. Watson GA, Rosengart MR, Zenati MS, Tsung A, Forsythe RM, Peitzman AB, et al. Nonoperative management of severe blunt splenic injury: are we getting better? J Trauma. 2006;61(5):1113–8; discussion 1118-9
36. Schurr MJ, Fabian TC, Gavant M, Croce MA, Kudsk KA, Minard G, et al. Management of blunt splenic trauma: computed tomographic contrast blush predicts failure of nonoperative management. J Trauma. 1995;39(3):507–12; discussion 512-3
37. Bhangu A, Nepogodiev D, Lal N, Bowley DM. Meta-analysis of predictive factors and outcomes for failure of non-operative management of blunt splenic trauma. Injury. 2012;43:1337–46.
38. Aseervatham R, Muller M. Blunt trauma to the spleen. Aust N Z J Surg. 2000;70:333–7.
39. Crawford RS, Tabbara M, Sheridan R, Spaniolas K, Velmahos GC. Early discharge after nonoperative management for splenic injuries: increased patient risk caused by late failure? Surgery. 2007;142:337–42.
40. Jeremitsky E, Smith RS, Ong AW. Starting the clock: defining nonoperative management of blunt splenic injury by time. Am J Surg. 2013;205:298–301.
41. Demetriades D, Rabinowitz B. Indications for operation in abdominal stab wounds. A prospective study of 651 patients. Ann Surg. 1987;205:129–32.
42. Velmahos GC, Demetriades D, Toutouzas KG, Sarkisyan G, Chan LS, Ishak R, et al. Selective nonoperative management in 1,856 patients with abdominal gunshot wounds: should routine laparotomy still be the standard of care? Ann Surg. 2001;234(3):395–402; discussion 402-3
43. Carlin AM, Tyburski JG, Wilson RF, Steffes C. Factors affecting the outcome of patients with splenic trauma. Am Surg. 2002;68(3):232–9.
44. Renz BM, Feliciano DV. Gunshot wounds to the right thoracoabdomen: a prospective study of nonoperative management. J Trauma. 1994;37:737–44.
45. Inaba K, Barmparas G, Foster A, Talving P, David J-S, Green D, et al. Selective nonoperative management of torso gunshot wounds: when is it safe to discharge? J Trauma. 2010;68:1301–4.
46. Haan JM, Bochicchio GV, Kramer N, Scalea TM. Nonoperative management of blunt splenic injury: a 5-year experience. J Trauma. 2005;58:492–8.
47. Haan J, Scott J, Boyd-Kranis RL, Ho S, Kramer M, Scalea TM. Admission angiography for blunt

splenic injury: advantages and pitfalls. J Trauma. 2001;51:1161–5.
48. Haan JM, Biffl W, Knudson MM, Davis KA, Oka T, Majercik S, et al. Splenic embolization revisited: a multicenter review. J Trauma Inj Infect Crit Care. 2004;56:542–7.
49. Frandon J, Rodière M, Arvieux C, Michoud M, Vendrell A, Broux C, et al. Blunt splenic injury: outcomes of proximal versus distal and combined splenic artery embolization. Diagn Interv Imaging. 2014;95:825–31.
50. Schnüriger B, Inaba K, Konstantinidis A, Lustenberger T, Chan LS, Demetriades D. Outcomes of proximal versus distal splenic artery embolization after trauma: a systematic review and meta-analysis. J Trauma. 2011;70:252–60.
51. Tugnoli G, Bianchi E, Biscardi A, Coniglio C, Isceri S, Simonetti L, et al. Nonoperative management of blunt splenic injury in adults: there is (still) a long way to go. The results of the Bologna-Maggiore Hospital trauma center experience and development of a clinical algorithm. Surg Today. 2015;45:1210–7.
52. Bessoud B, Denys A, Calmes JM, Madoff D, Qanadli S, Schnyder P, et al. Nonoperative management of traumatic splenic injuries: is there a role for proximal splenic artery embolization? Am J Roentgenol. 2006;186:779–85.
53. Brillantino A, Iacobellis F, Robustelli U, Villamaina E, Maglione F, Colletti O, et al. Non operative management of blunt splenic trauma: a prospective evaluation of a standardized treatment protocol. Eur J Trauma Emerg Surg. 2016;42:593–8.
54. Smith HE, Biffl WL, Majercik SD, Jednacz J, Lambiase R, Cioffi WG. Splenic artery embolization: have we gone too far? J Trauma. 2006;61:541–4; discussion 545-6
55. Capecci LM, Jeremitsky E, Smith RS, Philp F. Trauma centers with higher rates of angiography have a lesser incidence of splenectomy in the management of blunt splenic injury. Surgery. 2015;158:1020–4; discussion 1024-6
56. Zarzaur BL, Savage SA, Croce MA, Fabian TC. Trauma center angiography use in high-grade blunt splenic injuries: timing is everything. J Trauma Acute Care Surg. 2014;77:666–71.
57. Raikhlin A, Baerlocher MO, Asch MR, Myers A. Imaging and transcatheter arterial embolization for traumatic splenic injuries: review of the literature. Can J Surg. 2008;51:464–72.
58. Banerjee A, Duane TM, Wilson SP, Haney S, O'Neill PJ, Evans HL, et al. Trauma center variation in splenic artery embolization and spleen salvage: a multicenter analysis. J Trauma Acute Care Surg. 2013;75:69–74; discussion 74-5
59. Rosati C, Ata A, Siskin GP, Megna D, Bonville DJ, Stain SC. Management of splenic trauma: a single institution's 8-year experience. Am J Surg. 2015;209:308–14.
60. Requarth JA, D'Agostino RB Jr, Miller PR. Nonoperative management of adult blunt splenic injury with and without splenic artery embolotherapy: a meta-analysis. J Trauma Inj Infect Crit Care. 2011;71:898–903.
61. Davis KA, Fabian TC, Croce MA, Gavant ML, Flick PA, Minard G, et al. Improved success in nonoperative management of blunt splenic injuries: embolization of splenic artery pseudoaneurysms. J Trauma. 1998;44:1008–13; discussion 1013-5
62. Dehli T, Bagenholm A, Trasti NC, Monsen SA, Bartnes K, Bågenholm A, et al. The treatment of spleen injuries: a retrospective study. Scand J Trauma Resusc Emerg Med. 2015;23:85.
63. Yuan K-C, Wong Y-C, Lin B-C, Kang S-C, Liu E-H, Hsu Y-P. Negative catheter angiography after vascular contrast extravasations on computed tomography in blunt torso trauma: an experience review of a clinical dilemma. Scand J Trauma Resusc Emerg Med. 2012;20:46.
64. Alarhayem AQ, Myers JG, Dent D, Lamus D, Lopera J, Liao L, et al. "Blush at first sight": significance of computed tomographic and angiographic discrepancy in patients with blunt abdominal trauma. Am J Surg. 2015;210:1104. s
65. Gavant ML, Schurr M, Flick PA, Croce MA, Fabian TC, Gold RE. Predicting clinical outcome of nonsurgical management of blunt splenic injury: using CT to reveal abnormalities of splenic vasculature. Am J Roentgenol. 1997;168:207–12.
66. Skattum J, Naess PA, Eken T, Gaarder C. Refining the role of splenic angiographic embolization in high-grade splenic injuries. J Trauma Acute Care Surg. 2013;74:100–3; discussion 103-4
67. Miller PR, Chang MC, Hoth JJ, Mowery NT, Hildreth AN, Martin RS, et al. Prospective trial of angiography and embolization for all grade III to V blunt splenic injuries: nonoperative management success rate is significantly improved. J Am Coll Surg. 2014;218:644–8.
68. Chastang L, Bège T, Prudhomme M, Simonnet AC, Herrero A, Guillon F, et al. Is non-operative management of severe blunt splenic injury safer than embolization or surgery? Results from a French prospective multicenter study. J Visc Surg. 2015;152:85–91.
69. Ekeh AP, McCarthy MC, Woods RJ, Haley E. Complications arising from splenic embolization after blunt splenic trauma. Am J Surg. 2005;189:335–9.
70. Frandon J, Rodiere M, Arvieux C, Vendrell A, Boussat B, Sengel C, et al. Blunt splenic injury: are early adverse events related to trauma, nonoperative management, or surgery? Diagnostic Interv Radiol. 2015;21:327–33.
71. Demetriades D, Scalea TM, Degiannis E, Barmparas G, Konstantinidis A, Massahis J, et al. Blunt splenic trauma: splenectomy increases early infectious complications: a prospective multicenter study. J Trauma Acute Care Surg. 2012;72:229–34.
72. Kaseje N, Agarwal S, Burch M, Glantz A, Emhoff T, Burke P, et al. Short-term outcomes of splenectomy avoidance in trauma patients. Am J Surg. 2008;196:213–7.

73. Freitas G, Olufajo OA, Hammouda K, Lin E, Cooper Z, Havens JM, et al. Postdischarge complications following nonoperative management of blunt splenic injury. Am J Surg. 2016;211:744–9.
74. Wei B, Hemmila MR, Arbabi S, Taheri PA, Wahl WL, et al. Angioembolization reduces operative intervention for blunt splenic injury. J Trauma Inj Infect Crit Care. 2008;64:1472–7.
75. Ekeh AP, Khalaf S, Ilyas S, Kauffman S, Walusimbi M, McCarthy MC. Complications arising from splenic artery embolization: a review of an 11-year experience. Am J Surg. 2013;205:250–4.
76. Wu SC, Chen RJ, Yang AD, Tung CC, Lee KH. Complications associated with embolization in the treatment of blunt splenic injury. World J Surg. 2008;32:476–82.
77. Swaid F, Peleg K, Alfici R, Matter I, Olsha O, Ashkenazi I, et al. Concomitant hollow viscus injuries in patients with blunt hepatic and splenic injuries: an analysis of a National Trauma Registry database. Injury. 2014;45:1409–12.
78. Morrell DG, Chang FC, Helmer SD. Changing trends in the management of splenic injury. Am J Surg. 1995;170:686–9; discussion 690
79. Carter JW, Falco MH, Chopko MS, Flynn WJ, Wiles Iii CE, Guo WA. Do we really rely on fast for decision-making in the management of blunt abdominal trauma? Injury. 2015;46:817–21.
80. Garber BG, Yelle JD, Fairfull-Smith R, Lorimer JW, Carson C. Management of splenic injuries in a Canadian trauma centre. Can J Surg. 1996;39:474–80.
81. Garber BG, Mmath BP, Fairfull-Smith RJ, Yelle JD. Management of adult splenic injuries in Ontario: a population-based study. Can J Surg. 2000;43:283–8.
82. Pisters PW, Pachter HL. Autologous splenic transplantation for splenic trauma. Ann Surg. 1994;219:225–35.
83. Qu Y, Ren S, Li C, Qian S, Liu P. Management of postoperative complications following splenectomy. Int Surg. 2013;98:55–60.
84. Nasr WI, Collins CL, Kelly JJ. Feasibility of laparoscopic splenectomy in stable blunt trauma: a case series. J Trauma. 2004;57:887–9.
85. Hallfeldt KK, Trupka AW, Erhard J, Waldner H, Schweiberer L. Emergency laparoscopy for abdominal stab wounds. Surg Endosc. 1998;12:907–10.
86. Rostas JW, Manley J, Gonzalez RP, Brevard SB, Ahmed N, Frotan MA, et al. The safety of low molecular-weight heparin after blunt liver and spleen injuries. Am J Surg. 2015;210:31–4.
87. Murphy PB, Sothilingam N, Charyk Stewart T, Batey B, Moffat B, Gray DK, et al. Very early initiation of chemical venous thromboembolism prophylaxis after blunt solid organ injury is safe. Can J Surg. 2016;59:118–22.
88. Alejandro KV, Acosta JA, Rodríguez PA. Bleeding manifestations after early use of low-molecular-weight heparins in blunt splenic injuries. Am Surg. 2003;69:1006–9.
89. Joseph B, Pandit V, Harrison C, Lubin D, Kulvatunyou N, Zangbar B, et al. Early thromboembolic prophylaxis in patients with blunt solid abdominal organ injuries undergoing nonoperative management: is it safe? Am J Surg. 2015;209:194–8.
90. Weinberger J, Cipolle M. Optimal reversal of novel anticoagulants in trauma. Crit Care Clin. 2017;33:135–52.
91. Zarzaur BL, Vashi S, Magnotti LJ, Croce MA, Fabian TC. The real risk of splenectomy after discharge home following nonoperative management of blunt splenic injury. J Trauma. 2009;66:1531–8.
92. Savage SA, Zarzaur BL, Magnotti LJ, Weinberg JA, Maish GO, Bee TK, et al. The evolution of blunt splenic injury: resolution and progression. J Trauma. 2008;64:1085–91; discussion 1091-2
93. Meguid AA, Bair HA, Howells GA, Bendick PJ, Kerr HH, Villalba MR. Prospective evaluation of criteria for the nonoperative management of blunt splenic trauma. Am Surg. 2003;69:238–42; discussion 242-3
94. Riezzo I, Di Battista B, De Salvia A, Cantatore S, Neri M, Pomara C, et al. Delayed splenic rupture: dating the sub-capsular hemorrhage as a useful task to evaluate causal relationships with trauma. Forensic Sci Int. 2014;234:64–71.
95. Clancy AA, Tiruta C, Ashman D, Ball CG, Kirkpatrick AW. The song remains the same although the instruments are changing: complications following selective non-operative management of blunt spleen trauma: a retrospective review of patients at a level I trauma Centre from 1996 to 2007. J Trauma Manag Outcomes. 2012;6:4.
96. Haan JM, Boswell S, Stein D, Scalea TM. Follow-up abdominal CT is not necessary in low-grade splenic injury. Am Surg. 2007;73:13–8.
97. Muroya T, Ogura H, Shimizu K, Tasaki O, Kuwagata Y, Fuse T, et al. Delayed formation of splenic pseudoaneurysm following nonoperative management in blunt splenic injury: multi-institutional study in Osaka, Japan. J Trauma Acute Care Surg. 2013;75:417–20.
98. Uecker J, Pickett C, Dunn E. The role of follow-up radiographic studies in nonoperative management of spleen trauma. Am Surg. 2001;67:22–5.
99. Lyass S, Sela T, Lebensart PD, Muggia-Sullam M. Follow-up imaging studies of blunt splenic injury: do they influence management? Isr Med Assoc J. 2001;3:731–3.
100. Lynch JM, Meza MP, Newman B, Gardner MJ, Albanese CT. Computed tomography grade of splenic injury is predictive of the time required for radiographic healing. J Pediatr Surg. 1997;32:1093–6.
101. Unal E, Onur MR, Akpinar E, Ahmadov J, Karcaaltincaba M, Ozmen MN, et al. Imaging findings of splenic emergencies: a pictorial review. Insights Imaging. 2016;7:215–22.

102. Linet MS, Nyrén O, Gridley G, Adami HO, Buckland JD, McLaughlin JK, et al. Causes of death among patients surviving at least one year following splenectomy. Am J Surg. 1996;172:320–3.
103. Alonso M, Brathwaite C, García V, Patterson L, Scherer T, Stafford P, et al. Practice management guidelines for the nonoperative management of blunt injury to the liver and spleen. Chicago, IL: Eastern Association for the Surgery of Trauma; 2003.
104. Moore EE, Cogbill TH, Jurkovich GJ, Shackford SR, Malangoni MA, Champion HR. Organ injury scaling: spleen and liver (1994 revision). J Trauma. 1995;38:323–4.
105. Bairdain S, Litman HJ, Troy M, McMahon M, Almodovar H, Zurakowski D, et al. Twenty-years of splenic preservation at a level 1 pediatric trauma center. J Pediatr Surg. 2015;50:864–8.
106. Stylianos S. Evidence-based guidelines for resource utilization in children with isolated spleen or liver injury. The APSA trauma committee. J Pediatr Surg. 2000;35:164–9.
107. McVay MR, Kokoska ER, Jackson RJ, Smith SD. Throwing out the "grade" book: management of isolated spleen and liver injury based on hemodynamic status. J Pediatr Surg. 2008;43:1072–6.
108. Martin K, Vanhouwelingen L, Bütter A. The significance of pseudoaneurysms in the nonoperative management of pediatric blunt splenic trauma. J Pediatr Surg. 2011;46:933–7.
109. Li D, Yanchar N. Management of pediatric blunt splenic injuries in Canada-practices and opinions. J Pediatr Surg. 2009;44:997–1004.
110. Bond SJ, Eichelberger MR, Gotschall CS, Sivit CJ, Randolph JG. Nonoperative management of blunt hepatic and splenic injury in children. Ann Surg. 1996;223:286–9.
111. Muehrcke DD, Kim SH, McCabe CJ. Pediatric splenic trauma: predicting the success of nonoperative therapy. Am J Emerg Med. 1987;5:109–12.
112. Delius RE, Frankel W, Coran AG. A comparison between operative and nonoperative management of blunt injuries to the liver and spleen in adult and pediatric patients. Surgery. 1989;106:788–92; discussion 792-3
113. Lynch JM, Ford H, Gardner MJ, Weiner ES. Is early discharge following isolated splenic injury in the hemodynamically stable child possible? J Pediatr Surg. 1993;28:1403–7.
114. Konstantakos AK, Barnoski AL, Plaisier BR, Yowler CJ, Fallon WF, Malangoni MA. Optimizing the management of blunt splenic injury in adults and children. Surgery. 1999;126:805–13.
115. Upadhyaya P. Conservative management of splenic trauma: history and current trends. Pediatr Surg Int. 2003;19:617–27.
116. Rodrigues CJ, Sacchetti JC, Rodrigues AJ. Age-related changes in the elastic fiber network of the human splenic capsule. Lymphology. 1999;32:64–9.
117. Murphy R, Ghosh A. Towards evidence based emergency medicine: best BETs from the Manchester Royal Infirmary. The accuracy of abdominal ultrasound in paediatric trauma. Emerg Med J. 2001;18:208–9.
118. Scaife ER, Rollins MD, Barnhart DC, Downey EC, Black RE, Meyers RL, et al. The role of focused abdominal sonography for trauma (FAST) in pediatric trauma evaluation. J Pediatr Surg. 2013;48:1377–83.
119. Holmes JF, Gladman A, Chang CH. Performance of abdominal ultrasonography in pediatric blunt trauma patients: a meta-analysis. J Pediatr Surg. 2007;42:1588–94.
120. Mooney DP, Rothstein DH, Forbes PW. Variation in the management of pediatric splenic injuries in the United States. J Trauma Inj Infect Crit Care. 2006;61:330–3.
121. Todd SR, Arthur M, Newgard C, Hedges JR, Mullins RJ. Hospital factors associated with splenectomy for splenic injury: a national perspective. J Trauma. 2004;57:1065–71.
122. Notrica DM, Eubanks JW, Tuggle DW, Maxson RT, Letton RW, Garcia NM, et al. Nonoperative management of blunt liver and spleen injury in children: evaluation of the ATOMAC guideline using GRADE. J Trauma Acute Care Surg. 2015;79:683–93.
123. Narci A, Solak O, Turhan-Haktanir N, Ayçiçek A, Demir Y, Ela Y, et al. The prognostic importance of trauma scoring systems in pediatric patients. Pediatr Surg Int. 2009;25:25–30.
124. Richards JR, McGahan JP, Jones CD, Zhan S, Gerscovich EO. Ultrasound detection of blunt splenic injury. Injury. 2001;32:95–103.
125. Tataria M, Nance ML, Holmes JH 4th, Miller CC 3rd, Mattix KD, Brown RL, et al. Pediatric blunt abdominal injury: age is irrelevant and delayed operation is not detrimental. J Trauma. 2007;63:608–14.
126. Holmes JH 4th, Wiebe DJ, Tataria M, Mattix KD, Mooney DP, Scaife ER, et al. The failure of nonoperative management in pediatric solid organ injury: a multi-institutional experience. J Trauma. 2005;59:1309–13.
127. Sharma OP, Oswanski MF, Singer D, Raj SS, Daoud YAH. Assessment of nonoperative management of blunt spleen and liver trauma. Am Surg. 2005;71:379–86.
128. McIntyre LK, Schiff M, Jurkovich GJ. Failure of nonoperative management of splenic injuries: causes and consequences. Arch Surg. 2005;140:563–8; discussion 568
129. Cloutier DR, Baird TB, Gormley P, McCarten KM, Bussey JG, Luks FI. Pediatric splenic injuries with a contrast blush: successful nonoperative management without angiography and embolization. J Pediatr Surg. 2004;39:969–71.
130. Gross JL, Woll NL, Hanson CA, Pohl C, Scorpio RJ, Kennedy AP Jr, et al. Embolization for pediatric blunt splenic injury is an alternative to splenectomy when observation fails. J Trauma Acute Care Surg. 2013;75:421–5.
131. Kiankhooy A, Sartorelli KH, Vane DW, Bhave AD. Angiographic embolization is safe and effec-

tive therapy for blunt abdominal solid organ injury in children. J Trauma. 2010;68:526–31.
132. Skattum J, Gaarder C, Naess PA. Splenic artery embolisation in children and adolescents—an 8 year experience. Injury. 2014;45:160–3.
133. Mayglothling JA, Haan JM, Scalea TM. Blunt splenic injuries in the adolescent trauma population: the role of angiography and embolization. J Emerg Med. 2011;41:21–8.
134. Schuster T, Leissner G. Selective angioembolization in blunt solid organ injury in children and adolescents: review of recent literature and own experiences. Eur J Pediatr Surg. 2013;23:454–63.
135. van der Vlies CH, Saltzherr TP, Wilde JCH, van Delden OM, de Haan RJ, Goslings JC. The failure rate of nonoperative management in children with splenic or liver injury with contrast blush on computed tomography: a systematic review. J Pediatr Surg. 2010;45:1044–9.
136. Ben-Ishay O, Gutierrez IM, Pennington EC, Mooney DP. Transarterial embolization in children with blunt splenic injury results in postembolization syndrome: a matched case-control study. J Trauma Acute Care Surg. 2012;73:1558–63.
137. Akinkuolie AA, Lawal OO, Arowolo OA, Agbakwuru EA, Adesunkanmi ARK. Determinants of splenectomy in splenic injuries following blunt abdominal trauma. S Afr J Surg. 2010;48:15–9.
138. Polites SF, Zielinski MD, Zarroug AE, Wagie AE, Stylianos S, Habermann EB. Benchmarks for splenectomy in pediatric trauma: how are we doing? J Pediatr Surg. 2015;50:339–42.
139. Nwomeh BC, Nadler EP, Meza MP, Bron K, Gaines BA, Ford HR. Contrast extravasation predicts the need for operative intervention in children with blunt splenic trauma. J Trauma. 2004;56:537–41.
140. Jen HC, Tillou A, Cryer HG, Shew SB. Disparity in management and long-term outcomes of pediatric splenic injury in California. Ann Surg. 2010;251:1162–6.
141. Mohamed AA, Mahran KM, Zaazou MM. Blunt abdominal trauma requiring laparotomy in polytraumatized patients. Saudi Med J. 2010;31:43–8.
142. Lo A, Matheson A-M, Adams D. Impact of concomitant trauma in the management of blunt splenic injuries. N Z Med J. 2004;117:U1052.
143. Resende V, Petroianu A. Functions of the splenic remnant after subtotal splenectomy for treatment of severe splenic injuries. Am J Surg. 2003;185:311–5.
144. Keller MS, Sartorelli KH, Vane DW. Associated head injury should not prevent nonoperative management of spleen or liver injury in children. J Trauma. 1996;41:471–5.
145. St Peter SD, Aguayo P, Juang D, Sharp SW, Snyder CL, Holcomb GW, et al. Follow up of prospective validation of an abbreviated bedrest protocol in the management of blunt spleen and liver injury in children. J Pediatr Surg. 2013;48:2437–41.
146. Minarik L, Slim M, Rachlin S, Brudnicki A. Diagnostic imaging in the follow-up of nonoperative management of splenic trauma in children. Pediatr Surg Int. 2002;18:429–31.
147. Pachter HL, Guth AA, Hofstetter SR, Spencer FC. Changing patterns in the management of splenic trauma: the impact of nonoperative management. Ann Surg. 1998;227:708–9.
148. Zabolotny B, Hancock BJ, Postuma R, Wiseman N. Blunt splenic injuries in a Canadian pediatric population: the need for a management guideline. Can J Surg. 2002;45:358–62.
149. Leone G, Pizzigallo E. Bacterial infections following splenectomy for malignant and nonmalignant hematologic diseases. Mediterr J Hematol Infect Dis. 2015:7.
150. Skattum J, P a N, Gaarder C. Non-operative management and immune function after splenic injury. Br J Surg. 2012;99(Suppl 1):59–65.
151. Shatz DV. Vaccination practices among North American trauma surgeons in splenectomy for trauma. J Trauma. 2002;53:950–6.
152. Shatz DV, Romero-Steiner S, Elie CM, Holder PF, Carlone GM. Antibody responses in postsplenectomy trauma patients receiving the 23-valent pneumococcal polysaccharide vaccine at 14 versus 28 days postoperatively. J Trauma. 2002;53:1037–42.
153. ACIP Vaccine Recommendations. Centers for disease control and prevention, recommended immunization schedules, 2016.
154. Spelman D, Buttery J, Daley A, Isaacs D, Jennens I, Kakakios A, et al. Guidelines for the prevention of sepsis in asplenic and hyposplenic patients. Intern Med J. 2008;38:349–56.
155. Salvadori MI, Price VE. Preventing and treating infections in children with asplenia or hyposplenia. Paediatr Child Heal. 2014;19:271–4.
156. Schimmer JAG, Van Der Steeg AFW, Zuidema WP. Splenic function after angioembolization for splenic trauma in children and adults: a systematic review. Injury. 2016;47:525–30.

# Further Reading

Coccolini, F., Montori, G., Catena, F. et al. Splenic trauma: WSES classification and guidelines for adult and pediatric patients. World J Emerg Surg 12, 40 Thursday (2017).

# Bowel Trauma

**97**

Carlos A. Ordoñez, Michael W. Parra, and Yaset Caicedo

**Learning Goals**
- When a definitive laparotomy is performed for small bowel, colon, or combined intestinal injuries, the surgical management should be a primary repair or primary anastomosis.
- When severe small and/or large bowel injuries are associated with hemodynamic instability, damage control surgery principles should be applied, and a delayed intestinal reconstruction via a deferred anastomosis should be performed.
- The rate of ostomy for severe colon injuries should be less than 10%.

C. A. Ordoñez (✉)
Division of Trauma and Acute Care Surgery, Department of Surgery, Fundación Valle del Lili, Cali, Colombia

Division of Trauma and Acute Care Surgery, Department of Surgery, Universidad del Valle, Cali, Colombia

Universidad Icesi, Cali, Colombia

M. W. Parra
Department of Trauma Critical Care, Broward General Level I Trauma Center, Fort Lauderdale, FL, USA

Y. Caicedo
Centro de Investigaciones Clínicas (CIC), Fundación Valle del Lili, Cali, Colombia
e-mail: edgar.caicedo@fvl.org.co

## 97.1 Introduction

Hollow viscus injuries represent a significant portion of overall lesions sustained during penetrating trauma [1–3]. However, blunt injuries to the small bowel or colon are much less common [4]. Currently, isolated small or large bowel injuries are commonly managed via primary repair or primary anastomosis in patients undergoing initial definitive management or deferred anastomosis in patients requiring Damage Control Surgery. The traditional surgical dogma of ostomy has proven to be unnecessary and, in many instances, actually increases morbidity [5–7]. The focus of this chapter will be on the management of hollow viscus injuries via a management algorithm that includes principles of Damage Control Surgery.

## 97.2 Epidemiology

The abdominal area extends from the level of the nipples to the inguinal ligament anteriorly and from the tip of the scapula to the buttock crease posteriorly. The nature and severity of bowel injury associated with penetrating trauma ranges from minor bruising to complete devascularization of the compromised segment [8]. According to the mechanism of injury, gunshot or shotgun wounds are more likely to result in multiple injuries to the hollow viscera (>80%) compared to stab wounds (30%) [9]. Bullets usually cause pared perforations and are associated with areas of tissue damage and frank necrosis not only by direct contact but also by the dissipation of energy lateral to the path of the missile (blast effect). Because the small bowel occupies most of the true abdominal cavity, it is predisposed to greater injury when compared to the colon [10].

On the other hand, blunt trauma is typically associated with: crush injury to the bowel, blowout injuries secondary to sudden increase in intraluminal pressure, and/or shearing of the bowel off its mesentery from sudden deceleration [4, 11]. The Eastern Association for the Surgery of Trauma (EAST) Hollow Viscus Injury Study showed an overall incidence of bowel injuries of 3.1% of which 90% were small bowel [12].

## 97.3 Classification

Bowel injuries are classified as destructive and nondestructive lesions. Nondestructive injuries are wounds that involve less than 50% of the bowel wall circumference (AAST Grade I–II) or greater than 50% without transection (AAST Grade III). Destructive injuries are completely transected bowel (AAST Grade IV) with segmental tissue loss or devascularization (AAST Grade V) [8, 13] (Table 97.1).

**Table 97.1** AAST severity classification of small and large bowel injuries [13]

| Grade | Type | Description |
|---|---|---|
| I | Hematoma | Contusion or hematoma without devascularization |
| | Laceration | Partial thickness, no perforation |
| II | Laceration | Laceration <50% of circumference |
| III | Laceration | Laceration ≥50% of circumference without transection |
| IV | Laceration | Transection of the small or large bowel |
| V | Laceration Vascular | Transection of the small or large bowel with segmental tissue loss Devascularized segment |

The American Association for the Surgery of Trauma (AAST) Classification of Small and Large Bowel Injuries

## 97.4 Diagnosis

### 97.4.1 Clinical Presentation

A hollow viscus injury can be suspected by the mechanism of injury. Abdominal pain, although common, is not a specific diagnostic indicator of a bowel injury. Abdominal wall hematomas, abdominal distention, tenderness, and/or signs of peritoneal irritation are signs found during physical examination that can suggest the existence of an intestinal injury.

### 97.4.2 Initial Approach and Diagnosis

Initial management must be directed toward the stabilization of the patient according to Advanced Trauma Life Support (ATLS) guidelines and following Damage Control Resuscitation principles [14, 15]. Upon arrival, the choice between immediate surgical exploration or further imaging studies is dependent on the hemodynamic status of the patient. If the patient is hemodynamically stable or a transient responder, a computed tomography (CT) should be performed to determine the extent of the injuries [16, 17]. However, patients with peritoneal signs and/or hemodynamic instability (sustained systolic blood pressure ≤ 90 mmHg) should be transferred immediately to the operating room where the diagnosis and appropriate staging of hollow viscus injuries should be done during the initial laparotomy (Table 97.1) [13].

Abdominal CT is the test of choice to aid in the identification of intestinal trauma and associated vascular and/or solid organ injuries. CT findings suggestive of hollow viscus injury include: bowel wall thickening or edema, mesenteric air, pneumoperitoneum, discontinuity of the hollow viscus wall, extraluminal enteric contrast, free intra-abdominal fluid in the absence of a solid organ injury, intravenous contrast extravasation, and mesenteric hematomas [18–20]. CT is generally reserved for hemodynamically stable patients, but transient responders can benefit from this diagnostic tool if potential surgical therapy is not delayed.

This management algorithmic work-up allows for prompt identification of associated injuries that can be managed either by surgery, endovascular techniques, or nonoperatively [17].

## 97.5 Treatment

Patients with suspected bowel injuries should undergo surgical exploration. The exploration can be done open in hemodynamically unstable patients and laparoscopic in those patients who comply with the following [21, 22]:

- Hemodynamically stable.
- Surgeon is proficient in the technique.
- The institution has the equipment readily available.

During the initial exploratory laparotomy, the trauma surgeon should initially control all sources of ongoing surgical bleeding and bowel contamination [23]. Only then can he or she direct their attention to staging the involved injuries. If the patient develops hemodynamic instability during or prior to the procedure with a sustained systolic blood pressure ≤ 70 mmHg, regardless of aggressive damage control resuscitation, the placement of a Resuscitative Balloon Occlusion of the Aorta (REBOA) should be considered and placed in Zone 1 as an adjunct [24–26]. It is our general recommendation to always seek bowel anastomosis via a primary or deferred technique and leaving ostomies as a last resort. The surgical management of combined hollow viscus injuries should be as follows (Fig. 97.1):

- **Step 1**: The patient is transferred to the operating room for an exploratory laparotomy with ongoing hemostatic resuscitation. Complete bowel examination is performed from the gastroesophageal junction all the way down to the

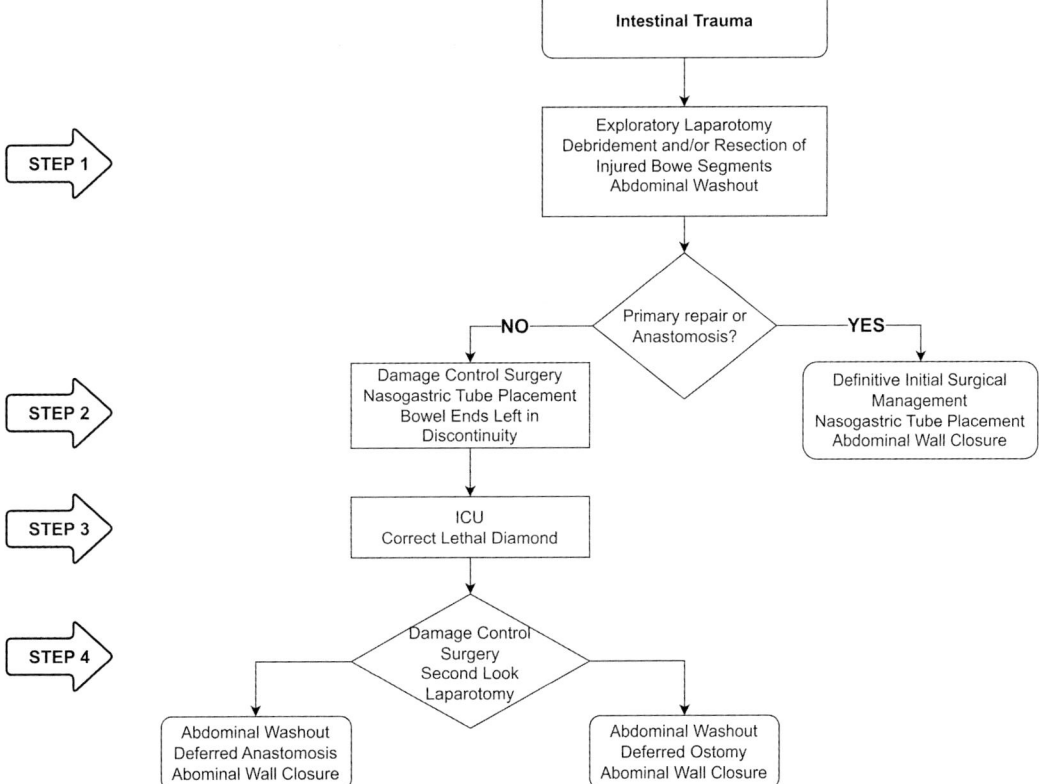

**Fig. 97.1** Surgical management algorithm of intestinal trauma

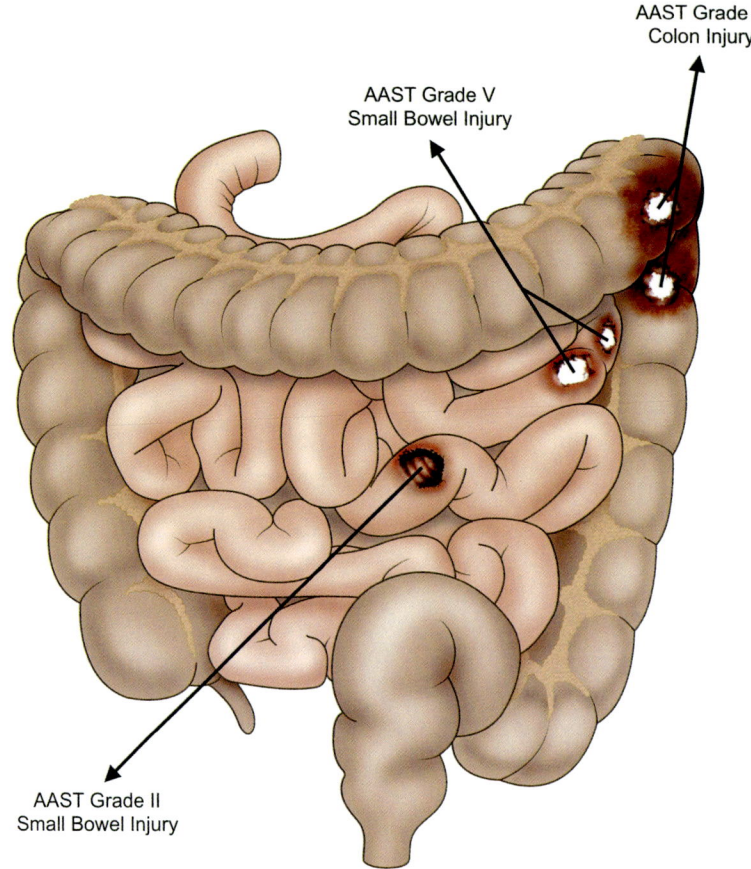

**Fig. 97.2** Combined penetrating hollow viscus injuries. Two small bowel injuries are seen (one is a AAST Grade V injury and the other is a AAST Grade II injury). In addition, two adjacent injuries are seen in the splenic flexure (AAST Grade V colon injury). (Illustration by Fabian R. Cabrera P. [28])

rectum to appropriately stage all small and large bowel injuries according to the AAST classification (Table 97.1 and Fig. 97.2).

The aim of the initial laparotomy is twofold:

- Immediate control of ongoing surgical bleeding of the mesentery.
- Control of bowel contamination.

Once these have been achieved, debridement, primary repair, and/or resection of all involved bowel segments are completed, followed by abdominal washout.

- **Step 2:** The surgeon must decide if the intestinal injuries meet the need for Damage Control Surgery which include: inability to correct the lethal diamond regardless of an aggressive Damage Control Resuscitation [15, 28], persistent hemodynamic instability, and associated severe solid organ/vascular injuries.
  - If so, bowel ends should be left in discontinuity (umbilical tape/lineal stapler) (Fig. 97.3), the anesthesiologist is instructed to place a nasogastric tube, Damage Control Resuscitation is continued, and the abdomen is left open with a negative pressure dressing.
  - If the patient does not meet the need for damage control surgery, then definitive laparotomy should be performed with primary anastomosis of all involved intestinal segments, the anesthesiologist is instructed to place a nasogastric tube, Damage Control Resuscitation is continued, and the abdominal wall is closed.

- **Step 3:** All patients are transferred immediately to the intensive care unit where ongoing correction of the lethal diamond is performed. To this end, the patient is rewarmed, and the

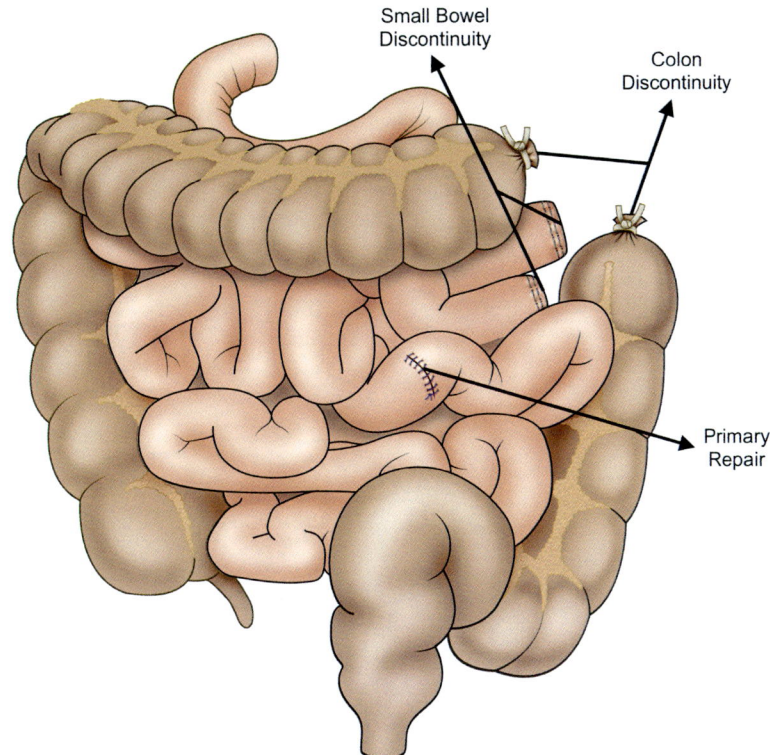

**Fig. 97.3** Damage control surgery for combined penetrating hollow viscus injuries. The AAST Grade II small bowel injury was managed via primary repair, while the AAST Grade V injury required segmental resection and was left in discontinuity. The complex colonic injury was also resected and left in discontinuity. (Illustration by Fabian R. Cabrera P. [28])

conglomerate of acidosis, coagulopathy, and hypocalcemia is reversed.
- **Step 4:** Patients that required Damage Control Surgery should be taken back to the operating room for a second look laparotomy after 24–48 h of aggressive hemostatic resuscitation. Four quadrant abdominal washout and reevaluation of the bowel viability are done. All missed or delayed bowel injuries are diagnosed, and definitive surgical management is contemplated. In most cases, bowel continuity is performed via deferred anastomosis of all bowel segments, and, in a few selected cases, deferred ostomies are performed at the surgeon's discretion (Fig. 97.4). Either of these options is followed by definitive abdominal wall closure.

Finally, these are the main take home messages for the reader regarding the surgical approach toward intestinal trauma:

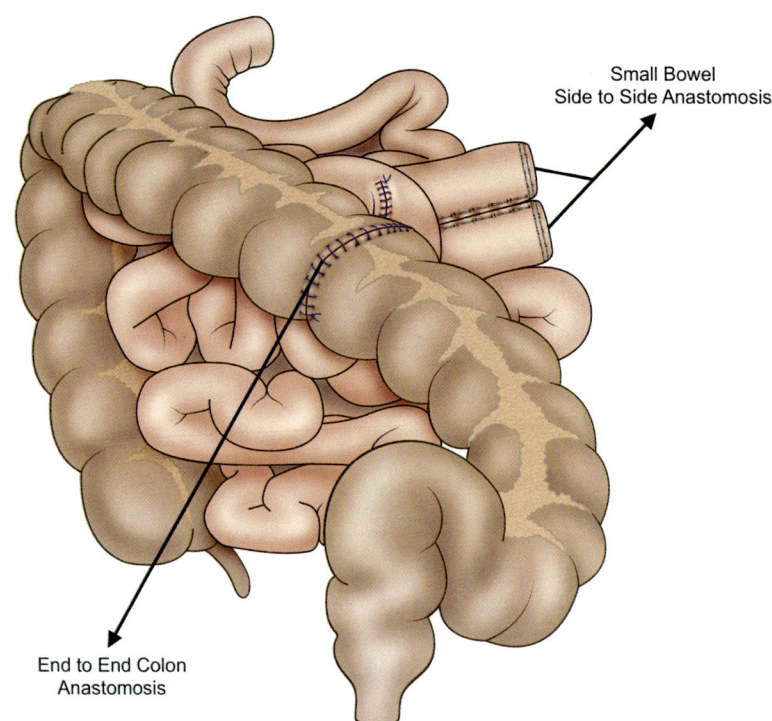

**Fig. 97.4** Definitive repair of combined penetrating hollow viscus injuries. The intestinal segments were re-anastomosed during subsequent follow-up damage control laparotomy. A stapled side-to-side functional end-to-end anastomosis was performed as definitive reconstructive management of the AAST Grade V small bowel injury, and a single-plane hand-sewn end-to-end anastomosis was performed as definitive reconstructive management of the complex colon injury. (Illustration by Fabian R. Cabrera P. [28])

## 97.6 Complications

Common systemic postoperative complications include renal dysfunction, pneumonia, sepsis, and thromboembolism. Complications specific to abdominal surgery include: incisional hernia, fascial dehiscence, enterocutaneous fistula, and organ/space surgical site infections. The incidence of complications ranges from 22 to 29 percent [7, 29].

## 97.7 Discussion

Successful management of bowel injuries includes restoring bowel wall integrity while at the same time limiting contamination from bowel contents [30, 31]. There is a general consensus among trauma surgeons that primary repair of hollow viscus injuries is indicated in most cases, but there are a few that differ from this mantra and advocate for a more traditional and conservative approach of opting for ostomies [32]. The

### Dos and Don'ts

**Dos**

- The first goal in the surgical approach of intestinal injuries is to control ongoing surgical hemorrhage and bowel contamination.
- Damage Control Surgery should be considered only in critically ill patients.
- Primary repair or primary anastomosis should be your go-to option in the surgical management of bowel injuries.
- Damage Control Surgery allows for optimization of the patient in the intensive care unit (ICU) after the first surgical intervention and opens the possibility for a deferred anastomosis during the follow-up take back.

**Don'ts**

- An ostomy should not be the primary surgical option offered to a patient with small bowel and/or colon injuries.

surgeon is then faced with the difficult decision of restoring bowel continuity in cases of combined hollow viscus injuries via primary or deferred anastomosis versus primary or deferred ostomy. To appropriately answer this conundrum, we performed a retrospective/observational study which included all patients with penetrating abdominal trauma with associated hollow viscus injuries between 2005 and 2015 at our regional Level I Trauma Center in Cali, Colombia. Patients were divided into two main groups according to the surgical course taken: Definitive Laparotomy (DL) Group and the Damage Control Surgery (DCS) Group. Clinical outcomes were compared among these groups [27]. A total of 95 patients were included. The most common mechanism of injury was gunshot wounds (94.7%). Forty-nine patients underwent DCS and 46 had DL. The DCS Group had significantly higher trauma severity scores when compared to the DL Group. The DCS Group also had significantly higher intraoperative bleeding and required more hemodynamic support (mechanical ventilation, inotropic medications, and total units of packed red blood cells (PRBC) transfused in 24 h). Forty-five (91.8%) patients underwent deferred anastomosis in the DCS group, and 41 (89.1%) patients underwent primary anastomosis in the DL Group. The DL Group required 5 (10.9%) ostomies (1 ileostomy/4 colostomy), while the DCS Group required 4 (8.2%) (1 ileostomy/3 colostomy) (Fig. 97.1). Reported complications included: anastomotic leak (9.7% in DL group and 17.7% in DCS group) and abdominal compartment syndrome (2.1% in DL Group and 28.5% in DCS Group). The mortality in the DCS Group was 7.4% (7) compared to 0% in the DL Group ($p = 0.013$).

### 97.7.1 Indications for Damage Control Surgery (DCS)

The underlying directive of DCS is that prolonged operations in trauma patients with profound physiologic derangements and complex injuries need to be avoided. The focus becomes control of surgical bleeding and bowel contamination [33, 34]. Once these goals have been achieved, the lethal diamond should be corrected. A recent Cochrane review found that DCS patient selection is heavily dependent on clinical judgment, and, although it certainly has improved overall survival in the severely injured, it has been unfortunately overused [35–37]. For these reasons, we believe that DCS should be reserved for those who really require and benefit from this technique and those who do not undergo definitive laparotomy. Performing DCS has been associated with postoperative complications including: incisional hernia, fascial dehiscence, evisceration, enterocutaneous fistula, and organ/space surgical site infections [12].

### 97.7.2 Combined Small and Large Bowel Injuries

The most commonly injured organ in penetrating abdominal trauma, regardless whether it be civilian or military, is the small bowel which accounts for 49 to 60% of all injuries. Although the critical care management of these patients has evolved considerably over the past decades, the principles of surgical management remain remarkably similar. This includes initial control of any significant bleeding, enteric spillage, and definitive management determined by the severity of the injury according to the AAST grading system. The preferred surgical methods are primary repair for minor injuries and limited bowel resection with primary anastomosis (preserving bowel length) for more extensive ones [38]. Small bowel ostomies are considered a secondary less appealing option especially in light of complications that ensue from its high output [39].

Although there are multiple studies regarding the management and outcomes of isolated penetrating small or large bowel trauma, the literature is limited in describing combined hollow viscus injuries [31, 40]. One of them is the study by Skube et al. who performed a retrospective review of the Department of Defense Trauma Registry from 2007 to 2012 which included all hollow viscus injuries endured by US soldiers during operations: Enduring Freedom, Iraqi

Freedom, and New Dawn. A total of 171 soldiers had small bowel injuries, and the most frequent concomitant injury was large bowel in 110 cases (64.3%). Fifty patients (29.2%) had a colostomy, 9 (5.3%) had an ileostomy, and 107 (62.6%) underwent Damage Control Surgery. The overall mortality rate was 1.8% ($n = 3$). The need for Damage Control Surgery occurred in 71.4% of patients with combined small and large bowel injuries which was significantly higher than those with only small bowel injuries (39.6%) ($p = 0.0013$). In addition, ostomies were significantly lower in the patients with only small bowel injuries (5.7%) when compared to those with combined injuries (39.7%) ($p < 0.0001$) [33].

### 97.7.3 Hand-Sewn Versus Staple Technique

The preferred surgical approach of a primary or delayed anastomosis in patients with a combined hollow viscus injury has been a topic of debate between those who favor a hand-sewn vs. those who favor a staple technique. Demetriades et al. found no difference between these techniques and their subsequent complications (anastomotic leak, intra-abdominal abscess, abdominal wall dehiscence, and mortality) [41]. This was further proven via a meta-analysis that reported similar results [42]. For this reason, we recommend that the surgical technique utilized by the surgeon for the anastomosis should be consistent with his or her experience and the availability of resources at hand.

### 97.7.4 Abdominal Closure

Early abdominal wall closure is a goal that should be in the forefront in patients undergoing DCS. In 2012, Burlew et al. found that those patients undergoing DCS who required multiple re-laparotomies and those who had a subsequent delay in abdominal wall closure had a higher incidence of postoperative complications [43]. These findings have been confirmed by recent publications in which the rate of adverse events significantly diminish when patients' abdomens are closed within the first 72 h [44].

Our experience in Cali, Colombia, over the past several years has been that more than 95% of all penetrating bowel injuries are managed with primary repair and/or resection followed by anastomosis. In the most severe cases of combined injuries, we have opted for definitive management using deferred anastomosis following damage control principles rather than the historical mainstay of bowel injury management via ostomies. For this reason, we propose a surgical management algorithm in which the general recommendation is to always seek bowel anastomosis via a primary or deferred technique leaving ostomies as a last resort (Fig. 97.1). These cases of last resort can be avoided by ensuring bowel vascularity, warranting minimal wall edema, limiting anastomotic tension, burring the anastomosis deep in the open abdomen, and performing abdominal wall closure as soon as possible.

## 97.8 Conclusion

Currently, isolated small or large bowel injuries are commonly managed via primary repair or primary anastomosis in patients undergoing initial definitive management or deferred anastomosis in patients requiring Damage Control Surgery. The traditional surgical dogma of ostomy has proven to be unnecessary and, in many instances, increases morbidity. Primary or deferred anastomosis even in the most severe cases should be the key surgical approach, and, by applying this strategy, the overall need for an ostomy (primary or deferred) can be reduced to less than 10%.

---

**Questions**
1. A patient with abdominal trauma is transferred to the operating room. During the surgical exploration, you see a jejunal laceration of less than 50% of its circumference. What is the AAST injury grade?
   A. AAST-I.
   B. AAST-II.**
   C. AAST-III.
   D. AAST-IV.

2. A 20-year-old is shot in the abdomen with a 0.38 caliber revolver. The entry wound is in the epigastrium to the left of the midline. He is hemodynamically stable, and the abdomen is moderately tender. Which of the following is the most appropriate next step in diagnosing the extent of the injuries?
   A. Close clinical observation.
   B. Serial e-FASTs.
   C. CT scan of the abdomen.**
   D. Diagnostic peritoneal lavage.

3. A 24-year-old woman was brought to the emergency department after being stabbed by her boyfriend. She arrived hemodynamically unstable, and she was transferred immediately to the operating room for an exploratory laparotomy. You find a colon injury that involves 20% of its circumference. She has responded appropriately to initial resuscitation efforts. How do you surgically manage this injury?
   A. Ostomy.
   B. Primary anastomosis.
   C. Primary repair.**
   D. Damage control.

4. Patient with a periumbilical gunshot wound to the abdomen with an exit flank wound around the right posterior axillary line. Initial blood pressure is 80/50 mm Hg and a pH of 7.2. Patient was taken immediately to the operating room for an exploratory laparotomy, and you find a threw and threw perforation of the transverse colon. Patient has required a total of 8 units of packed red blood cells and 6 units of fresh frozen plasma. How will you surgically manage this injury?
   A. Ostomy.
   B. Resection and primary anastomosis.
   C. Proximal and distal closure of the colon.**
   D. Wound packing.

5. Patient, who was involved in a high-speed car accident, arrives to the emergency department with multiple facial fractures and abdominal pain. He is hemodynamically unstable and is tender to palpation in all four quadrants of the abdomen. During laparotomy, you find multiple intestinal injuries. You repair a jejunum injury, but the colon injury was left in discontinuity. What is the best management approach for the abdominal wall?
   A. Bogota bag.
   B. Barker patch.
   C. Skin closure.
   D. VAC.**

6. Are the following complication common in patients with bowel injuries treated by damage control surgery? Except:
   A. Incisional hernia.
   B. Fascial dehiscence.
   C. Enterocutaneous fistula.
   D. Wound bleeding due to negative pressure wound therapy.**

7. A 53-year-old woman, restrained driver, sustains multiple injuries during a head-on automobile collision. Initial survey reveals closed fractures of both upper extremities, facial lacerations, and abdominal wall bruising. She is neurologically intact but complaining of severe abdominal pain. Blood pressure is 75/55 mm Hg and heart rate is 110 beats per minute. On physical exam, the abdomen is tender with guarding and rebound in all four quadrants. Which of the following would be the most appropriate study to evaluate her abdominal injuries?
   A. Chest X-ray.
   B. Abdominal CT scan.
   C. Diagnostic peritoneal lavage.
   D. Exploratory laparotomy.**

8. The same patient from question 7 was taken to the operating room for an

exploratory laparotomy. You find multiple intestinal injuries (3-small bowel and 1-colon), and she has not responded well to initial resuscitation maneuvers. You perform a damage control surgery and open abdomen. She is transferred postoperatively to the intensive care unit. Patient returns to the operating room 36 h later, and you perform a deferred anastomosis of her small bowel injuries. However, colon viability is questionable. What is your best surgical management option for this injury?
   A. Ostomy.
   B. Deferred anastomosis.
   C. Further intestinal resection/continue Damage Control Surgery.**
   D. Nonoperative management.
9. Regarding primary or deferred anastomosis for intestinal trauma, which of the following statements is correct?
   A. Stapled anastomosis has a higher rate of complications than a hand-sewn anastomosis.
   B. Hand-sewn anastomosis has a higher rate of complications than a stapled anastomosis.
   C. There is not difference between a hand-sewn or a stapled anastomosis regarding their complications rates.**
10. Are the following surgical approaches indicated for bowel trauma= Except:
    A. Colostomy.
    B. Primary repair.
    C. Primary anastomosis.
    D. Ileostomy.**

## References

1. Cardi M, Ibrahim K, Alizai SW, Mohammad H, Garatti M, Rainone A, et al. Injury patterns and causes of death in 953 patients with penetrating abdominal war wounds in a civilian independent non-governmental organization hospital in Lashkargah, Afghanistan. World J Emerg Surg. 2019;14:51. https://doi.org/10.1186/s13017-019-0272-z.
2. Parra-Romero G, Contreras-Cantero G, Orozco-Guibaldo D, Domínguez-Estrada A, del Campo J d JMM, Bravo-Cuéllar L. Abdominal trauma: experience of 4961 cases in western Mexico. Cir Cir (English Ed). 2019;87:183–9. https://doi.org/10.24875/CIRU.18000509.
3. Oosthuizen GV, Kong VY, Estherhuizen T, Bruce JL, Laing GL, Odendaal JJ, et al. The impact of mechanism on the management and outcome of penetrating colonic trauma. Ann R Coll Surg Engl. 2018;100:152–6. https://doi.org/10.1308/rcsann.2017.0147.
4. Iaselli F, Mazzei MA, Firetto C, D'Elia D, Squitieri NC, Biondetti PR, et al. Bowel and mesenteric injuries from blunt abdominal trauma: a review. Radiol Med. 2015;120:21–32. https://doi.org/10.1007/s11547-014-0487-8.
5. Cullinane DC, Jawa RS, Como JJ, Moore AE, Morris DS, Cheriyan J, et al. Management of penetrating intraperitoneal colon injuries: a meta-analysis and practice management guideline from the Eastern Association for the Surgery of Trauma. J Trauma Acute Care Surg. 2019;86:505–15. https://doi.org/10.1097/TA.0000000000002146.
6. Ahern DP, Kelly ME, Courtney D, Rausa E, Winter DC. The management of penetrating rectal and anal trauma: a systematic review. Injury. 2017;48:1133–8. https://doi.org/10.1016/j.injury.2017.03.002.
7. Demetriades D, Murray JA, Chan L, Ordoñez C, Bowley D, Nagy KK, et al. Penetrating colon injuries requiring resection: diversion or primary anastomosis? An AAST prospective multicenter study. J Trauma Inj Infect Crit Care. 2001;50:765–75. https://doi.org/10.1097/00005373-200105000-00001.
8. Ashley SW, Cance WG, Chen J, Jurkovich GJ, Napolitano LM, Riall TS. ACS Surgery (7th edition) Principles and Practice. 2014;2. Published by Decker Inc. ISBN 0-615-85974-7.
9. Gardner J. Blunt and penetrating trauma to the abdomen. Emerg Surg. 2005;23:223–8. https://doi.org/10.1385/1-59259-886-2:095.
10. Moore EE, Feliciano D V, Mattox KL. Trauma. 2017.
11. Dhillon RS, Barrios C, Lau C, Pham J, Bernal N, Kong A, et al. Seatbelt sign as an indication for four-vessel computed tomography angiogram of the neck to diagnose blunt carotid artery and other cervical vascular injuries. Am Surg. 2013;79:1001–4.
12. George MJ, Adams SD, McNutt MK, Love JD, Albarado R, Moore LJ, et al. The effect of damage control laparotomy on major abdominal complications: a matched analysis. Am J Surg. 2018;216:56–9. https://doi.org/10.1016/j.amjsurg.2017.10.044.
13. Moore E, Cogbill T, Malangoni M, Jurkovich G, Champion H, Gennarelli T, et al. Organ injury scaling, II: pancreas, duodenum, small bowel, colon and rectum. J Trauma. 1990;30:1427–9.
14. Advanced trauma life support (ATLS): 10th Edition. 2018. https://doi.org/10.1111/j.1365-2044.1993.tb07026.x.
15. Ordoñez CA, Parra MW, Serna JJ, Rodríguez HF, García AF, Salcedo A, et al. Damage control resusci-

16. Shanmuganathan K, Mirvis SE, Chiu WC, Killeen KL, Hogan GJF, Scalea TM. Penetrating torso trauma: triple-contrast helical CT in peritoneal violation and organ injury - a prospective study in 200 patients. Radiology. 2004;231:775–84. https://doi.org/10.1148/radiol.2313030126.
17. Ordoñez CA, Parra MW, Holguín A, García C, Guzmán-Rodríguez M, Padilla N, et al. Whole-body computed tomography is safe, effective and efficient in the severely injured hemodynamically unstable trauma patient. Colomb Med. 2020;51:e4054362. https://doi.org/10.25100/cm.v51i4.4362.
18. Kim HC, Shin HC, Park SJ, Il PS, Kim HH, Bae WK, et al. Traumatic bowel perforation: analysis of CT findings according to the perforation site and the elapsed time since accident. Clin Imaging. 2004;28:334–9. https://doi.org/10.1016/S0899-7071(03)00244-4.
19. Baron BJ, Benabbas R, Kohler C, Biggs C, Roudnitsky V, Paladino L, et al. Accuracy of computed tomography in diagnosis of intra-abdominal injuries in stable patients with anterior abdominal stab wounds: a systematic review and meta-analysis. Acad Emerg Med. 2018;25:744–57. https://doi.org/10.1111/acem.13380.
20. LeBedis CA, Anderson SW, Soto JA. CT imaging of blunt traumatic bowel and mesenteric injuries. Radiol Clin N Am. 2012;50:123–36. https://doi.org/10.1016/j.rcl.2011.08.003.
21. Matsevych OY, Koto MZ, Aldous C. Laparoscopic-assisted approach for penetrating abdominal trauma: a solution for multiple bowel injuries. Int J Surg. 2017;44:94–8. https://doi.org/10.1016/j.ijsu.2017.06.040.
22. Koto MZ, Matsevych OY, Aldous C. Laparoscopic-assisted approach for penetrating abdominal trauma: an underutilized technique. J Laparoendosc Adv Surg Tech. 2017;27:1065–8. https://doi.org/10.1089/lap.2016.0368.
23. Ordoñez C, Pino L, Badiel M, Sanchez A, Loaiza J, Ramirez O, et al. The 1-2-3 approach to abdominal packing. World J Surg. 2012;36:2761–6. https://doi.org/10.1007/s00268-012-1745-3.
24. Du Bose JJ, Scalea TM, Brenner M, Skiada D, Inaba K, Cannon J, et al. The AAST prospective Aortic Occlusion for Resuscitation in Trauma and Acute Care Surgery (AORTA) registry: Data on contemporary utilization and outcomes of aortic occlusion and resuscitative balloon occlusion of the aorta (REBOA). J Trauma Acute Care Surg. 2016;81(3):409–19. https://doi.org/10.1097/TA.0000000000001079.
25. Reva VA, Matsumura Y, Hörer T, Sveklov DA, Denisov AV, Telickiy SY, et al. Resuscitative endovascular balloon occlusion of the aorta: what is the optimum occlusion time in an ovine model of hemorrhagic shock? Eur J Trauma Emerg Surg. 2018;44:511–8. https://doi.org/10.1007/s00068-016-0732-z.
26. Ordoñez CA, Rodríguez F, Orlas CP, Parra MW, Caicedo Y, Guzmán M, et al. The critical threshold value of systolic blood pressure for aortic occlusion in trauma patients in profound hemorrhagic shock. J Trauma Acute Care Surg. 2020;89:1107–13. https://doi.org/10.1097/TA.0000000000002935.
27. Ordóñez CA, Parra MW, Caicedo Y, Padilla N, Angamarca E, Serna JJ, et al. Damage control surgical management of combined small and large bowel injuries in penetrating trauma: are ostomies still pertinent? Colomb Med. 2021;52(2):e4114425.
28. Ditzel RM, Anderson JL, Eisenhart WJ, Rankin CJ, DeFeo DR, Oak S, et al. A review of transfusion- and trauma-induced hypocalcemia: is it time to change the lethal triad to the lethal diamond? J Trauma Acute Care Surg. 2020;88:434–9. https://doi.org/10.1097/TA.0000000000002570.
29. Fakhry SM, Watts DD, Luchette FA. Current diagnostic approaches lack sensitivity in the diagnosis of perforated blunt small bowel injury: analysis from 275,557 trauma admissions from the East multi-institutional HVI trial. J Trauma Inj Infect Crit Care. 2003;54:295–306. https://doi.org/10.1097/01.TA.0000046256.80836.AA.
30. Ordoñez C, García A, Parra MW, Scavo D, Pino LF, Millán M, et al. Complex penetrating duodenal injuries: less is better. J Trauma Acute Care Surg. 2014;76:1177–83. https://doi.org/10.1097/TA.0000000000000214.
31. Ordoñez CA, Pino LF, Badiel M, Sánchez AI, Loaiza J, Ballestas L, et al. Safety of performing a delayed anastomosis during damage control laparotomy in patients with destructive colon injuries. J Trauma Inj Infect Crit Care. 2011;71:1512–8. https://doi.org/10.1097/TA.0b013e31823d0691.
32. Velmahos GC, Degiannis E, Doll D. Penetrating Trauma. 2012. https://doi.org/10.1213/ane.0b013e3182572adb.
33. Skube ME, Mallery Q, Lusczek E, Elterman J, Spott MA, Beilman GJ. Characteristics of combat-associated small bowel injuries. Mil Med. 2018;183:e454–9. https://doi.org/10.1093/milmed/usy009.
34. Roberts DJ, Stelfox HT, Moore LJ, Cotton BA, Holcomb JB, Harvin JA. Accuracy of published indications for predicting use of damage control during laparotomy for trauma. J Surg Res. 2020;248:45–55. https://doi.org/10.1016/j.jss.2019.11.010.
35. Weinberg JA, Croce MA. Penetrating injuries to the stomach, duodenum, and small bowel. Curr Trauma Rep. 2015;1:107–12. https://doi.org/10.1007/s40719-015-0010-2.
36. Weale R, Kong V, Buitendag J, Ras A, Blodgett J, Laing G, et al. Damage control or definitive repair? A retrospective review of abdominal trauma at a major trauma center in South Africa. Trauma Surg Acute Care Open. 2019;4:1–5. https://doi.org/10.1136/tsaco-2018-000235.
37. Nelson RL, Singer M. Primary repair for penetrating colon injuries. Cochrane Database Syst Rev. 2009;(3):CD002247. https://doi.org/10.1002/14651858.CD002247.

38. Urbanavičius L. How to assess intestinal viability during surgery: a review of techniques. World J Gastrointest Surg. 2011;3:59. https://doi.org/10.4240/wjgs.v3.i5.59.
39. Siddharth BR, Keerthi MSS, Naidu SB, Venkanna M. Penetrating injuries to the abdomen: a single institutional experience with review of literature. Indian J Surg. 2017;79:196–200. https://doi.org/10.1007/s12262-016-1459-0.
40. Cleary RK, Pomerantz RA, Lampman RM. Colon and rectal injuries. Dis Colon Rectum. 2006;49:1203–22. https://doi.org/10.1007/s10350-006-0620-y.
41. Demetriades D, Murray JA, Chan LS, Ordoñez C, Bowley D, Nagy KK, et al. Handsewn versus stapled anastomosis in penetrating colon injuries requiring resection: a multicenter study. J Trauma. 2002;52:117–21. https://doi.org/10.1097/00005373-200201000-00020.
42. Naumann DN, Bhangu A, Kelly M, Bowley DM. Stapled versus handsewn intestinal anastomosis in emergency laparotomy: a systemic review and meta-analysis. Surgery (United States). 2015;157:609–18. https://doi.org/10.1016/j.surg.2014.09.030.
43. Burlew CC, Moore EE, Cuschieri J, Jurkovich GJ, Codner P, Crowell K, et al. Sew it up! A western trauma association multi-institutional study of enteric injury management in the postinjury open abdomen. J Trauma Inj Infect Crit Care. 2011;70:273–7. https://doi.org/10.1097/TA.0b013e3182050eb7.
44. Loftus TJ, Efron PA, Bala TM, Rosenthal MD, Croft CA, Walters MS, et al. The impact of standardized protocol implementation for surgical damage control and temporary abdominal closure after emergent laparotomy. J Trauma Acute Care Surg. 2019;86:670–8. https://doi.org/10.1097/TA.0000000000002170.

# Kidney and Urotrauma

**98**

Federico Coccolini, Camilla Cremonini, and Massimo Chiarugi

**Learning Goals**
- Know that the hemodynamic status and the injury grade drive the decisional algorithm and the management of kidney and urologic trauma.
- Choose the most appropriate diagnostic-therapeutic strategy in case of kidney or urinary tract trauma.
- Know that nonoperative management may rely on some adjuncts as interventional radiology, endoscopic stenting, and percutaneous drainage, also useful in treating eventual complications.
- Nonoperative management may be the first phase inside a step-up treatment, with a planned delayed surgery.

## 98.1 Introduction

The incidence of genitourinary trauma is approximately 10%, and it usually involves males more frequently than females (3:1) [1–3]. Over the last decades, there has been a move toward a minimally invasive approach in the treatment of traumatic lesions. Across the years, nonoperative management (NOM) allowed trauma physicians to successfully treat an increasing number of traumatic injuries achieving good results in terms of outcomes, also thanks to the progressive introduction and development of new technologies as interventional endovascular procedures. The majority of genitourinary injuries, especially those caused by blunt trauma, can be managed nonoperative. As for other intra-abdominal organs, the decision process is based on the physiological status of the patient as well as on the anatomic grade of the injury and associated injuries [4]. A multidisciplinary approach (especially involving trauma surgeons and urologist) is cardinal to improve outcomes when dealing with urinary tract injuries.

### 98.1.1 Epidemiology and Mechanism of Injury

#### 98.1.1.1 Kidney

The kidney is the most frequently injured genitourinary organ after trauma. Renal trauma occurs in 1–3% of all trauma cases and in up to 10% of abdominal trauma [1, 3, 5]. Kidney injuries are often consequences of blunt trauma, that is, the predominant mechanism of injury (>90%), while penetrating injuries such as stab and gunshot wounds are a less common mechanism of injury [2, 4]. However, these percent-

F. Coccolini (✉) · C. Cremonini · M. Chiarugi
General Emergency and Trauma Surgery Department,
Pisa University Hospital, Pisa, Italy

ages vary between different geographic areas and healthcare systems.

The kidney is located deeply in the retroperitoneum, enclosed in a fibrous capsule that plays a key role in effectively containing bleeding and urinary leaks and should be preserved as much as possible during kidney mobilization and dissection. The renal capsule is surrounded by adipose tissue or perirenal fat, wrapped by the anterior (Gerota's fascia) and posterior (Zuckerkandl's fascia) leaves of the renal fascia. The kidney is kept in place only by the fibro-adipose fascia and the vascular pedicles and hence is vulnerable to blunt mechanism, especially associated with rapid deceleration.

- *Blunt trauma* may cause renal damage by direct blow to the organ or in case of rapid deceleration from high velocity. This specific mechanism is usually responsible of vascular pedicle and ureteropelvic junction injuries [2]. Rapid deceleration can stretch the renal vessels hence hesitating in a rare type of lesion: an isolated renal artery transection or divulsion [4]. Other common blunt mechanisms are fall from height, assault, skiing, and traffic accidents. Blunt injuries are often minor (75% of cases) and can be successfully managed with NOM in most of cases. Operative treatment (OM) is required in only 10% of blunt renal trauma.
- *Penetrating trauma*, either by stab and gunshot wounds, is related to higher incidence of major renal injuries than blunt mechanism (up to 70%) [2]. Renal injuries due to penetrating trauma tend to be associated with lesions of other intra-abdominal organs and are more likely to require surgical intervention [2, 4].

Pediatric kidneys are more vulnerable to injury when compared to adults for several anatomical reasons: relatively larger size of the organ in relation to the abdominal volume and lack of perinephric fat, thinner abdominal muscles, and lack of ossification of the rib cage [4–6]. According to some authors, the kidney is the most frequently injured intra-abdominal organ in the pediatric population [5]. Some injuries, like laceration of the renal pelvis or the ureteropelvic junction avulsion, are more frequent in children, but almost 85% of all pediatric kidney injuries due to blunt trauma are minor and are successfully treated with NOM.

### 98.1.1.2 Ureter

Ureteral injuries are rare, and the most common mechanism of injury is penetrating trauma (around 80% of cases). A damage to the ureter, in fact, occurs in less than 1% of blunt trauma and in approximately 4% of penetrating abdominal trauma [5]. Being caused most commonly by penetrating trauma (especially gunshot wounds), ureteral injuries are often associated with other intra-abdominal organ lesions [4]. Blunt trauma may cause damage to the ureter with high velocity deceleration mechanism: the most frequently injured area is the ureteropelvic junction [7, 8]. In general, injuries occur more commonly in the upper third of the ureter than in the middle or in the lower third [9].

### 98.1.1.3 Bladder

Blunt trauma is the most common cause of bladder injuries (65–80%). Common blunt mechanisms are sudden compression of a full bladder, shear forces, or, lastly, bone fragments in case of pelvic fracture. Considering the high amount of energy necessary to damage the bladder, it is not unexpected that the majority of bladder injuries (60–90%) are associated with pelvic fractures; nevertheless, patients with pelvic fracture present a bladder injury in 6–8% of cases [4, 8]. Bladder injuries may be *intraperitoneal* or *extraperitoneal* (see the paragraph "Classification") considering the involved portion of the organ. Intraperitoneal rupture is less frequent (around 15–40% of cases), and it usually occurs after direct application of blunt forces over a distended urinary bladder that cause a sudden increase in the intraluminal pressure and a rupture of the weakest part, the dome [7, 8]. Extraperitoneal rupture is the most common type, presenting in 60–90% of cases, and is seen almost exclusively associated with pelvic fractures [8]. When a pelvic ring fracture occurs, the shearing forces of the disruption may tear the bladder by stretching its ligamentous attachments [8, 10]. The bladder can also be injured by a sharp bony fragment of the fractured pelvic ring. Combined intra-extraperitoneal bladder ruptures (CBR) are found in 5–12% of all bladder ruptures [4, 8, 10].

#### 98.1.1.4 Urethra

Injuries to the urethra are uncommon, are more frequent in males, and are due to blunt trauma in 90% of cases [7, 11]. Urethral injuries can be divided in *anterior* or *posterior* ones (see the paragraph "Classification"). Anterior injuries involve the penile and the bulbar urethra. Posterior injuries instead involve the membranous and the prostatic urethra, those proximal to the perineal membrane.

Posterior urethral injuries are usually related to pelvic fracture and may be present in up to 5–10% of pelvic fractures [5]. The mechanism beneath consist of a shear of the puboprostatic ligaments: the consequent hematoma of the retropubic and peri-vesical space can be documented at the CT scan and is highly predictive of urethral injuries [8]. The site and type of pelvic fracture predicts the risk of urethral injury: in case of pubic symphysis involvement, every 1 mm of diastasis increase by 10% the risk of urethral injuries [12]. The anterior urethra is more commonly injured in case of straddle trauma by direct compression of the urethra itself against the inferior pubic arch. Penetrating trauma is a rare cause of injury both for anterior and posterior urethra [4].

Female urethral injuries are extremely rare due to its short size and commonly associated with pelvic injuries and rectal/vaginal lesions [4].

### 98.1.2 Classification

As for traumatic injuries to other organs, the AAST-OIS (American Association of Surgery of Trauma—Organ Injury Scale) classification and its revisions describe the anatomical aspect and extent of different types of damage to the kidney, ureter, bladder, and urethra [13–15] (Table 98.1). This classification represented a cornerstone of trauma injuries management and, since its introduction in 1989, has been effectively used in the treatment decision-process of several organs damaged, including the kidney. For other organs, such as the ureter, bladder, and urethra, the AAST system has been less utilized. Injuries to these organs are, in fact, difficult to be graded using available imaging approaches that often do not provide the necessary data to stratify the damage [5].

#### 98.1.2.1 Kidney

The AAST classification describes different types of renal injuries and their extent, ranging from hematoma or subcapsular hematoma (grade I) to completely shattered kidney (Grade V; Table 98.1). As for other organs in the last decade (i.e., liver, spleen), NOM has presented progressively increasing success rates in patients who presented severe traumatic renal injuries but were hemodynamically stable. These results, along with significant advances in minimally invasive technologies, showed how physiology as well as anatomy is important. The World Society of Emergency Surgery (WSES) proposed a classification system based not only on the anatomical aspect of the injury but also on the physiologic status of the patient [4].

Kidney injuries can be divided into four classes according to the WSES classification that considers the AAST-OIS classification and the hemodynamic status (Table 98.2):

- Minor (WSES class I).
- Moderate (WSES class II).
- Severe (WSES class III and IV).

#### 98.1.2.2 Urinary Tract

**Ureteral injuries** are graded by the AAST system considering the extent of contusion/laceration. Determining the grade is important in planning the treatment.

The AAST-OIS classification describes five grades of **bladder injuries**, ranging from bladder contusion to bladder neck avulsion (Table 98.1). Another classification system [10] does not take into account the size of the laceration but only its

**Table 98.1** AAST-OIS injury scale

| Grade | Injury type | Injury description |
|---|---|---|
| *Kidney injury scale* | | |
| I | Contusion | Microscopic or gross hematuria, urologic studies normal |
| | Hematoma | Subcapsular, non-expanding without parenchymal laceration |
| II | Hematoma | Non-expanding peri-renal hematoma confined to renal retroperitoneum |
| | Laceration | <1 cm parenchymal depth of renal cortex without urinary extravasation |
| III | Laceration | >1 cm parenchymal depth of renal cortex without collecting system rupture or urinary extravasation |
| IV | Laceration | Parenchymal laceration extending through the renal cortex, medulla, and collecting system |
| | Vascular | Main renal artery or vein injury with contained hemorrhage |
| V | Laceration | Completely shattered kidney |
| | Vascular | Avulsion of renal hilum that devascularizes kidney |
| *Ureter injury scale* | | |
| I | Hematoma | Contusion or hematoma without devascularization |
| II | Laceration | ≤50% transection |
| III | Laceration | >50% transection |
| IV | Laceration | Complete transection with 2 cm devascularization |
| V | Laceration | Avulsion of renal hilum that devascularizes kidney |
| *Bladder injury scale* | | |
| I | Hematoma | Contusion, intramural hematoma |
| | Laceration | Partial thickness |
| II | Laceration | Extraperitoneal bladder wall laceration ≤2 cm |
| III | Laceration | Extraperitoneal (>2 cm) or intraperitoneal (≤2 cm) bladder wall lacerations |
| IV | Laceration | Intraperitoneal bladder wall laceration >2 cm |
| V | Laceration | Intraperitoneal or extraperitoneal bladder wall laceration extending into the bladder neck or ureteral orifice (trigone) |
| *Urethral injury scale* | | |
| I | Contusion | Blood at urethral meatus; urethrography normal |
| II | Stretch injury | Elongation of urethra without extravasation on urethrography |
| III | Partial disruption | Extravasation of urethrographic contrast medium at injury site, with contrast visualized in the bladder |
| IV | Complete disruption | Extravasation of urethrographic contrast medium at injury site without visualization in the bladder; <2 cm of urethral separation |
| V | Complete disruption | Complete transection with >2 cm urethral separation or extension into the prostate or vagina |

Advance one grade for multiple injuries up to grade III
From: Moore E.E., et al. "Scaling System for Organ-Specific Injuries." p. Table 19–22, 2007, [Online]. Available: http://www.aast.org

**Table 98.2** WSES kidney trauma classification

| | WSES grade | AAST | Hemodynamic |
|---|---|---|---|
| Minor | WSES grade I | I–II | Stable |
| Moderate | WSES grade II | III or segmental vascular injuries | Stable |
| Severe | WSES grade III | IV–V or any grade parenchymal lesion with main vessel dissection/occlusion | Stable |
| | WSES grade IV | Any | Unstable |

*WSES* World Society of Emergency Surgery, *AAST* American Association for the Surgery of Trauma
F. Coccolini et al., "Kidney and urotrauma: WSES-AAST guidelines," World J. Emerg. Surg., vol. 14, no. 1, 2019

site, being more suitable and easier to be determined using radiological imaging techniques. This classification identifies four types:

- Bladder contusion.
- Intraperitoneal bladder rupture (IBR).
- Extraperitoneal bladder rupture (EBR).
- Combined bladder rupture (CBR).

The EBR can be further classified into two groups, simple and complex [16]:

- In the simple EBR, the urinary extravasation is confined to the extraperitoneal pelvic region.
- In complex EBR, the urinary extravasation can widely extend into the abdominal wall, the penis, the scrotum, and the perineum due to the disruption of fascial planes.

Several classifications systems exist to describe **urethral injuries:** the Colapinto and McCallum classification [17] has been used per years, but it only addresses posterior urethral injuries. The new Goldman classification [18] describes both anterior and posterior injuries, discerns between partial or complete lesions, and also addresses combined injuries of urethra and bladder, determining five types of damage. The imperative aspect that needs to be assessed is whether the injury is a partial or complete disruption of the anterior or the posterior urethra and if the damage involves the bladder neck or the rectum. All of these classifications are based on the aspect of the urethra at the retrograde urethrography [16].

## 98.2 Diagnosis

### 98.2.1 Clinical Presentation

The initial evaluation of a trauma patient follows the ATLS principles. The hemodynamic status is the key aspect that should drive the first management choices and diagnostic procedures. During the evaluation of a hemodynamically stable trauma patient, several factors should be investigated: mechanism of injury; an accurate abdominal, pelvic, and perineal examination; anamnestic data (solitary kidney, previous renal injuries or surgery; ureteropelvic obstruction; and kidney diseases like tumor or calculi). Preexisting renal abnormalities may increase the risk of injury, making the kidney more susceptible to trauma damage [11]. Furthermore, a solitary kidney should always be recognized before performing a nephrectomy in a trauma laparotomy.

Hematuria, gross or micro (defined as >3 red blood cells [RBC] per high-power field [HPF]), is an indicator of renal and urinary tract trauma, being frequently present (88–95%), but it does not predict the grade of injury [4, 19]. In fact, hematuria may be absent in case of renal pedicle avulsion or thrombosis of renal arteries, while renal contusion can present with macro-hematuria [6, 19].

Clinical examination should also investigate other findings that are suggestive of renal trauma: flank/abdominal pain, tenderness, contusion (ecchymosis or abrasions), or palpable mass.

Ureteral injuries may be subtle in presentation, thus a high index of suspicion is critical: hematuria is a common finding but may be absent in up to 45% of cases [5]. Bladder injuries frequently present with gross hematuria (95%), and the combination of pelvic fracture and macro-hematuria is a strong predictor of bladder rupture [5, 11]. Bladder rupture may also present with suprapubic or perineal ecchymosis, inability to void, and abdominal pain/distension [5]. These same symptoms, associated with blood from the meatus, scrotal hematoma, and superiorly displaced prostate on rectal examination, also suggest a possible urethral injury.

### 98.2.2 Diagnostic Procedures

The diagnostic procedures performed on a trauma patient upon admission are strictly planned according to the hemodynamic status of the patient itself [4].

The **E-FAST** (extended-focused assessment with sonography for trauma) is highly sensitive in rapidly detecting free intra-abdominal fluid, but its sensitivity and specificity decrease in diagnosing specific organ injuries, especially renal and urinary ones [4]. Ultrasonography may be used for follow-up evaluation of stable injuries, urinoma, and retroperitoneal hematomas [11].

The following patients should be investigated with appropriate urological imaging (i.e., CT scan with delayed urographic phase), in the suspect of renal or urinary tract trauma [5, 11]:

1. Blunt trauma and gross hematuria (always remember possible bladder lesions by pelvic trauma).
2. Blunt trauma with micro-hematuria and shock.
3. Major deceleration mechanism.
4. Penetrating trauma in the flank, back, or abdomen regardless the presence or degree of hematuria.
5. Other signs/symptoms that suggest a lower urinary tract injury (see above).

Over the years, **CT scan** with intravenous contrast became the gold standard in the evaluation of stable or stabilized trauma patients and, more specifically, replaced intravenous pyelography (IVP) in the primary diagnosis of renal and urinary tract injuries [4, 5, 11]. The standard execution of a CT scan, during the arterial and venous phases (20–30 s and 70–80 s of delayed images acquisition, respectively), allows to identify renal parenchymal injuries and vascular lesions. Usually, the kidney excretive phase (>80 s) is needed to properly complete the evaluation and staging of renal injuries [6]. The delayed excretory phase (urographic phase at 5–10 min of delay) is viable in diagnosing urinary tract injuries and detecting urinary extravasation [6, 19, 20].

Nevertheless, kidney and ureter are usually evaluated with CT scan, while lower urinary tract is better assessed with retrograde cystography/urethrography. Hence, different diagnostic procedures may be used according to the suspected injury site (Table 98.3).

**Table 98.3** Imaging techniques in kidney and urotrauma

| Organ | Imaging modalities of choice |
|---|---|
| Kidney | CT scan with urographic phase |
|  | IVU |
| Ureter | CT scan with urographic phase |
|  | Retrograde pyelography/IVU |
| Bladder | Retrograde cystography |
|  | CT scan with urographic phase |
| Urethra | Retrograde urethrography |
|  | Urethroscopy |

### 98.2.2.1 Kidney

**E-FAST** has low sensitivity in diagnosing kidney injuries, due to the anatomical location of the organ [11]. Other ultrasonography imaging modalities, such as contrast-enhanced ultrasound (CEUS) and eco-Doppler, are not routinely used during primary evaluation of a trauma patient but, in case of hemodynamic stability, can be performed as an alternative to CT scan in *pregnant women* or in the *pediatric population* [4]. Several studies have shown good results and effectiveness of CEUS in detecting extravasation, thrombosis, pseudoaneurysm (PSA), and post-traumatic arteriovenous fistulas [4, 21, 22]. CEUS also seems to increase the accuracy of E-FAST in hemodynamically stable patients with suspected renal injury [4, 21, 23].

**CT scan** has become, over the years, the gold standard for precise evaluation and grading of renal injuries in stable patients [5, 11]. CT imaging, with its *arterial, venous, and nephrogenic phases*, is both sensitive and specific for demonstrating parenchymal contusion or lacerations (also defining the depth and the extension), devitalized segments, subcapsular hematoma, contrast extravasation (Fig. 98.1), and other vascular injuries (arterial or venous) such as lacerations or thrombosis. A lack of contrast enhancement of the kidney or a central para-hilar hematoma may suggest a pedicle injury; the "rim sign" (a thin rim of subcapsular cortex) indicates a renal vascular compromise as an arterial occlusion (also suggested by the "cut off sign": sudden stop of a contrast-opacified renal artery) and consequent infarction [24]. The *delayed excretory phase*

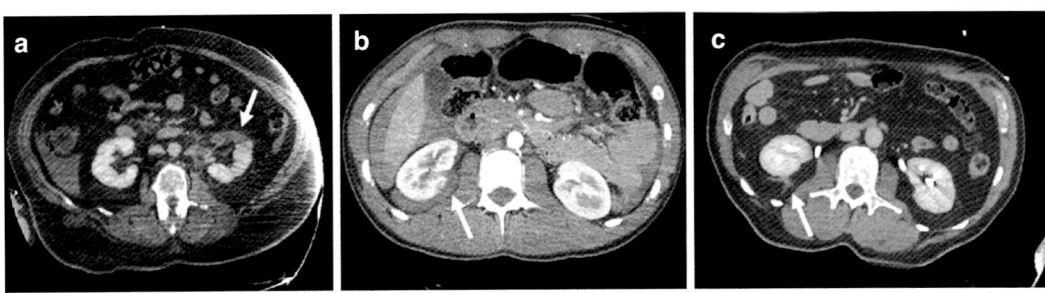

**Fig. 98.1** CT scan imaging of renal trauma: (**a**) renal contusion (AAST Grade I, white arrow); (**b**) renal laceration (AAST Grade II, white arrow) with peri-renal hematoma; (**c**) urinary extravasation (white arrow)

(urographic) allows visualization of the renal collecting system, the pelvis, and the ureter detecting urinary extravasation. CT scan is also viable in evaluating the perinephric space (i.e., perinephric hematomas that need to be distinguished from subcapsular hematoma [25]) and the retroperitoneum and in diagnosing possible associated intra-abdominal injuries (liver, spleen, etc.).

**Intravenous urography** (IVU) or pyelography (IVP), consisting in an intravenous injection of ionic or nonionic contrast followed by an serial abdominal radiograph 2–15 min later, has been largely replaced by CT scan in most clinical settings [4, 5, 11]. Nevertheless, IVU is still used in some low-resources areas or infrastructure or when CT scan is not available, but a urinary tract injury is suspected. IVU can document the presence of both kidneys, gives general information of parenchymal injuries, and outlines the collecting system detecting eventual urinary extravasation. Finally, a one shot intraoperative IVU may be useful in unstable patients directly taken to the OR, when a kidney injury is discovered or suspected.

On the other hand, IVU is not able to provide precise staging, and its findings are nonspecific: false negative ranges between 37 and 75%, and up to 20% of patients with severe renal injuries may have a normal IVP [5, 26]. Retrograde ureteropyelogram plays a limited role but may be performed aiming to evaluate and treat concomitant ureteral injuries [5].

### 98.2.2.2 Pediatric Kidney Trauma

Kidney injuries in the pediatric population deserve special mention. As for adults, the degree of hematuria does not correlate with the grade of kidney injury, but macro-hematuria seems to be more related to major renal injuries [4, 27]. An aggressive imaging approach in children is emphasized by their ability to maintain a normal systolic pressure despite significant blood loss: according to some studies, signs of shock will present only in around 5% of pediatric patients with a severe renal damage [5]. On the other hand, to decrease the radiological exposition of children, it is important to select appropriate factors that demand a CT scan imaging. Traditionally, all pediatric patients with any degree of hematuria after blunt trauma were scanned [19], but nowadays the criteria changed: most authors suggest to perform a CT scan in all children that sustained a blunt trauma and present micro-hematuria >50 RBC/HPF regardless of hemodynamic parameters [6, 27]. Other factors, such as mechanism of injury, its energy, and other physical findings (flank hematoma, ribs fractures, drop in the hematocrit associated with hematuria), should be considered when planning the imaging technique [4, 6, 27, 28]. Hemodynamically stable children that present mild symptoms, micro-hematuria <50 RBC/HPF, and no other indications for CT scan may be evaluated with ultrasound and/or CEUS and/or Doppler [4].

### 98.2.2.3 Ureter

In diagnosing a suspected ureteral injury, ultrasound plays no role. Again, CT scan with delayed excretory phase is the imaging method of choice when investigating a ureteral injury [9, 11, 29]. Suggestive radiological signs of an injury to the ureter or to the ureteropelvic junction are low density retroperitoneal fluid, perirenal hematoma with extravasation of contrast in the peri-nephric space, peri-ureteral hematoma, partial or complete obstruction of the ureteral lumen, lack of contrast in the distal ureter, and extravasation of contrast [5, 29]. An important distinction that must be made with imaging is between transection and lacerations: in case of transection, distal ureter will not be opacified; otherwise, contrast will be present in the distal ureter [8]. Transections require surgical operations, whereas some lacerations can be treated with ureteral stenting. If the CT scan provides equivocal findings, an ascending urography (retrograde pyelogram) or an IVP may be considered as next imaging modalities [4, 9].

Delayed diagnosis of ureteral damage is related to increased morbidity and mortality, hence the importance of an early diagnosis in order to avoid missed injuries [9].

A direct inspection of the ureter is indicated in case of a trauma laparotomy performed in patients with suspected ureteral injuries without preoperative imaging: the aid of a single shot IVU or the extravasation of a renally excreted intravenous dye (methylene blue or indigo carmine) may help identify the site of the damage [11].

#### 98.2.2.4 Bladder

**Retrograde cystography (RC)**, either with conventional plain films or CT technique, represents the gold standard imaging for the diagnosis of bladder injuries [4, 5, 11, 16]. The procedure consists in filling the bladder with a minimum of 350–400 ml of contrast via a Foley catheter, and it usually requires a plain film before (as a scout radiograph), a full-bladder film, and a post-emptying film in order to obtain the highest diagnostic accuracy. In case of a suspected urethral injury, a retrograde urethrogram with contrast should be performed before placing a Foley catheter. The post-drainage image, showing a contrast extravasation behind an empty bladder, may be the diagnostic scout in about 10% of cases [16]. The CT scan cystography is equally effective and accurate in detecting and staging a bladder injury, showing a sensitivity and specificity of 95% and

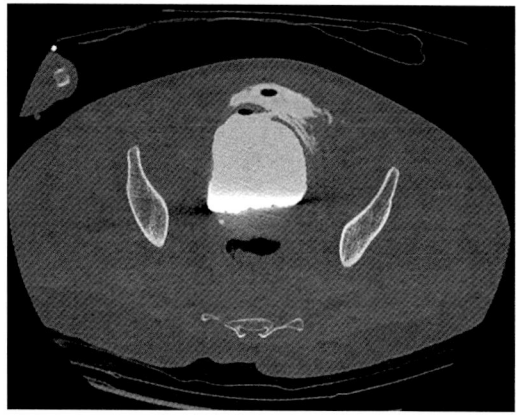

**Fig. 98.2** SEQ Figure \* ARABIC 2. Extraperitoneal bladder rupture with contrast extravasation

100%, respectively [4, 5, 11]. If possible, CT scan cystography should be preferred, considering its accuracy, the speed of execution, and the absence of need of post-emptying scout [4, 5].

**Intravenous contrast-enhanced CT scan** with urographic phase may be diagnostic, especially in trauma patients undergone CT to investigate other intra-abdominal injuries. This imaging technique is, however, less sensitive and specific than RC in detecting bladder injuries, due to the low intravesical pressure obtained with passive bladder filling with contrast-opacified urine by clamping the Foley catheter [4, 5, 8].

If the suspected bladder injury is associated to a pelvic bleeding amenable to angiography/angioembolization (AG/AE), the RC should be postponed; hence, the AG/AE may be completed without being affected in accuracy [4] (Fig. 98.2).

As for the ureter, direct inspection of the bladder is indicated in case of a trauma laparotomy performed in patients with suspected bladder injuries without preoperative imaging: the aid of a single shot IVU or the extravasation of a renally excreted intravenous dye (methylene blue or indigo carmine) may help identify the site of the damage [11].

#### 98.2.2.5 Urethra

In case the trauma patients present the above-mentioned symptoms, suggesting a urethral injury (i.e., blood from the meatus), two imaging techniques may be used in order to investigate it:

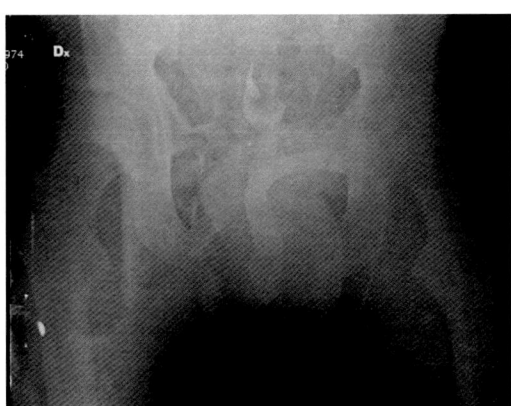

**Fig. 98.3** SEQ Figure \* ARABIC 3. Anterior urethral injury with extravasation of contrast, in a patient with severe pelvic fracture

**retrograde urethrography (RUG)** and **selective urethroscopy**. The first one is the procedure of choice if a urethral injury is suspected. Selective urethroscopy may be preferred in case of a penile lesion [4, 8, 11, 16] (Fig. 98.3).

RUG is performed instilling 10 ml of iodine contrast via a catheter inserted just at the urethral meatus, to avoid maneuvers that can further complicate the injury itself. Then, a radiograph of the lower abdomen is obtained, and it allows the physician not only to diagnose a damage to the urethra but also to distinguish between a complete and an incomplete rupture. An incomplete lesion is seen as an extravasation of contrast that also fills the bladder; complete injuries are associated with no presence of contrast inside the bladder [4]. In case of suspected urethral injuries, no bladder catheter should be positioned until a negative RUG is obtained: otherwise, positioning a suprapubic catheter should be considered (i.e., hemodynamic unstable patients directly taken to the OR) [4]. Considering that 10–15% of patients with an urethral injury due to a pelvic fracture also have an associated bladder damage, a retrograde cystography should be performed after a RUG via a Foley catheter (if the RUG was negative) or via a suprapubic catheter (if RUG showed an urethral rupture) [5]. The cystogram may be also obtained using the CT modality during an abdominal CT scan (CT cystogram) instead of the standard oblique X-rays [5].

## 98.3 Kidney Trauma: Management

### 98.3.1 Kidney: Nonoperative Management (NOM)

The management of renal trauma, as for other injured intra-abdominal organs, underwent a progressive shift toward nonoperative management (NOM) during the last few decades. Thanks to the increasing progress showed by technologies and minimally invasive procedures, NOM gained more and more consent showing good results even in high-grade injuries [3].

The majority of *blunt injuries* can be approached with NOM since these lesions are minor in most cases: several studies documented how NOM led to a lower rate of nephrectomies and a lower length of hospital stay without any apparent increase in complications rate [2, 30, 31].

NOM of *penetrating injuries* was once an unthinkable concept: isolated penetrating renal injuries are rare, being usually associated with other intra-abdominal injuries and hemodynamic instability. Recently, due to the improved imaging techniques that have allowed a proper staging, NOM is now considered as a safe treatment option in selected patients with renal trauma, with good outcomes and higher renal preservation rates [2, 4, 32, 33]. Hence, a significant proportion of penetrating renal trauma can be safely managed with NOM [34]: reported success rates of NOM in penetrating injuries are, respectively, around 50% and 40% in stab wounds (SWs) and gunshot wounds [2, 4, 35, 36]. The site of penetration can also be considered in the management decision: conservative treatment can be the successful strategy in around 88% of SWs posterior to anterior axillary line [11].

The hemodynamic status of the patient alongside the anatomic aspect of the injury are key factors in driving the management decision. WSES-AAST guidelines combined these two aspects in their classification (Table 98.2) and provided an algorithm for the management of renal and urological trauma (Figs. 98.4 and 98.6): NOM should be the first-line treatment in all hemodynamically stable patients with no other indications

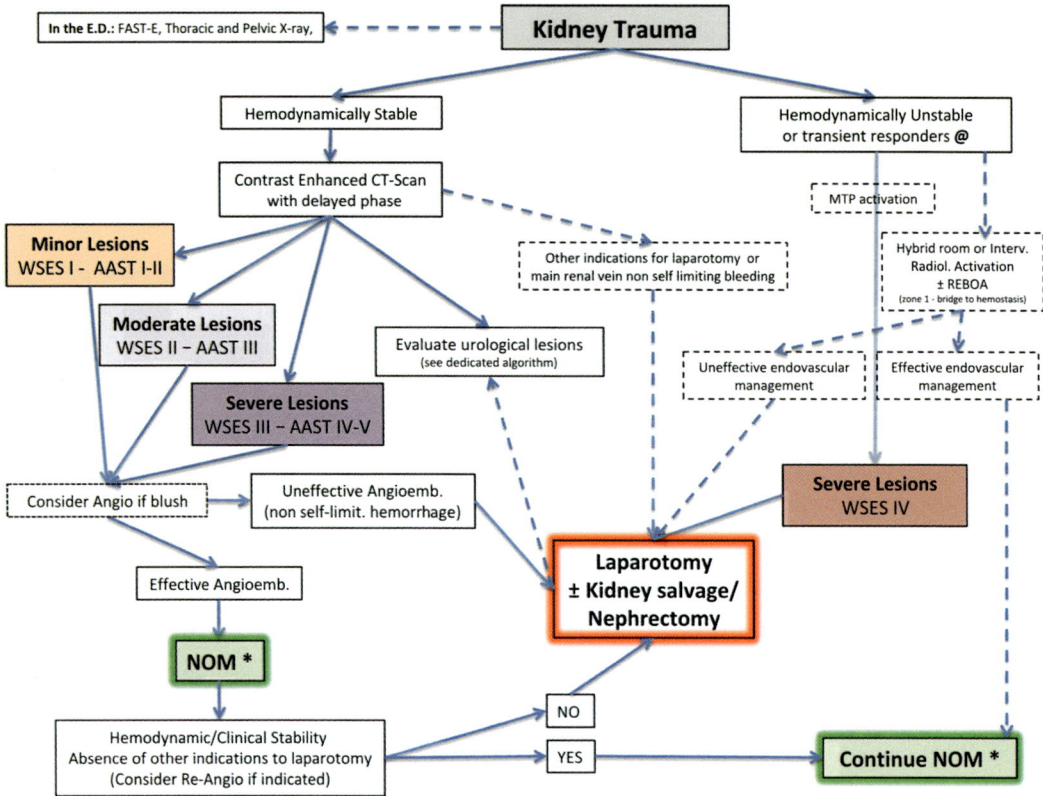

**Fig. 98.4** WSES, World Society of Emergency Surgery; AAST, American Association for the Surgery of Trauma. F. Coccolini et al., "Kidney and urotrauma: WSES-AAST guidelines," World J. Emerg. Surg., vol. 14, no. 1, 2019

for surgery, regardless the severity of the renal injury (AAST grade I to V) [4, 5, 37, 38]. Even patients with urinary extravasation or a shattered kidney, if hemodynamically stable, may be effectively managed with conservative treatment.

In stable patients, an accurate staging of the damage extent with **CT scan** with intravenous contrast and delayed urographic phase is fundamental in order to properly grade the injury and plan the treatment modalities [35, 37, 39]. Since several authors consider inaccurate staging a relative indication to surgery [4, 6, 36, 40], CT scan with urographic phase plays a key role in selecting stable patients for NOM and in identifying patients at high risk for NOM failure [4].

In case of moderate/severe injuries, the presence of at least two of the following criteria suggests high risk of **NOM failure**:

1. Contrast blush.
2. Perirenal hematoma >3.5 cm.
3. Medial laceration with medial urinary extravasation.
4. Lack of contrast in the ureter (suggesting a complete ureteropelvic junction avulsion).

Conservative management relies on close monitoring, clinical observation, repeated examinations, and trained surgeons that are essential factors. In fact, NOM can be considered as treatment in severe injuries or in transient responder patients only in selected settings, where adequate resuscitation, ICU monitoring, operative room, surgical and interventional expertise are rapidly available [4]. Patients treated nonoperatively need to be monitored due to the risk of bleeding or complications.

Considering that urinary extravasation usually resolves spontaneously in around 80–90% of patients and that Gerota's fascia plays a key role containing bleeding and urinary leak, a conservative treatment is a reasonable strategy if the hemodynamical stability is maintained. A nonoperative strategy can also comprehend *minimally invasive techniques as adjuncts*:

- Angiography/angioembolization.
- Endoscopic stent.
- Percutaneous drainage.

These adjunctive procedures can be used as first-line treatment in the acute setting, inside a conservative strategy, or as management options in case of complications (i.e., delayed pseudo-aneurism). Conservative management, for example, may result in non-resolving urinomas that can be treated with ureteral stenting or percutaneous drainage [37, 39] (Fig. 98.5).

Summarizing, *in the absence of other indications for laparotomy* and *in hemodynamically stable patients*, **NOM is feasible** in some specific situations that are not "per se" contraindications of a conservative approach [35, 41]:

- Isolated urinary extravasation.
- Prerenal hematoma.
- Renal fragmentation or a shattered kidney (Fig. 98.6b).
- Damage to the renal pelvis and ureteropelvic junction injuries.
- Penetrating lateral kidney injury.

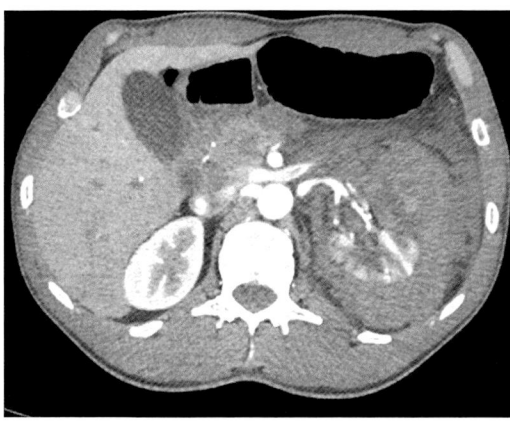

**Fig. 98.5** SEQ Figure \* ARABIC 5. AAST grade V renal injury ("shattered kidney")

In a hemodynamically stable patient, a shattered kidney or even a total avulsion of the ureteropelvic junction are not indications for an urgent operation [35]. These two and other conditions may require a delayed planned treatment, either with minimally invasive technique (i.e., endoscopic stenting, percutaneous drainage) or open repair that definitively treat the damage or some eventual complications, outside the acute setting [37, 39]. Whenever the damage is not amenable of repairing, the kidney should be removed. In some situations, in fact, NOM should be considered as an *intermediate treatment or part of a planned step-up approach* (Table 98.4).

### 98.3.1.1 Angiography and/or Angioembolization (AG/AE)

Angiography and angioembolization play an important role as extensions of conservative management, showing lower complication rates than surgical approach [42]. In hemodynamically stable patients, *indications* to AG and eventual AE in case of renal trauma are the following [4, 43]:

- Segmental arterial injuries and other vascular anomalies detected at the CT scan (i.e., active contrast extravasation, pseudo-aneurism, arteriovenous fistula).
- Gross non-self-limiting hematuria.
- Extended perirenal hematoma.

Rates of AE success in blunt renal trauma reported in the literature range between 63 and 100% [4, 42], [43]. Conditions that have been described as *risk factors for AE failure* are the following [4, 44]:

- Age.
- Volume of blood products transfused in the first 24 h.
- Expertise of the center.
- Penetrating trauma.

Others, such as ISS or low hemoglobin level, are not associated with higher failure

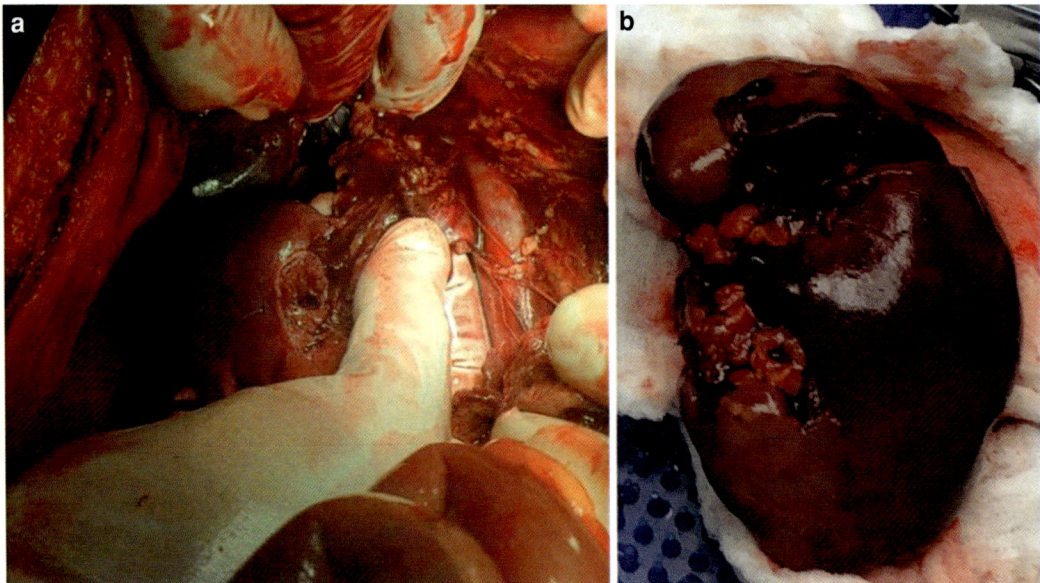

**Fig. 98.6** (**a**) Renal laceration with associated renal vein injury (fingers are clamping the vein to attempt a repair); (**b**) renal laceration due to penetrating trauma

**Table 98.4** Indications to surgical exploration in renal trauma

| Absolute | Relative |
|---|---|
| 1. Uncontrollable life-threatening hemorrhage | 1. Ureteropelvic junction injuries |
| 2. Pulsating/expanding retroperitoneal hematoma identified intraoperatively | 2. Extensive tissue damage (high proportion of devascularized parenchyma) |
| 3. Renal vein lesion with non-self-limiting hemorrhage (usually delayed interventions) | 3. Shattered kidney |
| | 4. Urinary extravasation |

rate of AE. Nevertheless, anatomical grade of damage seems related to a higher need of repeating AE but not to an overall AE failure [44]. A repeated AE can be considered as treatment in case of rebleeding or failure of first AE in patients that remains hemodynamically stable [4].

When indicated, angioembolization should be performed as *super-selectively* as possible, in order to limit the extension of devascularized parenchymal tissue and preserve renal function [37].

Angiography may be negative after detection of a contrast extravasation at the CT scan in around 30% of blunt renal trauma [45]: in these cases prophylactic angioembolization is not indicated [4].

Angiography also finds indication in the treatment of hemodynamically stable patients with severe blunt trauma (i.e., shattered kidney) and main renal artery injuries (i.e., dissection or occlusion): embolization or endovascular stenting may be adopted as strategies in order to treat these injury patterns in selected centers and patients [4]. Percutaneous revascularization with stents showed better results than surgical operation on renal function [46], when warm ischemia time is less than 120 min.

Renal hilum avulsion and especially main renal vein injuries requires surgical management [4].

### 98.3.2 Kidney Trauma: Operative Management

Operative management (OM) should be adopted as treatment of choice in all hemodynamically unstable or nonresponder patients (WSES IV) and in case of other indications to surgery (i.e., hollow viscous injury, see Liver chapter, Table 98.3).

Table 98.4 summarizes absolute and relative indications to surgical renal exploration.

Due to the lack of consensus in the literature regarding the relative indications presented in Table 98.4, the approved general trend is to approach these situations conservatively, if the hemodynamic status remains within the normality range and other viable solution to the anatomical damage exist. As already mentioned above, most of the situations considered as relative indications to surgery heal spontaneously and may be successfully treated with NOM and associated minimally invasive techniques (AE, percutaneous drainage, or endoscopic procedures).

Sometimes there is the need of *late planned surgery* in case of failure of conservative strategies, if the injury is not amenable to endovascular/endoscopic/percutaneous techniques or due to some complications [4, 11]. For example, devascularized renal tissue is not an indication for OM itself but can cause hypertension due to a high renin-angiotensin-aldosterone cascade activation. In case of hypertension nonresponsive to medical treatment and functional contralateral kidney, nephrectomy may be indicated [4, 11].

Retroperitoneal hematomas intra-operatively discovered and not adequately studied require surgical exploration if [4, 5, 11, 34]:

1. They are expanding or pulsatile.
2. They seem to be the only cause of hemodynamic instability.
3. Caused by penetrating trauma.

Renal exploration should not be performed routinely during a laparotomy carried out for other traumatic abdominal injuries in patients with associated renal injuries that do not require surgery, as opening the renal fascia increases the probabilities of nephrectomy [34]. An intraoperative IVP may also be considered in case of a suspected renal injury in patients without preoperative scanning.

Some surgical tips:

1. In unstable patients directly taken to the OR, a rapid palpatory assessment of the presence and dimension of the contralateral kidney is fundamental when suspecting a major renal injury probably requiring a nephrectomy.
2. Major renal artery laceration or severe parenchymal disruption that cause hemodynamical instability often require nephrectomy as surgical treatment (10% of cases, [34]). Some arterial injuries may be amenable to surgical repair, with success rate of 25–35%, and this strategy should be attempted especially in patients with solitary kidney or in those with bilateral renal injuries [4].
3. During exploratory laparotomy for renal trauma, two approaches have been described [5, 34]:

    - Exposing the kidney, its pelvis, and blood supply through a medial visceral rotation (Cattle-Braash or Mattox maneuver, right and left, respectively) and with direct incision of Gerota's fascia. This approach is the preferred one in case the patients are unstable and the renal damage appears to be too extensive.
    - Achieve a vascular control firstly, before opening Gerota's fascia, through an incision of the peritoneum above the aorta. This approach may be used in case of stable patients with injuries amenable to kidney-sparing operations but must be performed with caution.

4. Surgical steps to follow to repair renal injuries [5, 11, 34]:

    - Control the bleeding with electrocautery, suture ligation, or large transfix stitches.
    - Remove sharply any devitalized tissue.
    - Close collecting system injuries with watertight absorbable monofilament suture.
    - If possible, close the renal capsule above the injury, with a pledgeted not-absorbable suture. If it's not possible to repair the capsule due to a large damage, consider closing it with the interposition of hemostatic bolsters or an omental flap.

5. Some polar injuries not amenable of repair may be treated with partial nephrectomy.

6. An intraoperative injection of methylene blue inside the renal pelvis helps to check for eventual persistent urinary leak that need to be repaired.
7. At the end of the operation, in case of other intra-abdominal associated injuries, an omental flap over the kidney should be placed in order to separate it from the surrounding structures and to eventually protect other sutures/anastomosis from the urinary leak that increases the possibility of disruption [34].

Resuscitative Endovascular Balloon Occlusion of the Aorta (REBOA) may be considered as a bridge to more definitive treatment (as surgical repair) in hemodynamically unstable patients, as for other intra-abdominal injuries [4].

### 98.3.3 Renal Trauma Complications

Complications after renal trauma may be divided in early and late according to the timing of presentation (within or after 1 month later to the trauma). Minor injuries (AAST grade 1 ore 2) usually heal without sequelae [8].

- **Urinomas** are the most common complication after renal trauma and they usually occur in case of not-self-resolving urinary extravasation (10–20% of cases [8]). They can be managed with conservative treatment consisting in ureteral stenting with or without percutaneous drainage [34]. Same strategy can be followed in case of infected urinomas or peri-nephric abscess [11].
- Vascular anomalies such as **pseudo-aneurism (PSA) or arteriovenous fistula** are amenable to angiographic treatment (embolization) [4, 34].
- **Delayed bleeding** may occur within 2 weeks, is usually caused by PSA or fistula rupture, and can be treated with angioembolization [11].
- **Hypertension** occurs in around 5% of cases [1, 11]. Significant devascularization and consequent scaring of renal parenchyma, renal compression by a subcapsular hematoma (Page kidney), and chronic occlusion or constriction of the renal artery (Goldblatt kidney) are all mechanism of post-traumatic hypertension. The decreased blood flow following these mechanisms cause an important activation of the renin-angiotensin-aldosterone cascade. The consequent hypertension may be medically treated in the majority of cases; in case of hypertension not responsive to medical treatment, a delayed nephrectomy may be considered [4, 34].
- **Other complications** that can follow renal trauma are hydroureteronephrosis, renal lithiasis, and chronic pyelonephritis [1].

## 98.4 Urinary Tract Injuries: Management

### 98.4.1 Ureteral Trauma

Several factors influence the management decision process in case of ureteral trauma: AAST grade and site of the injury, associated injuries, and whether the ureteral lesion is discovered during a CT scan, a trauma laparotomy performed in an unstable patient or in a delayed setting (i.e., late presentation) [9]. The main goal of ureteral injury management is preserving the renal function allowing urinary flow and preventing urinoma formation (Fig. 98.7).

Considering only stable patients with no other indications for laparotomy, AAST grade I and II (contusion and partial laceration) can be successfully managed with nonoperative treatment and/or ureteral stenting in most cases [4, 9, 11]. A nephrostomy tube may be necessary in case the stenting procedure is unsuccessful.

A direct inspection of the ureter is indicated in case of a trauma laparotomy performed in patients with suspected ureteral injuries without preoperative imaging: the aid of a single shot IVU or the extravasation of a renally excreted intravenous dye (methylene blue or indigo carmine) may help identify the site of the damage [11].

Once diagnosed, a ureteral injury should be repaired whenever possible. Ureteral injury repair depends on the hemodynamic status of the

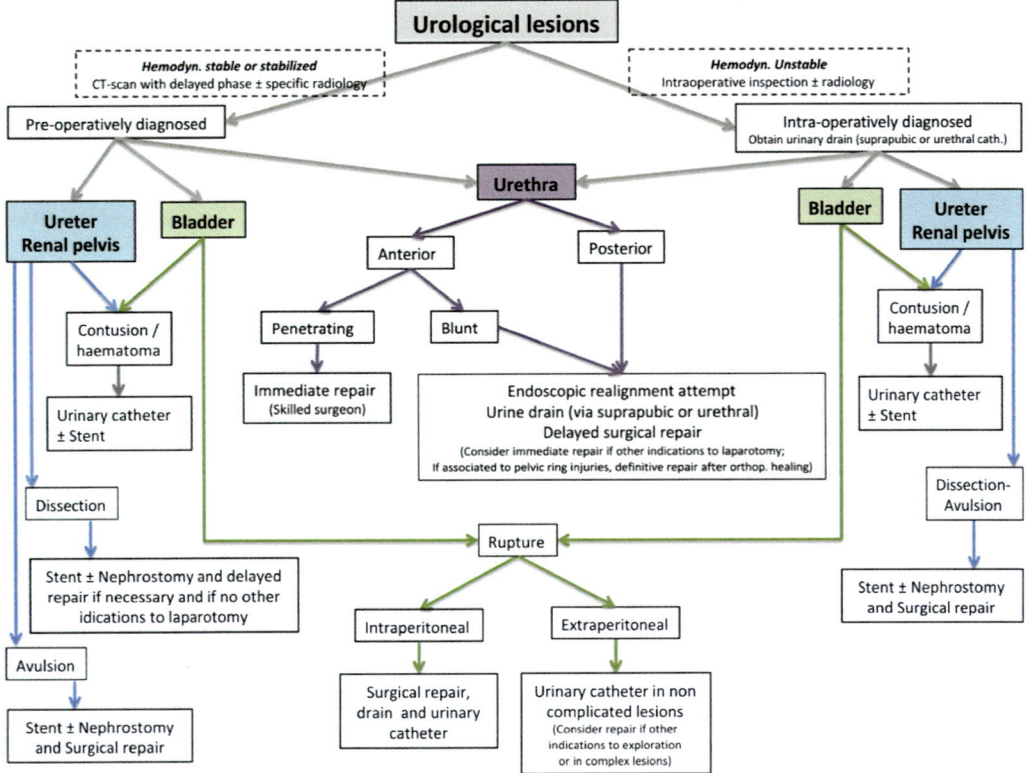

**Fig. 98.7** WSES World Society of Emergency Surgery, AAST American Association for the Surgery of Trauma. F. Coccolini et al., "Kidney and urotrauma: WSES-AAST guidelines," World J. Emerg. Surg., vol. 14, no. 1, 2019

patient, on the site of injury and on the extent of damage [11, 34]. Anyway, there are some general principles that need to be remembered:

- Debridement of devitalized tissue in order to have vital margins but paying attention to not waste tissue and consequently to impair potential repair.
- Avoiding excessive dissection of the tissue surrounding the ureter during mobilization since this can cause a reduction of the blood supply and consequent ischemia.
- Spatulation of ureteral ends to reduce the risk of strictures.
- Performing a tension free, watertight, absorbable suture over a double J stent, which also helps in reducing the risk of stenosis.
- Eventual separation of the ureteral anastomosis from the surrounding tissues with the interposition of omentum.

In case of hemodynamical instability and damage control surgery need, a temporary strategy must be adopted: ligate the damaged ureter (both ends in case of transection), proceed with resuscitation, and delay definitive repair. Urinary diversion may be obtained through a temporary percutaneous nephrostomy tube.

Finally, different type of repair may be attempted according to the location (Table 98.5).

Ureteral reimplant with Boari flap or "psoas hitch" are useful techniques that can be used in case of injuries of the lower and middle (more rarely) third of the ureter when the tissue loss makes impossible to perform a direct anastomosis or reimplant into the bladder without tension [5, 9, 11, 34].

In the postoperative period, the bladder catheter should be removed first, followed 2–3 days later by the abdominal drain if the output is low, and there are no urinary leaks. Ureteral stents

**Table 98.5** Surgical repair options, based on location and tissue loss

| Upper third | Ureteroureterostomy (preferred) |
|---|---|
| | Ureteropyelostomy |
| Middle third | Ureteroureterostomy (preferred) |
| | (Ureteral reimplant with Boari flap or "psoas hitch") |
| Lower third | Direct reimplantation of the ureter (ureteroneocystostomy) |
| | Ureteral reimplant with "psoas hitch" |
| | Ureteral reimplant with Boari flap |

should be left in place for 4–6 weeks after the repair, followed by an IVP or a retrograde pyelography to check the patency of the anastomosis or for urinary leak. An IVP or a RP should be repeated after 3 months [11, 34].

In case of delayed diagnosis or presentation of an incomplete ureteral injury, a stent placement should be attempted; if unsuccessful, a planned surgical repair should be considered [4].

#### 98.4.1.1 Ureteral Trauma Complications

Common complications that can rise after ureteral trauma are urinary leak and consequent urinomas, periureteral abscess, and ureteral strictures. Most of this complication is preventable with proper early diagnosis, stenting, eventual nephrostomy tube, or surgical repair [9]. These complications are also treatable with the same techniques abovementioned.

### 98.4.2 Bladder Trauma

Bladder contusion can be managed with observation and conservative management without any specific treatment. For other types of damage, the injury location and the extent of damage influence the type of treatment required:

- All *penetrating injuries* and *intraperitoneal bladder rupture* (IBR) require surgical exploration and operative repair; the most common injury site of IBR is the dome. The repair can be performed with a single- or double-layer absorbable suture [5, 34]. In case of an isolated IBR, the repair may be attempted with laparoscopic technique [4]. Combined bladder rupture (CBR) usually needs to be surgically repaired [34].
- Extraperitoneal bladder rupture (EBR) can usually be managed with bladder catheter left in place for 7–10 days; hence, in case of no other indications for surgery, EBR is amenable to NOM, with clinical observation, laboratory exams, and antibiotic therapy. If urinary leak persist, another 10 days of catheter and a repeated cystogram are recommended [5]. The success rate in such cases is around 90% with most patients completely healed within 3 weeks [11]. In some cases, conservative management may be unsuccessful, and if urinary extravasation persists, surgical repair can be considered.
- In case of *complex EBR* (i.e., injuries to the bladder neck) and *EBR associated with other injuries* requiring surgery (rectal/vaginal lesions or pelvic ring fractures that need fixation), operative repair is indicated.

Postoperative care of the patients usually requires maintenance of the Foley catheter for 7–10 days, and abdominal drain should be removed first. Retrograde cystography can be performed in order to exclude urinary leakage before urinary catheter removal [34]. In the pediatric population, positioning of a suprapubic catheter after bladder repair is recommended [4].

In case of hemodynamic instability and need of damage control strategies, the bladder repair can be delayed and a bladder or suprapubic catheter can be placed as a temporary strategy to divert urinary flow [4].

A suprapubic catheter can replace a urethral catheter if the patient presents suspected associated injuries to the perineum or to the urethra [4].

### 98.4.3 Urethral Trauma

Management of urethral trauma requires taking into account several factors [5]:

- Hemodynamic stability of the patient.
- Mechanism of injury (penetrating vs. blunt).

- Site of injury (anterior, posterior, combined; see Goldman classification).
- Extent of damage (partial, complete, grade of tissue loss).
- Associated injuries.

In case of perineal trauma or suspected urethral injuries, urinary drainage should be obtained as soon as possible. A retrograde urethrography (RU) should be performed in order to detect such injuries and to decide between a transurethral and a suprapubic catheter: the latter one is indicated in case of contrast extravasation at the urethrogram or in case of hemodynamically unstable patients with suspect perineal damage directly taken to the OR [4]. Positioning a suprapubic catheter may not be easy, especially in case of associated hematoma or hypotension with consequent poor bladder filling: in such cases, it may be placed in an ultrasound-guided fashion way [47] or in alternative with open technique during surgical exploration.

Another treatment option of an injured urethra consists in primary realignment of the urethra with endoscopic approach (i.e., flexible cystoscope) [5].

In case of NOM, standard care comprehends maintenance of the transurethral or suprapubic catheter for at least 2 weeks and a retrograde urethrography prior to eventual catheter removal.

**Blunt Injuries**
- *Incomplete anterior urethral injuries:* may be managed conservatively with the placement of a transurethral catheter or supra-pubic diversion. Endoscopic realignment and catheterization should be considered before surgery. If NOM and these techniques fail, a delayed surgical repair (urethroplasty) should be planned [4, 5].
- *Complete anterior urethral injuries:* data are somehow contradictory, with suprapubic catheter and endoscopic realignment being the two most adopted strategies in the acute setting, followed by planned urethroplasty (usually after 3 months). Acute attempts of repair are not recommended. The definitive surgical repair rely on the necessity of an accurate evaluation of damage extension [4, 5, 48].
- *Incomplete posterior urethral injuries:* may be initially treated with conservative management (urinary diversion or endoscopic realignment), and delaying surgical definitive repair after 14 days, if there are no other indications for laparotomy.
- *Complete posterior urethral injuries:* immediate endoscopic realignment is the preferred option of treatment, since it is associated with good outcomes and results [4, 5]. If unsuccessful, positioning of a suprapubic catheter is another viable option, whereas surgical definitive urethroplasty should be delayed at least 14 days after the injury time.
- *Blunt posterior injuries*, in a hemodynamically unstable patient or in case of other abdominal injuries requiring surgery, should be treated as already described, with immediate urinary diversion and delayed planned surgical repair [4].
- *Posterior urethral injuries* associated to pelvic fractures should be treated with definitive surgical repair after the pelvic damage has healed [4].

### 98.4.3.1 Penetrating Injuries

Penetrating injuries of the urethra, either anterior or posterior, usually require operative management. In both cases (anterior and posterior), the management decision is primarily taken considering the hemodynamic status of the patient and the rapid availability of an experienced urologist.

In case of hemodynamic stability and if an expert urologist is available, a prompt operative repair is recommended. Otherwise, if patient's condition is unstable, there is the necessity of damage control procedures, or if the surgical repair is not feasible due to extensive tissue damage, the surgeon should adopt the following strategy [4, 11]:

- Temporary urinary diversion via suprapubic catheter.
- Eventual marsupialization of the urethra (in case of large anatomic defect).
- Delayed urethroplasty or reconstruction with graft if needed (usually 3 months after the injury).

## Urethral Trauma Complications

A *multidisciplinary approach* of urethral trauma management is imperative to combine different expertise and obtain good outcomes: the aim is to proper select strategies that minimize adverse events such as urethral strictures, incontinence, and impotence.

Primary open realignment or primary open anastomosis showed higher rates of the above-mentioned complications [4], whereas endoscopic realignment and suprapubic catheterization showed good results [5, 11, 37]. Strictures may be treated with endoscopic procedures or planned urethroplasty.

> **Dos and Don'ts**
>
> **Renal Trauma:**
> - Always consider NOM as a first strategy in hemodynamically stable patients and in transient responder if treated in a level I trauma center.
> - *Do not* base the management decision only on the anatomical severity of the injury.
> - Consider AG/AE, endoscopic stenting, and percutaneous drainage as precious adjuncts to NOM.
>
> **Urinary Tract Trauma:**
> - Remember to consider minimally invasive techniques (endoscopic or drainage) as nonoperative strategies to treat or to temporary manage certain injuries.
> - Consider a step-up strategy with planned delayed surgical treatment;
> - *Do not* forget that the treatment of urinary tract trauma needs to be multidisciplinary.

## 98.5 Follow-Up

Follow up varies according to injury grade and clinical conditions of the patient.

Minor injuries (AAST grade I and II) rarely are followed by clinical sequelae and do not require follow-up imaging [4]. In moderate and severe lesions, imaging follow-up is tailored on patient injury pattern and clinical status; contrast-enhanced CT scan with excretory phase is recommended in patients with severe renal injuries within 48 h after trauma or in patients with moderate injuries without urinary extravasation but with a worsening clinical status [49]. Ultrasound with or without contrast may be a valid alternative and represent the first choice in the pediatric patient.

CT scan with urographic phase is also indicated in case of ureteral and bladder injuries, whereas urethroscopy or urethrogram are the recommended imaging methods in case of urethral trauma [4].

Return to normal physical activity and sports is not recommended until microscopic hematuria is resolved. While minor/moderate injuries may require 2–6 weeks of rest, severe trauma may necessitate of 6–12 months away from sport activity [4].

> **Take-Home Messages**
> - Kidney is the most common injured genitourinary organ in case of abdominal trauma; the majority of injuries can be managed nonoperatively.
> - Ureteral trauma occurs more frequently after penetrating trauma, requiring high index of suspicion, with a grade- and site-dependent repair.
> - Injuries to the bladder may be associated with pelvic fractures; intraperitoneal lesions require a surgical repair, extraperitoneal ones may be treated conservatively.
> - Urethral lesions may be managed with conservative treatment and realignment (with catheter or endoscopic technique), delaying the eventual urethroplasty.
> - Adjunctive techniques like endoscopic stenting or percutaneous drainage may be used inside a nonoperative strategy.

## Multiple Choice Questions

1. Kidney trauma:
   A. Is the most frequent type of genitourinary trauma and is usually due to blunt mechanism.
   B. May be caused by direct blow to the organ or in case of rapid deceleration.
   C. Is better diagnosed with contrast enhanced CT scan in hemodynamically stable patients.
   D. **All of the above.**

2. Post-traumatic bladder injuries:
   A. **Can be classified according to the rupture site in intraperitoneal, extraperitoneal, and combined.**
   B. Are rarely associated to pelvic fracture.
   C. Are most frequently intraperitoneal.
   D. Needs to be diagnosed with CT scan (urographic phase), which is the most sensitive method for these injuries.

3. Hematuria.
   A. Is not a reliable indicator of kidney or urinary tract trauma being frequently absent.
   B. **Is a common clinical finding in case of genitourinary trauma being present in up to 90% of cases.**
   C. Accurately predict the grade of renal injury.
   D. Is usually due to ureteral injuries.

4. In which of the following cases genitourinary tract must be suspected?
   A. Blunt trauma and gross hematuria.
   B. Major deceleration mechanism.
   C. Penetrating trauma in the flank, back, or abdomen regardless the presence or degree of hematuria.
   D. **All of the above.**

5. Retrograde urethrography-cystography.
   A. Plays no role in the acute setting in case of suspected genitourinary trauma.
   B. Has too low sensitivity and specificity to detect bladder injuries.
   C. **Is the imaging of choice if an urethral or a bladder injury is suspected.**
   D. Is useless if the aim is to distinguish between a complete and an incomplete urethral rupture.

6. Select the wrong sentence:
   A. Most renal injuries, even severe ones, may be managed conservatively with NOM.
   B. NOM should be the first line treatment in all hemodynamically stable patients with no other indications for surgery, regardless the severity of the renal injury (AAST grade I to V).
   C. **All penetrating injuries need to be operatively managed, being frequently associated with other intra-abdominal organ injuries.**
   D. NOM may be a first strategy in case of a shattered kidney or a ureteropelvic junction injury, in a hemodynamically stable patient.

7. Angiography and angioembolization (select the wrong one):
   A. **Are rarely indicated in case of renal trauma and has been replaced by innovative operative techniques.**
   B. Play an important role as extensions of conservative management, showing lower complication rates than surgical approach.
   C. When indicated, angioembolization should be performed as *sub-selectively* as possible, in order to limit the extension of devascularized parenchymal tissue.
   D. Allow to treat renal artery injury such as thrombosis or dissection with minimally invasive technique (endovascular stenting).

8. In case of operative management of renal trauma:
   A. Renal exploration should be performed routinely during a laparotomy carried out for other traumatic abdominal injuries in patients with associated renal injuries that do not require surgery.
   B. Expanding or pulsatile retroperitoneal hematomas intraoperatively

discovered and not adequately studied do not require surgical exploration.
C. **When attempting a kidney injury repair, follow the step of debridement of necrotic tissue, watertight absorbable suture, and closure the capsule above it.**
D. The most common surgical procedure performed is nephrectomy (90% of cases).

9. Select the correct sentence:
   A. The site of the ureteral injury does not affect the choice of the surgical procedure.
   B. **Extraperitoneal bladder rupture (EBR) can usually be managed with bladder catheter left in place for 10 days.**
   C. Penetrating bladder injuries and intraperitoneal ones should be managed with nonoperative management, drainage, or endoscopic treatment.
   D. Perform extensive dissection of the tissue surrounding the ureter during mobilization.

10. In case of urethral injuries:
    A. Their management requires taking consideration of several factors including hemodynamic status of the patient, site, and mechanism of injury, extent of damage, and associated injuries.
    B. A treatment option consists in primary realignment of the urethra with endoscopic instrumentation and eventual delayed definitive repair.
    C. A multidisciplinary approach of urethral trauma management is imperative in order to combine different expertise and obtain good outcomes.
    D. **All of the above.**

## References

1. Petrone P, Perez-Calvo J, Brathwaite CEM, Islam S, Joseph AK. Traumatic kidney injuries: a systematic review and meta-analysis. Int J Surg. 2020;74:13–21. https://doi.org/10.1016/j.ijsu.2019.12.013.
2. Gourgiotis S, Germanos S, Dimopoulos N, Vougas V, Anastasiou T, Baratsis S. Renal injury: 5-year experience and literature review. Urol Int. 2006;77(2):97–103. https://doi.org/10.1159/000093899.
3. Glykas I, Fragkoulis C, Paizis T, Papadopoulos G, Stathouros G, Ntoumas K. Conservative management of grade 4 and 5 renal injuries: a high-volume trauma center experience. Urol J. 2021;88(4):287–91. https://doi.org/10.1177/03915603211022293.
4. Coccolini F, et al. Kidney and uro-trauma: WSES-AAST guidelines. World J Emerg Surg. 2019;14(1):54. https://doi.org/10.1186/s13017-019-0274-x.
5. Kim F, Donalisio da Silva R. Genitourinary trauma. In: Moore EE, Feliciano DV, Mattox KL, editors. Trauma. 8th ed. New York: McGraw-Hill Education; 2017. p. 693–729.
6. Brandes SB, Mcaninch JW. Renal trauma: a practical guide to evaluation and management. Artic ScientificWorldJournal. 2004;4(S1):31–40. https://doi.org/10.1100/tsw.2004.
7. Zinman LN, Vanni AJ. Surgical management of urologic trauma and iatrogenic injuries. Surg Clin N Am. 2016;96(3):425–39. https://doi.org/10.1016/j.suc.2016.02.002.
8. Ramchandani P, Buckler PM. Imaging of genitourinary trauma. AJR Am J Roentgenol. 2009;192(6):1514–23. https://doi.org/10.2214/AJR.09.2470.
9. Pereira BMT, et al. A review of ureteral injuries after external trauma. Scand J Trauma Resusc Emerg Med. 2010;18(1):6. https://doi.org/10.1186/1757-7241-18-6.
10. Gomez RG, et al. Consensus statement on bladder injuries. BJU Int. 2004;94(1):27–32. https://doi.org/10.1111/j.1464-410X.2004.04896.x.
11. Santucci RA, Bartley JM. Urologic trauma guidelines: a 21st century update. Nat Rev Urol. 2010;7(9):510–9. https://doi.org/10.1038/nrurol.2010.119.
12. Basta AM, Blackmore CC, Wessells H. Predicting urethral injury from pelvic fracture patterns in male patients with blunt trauma. J Urol. 2007;177(2):571–5. https://doi.org/10.1016/j.juro.2006.09.040.
13. Moore EE, Cogbill TH, Malangoni M, Jurkovich GJ, Howard M Champion R. Scaling system for organ specific injuries. p. Table 19–22, 2007. http://www.aast.org.
14. Moore EE, et al. Organ injury scaling: spleen, liver, and kidney. J Trauma Inj Infect Crit Care. 1989;29(12):1664–6. https://doi.org/10.1097/00005373-198912000-00013.

15. Kozar RA, et al. Organ injury scaling 2018 update: spleen, liver, and kidney. J Trauma Acute Care Surg. 2018;85(6):1119–22. https://doi.org/10.1097/TA.0000000000002058.
16. Sandler CM, Goldman SM, Kawashima A. Lower urinary tract trauma. World J Urol. 1998;16(1):69–75. https://doi.org/10.1007/s003450050028.
17. Colapinto V, McCallum RW. Injury to the male posterior urethra in fractured pelvis: a new classification. J Urol. 1977;118(4):575–80. https://doi.org/10.1016/S0022-5347(17)58110-0.
18. Goldman SM, Sandler CM, Corriere JN, McGuire EJ. Blunt urethral trauma: a unified, anatomical mechanical classification. J Urol. 1997;157(1):85–9. https://doi.org/10.1016/S0022-5347(01)65291-1.
19. Smith JK, Kenney PJ. Imaging of renal trauma. Radiol Clin North Am. 2003;41(5):1019–35. https://doi.org/10.1016/S0033-8389(03)00075-7.
20. Kawashima A. et al. Education exhibit imaging of renal trauma: a comprehensive review 1 learning objectives for test 1. www.rsna.org.
21. Armstrong LB, et al. Contrast enhanced ultrasound for the evaluation of blunt pediatric abdominal trauma. J Pediatr Surg. 2018;53(3):548–52. https://doi.org/10.1016/j.jpedsurg.2017.03.042.
22. Miele V, Piccolo CL, Galluzzo M, Ianniello S, Sessa B, Trinci M. Contrast-enhanced ultrasound (CEUS) in blunt abdominal trauma. Br J Radiol. 2016;89(1061):20150823. https://doi.org/10.1259/bjr.20150823.
23. Regine G, et al. L'Ecografia con MdC di II generazione nella valutazione del trauma renale. Radiol Med. 2007;112(4)):581–7. https://doi.org/10.1007/s11547-007-0164-2.
24. Hsiao PJ, Wu TJ, Lin SH. Cortical rim sign and acute renal infarction. CMAJ. 2010;182(8):E313. https://doi.org/10.1503/cmaj.091110.
25. Dayal M, Gamanagatti S, Kumar A. Imaging in renal trauma. World J Radiol. 2013;5(8):275–84. https://doi.org/10.4329/wjr.v5.i8.275.
26. Obenauer S, Plothe KD, Ringert RH, Heuser M. Imaging of genitourinary trauma. Scand J Urol Nephrol. 2006;40(5):416–22. https://doi.org/10.1080/00365590600796642.
27. Fernández-Ibieta M. Renal trauma in pediatrics: a current review. Urology. 2018;113:171–8. https://doi.org/10.1016/j.urology.2017.09.030.
28. Nguyen MM, Das S. Pediatric renal trauma. Urology. 2002;59(5):762–6. https://doi.org/10.1016/S0090-4295(02)01548-0.
29. Ortega SJ, Netto FS, Hamilton P, Chu P, Tien HC. CT scanning for diagnosing blunt ureteral and ureteropelvic junction injuries. BMC Urol. 2008;8:3. https://doi.org/10.1186/1471-2490-8-3.
30. Sujenthiran A, et al. Is nonoperative management the best first-line option for high-grade renal trauma? A systematic review. Eur Urol Focus. 2019;5(2):290–300. https://doi.org/10.1016/j.euf.2017.04.011.
31. Mingoli A, et al. Therapeutics and clinical risk management dovepress operative and nonoperative management for renal trauma: comparison of outcomes. A systematic review and meta-analysis. Ther Clin Risk Manag. 2017;13:1127–38. https://doi.org/10.2147/TCRM.S139194.
32. DuBose J, Inaba K, Teixeira PGR, Pepe A, Dunham MB, McKenney M. Selective non-operative management of solid organ injury following abdominal gunshot wounds. Injury. 2007;38(9):1084–90. https://doi.org/10.1016/j.injury.2007.02.030.
33. Moolman C, Navsaria PH, Lazarus J, Pontin A, Nicol AJ. Nonoperative management of penetrating kidney injuries: a prospective audit. J Urol. 2012;188(1):169–73. https://doi.org/10.1016/j.juro.2012.03.009.
34. Best C, Varga S. Urological trauma. In: Demetriades D, Inaba K, Velmahos G, editors. Atlas of surgical techniques in trauma. Cambridge: Cambridge University Press; 2015. p. 228–39.
35. Santucci RA, Fisher MB. The literature increasingly supports expectant (conservative) management of renal trauma - a systematic review. J Trauma. 2005;59(2):J493–503. https://doi.org/10.1097/01.ta.0000179956.55078.c0.
36. Demetriades D, et al. Selective nonoperative management of penetrating abdominal solid organ injuries. Am Surg. 2006;244(4):620–8. https://doi.org/10.1097/01.sla.0000237743.22633.01.
37. Morey AF, et al. Urotrauma: AUA guideline. J Urol. 2014;192(2):327–35. https://doi.org/10.1016/j.juro.2014.05.004.
38. Morey AF, Broghammer JA, Hollowell CMP, Mckibben MJ, Souter L. Urotrauma guideline 2020: aua guideline. J Urol. 2020;205(1):30–5. https://doi.org/10.1097/JU.0000000000001408.
39. Stein DM, Santucci RA. An update on urotrauma. Curr Opin Urol. 2015;25(4):323–30. https://doi.org/10.1097/MOU.0000000000000184.
40. Shewakramani S, Reed KC. Genitourinary trauma. Emerg Med Clin North Am. 2011;29(3):501–18. https://doi.org/10.1016/j.emc.2011.04.009.
41. Buckley JC, McAninch JW. Selective management of isolated and nonisolated grade IV renal injuries. J Urol. 2006;176(6):2498–502. https://doi.org/10.1016/j.juro.2006.07.141.
42. Muller A, Rouvière O. Renal artery embolization-indications, technical approaches and outcomes. Nat Rev Nephrol. 2015;11(5):288–301. https://doi.org/10.1038/nrneph.2014.231.
43. Breyer BN, McAninch JW, Elliott SP, Master VA. Minimally invasive endovascular techniques to treat acute renal hemorrhage. J Urol. 2008;179(6):2248–53. https://doi.org/10.1016/j.juro.2008.01.104.
44. Hotaling JM, Sorensen MD, Smith TG, Rivara FP, Wessells H, Voelzke BB. Analysis of diagnostic angiography and angioembolization in the acute management of renal trauma using a national data set. J Urol. 2011;185(4):1316–20. https://doi.org/10.1016/j.juro.2010.12.003.
45. Yuan KC, Wong YC, Lin BC, Kang SC, Liu EH, Hsu YP. Negative catheter angiography after

vascular contrast extravasations on computed tomography in blunt torso trauma: an experience review of a clinical dilemma. Scand J Trauma Resusc Emerg Med. 2012;20:46. https://doi.org/10.1186/1757-7241-20-46.
46. Lopera JE, Suri R, Kroma G, Gadani S, Dolmatch B. Traumatic occlusion and dissection of the main renal artery: endovascular treatment. J Vasc Interv Radiol. 2011;22(11):1570–4. https://doi.org/10.1016/j.jvir.2011.08.002.
47. Mundy AR, Andrich DE. Urethral trauma. Part I: introduction, history, anatomy, pathology, assessment and emergency management. BJU Int. 2011;108(3):310–27. https://doi.org/10.1111/j.1464-410X.2011.10339.x.
48. Brandes S. Initial management of anterior and posterior urethral injuries. Urol Clin North Am. 2006;33(1):87–95. https://doi.org/10.1016/j.ucl.2005.10.001.
49. McCombie SP, et al. The conservative management of renal trauma: a literature review and practical clinical guideline from Australia and New Zealand. BJU Int. 2014;114(Suppl 1):13–21. https://doi.org/10.1111/bju.12902.

# Duodeno-Pancreatic and Extrahepatic Biliary Trauma

Gennaro Perrone, Alfredo Annicchiarico, Elena Bonati, and Fausto Catena

**Learning Goals**
- Know the incidence, the mechanism of damage, and the clinical presentation of duodeno-pancreatic and extra-hepatic biliary trauma.
- Establish the early management of a patient given his hemodynamic conditions; choose the most correct diagnostic tests and identify patients who are candidates for NOM.
- Identify the most correct surgical strategies for the patient in relation to the severity of the injuries.

## 99.1 Introduction

Duodeno-pancreatic and extrahepatic biliary trauma are traumatic lesions of the duodenum, pancreas, and extrahepatic biliary tree that very often occur in the context of major multi-organ traumas that often requires multidisciplinary management. The emergency surgeon plays a key role in the initial management, but, often following surgical reconstructions with hepato-pancreato-biliary (HPB), surgeons are required. Endoscopists, interventional radiologists, and gastroenterologists are essential not only in the early diagnosis and management of trauma but also in nonoperative management (NOM) and in the treatment of complications and long-term sequelae. Mortality and morbidity increase enormously with time in these traumas; hence, the management should be as early as possible.

## 99.2 Epidemiology

Although duodenal trauma is very rare, ranging from 0.2 to 0.6% of all trauma patients and 1–4.7% of all abdominal trauma, their lethality remains very high with a mortality of up to 20% [38, 41, 47]. This is mainly due to the fact that duodenal trauma is often associated with other lesions, such as pancreatic, biliary, or vascular injuries, and this can lead greater difficulties not only in the treatment but also in the diagnosis.

Injuries treated quickly and promptly diagnosed offer greater success, while those with delayed recognition are more often associated with poor outcome. Pancreatic trauma is rare with an incidence of less than 1% in all traumas and 3.7–11% of abdominal traumas [28, 35, 47]. As in duodenal trauma, the outcome of these can be worsened by the retroperitoneal localization which can weaken signs and symptoms of injury delaying diagnosis and treatment.

Extrahepatic biliary traumas are rarer and occur in 0.1% of adult trauma. As well as the others, these are also associated with other injuries in most traumas. Isolated lesions are extremely rare and occur only in 2–3% of cases of extrahepatic biliary lesions [19, 39, 46].

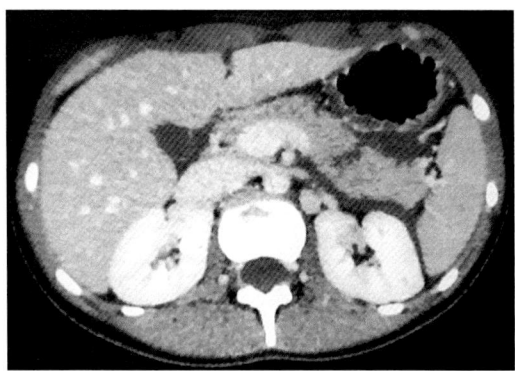

**Fig. 99.1** CT scan image of body pancreatic injury (AAST Grade III)

## 99.3 Etiology

Penetrating trauma, such as gunshot and stab wounds, are the most common causes in adult duodenal injuries although blunt traumas may cause duodenal lesions when its compression into the lumbar spine is determined. Pancreatic penetrating injuries are more frequent in series from North America, Africa, and among military involved in wars, but car or bicycle crashes remain the most common causes of pancreatic injuries in adults and children. This gland, along with duodenum, is placed in the retroperitoneum in front of the vertebral column, and blunt traumas can cause its rupture (Fig. 99.1). A classic example can be the "Chance Fracture," typically caused by seat belt injuries in which vertebral fracture is made from an excessive flexion of the spine. In around half of cases, there is an associated abdominal injury such as a splenic rupture, small bowel injury, pancreatic injury, or mesenteric tear [28, 38, 41, 49]. In extrahepatic biliary, blunt trauma is the most frequent except for the gallbladder which is more frequently associated with penetrating trauma [19, 39, 46].

## 99.4 Classification

The American Association for the Surgery of Trauma (AAST) has proposed a grading system for both duodenal, pancreatic, and extrahepatic biliary tree lesions. In AAST the injuries are graded from I to V with increasing severity and are described indicating degree and description of the lesion. In pancreatic and duodenal traumas, the type of injury is also described distinguishing between hematoma, laceration, or vascular lesion [30, 31] (Tables 99.1, 99.2, and 99.3). World Society of Emergency Surgery (WSES) revised the guidelines for pancreatic, duodenal, and extrahepatic biliary traumas by proposing a classification in four classes that considers both the AAST classification and the hemodynamic status. The final grade of the lesion depends on the higher-grade lesion among the various lesions. WSES guidelines divided the severity of the lesions into three grades: minor (WSES Class I), moderate (WSES Class II), and severe (WSES Class III–IV) (Table 99.4) [9].

**Table 99.1** The grading system proposed by the American Association for the Surgery of Trauma Society (AAST) for extrahepatic biliary trauma [31]

| Grade[a] | Description of injury |
|---|---|
| I | Gallbladder contusion/hematoma<br>Portal triad contusion |
| II | Partial gallbladder avulsion from liver bed; cystic duct intact<br>Laceration or perforation of the gallbladder |
| III | Complete gallbladder avulsion from liver bed<br>Cystic duct laceration |
| IV | Partial or complete right hepatic duct laceration<br>Partial or complete left hepatic duct laceration<br>Partial common hepatic duct laceration (<50%)<br>Partial common bile duct laceration (<50%) |
| V | >50% transection of common hepatic duct<br>>50% transection of common bile duct<br>Combined right and left hepatic duct injuries<br>Intraduodenal or intrapancreatic bile duct injuries |

[a] Advance one grade for multiple injuries up to grade III

**Table 99.2** The grading system proposed by the American Association for the Surgery of Trauma Society (AAST) for Duodenal trauma [30]

| Grade[a] | Type of injury | Description of injury |
|---|---|---|
| I | Hematoma<br>Laceration | Involving single portion of duodenum<br>Partial thickness, no perforation |
| II | Hematoma<br>Laceration | Involving more than one portion<br>Disruption <50% of circumference |
| III | Laceration | Disruption 50–75% of circumference of D2<br>Disruption 50–100% of circumference of D1, D3, D4 |
| IV | Laceration | Disruption >75% of circumference of D2<br>Involving ampulla or distal common bile duct |
| V | Laceration<br>Vascular | Massive disruption of duodeno-pancreatic complex<br>Devascularization of duodenum |

*D1* first position of duodenum, *D2* second portion of duodenum, *D3* third portion of duodenum, *D4* fourth portion of duodenum

[a] Advance one grade for multiple injuries up to grade III

**Table 99.3** The grading system proposed by the American Association for the Surgery of Trauma Society (AAST) for pancreatic trauma [30]

| Grade[a] | Type of injury | Description of injury |
|---|---|---|
| I | Hematoma<br>Laceration | Minor contusion without duct injury<br>Superficial laceration without duct injury |
| II | Hematoma<br>Laceration | Major contusion without duct injury or tissue loss<br>Major laceration without duct injury or tissue loss |
| III | Laceration | Distal transection or parenchymal injury with duct injury |
| IV | Laceration | Proximal[b] transection or parenchymal injury involving ampulla |
| V | Laceration | Massive disruption of pancreatic head |

[a] Advance one grade for multiple injuries up to grade III
[b] Proximal pancreas is to the patients' right of the superior mesenteric vein

**Table 99.4** The grading system proposed by the World Society of Emergency Surgery (WSES) considering both AAST grade and hemodynamic status of patients [9]

| Grade | WSES class | Organ | AAST grade |
|---|---|---|---|
| Minor | WSES class I | Pancreas<br>Duodenum<br>Extrahepatic biliary tree | I–II<br>I<br>I–II–III |
| Moderate | WSES class II | Pancreas<br>Duodenum<br>Extrahepatic biliary tree | III<br>II<br>IV |
| Severe | WSES class III | Pancreas<br>Duodenum<br>Extrahepatic biliary tree | IV–V<br>III–IV–V<br>V |
| Severe | WSES class IV | Any[a] | Any[a] |

[a] In hemodynamically unstable patients

## 99.5 Diagnosis

In penetrating traumas, multiple organs are generally involved, and the inspection of the wounds with the evaluation of the direction of knife or bullet or the simple assessment of abdomen tenderness can give information on the organs involved. Penetrating trauma or hemodynamic instability often forces the exploratory laparotomy, and, in this step, control of bleeding is crucial. When hemostasis has been performed, careful exploration of the other organs should be made to identify any other possible lesions. When intraoperative findings such as hepatic flexure, transverse, gastric, or liver injuries are manifested or signs, such as saponification, bilomas, or bruised duodenum, are present, a duodenum-pancreatic injury or a lesion of the external biliary tract should be supposed, and this often imposes a complete kocherization of duodenum. In less severe degrees of blunt traumas and hemodynamic stable patients, nonoperative management (NOM) can be considered, so early diagnosis of duodeno-pancreatic lesions is the real challenge. The onset of symptoms generally occurs in 6–24 h after injury but has been reported as late as 5 days after traumas [15, 40]. Patients may have vague and poorly defined symptoms with abdominal pain, especially in the upper quadrants, or back pain. In blunt trauma, impact signs such as rib fractures, bruising, ecchymosis, upper lumbar spine lesions, and seat belt injuries may suggest involvement of the pancreas or duodenum. Lipases and amylases dosage can help in the diagnosis but, by themselves, do not allow to establish the presence or absence of a duodenum-pancreatic lesion. Amylase levels are neither specific nor sensitive for diagnosis and can raise in head, hepatic, and bowel injuries, while serum lipases are more specific [21, 29]. Nowadays, repeated and combined measurements of both amylases and lipases are useful for clinical evaluation and, if elevated, are indications for further investigations [9]. The presence of free fluid in the abdomen on Extended Focused Assessment with Sonography for Trauma (E-FAST) may suggest the presence of a perforation, but, in a hemodynamically stable patient, CT scan remains the gold-standard exam [8] (Figs. 99.2 and 99.3). The presence of free fluid, peripancreatic collections, or retroperitoneal free air can be indicative of a duodenal-pancreatic lesion even if, in early hours, a variable percentage of cases can be misdiagnosed resulting in delayed manifestations [11]. On CT scan images, pancreas can appear normal up to 40% of patients with acute blunt injuries, especially when imaging is done within

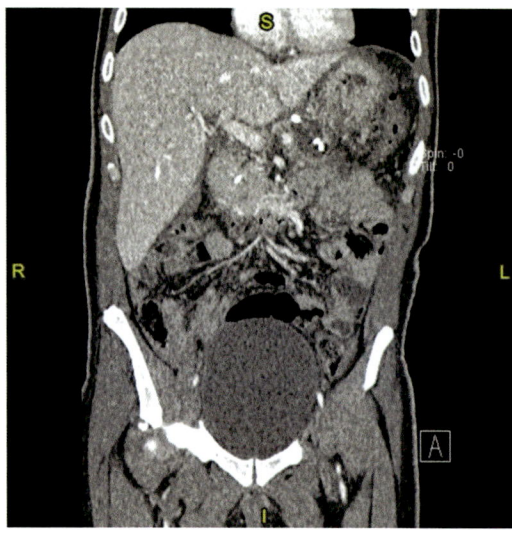

**Fig. 99.2** Body pancreatic hematoma in blunt trauma

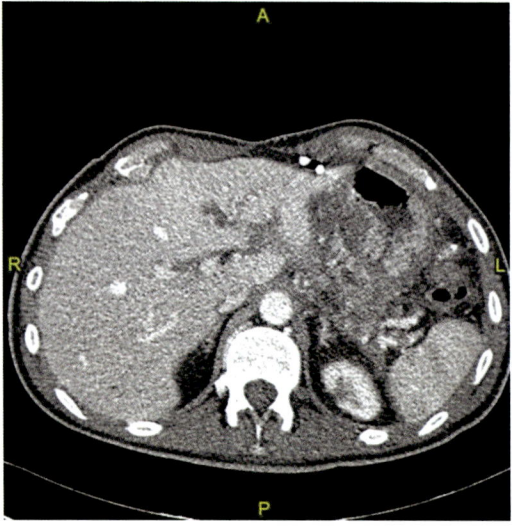

**Fig. 99.3** Body pancreatic hematoma associated to SII-SIII liver hematoma, SII-SIII-SIV lacerations, and spleen laceration

the first 12 h [37]. Diagnosis often derives from a combination of clinical elements, laboratory exams, and radiological findings, and often, in patients with high clinical suspicion, a new CT-Scan with specific pancreatic phase at 12–24 h should be performed [9]. Endoscopic retrograde cholangiopancreatography (ERCP), in hemodynamically stable patients, is useful in identification and characterization of minor pancreatic lesions or biliary leaks. ERCP also offers some help in treatments of isolated biliary lesions and follow-up, even if its use is limited in the early stages of trauma and in suspected duodenal perforations [37]. Magnetic resonance cholangiopancreatography (MRCP) is a minimally invasive diagnostic modality which, like the ERCP, can be considered a second level examination. MRCP is useful in the follow-up of parenchymal damage and minor ductal injuries, providing high-quality images of the pancreatic and biliary ducts (Figs. 99.4 and 99.5). Secretin administration may help in diagnosis of pancreatic leakages by improving ductal visualization, particularly of non-dilated ducts [36]. Both ERCP and MRCP are exams performed in the late phases of the trauma's workup and generally after 48 h. They are useful in defining the chances of NOM or in the operative planning in selected hemodynamically stable patients [9]. Diagnostic Peritoneal Lavage (DPL) has a sensibility higher than 99% for the presence of hemoperitoneum, but the ability to recognize early retroperitoneal organ injuries is very low. Although DPL alone has been associated with a high number of unnecessary laparotomies [4], we must emphasize that a negative laparotomy could still lead to fewer complications when compared to a late identification of a duodenal-pancreatic lesions. The specificity of DPL is very low, and in recent years its use has in fact been progressively replaced by E-FAST and CT scan. Duodeno-pancreatic and biliary tract injuries occur within the context of multiple lesions for which an emergency exploratory laparotomy is often required. Recently, Coccolini et al. proposed the new WSES-ASST guidelines in which the diagnostic algorithm is based on the severity of the lesions. CT differentiates the severity of stable patients in WSES grades, and tests such as ERCP and MRCP can be used later to define NOM or surgical planning. Hemodynamically unstable patients or with free air, peritonitis, or evisceration on CT-Scan always require an accurate surgical exploration [9] (Fig. 99.6).

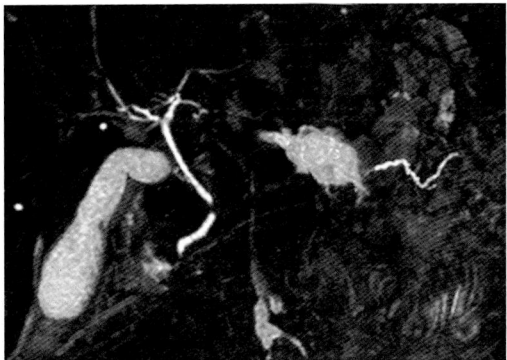

**Fig. 99.5** A follow-up MRCP shows a Wirsung stent associated with a pseudocystic lesion of the body-tail of the pancreas

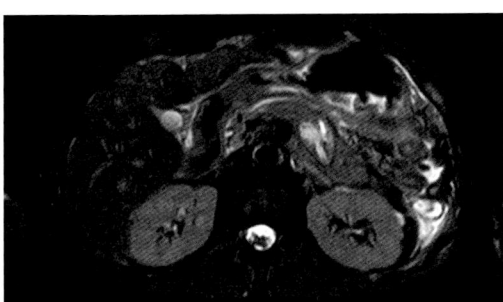

**Fig. 99.4** Pseudocystic lesion of the body-tail of the pancreas due to blunt trauma

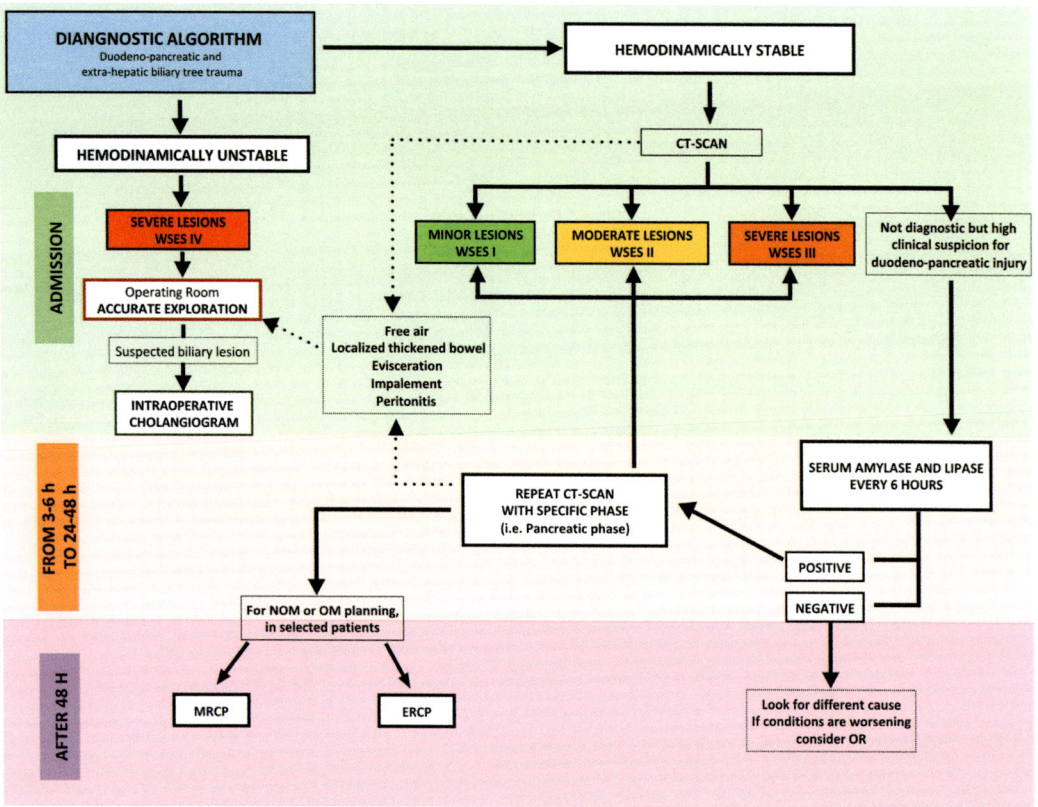

**Fig. 99.6** Diagnostic algorithm proposed by World Society of Emergency Surgery based both on severity of lesions at CT scan and hemodynamic status [9]. *NOM* nonoperative management, *OM* operative management, *MRCP* magnetic resonance cholangiopancreatography, *ERCP* endoscopic retrograde cholangiopancreatography

## 99.6 Treatment

Given that most of duodeno-pancreatic and extra-hepatic biliary traumas are often associated with other injuries, surgical treatment is often mandatory. On the contrary, in minor traumas, stable or stabilized patients, and isolated/low-grade injuries, nonoperative management (NOM) may be considered.

### 99.6.1 Nonoperative Management

In a blunt trauma of duodenum, the energy transmission to the mucosa and submucosa can cause a break of vascular submucosal plexus which can lead to an intramural hematoma. In previous series, it had already been described that the surgical approach in these cases could lead to an increase in complication rate and hospital stay [17]. NOM should be based on seriates laboratory tests, bowel rest, nasogastric tube decompression, and parenteral nutrition. Duodenal obstruction, due to hematoma, is not a contraindication to NOM and generally resolves within 14 days. Otherwise, treatment could be made both in open and laparoscopically though percutaneous drainage could be viable alternatives [9, 25, 33].

In most minor pancreatic hematoma and surface lacerations (AAST Grade 1), NOM can be effective both in adults and children. In pancreatic blunt trauma in which pancreatic ducts are involved (AAST grade 2), the site of injury influences management enormously. In lesions of pancreatic tail or distal to the superior mesenteric vein, distal pancreatectomy, with or without splenectomy, is associated with a shorter period of complete resolution, while NOM is reserved only to lesions in very proximal pancreatic body injuries [13, 20].

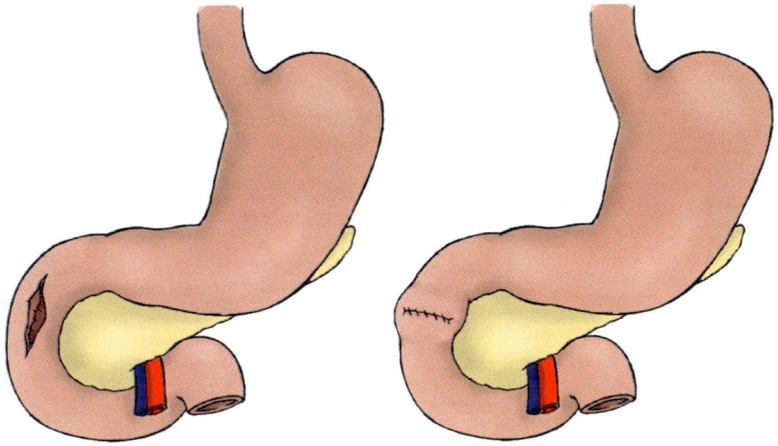

Fig. 99.7 Direct duodenal repair

Although literature about NOM in extrahepatic biliary trauma is scarce, few small cases series have demonstrated NOM to be successful in both adult and pediatric patients. Hemodynamically stable patients, with isolated gallbladder wall hematoma or contusion (AAST Grade 1), could be usefully treated with NOM [39, 44, 46]. Abdominal bile collections can be drained through percutaneous drains, and the ERCP with stent placement should be mandatory to address ductal lacerations and to promote biliary flow in duodenum.

The latest WSES-AAST guidelines, in duodenal wall (WSES I-II/AAST I-II) and gallbladder (AAST I) hematomas and in very proximal pancreatic body injuries with ductal involvement (AAST III), consider NOM feasible only in isolated lesions and in hemodynamically stable patients [9].

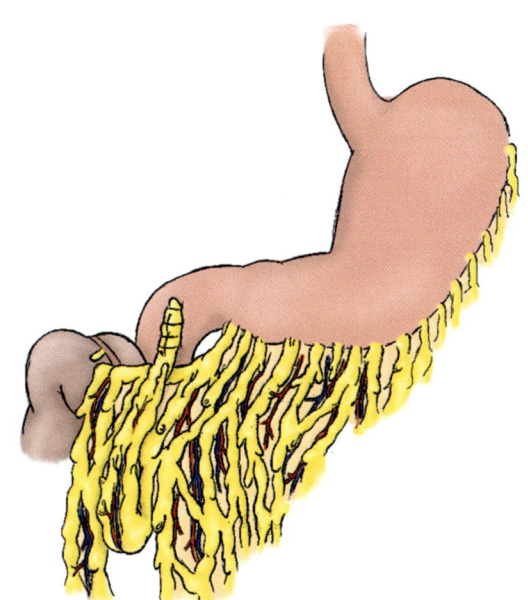

Fig. 99.8 Omental patch

## 99.6.2 Operative Management

In most traumas, especially in major ones with associated injuries, in hemodynamically unstable patients, and in patients with evident signs of peritonitis, perforation, evisceration, or penetrating wounds, the emergency/urgent surgical approach is mandatory, but technique is highly dependent on the extent of the injury. Stopping the bleeding remains the first aim to be carried out, followed by an adequate debridement of the duodenal walls around the laceration back to vital tissue. Direct duodenal repair can be performed in one–two layers of resorbable or non-resorbable suture, and, in order to avoid stenosis of the duodenal lumen, a transverse rather than longitudinal repair may be required (Fig. 99.7). Segmental resection and primary end-to-end duodenoduodenostomy are usually feasible when dealing with injuries to DI, DIII, or DIV, but if the injury is in the second part of duodenum, the ampulla of Vater should be carefully identified [14]. An omental patch and serosal patch may be useful in those cases where the loss of duodenal tissue cannot be primarily repaired (Fig. 99.8). These techniques are successfully utilized by placing omentum or a small bowel loop on the defect and fixed by stitches [14, 48]. In all duodenal repairs,

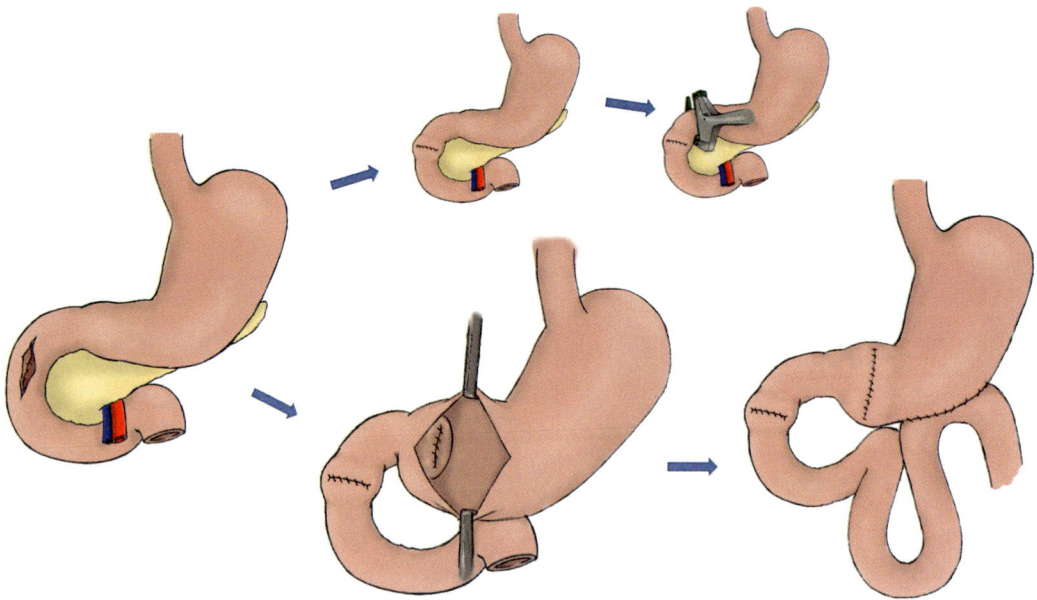

**Fig. 99.9** Pyloric exclusion: the pylorus can be stapled without section or, by a gastrotomy, sutured internally with absorbable stitches. Gastric contents can be diverted through a gastrojejunostomy

nasogastric tube decompression and drainage placement are suggested.

A range of techniques have been deployed in the largest trauma centers in the presence of high-grade trauma when pancreas is involved, and duodenal repair is complex. In these cases, the risk of pancreatic fistula is higher, and the exclusion of gastric secretions from the duodenum with different techniques can allow better healing in a shorter time. An approach to duodenal trauma was described by Stone and Fabian in the "triple ostomy" technique consisting of jejunostomy, gastrostomy, and duodenostomy especially for higher-grade trauma in the second duodenal portion [45]. Furthermore, in 1974, Berne had already presented the concept of "duodenal diverticulization" whose essential components included gastric antrectomy, duodenostomy, gastrojejunostomy, and drainage [5].

These two techniques have now been largely left behind in favor of pyloric exclusion (PE). In PE, the gastric contents can be diverted through a gastrojejunostomy, and the pylorus can be stapled without section or, by a gastrotomy, sutured internally with absorbable stitches so that it can spontaneously open a few weeks later or reopened endoscopically [27] (Fig. 99.9). Nevertheless, many surgeons prefer a gastric emptying via a suction tube along with parenteral or enteral nutrition. In grades III, IV, and V, complex reconstruction techniques are often required. In lesions of D1 or D2 but proximal to the papilla, antrectomy and gastrojejunostomy is a feasible, instead, when the ampulla is involved or the lesion is distal to it, a Roux-en-Y duodenojejunostomy should be performed with the proximal stump. In complete destruction of the duodenum-pancreatic complex and associated devascularization (Grade 4), pancreaticoduodenectomy should be considered. Although class IV and V injuries require complex reconstructions in about half of cases, staged procedures have been suggested to improve outcomes, and support of hepatobiliary surgeons should be considered case by case [10, 25].

Many duodenal injuries discovered at laparotomy are AAST Grade 1 and 2 and can be repaired primarily, and, in some series, up to 60% of patients with duodenal lesions, regardless of severity, can be repaired with primary duodenorraphy [16]. The most modern studies are in fact "pressing" toward direct repair even in large and high-grade lesions when feasible. The more conservative techniques are in fact related to a lower mortality and a better outcome compared to the more complex reconstruction procedures that must be reserved only when primary repair is not possible [12, 34]. In all hemodynamically unstable patients with pancreatic lesions or in those in whom the NOM is not allowed, immediate operational management is mandatory. Damage Control Surgery (DCS) should be considered in the presence of patients in shock and with massive bleeding. The surgical strategy is strictly dependent on the degree, extent, and location of the lesion. During surgical exploration, the pancreas must be well visualized, and the status of the main ducts evaluated. The opening of the gastrocolic ligament together with the Kocher maneuver allows the exposure of the anterior aspect of the gland, while the lateral mobilization of the spleen and the dissection of the splenic flexure of the colon allow visualization and manual palpation of the body and tail [2]. Most pancreatic lesions in which the ducts are not involved can be treated with drainage placement alone, and laceration repairing may be associated with an increased risk of pseudocyst formation [24]. It is well established that pancreatic lesions with interruption of the main ducts at or to the left of the superior mesenteric vein (SMV) must be treated with distal pancreatectomy with or without spleen preservation [9]. The management of the pancreatic stump is more uncertain, although in the past it was thought that selective ligation of the pancreatic duct significantly reduced leaks [6]; a recent series of 704 pancreatic traumas questioned its usefulness [7]. The management of pancreatic head is much less standardized with higher morbidity and mortality rates. Often, especially in multi-organ injuries, drain positioning alone is the best option. When conditions are favorable, a duodeno-preserving total pancreatectomy or a subtotal pancreatectomy with a pancreaticojejunostomy of the distal stump may be performed, but the remaining pancreatic tissue can result in severe exocrine and endocrine dysfunction.

Except for gallbladder hematomas (Grade 1) for which NOM is possible, cholecystectomy is the intervention of choice in all gallbladder lesions. Gallbladder is involved in about 30–60% of all extrahepatic biliary injuries, and most are an intraoperative finding. Cystic duct and main bile ducts injuries (Grades 3–5) generally occur in conjunction with lesions of the pancreas, duodenum, and liver, and treatment is strictly dependent on the severity of the lesions. Among the most appropriate surgical alternatives, primary repair over a T-tube can be useful especially in lesions where the laceration is partial but may result in strictures and need for reconstructive surgery. In most of complete duct lesions, a Roux-en-Y hepaticojejunostomy or a choledochojejunostomy remains the only alternatives.

The new WSES-AAST guidelines highlighted the various therapeutic alternatives according to the degree of the lesion and the stability of the patient [9] (Fig. 99.10).

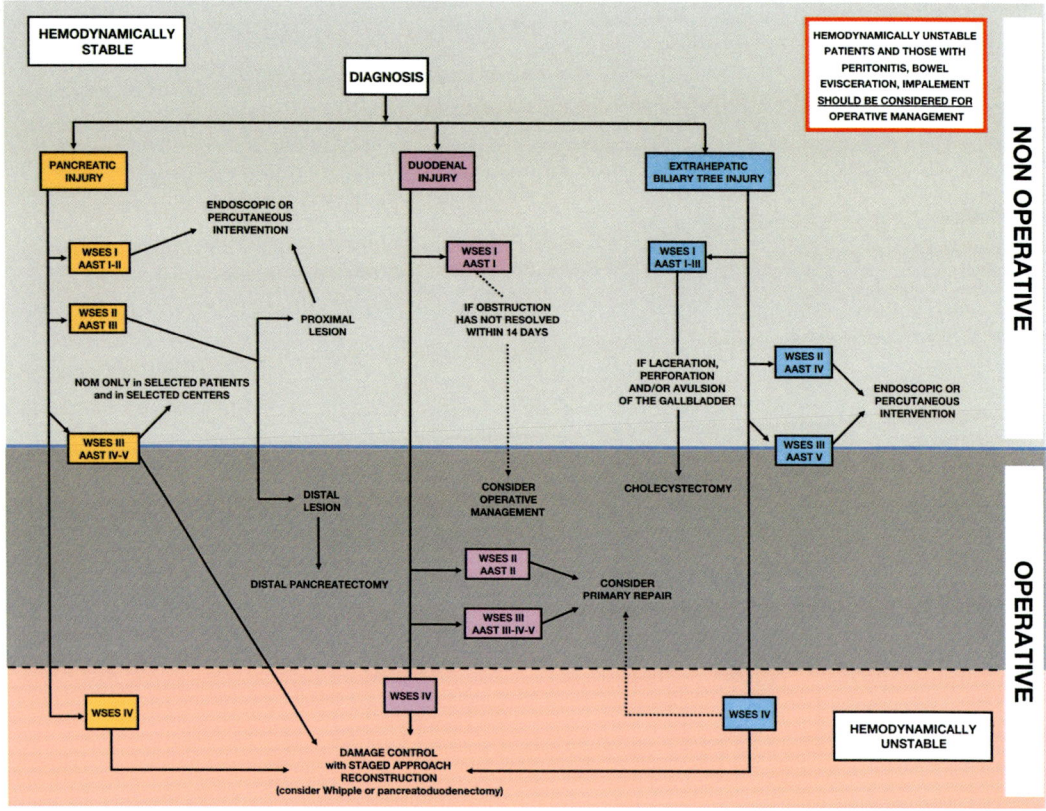

**Fig. 99.10** The WSES-AAST proposed management algorithm duodeno-pancreatic and extrahepatic biliary tree traumatic lesions [9]. *NOM* nonoperative management

## 99.7 Outcomes and Complications

The management of duodenal-pancreatic trauma is often complex, and, in most patients, other organs are also involved; therefore, the mortality rates remain very high. The overall mortality rate of duodenal injuries continues to be significant, up to an average of 17%. Major complications reported after a duodenal trauma are duodenal fistula, intra-abdominal abscess, pancreatitis, obstruction, and bile duct fistula. Overall mortality of duodenal injuries is significant up to an average of 17%, but it is linked to associated vascular or pancreatic lesion. When other causes are excluded, mortality to duodenal injury itself is probably less than 5% [3, 10, 14, 42]. Among most important factors influencing morbidity and mortality are mechanism of trauma (blunt or penetrating), delayed diagnosis, localization, and size of lesion [42]. Generally, mortality in penetrating trauma is higher than in closed trauma, respectively, 25–28% and 12–15%. High mortality is often conditioned by injury to adjacent organs and great vessels, especially in penetrating injuries as well as the complications deriving from the treatment (dehiscence, sepsis, and multi-organ failure) [3, 14, 42]. In the multicenter series by Cogbill et al., the mortality rate for blunt trauma was higher (14.4%) than penetrating ones (3.6%), and this difference was mostly attributed to a delayed diagnosis of blunt duodenal injury [10].

The size of the defect as well the location is pivotal in the choice of reconstruction. Penetrating injuries result in less tissue loss and, if identified early, better management. Snyder et al. demonstrated lower mortality and morbidity in patients with duodenal lacerations of less than 75% [42]. Furthermore, the technical difficulties resulting from lesions of D2, containing the ampulla of Vater and the pancreatic head, force the surgeons to perform more complex surgical procedures with consequent longer recovery and higher mortality rates [14]. Time to diagnosis plays a key role in conditioning the prognosis of duodenal-pancreatic trauma, especially for blunt trauma. Delayed diagnosis has been shown to be one of the fundamental outcome factors; in fact, in these cases, the mortality seems to double with greater possibility of duodenal fistula formation [10, 22]. Mortality rate in pancreatic blunt injury is less than 10% while in penetrating ones is about 15–20% and most caused by unstoppable bleeding. Morbidity is much higher, ranges from 11 to 62%, and derives from major complications such as pseudocyst formation, pancreatic fistula, abscesses or intra-abdominal sepsis, and post-traumatic pancreatitis [1, 18, 23, 43, 47]. Time of diagnosis also plays an important role; in pancreatic injury, up to 40% of pancreatic lesions can be misdiagnosed on CT scans within 12 h influencing the outcome [11, 37]. Post-traumatic glucose intolerance is common in all critical patients, but persistent new-onset endocrine or exocrine dysfunction after traumatic distal pancreatectomy is very low (<4%), and insulin is more frequently required in proximal pancreatic resections or Whipple procedure [26, 32].

> **Dos and Don'ts**
> - In minor traumas, stable or stabilized patients, and isolated/low-grade injuries of duodenum, pancreas, and extrahepatic biliary tree (AAST Grade 1), non-operative management (NOM) may be considered.
> - Duodeno-pancreatic and extrahepatic biliary trauma are traumatic lesions that often occur in the context of major multi-organ lesions. Surgical treatment is strictly dependent on the extent and location (including, for example, the ampulla of Vater or the pancreatic head) of the lesion and can range from simple washing and drainage to more invasive approaches such as duodenopancreatectomy.
> - In hemodynamically unstable patients and in patients with evident signs of peritonitis, perforation, evisceration, or penetrating wounds, the emergency/urgent surgical exploration is mandatory, and the technique is highly dependent on the extent of the injury.
> - In emergency setting, stopping the bleeding remains the first aim to be carried out, and Damage Control Surgery (DCS) should be considered.

> **Take-Home Messages**
> - Duodeno-pancreatic and extrahepatic biliary trauma are rare and often associated to other lesions.
> - Hemodynamic status of the patient determines management strategy.
> - In the diagnosis, CT scan is crucial in assessing the degree of injury.
> - In isolated pancreatic, duodenal, and gallbladder hematomas, NOM can be considered with close clinical monitoring.
> - In unstable patients, the surgical approach is mandatory, and the surgical strategy depends on the degree of the lesion.

> **Questions**
> 1. Report the grade of a duodenal injury involving 90% of the circumference of D1 according to the American Association for the Surgery of Trauma Society (AAST) for Duodenal trauma:
>    A. II Grade.
>    B. **III Grade.**
>    C. IV Grade.
>    D. V Grade.

2. Report the grade of major pancreatic laceration without duct injury according to the American Association for the Surgery of Trauma Society (AAST) for Pancreatic trauma:
   A. I Grade.
   B. **II Grade.**
   C. III Grade.
   D. IV Grade.
3. Report the grade of a complete gallbladder avulsion from liver bed associated with a complete left hepatic duct laceration according to the American Association for the Surgery of Trauma Society (AAST) for extrahepatic biliary trauma:
   A. II Grade.
   B. III Grade.
   C. **IV Grade.**
   D. V Grade.
4. Report the grade of a major contusion of the pancreas tail associated with a parenchymal injury involving the ampulla:
   A. II Grade.
   B. III Grade.
   C. **IV Grade.**
   D. V Grade.
5. Report the class of major pancreatic laceration without duct injury in a hemodynamically unstable patient according to World Society of Emergency Surgery (WSES) classification:
   A. Class I.
   B. Class II.
   C. Class III.
   D. **Class IV.**
6. Choose the truest one from the following statements:
   A. The cooperation between the various professional figures (endoscopist, radiologist, gastroenterologist) is sufficient in the management of hepato-pancreatic-biliary traumas, making the figure of a dedicated HPB surgeon superfluous.
   B. Mortality from these injuries is still very high and is generally associated with single injuries to vital organs.
   C. **Often a duodenal trauma is associated with lesions of the pancreas, biliary, or vascular tract; therefore, the figure of a dedicated HPB surgeon becomes fundamental even when nonoperative management (NOM) is chosen.**
   D. Extrahepatic biliary traumas are often associated with other lesions and are more frequent than pancreatic or duodenal lesions.
7. Define which diagnostic exam still represents the gold standard in a hemodynamically stable patient with suspected duodenal-pancreatic trauma:
   A. **CT-Scan.**
   B. Eco-Fast.
   C. Magnetic resonance cholangiopancreatography (MRCP).
   D. Diagnostic peritoneal lavage (DPL).
8. A 17-year-old boy reported a superficial laceration of pancreatic tail without ducts injury in a car accident. CT scan of the abdomen reports peripancreatic edema, edema of the mesentery, and absence of free air. The patient is hemodynamically stable, has elevated amylase and lipase, and has severe abdominal pain. Define the most appropriate therapeutic management:
   A. Diagnostic Peritoneal Lavage (DPL).
   B. **Nonoperative Management (NOM).**
   C. Explorative Laparotomy.
   D. Distal pancreatectomy.
9. A 47-year-old man is stabbed in a brawl. The patient is hemodynamically stable, but CT-Scan reveal periduodenal free air, free fluid in the Douglas, and a complete laceration of the first duodenal portion, immediately after the pylorus. Choose the most appropriate therapeutic management:

A. Nonoperative management (NOM).
B. Pancreatoduodenectomy.
C. **Exploratory laparotomy, antrectomy, and gastrojejunostomy.**
D. Pyloric exclusion (PE).

10. After a simple bicycle accident, a 19-year-old girl does a CT scan of the abdomen for abdominal pain showing a gallbladder hematoma with no signs of perforation and a mild pancreatic contusion. Immediately after the examination, the patient becomes hemodynamically unstable, and intubation becomes necessary. Choose the most appropriate therapeutic management:
    A. **Exploratory laparotomy.**
    B. Nonoperative management (NOM) with fluid infusions, amine support, and mechanical ventilation.
    C. Magnetic resonance cholangiopancreatography (MRCP).
    D. Diagnostic Peritoneal Lavage (DPL).

# References

1. Ahmed N, Vernick JJ. Pancreatic injury. South Med J. 2009;102(12):1253–6.
2. Asensio JA, Demetriades D, Berne JD, Falabella A, Gomez H, Murray J, Cornwell EE 3rd, Velmahos G, Belzberg H, Shoemaker W, Berne TV. A unified approach to the surgical exposure of pancreatic and duodenal injuries. Am J Surg. 1997;174(1):54–60.
3. Asensio JA, Feliciano DV, Britt LD, Kerstein MD. Management of duodenal injuries. Curr Probl Surg. 1993;30(11):1023–93.
4. Bain IM, Kirby RM. 10 year experience of splenic injury: an increasing place for conservative management after blunt trauma. Injury. 1998;29(3):177–82.
5. Berne CJ, Donovan AJ, White EJ, Yellin AE. Duodenal "diverticulization" for duodenal and pancreatic injury. Am J Surg. 1974;127(5):503–7.
6. Bilimoria MM, Cormier JN, Mun Y, Lee JE, Evans DB, Pisters PW. Pancreatic leak after left pancreatectomy is reduced following main pancreatic duct ligation. Br J Surg. 2003;90(2):190–6.
7. Byrge N, Heilbrun M, Winkler N, Sommers D, Evans H, Cattin LM, Scalea T, Stein DM, Neideen T, Walsh P, Sims CA, Brahmbhatt TS, Galante JM, Phan HH, Malhotra A, Stovall RT, Jurkovich GJ, Coimbra R, Berndtson AE, O'Callaghan TA, Gaspard SF, Schreiber MA, Cook MR, Demetriades D, Rivera O, Velmahos GC, Zhao T, Park PK, Machado-Aranda D, Ahmad S, Lewis J, Hoff WS, Suleiman G, Sperry J, Zolin S, Carrick MM, Mallory GR, Nunez J, Colonna A, Enniss T, Nirula R. An AAST-MITC analysis of pancreatic trauma: staple or sew? Resect or drain? J Trauma Acute Care Surg. 2018;85(3):435–43.
8. Cinquantini F, Tugnoli G, Piccinini A, Coniglio C, Mannone S, Biscardi A, Gordini G, Di Saverio S. Educational review of predictive value and findings of computed tomography scan in diagnosing bowel and mesenteric injuries after blunt trauma: correlation with trauma surgery findings in 163 patients. Can Assoc Radiol J. 2017;68(3):276–85.
9. Coccolini F, Kobayashi L, Kluger Y, Moore EE, Ansaloni L, Biffl W, Leppaniemi A, Augustin G, Reva V, Wani I, Kirkpatrick A, Abu-Zidan F, Cicuttin E, Fraga GP, Ordonez C, Pikoulis E, Sibilla MG, Maier R, Matsumura Y, Masiakos PT, Khokha V, Mefire AC, Ivatury R, Favi F, Manchev V, Sartelli M, Machado F, Matsumoto J, Chiarugi M, Arvieux C, Catena F, Coimbra R. Duodeno-pancreatic and extrahepatic biliary tree trauma: WSES-AAST guidelines. World J Emerg Surg. 2019;14:56.
10. Cogbill TH, Moore EE, Feliciano DV, Hoyt DB, Jurkovich GJ, Morris JA, Mucha P Jr, Ross SE, Strutt PJ, Moore FA, et al. Conservative management of duodenal trauma: a multicenter perspective. J Trauma. 1990;30(12):1469–75.
11. Elbanna KY, Mohammed MF, Huang SC, Mak D, Dawe JP, Joos E, Wong H, Khosa F, Nicolaou S. Delayed manifestations of abdominal trauma: follow-up abdominopelvic CT in posttraumatic patients. Abdom Radiol (NY). 2018;43(7):1642–55.
12. Ferrada P, Wolfe L, Duchesne J, Fraga GP, Benjamin E, Alvarez A, Campbell A, Wybourn C, Garcia A, Morales C, Correa J, Pereira BM, Ribeiro M, Quiodettis M, Peck G, Salamea JC, Kruger VF, Ivatury RR, Scalea T. Management of duodenal trauma: a retrospective review from the Panamerican trauma society. J Trauma Acute Care Surg. 2019;86(3):392–6.
13. Iqbal CW, St Peter SD, Tsao K, Cullinane DC, Gourlay DM, Ponsky TA, Wulkan ML, Adibe OO. Operative vs nonoperative management for blunt pancreatic transection in children: multi-institutional outcomes. J Am Coll Surg. 2014;218(2):157–62.
14. Ivatury RR, Gaudino J, Ascer E, Nallathambi M, Ramirez-Schon G, Stahl WM. Treatment of penetrating duodenal injuries: primary repair vs. repair with decompressive enterostomy/serosal patch. J Trauma. 1985;25(4):337–41.
15. Jain P, Parelkar S, Shah H, Sanghvi B. Laparoscopic partial splenectomy for splenic epidermoid cyst. J Laparoendosc Adv Surg Tech A. 2008;18(6):899–902.
16. Jansen M, Du Toit DF, Warren BL. Duodenal injuries: surgical management adapted to circumstances. Injury. 2002;33(7):611–5.

17. Jewett TC Jr, Caldarola V, Karp MP, Allen JE, Cooney DR. Intramural hematoma of the duodenum. Arch Surg. 1988;123(1):54–8.
18. Jones RC. Management of pancreatic trauma. Am J Surg. 1985;150(6):698–704.
19. Jurkovich GJ, Hoyt DB, Moore FA, Ney AL, Morris JA Jr, Scalea TM, Pachter HL, Davis JW. Portal triad injuries. J Trauma. 1995;39(3):426–34.
20. Lin BC, Chen RJ, Fang JF, Hsu YP, Kao YC, Kao JL. Management of blunt major pancreatic injury. J Trauma. 2004;56(4):774–8.
21. Linsenmaier U, Wirth S, Reiser M, Körner M. Diagnosis and classification of pancreatic and duodenal injuries in emergency radiology. Radiographics. 2008;28(6):1591–602.
22. Lucas CE, Ledgerwood AM. Factors influencing outcome after blunt duodenal injury. J Trauma. 1975;15(10):839–46.
23. Madiba TE, Mokoena TR. Favourable prognosis after surgical drainage of gunshot, stab or blunt trauma of the pancreas. Br J Surg. 1995;82(9):1236–9.
24. Malgras B, Douard R, Siauve N, Wind P. Management of left pancreatic trauma. Am Surg. 2011;77(1):1–9.
25. Malhotra A, Biffl WL, Moore EE, Schreiber M, Albrecht RA, Cohen M, Croce M, Karmy-Jones R, Namias N, Rowell S, Shatz DV, Brasel KJ. Western trauma association critical decisions in trauma: diagnosis and management of duodenal injuries. J Trauma Acute Care Surg. 2015;79(6):1096–101.
26. Mansfield N, Inaba K, Berg R, Beale E, Benjamin E, Lam L, Matsushima K, Demetriades D. Early pancreatic dysfunction after resection in trauma: an 18-year report from a level I trauma center. J Trauma Acute Care Surg. 2017;82(3):528–33.
27. Martin TD, Feliciano DV, Mattox KL, Jordan GL Jr. Severe duodenal injuries. Treatment with pyloric exclusion and gastrojejunostomy. Arch Surg. 1983;118(5):631–5.
28. Menahem B, Lim C, Lahat E, Salloum C, Osseis M, Lacaze L, Compagnon P, Pascal G, Azoulay D. Conservative and surgical management of pancreatic trauma in adult patients. Hepatobiliary Surg Nutr. 2016;5(6):470–7.
29. Mitra B, Fitzgerald M, Raoofi M, Tan GA, Spencer JC, Atkin C. Serum lipase for assessment of pancreatic trauma. Eur J Trauma Emerg Surg. 2014;40(3):309–13.
30. Moore EE, Cogbill TH, Malangoni MA, Jurkovich GJ, Champion HR, Gennarelli TA, McAninch JW, Pachter HL, Shackford SR, Trafton PG. Organ injury scaling, II: pancreas, duodenum, small bowel, colon, and rectum. J Trauma. 1990;30(11):1427–9.
31. Moore EE, Jurkovich GJ, Knudson MM, Cogbill TH, Malangoni MA, Champion HR, Shackford SR. Organ injury scaling. VI: Extrahepatic biliary, esophagus, stomach, vulva, vagina, uterus (nonpregnant), uterus (pregnant), fallopian tube, and ovary. J Trauma. 1995;39(6):1069–70.
32. Morita T, Takasu O, Sakamoto T, Mori S, Nakamura A, Nabeta M, Hirayu N, Moroki M, Yamashita N. Long-term outcomes of pancreatic function following pancreatic trauma. Kurume Med J. 2017;63(3.4):53–60.
33. Nolan GJ, Bendinelli C, Gani J. Laparoscopic drainage of an intramural duodenal haematoma: a novel technique and review of the literature. World J Emerg Surg. 2011;6(1):42.
34. Ordoñez C, García A, Parra MW, Scavo D, Pino LF, Millán M, Badiel M, Sanjuán J, Rodriguez F, Ferrada R, Puyana JC. Complex penetrating duodenal injuries: less is better. J Trauma Acute Care Surg. 2014;76(5):1177–83.
35. Pata G, Casella C, Di Betta E, Grazioli L, Salerni B. Extension of nonoperative management of blunt pancreatic trauma to include grade III injuries: a safety analysis. World J Surg. 2009;33(8):1611–7.
36. Ragozzino A, Manfredi R, Scaglione M, De Ritis R, Romano S, Rotondo A. The use of MRCP in the detection of pancreatic injuries after blunt trauma. Emerg Radiol. 2003;10(1):14–8.
37. Rekhi S, Anderson SW, Rhea JT, Soto JA. Imaging of blunt pancreatic trauma. Emerg Radiol. 2010;17(1):13–9.
38. Rickard MJ, Brohi K, Bautz PC. Pancreatic and duodenal injuries: keep it simple. ANZ J Surg. 2005;75(7):581–6.
39. Sawaya DE Jr, Johnson LW, Sittig K, McDonald JC, Zibari GB. Iatrogenic and noniatrogenic extrahepatic biliary tract injuries: a multi-institutional review. Am Surg. 2001;67(5):473–7.
40. Schneider R, Moebius C, Thelen A, Jonas S. Duodenal perforation after blunt abdominal trauma. Zentralbl Chir. 2009;134(6):567–9.
41. Siboni S, Kwon E, Benjamin E, Inaba K, Demetriades D. Isolated blunt pancreatic trauma: a benign injury? J Trauma Acute Care Surg. 2016;81(5):855–9.
42. Snyder WH 3rd, Weigelt JA, Watkins WL, Bietz DS. The surgical management of duodenal trauma. Precepts based on a review of 247 cases. Arch Surg. 1980;115(4):422–9.
43. Sorensen VJ, Obeid FN, Horst HM, Bivins BA. Penetrating pancreatic injuries, 1978-1983. Am Surg. 1986;52(7):354–8.
44. Soukup ES, Russell KW, Metzger R, Scaife ER, Barnhart DC, Rollins MD. Treatment and outcome of traumatic biliary injuries in children. J Pediatr Surg. 2014;49(2):345–8.
45. Stone HH, Fabian TC. Management of duodenal wounds. J Trauma. 1979;19(5):334–9.
46. Thomson BN, Nardino B, Gumm K, Robertson AJ, Knowles BP, Collier NA, Judson R. Management of blunt and penetrating biliary tract trauma. J Trauma Acute Care Surg. 2012;72(6):1620–5.
47. Vasquez JC, Coimbra R, Hoyt DB, Fortlage D. Management of penetrating pancreatic trauma: an 11-year experience of a level-1 trauma center. Injury. 2001;32(10):753–9.
48. Vaughan GD 3rd, Frazier OH, Graham DY, Mattox KL, Petmecky FF, Jordan GL Jr. The use of pyloric exclusion in the management of severe duodenal injuries. Am J Surg. 1977;134(6):785–90.

49. Vertrees A, Elster E, Jindal RM, Ricordi C, Shriver C. Surgical management of modern combat-related pancreatic injuries: traditional management and unique strategies. Mil Med. 2014;179(3):315–9.

## Further Reading

Byrge N, Heilbrun M, Winkler N, Sommers D, Evans H, Cattin LM, Scalea T, Stein DM, Neideen T, Walsh P, Sims CA, Brahmbhatt TS, Galante JM, Phan HH, Malhotra A, Stovall RT, Jurkovich GJ, Coimbra R, Berndtson AE, O'Callaghan TA, Gaspard SF, Schreiber MA, Cook MR, Demetriades D, Rivera O, Velmahos GC, Zhao T, Park PK, Machado-Aranda D, Ahmad S, Lewis J, Hoff WS, Suleiman G, Sperry J, Zolin S, Carrick MM, Mallory GR, Nunez J, Colonna A, Enniss T, Nirula R. An AAST-MITC analysis of pancreatic trauma: Staple or sew? Resect or drain? J Trauma Acute Care Surg. 2018;85(3):435–43. https://doi.org/10.1097/TA.0000000000001987.

Coccolini F, Kobayashi L, Kluger Y, Moore EE, Ansaloni L, Biffl W, Leppaniemi A, Augustin G, Reva V, Wani I, Kirkpatrick A, Abu-Zidan F, Cicuttin E, Fraga GP, Ordonez C, Pikoulis E, Sibilla MG, Maier R, Matsumura Y, Masiakos PT, Khokha V, Mefire AC, Ivatury R, Favi F, Manchev V, Sartelli M, Machado F, Matsumoto J, Chiarugi M, Arvieux C, Catena F, Coimbra R. WSES-AAST Expert Panel. Duodeno-pancreatic and extrahepatic biliary tree trauma: WSES-AAST guidelines. World J Emerg Surg. 2019;14:56. https://doi.org/10.1186/s13017-019-0278-6. PMID: 31867050; PMCID: PMC6907251

Ho VP, Patel NJ, Bokhari F, Madbak FG, Hambley JE, Yon JR, Robinson BR, Nagy K, Armen SB, Kingsley S, Gupta S, Starr FL, Moore HR 3rd, Oliphant UJ, Haut ER, Como JJ. Management of adult pancreatic injuries: A practice management guideline from the Eastern Association for the Surgery of Trauma. J Trauma Acute Care Surg. 2017;82(1):185–99. https://doi.org/10.1097/TA.0000000000001300.

Pereira R, Vo T, Slater K. Extrahepatic bile duct injury in blunt trauma: a systematic review. J Trauma Acute Care Surg. 2019;86(5):896–901. https://doi.org/10.1097/TA.0000000000002186.

Potoka DA, Gaines BA, Leppäniemi A, Peitzman AB. Management of blunt pancreatic trauma: what's new? Eur J Trauma Emerg Surg. 2015;41(3):239–50. https://doi.org/10.1007/s00068-015-0510-3. Epub 2015 Mar 17

Søreide K, Weiser TG, Parks RW. Clinical update on management of pancreatic trauma. HPB (Oxford). 2018;20(12):1099–108. https://doi.org/10.1016/j.hpb.2018.05.009. Epub 2018 Jul 11

Streith L, Silverberg J, Kirkpatrick AW, Hameed SM, Bathe OF, Ball CG. Optimal treatments for hepato-pancreato-biliary trauma in severely injured patients: a narrative scoping review. Can J Surg. 2020;63(5):E431–4. https://doi.org/10.1503/cjs.013919. PMID: 33009897; PMCID: PMC7608711

Zakaria HM, Oteem A, Gaballa NK, Hegazy O, Nada A, Zakareya T, Omar H, Abdelkawy H, Abdeldayem H, Gad EH. Risk factors and management of different types of biliary injuries in blunt abdominal trauma: Single-center retrospective cohort study. Ann Med Surg (Lond). 2020;52:36–43. https://doi.org/10.1016/j.amsu.2020.02.009. PMID: 32211187; PMCID: PMC7082429.

# Abdominal Vascular Trauma

Franchesca J. Hwang, Jarrett E. Santorelli, Leslie M. Kobayashi, and Raul Coimbra

## 100.1 Introduction

> **Learning Goals (Listing the Chapter Core Messages)**
> - To recognize and diagnose AVI expeditiously.
> - To be able to obtain appropriate operative exposure to treat AVI.
> - To be able to control hemorrhage and determine which treatment of injured vessels is optimal depending on the extent of the injury, concomitant injuries, and stability of the patient.

### 100.1.1 Epidemiology

Abdominal vascular trauma is responsible for extremely high mortality and morbidity affecting all age groups in both civilian and military settings. However, it is seen most frequently in adult males and is less common among geriatric and pediatric populations [1–3]. The majority of AVI, up to 70–90%, are due to penetrating trauma [1, 4]. The most common mechanisms of injury are gunshot wounds (GSW) followed by stab wounds (SW), while blunt causes are most frequently due to motor vehicle collisions (MVC) [1, 5]. In contrast to adults, blunt causes of AVI are most common in the pediatric population where MVC is the most frequent etiology [6]. AVI is seen less frequently in military compared to civilian settings likely due to both high on-scene mortality and the protective effect of body armor [7]. The predominant mechanism of injury also varies geographically with penetrating mechanisms due to interpersonal violence being common in the United States, South America, and Africa and blunt mechanisms predominating in Europe, Asia, and Australia [1–3, 8].

Arterial and venous structures are injured with relatively equal frequency [1, 3, 4, 9]. The iliac artery (IA), renal artery (RA), and abdominal aorta (AA) are the most frequently damaged arterial vessels, while the inferior vena cava (IVC) and iliac veins are the most commonly injured venous structure [1, 4, 9, 10]. Both intra-abdominal and extra-abdominal injuries are commonly associated with AVI. A half to a third of patients have bowel or liver injuries, or both [4, 11]. Less commonly injured organs include the spleen, pancreas, and the genitourinary system in

F. J. Hwang · J. E. Santorelli · L. M. Kobayashi
University of California San Diego,
San Diego, CA, USA
e-mail: fjhwang@health.ucsd.edu;
franchesca.hwang@nyulangone.org;
jsantorelli@health.ucsd.edu; lkobayashi@ucsd.edu

R. Coimbra (✉)
Riverside University Health System Medical Center,
Loma Linda University School of Medicine,
Moreno Valley, CA, USA
e-mail: r.coimbra@ruhealth.org

10–20% of cases [4, 11]. Common extra-abdominal injuries include traumatic brain or spinal cord, thoracic, and orthopedic injuries. About half of blunt abdominal aortic injuries (BAAI) have associated lumbar spine, rib, or pelvic fractures [12–14]. More than three quarters of blunt iliac vascular injuries have associated severe pelvic injuries [15].

## 100.2 Diagnosis

### 100.2.1 Clinical Presentation

Any patients who are hemodynamically (HD) unstable or have peritonitis with abdominal or pelvic trauma need immediate surgical exploration and should be presumed to have major AVI until proven otherwise. HD stability does not rule out a major AVI as almost one-third of patients with AVI are stable upon admission [16]. After peritonitis, other physical exam findings associated with AVI include abdominal wounds from GSW/SW, seatbelt signs, pelvic instability, perineal injuries, and gross hematuria. Bilateral femoral pulses should be assessed to exclude common or external iliac artery injuries. Laboratory findings are not specific, and anemia is usually not seen immediately. Early laboratory findings suggestive of significant blood loss are metabolic acidosis and coagulopathy; however, their absence does not exclude AVI.

### 100.2.2 Tests

Imaging studies useful in diagnosing AVI include X-rays, Focused Assessment with Sonography for Trauma (FAST), and CTA. Plain X-rays of the pelvis are adjuncts of the primary survey and can be used to rapidly diagnose unstable pelvic fractures, often associated with iliac vessel injuries. FAST, although having low sensitivity (~40%) and high operator variability, has a high specificity of 90% in blunt abdominal trauma [17]. FAST carries a false-negative rate of almost 50% in patients with abdominal or pelvic hemorrhages, and, in zone I, II, and III injuries, the false-negative rate reaches 37%, 45%, and 61% [18].

In contrast, CTA can be used to identify AVI with a high degree of sensitivity and specificity. It can be utilized to identify active extravasation, occlusion, dissection, pseudoaneurysm, arteriovenous fistulas, and focal narrowing secondary to intimal injuries in both intraperitoneal and retroperitoneal areas. Utilization of arterial, portal and delayed venous phase can help differentiate arterial versus venous hemorrhage, which can be helpful in making decisions for open or endovascular treatment [19–22]. However, CTA should only be considered in HD stable patients, and immediate operative exploration should not be delayed for diagnostic imaging in unstable patients suspected of AVI.

## 100.3 Treatment

### 100.3.1 Nonoperative Management (NOM)

NOM of blunt abdominal vascular injury has been described in the literature. Awake, alert, HD stable patients with benign abdominal exams and low suspicion for other intra-abdominal injuries may be considered for NOM. A multicenter study on blunt abdominal aortic injury (BAAI) demonstrated that NOM was successful in those with intimal tears without any external aortic contour abnormality [23]. NOM of BAAI includes strict blood pressure control and antiplatelet therapy with close follow-up [23]. Continued monitoring with serial exams for any bleeding or ischemia is critical. Any changes in patient's hemodynamics or physical exam should prompt further evaluation and possible surgical intervention.

Endovascular management of AVI should only be considered in stable patients without associated surgical injuries. The most support for effective endovascular treatment is for bleeding associated with pelvic fractures. In low grade injuries of the renal and iliac arteries, endovascular treatment is also effective [24]. Less data exist for endovascular treatment of Zone I AVI; however, it may be effective particularly in difficult-to-access areas such as the supraceliac aorta, celiac trunk, and proximal SMA [12, 25]. A retrospective National Trauma Databank study demonstrated a decrease in mortality after BAAI since the early 2000s, with an increase in utilization of endovascular treatment [26]. A few small series of endovascular repairs of celiac and SMA injuries generally demonstrated lower mortality, shorter hospital and intensive care unit length of stay, and fewer ischemic complications [9, 24, 27–30]. It is essential to closely monitor patients following endovascular treatment and rapidly convert to open repair, to control hemorrhage or treat associated intra-abdominal injuries or ischemic complications. Endovascular approaches cannot address associated injuries, and existing studies have very limited long-term outcomes. In addition, the time from diagnosis to intervention can be quite lengthy. At present, given current limitations and lack of long-term outcome evidence, endovascular therapy remains impractical for most patients with AVI [16, 25].

REBOA is a minimally invasive option for aortic occlusion and temporary hemorrhage control in HD unstable patients prior to definitive open or endovascular treatment of bleeding. It can be placed in Zone I (between the left subclavian artery and the celiac trunk) for suspected abdominal hemorrhage and in Zone III (between the renal artery and aortic bifurcation) for suspected pelvic hemorrhage. Newer REBOA versions with smaller introducer sheaths are preferred as older models were associated with a high rate of ischemic complications [31–33]. Survival rates with REBOA range from 33% to 66% with the highest survival rates noted in patients with Zone III deployment for control of pelvic hemorrhage [33–35].

### 100.3.2 Open Surgical Treatment

Exploratory laparotomy should not be delayed for any trauma patients with HD instability or peritonitis. At any point, if the patient has cardiopulmonary arrest or is profoundly hypotensive, a resuscitative thoracotomy should be performed for cross clamping of the aorta prior to exploratory laparotomy. In patients suspected to have unstable pelvic fractures, it is advised to leave room in the suprapubic area for a separate incision for pre-peritoneal packing (PPP). Expeditious evacuation of hemoperitoneum followed by packing of all four quadrants with laparotomy pads should be performed. While resuscitation continues, the abdomen is explored with sequential unpacking from the least injured areas to the most injured areas and repacked as needed. If adequate exposure is not obtained, extending the incision more cephalad or caudad or adding a subcostal incision may optimize exposure. If torrential bleeding is encountered, supraceliac control of the aorta or aortic clamping from a left anterolateral thoracotomy may be necessary.

AVI can be categorized into three retroperitoneal zones with its respective vessels.

- **Zone I** (central): aorta, IVC, celiac trunk, superior mesenteric artery (SMA), inferior mesenteric artery (IMA), portal vein (PV)/superior mesenteric vein (SMV)
- **Zone II** (lateral/perinephric): renal arteries/veins
- **Zone III** (pelvic): iliac arteries/veins

All Zone I injuries must be explored in both penetrating and blunt trauma. The best exposure of the aorta and its major branches and left-sided Zone II is achieved via the "Mattox maneuver" or left visceral rotation. The left colon is mobilized medially by dividing the white line of Toldt; this is extended around the spleen and the pancreatic tail. Depending on the location of the injury, it may also be necessary to mobilize the left kidney. To obtain supraceliac aortic control, the left crus of the diaphragm may need to be divided. For IVC injury or right-sided Zone II exposure, the "Cattell-Braasch maneuver," or right medial visceral rotation, is performed. The right colon is medialized by taking down the white line of Toldt, and the duodenum is fully Kocherized.

In *penetrating* trauma, all Zone II hematomas should be explored, while only expanding or pulsatile hematomas in *blunt* trauma need to be

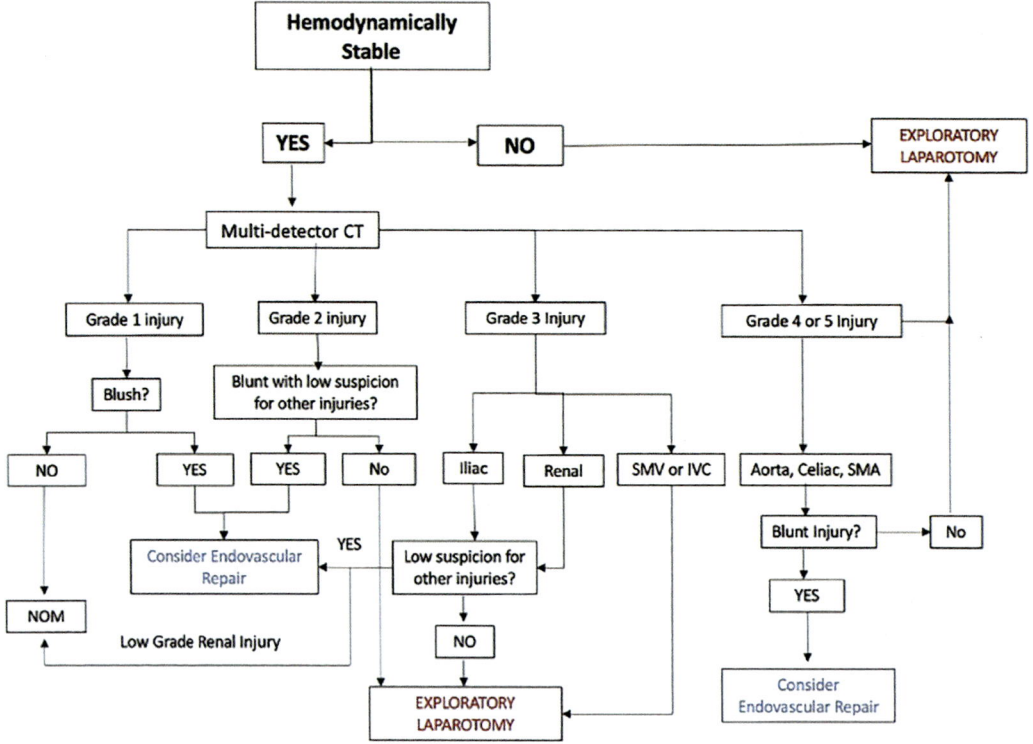

**Fig. 100.1** Diagnosis and management of abdominal vascular injuries [36]

explored. Similarly, only penetrating or pulsatile/expanding blunt Zone III hematomas need to be explored. Distal femoral pulses should be assessed in patients with abdominal or pelvic trauma to rule out iliac artery injuries during the initial evaluation. If no distal pulses are present or there is a pulse deficit, the ipsilateral Zone III needs to be explored. For *blunt* Zone III hemorrhage associated with pelvic fractures, PPP can be performed to effectively tamponade both arterial and venous bleeding as a temporizing measure prior to angioembolization or pelvic fixation. The algorithm for the diagnosis and management of AVI developed by the AAST-WSES is shown in Fig. 100.1 [36]. The following section describes the step-by-step management of individual AVI, summarized in Table 100.1.

### 100.3.2.1 Aorta

AA injuries can be divided by injury location into supraceliac, suprarenal, and infrarenal. Contained injuries present with Zone I hematomas. In the setting of uncontained hemorrhage, proximal control can be rapidly obtained by placing a vascular clamp, an aortic occluder, or sponge sticks at the diaphragmatic hiatus. Division of the gastrohepatic ligament and retraction of the stomach and the esophagus to the left may be required to expose the AA for formal control with clamps or vessel loops. If these maneuvers fail, left anterolateral thoracotomy is performed to control the aorta above the diaphragm. Proximal AA exposure is then obtained via the Mattox maneuver. Infrarenal AA injuries can be exposed by dividing the ligament of Treitz similarly to open exposure of an abdominal aortic aneurysm. Depending on the location and the severity of the injuries, in addition to the stability of the patient, treatment options include primary repair, patch angioplasty with either native or prosthetic grafts, interposition graft, or ligation and extra-anatomical bypass [12]. Primary repair with monofilament suture is recommended; however, if there is tension or stenosis, a native vein or synthetic patch or an inter-

**Table 100.1** Treatment of AVI

| | |
|---|---|
| *Arterial Injury* | |
| Aorta | Primary repair vs. patch angioplasty or interposition graft. For stable BAAI, consider endovascular repair |
| Celiac | Primary repair vs. ligation |
| SMA | Primary repair vs. TIVS of proximal vessel. Primary repair vs. ligation of distal branch vessel |
| Renal | Primary repair vs. nephrectomy if normal contralateral kidney. Repair if solitary kidney or atrophic contralateral kidney |
| Iliac | Primary repair vs. TIVS of common/external iliac artery. Primary repair vs. ligation of internal iliac artery |
| *Venous injury* | |
| Suprarenal IVC | Repair vs. TIVS |
| Infrarenal IVC | Primary repair vs. ligation if large/destructive injury |
| Retrohepatic IVC | Repair |
| SMV/portal vein | Primary repair vs. ligation if large/destructive injury |
| Common/external iliac vein | Primary repair vs. ligation if large/destructive injury |
| Renal vein | Primary repair vs. ligation of left if distal to gonadal vein. Primary repair vs. nephrectomy of right |
| Internal iliac vein | Ligate |

Sources: WTA Critical Decisions in Trauma: Management of abdominal vascular trauma and AAST-WSES guidelines on diagnosis and management of abdominal vascular injuries [36, 56]

position graft should be used. In the setting of gross contamination, synthetic material should be avoided [16]. If the patient is unstable or has complex injuries, a temporary intravascular shunt (TIVS) with delayed definitive repair should be utilized [37].

### 100.3.2.2 IVC

The infrahepatic IVC can be exposed with the Cattell-Braasch maneuver, as described previously. It is essential to communicate closely with the anesthesia team, so the resuscitation continues, and fluid administration is switched to upper extremity IVs, internal jugular, or subclavian central lines, rather than a femoral venous catheter. Primary repairs are usually feasible (see Fig. 100.2). Posterior injuries need to be ruled out by rotating the vena cava anteriorly, taking caution not to cause bleeding from the posterior lumbar veins. For larger defects or for those injuries in which primary repair would cause tension or significant stenosis, patch repair can be utilized. If the patient is unstable, the *infrarenal* IVC can be ligated. If IVC ligation is performed, lower extremity fasciotomies should be considered and the legs wrapped and elevated to decrease edema postoperatively. *Suprarenal* IVC

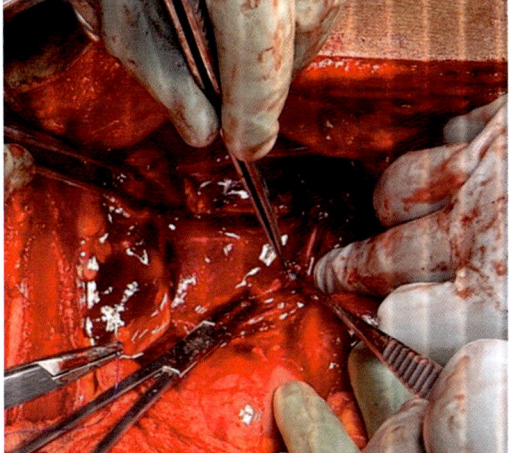
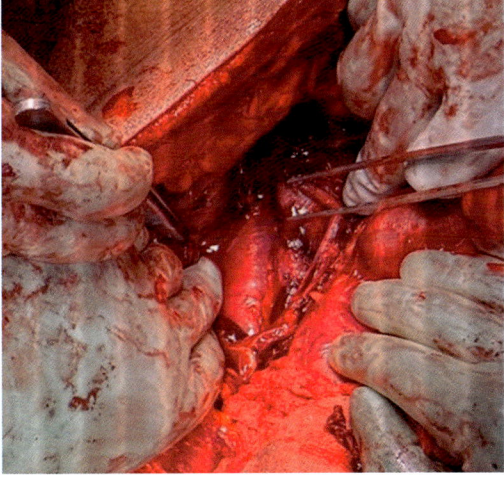

**Fig. 100.2** Intra-operative images of an infrahepatic IVC injury due to SW. Images show the anterior wall injury pre and post repair

injuries in HD unstable patients can be shunted prior to definitive repair.

For hemorrhage near or from the liver, a Pringle maneuver should be utilized immediately. If the bleeding does not slow down with this maneuver, retrohepatic IVC injury should be suspected. This injury is associated with an extremely high mortality rate up to 70% [38]. The falciform and the triangular ligaments are divided, and the liver is medialized to improve exposure of the IVC. Care should be taken not to injure the short hepatic veins during the mobilization. If the injury is small, primary venorraphy can be done. For large or multiple injuries, two maneuvers can be considered: placing an atriocaval shunt, also known as the Shrock Shunt, or total hepatic isolation, also known as the Heaney Maneuver. The atrio-caval shunt is accomplished by passing a large-bore chest tube from the right atrium to the infrahepatic suprarenal vena cava. Extra holes cut into the chest tube are necessary to allow blood from the infrahepatic IVC to drain into the right atrium. This maneuver requires opening the chest via median sternotomy. Total hepatic isolation requires a Pringle maneuver, clamping the suprahepatic IVC, which can be done below or above the diaphragm, clamping the infrahepatic suprarenal IVC and cross clamping of the supra celiac aorta. This maneuver will often cause cardiac arrest from the drop in the preload. Both maneuvers are temporizing measures to control bleeding while appropriate exposure, identification, and repair are performed, and they should be done as early as possible after retrohepatic IVC injury is suspected.

### 100.3.2.3 Celiac Artery

Exposure of the celiac trunk and its branches is facilitated by a left medial visceral rotation. For proximal control, division of the median arcuate ligament and the left crus of the diaphragm may be necessary. Small injuries can be treated with primary repair; for complex injuries or in hemodynamically unstable patients, the celiac trunk can be ligated safely as long as the SMA is intact in patents. After ligation of the celiac trunk, ischemia and necrosis of gallbladder has been described; therefore, cholecystectomy is recommended [39].

### 100.3.2.4 SMA

The proximal SMA can be approached via left medial visceral rotation with distal control achieved by opening the root of the mesentery below the pancreas or by dividing the ligament of Treitz. Extended Kocherization of the duodenum may be necessary. Primary repair of the SMA is recommended if possible. In larger defects, patch angioplasty or interposition graft can be considered. However, in unstable patients, proximal SMA injuries should be shunted, and distal injuries ligated. If the proximal SMA is ligated, temporary abdominal closure (TAC) is recommended due to the high risk of bowel ischemia and necrosis (Fig. 100.3) as well as abdominal compartment syndrome [40].

### 100.3.2.5 IMA

IMA injuries can be approached by elevating the transverse colon and incising the ligament of Treitz. The IMA is located just distal to the left renal vein crossing the aorta, about 3–4 cm above the aortic bifurcation. Direct approach and repair can be done, if possible, but ligation of IMA is generally well tolerated. Nonetheless, a high index of suspicion for colon or rectal ischemia should be maintained in older patients or those with extensive atherosclerotic disease after IMA ligation.

### 100.3.2.6 PV/SMV

Initial control of a PV injury is done with a Pringle maneuver until further dissection of the hepatoduodenal ligament is achieved. The proximal and distal control may be challenging if the porta hepatitis length is short; extra length or access to SMV injuries can be obtained by dividing the neck of the pancreas, wide Kocherization, or a Cattell-Braasch maneuver. PV injuries can be treated with any of the following, depending on the extent of the injury, the stability of the patient, and concomitant injuries: primary repair, resection and anastomosis, interposition graft, or ligation. Ligation of the PV can be tolerated with a patent hepatic artery but carries a high mortality

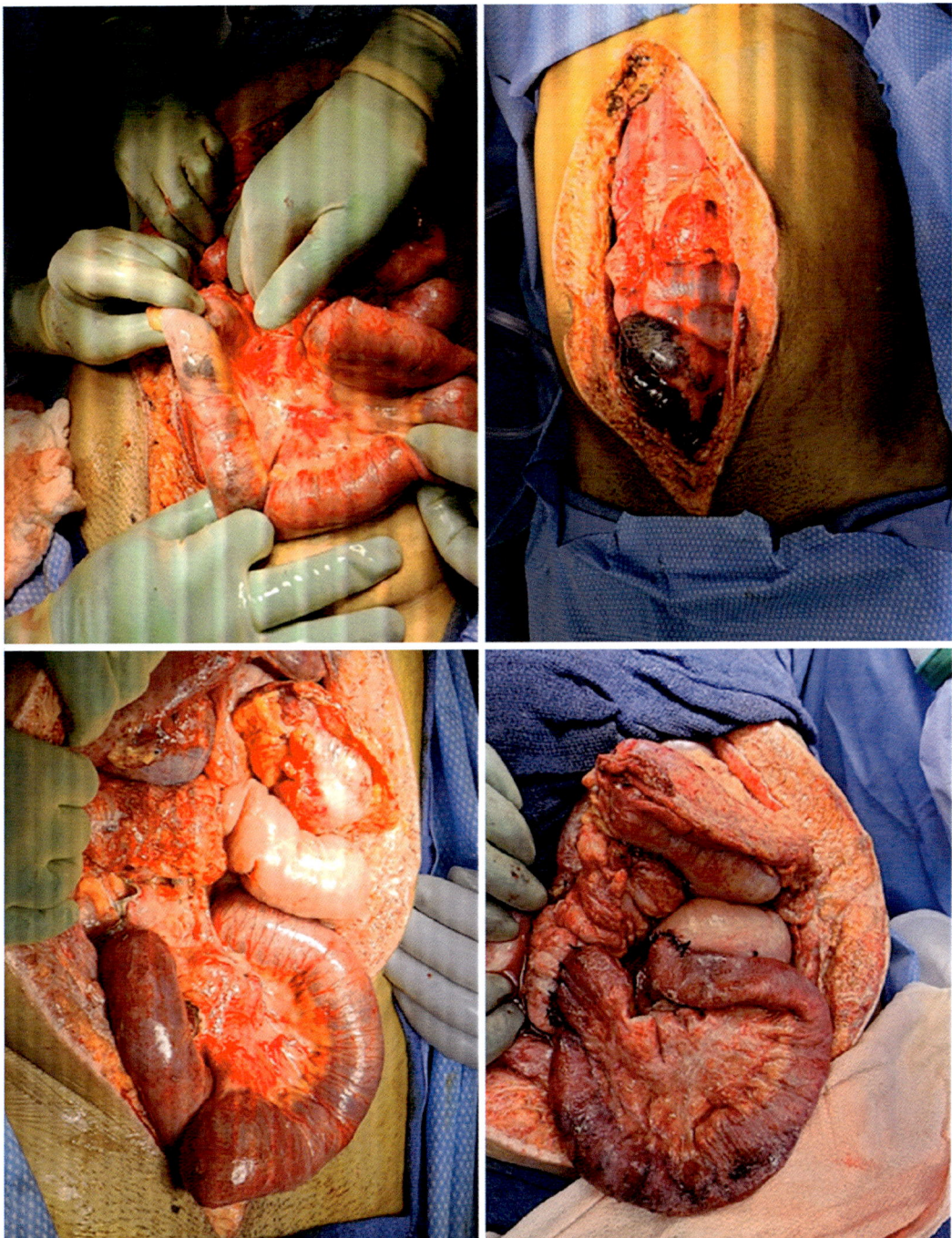

**Fig. 100.3** The pictures demonstrate delayed small bowel ischemia following SMV injury due to GSW. Pictures are taken during the first, second, third, and fourth returns to the operating room, all 1 day apart

ranging from 20% to 90% [24, 41]. If ligation is deemed necessary, it needs to be done early. PV ligation may be followed by systemic hypotension and splanchnic hypertension, for which close communication with the anesthesia team for more aggressive volume resuscitation is crucial. SMV injuries can be either repaired or ligated. Studies have shown a survival benefit with repair over ligation; however, the patients who underwent repair had less severe injuries and fewer associated injuries [42]. In both PV and SMV injuries, TIVS can be considered as an alternative to ligation [43].

For both repairs and ligations of the SMV and PV, TAC with planned return to the operating room is highly recommended, given the risk of bowel edema from venous congestion, bowel ischemia, and abdominal compartment syndrome. It may be necessary to return to the operating room multiple times as delayed bowel ischemia may occur (see Fig. 100.3).

### 100.3.2.7 Renal Arteries/Veins

The renal vessels can be approached through a medial visceral rotation with or without kidney mobilization. Once Gerota's fascia is opened from the lateral aspect, the kidney can be elevated, and the renal hilum can be exposed further for manual compression or proximal control with clamps or vessels loops. Small injuries can be primarily repaired or resected and re-anastomosed if patients are stable. For larger renal arterial injuries or if patients are unstable, nephrectomy should be performed after confirming that the contralateral kidney is intact and normal. Renal salvage can be attempted if bilateral kidneys are injured, but the patient's hemodynamics and concomitant injuries will determine the feasibility. Outcomes after renal salvage are generally worse when compared to immediate nephrectomy [44, 45]. If the left renal vein is injured distal to the gonadal vein, it can be safely ligated as the left renal outflow is maintained via the gonadal vein. If the right renal vein is injured and is to be ligated, right nephrectomy is necessary. In stable blunt trauma, intimal flaps in the renal artery causing thrombosis or occlusion can be treated with endovascular stenting if the injury is identified early; if the arterial patency is not restored, nephrectomy may still be necessary [46].

### 100.3.2.8 Iliac Arteries/Veins

Displacement of the small bowel to the right and division of the posterior peritoneum over the aortic bifurcation will provide exposure of the iliac vessels. More proximal control of the aorta may be necessary by incising the peritoneum over the aorta just distal to the duodenum. During the dissection to obtain proximal and distal control, it is imperative to identify and preserve the ureter, which courses over the IA at the level of the iliac bifurcation. Small injuries can be repaired primarily, while larger ones may need resection and end-to-end anastomosis. If under tension, vein or PTFE interposition grafts are utilized. In grossly contaminated fields, vein grafts should be used over synthetic grafts, if possible, as the synthetic grafts may develop blowout later from infection. Ligation of the common and external IA with subsequent extra-anatomic femoral-femoral or axillary-femoral bypasses in a completely noncontaminated field can be considered if the patient is stable [47]. In damage control settings, TIVS can be utilized to maintain perfusion to the lower extremity for destructive common and external IA injuries. Once resuscitation is adequate, the injuries can be repaired definitively. When compared to ligation, TIVS is associated with reduced risk of amputation and reduced need for fasciotomies of the lower extremities [48]. Injuries to the internal iliac artery can be ligated with few complications due to rich pelvic collateralization.

Access to iliac vein is limited by the overlying common IA. Transection of the IA to identify and repair the iliac vein injury has been historically described but is not recommended. Primary repair of small venous injuries is recommended; for larger injuries, vein patch or a vein interposition graft may be considered. If repair results in significant stenosis, anticoagulation may be necessary to prevent delayed thrombosis. For unstable patients, ligation of the iliac vein is generally well tolerated with few adverse outcomes [49].

### 100.3.3 Prognosis

Despite medical and surgical advances, mortality from AVI remains high, ranging 20–80% and increases in the presence of associated injuries [16, 50, 51]. Early mortality is due to rapid exsanguination and late deaths from multi-organ failure. Mortality in AVI increases with age; 2–12% in children, 13–29% in adults, and over 43% in the elderly [2, 3, 8, 24, 26, 52, 53]. Risk factors for mortality include shock (systolic blood pressure ≤90 mmHg) on presentation, metabolic acidosis (base deficit less than −15), hypothermia (temperature < 34 °C), coagulopathy, need for either resuscitative thoracotomy or damage control procedures, massive transfusion, number of injured vessels, and more advanced American Association for the Surgery of Trauma-Organ Injury Scale (AAST-OIS) grade and Injury Severity Score (ISS) [4, 39, 42, 47, 50, 54, 55]. The vessels associated with the highest mortality are the AA (80–100%), hepatic veins and/or retrohepatic IVC (90%), SMA (80%), and PV (70%) [4, 12, 16, 55, 56].

---

**Dos and Don'ts**

**Dos**

- Patients presenting with shock or peritonitis should be taken emergently for laparotomy as risk of AVI is high.
- All retroperitoneal hematomas resulting from penetrating trauma and all Zone I hematomas regardless of mechanism of injury should be explored.
- REBOA with Zone III deployment can be considered in transient responders and hemodynamically unstable patients with pelvic injury to allow resuscitation prior to definitive open or endovascular control.
- Pre-peritoneal packing (PPP) supplemented with angiography should be used for hemodynamic instability associated with severe pelvic fractures without another significant source of bleeding.
- After initial vascular control, it is reasonable to consider definitive reconstruction including primary repair, patch angioplasty, resection with primary anastomosis, and resection with interposition graft in stable, well-resuscitated patients.
- In stable patients with isolated vascular injuries from blunt mechanism without associated injuries, endovascular repair may be considered.

**Don'ts**

- Conservative management should **not** be performed in the setting of penetrating injury.
- **Don't** perform a complicated vascular reconstruction during the initial procedure if the patient is unstable.
- After ligating the celiac, SMA, IMA, or PV/SMV, do **not** perform abdominal closure during the index operation due to concern for developing mesenteric ischemia and abdominal compartment syndrome.

---

**Take-Home Messages**

- AVI remains rare but continues to have high morbidity and mortality despite evolving technologies.
- Unstable patients with signs of abdominal or pelvic trauma and patients with peritonitis should be suspected to have major AVIs and taken immediately for surgical exploration.
- CTA is recommended for screening stable patients who have signs of abdominal trauma.
- In patients who remain unstable and in those with significant physiological

- derangements, damage control techniques should be employed including vessel ligation, TIVS, and TAC.
- Emerging technology including REBOA and endovascular interventions are being used with increasing frequency; however, open surgical repair remains the gold standard for treatment of AVI.

## Questions

1. A 42-year-old male who was working at a construction site fell off a roof which was about 20 ft high. He is hemodynamically stable. He is found to have a left renal artery injury with an intimal flap with evidence of thrombosis. Which of the following statements regarding renal vascular injuries is **TRUE**?
    A. The patient needs nephrectomy immediately.
    B. Complications occur more frequently after nephrectomy than nephorraphy.
    C. Acute renal failure after nephrectomy is usually irreversible.
    D. **Endovascular stenting is a viable option for this patient.**
2. Which of the following statements is **TRUE** regarding iliac vessel injuries?
    A. Mortality from iliac vessel injuries is low.
    B. **Temporary intravascular shunts should be used in damage control settings.**
    C. An internal iliac artery injury needs to be repaired rather than ligated due to a high rate of complications.
    D. Iliac vein injuries most commonly occur in isolation and associated injuries are rare.
3. Which of the following intraoperative findings does **NOT** need surgical exploration?
    A. Zone I hematoma following blunt trauma.
    B. Zone I hematoma following penetrating trauma.
    C. **Zone II hematoma following blunt trauma.**
    D. Zone III hematoma following penetrating trauma.
4. Of the following scenarios, which is **NOT** an indication for temporary abdominal closure?
    A. A 45-year-old male with an external iliac artery transection requiring an intravascular shunt placement.
    B. A 23-year-old female with proximal superior mesenteric artery injury requiring ligation and repair of multiple small bowel injuries.
    C. A 39-year-old female with destructive infrarenal aortic injury not amenable to primary repair in addition to multiple small and large bowel injuries.
    D. **A 63-year-old male with left renal vein injury distal to the gonadal vein requiring ligation.**
5. Which of the following statements regarding abdominal vascular trauma is **TRUE**?
    A. **Stable patients with mild blunt abdominal aortic injuries can be observed with strict blood pressure control, if there is low suspicion for concomitant intra-abdominal injuries.**
    B. The mortality from abdominal vascular injury has decreased in recent years due to medical and surgical advances.
    C. A patient presenting after penetrating pelvic trauma with no distal pulses should undergo CT angiogram to evaluate for the exact location of the injuries regardless of hemodynamic stability.
    D. The most commonly injured vessels in the abdomen following blunt trauma are the celiac trunk and superior mesenteric artery/vein.

6. Who among the following patients needs exploratory laparotomy immediately?
   A. A 62-year-old male, who tripped and fell down 10 stairs, is found to have multiple left-sided rib fractures and is found to have intimal flap of the abdominal aorta.
   B. **A 32-year-old female, who was a restrained driver in a high-speed motor vehicle collision, was initially hypotensive but responded to IV fluids. On exam, she has abrasions across the lower abdomen and is tender on exam.**
   C. A 24-year-old male motorcyclist after a crash on a highway with an open book fracture on initial pelvis X-ray. He is tachycardic to 110 s and blood pressure is 130/80 with palpable distal pulses in his feet.
   D. A 17-year-old female, a restrained passenger, T-boned at an intersection, who presents with a right hemopneumothorax and is found to have a large perinephric retroperitoneal hematoma. HR 110, BP 110/70.
7. Which of the following surgical exposures/maneuvers is correctly paired with the suspected injuries?
   A. Mattox maneuver—IVC injury.
   B. Cattell-Braasch maneuver—left renal injury.
   C. Pringle maneuver—celiac artery.
   D. **Kocherization—SMV injury**.
8. As you are performing exploratory laparotomy on a 24-year-old male involved in a highway speed motorcycle collision with hemodynamic instability and peritonitis, you encounter a large amount of bleeding upon entering the abdominal cavity. The blood pressure drops to 40/20. You should perform the following maneuvers immediately **EXCEPT**:
   A. Pack all four quadrants with laparotomy pads.
   B. Clamp or occlude the supraceliac aorta.
   C. **Eviscerate the small bowel to assess the location of the bleeding.**
   D. Perform left anterolateral thoracotomy for aortic cross clamping and cardiac massage if the patient arrests.
9. You are performing exploratory laparotomy on a 17-year-old after a stab wound to the back, who presents with hemodynamic instability. After you pack, you notice hemorrhage from the right side of the abdomen. The following statements are true in this situation **EXCEPT**:
   A. You perform a Pringle maneuver immediately for hemorrhage from the liver.
   B. An atrio-caval shunt, or Shrock shunt, can be considered for *retrohepatic* IVC injury to control bleeding.
   C. You identify a destructive *infrarenal* IVC injury, and due to the patient's ongoing hemodynamic instability, you ligate the IVC and perform lower extremity fasciotomies.
   D. **For *suprarenal* IVC injury in hemodynamic instability, ligation should be done immediately.**
10. Which of the following statements is **TRUE**?
    A. Mortality in abdominal vascular injury decreases with age.
    B. **Pre-peritoneal packing with angiography should be considered for patients with isolated pelvic fractures and hemodynamic instability.**
    C. Performing complicated vascular reconstruction during an index operation is advised for unstable patients to limit reoperations.
    D. REBOA with Zone II deployment can be utilized as a temporizing measure for hemodynamically unstable patients with pelvic injury.

# References

1. Barmparas G, Inaba K, Talving P, David JS, Lam L, Plurad D, et al. Pediatric vs adult vascular trauma: a National Trauma Databank review. J Pediatr Surg. 2010;45(7):1404–12.
2. Konstantinidis A, Inaba K, Dubose J, Barmparas G, Lam L, Plurad D, et al. Vascular trauma in geriatric patients: a National Trauma Databank review. J Trauma. 2011;71(4):909–16.
3. DuBose JJ, Savage SA, Fabian TC, Menaker J, Scalea T, Holcomb JB, et al. The American Association for the Surgery of Trauma PROspective Observational Vascular Injury Treatment (PROOVIT) registry: multicenter data on modern vascular injury diagnosis, management, and outcomes. J Trauma Acute Care Surg. 2015;78(2):215–22; discussion 22–3.
4. Asensio JA, Chahwan S, Hanpeter D, Demetriades D, Forno W, Gambaro E, et al. Operative management and outcome of 302 abdominal vascular injuries. Am J Surg. 2000;180(6):528–33; discussion 33–4.
5. Kobayashi LM, Costantini TW, Hamel MG, Dierksheide JE, Coimbra R. Abdominal vascular trauma. Trauma Surg Acute Care Open. 2016;1(1):e000015.
6. Wang SK, Severance S, Troja W, Drucker N, Gray BW, et al. Operative traumatic aortic injuries at an urban pediatric hospital. Am Surg. 2020;87(6):965–70.
7. Stannard A, Brown K, Benson C, Clasper J, Midwinter M, Tai NR. Outcome after vascular trauma in a deployed military trauma system. Br J Surg. 2011;98(2):228–34.
8. Markov NP, DuBose JJ, Scott D, Propper BW, Clouse WD, Thompson B, et al. Anatomic distribution and mortality of arterial injury in the wars in Afghanistan and Iraq with comparison to a civilian benchmark. J Vasc Surg. 2012;56(3):728–36.
9. Chang R, Fox EE, Greene TJ, Eastridge BJ, Gilani R, Chung KK, et al. Multicenter retrospective study of noncompressible torso hemorrhage: anatomic locations of bleeding and comparison of endovascular versus open approach. J Trauma Acute Care Surg. 2017;83(1):11–8.
10. Clouse WD, Rasmussen TE, Peck MA, Eliason JL, Cox MW, Bowser AN, et al. In-theater management of vascular injury: 2 years of the Balad Vascular Registry. J Am Coll Surg. 2007;204(4):625–32.
11. Oliver JC, Bekker W, Edu S, Nicol AJ, Navsaria PH. A ten year review of civilian iliac vessel injuries from a single trauma centre. Eur J Vasc Endovasc Surg. 2012;44(2):199–202.
12. de Mestral C, Dueck AD, Gomez D, Haas B, Nathens AB. Associated injuries, management, and outcomes of blunt abdominal aortic injury. J Vasc Surg. 2012;56(3):656–60.
13. Inaba K, Kirkpatrick AW, Finkelstein J, Murphy J, Brenneman FD, Boulanger BR, et al. Blunt abdominal aortic trauma in association with thoracolumbar spine fractures. Injury. 2001;32(3):201–7.
14. Sheehan BM, Grigorian A, de Virgilio C, Fujitani RM, Kabutey NK, Lekawa M, et al. Predictors of blunt abdominal aortic injury in trauma patients and mortality analysis. J Vasc Surg. 2020;71(6):1858–66.
15. Lauerman MH, Rybin D, Doros G, Kalish J, Hamburg N, Eberhardt RT, et al. Characterization and outcomes of iliac vessel injury in the 21st century: a review of the National Trauma Data Bank. Vasc Endovasc Surg. 2013;47(5):325–30.
16. Deree J, Shenvi E, Fortlage D, Stout P, Potenza B, Hoyt DB, et al. Patient factors and operating room resuscitation predict mortality in traumatic abdominal aortic injury: a 20-year analysis. J Vasc Surg. 2007;45(3):493–7.
17. Miller MT, Pasquale MD, Bromberg WJ, Wasser TE, Cox J. Not so FAST. J Trauma. 2003;54(1):52–9; discussion 59–60.
18. Do WS, Chang R, Fox EE, Wade CE, Holcomb JB, Martin MJ. Too fast, or not fast enough? The FAST exam in patients with non-compressible torso hemorrhage. Am J Surg. 2019;217(5):882–6.
19. Tsai R, Raptis C, Schuerer DJ, Mellnick VM. CT appearance of traumatic inferior vena cava injury. AJR Am J Roentgenol. 2016;207(4):705–11.
20. Beyer C, Zakaluzny S, Humphries M, Shatz D. Multidisciplinary management of blunt renal artery injury with endovascular therapy in the setting of polytrauma: a case report and review of the literature. Ann Vasc Surg. 2017;38(318):e11–6.
21. Costantini TW, Coimbra R, Holcomb JB, Podbielski JM, Catalano R, Blackburn A, et al. Current management of hemorrhage from severe pelvic fractures: results of an American association for the surgery of trauma multi-institutional trial. J Trauma Acute Care Surg. 2016;80(5):717–23.
22. Kertesz JL, Anderson SW, Murakami AM, Pieroni S, Rhea JT, Soto JA. Detection of vascular injuries in patients with blunt pelvic trauma by using 64-channel multidetector CT. Radiographics. 2009;29(1):151–64.
23. Shalhub S, Starnes BW, Brenner ML, Biffl WL, Azizzadeh A, et al. Blunt abdominal aortic injury: a Western Trauma Association multicenter study. J Trauma Acute Care Surg. 2014;77(6):879–85. discussion 885.
24. Branco BC, DuBose JJ, Zhan LX, Hughes JD, Goshima KR, Rhee P, et al. Trends and outcomes of endovascular therapy in the management of civilian vascular injuries. J Vasc Surg. 2014;60(5):1297–307.e1.
25. Berthet JP, Marty-Ane CH, Veerapen R, Picard E, Mary H, Alric P. Dissection of the abdominal aorta in blunt trauma:endovascular or conventional surgical management. J Vasc Surgery. 2003;38(5):997–1003.
26. Branco BC, Naik-Mathuria B, Montero-Baker M, Gilani R, West CA, Mills JL Sr, et al. Increasing use of endovascular therapy in pediatric arterial trauma. J Vasc Surg. 2017;66(4):1175–83.e1.
27. Richmond BK, Judhan R, Sherrill W, Yacoub M, AbuRahma AF, Knackstedt K, et al. Trends and outcomes in the operative management of traumatic vascular injuries: a comparison of open versus endovascular approaches. Am Surg. 2017;83(5):495–501.

28. Hagiwara A, Takasu A. Transcatheter arterial embolization is effective for mesenteric arterial hemorrhage in trauma. Emerg Radiol. 2009;16(5):403–6.
29. Demirel S, Winter C, Rapprich B, Weigand H, Gamstatter G. Stab injury of the superior mesenteric artery with life threatening bleeding - endovascular treatment with an unusual technique. Vasa. 2010;39(3):268–70.
30. Ghelfi J, Frandon J, Barbois S, Vendrell A, Rodiere M, Sengel C, et al. Arterial embolization in the management of mesenteric bleeding secondary to blunt abdominal trauma. Cardiovasc Intervent Radiol. 2016;39(5):683–9.
31. Saito N, Matsumoto H, Yagi T, Hara Y, Hayashida K, Motomura T, et al. Evaluation of the safety and feasibility of resuscitative endovascular balloon occlusion of the aorta. J Trauma Acute Care Surg. 2015;78(5):897–903; discussion 4.
32. Matsumura Y, Matsumoto J, Kondo H, Idoguchi K, Ishida T, Kon Y, et al. Fewer REBOA complications with smaller devices and partial occlusion: evidence from a multicentre registry in Japan. Emerg Med J. 2017;34(12):793–9.
33. DuBose JJ, Scalea TM, Brenner M, Skiada D, Inaba K, Cannon J, et al. The AAST prospective Aortic Occlusion for Resuscitation in Trauma and Acute Care Surgery (AORTA) registry: data on contemporary utilization and outcomes of aortic occlusion and resuscitative balloon occlusion of the aorta (REBOA). J Trauma Acute Care Surg. 2016;81(3):409–19.
34. Morrison JJ, Galgon RE, Jansen JO, Cannon JW, Rasmussen TE, Eliason JL. A systematic review of the use of resuscitative endovascular balloon occlusion of the aorta in the management of hemorrhagic shock. J Trauma Acute Care Surg. 2016;80(2):324–34.
35. Moore LJ, Martin CD, Harvin JA, Wade CE, Holcomb JB. Resuscitative endovascular balloon occlusion of the aorta for control of noncompressible truncal hemorrhage in the abdomen and pelvis. Am J Surg. 2016;212(6):1222–30.
36. Kobayashi L, Coimbra R, Goes AMO Jr, Reva V, Santorelli J, et al. American Association for the Surgery of Trauma–World Society of Emergency Surgery guidelines on diagnosis and management of abdominal vascular injuries. J Trauma Acute Care Surg. 2020;89(6):1197–211.
37. Inaba K, Aksoy H, Seamon MJ, Marks JA, Duchesne J, Schroll R, et al. Multicenter evaluation of temporary intravascular shunt use in vascular trauma. J Trauma Acute Care Surg. 2016;80(3):359–64; discussion 64–5.
38. Hansen CJ, Bernadas C, West MA, Ney AL, Muehlstedt S, Cohen M, et al. Abdominal vena caval injuries: outcomes remain dismal. Surgery. 2000;128(4):572–8.
39. Asensio JA, Petrone P, Kimbrell B, Kuncir E. Lessons learned in the management of thirteen celiac axis injuries. South Med J. 2005;98(4):462–6.
40. Asensio JA, Britt LD, Borzotta A, Peitzman A, Miller FB, Mackersie RC, et al. Multiinstitutional experience with the management of superior mesenteric artery injuries. J Am Coll Surg. 2001;193(4):354–65; discussion 65–6.
41. Coimbra R, Filho AR, Nesser RA, Rasslan S. Outcome from traumatic injury of the portal and superior mesenteric veins. Vasc Endovasc Surg. 2004;38(3):249–55.
42. Asensio JA, Petrone P, Garcia-Nunez L, Healy M, Martin M, Kuncir E. Superior mesenteric venous injuries: to ligate or to repair remains the question. J Trauma. 2007;62(3):668–75; discussion 75.
43. Fraga GP, Bansal V, Fortlage D, Coimbra R. A 20-year experience with portal and superior mesenteric venous injuries: has anything changed? Eur J Vasc Endovasc Surg. 2009;37(1):87–91.
44. Pereira BMT, Chiara O, Ramponi F, Weber DG, Cimbanassi S, De Simone B, et al. WSES position paper on vascular emergency surgery. World J Emerg Surg. 2015;10:49.
45. Knudson MM, Harrison PB, Hoyt DB, Shatz DV, Sietlow SP, Bergstein JM, et al. Outcome after major renovascular injuries: a Western Trauma Association multicenter report. J Trauma. 2000;49(6):1116–22.
46. Lopera JE, Suri R, Kroma G, Gadani S, Dolmatch B. Traumatic occlusion and dissection of the main renal artery: endovascular treatment. J Vasc Interv Radiol. 2011;22(11):1570–4.
47. Asensio JA, Petrone P, Roldan G, Kuncir E, Rowe VL, Chan L, et al. Analysis of 185 iliac vessel injuries: risk factors and predictors of outcome. Arch Surg. 2003;138(11):1187–93; discussion 93–4.
48. Ball CG, Feliciano DV. Damage control techniques for common and external iliac artery injuries: have temporary intravascular shunts replaced the need for ligation? J Trauma. 2010;68(5):1117–20.
49. Magee GA, Cho J, Matsushima K, Strumwasser A, Inaba K, Jazaeri O, et al. Isolated iliac vascular injuries and outcome of repair versus ligation of isolated iliac vein injury. J Vasc Surg. 2018;67(1):254–61.
50. Paul JS, Webb TP, Aprahamian C, Weigelt JA. Intraabdominal vascular injury: are we getting any better? J Trauma. 2010;69(6):1393–7.
51. Altoijry A, Lindsay TF, Johnston KW, Mamdani M, Al-Omran M. Vascular-injury-related in-hospital mortality in Ontario between 1991 and 2009. J Int Med Res. 2021;49(1):300060520987728.
52. Villamaria CY, Morrison JJ, Fitzpatrick CM, Cannon JW, Rasmussen TE. Wartime vascular injuries in the pediatric population of Iraq and Afghanistan: 2002–2011. J Pediatr Surg. 2014;49(3):428–32.
53. Corneille MG, Gallup TM, Villa C, Richa JM, Wolf SE, Myers JG, et al. Pediatric vascular injuries: acute management and early outcomes. J Trauma. 2011;70(4):823–8.
54. Coimbra R, Hoyt D, Winchell R, Simons R, Fortlage D, Garcia J. The ongoing challenge of retroperitoneal vascular injuries. Am J Surg. 1996;172(5):541–4; discussion 545.
55. Tyburski JG, Wilson RF, Dente C, Steffes C, Carlin AM. Factors affecting mortality rates in patients

with abdominal vascular injuries. J Trauma. 2001;50(6):1020–6.
56. Feliciano D, Moore E, Biffl W. Western Trauma Association Critical Decisions in Trauma: management of abdominal vascular trauma. J Trauma Acute Care Surg. 2015;79(6):1079–88.

## Further Reading

Feliciano D, Moore E, Biffl W. Western Trauma Association Critical Decisions in Trauma: management of abdominal vascular trauma. J Trauma Acute Care Surg. 2015;79(6):1079–88.

Kobayashi L, Coimbra R, Goes AMO Jr, Reva V, Santorelli J, et al. American Association for the Surgery of Trauma–World Society of Emergency Surgery guidelines on diagnosis and management of abdominal vascular injuries. J Trauma Acute Care Surg. 2020;89(6):1197–211.

Pereira BMT, Chiara O, Ramponi F, Weber DG, Cimbanassi S, De Simone B, et al. WSES position paper on vascular emergency surgery. World J Emerg Surg. 2015;10:49.

# Genital and Anorectal Trauma

**101**

Thobekile Nomcebo Shangase, Feroz Ganchi, and Timothy Craig Hardcastle

**Learning Goals**
- Understand the anatomic and mechanism of injury aspects of injury to the external genitalia and the anorectal region.
- Develop a diagnostic approach and understanding of the appropriate use of other investigations to determine the severity of each injury.
- Apply the management principles for external genital, nongravid uterine, and anorectal injury.

## 101.1 Introduction: Epidemiology and Background Information

Genital and anorectal injuries are not common; however, they are not rare and affect both males and females with a male predominance [1]. According to the largest study by Petrone from 2013, the overall incidence is approximately 0.1% [2]. Blunt trauma accounts for majority of the cases overall, with pedestrian-vehicle collisions resulting in pelvic fracture and saddle injuries (motor-cyclists and animal-related) the most frequent. Penetrating trauma accounts for minority of the cases (gunshot, stabs, but not forgetting sexual assault and impalement) however may predominate in countries with high rates of penetrating trauma [2]. Morbidity and mortality are reduced by early recognition and appropriate management, although major injury with massive bleeding contributes to up to 25% pre-admission death, especially with compound pelvic fracture [1]. Petrone reported a mortality rate in a comprehensive review of between 7% and 60% [1].

## 101.2 Anatomy of the Anorectal and Genital Structures

The perineum is the region of the body below the pelvic diaphragm [3, 4]. With lower limbs abducted, it is a diamond-shaped area between the thighs and is divided into two triangles by a

T. N. Shangase · F. Ganchi
Trauma Service, Inkosi Albert Luthuli Central Hospital, Durban, South Africa

Department of Surgery, University of KwaZulu-Natal, Durban, South Africa

T. C. Hardcastle (✉)
Trauma Service, Inkosi Albert Luthuli Central Hospital, Durban, South Africa

Department of Surgery, University of KwaZulu-Natal, Durban, South Africa

Faculty of Health Sciences, Durban University of Technology, Durban, South Africa
e-mail: hardcastle@ukzn.ac.za

© The Author(s), under exclusive license to Springer Nature Switzerland AG 2023
F. Coccolini, F. Catena (eds.), *Textbook of Emergency General Surgery*,
https://doi.org/10.1007/978-3-031-22599-4_101

transverse line joining the two ischial tuberosities. This line divides the perineum into the posterior anal triangle consisting of the anal canal and anus and anteriorly located urogenital triangle where the root of scrotum and penis is found in males and the vulva in females. Other important structures in this region include the perineal body and the anococcygeal body. The roof of the entire perineum is the levator ani muscles which form the so-called pelvic diaphragm.

Within the urogenital triangle, a number of fascial layers and pouches are found, namely, the superficial and deep fascia forming the perineal pouches. These are relevant in trauma as potential sources of fluid collection and infection following injury (see Figs. 101.1 and 101.2: male and female sagittal anatomical drawings).

Similarly, the anal triangle contains the ischio-anal fossae (also known as the ischiorectal fossae). The pudendal canal is found here, and the pudendal artery, vein, and nerve enter this canal. The anal canal forms the terminal part of the large intestine and terminates at the anus. This region has an external voluntary sphincter and an internal involuntary sphincter. Within the canal, the inferior comb-shaped limit of the anal valves forms an irregular line, the pectinate (dentate) line, the junction of the superior part, and the inferior part. This is relevant from the perspective of the blood and nerve supply, namely, the superior part is supplied by the superior rectal artery (from the inferior mesenteric artery) and the middle rectal artery (from the internal iliacs). It has visceral innervation, from the hypogastric plexus. On the other hand, the inferior part is fed by the inferior rectal arteries from below the sphincters. The region has somatic innervation, coming from the inferior rectal nerves. There is a potential "watershed" area of poor blood supply between these two vascular trees.

The male perineum consists of external genitalia, perineal muscles, and anal canal. The external genitalia include the distal (anterior) male urethra in the tissues, the scrotum housing the testes and epididymis, and the penis. Blood supply to the anterior aspect is via the anterior

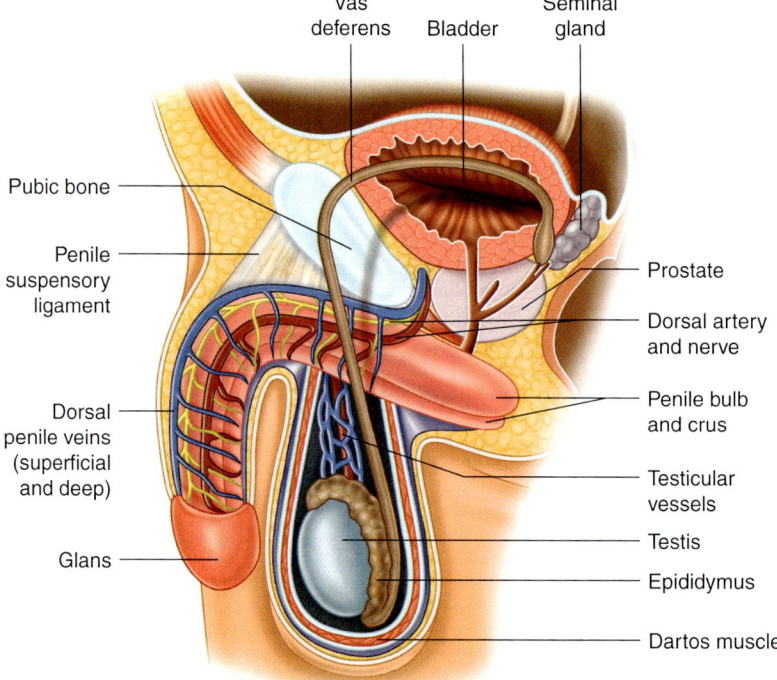

**Fig. 101.1** Anatomy of the male genitalia. (Drawn by Jonathan Hardcastle)

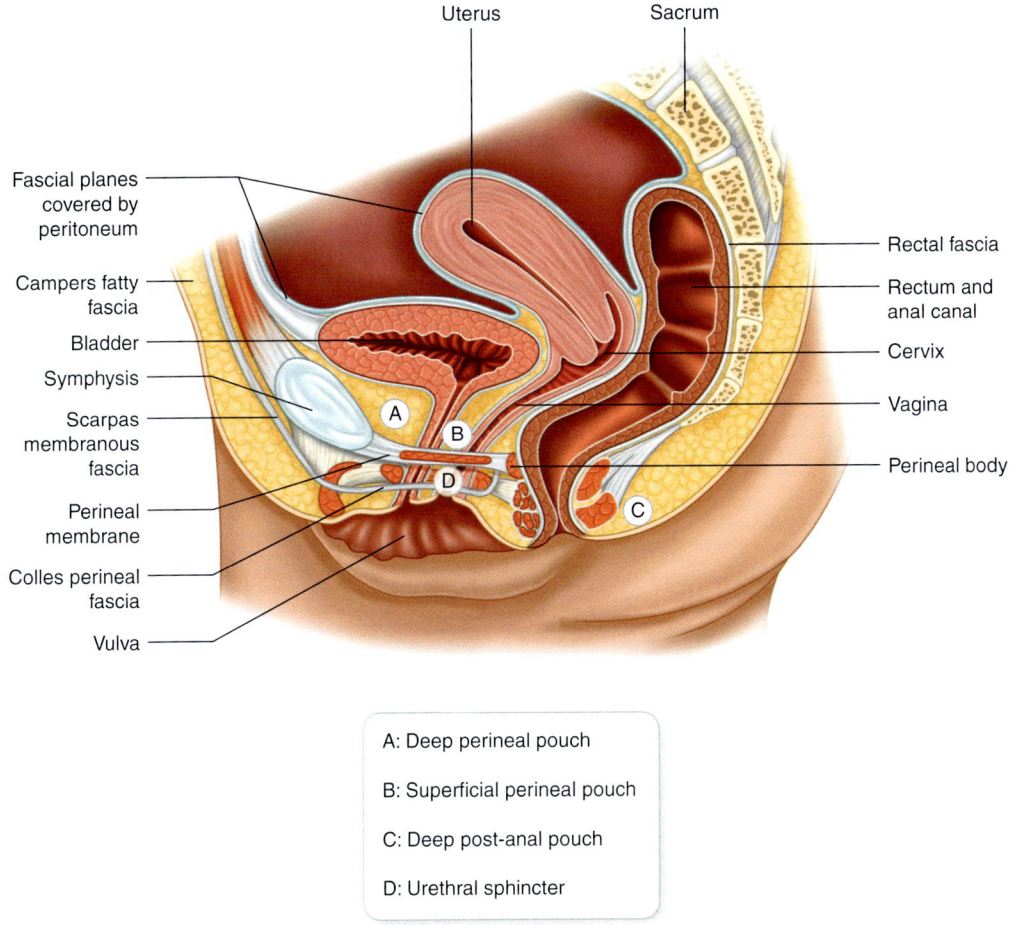

**Fig. 101.2** Anatomy of the female perineum, fascial planes, and associated internal organs. (Image drawn by Jenna Kershaw Hardcastle)

scrotal arteries, while the posterior aspect is via the posterior scrotal arteries and branches from cremasteric arteries.

Innervation of this aspect of the perineum is the anterior and posterior scrotal nerves. The penis functions as the outlet for urine and semen and has three cylindrical bodies of erectile cavernous tissue, with the urethra enclosed within one of these cylinders. The penile blood supply is from the dorsal arteries of the penis, deep arteries of the penis, and the arteries of the bulb of the penis, which includes the superficial and deep branches of external pudendal vessels. The innervation is from the pudendal nerve. The main perineal muscles are the superficial transverse perineal, ischiocavernosus, and bulbospongiosus. The prostatic and membranous (posterior) urethra is suspended by the puboprostatic ligaments and is liable to injury during pelvic fractures.

The female perineum externally is the vulva or pudendum which includes the mons pubis, labia majora, labia minora, clitoris, bulbs of the vestibule, and greater and lesser vestibular glands. The blood supply is from the external and internal pudendal arteries and the innervation via the anterior and posterior labial nerves. Similar to the male, the perineal muscles consist of the superficial transverse perineal, ischiocavernosus, and bulbospongiosus. Through these muscle layers run the urethra and the vagina anteriorly and the anal canal posteriorly.

## 101.3 Injury to the Male External Genitalia: Blunt and Penetrating (See Flowchart 101.1—Penetrating)

The external male genitalia are at risk of injury due to a number of mechanisms, in the case of blunt injury from direct blows, crush injury, or from the so-called Zipper (or entrapment) injury, while penetrating trauma includes most commonly ballistic injury, knife wounds, and other impalement or amputation injury [5]. Human bites and self-mutilation/amputation of the penis during assaults are also reported [5, 6]. Scrotal involvement is found in approximately 2% of penetrating trauma [6].

Blunt injury can cause testicular disruption, a degree of torsion or tearing of the tunica vaginalis, degloving of the penile or scrotal skin, or rupture of the corpus of the penis [5, 6] (Fig. 101.3).

**Diagnosis** Following initial patient-centered resuscitation, with clinical examination of obvious visible injuries, the next modality that may be

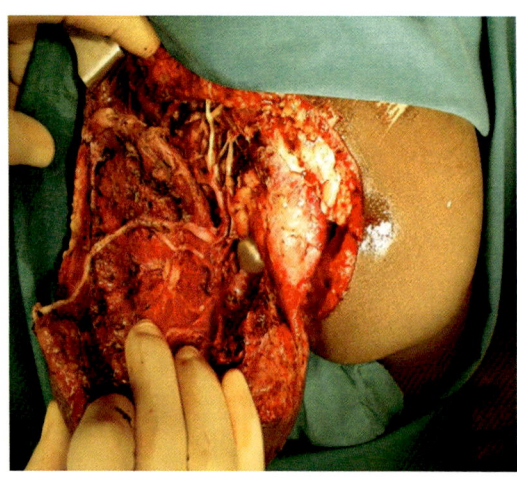

**Fig. 101.3** Complex perineal and buttock blunt injury that required hemipelvectomy as management

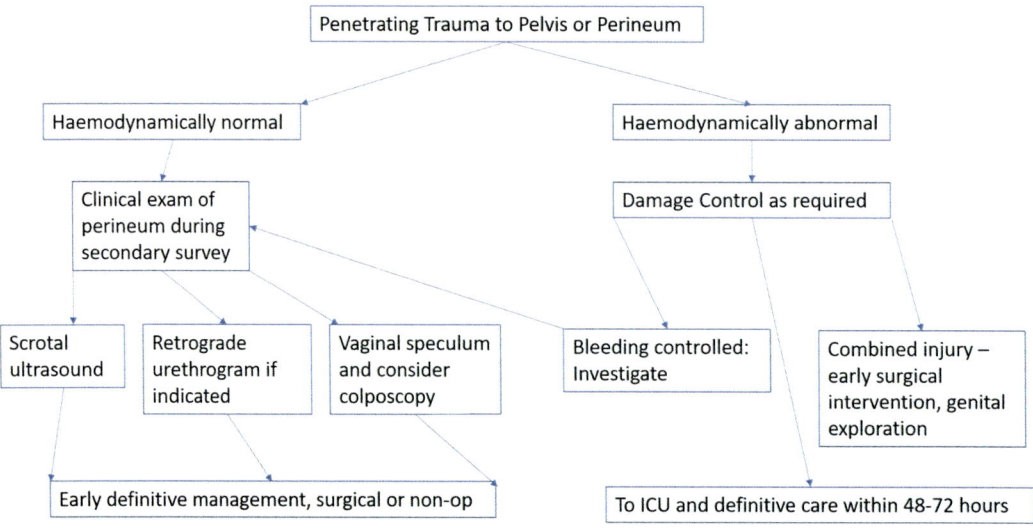

**Flowchart 101.1** General approach to penetrating trauma to perineum

employed to assess the testes is ultrasound [7]. This may assist in distinguishing between torsion, disruption, and a hematoma.

**Management** Due to good blood supply to the scrotum, debridement and suturing usually suffice, with low rates of wound complications. If there is extensive skin loss, split skin grafting is associated with good outcomes. If the tunica vaginalis of the testis is disrupted, debride and close the capsule to prevent host reaction against the testis, using an absorbable suture [5–7]. In the presence of loss of scrotal skin and an exposed testicle, pouches can be created in the proximal thigh skin to busy the testis and spermatic cord with subsequent approximation under a soft-tissue bridge. Testicular function is usually spared.

Most cases of penetrating urethral injury are best managed with exploration and direct suture repair with injury to the urethra proper repaired over a Silastic Foley catheter to act as a stent. Use of absorbable sutures is currently the preferred repair option, ensuring a watertight closure of the corpus cavernosum [5–8].

Penile injury mostly only involves the external skin and subcutaneous fascia due to degloving type injury from blunt trauma. These skin defects of the penile shaft can usually be debrided and sutured primarily with or without circumcision [5, 6, 9]. If there is clinical evidence that the corpora cavernosa have been penetrated, then exploration is recommended. Ideally, preoperatively, a retrograde urethrogram can be performed to exclude urethral perforation, with urethral catheter placement as a stent to enable identification of the defects during repair [8]. Avoidance of a false tract is important, however. The corpora cavernosa should be repaired in a watertight fashion using absorbable sutures to avoid the complications of penile deformity and inability to achieve an erection. The same principles apply to "penile fracture" with early repair currently advocated. Penile amputation requires hemostasis followed by referral to urological experts for attempts at reattachment in the following order:

corpora cavernosa, dorsal vessels, followed by nerve repair using microsurgical techniques. Outcomes are variable from a functional perspective.

Injury to the foreskin is simply treated by circumcision and injury to the glans penis by debridement and suture, avoiding stenosis of the urethral meatus. Human bites often present late, and antibiotic cover (including anaerobic cover) with secondary intention healing (open wound care) is advised [5, 6].

## 101.4 Injury to the Female External Genitalia (See Also Flowchart 101.1 for General Approach)

These are uncommon injuries accounting for less than 5% of injuries sustained by female trauma patients. Most of these injuries are associated with pelvic fractures caused by blunt trauma; the remainder of the injuries is from penetrating trauma (gunshot and stab wounds), accidental impalement, and sexual assault [10–12]. Although genital injuries alone rarely result in death, if not properly managed, chronic discomfort, dyspareunia, infertility, or fistula formation may result [13]. Iatrogenic- and obstetrics-related injuries will not be discussed in this section.

These injuries are categorized into saddle injuries, sexual assault, and impalement (accidental) injuries [11, 12].

**Straddle injuries** are defined as injuries that occur when a female hits the vulva/perineum on an object, and a force generated by her body weight causes the injury. Waterskiing, gymnastics, and cycling seem to be common causes of these injuries [13].

***Diagnosis*** relies on clinical examination. Sedation and analgesia may be required to adequately examine the patient; some patients may require examination under general anesthesia. Vaginal speculum examination and perianal examination is essential as internal injury is common [11].

**Table 101.1** Vulva injury grading AAST

I. Hematoma or contusion
II. Superficial laceration involving the skin only
III. Deep laceration extending to the fat and subcutaneous tissue
IV. Avulsion of skin, fat, or muscle
V. Injury to adjacent organ

**Table 101.2** Vaginal injury grading AAST

I. Contusion or hematoma
II. Superficial laceration involving mucosa
III. Deep laceration extending into submucosal fat or muscle
IV. Complex laceration extending to the cervix or peritoneum
V. Laceration extending to adjacent organs

On examination, it is helpful to grade the injuries according to American Association for the Surgery of Trauma (AAST) grading (see Tables 101.1 and 101.2). Most injuries are grades I–III [10, 11].

***Investigation*** Primary and secondary survey remains the same for all polytrauma patients, and then the focus moves to specific injuries, best examined in the Lloyd-Davies or lithotomy position.

***Management*** Accepted trauma management principles focusing on the whole patient must be used, only when the patient is stable are minor injuries addressed. Clean and repair the injuries under local or general anesthesia, depending on the injury grade and patient's hemodynamic stability. Minor injuries and small hematomas are treated by means of analgesics, soothing soaks, and intermittent ice packs to reduce swelling [13].

Stable patients have their more extensive injuries primarily repaired under local anesthesia for a low grade injury, while high grade injuries (AAST Grade III–V) are best repaired in the operation room under general anesthesia with appropriate consent for the procedure. Appropriate instruments and head lights are essential. The female urethra is short, and, since there is no prostatic membranous component, urethral injury in females is rare, although avulsion from the bladder neck is reported [12, 13]. Large vulvar hematomas should be drained and hemostasis obtained [13]. Repair over a closed suction drain may be required.

Hemodynamically unstable patients are taken to the operation room immediately. If a pelvic fracture is present and a pelvic binder is in situ, lithotomy position is contraindicated. The pelvic binder is left in situ, and in a supine position legs are gently separated, and then the procedure of choice is to pack the vagina with swabs. As with any other damage control approach, the patient is then transferred to ICU for further resuscitation (or to the interventional suite for embolization if available) and then may return for definitive surgical repair when more stable, ideally within 48 h.

**Sexual Assault Injuries** These are injuries that occur post sexual assault to the anogenital area. These injuries can be classified as: *external* injuries involving the labia majora, labia minora in 53%, perineum, and posterior fourchette; *internal* injuries involving the fossa navicularis, hymen, vagina, or cervix; and finally *perianal* injuries involving the anus and distal rectum [13].

***Diagnosis*** Injury types are described as tears, abrasions, ecchymoses, redness, and swelling. Prevalence of these injuries varies depending on type of examination, from 5% for direct visualization to 87% with colposcopic examination [14]. Vaginal and vulval injuries are also graded via the appropriate AAST grading system and managed accordingly. A chaperone in the room is advised.

***Management*** of these patients requires multidisciplinary approach involving social workers, psychologist, gynecologists, and special police units where appropriate. The general principles for initial assessment and resuscitation are used in patient care, and then specific injuries are managed as per their grading as described in the above section. Crime kits should be used when necessary. Surgical intervention is required less often than with impalement or other blunt/penetrating injury [13].

**Impalement Injuries** Accidental impalement occurs when a patient accidentally fall onto a sharp object and causes injury into the torso involving both anorectal and genital area [13]. These injuries are relatively rare and may be complicated, due to small tunnel-like tracts with sepsis a major risk.

*Diagnosis* General ATLS principles are followed for these patients and hemodynamically stable, a full history is taken, and then a thorough physical examination performed. Commonly, the patient can present with hematuria, vaginal bleeding, vaginal discharge, pain, or rectal bleeding [13].

**Management**
Appropriate antibiotics and tetanus toxoid must be administered, and the patient ideally prepared for the operation room (consent for sigmoidoscope, EUA, Laparotomy, defunctioning colostomy, and debridement must be obtained, depending on the injury patterns identified).

Examination is generally done under general anesthesia in the operating room. Sigmoidoscopy without laparotomy is performed if the patient is not peritonitic or has no other indication for laparotomy. Diverting colostomy is fashioned if a rectal injury is diagnosed on sigmoidoscope, while distal anal injury may be repaired without diversion. Any lacerations to the anogenital area are irrigated and repaired in layers with absorbable suture material, preferably using interrupted sutures. Drains are left in situ for extensive, complex injuries.

## 101.5 Injury to the Nongravid Uterus

Reports of injury to the nongravid uterus are few and far between [15]. Injury due to blunt trauma is extremely rare, and the few reported cases are usually after penetrating trauma, most often due to bullet wounds. In blunt trauma, the compounding factor often reported is related to the presence of large fibroids of the uterus [15, 16]. Management is hemostasis and suture-control of bleeders—if this is not successful, the option of a "damage-control" hysterectomy must be considered.

## 101.6 Injury to the Male Perineum and Anal Canal Due to Blunt Trauma

These injuries usually result from motor vehicle collisions or fall from a height, with straddle-type injury also common. The history should increase index of suspicion regarding anal injuries. Clinical examination findings are the most important to guide treatment, and, after initial patient-centered resuscitation following standard principles, the perineum and anal canal are best examined by inspection and palpation which includes per rectum examination, usually toward the end of primary survey if placing a catheter or during secondary survey. If the patient is in the operation room for other reasons, then placing the patient in the Lloyd-Davies position is an advantage for surgical access.

Special investigations that may assist in planning of treatment include rigid proctoscopy, rigid or flexible sigmoidoscopy to exclude a more proximal rectal injury, and on occasion CT scan with per rectal contrast or even MRI; however, this is not routinely necessary in the absence of pelvic fractures [17].

Management recommendations are to repair only if easily accessible. Anal mucosa-only injuries can be sutured to repair the defect. For more extensive injury involving the sphincters, the empirical use of fecal diversion (Sigmoid colostomy) is recommended and later secondary intention healing. As a rule, there is no need for rectal or anal canal washouts; however, in severely contaminated blunt wounds, repeated debridement at an early stage is advised, especially if there is plant or animal material as contaminants [17]. The use of negative pressure wound care and extensive topical washes are recommended.

Broad spectrum antimicrobial cover that includes anaerobic cover is advised.

Sphincter repair is indicated with a localized defect in the external anal sphincter provided the healthy sphincter is capable of vigorous contraction. Prone, jack-knife, or lithotomy position may be used. The actual incision for the procedure is dependent on the precise site of the defect. Various techniques have been described. In severe injury usually confirmed on MRI, reconstruction of the anorectum by repair of its circular smooth muscle fibers and mucosa may have to be combined with sphincter repair. Especially where there is a recto-vaginal or recto-vesical fistula present, this should be repaired with tissue interposition. Otherwise, a gracilis sphincteroplasty or a synthetic repair may be required for more extensive injury [17].

### 101.6.1 Penetrating Injury to the Rectum and Anus: Modern Evidence-Based Approaches (See Flowchart 101.2)

In this section, extraperitoneal rectal injury and proximal anal canal injury, which are a potential source of missed injury, are included. Anorectal penetrating trauma is mostly seen in pelvic ballistic injury but occasionally in impalement cases as well. The common injury patterns include transpelvic or buttock penetrating wounds from bullets, mostly low energy rounds, knife wounds to the buttocks, and implement on fence-spikes or construction rebars [17].

Traditionally, the concepts of management were very aggressive based on experience from the Second World War and Vietnam [17]. This included defunctioning of the colon (loop-colostomy) above the injury, distal rectal washout, and pararectal drains. More recent literature from high-trauma countries has shown that less invasive approaches work just as well for the extraperitoneal injury in the civilian practice, namely a simple open or laparoscopic loop colostomy (either option allows for excluding intra-peritoneal injury), with no improvement in healing with distal rectal washouts or pararectal drains [18, 19]. Both literatures from South Africa and from the USA support the more conservative management approach, and there is a recent EAST-guideline with similar recommendations [18–22]. A subsequent large multicenter study confirmed these findings and showed that distal washout and drains increased complications threefold [21]. For the anal canal, the

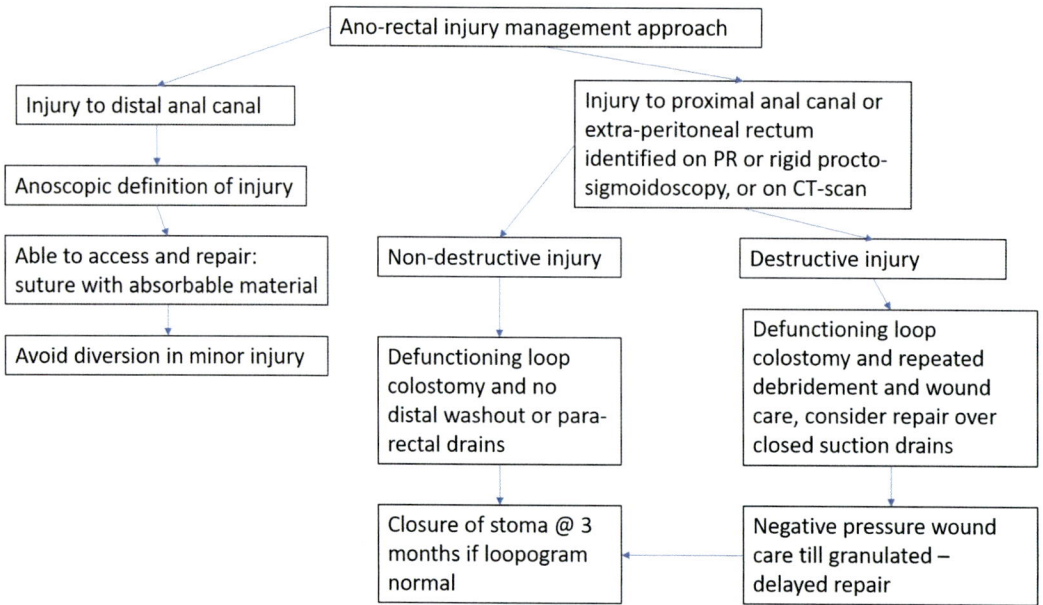

**Flowchart 101.2** Anorectal injury approach

options include primary repair of injuries that are accessible via anoscope using an absorbable suture or allowing secondary healing for those injuries not amenable to suture that are very distal, with later reconstruction including the sphincters, usually after endo-anal MRI clarification of the extent of sphincter injury, avoiding diversion if possible; however, the evidence-base is very weak [17, 23].

### 101.6.2 Male Proximal Urethral Injuries (See Flowchart 101.3)

Urethral injuries in blunt trauma are usually associated with pelvic fractures or straddle injury. Blood at the urethral meatus, or frank hematuria, should alert the clinician to a suspected urethral injury or bladder injury. Confirmation of the injury is by retrograde urethrography, which is, however, not an emergency procedure, should a gentle catheter attempt be successful. The AIS organ injury scale is detailed in Table 101.3 and is useful to guide the treatment options. Differentiation into anterior and posterior rupture and the completeness thereof is important for management [24]. Current recommendations include one attempt at gentle catheter placement using the largest available Silastic balloon catheter (ideally a three-way device), and if successful this is adequate early treatment, especially for anterior rupture to avoid stricturing; however, this is only successful in about 30–60% of cases [24, 25].

Recommended management options following blunt trauma are immediate or early endoscopic alignment, either transurethral or via the bladder or both [24–29]. If this is not possible, early open approaches are considered acceptable, using a double-urethral sound [Davis] technique (with or without magnetic tips) to perform retrograde catheter placement via a surgical tie placed onto the tip of the urethral sound once the urethral tract has been defined, and catheter is pulled though into the bladder under vision, thus avoiding any pelvic hematoma altogether, preventing conversion of a closed pelvic fracture into an open fracture (see Fig. 101.4) [8, 27, 28]. Retrograde pericatheter urethrograms are performed to ensure healing has occurred at around 6 weeks [26]. If not successful, urinary diversion

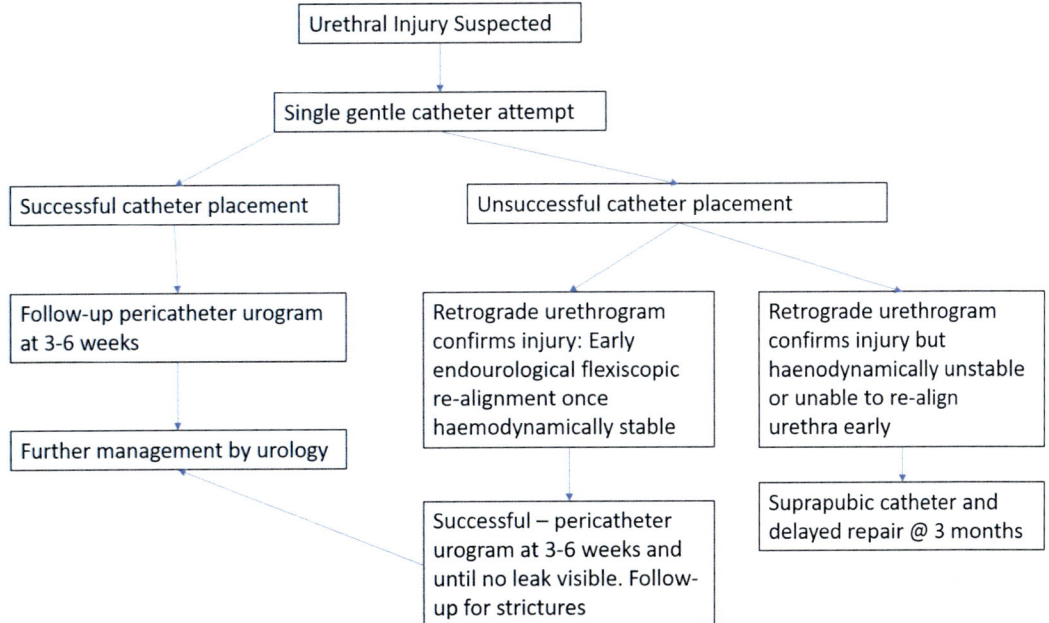

**Flowchart 101.3** Urethral injury

**Table 101.3** Urethra injury scale

| Grade | Injury type | Injury description |
|---|---|---|
| 1 | Contusion | Blood at urethral meatus. Urethrography negative |
| 2 | Stretch injury | Elongation of urethra without extravasation on urethrography |
| 3 | Partial disruption | Extravasation of urethrography contrast at injury site with visualization in the bladder |
| 4 | Complete disruption | Extravasation of urethrography contrast at injury site without visualization in the bladder, <2 cm of urethral separation |
| 5 | Complete disruption | Complete transection with >2 cm urethral separation or extension into the prostate or vagina |

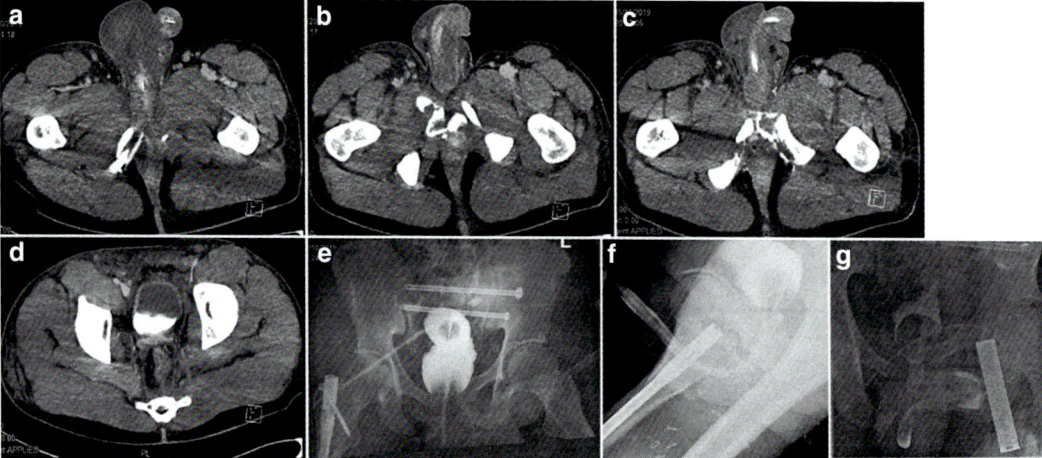

**Fig. 101.4** Complex pelvic injury with posterior urethral rupture: (**a**) shows catheter placed outside the bladder with complete urethral injury; (**b, c**) demonstrates extravasation of contrast and (**d**) the intact bladder. (**e**) Shows the large transurethral catheter and suprapubic catheter placed using the magnetic-sound technique at surgery on post-injury day 3. (**f**) Shows the 3-week para-catheter retrograde urethrogram with a small residual leak and (**g**) at 8 weeks with no residual leak. The catheter was removed at 10 weeks, and further management consists of stricture management as needed. This technique avoids prolonged suprapubic catheter and delayed repair in systems with limited access to elective surgery, such as in lower- and middle-income countries

(suprapubic catheterization) and either subsequent realignment via endoscopy (8–10 days, especially with a large hematoma) or deferred urethroplasty (>3 months) may suffice [28, 29]. Absolute indications for early surgical repair are injuries with associated rectal or bladder neck injuries and those where there is wide separation of the defect in the urethra. Early alignment does not impact negatively on erectile function or continence. It also lessens the severity of strictures, which occur in 50% of those with early realignment but in 100% of those with delayed repair [25, 29].

**Dos and Don'ts**
- Do assess the entire patient using standard approaches to trauma patients.
- Do examine the perineum as missed injury is common.
- Do assess for sexual assault and record the findings carefully.
- Do offer early injury classification and operative management.
- Do cover with appropriate antimicrobials and Sitz baths if indicated.

- Do not try to obtain male urethral catheterization if first attempt is difficult.
- Do try to ensure early urethral repair if feasible and experts are available.
- Do use suprapubic catheter and sigmoid loop colostomy liberally.
- Do not be overly aggressive with pararectal drains and distal rectal washouts.

**Take-Home Points**
- Perineal injury is uncommon but occurs in both adults and children.
- Mechanisms include penetrating (weapons or impalement) and blunt (pelvic fracture, straddle) or sexual assault.
- Missed injury is not uncommon.
- Early intervention once resuscitation is complete is essential.
- Operative management is mostly early and conservative unless expert urologist cover is unavailable where suprapubic catheterization is the default.
- Sepsis is a common complication and requires debridement and appropriate antimicrobials.

**Multiple Choice Questions**

1. The most common injuries to the genitalia and anorectal regions are as a result of:
   A. Blast injury
   B. **Blunt trauma**
   C. Burns
   D. Penetrating injury
2. The roof of the perineum is anatomically:
   A. External sphincter muscle
   B. Internal Sphincter muscle
   C. **Levator ani muscles**
   D. Puborectalis muscle
3. Regarding blunt scrotal injury—after clinical examination, the most important additional investigation is:
   A. Angiography of the penis
   B. Contrast urethrogram
   C. Plain film X-ray of the pelvis
   D. **Ultrasound of the scrotum**
4. A male is working on a conveyor belt and the crotch of his pants gets caught in the mechanism. This mechanism of injury will **most likely** lead to:
   A. Fracture of the pelvis
   B. Open fracture of the femur
   C. **Penile or scrotal degloving injury**
   D. Vascular and nerve injury
5. A motorcyclist is injured in a head-on collision and flies over the handlebars hitting the center point. He is found to have bilateral pubic rami fractures. The likely urethral injury will be:
   A. **Anterior urethral injury**
   B. Meatal laceration
   C. Membranous urethral injury
   D. Posterior urethral injury
6. In the case of an impalement injury, the most concerning risk subsequently is:
   A. Bleeding
   B. Anorectal fistula
   C. Sexual dysfunction
   D. **Sepsis**
7. Injury to the nongravid uterus in cases of blunt trauma is commonly associated with:
   A. Cervical hyperplasia
   B. **Large fibroids**
   C. Previous caesarean section
   D. Ovarian cysts
8. Modern management of acute blunt urethral injury due to pelvic fractures espouses:
   A. **Early transurethral endoscopic realignment**
   B. Open repair of the urethra after hematoma evacuation

C. Suprapubic catheter and routine delayed repair
D. Radiologically guided realignment of the urethra

9. A man presents after sustaining a trans-axial low energy gunshot wound involving both buttocks, and there is blood present on the rectal examination. Best management if there is *no peritoneal breach* and the defect is not accessible is:
   A. **Defunctioning loop colostomy of the sigmoid colon**
   B. Defunctioning end colostomy and Hartman procedure
   C. Laparotomy, rectal mobilization, and primary repair
   D. Rectal washout and drain with colostomy

10. When assessing an anal canal injury, the one relative *contraindication to primary repair* and avoidance of fecal diversion is:
    A. Anal canal full thickness injury
    B. **Involvement of internal sphincter**
    C. Ischiorectal fossa contamination
    D. Puborectalis muscle involvement

# References

1. Petrone P, Velandia WR, Dziakova J, Marini CP. Treatment of complex perineal trauma. A review of the literature. Cir Esp. 2016;94(6):313–22. https://doi.org/10.1016/j.ciresp.2015.11.010.
2. Petrone P, Inaba K, Wasserberg N, Teixeira PG, Sarkisyan G, Dubose JJ, et al. Perineal injuries at a large urban trauma center: injury patterns and outcomes. Am Surg. 2009;75:317–20.
3. Moore KL, Agur AMR, Dalley AF. Chapter 3, Pelvis and perineum. In: Essential clinical anatomy. 4th ed. Baltimore, MD: Lippincott Williams and Wilkins; 2011. ISBN 978-0781799157
4. Boffard KD. Chapter 9.8: The urogenital System. In: Boffard KD, editor. Manual of definitive trauma care. 5th ed. Boca Raton, FL: CRC Press; 2019. ISBN: 9780367244682.
5. McCormick CS, Dumais MG, Johnsen NV, Voelzke BB, Hagedorn JC. Male genital trauma at a level 1 trauma center. World J Urol. 2020;38(12):3283–9. https://doi.org/10.1007/s00345-020-03115-0.
6. Bjurlin MA, Kim DY, Zhao LC, Palmer CJ, Cohn MR, Vidal PP, et al. Clinical characteristics and surgical outcomes of penetrating external genital injuries. J Trauma Acute Care Surg. 2013;74:839–44.
7. Van der Horst C, Martinez Portillo FJ, Seif C, Groth W, Junemann KP. Male genital injury: diagnostics and treatment. Br J Urol Int. 2004;93:927–30. https://doi.org/10.1111/j.14eA-410X.20Q4.O4757.x.
8. Coburn M. Chapter 36, Genitourinary trauma. In: Mattox KL, Moore EE, Feliciano DV, editors. Trauma. 7th ed. New York: McGraw-Hill; 2013. ISBN: 978-0-07-171784-7.
9. Phonsombat S, Master VA, McAninch JW. Penetrating external genital trauma: a 30-year single institution experience. J Urol. 2008;180:192–5.
10. Goldman HB, Idom CB Jr, Dmochowski RR. Traumatic injuries of the female external genitalia and their association with urological injuries. J Urol. 1998;159(3):956–9.
11. Wright JL, Wessels H. Chapter 10: Urinary and genital trauma. In: Hanno PM, Guzzo TJ, Malkowicz SB, Wein AJ, editors. Penn clinical manual of urology. 2nd ed. Philadelphia, PA: Saunders; 2007. p. 283–309. ISBN: 9781455753598.
12. Lopez HN, Focseneanu MA, Merritt DF. Genital injuries acute evaluation and management. Best Pract Res Clin Obstet Gynaecol. 2018;48:28–39. https://doi.org/10.1016/j.bpobgyn.2017.09.009.
13. Gambhir S, Grigorian A, Schubl S, Barrios C, Bernal N, Joe V, et al. Analysis of non-obstetric vaginal and vulvar trauma: risk factors for operative intervention. Updat Surg. 2019;71(4):735–40. https://doi.org/10.1007/s13304-019-00679-4.
14. Sommers MS. Defining patterns of genital injury from sexual assault: a Review. Trauma Violence Abuse. 2007;8(3):270–80. https://doi.org/10.1177/1524838007303194.
15. Hardcastle TC, Van der Merwe J, Cooper C, Grieve C. Non-gravid uterine trauma. Injury Extra. 2008;39:267–9.
16. Sule AZ. Traumatic rupture of uterine fibroid: an uncommon cause of post traumatic haemoperitoneum. West Afr J Med. 2000;19(2):158–9.
17. Herzig DO. Care of the patient with anorectal trauma. Clin Colon Rectal Surg. 2012;25:210–3. https://doi.org/10.1055/s-0032-1329391.
18. Navsaria PH, Edu S, Nicol AJ. Civilian extraperitoneal rectal gunshot wounds: surgical management made simpler. World J Surg. 2007;31:1345–51. https://doi.org/10.1007/s00268-007-9045-z.
19. Navsaria PH, Graham R, Nicol A. A new approach to extraperitoneal rectal injuries: laparoscopy and diverting loop sigmoid colostomy. J Trauma. 2001;51(3):532–5.
20. Bosarge PL, Como JJ, Fox N, Falck-Ytter Y, Haut ER, Dorian HA, et al. Management of penetrating extraperitoneal rectal injuries: an Eastern Association for the Surgery of Trauma practice management guideline. J Trauma Acute Care Surg. 2016;80:546–51.
21. Brown CVR, Teixeira PG, Furay E, Sharpe JP, Musonza T, Holcolm J, et al. Contemporary manage-

ment of rectal injuries at Level I trauma centers: the results of an American Association for the Surgery of Trauma multi-institutional study. J Trauma Acute Care Surg. 2018;84:225–33.
22. Clemens MS, Peace KM, Yi F. Rectal trauma: evidence-based practices. Clin Colon Rectal Surg. 2018;31:17–23. https://doi.org/10.1055/s-0037-1602182.
23. Ahern DP, Kelly ME, Courtney D, Rausa E, Winter DC. The management of penetrating rectal and anal trauma: a systematic review. Injury. 2017;48:1133–8. https://doi.org/10.1016/j.injury.2017.03.002.
24. Mouraviev VB, Coburn M, Santucci RA. The treatment of posterior urethral disruption associated with pelvic fractures: comparative experience of early realignment versus delayed urethroplasty. J Urol. 2005;173(3):873–6.
25. Fu Q, Zhang Y, Barbagli G, Zhang J, Xie H, Sa Y, et al. Factors that influence the outcome of open urethroplasty for pelvis fracture urethral defect (PFUD): an observational study from a single high-volume tertiary care center World. J Urol. 2015;33:2169–75. https://doi.org/10.1007/s00345-015-1533-4.
26. El Darawany HM. Endoscopic urethral realignment of traumatic urethral disruption: a monocentric experience. Urol Ann. 2018;10(1):47–51. https://doi.org/10.4103/UA.UA_151_17.
27. Shrinivas RP, Dubey D. Primary urethral realignment should be the preferred option for the initial management of posterior urethral injuries. Indian J Urol. 2010;26(2):310–3. https://doi.org/10.4103/0970-1591.65416.
28. Lumen N, Kuehhas FE, Djakovic N, Kitrey ND, Serafetinidis E, Sharma DM. Review of the current management of lower urinary tract injuries by the EAU Trauma Guidelines Panel. Eur Urol. 2015;67(5):925–9. https://doi.org/10.1016/j.eururo.2014.12.035.
29. Dixon AN, Webb JC, Wenzel JL, Wolf JS Jr, Osterberg EC. Current management of pelvic fracture urethral injuries: to realign or not? Transl Androl Urol. 2018;7(4):593–602. https://doi.org/10.21037/tau.2018.01.14.

## Further Reading

Ahern DP, Kelly ME, Courtney D, Rausa E, Winter DC. The management of penetrating rectal and anal trauma: a systematic review. Injury. 2017;48:1133–8. https://doi.org/10.1016/j.injury.2017.03.002.

Boffard KD. Chapter 9.8: The urogenital System. In: Boffard KD, editor. Manual of definitive trauma care. 5th ed. Boca Raton, FL: CRC Press; 2019. ISBN: 9780367244682.

Bosarge PL, Como JJ, Fox N, Falck-Ytter Y, Haut ER, Dorian HA, et al. Management of penetrating extraperitoneal rectal injuries: an Eastern Association for the Surgery of Trauma practice management guideline. J Trauma Acute Care Surg. 2016;80:546–51.

Coburn M. Chapter 36, Genitourinary trauma. In: Mattox KL, Moore EE, Feliciano DV, editors. Trauma. 7th ed. New York: McGraw-Hill; 2013. ISBN: 978-0-07-171784-7.

Lopez HN, Focseneanu MA, Merritt DF. Genital injuries acute evaluation and management. Best Pract Res Clin Obstet Gynaecol. 2018;48:28–39. https://doi.org/10.1016/j.bpobgyn.2017.09.009.

Mouraviev VB, Coburn M, Santucci RA. The treatment of posterior urethral disruption associated with pelvic fractures: comparative experience of early realignment versus delayed urethroplasty. J Urol. 2005;173(3):873–6.

# Pelvic Trauma

## 102

Philip F. Stahel and Vincent P. Stahel

## 102.1 Introduction

**Learning Goals**
- Explain the mechanism-based classification of pelvic ring injuries and its correlation to the risk of hemorrhage and adverse patient outcomes.
- Describe the acute management strategies for patients with bleeding pelvic fractures.
- Recognize patients who are candidates for "damage control" external fixation and pelvic packing.
- Establish the concepts of initial stabilization and resuscitation with delayed scheduled definitive fixation of unstable pelvic ring injuries.

### 102.1.1 Epidemiology

Traumatic disruptions of the pelvic ring result from high-energy trauma mechanisms and represent a major source of life-threatening hemorrhage and preventable postinjury mortality in young trauma patients [1]. The main root cause of adverse outcomes is represented by the "occult" bleeding sources in the retroperitoneal space. While isolated pelvic ring injuries have a reported mortality of around 5%, the risk of death dramatically increases to 50–60% in polytrauma patients [2]. Patients who survive the injury are confronted with long-term rehabilitation and residual functional impairment related to gait and mobility, urogenital and neurological injuries, and chronic pain [3, 4].

### 102.1.2 Etiology

Most pelvic ring injuries are caused by blunt trauma forces. In the elderly patient population, same-level falls are the most frequent cause of stable pelvic fracture patterns. In contrast, in young patients, high-energy deceleration forces are required to disrupt the pelvic ring, mainly due to motor vehicle and motorcycle crashes, ATV and equestrian accidents, and falls from height [5]. The posterior sacroiliac ligamentous complex represents the strongest ligaments in the human body. Kinetic studies have revealed that an energy of around 150–200 G-forces is required to disrupt the integrity of the posterior pelvic ring [5]. Penetrating injuries rarely lead to unstable pelvic ring injuries.

P. F. Stahel (✉)
Department of Surgery, East Carolina University, Brody School of Medicine, Greenville, NC, USA

V. P. Stahel
University of Colorado (CU) Boulder, Boulder, CO, USA

### 102.1.3 Classification

The biomechanical stability of the pelvic ring relies on the integrity of the pubic symphysis and the posterior ligamentous complex. High-energy translational, rotational, and vertical shearing forces are required to disrupt the integrity and stability of the pelvic ring, leading to potentially exsanguinating retroperitoneal hemorrhage from venous presacral and paravesical plexus and cancellous bone from associated sacral fractures [6]. The vector of the impacting force has been shown to drive specific patterns of pelvic ring disruptions and determine their underlying extent of biomechanical instability and risk of associated bleeding. In the twenty-first century, the most widely used classification systems that serve as a basis for therapeutic decision-making include the alpha-numeric AO/OTA classification—which is historically based on the classification by Marvin Tile—and the mechanistic classification by Young and Burgess [7].

#### 102.1.3.1 History of Pelvic Fracture Classification

The first clinically relevant systematic classification of pelvic fractures was described in 1961 by Pennal and Sutherland, based on the mechanism of injury [8]. This system defines three distinct categories of pelvic ring injuries—(1) avulsion fractures, (2) "stable" fractures, and (3) "unstable" fractures—and attempts to correlate injury severity with outcomes. In 1980, Pennal and Tile introduced the aspect of fracture stability to the original Pennal/Sutherland classification and incorporated mechanisms and vectors of injury [9]. Furthermore, the Pennal/Tile classification served as a basis for therapeutic decision-making and management protocols of pelvic ring injuries. Currently used classification systems are largely based on the seminal historic publications by Tile, Pennal, and Sutherland [8].

#### 102.1.3.2 The Young and Burgess Classification (1990)

The classification by Young and Burgess is essentially based on the historic description by Pennal and Sutherland description. This mechanistic classification system is clinically relevant in the acute trauma setting by reflecting on the injury severity and taking into account the main vectors of impacting forces [10, 11].

In brief, *anteroposterior compression (APC)* mechanisms induce a gradual disruption of the pubic symphysis with an external rotation deformity of the injured hemipelvis ("open book"), leading to hinging forces on the sacroiliac (SI) joints and consecutive disruption of the anterior and posterior SI-ligaments. In contrast, *lateral compression (LC)* injuries lead to an internal rotation deformity of the injured hemipelvis and to gradual disruption of the SI-ligament complex by compressing forces, as opposed to the tensile forces resulting from APC injuries. While most high-energy pelvic ring injuries are based on predicted APC- and LC-type mechanisms, a rare, yet more lethal, entity is represented by *vertical shear (VS)* injuries due to massive axial loading forces, including high-speed acceleration/deceleration collisions and falls from significant heights. Vertical shear injuries are characterized by a complete unilateral disruption of the anterior and posterior pelvic ring, leading to external rotation and vertical translation of the injured hemipelvis. Any injury mechanism with multiple vectors which do not follow the standard mechanisms of APC, LC, or VS forces can be classified as a *combined mechanism (CM)* injury, which is typically highly unstable and associated with major retroperitoneal hemorrhage.

#### 102.1.3.3 The AO/OTA Classification (2018)

The "classic" AO/OTA classification for pelvic ring injuries is based on Marvin Tile's original classification system. A revised comprehensive version of the AO/OTA classification was recently published in 2018 [12]. In essence, the pelvic region is designated by the number 61, followed by an alphanumeric classification in ascending order by severity of injury (i.e., A > B > C and 1 > 2 > 3). While A-type injuries are considered stable fracture patterns, including the low-energy mechanisms seen in the elderly population after a same-level fall, B-type injuries are rotationally unstable, whereas C-type injuries reflect a complete pelvic ring disruptions with rotational and vertical instability. Aside from the simple anatomic/descriptive alpha-numeric designation, the recent revised 2018 AO/OTA compendium relies largely on the mechanistic classification by Young and Burgess (Fig. 102.1).

### 102.1.3.4 The WSES Classification (2017)

A shortcoming of the conventional classification systems (Tile, Young and Burgess, AO/OTA) is related to the lack of a predictive correlation between the anatomic and mechanistic criteria with the physiologic and hemodynamic response in patients with pelvic ring disruptions. To overcome this limitation, the *World Society of Emergency Surgery* (WSES) recently published an innovative classification in 2017 which is based on a combination of the classification by Young and Burgess in conjunction with hemodynamic stability, based on ATLS® guidelines (Table 102.1) [13]. The WSES classification stratifies pelvic ring injuries into three grades of severity:

1. *Minor* pelvic ring injuries (*WSES grade 1*): Mechanically (APC-1, LC-1) and hemodynamically stable injury patterns.

**Fig. 102.1** Comparison of the AO/OTA and Young and Burgess classification systems for pelvic ring injuries, based on injury mechanism and pelvic ring stability

| AO/OTA (Tile) | Young&Burgess | Description |
|---|---|---|
| **A-type:** Stable pelvic ring 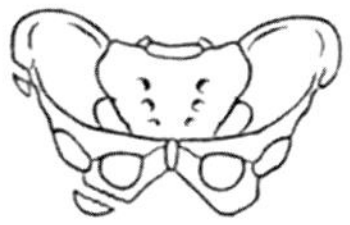 | • APC-1<br>• LC-1 | Iliac wing Fx;<br>Pubic rami Fx;<br>Pubic symphysis sprain (<2.5cm) |
| **B-type:** Rotationally unstable, vertically stable 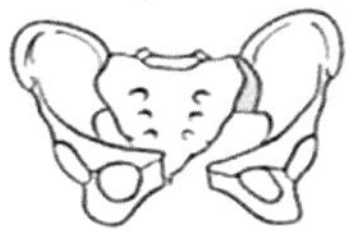 | • APC-2 | Pubic symphysis disruption (>2.5cm) *"Open book" injury* |
| 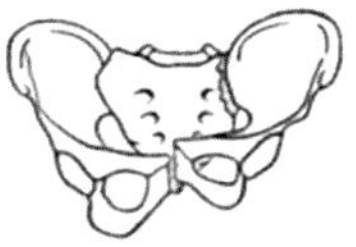 | • LC-2 | Unstable lateral compression injuries *"Crescent" Fx* *"Bucket handle" Fx* |
| 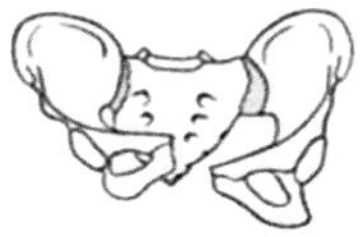 | • LC-3 | Combined B1/B2 type, bilaterally unstable *"Windswept pelvis"* |
| **C-type:** Rotationally AND vertically unstable 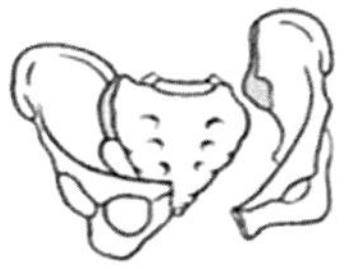 | • APC-3<br>• VS<br>• CM | Complete detachment of hemipelvis, uni-/ or bilateral, posterior injury through SI-joint or sacrum *"Vertical shear" injury* |

**Table 102.1** WSES pelvic injury severity classification

|  | WSES grade | Young-Burgess classification | Haemodynamic | Mechanic | CT-scan | First-line treatment |
|---|---|---|---|---|---|---|
| Minor | WSES grade I | APC I or LC I | Stable | Stable | Yes | Non-operative management (NOM) |
| Moderate | WSES grade II | LC II/III or APC II/III | Stable | Unstable | Yes | Pelvic binder in the field ± Angioembolization (if blush on CT-scan) Operative management (OM): Anterior external fixation[a] |
|  | WSES grade III | VS or CM | Stable | Unstable | Yes | Pelvic Binder in the field ± Angioembolization (if blush at CT-scan) Operative management (OM): C-clamp[a] |
| Severe | WSES grade IV | Any injury type associated with hemodynamic instability | Unstable | Irrelevant | No | Pelvic binder in the field Preperitoneal pelvic packing ± Mechanical fixation ± REBOA ± Angioembolization |

*Adopted with permission from: Coccolini F et al., World J. Emerg. Surg. 2017, 12:5. (Creative Commons 4.0 International License)*
*LC* lateral compression, *APC* antero-posterior compression, *VS* vertical shear, *CM* combined mechanism, *NOM* non-operative management, *OM* operative management, *REBOA* resuscitative endovascular balloon occlusion of the aorta
[a] Patients who are hemodynamically stable and mechanically unstable with no other lesions requiring treatment and with a negative CT-scan can proceed directly to definitive mechanical stabilization

2. *Moderate* pelvic ring injuries: Mechanically unstable (*WSES grade 2*: LC-2, LC-3, APC-2, APC-3; *WSES grade 3*: VS or CM) with hemodynamic stability and/or adequate response to resuscitation ("responders").
3. *Severe* pelvic ring injuries (*WSES grade 4*): Any hemodynamically unstable injury pattern with patients at risk for acute exsanguinating hemorrhage, independent of the mechanistic fracture classification ("nonresponders").

Based on this innovative anatomic/physiologic classification, the WSES recently published international expert consensus guidelines to provide a classification-based decision-making algorithm for the management of patients with bleeding pelvic ring injuries (Fig. 102.2) [13].

### 102.1.4 Pathophysiology

The traumatic hemorrhage in high-energy pelvic ring disruptions relates in large part to venous bleeding sources in the retroperitoneal space (>90%) and rarely to arterial bleeding sources (<10%) [14]. The main pelvic bleeding sources originate from extensive retroperitoneal plexuses and cancellous bone bleeding from the posterior pelvic elements (sacral fractures, SI-joint disruption) [14]. In addition, about one-third of all patients with traumatic pelvic ring disruptions are coagulopathic on admission, and the presence of coagulopathy is associated with significantly increased postinjury mortality from exsanguinating hemorrhage [15, 16].

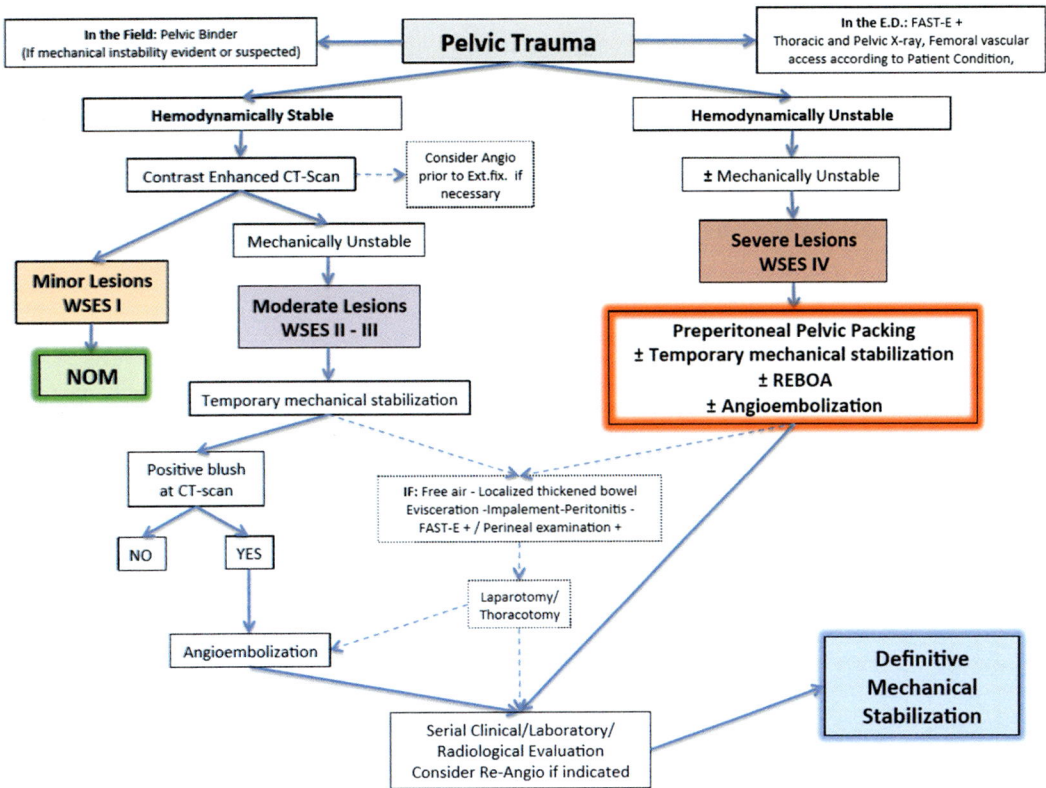

**Fig. 102.2** International consensus guideline by the World Society for Emergency Surgery (WSES) for the acute management of pelvic ring injuries. Adopted with permission from: Coccolini F et al., World J. Emerg. Surg. 2017, 12:5. (Creative Commons 4.0 International License)

## 102.2 Diagnosis

### 102.2.1 Clinical Presentation

Patients with severe traumatic pelvic ring injuries subsequent to high-energy trauma mechanisms typically present with clinical signs of shock, as traditionally described in the ATLS manual ("clinical windows to the microcirculation") [5]. Unstable pelvic ring injuries are challenging to diagnose by clinical examination alone. In extreme cases with complete pelvic ring disruption, a palpable diastasis of the pubic symphysis may be found in conjunction with local point tenderness over the anterior pelvic ring. The sensitivity of a posterior pelvic ring exam is extremely low. Many polytrauma patients present with distracting injuries and may not be able to reliably describe posterior tenderness on palpation over the sacrum and SI-joint. In vertical shear injuries, limb shortening and external rotation may be evident on the side of the vertical hemipelvis displacement. Documentation of peripheral neurovascular status is imperative due to the high risk of associated vascular trauma and lumbosacral plexus injuries. Finally, there is a high incidence of urologic injuries including traumatic bladder rupture and urethral rupture. A scrotal hematoma, blood at the meatus urethrae, and perineal ecchymosis are subtle indicators of anterior pelvic ring injuries and potential associated urogenital trauma. Finally, a rectal and vaginal exam is mandatory to detect an occult open pelvic fracture [5].

## 102.2.2 Tests

### 102.2.2.1 Laboratory Tests

Serum lactate and base deficit represent sensitive markers for early recognition of occult hemorrhage and "hidden shock" [17, 18]. The amount of lactate produced by anaerobic glycolysis is an indirect marker of oxygen debt, tissue hypoperfusion, and the severity of hemorrhagic shock. In addition, base deficit values derived from arterial blood gas analysis provide an indirect estimation of global tissue acidosis from impaired tissue perfusion. A landmark study from the 1990s on multiple injured patients correlated lactate clearance with survival [17]. The study results demonstrated a 100% survival rate in patients whose lactate levels returned to the normal range ($\leq 2$ mmol/L) within 24 h, whereas survival decreased to just above 10% in those patients with elevated lactate levels above 2 mmol/L for more than 48 h postinjury. Similar to the predictive value of lactate levels, the initial base deficit has been established as a potent independent predictor of mortality in patients with traumatic-hemorrhagic shock [18]. The extent of base deficit has been stratified into three categories of severity (mild, −3 to −5 mEq/L; moderate, −6 to −9 mEq/L; severe, less than −10 mEq/L), and a significant correlation has been demonstrated between the admission base deficit and transfusion requirements within the first 24 h and the risk of post-traumatic organ failure and postinjury death. In contrast to the predictive value of lactate and base deficit, other traditional laboratory tests, including hemoglobin and hematocrit, are *not* sensitive in reflecting the extent of pelvic hemorrhage or predictive of patient outcomes [14].

The presence of postinjury coagulopathy is best determined with bedside "point-of-care" testing by thromboelastography (TEG) or rotational thromboelastometry (ROTEM). These real-time diagnostic methods allow for a targeted resuscitation from traumatic-hemorrhagic shock and coagulopathy with blood products and improved survival rates [15, 16, 19].

### 102.2.2.2 Diagnostic Imaging

Standard diagnostic imaging for trauma patients include a plain anteroposterior pelvic radiograph in the ED trauma bay to screen for a pelvic fracture, per ATLS® protocol [5]. In the presence of a pelvic fracture, additional inlet and outlet radiographs must be obtained to assess the integrity of the pelvic ring and to determine the extent of vertical and rotational displacement in case of pelvic ring disruptions. In addition, most trauma patients with significant injury mechanisms undergo standard radiographic assessment by a multislice CT (MSCT) scanning, which includes the abdomen/pelvic region, if indicated. The MSCT allows to obtain two-dimensional and three-dimensional reconstruction images of the pelvis.

## 102.3 Treatment

### 102.3.1 Medical Treatment

#### 102.3.1.1 Volume Resuscitation

Patients with traumatic-hemorrhagic shock from bleeding pelvic fractures undergo fluid resuscitation and blood product replacement, including mass transfusion protocol (MTP), if indicated. Recent randomized prospective trials revealed that the use of goal-directed, TEG-guided resuscitation strategies resulted in improved postinjury survival rates compared to standard mass transfusion protocols guided by conventional laboratory testing [19]. The specific aspects of volume resuscitation in trauma patients are described in detail elsewhere in this textbook.

#### 102.3.1.2 Pelvic Binders

The application of pelvic binders or circumferential sheets represents a life-saving measure for acute bleeding control in patients with unstable pelvic ring disruptions [20, 21]. Experimental human cadaveric studies have demonstrated that circumferential sheets are equivalent in providing temporary biomechanical stability in unstable pelvic ring injuries to commercial pelvic binders and external pelvic fixation [22]. In addition, systematic reviews have demonstrated the effectiveness of pelvic binders in the temporary restoration adequate blood pressure in hemodynamically unstable pelvic ring disruptions [23]. Due to the potential risk of soft tissue complications from prolonged compression by pelvic binders, it is recommended to remove pelvic binders as soon as physiologically justifiable and to consider replacing binders by early external pelvic fixation, if indicated (see below).

### 102.3.1.3 REBOA

For patients with exsanguinating hemorrhage "*in extremis*," the option of a resuscitative endovascular balloon occlusion of the aorta (REBOA) has recently resurged as a valid alternative to the classic "ED thoracotomy" (EDT) with cross-clamping of the aorta [24, 25]. The REBOA procedure allows for a minimally invasive (percutaneous) modality of temporary hemorrhage control in hypotensive trauma patients with a systolic blood pressure <80 mmHg on presentation. In brief, the REBOA technique consists of a percutaneous femoral arterial cannulation with a size 7 Charrière/French gauge balloon catheter, either by direct arterial palpation or by ultrasound-guided cannulation. The approximate distance of catheter insertion is measured externally with the bottom of the balloon located at the umbilicus. This estimated distance should be documented prior to catheter insertion. The balloon catheter is then advanced to zone III of the aorta, i.e., just proximal to the aortic bifurcation and distal the most caudal renal artery. Before balloon inflation, vital signs are again verified and documented. The balloon is then gradually inflated using a mixture of saline and contrast dye, with a maximal inflation volume of 24 cc, whereas typical volumes for aortic occlusion are around or less than 15 cc. Documentation after balloon inflation includes vital signs, catheter insertion depth, and exact time of inflation. If available, radiologic imaging is used to confirm proper catheter placement in aortic zone III (Fig. 102.3) [1]. Patients are then taken to the operating room for emergent surgical bleeding control, including external fixation and pelvic packing, if indicated

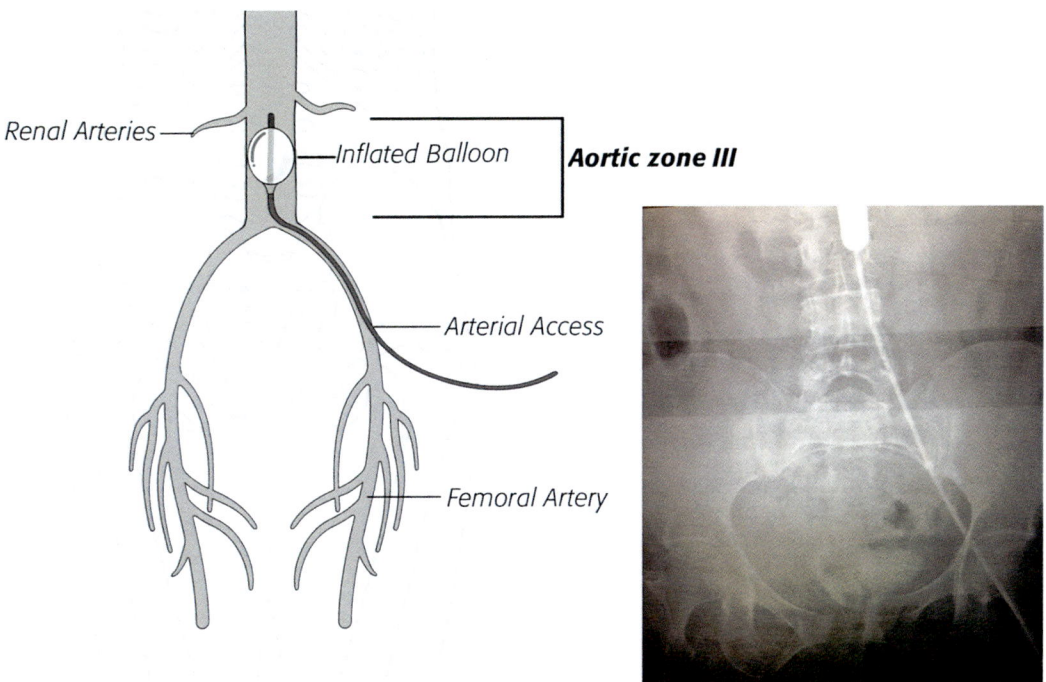

**Fig. 102.3** Schematic depiction of the REBOA application for temporary bleeding control in hemodynamically unstable pelvic fractures. (Image © Philip F. Stahel & Ernest E. Moore, 2017)

(see below). The intuitive advantages of endovascular techniques over resuscitative thoracotomies have to be balanced against a technical learning curve for REBOA with an associated risk of severe iatrogenic complications.

### 102.3.1.4 Angioembolization

Historically, interventional angioembolization represented the main technical option for obtaining bleeding control in hemodynamically unstable pelvic fractures [26]. However, the pertinent literature suggests that arterial injuries represent less than 10% of bleeding sources associated with pelvic fractures, and only around 2% overall are successfully coiled [14]. In addition, the average time of more than 2 h from the decision to proceeding to interventional radiology until successful embolization is achieved introduces and unjustified time delay in the resuscitation of critically injured patients during the "golden hour" for patients at risk [5]. Recent evidence suggests that the proactive protocolized approach of initial pelvic packing and external fixation, followed by secondary angioembolization in case of ongoing bleeding, provides superior patient outcomes and decreased blood product transfusions [27–29]. Furthermore, pelvic packing precludes from the risk of iatrogenic interventional complications, such as perineal necrosis, resulting from the traditional pre-emptive coiling of internal iliac arteries [30].

## 102.3.2 Surgical Treatment

### 102.3.2.1 External Pelvic Fixation

External fixation of the pelvic ring represents an effective resuscitative tool and "damage control" strategy for acute hemorrhage control by decreasing the extent of retroperitoneal bleeding through closure and reduction of the pelvic ring and adjunctive stability by external fixation [31]. Furthermore, pelvic packing has been shown to be effective only in conjunction with external fixation, in order to provide a counter-pressure from the pelvic ring to the applied lap sponges in the retroperitoneal space [31]. As part of the acute resuscitation strategy, any unstable pelvic ring injury with associated disruption of posterior element stability (WSES grade 2 and 3), particularly in conjunction with hemodynamic instability (WSES grade 4), should be considered for temporary external pelvic fixation [13].

From a technical decision-making perspective, most APC- or LC-equivalent injury patterns are preferably stabilized by anterior external fixation, either through the iliac crest route or through a fluoroscopy-guided supraacetabular route [31]. Anterior pelvic external fixation allows for a closed reduction of the externally malrotated hemipelvis in APC-2 and APC-3 injuries ("close the book") and for a provisional reduction and retention of the internally malrotated hemipelvis in LC-2 and LC-3 injury patterns. In contrast to the fast application of a "damage control" iliac crest frame, the supraacetabular route for external fixation allows for improved stability of the external fixator frame, however, at the cost of requiring strict fluoroscopy-guided pin placement with dedicated views of the supraacetabular corridor [31]. In contrast to APC- and LC-injury patterns, vertical shear (VS) injuries are inadequately stabilized by anterior external fixation frames, due to the complete instability of the posterior elements through the iliosacral joint. For these rare injury patterns, the pelvic "C-clamp" has been shown to provide temporary stabilization of the posterior pelvic elements with effective control of associated retroperitoneal hemorrhage [32]. However, the use of a C-clamp should be restricted to selected indications (VS injuries with exsanguinating hemorrhage) and to adequately trained orthopedic trauma surgeons in order to mitigate the risk of serious intraoperative complications associated with inconsiderate C-clamp application. Skeletal traction represents an optional minimal-invasive measure of temporary pelvic ring stabilization in VS-type injuries which provides temporary relative stability and restoration of vertical hemipelvis displacement. The main downside of skeletal traction relates to patient immobilization in supine position which impedes the appropriate patient positioning for the care of associated injuries. Finally, the proactive modality of acute placement of a percutaneous "antishock" iliosacral screw has been described as a technique to rapidly stabilize the posterior pelvic ring as an adjunct to anterior pelvic external fixation [33].

### 102.3.2.2 Pelvic Packing

Pelvic packing was initially described in the 1980s and 1990s in Hannover, Germany, and Zurich, Switzerland, as a technique of transabdominal open pelvic packing through a "damage control" explorative laparotomy [34, 35]. These early studies demonstrated that severely injured patients with associated pelvic ring injuries have improved outcomes by early surgical "damage control" intervention, including temporary external fixation of unstable pelvic fractures, transabdominal pelvic packing, and surgical bleeding control. The pelvic packing technique was later modified in Denver, Colorado, to a concept of "direct" preperitoneal pelvic packing (PPP) by applying a distinct surgical technique through a suprapubic midline incision that allows packing directly into the space of Retzius, without the necessity of opening the retroperitoneal compartment through a laparotomy [28]. When using the new PPP technique, a midline laparotomy can still be performed through a separate proximal midline incision, if a laparotomy is indicated simultaneously for the management of associated intraabdominal bleeding sources. Importantly, the technique of using two separate midline incisions for pelvic packing and explorative laparotomy appears to be safe with regard to the potential risk of postoperative infections subsequent to pelvic depacking and delayed definitive orthopedic fracture fixation. Recent studies demonstrated that the pelvic packing protocol incorporated as part of a standardized institutional guidelines led to a significant decrease in blood product utilization and to improved patient outcomes [30]. The current pertinent literature supports the notion that pelvic packing represents an effective technique for acute hemorrhage control that is associated with a significantly reduced mortality compared to conventional measures without pelvic packing [13, 14].

### 102.3.3 Outcomes

More than 10-year follow-up data from high-volume level I trauma centers with a protocolized pelvic packing strategy revealed that the postinjury mortality from acute exsanguinating pelvic hemorrhage was reduced to 2% after resuscitative measures that include PPP and external pelvic fixation [30]. Definitive surgical pelvic ring fixation is typically performed subsequent to successful resuscitation from hemorrhage shock and associated life-threatening injuries [33]. In this regard, the recent literature demonstrates that there is no increased postoperative infection rate subsequent to open reduction and internal fixation of pelvic ring injuries with preceding pelvic packing and depacking, which corroborates the safety of the PPP protocol [36]. Due to the proven benefits of improving patient outcomes, pelvic packing was introduced into the recommended management algorithm of the 10th edition of the ATLS® manual (Fig. 102.4) [5].

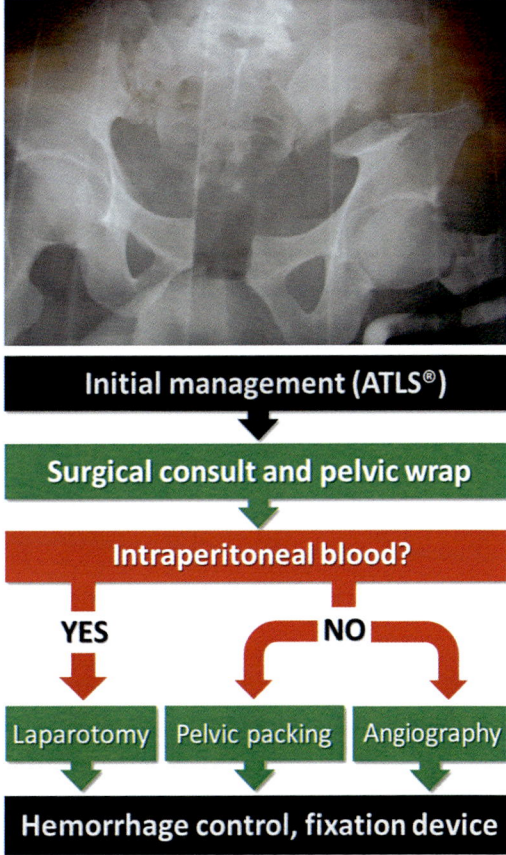

**Fig. 102.4** Advanced Trauma Life Support (ATLS®) decision-making algorithm for the acute management of patients with hemodynamically unstable pelvic ring injuries

### Dos and Don'ts
- Maintain a high level of suspicion for significant occult retroperitoneal hemorrhage with "hidden shock" in patients with high-energy pelvic ring injuries.
- Avoid a delay to definitive bleeding control, by applying proactive strategies including "damage control" pelvic external fixation and pelvic packing.
- Utilize point-of-care testing by thromboelastography and lactate and base deficit as sensitive laboratory parameters of choice to determine the patients' response to resuscitation.

### Take-Home Messages
- High-energy pelvic ring disruptions are associated with major blood loss from retroperitoneal bleeding sources and continue to represent a global cause of potentially preventable postinjury mortality from exsanguinating hemorrhage.
- Resuscitative endovascular balloon occlusion of the aorta (REBOA) represents an effective and rapid bedside procedure in the emergency department for temporary bleeding control in hypotensive patients with bleeding pelvic fractures.
- Injury mechanism-based classification systems are essential for understanding the severity of pelvic ring disruptions and to guide in therapeutic decision-making.
- A protocolized approach of early external fixation with direct preperitoneal pelvic packing and delayed angioembolization in case of ongoing hemodynamic instability has been shown to significantly reduce postinjury mortality from acute exsanguinating hemorrhage.
- Recently published international expert consensus guidelines provide standardized algorithms for multidisciplinary care and classification-based decision-making toward improving outcomes for patients with severe pelvic ring disruptions.

### Multiple Choice Questions
1. The high mortality of acute pelvic ring disruptions is mainly attributed to:
   A. Associated bowel injuries
   B. Open fractures
   C. Sepsis
   D. **Hemorrhage**
2. Pelvic ring injuries are described by injury mechanism using the following classification system:
   A. **Young and Burgess**
   B. Tile
   C. AO
   D. All of the above
3. Which statement about pelvic binders is correct:
   A. The use of pelvic binders is restricted to the inpatient setting
   B. **Plain sheets can replace commercial pelvic binders**
   C. Pelvic binders should be left in place as long as possible
   D. Pelvic binders are exclusively indicated for "open book" injuries
4. Which is the most sensitive indicator of pelvic hemorrhage:
   A. AO fracture classification
   B. Systolic blood pressure on ED arrival
   C. **Lactate or base deficit**
   D. Hemoglobin or hematocrit
5. What are potential measures of pelvic hemorrhage control:
   A. Angioembolization
   B. Pelvic packing
   C. REBOA
   D. **All of the above**
6. The standard diagnostic workup of pelvic ring injuries includes all of the following, except:
   A. Anteroposterior pelvic radiograph
   B. CT scan
   C. **MRI**
   D. Inlet/outlet views

7. The following statement about pelvic hemorrhage is correct:
   A. Point-of-care resuscitation by TEG or ROTEM does not require blood product administration.
   B. **"Hidden shock" is recognized by base deficit and lactate levels.**
   C. REBOA can be used for definitive pelvic hemorrhage control.
   D. Absence of hypotension indicates a low level of concern for retroperitoneal bleeding.
8. Which of the following treatments has been proven to effectively reduce mortality in hemodynamically unstable pelvic ring injuries:
   A. Mass transfusion protocols
   B. Early pelvic fracture fixation
   C. **Pelvic packing with external fixation**
   D. Tranexamic acid administration
9. The WSES guideline is based on the following parameters:
   A. Anatomic pelvic ring classification (Tile)
   B. Mechanistic pelvic ring classification (Young and Burgess)
   C. Hemodynamic stability (ATLS® protocol)
   D. **Young and Burgess classification and ATLS® protocol**
10. The following statement about pelvic packing is wrong:
    A. **Pelvic packing increases the risk of surgical site infections after pelvic depacking and definitive fracture fixation.**
    B. Pelvic packing achieves faster hemorrhage control than angioembolization.
    C. Pelvic packing is most effective when performed with adjunctive external fixation.
    D. Pelvic packing represents a recommended treatment option in the ATLS® protocol.

## References

1. Stahel PF, Burlew CC, Moore EE. Current trends in the management of hemodynamically unstable pelvic ring injuries. Curr Opin Crit Care. 2017;23(6):511–9.
2. Chen HT, Wang YC, Hsieh CC, Su LT, Wu SC, Lo YS, Chang CC, Tsai CH. Trends and predictors of mortality in unstable pelvic ring fracture: a 10-year experience with a multidisciplinary institutional protocol. World J Emerg Surg. 2019;14:61.
3. Hermans E, Brouwers L, van Gent T, Biert J, de Jongh MAC, Lansink KWW, Edwards MJR. Quality of life after pelvic ring fractures: long-term outcomes. A multicentre study. Injury. 2019;50(6):1216–22.
4. Banierink H, Reininga IHF, Heineman E, Wendt KW, Ten Duis K, Ijpma FFA. Long-term physical functioning and quality of life after pelvic ring injuries. Arch Orthop Trauma Surg. 2019;139(9):1225–33.
5. American College of Surgeons Committee on Trauma. Advanced trauma life support (ATLS) student course manual. 10th ed. Chicago, IL: ACS-COT; 2018.
6. Stahel PF, Moore EE. Modern strategies for the management of high-energy pelvic fractures in the twenty-first century. In: Aseni P, De Carlis L, Mazzola A, Grande AM, editors. Operative techniques and recent advances in acute care and emergency surgery. Heidelberg: Springer; 2019. p. 261–71.
7. Fakler JKM, Stahel PF, Lundy DW. Classification of pelvic ring injuries. In: Smith WR, Ziran BH, Morgan SJ, editors. Fractures of the pelvis and acetabulum. New York: Informa Healthcare; 2007. p. 11–25.
8. Stahel PF, Hammerberg EM. History of pelvic fracture management: a review. World J Emerg Surg. 2016;11:18.
9. Tile M. Acute pelvic fractures: I. Causation and classification. J Am Acad Orthop Surg. 1996;4(3):143–51.
10. Burgess AR, Eastridge BJ, Young JW, et al. Pelvic ring disruptions: effective classification system and treatment protocols. J Trauma. 1990;30(70):848–56.
11. Young JW, Resnik CS. Fracture of the pelvis: current concepts of classification. Am J Roentgenol. 1990;155(6):1169–75.
12. Meinberg EG, Agel J, Roberts CS, Karam MD, Kellam JF. Fracture and dislocation classification compendium - 2018. J Orthop Trauma. 2018;32(Suppl 1):S1–170.
13. Coccolini F, Stahel PF, Montori G, et al. Pelvic trauma: WSES classification and guidelines. World J Emerg Surg. 2017;12:5.
14. Rossaint R, Bouillon B, Cerny V, et al. Management of bleeding following major trauma: an updated European guideline. Crit Care. 2010;14(2):R52.
15. Kashuk JL, Moore EE, Sawyer M, et al. Postinjury coagulopathy management: goal directed resuscitation via POC thrombelastography. Ann Surg. 2010;251(4):604–14.
16. Stahel PF, Moore EE, Schreier SL, Flierl MA, Kashuk JL. Transfusion strategies in postinjury coagulopathy. Curr Opin Anaesthesiol. 2009;22(2):289–98.

17. Abramson D, Scalea TM, Hitchcock R, Trooskin SZ, Henry SM, Greenspan J. Lactate clearance and survival following injury. J Trauma. 1993;35(4):584–8; discussion 588–9.
18. Davis JW, Parks SN, Kaups KL, Gladen HE, O'Donnell-Nicol S. Admission base deficit predicts transfusion requirements and risk of complications. J Trauma. 1996;41(5):769–74.
19. Gonzalez E, Moore EE, Moore HB, et al. Goal-directed hemostatic resuscitation of trauma-induced coagulopathy: a pragmatic randomized clinical trial comparing a viscoelastic assay to conventional coagulation assays. Ann Surg. 2016;263(6):1051–9.
20. McCreary D, Cheng C, Lin ZC, Nehme Z, Fitzgerald M, Mitra B. Haemodynamics as a determinant of need for pre-hospital application of a pelvic circumferential compression device in adult trauma patients. Injury. 2020;51(1):4–9.
21. Jarvis S, Salottolo K, Meinig R, et al. Utilization of pre-hospital pelvic circumferential compression devices for pelvic fractures: survey of U.S. level I trauma centers. Patient Saf Surg. 2020;14:12.
22. Prasarn ML, Conrad B, Small J, Horodyski M, Rechtine GR. Comparison of circumferential pelvic sheeting versus the T-POD on unstable pelvic injuries: a cadaveric study of stability. Injury. 2013;44(12):1756–9.
23. Bakhshayesh P, Boutefnouchet T, Tötterman A. Effectiveness of non-invasive external pelvic compression: a systematic review of the literature. Scand J Trauma Resusc Emerg Med. 2016;24:73.
24. Coccolini F, Ceresoli M, McGreevy DT, et al. Aortic balloon occlusion (REBOA) in pelvic ring injuries: preliminary results of the ABO Trauma Registry. Updat Surg. 2020;72(2):527–36.
25. Jarvis S, Kelly M, Mains C, et al. A descriptive survey on the use of resuscitative endovascular balloon occlusion of the aorta (REBOA) for pelvic fractures at US level I trauma centers. Patient Saf Surg. 2019; 13:43.
26. Rossaint R, Duranteau J, Stahel PF, Spahn DR. Nonsurgical treatment of major bleeding. Anesthesiol Clin. 2007;25(1):35–48.
27. Osborn PM, Smith WR, Moore EE, Cothren CC, Morgan SJ, Williams AE, Stahel PF. Direct retroperitoneal pelvic packing versus pelvic angiography: a comparison of two management protocols for haemodynamically unstable pelvic fractures. Injury. 2009;40(1):54–60.
28. Burlew CC, Moore EE, Smith WR, Johnson JL, Biffl WL, Barnett CC, Stahel PF. Preperitoneal pelvic packing/external fixation with secondary angioembolization: optimal care for life-threatening hemorrhage from unstable pelvic fractures. J Am Coll Surg. 2011;212(4):628–35.
29. Chiara O, di Fratta E, Mariani A, et al. Efficacy of extra-peritoneal pelvic packing in hemodynamically unstable pelvic fractures, a Propensity Score Analysis. World J Emerg Surg. 2016;11:22.
30. Burlew CC, Moore EE, Stahel PF, et al. Preperitoneal pelvic packing reduces mortality in patients with life-threatening hemorrhage due to unstable pelvic fractures. J Trauma Acute Care Surg. 2017;82(2):233–42.
31. Stahel PF, Mauffrey C, Smith WR, et al. External fixation for acute pelvic ring injuries: decision making and technical options. J Trauma Acute Care Surg. 2013;75(5):882–7.
32. Lustenberger T, Meier C, Benninger E, Lenzlinger PM, Keel MJ. C-clamp and pelvic packing for control of hemorrhage in patients with pelvic ring disruption. J Emerg Trauma Shock. 2011;4(4):477–82.
33. Stahel PF, Auston DA. Pelvic ring injuries. In: Pape HC, Moore EE, Borrelli J, Stahel PF, Pfeifer R, editors. Textbook of polytrauma management: a multidisciplinary approach. Springer-Nature; 2021.
34. Pohlemann T, Culemann U, Gansslen A, Tscherne H. Severe pelvic injury with pelvic mass hemorrhage: determining severity of hemorrhage and clinical experience with emergency stabilization [German]. Unfallchirurg. 1996;99(10):734–43.
35. Ertel W, Keel M, Eid K, Platz A, Trentz O. Control of severe hemorrhage using C-clamp and pelvic packing in multiply injured patients with pelvic ring disruption. J Orthop Trauma. 2001;15(7):468–74.
36. Stahel PF, Moore EE, Burlew CC, et al. Preperitoneal pelvic packing is not associated with an increased risk of surgical site infections after internal anterior pelvic ring fixation. J Orthop Trauma. 2019;33:601–7.

# Ruptured Abdominal Aortic Aneurysm (rAAA)

## 103

Tal M. Hörer

> **Learning Goals**
> - Understand the background of ruptured abdominal aortic aneurysm and its etiology and pathology.
> - Discuss the diagnostic strategies and clinical decision-making process.
> - Discuss the treatment options and possibilities.

## 103.1 Introduction and Overview

### 103.1.1 Etiology and Epidemiology

Abdominal aortic aneurysm (AAA) involves widening of the aortic wall (all three layers, meaning a true aneurysm); an aorta is considered pathologic when it exceeds 1.5 times the diameter of the normal aorta. The process of widening the abdominal aorta may lead to rupture (rAAA)

---

T. M. Hörer (✉)
Vascular Unit, Department of Cardiothoracic and Vascular Surgery and Department of General Surgery, Faculty of Life Science, Örebro University Hospital and University, Örebro, Sweden

Visiting Professor and Attending Vascular Surgeon at the Carmel Hospital, Technion Institute Medical Faculty, Haifa, Israel
e-mail: tal.horer@regionorebrolan.se;
http://www.jevtm.com

and death [1–3]. The incidence of AAA is reported to be around 4–8% for men aged over 65, with a lower incidence for women and varies worldwide (1–2%). Known risk factors include smoking, hypertension, male gender, and age greater than 60 and Caucasian ethnicity [2, 4–6]. In general, the larger the aneurysm, the greater is the risk it might rupture, but the risk of rupture of small AAAs (up to 4 cm) is very low (Fig. 103.1) [5, 7–9]. Rupture of the abdominal aorta carries extreme risk and very high morality [9–12]. The mortality for rAAA surgery is estimated to be around 40% but ranges from about 25% to 60%, depending on patient group, methods, and reporting center [5, 10, 13]. This is the main reason why abdominal aneurysms should be treated electively, with a mortality rate as low as 1–4% [5, 14–16].

The risk of rupture increases exponentially with aneurysms over 50 mm diameter in women and 55 mm in men, or when the growth rate is more than 5 mm per year, as reported in large population studies, meta-analyses, and major vascular guidelines [1, 2, 5, 7, 14, 17, 18]. These data are based on atherosclerotic aneurysms in general, and there are less clear data on size and risk of rupture in other types of AAA, such as mycotic (inflammatory or infected) AAA, ulcerous or connective tissue-related AAA or post-dissection AAA, or in traumatic pseudoaneurysm [2, 5, 8]. The form of the aneurysm is important (fusiform, oval,

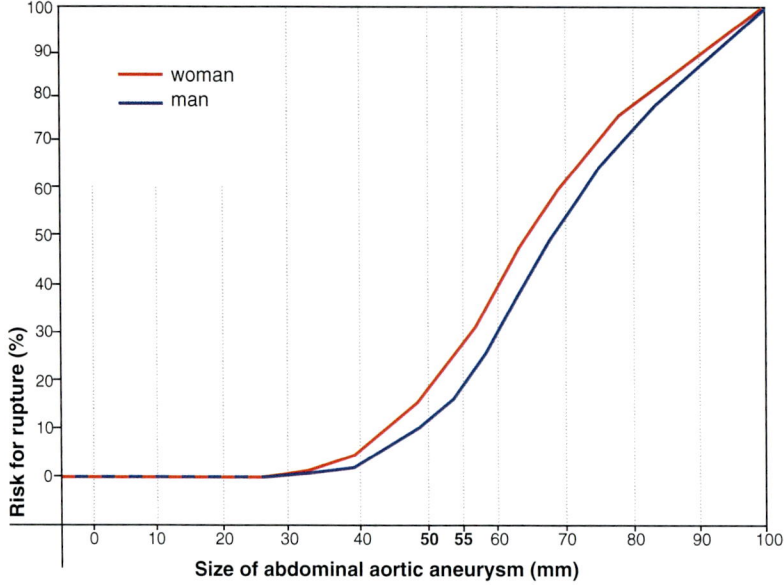

**Fig. 103.1** General illustration of the estimated annual risk of abdominal aortic aneurysm rupture in men (blue) and women (red). Small aneurysms can rupture but, as size increases, in general to a diameter over 50–55 mm, the annual risk increases considerably. Many variables, such as aortic correct sizing, form of aneurysm, and biological age and surgical risk, are important when considering repair. This graph is for illustrative purpose only and based on published and register data as well as the author's hospital cohort and experience

thrombus load, ulceration, etc.) since it is believed that increased localized pressure on the aortic wall plays a central role in the risk of rupture. Even here, recommendations are based on expert opinion, and there are no clear data on the risk of rupture and relation to size in these pathologies [5]. It is commonly believed by clinicians worldwide that penetrating or circular aneurysms, and mycotic ones, may rupture in even smaller sizes (as small as 35–40 mm). In general, in patients with AAAs of more than 30–40 mm, there should be vascular consultation to estimate risk and decide on follow-up. Genetic factors and familial anamnesis play a central role in risk of aneurysm and rupture and should be investigated as needed during the routine checkup for AAA [3].

The recommended follow-up by computed tomographic angiography (CTA) or ultrasound should be conducted annually up to a size of 40–45 mm of the aneurysm but also depends, as stated, on its growth rate and format [1, 5, 18]. This chapter concentrates on ruptured abdominal aortic aneurysm diagnosis and treatment.

### 103.1.2 Classifications and Mechanisms of AAA and rAAA

There are several classifications of aortic aneurysms, depending on their location and extent [3, 14, 19–22]. Iliac aneurysms can be isolated or form part of aortoiliac aneurysms or other visceral aneurysms. If the aneurysms involve the thoracic aorta, they are called thoracoabdominal aneurysms, but rupture of these aneurysms is beyond the scope of this chapter. Isolated AAAs can be infrarenal, pararenal, or para-visceral (Fig. 103.2), while the majority of treated rAAAs are infrarenal. The definition of extent of the aneurysm is crucial when discussing treatment options. The more extensive the aneurysm (i.e., pararenal and more cranially, thoracoabdominal), the more complicated and time-consuming is its repair, and

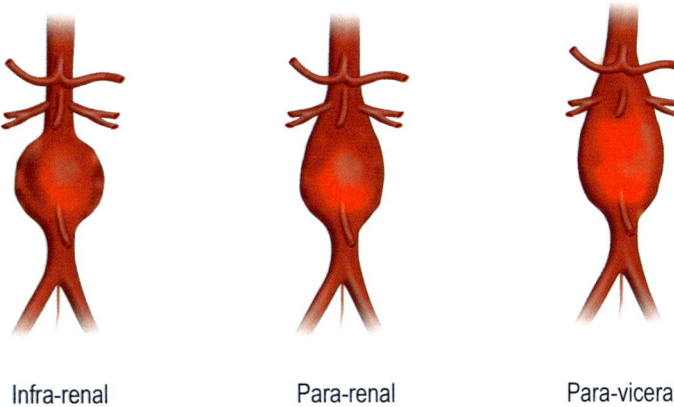

**Fig. 103.2** Illustrations of the normal anatomy of aortic and abdominal aneurysms. There are many configurations and annotations of AAA, but they can simply be called infrarenal, pararenal, and para-visceral abdominal aneurysms. The extent of the aneurysm is important when considering repair of ruptured and non-ruptured aneurysms. Infrarenal aneurysms are considered clinically as easy to repair electively and when ruptured. More extensive aneurysms demand a highly experienced team for both elective and acute repair

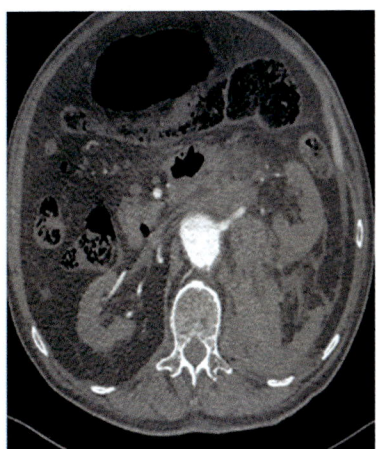
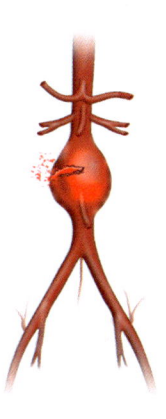
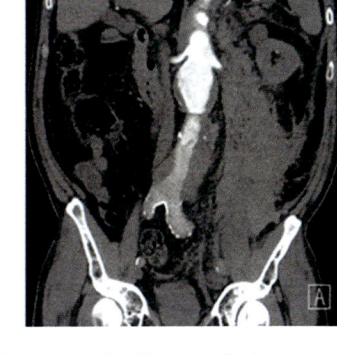

**Fig. 103.3** Aortic rupture can be in different, unpredictable parts of the aneurysm, but are probably at the weakest part of the aortic wall. The rupture may be limited, or contained, or free with massive bleeding, usually into retroperitoneal space. The computed tomographic angiography (CTA) seen here shows a large retroperitoneal hematoma

patient survival in the case of rupture is lower than for an isolated infrarenal aneurysm [3, 5].

Rupture (Fig. 103.3) is defined as a sudden disruption of the aneurysm wall, with limited bleeding in the aortic wall and surrounding tissue or extensive bleeding into the retroperitoneal or/and the peritoneal space. Free rupture leads to death within a short period of time. It is estimated that around 50% of rAAA patients die at the scene of rupture [3, 5, 23]. The term "contained rAAA" is controversial but clinically useful when observing patients with a limited (small) amount of blood outside the aneurysm wall. Most rAAAs are in men of advanced age, with an aneurysm size of more than 55 mm, which gives a foundation for treatment guidelines.

There is no medical treatment to prevent growing AAA or rupture, but there are some data showing that diabetes, and possibly anti-diabetes medications, might have some protective effect, since the prevalence of AAA is lower in diabetics [3, 23, 24]. The mortality of women with rAAA is higher than that of men, but to date there is no clear explanation for this [25, 26]. The mechanism of rupture is not completely clear, but rAAA is considered to follow a process of weakening of the vessel wall due to atherosclerotic plaque and then a widening of the wall until the intra-vessel tension causes disruption of the wall and accumulation of blood in the periaortic retroperitoneal space. It is believed that the atherosclerosis burden and disturbed balance between different vascular wall elements and connective tissue contribute to rAAA [2, 27–29]. There are some limited data on risk of rupture and pressure estimates from different models, but no measurement methods are yet in clinical use [30]. At times, imaging reveals atherosclerotic plaque at the site of rupture, and the rupture might be called a "plaque rupture." Ultrasound and CTA are the methods of choice for aneurysm size control, but sizes differ by some millimeters due to varying measurement modalities. In general, CTA sizing will show an around 3–5 mm larger diameter than ultrasound. The most common and least operator-dependent form of measuring is of the CTA external wall to external wall maximal diameter (in mm), which should be performed on multiple planes to obtain a correct measurement. A 1 mm CTA series or less is recommended for optimal endovascular treatment planning (as discussed later in this chapter).

## 103.2 Diagnosis and Clinical Presentation of rAAA

The most reliable method of rAAA diagnosis and the gold standard for detecting rAAA is CTA [5, 22]. Diagnosis of rAAA is sometimes clear-cut, but at times extremely difficult clinically, as the symptoms might be nonspecific. On admission, a patient with a known AAA and abdominal and back pain should be suspected of having suffered a rupture, and emergency CTA should be performed without delay. Typical symptoms of rAAA are abdominal pain, referred back pain, circulatory shock, and hemodynamic collapse (systolic blood pressure below 90–100 mmHg or less, tachycardia, tachypnea, cold sweat, etc.), but some patients may have diffuse symptoms that are more suggestive of gastrointestinal problems or urinary infections. At times, abdominal and back pain that is "out of proportion" might be the initial presentation. Clinical status may include a tender, swollen, tympanic abdomen. Usually, palpation of the aneurysm is not easy when ruptured, and it causes severe local and referred back pain. Some patients might complain of unilateral lower back pain due to the hematoma's mechanical pressure on the psoas muscle. In extremis, patients arrive with pending arrest (systolic blood pressure under 40–50 mmHg or mean arterial pressure under 40), with no measurable blood pressure, or in cardiac arrest. Laboratory testing might reveal a typical hemodynamic shock situation with low hemoglobin, acidosis, high white-cell count, hypocalcemia, hypokalemia, high creatinine and urea, etc. As typical of shock, low urine production (less than 30 mL/h) is expected in most cases.

The Hardman signs have been used traditionally as predictors of mortality and include high age (over 80), loss of consciousness, ECG changes or arrhythmia, high creatinine, and low blood pressure (shock) [31]. Patients with all-positive Hardeman scores have an exceptionally low survival rate [31], but other predictors might be highly important, such as ongoing cardiopulmonary resuscitation (CPR), low pH (less than 6.9), and length of circulatory collapse. All these factors are regarded as negative predictors of survival. Once a rupture is diagnosed, sizing of the aneurysm is meaningless, and the most crucial information for treatment planning is anamnesis, patient status, and the extent of the aneurysm. The will of the patient (and family) and life quality are of the utmost importance in the decision path regarding curative or palliative treatment.

The gold standard of diagnosis in rAAA is, as stated, emergency CTA in the arterial phase, showing disruption of the AAA wall, with limited or extensive hematoma with or without extravasation (Fig. 103.3) [5, 22]. At times, just a small volume of blood can be detected near the aneurysm wall; a swollen, irregular vessel wall may indicate ruptured or near-ruptured (symptomatic) AAA, which is considered to be a pre-rupture condition and should be treated promptly. CTA images of 0.6–1 mm thick should be produced, with a dedicated protocol for rAAA if possible, with a highly concentrated contrast medium of about 100–120 mL contrast fluid (calculated by the CTA program, per body weight in modern apparatuses). CTA should be initiated as soon as possible and should not be delayed. In general, the procedure can be performed in a few minutes, and its main limitations are related to transfer to the CT suite (which depends on local hospital organization). Another important issue is the transfer of the patient to the CT table and then to the surgical or hybrid suite. Ultra-modern facilities may offer hybrid Gentry (CT on rails) at the hybrid suite, which might reduce transfer time and the risk of transferring unstable patients. At time of writing, however, there are very few, if any, Gentry CT hybrid emergency angio suites installed in the world that are used in the case of rAAA. Some data on these and other modalities are updated on the EVTM society website and journal (www.jevtm.com) [32, 33].

The question of high creatinine, renal function and performing CTA is not relevant for patients with a strongly suspected rAAA, since the procedure is an emergency and potentially lifesaving and should not be delayed. In rAAA, time is of tremendous importance, especially if the patient is hemodynamically unstable, and—as imaging is being undertaken—the next step in the chain of treatment must be prepared to prevent any further delay. Once a CTA shows an rAAA, the main decision is whether the patient should be operated on (endo or open). The most important issues to consider are benefit of surgery and life quality and, of course, the will of the patient. In the author's center, as in others, we check if the patient is physically active and has a life expectancy of more than 6–12 months, if the patient wants to go through surgery and if the patient has major comorbidities that might cause reconsideration of the surgical alternative (i.e., if the patient is nonmobile or has had a cerebral vascular event or stroke). The family is obviously consulted whenever possible. Parallel to all this, the vascular surgeon should make a rapid decision on whether to perform an Endovascular Aortic Repair (EVAR) or open surgery (OS) [5, 13, 22, 34]. There are many factors influencing this decision, but the major ones are surgical experience, center organization, and team 24/7 availability. It is probably better to transfer the patient, if possible, to a major center with a high volume of aortic endovascular or open procedures for best results as high surgical volume is correlated with the survival of rAAA patients [5].

It should be emphasized again that the most important questions are the following: What is best for this specific patient? Can you help the patient by repair? What does the patient want? Can we perform the procedure, or do we need to transfer the patient? Is palliative treatment a better option for the patient here and now? Especially when meeting an rAAA patient, your own ego should be put aside, and you must consider what is best for the patient.

## 103.3 Treatment of rAAA

Ongoing CPR and high-age patients will usually not survive any of the treatment options, but there are exceptions in the author's center (and other centers), which are critical in deciding whether or not to go ahead with treatment upon diagnosis. Before initiating treatment, we recommend that a highly experienced vascular surgeon should be consulted, meet the patients and take the decision (see Flowchart 103.1). Patients with rAAA have no margin of error, and it should be emphasized again that treatment should be only conducted by a highly experienced team. The majority of rAAA patients will die without surgical treatment, but some with contained or minimal hematoma might survive (as said, these are exceptions). A few patients with limited rAAA have managed to live for weeks or months after rAAA (author's personal experience), but the general rule is that

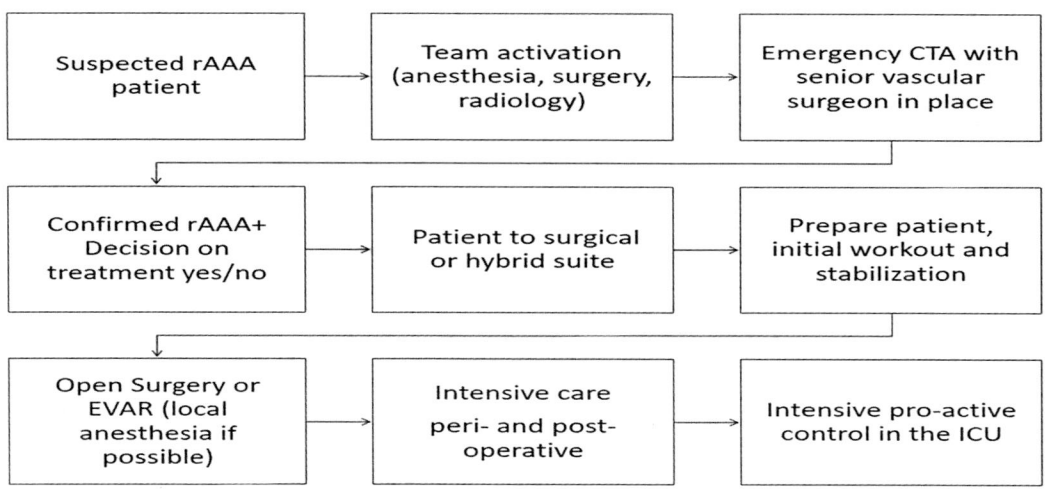

**Flowchart 103.1** A general schematic presentation of the steps to follow from arrival of a patient with suspected rAAA through to the postoperative intensive care unit

rAAA is a direct life-threatening situation with extremely high mortality.

There are only two treatment options for rAAA: OS and EVAR. Both are good options, and the choice between them depends heavily on center and surgeon experience [5, 10, 13, 35, 36]. It is well accepted by experts that both volume of elective aorta surgery and intensive-care availability and quality affect results. The goal of treatment is to prevent death, and OS or EVAR should be initiated immediately upon diagnosis. Several randomized control studies of EVAR vs. OS treatments for rAAA generally show short-term positive effects of EVAR but no effect on mortality after 3–5 years. These studies have been criticized for not randomizing all patients and for not fully following protocols and experiences in the last 5–10 years, i.e., for being outdated. Even if historical data show the same long-term results for OS and EVAR in rAAA, newer data show better survival for EVAR [10, 37], and it is now recommended in major guidelines that EVAR should be performed in the majority of cases of infrarenal rAAA, even among younger patients [5, 38]. There is an ongoing debate about younger patients (<65 year old) and the belief that they might be better served by open surgery. The individual decision is, as stated, highly dependent on the center and its experience. In the author's center (Örebro University Hospital, Sweden), however, EVAR has been performed on 100% of ruptured patients, from 2009, with a very low exclusion rate and an acceptable mortality of around 24–28%. EVAR, as part of the Endovascular Resuscitation and Trauma Management concept (EVTM) is now practiced to varying degrees in other centers worldwide [13, 38].

### 103.3.1 Open Surgery

Midline laparotomy under general anesthesia is the gold standard incision for rAAA. The main goal is to get fast access to the aortic neck for aortic clamping, followed by open aortic or aorta bi-iliac interposition grafting (with a tube graft or aorta-bi-iliac graft). Clamping is preferably performed in the infrarenal aortic area, but at times suprarenal clamping is needed when the aortic neck is short or atherosclerotic and with thrombus (Fig. 103.3). Since the patients might be hemodynamically unstable, massive transfusion and vasopressors are needed to maintain blood pressure, and, on introduction of anesthesia, hemodynamic collapse should be anticipated. Once in the abdomen, major bleeding might be seen, and extensive scoping of blood is performed to enhance fast dissection under the mesentery sac toward the infrarenal aorta. A table retractor (such as Omni-Tract or Martin Arm) may facilitate visualization of the open abdomen and should be used. Cell-saver should be used when possible, enhancing auto-transfusion. Care should be taken to avoid injury to organs or vessels (i.e., renal vein or arteries) during dissection. The infrarenal or suprarenal aorta is dissected for proximal surgical control. Once aortic clamping is achieved, dissection of the iliac bifurcation is performed, bilaterally as needed, and clamped, and the aortic sac is opened for repair by interposition grafting. Once the sac is opened, bleeding from the lumbar arteries is controlled by large surgical nonabsorbable sutures. An aortic synthetic graft is fitted with continuous sutures, and the proximal anastomosis is checked for leakage as the aorta is gradually de-clamped. Retrograde iliac flow should be checked as thrombosis might occur. Distal status (flow to the iliac arteries and distally) should be confirmed. During repair, massive blood products should be given to maintain hemodynamic stability. Usually, massive vasopressor transfusion is also needed for unstable patients. Products like calcium and bicarbonate might be needed to correct acidosis and coagulation.

A hybrid option for repair is the use of an aortic balloon for proximal control before opening the abdomen (aneurysm). Via a puncture in the femoral artery and vascular access via an introducer, an aortic balloon is advanced to the aorta (even suprarenal if needed) for temporary hemodynamic stabilization. The purpose of the balloon is to facilitate open repair. The balloon can be used for total occlusion or even for partial occlusion, just to obtain temporary hemodynamic stabilization until repair is initiated. The balloon can be replaced by surgical clamping, or repair can be performed with the balloon in place and then removed just before the proximal anastomosis is completed. The use of aortic balloon for occlusion in rAAA and open surgery is not in widespread use but can, if needed, be used in centers with endovascular experience.

After repair and evacuation of free blood, the abdomen is closed. The abdominal fascia and skin are closed, and, in selected cases, because of massive bleeding and swelling, the abdomen may be left open (Bogota bag or vacuum-assisted cover), with closure following later in the postoperative period. Once surgery is terminated, the distal status of the extremities should be checked and supportive intensive care initiated (respiratory, metabolic, etc.). Postoperative intensive care (in an intensive care unit, ICU) aims at reducing hemodynamic shock and surgical insult and correcting the metabolic and respiratory acidosis and fluid balance after massive transfusion. CTA control is usually not performed but should be considered on the first or second postoperative day. Abdominal hypertension and abdominal compartment syndrome (ACS) might follow rAAA and should be monitored by measurements of the intra-abdominal pressure via a Foley manometer and by following the guidelines for ACS with decompression if needed [39–41]. A proactive approach is to be recommended, with decompressive laparotomy on signs of organ failure (as urine production) or very high abdominal pressure (above 20 mmHg) [13, 42]. Early, aggressive treatment of signs of infection, abscess formation, lung inflammation, and cardiac complications are usually indicated as the majority of patients with rAAA will develop complications. Considering the physiological impact of rAAA on elderly patients, there are no wide margins and expectancy times, and daily evaluation is needed in the first few postoperative days. As OS for rAAA has not changed in the last decades and there is a widely available literature on the subject, the author refers to operative textbooks for more detailed information on the technique.

### 103.3.2 Endovascular Surgery

EVAR can be performed in a standard way with a bi-iliac endo-graft, but, in selected cases, a straight endo-graft has been used [13, 35, 43]. The main idea is to land in a proximal and distal "normal" vessel without significant thrombus or atherosclerosis, but this is a very challenging target at times given the extent of disease. Correct landing vessel part with the endo-graft will prevent endo-leakage to the aneurysm and thereby exclude the rAAA and offer definitive treatment

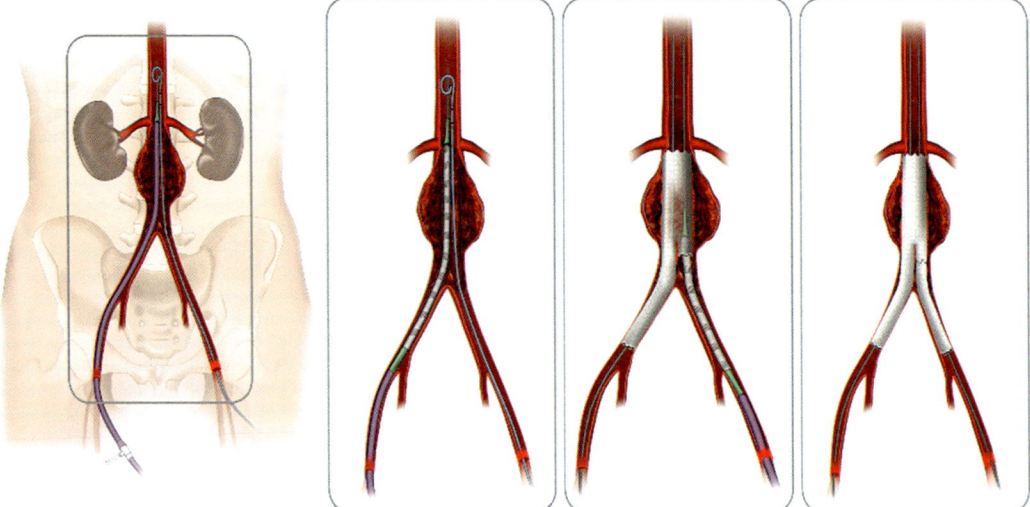

**Fig. 103.4** Endovascular Aortic Repair (EVAR) illustrated in an infrarenal aneurysm. Bilateral femoral artery access gained and angiography for anatomical orientation to follow. Endo-graft from one side deployed below the renal arteries, followed by extensions on the contralateral side, as the aneurysm is excluded. Simple EVAR procedure for rAAA may take only a very short time in experienced hands but is very much dependent on the anatomic and vascular access

(Fig. 103.4). Treatment starts with fast evaluation and CTA measurements by a highly experienced surgeon. Complete evaluation and selection of endo-grafts and strategies can be performed in minutes and are essential to successful treatment. While measurements are being taken, the patient should be moved to the semi-hybrid or hybrid surgical suite and prepared for surgery by a highly experienced team of anesthetists. In the author's center, it is recommended not to give fluids or blood before EVAR for rAAA is completed, while maintaining a mean arterial pressure (MAP) of over 50–60 mmHg or a systolic pressure of over 70–80 mmHg. There is now some limited evidence that treatment under local anesthesia is preferable. Some of the patients might be confused or have lost consciousness and should then be intubated. In the author's' center, most rAAAs are performed under local anesthesia [13, 34]. The main concern in performing EVAR for rAAA is finding the correct "landing zone" under the renal arteries and in the iliac vessels. Oversizing of the endo-graft in the neck (proximal sealing zone) depends on the graft itself but should be around 20–30%. The same applies to the iliac vessels. While the patient is prepared by the team of anesthesiologists, draping should be performed in parallel, with no time delay. There are no "stable" rupture patients, only patients who are about to become unstable. All patients should be given a prophylactic antibiotic, but we do not recommend anticoagulation before the end of the surgical procedure. Vascular access is gained on both femoral arteries percutaneously by ultrasound under local anesthesia, and catheters and wires advanced to the descending aorta are replaced by a large bore introducer as needed for delivery of the endo-graft (stent-graft). There are different types of systems, but all aim to exclude the aneurysm with an aortic-bi-iliac endo-graft. When the graft is in place, positioned and deployed, the contralateral graft is inserted. Positioning of the graft is achieved by contrast injection. Completion control by angiography is performed to ensure that the rupture is excluded. Intensive care and blood transfusion should be given to replace lost blood volume. A standard EVAR for rupture can be performed within 30–40 min and depends very much on the aortic and iliac anatomy. If the patient is hemodynamically unstable before or during surgery, an aortic occlusion balloon can be used for tempo-

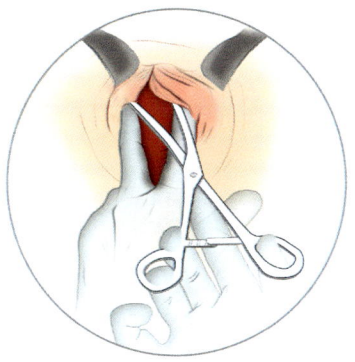 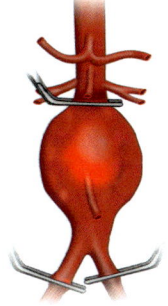 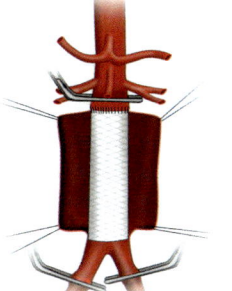 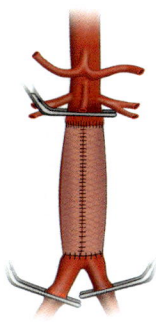

**Fig. 103.5** Illustration of the principles of open repair of a rAAA (with a tube graft in this example). Surgical dissection to the aortic renal arteries level is performed for proximal aortic control followed by iliac arteries dissection and clamping. This is followed by replacement of the aneurysmatic aorta with a synthetic interposition graft. At times, an aortic occlusion balloon might help achieve proximal control of the aorta flow. This can be used in open repair as part of a hybrid procedure. The balloon can be inflated temporarily, and then partially if needed, during anastomosis control. This is an adjunct method for bleeding control in both open and endovascular treatment and should be used only with hemodynamic instable patients

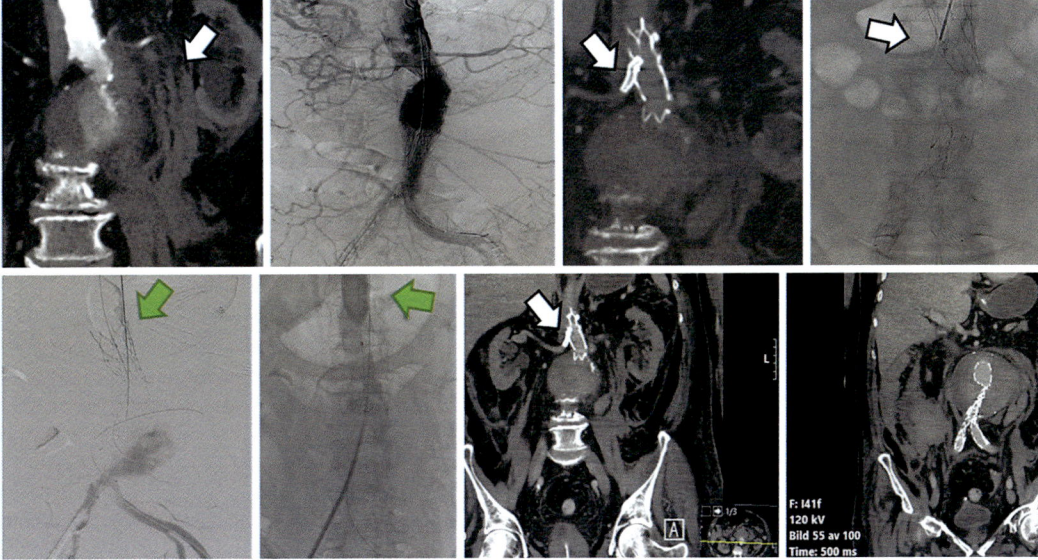

**Fig. 103.6** Some advanced methods in rAAA EVAR. Chimney or parallel grafts can be used to extend the endo-graft landing zone (white arrow). Aortic balloon occlusion can be useful for temporary stabilization during the procedure (green arrow)

rary stabilization (Fig. 103.5). It is highly recommended for the balloon only to be used if needed and for as a short time as possible. Parallel grafts, off-the-shelf grafts, or surgeon-modified grafts can be used in very experienced hands. In selected patients with contained ruptures, complex repair with multiple solutions can be performed, but these procedures are time-consuming even in highly experienced hands (Fig. 103.6). Other solutions include use of embolization agents and coils or plugs for endo-leak prevention. Such advanced techniques are beyond the scope of this chapter. Closure of the vascular access is achieved by a closing device, fascia suture, or surgical cutdown. It is important to validate the distal-leg status for any signs of ischemia and proceed to a surgical solution directly if needed. ICU care for at least 2–3 days is essential for all rAAA patients [32, 44].

### 103.3.3 Complications

The majority of rAAA patients will be in some degree of hemodynamic shock, and some will develop abdominal compartment syndrome, lung inflammation, cardiac infarct, or other complications. The open abdomen, blood loss, and surgical insult in these elderly populations may complicate the postoperative process through hyper-activation of the coagulation and inflammatory systems. Endovascular access might cause thrombosis and dissections or embolus formation or bleeding of the access site. The lower extremities should be inspected directly after surgery and at regular intervals (hourly) in the ICU in the first 1–3 days. In general, major complications should be anticipated in patients with rAAA and decision-making during postoperative care needs to be proactive.

> **Dos and Don'ts**
> **Dos**
> - Once suspected rAAA, do immediate CTA and activate the vascular and anesthesia team.
> - Carefully consider whether to operate (EVAR or open)—what is best for the patient?
> - Communicate with the patient and ask what they want.
> - Communicate with the anesthetic and ICU team during and after treatment.
> - Treatment should be done by a highly experienced team.
> - Do open surgery if this is what your institute does best.
> - Do EVAR if this is what your institute does best.
> - Adopt an emergency procedure as there is no time for any delay. Every minute counts.
>
> **Don'ts**
> - Limit intravenous fluids as far as possible until the aneurysm is excluded.
> - Use aortic balloon occlusion only if hemodynamic instability occurs.
> - Resuscitation and intensive care start before surgery and continues into the days after. Do not lean back and relax until the patient is out of danger: "It's not over until it's over!"
> - Don't let your ego lead you. Call on the help of experienced people.

> **Take-Home Messages**
> - rAAA is an immediate life-threatening situation, and the medical team should act immediately. High levels of experience of all team members are essential to successful treatment.
> - CTA is the diagnostic method of choice, and open surgery and EVAR are the only two operative options possible.
> - EVAR is probably to be preferred in centers experienced in endovascular procedures. Palliative treatment is an option to be considered.
> - Treatment should be performed by a highly experienced team, and multidisciplinary collaboration is extremely important.
> - Definitive treatment is exclusion of the aneurysm by open or endovascular methods or both, and the provision of aggressive postoperative intensive care, avoiding complications like abdominal compartment syndrome among others.

**Multiple Choice Questions (Please Choose the *Best*, and Give Only *One* Answer)**

1. The diagnosis of rAAA is based on the following radiological finding on CT:
   A. Interruption of the aortic wall with or without active extravasation and blood around the aorta.
   B. Major AAA on CT with abdominal pain as well as pain on abdominal palpation.
   C. Known AAA and abdominal and/or back pain with irregularity on the para-aortic contrast CT around the aorta.
   D. Free contrast (blood) on CTA with or without AAA.
   Correct Answer: A

2. The risk of rupture is correlated with the size of aneurysm and should be considered for treatment (as per guidelines) in the following range:
   A. AAA of 50 mm in women and 55 mm in man.
   B. AAA of more than 50 mm.
   C. Depends on location as infrarenal or para-visceral but about 50 mm.
   D. Is not correlated with size when more than 40 mm.
   Correct Answer: A

3. rAAA should be treated:
   A. In all patients; there is a chance of a good outcome.
   B. When there is a good chance of survival and good quality of life, which depends on many factors, such as patient general status, age, comorbidities, and state on arrival at the hospital.
   C. Treatment should be immediate if the patient is hemodynamically unstable.
   D. Treatment should always be initiated on diagnosis, in all patients.
   Correct Answer: B

4. rAAA treatment of choice is (as guided by major guidelines):
   A. Endovascular
   B. Open surgery
   C. Endovascular or open surgery, depends on the center's volumes and experience and patient's older and clinical status
   D. Depends on the patient's status
   Correct Answer: C

5. The major parameters that might affect the results of treatment of an rAAA patient:
   A. High creatinine, high age, loss of consciousness, blood pressure, CPR
   B. Size of the aneurysm
   C. Patient's mental status on arrival
   D. Hemoglobin and hematocrit
   Correct Answer: A

6. Please choose the most proper claim:
   A. The anatomical appearance (such as angulation of the iliac vessels) of the aneurysm has a crucial effect on the open surgical option.
   B. A very long aortic neck is needed for successful rAAA treatment by EVAR.
   C. Only simple rAAAs are possible to treat by EVAR.
   D. Anatomical appearances, such as iliac angulation and iliac size as well as the aortic neck, are crucial for planning of rAAA by EVAR.
   Correct Answer: D

7. Stable rAAA is defined as:
   A. All patients with systolic blood pressure above 90 mmHg.
   B. All patients who can communicate and did not lose consciousness.
   C. There are "no stable rAAAs," but the patient's blood pressure might remain stable in contained ruptures; rAAA patients should be considered as potentially instable.

    D. Patients who did not have an episode of systolic blood pressure under 90 mmHg.

    Correct Answer: C

8. The size of the aneurysm is:
    A. Crucial for treatment options.
    B. Not that important; other parameters, such as iliac vessel size and aortic neck, are more important.
    C. Important for planning of the treatment.
    D. Important to define on diagnosis by CT.

    Correct Answer: B

9. A typical rAAA patient has the following clinical image:
    A. Pale, tachycardia, abdominal and back pain, distended abdomen.
    B. Low urine output and chest pain.
    C. Low back pain and hyperventilation as well as low saturation.
    D. Right side abdominal pain and pain on palpation of the abdomen, fever.

    Correct Answer: A

10. This might be the best way to proceed when you suspect clinically an rAAA in a patient with stable parameters:
    A. Go with the patient to the CT and then to the surgical or hybrid suite.
    B. Go directly to surgery.
    C. Stay in the ER and get a full diagnosis and anamnesis.
    D. Send the patient to the CT (within the coming hours) and wait for information from radiology.

    Correct Answer: A

# References

1. Bergqvist D, Mani K, Troeng T, Wanhainen A. Treatment of aortic aneurysms registered in Swedvasc: development reflected in a national vascular registry with an almost 100% coverage. Gefasschirurgie. 2018;23(5):340–5.
2. Aggarwal S, Qamar A, Sharma V, Sharma A. Abdominal aortic aneurysm: a comprehensive review. Exp Clin Cardiol. 2011;16(1):11–5.
3. Sakalihasan N, Michel JB, Katsargyris A, Kuivaniemi H, Defraigne JO, Nchimi A, et al. Abdominal aortic aneurysms. Nat Rev Dis Primers. 2018;4(1):34.
4. Nordon IM, Hinchliffe RJ, Loftus IM, Thompson MM. Pathophysiology and epidemiology of abdominal aortic aneurysms. Nat Rev Cardiol. 2011;8(2): 92–102.
5. Wanhainen A, Verzini F, Van Herzeele I, Allaire E, Bown M, Cohnert T, et al. Editor's Choice - European Society for Vascular Surgery (ESVS) 2019 clinical practice guidelines on the management of abdominal aorto-iliac artery aneurysms. Eur J Vasc Endovasc Surg. 2019;57(1):8–93.
6. Cabellon S Jr, Moncrief CL, Pierre DR, Cavanaugh DG. Incidence of abdominal aortic aneurysms in patients with atheromatous arterial disease. Am J Surg. 1983;146(5):575–6.
7. Powell JT, Greenhalgh RM. Clinical practice. Small abdominal aortic aneurysms. N Engl J Med. 2003;348(19):1895–901.
8. Powell JT, Sweeting MJ, Brown LC, Gotensparre SM, Fowkes FG, Thompson SG. Systematic review and meta-analysis of growth rates of small abdominal aortic aneurysms. Br J Surg. 2011;98(5):609–18.
9. Lederle FA, Johnson GR, Wilson SE, Ballard DJ, Jordan WD Jr, Blebea J, et al. Rupture rate of large abdominal aortic aneurysms in patients refusing or unfit for elective repair. JAMA. 2002;287(22): 2968–72.
10. Roosendaal LC, Kramer GM, Wiersema AM, Wisselink W, Jongkind V. Outcome of ruptured abdominal aortic aneurysm repair in octogenarians: a systematic review and meta-analysis. Eur J Vasc Endovasc Surg. 2020;59(1):16–22.
11. Sweeting MJ, Ulug P, Powell JT, Desgranges P, Balm R, Ruptured Aneurysm Trials. Ruptured Aneurysm Trials: the importance of longer-term outcomes and meta-analysis for 1-year mortality. Eur J Vasc Endovasc Surg. 2015;50(3):297–302.
12. Shahidi S, Schroeder TV, Carstensen M, Sillesen H. Outcome and survival of patients aged 75 years and older compared to younger patients after ruptured abdominal aortic aneurysm repair: do the results justify the effort? Ann Vasc Surg. 2009;23(4):469–77.
13. Mayer D, Aeschbacher S, Pfammatter T, Veith FJ, Norgren L, Magnuson A, et al. Complete replacement of open repair for ruptured abdominal aortic aneurysms by endovascular aneurysm repair: a two-center 14-year experience. Ann Surg. 2012;256(5):688–95; discussion 95–6.
14. Wanhainen A, Bergqvist D, Boman K, Nilsson TK, Rutegard J, Bjorck M. Risk factors associated with abdominal aortic aneurysm: a population-based study with historical and current data. J Vasc Surg. 2005;41(3):390–6.
15. Mortality results for randomised controlled trial of early elective surgery or ultrasonographic surveillance for small abdominal aortic aneurysms. The UK Small Aneurysm Trial Participants. Lancet. 1998;352(9141):1649–55.

16. Harris LM, Faggioli GL, Fiedler R, Curl GR, Ricotta JJ. Ruptured abdominal aortic aneurysms: factors affecting mortality rates. J Vasc Surg. 1991;14(6):812–8; discussion 9–20.
17. Budtz-Lilly J, Wanhainen A, Mani K. Outcomes of endovascular aortic repair in the modern era. J Cardiovasc Surg. 2018;59(2):180–9.
18. Gunnarsson K, Wanhainen A, Djavani Gidlund K, Bjorck M, Mani K. Endovascular versus open repair as primary strategy for ruptured abdominal aortic aneurysm: a national population-based study. Eur J Vasc Endovasc Surg. 2016;51(1):22–8.
19. Svensjo S, Bjorck M, Wanhainen A. Editor's choice: Five-year outcomes in men screened for abdominal aortic aneurysm at 65 years of age: a population-based cohort study. Eur J Vasc Endovasc Surg. 2014;47(1):37–44.
20. Johnston KW, Rutherford RB, Tilson MD, Shah DM, Hollier L, Stanley JC. Suggested standards for reporting on arterial aneurysms. Subcommittee on Reporting Standards for Arterial Aneurysms, Ad Hoc Committee on Reporting Standards, Society for Vascular Surgery and North American Chapter, International Society for Cardiovascular Surgery. J Vasc Surg. 1991;13(3):452–8.
21. Rogers IS, Massaro JM, Truong QA, Mahabadi AA, Kriegel MF, Fox CS, et al. Distribution, determinants, and normal reference values of thoracic and abdominal aortic diameters by computed tomography (from the Framingham Heart Study). Am J Cardiol. 2013;111(10):1510–6.
22. Moll FL, Powell JT, Fraedrich G, Verzini F, Haulon S, Waltham M, et al. Management of abdominal aortic aneurysms clinical practice guidelines of the European Society for Vascular Surgery. Eur J Vasc Endovasc Surg. 2011;41(Suppl 1):S1–S58.
23. Grondal N, Sogaard R, Lindholt JS. Baseline prevalence of abdominal aortic aneurysm, peripheral arterial disease and hypertension in men aged 65–74 years from a population screening study (VIVA trial). Br J Surg. 2015;102(8):902–6.
24. Sweeting MJ, Thompson SG, Brown LC, Powell JT, RESCAN Collaborators. Meta-analysis of individual patient data to examine factors affecting growth and rupture of small abdominal aortic aneurysms. Br J Surg. 2012;99(5):655–65.
25. Truong C, Kugler NW, Rossi PJ, Patel PJ, Hieb RA, Brown KR, et al. Sex-dependent outcomes following elective endovascular aortic repair. J Surg Res. 2018;229:177–85.
26. Ulug P, Sweeting MJ, von Allmen RS, Thompson SG, Powell JT, SWAN Collaborators. Morphological suitability for endovascular repair, non-intervention rates, and operative mortality in women and men assessed for intact abdominal aortic aneurysm repair: systematic reviews with meta-analysis. Lancet. 2017;389(10088):2482–91.
27. Talvitie M, Lindquist Liljeqvist M, Siika A, Hultgren R, Roy J. Localized hyperattenuations in the intraluminal thrombus may predict rupture of abdominal aortic aneurysms. J Vasc Interv Radiol. 2018;29(1):144–5.
28. Siika A, Lindquist Liljeqvist M, Hultgren R, Gasser TC, Roy J. Aortic lumen area is increased in ruptured abdominal aortic aneurysms and correlates to biomechanical rupture risk. J Endovasc Ther. 2018;25(6):750–6.
29. Lindquist Liljeqvist M, Silveira A, Hultgren R, Frebelius S, Lengquist M, Engstrom J, et al. Neutrophil elastase-derived fibrin degradation products indicate presence of abdominal aortic aneurysms and correlate with intraluminal thrombus volume. Thromb Haemost. 2018;118(2):329–39.
30. Stevens RRF, Grytsan A, Biasetti J, Roy J, Lindquist Liljeqvist M, Gasser TC. Biomechanical changes during abdominal aortic aneurysm growth. PLoS One. 2017;12(11):e0187421.
31. Tambyraja AL, Fraser SC, Murie JA, Chalmers RT. Validity of the Glasgow Aneurysm Score and the Hardman Index in predicting outcome after ruptured abdominal aortic aneurysm repair. Br J Surg. 2005;92(5):570–3.
32. EndoVascular resuscitation and Trauma Management (EVTM) textbook. Springer; 2019.
33. Rasmussen TE. Journal of Endovascular Resuscitation and Trauma Management (JEVTM). 2017; 1(1):3.
34. Veith FJ, Lachat M, Mayer D, Malina M, Holst J, Mehta M, et al. Collected world and single center experience with endovascular treatment of ruptured abdominal aortic aneurysms. Ann Surg. 2009;250(5):818–24.
35. Veith FJ, Gargiulo NJ III, Ohki T. Endovascular treatment of ruptured infrarenal aortic and iliac aneurysms. Acta Chir Belg. 2003;103(6):555–62.
36. Lederle FA, Kyriakides TC, Stroupe KT, Freischlag JA, Padberg FT Jr, Matsumura JS, et al. Open versus endovascular repair of abdominal aortic aneurysm. N Engl J Med. 2019;380(22):2126–35.
37. IMPROVE Trial Investigators. Comparative clinical effectiveness and cost effectiveness of endovascular strategy v open repair for ruptured abdominal aortic aneurysm: three year results of the IMPROVE randomised trial. BMJ. 2017;359:j4859.
38. Horer T. Resuscitative endovascular balloon occlusion of the aorta (REBOA) and endovascular resuscitation and trauma management (EVTM): a paradigm shift regarding hemodynamic instability. Eur J Trauma Emerg Surg. 2018;44(4):487–9.
39. Ganeshanantham G, Walsh SR, Varty K. Abdominal compartment syndrome in vascular surgery - a review. Int J Surg. 2010;8(3):181–5.
40. Malbrain ML, Cheatham ML, Kirkpatrick A, Sugrue M, Parr M, De Waele J, et al. Results from the International Conference of Experts on Intra-abdominal Hypertension and Abdominal Compartment Syndrome. I. Definitions. Intens Care Med. 2006;32(11):1722–32.

41. Mayer D, Veith FJ, Lachat M, Pfammatter T, Hechelhammer L, Rancic Z. Abdominal compartment syndrome. Minerva Chir. 2010;65(3):329–46.
42. Sa P, Oliveira-Pinto J, Mansilha A. Abdominal compartment syndrome after r-EVAR: a systematic review with meta-analysis on incidence and mortality. Int Angiol. 2020;39(5):411–21.
43. Mayer D, Pfammatter T, Rancic Z, Hechelhammer L, Wilhelm M, Veith FJ, et al. 10 years of emergency endovascular aneurysm repair for ruptured abdominal aortoiliac aneurysms: lessons learned. Ann Surg. 2009;249(3):510–5.
44. Tal H. Top Stent manual. 1st ed. Sweden: Örebro University Hospital; 2017.

# Visceral Artery Aneurysms

## 104

Jonathan Parks and George C. Velmahos

## 104.1 Introduction

Visceral artery aneurysms (VAAs) consist of aneurysms of the splanchnic circulation, namely, the splenic, hepatic, celiac, superior, and inferior mesenteric and gastroduodenal arteries and the pancreaticoduodenal arcade. VAAs are relatively rare and typically asymptomatic until rupture, which carries an estimated mortality of 25%.

Historically, the insidious nature of these aneurysms stymied our understanding of their natural history. As the utilization of cross-sectional imaging has expanded, though, the discovery of incidental asymptomatic aneurysms has risen dramatically. This opportunity to learn how and when to treat VAAs has led to several advances in endovascular treatment. Still, several questions remain, and the risk factors for rupture are not well understood.

Here, we describe the pathogenesis of VAAs and what is known about risk factors for rupture. Additionally, we discuss the presenting signs and symptoms of ruptured aneurysms. Finally, we review the indications for treatment of VAAs, the various surgical techniques for repair, as well as the possible complications and their management.

> **Learning Goals**
> - To understand the natural history of visceral artery aneurysms.
> - To be able to identify VAAs at risk for rupture that warrant repair.
> - To learn how to evaluate a patient with a VAA and select a surgical approach for repair.

### 104.1.1 Epidemiology

Visceral artery aneurysms (VAAs) are a rare entity, with reported incidence rates of 0.01–0.2% [1]. Since most VAAs are asymptomatic, their true prevalence is unknown. Autopsy series looking specifically for the presence of VAAs estimate the prevalence to be between 0.1% and 2% [2–5]. Of all intraabdominal arterial aneurysms, only 5% affect the visceral arteries [6].

Of VAAs, splenic artery aneurysms (SAAs) are the most common type and comprise approximately 60% [7]. They are four times more likely to occur in women. SAAs in men, however, are three times more likely to rupture [8]. SAAs are more common in multiparous women and pres-

J. Parks (✉) · G. C. Velmahos
Division of Trauma, Emergency Surgery and Surgical Critical Care, Massachusetts General Hospital and Harvard Medical School, Boston, MA, USA
e-mail: jjparks@mgh.harvard.edu; gvelmahos@mgh.harvard.edu

ent in 9–50% of patients with cirrhosis [9]. Pseudoaneurysms of the splenic artery are also rare, with only a few reported cases in the literature [8–11].

After SAA, hepatic artery aneurysm (HAA) is the second most common type of VAA, accounting for approximately 20% [12, 13]. They are more often identified during the sixth decade of life with a 3:2 male predominance [14]. Over 70% of patients with HAA have concomitant visceral aneurysms. Other nonvisceral aneurysms occur in 40% of patients, abdominal aortic aneurysms being the most common type. Thirty percent of patients have other VAAs, with SAA occurring most frequently [14]. Pseudoaneurysms of the hepatic artery caused by iatrogenic injury from percutaneous and endoscopic procedures in the biliary tree comprise an increasingly large proportion, accounting for 25–80% of all HAAs [15, 16].

VAAs are less frequently found in other abdominal vessels. Aneurysms of the superior mesenteric, celiac, gastric, gastroepiploic, gastroduodenal, and pancreaticoduodenal arteries each constitute less than 5% of all VAAs [7, 17, 18]. Jejunal, ileal, and colic branch aneurysms together account for less than 3% of VAAs (Fig. 104.1) [18].

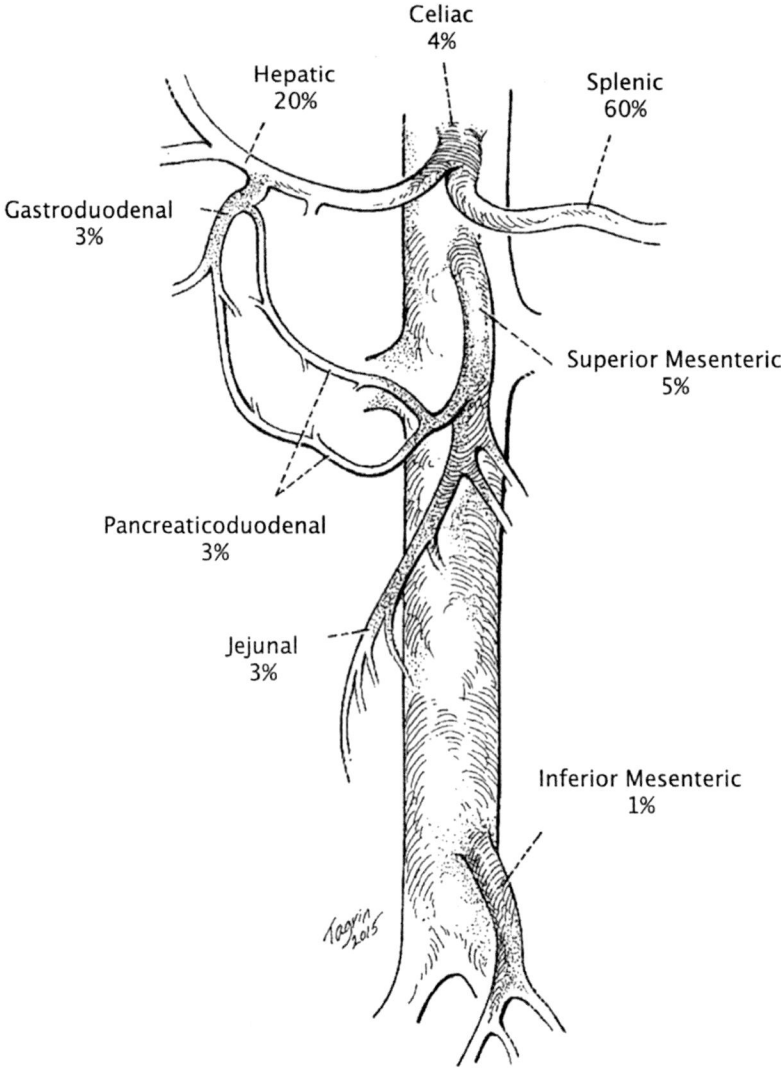

**Fig. 104.1** Distribution of aneurysms throughout the splanchnic circulation. From

The incidence of all VAAs is rising due to the growing availability and utilization of cross-sectional imaging. Historically, VAAs were only identified after becoming symptomatic or rupturing. The widespread use of and reliance on modern imaging modalities has increased the identification of incidental asymptomatic visceral aneurysms [19]. Ultimately, this has improved the understanding of the natural history of VAAs and led to advancements in their treatment [13].

## 104.1.2 Etiology

As many VAAs are asymptomatic and evident only after rupturing, their etiology is poorly understood. Generally, true aneurysms are degenerative, with reduction of smooth muscle, disruption of elastic fibers, and deficiency of the media leading to attenuation of the vessel wall. Consequently, associated conditions related to aneurysmal growth include atherosclerosis, fibromuscular dysplasia, collagen vascular disease, and congenital connective tissue disorders. Whereas true aneurysms develop in this manner, the majority of pseudoaneurysms are caused by trauma or iatrogenic injury [6].

Apart from the general causes of aneurysms, SAAs can arise from pancreatitis, portal hypertension, or pregnancy. In pancreatitis, severe local inflammation can drive local degradation of the splenic arterial wall [20]. The hyperdynamic circulation seen with portal hypertension often contributes to splenic aneurysm growth [18, 21]. Multiparous patients are at higher risk of developing SAAs, which may be due to estrogen and progesterone receptors in the wall of the artery [20].

Historically, the most common primary cause of HAA was bacterial endocarditis. As the incidence of endocarditis has fallen, mycotic HAAs are now rarely seen [22]. Currently, several chronic inflammatory conditions are correlated with HAAs, including hypertension, peptic ulcer disease, gastritis, coronary artery disease, peripheral arterial disease, chronic obstructive pulmonary disease, and obesity. Tobacco and alcohol use is recorded in two-thirds of patients [14].

SMAAs are largely caused by either infection or dissection. Subacute bacterial endocarditis or nonhemolytic streptococcus is usually responsible for mycotic SMAAs [23]. Dissection leading to SMAA can either originate directly at the SMA or its branches or continue as an extension of a larger aortic dissection. Atherosclerosis is responsible for another 25% of cases. Pancreatitis and trauma can lead to pseudoaneurysm formation [24, 25].

In the early twentieth century, infection from either syphilis or tuberculosis was the most frequent cause of celiac artery aneurysm (CAA). These cases were typically diagnosed at autopsy following rupture [6, 26]. Most contemporary CAAs are asymptomatic and often result from atherosclerosis and medial degeneration. Roughly 15% of CAAs are associated with either extension of an aortic dissection or a primary dissection of the celiac axis [21].

Aneurysms of the pancreatic and duodenal vessels are often associated with celiac stenosis or complete occlusion [17]. Aneurysmal growth is attributed to the maturation of collateral flow to the liver through these thin-walled vessels [21].

The study of the remainder of VAA subtypes is limited to small case series and individual case reports, hindering the ability to make generalizations about their origins.

## 104.1.3 Classification

VAAs are described by their anatomic location, size, and type (true aneurysm versus pseudoaneurysm). A vessel is considered aneurysmal when its diameter is 1.5 times that of the native vessel on axial imaging [21].

## 104.1.4 Pathophysiology

The evolution of VAAs and the characteristics that predispose rupture are poorly understood on account of their scarcity and occult nature [6]. A significant portion of VAAs are identified only after becoming symptomatic. The widespread availability of advanced abdominal imaging, though, has facilitated the early identification of incidental asymptomatic visceral aneurysms and is responsible for the increasing incidence of VAAs [19]. The serial imaging routinely performed on asymptomatic VAAs has provided more recent insight on how they mature.

For most aneurysm types, size poorly correlates with rupture risk; small aneurysms can rupture too [27]. Most VAAs enlarge slowly. In a recent retrospective study of 250 small VAAs, more than 90% remained stable over 36 months, while 8.7% grew in size and only 1.5% grew to be larger than 2.5 cm in size [21]. Generally, mycotic aneurysms are at a higher risk of rupture; these are increasingly rare. Pseudoaneurysms also carry a higher rupture potential than true aneurysms [13].

Asymptomatic SAAs rupture at a rate of 2% [28]. The mortality related to a SAA rupture is estimated to be 25%. In SAAs recognized during pregnancy, the risk of rupture is as high as 95%, which carries extremely high mortality for the mother and fetus [6, 29, 30]. Any SAA identified in a woman of child-bearing age should be repaired regardless of size.

The majority of ruptured HAAs are over 2 cm in size. Ruptured HAAs carry a mortality rate of 30–40% [6]. HAAs of nonatherosclerotic origin may be at an increased risk of rupture, with one notable series demonstrating a 50% rupture rate in HAAs from other causes, particularly fibromuscular dysplasia, polyarteritis nodosa, and endocarditis [14]. The majority of hepatic artery pseudoaneurysms are symptomatic at presentation, with gastrointestinal bleeding or hemobilia.

Symptoms from VAAs are usually related to rupture. Patients present with abdominal pain, peritonitis, or gastrointestinal bleeding from the upper or lower GI tract. In later stages, presentation will include evidence of hemorrhagic shock. Suspicion for VAA should be present in patients presenting with new onset abdominal pain, particularly those with a history of conditions that are known to be associated with VAAs, such as cirrhosis, pancreatitis, collagen vascular disease, or pregnancy.

Up to a quarter of patients with ruptured SAAs may present with a "double rupture" phenomenon, in which bleeding occurs first in the lesser sac. The patient will initially present with evidence of bleeding and shock but then recover once tamponade occurs in the retrogastric space. Later, the patient will decompensate as the lesser sac tamponade is lost and free intraperitoneal hemorrhage occurs [18].

Rather than presenting with peritonitis and hemoperitoneum, ruptured hepatic artery pseudoaneurysms typically manifest with gastrointestinal bleeding, hemobilia, or fever from cholangitis, as clots can obstruct the biliary tree. Similarly, ruptured gastric and gastroepiploic aneurysms present more commonly with hematemesis and gastrointestinal bleeding [18, 31]. SMAAs may present with a mobile pulsatile mass [23].

Considering that many aneurysms present at rupture and that ruptured SAAs carry a significant mortality risk, an aggressive approach to their diagnosis and management is essential [6].

## 104.2 Diagnosis

### 104.2.1 Clinical Presentation

The primary significance of any aneurysm is the ever-present risk for spontaneous rupture. While the majority of VAAs are asymptomatic, nearly 25% are diagnosed at rupture. The reported mortality rate after diagnosis is 10%, though the true mortality rate from undiagnosed ruptured VAAs is likely higher [6].

### 104.2.2 Tests

Multiple imaging modalities are available for the diagnosis and monitoring of VAAs. Computed tomography angiography (CTA) is widely considered the radiographic modality of choice for all types of VAA (Fig. 104.2). Alternatively, contrast-enhanced ultrasonography can track aneurysm size longitudinally even if limited by bowel gas and body habitus. Additionally, ultrasonography has poor sensitivity for aneurysms

**Fig. 104.2** CT imaging of various visceral artery aneurysms. (**a**) Splenic artery aneurysm 3D reconstruction [32]. (**b**) Post-traumatic hepatic artery pseudoaneurysm [33]. (**c**) Celiac artery aneurysm 3D reconstruction [34]. (**d**) Axial view of CAA [34]. (**e**) Coronal view of IMA aneurysm [35]. (**f**) 3D reconstruction of IMA aneurysm [35]

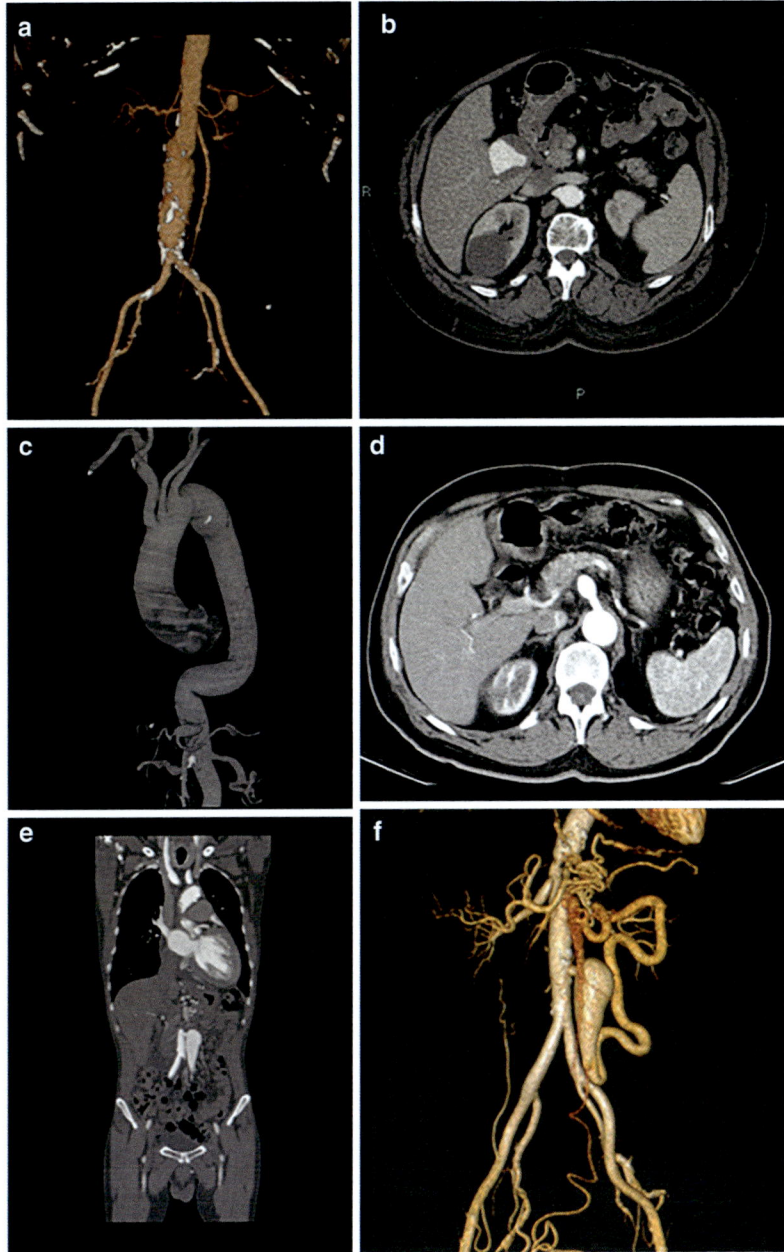

smaller than 3 cm [36]. Magnetic resonance angiography (MRA) is used for surveillance before and after repair. It produces images similar in quality to CTA and should not be used in emergent situations [36].

Given the nonspecific presenting symptoms of a ruptured VAA, any suspicion for bleeding in a patient with a new onset abdominal pain should prompt rapid evaluation. Beyond immediate efforts toward resuscitation, laboratory studies including a hemoglobin level, blood gas with base deficit, serum electrolyte panel, coagulation studies, and blood type and crossmatch should be performed. If the patient is hemodynamically stable, CTA of the abdomen should be obtained expeditiously [37].

> **Differential Diagnosis**
> Unfortunately, patients with VAAs present with nonspecific symptoms, such as abdominal pain, bloating, or nausea. The differential diagnosis is broad. VAAs can mimic more common disease processes including biliary obstruction, pancreatitis, and gastrointestinal bleeding from other causes. A medical history that includes associated conditions may be the only indication that a VAA is present before imaging is performed.

## 104.3 Treatment

### 104.3.1 Medical Treatment

There are currently no medical options for the treatment of VAAs.

### 104.3.2 Surgical Treatment

The objective of surgical repair for VAAs is to exclude the aneurysm for systemic circulation to prevent growth and rupture while maintaining perfusion to the end organs involved. The surgical approach depends largely on the specific type and location of the aneurysm, as well as the underlying clinical condition of the patient. Both open and endovascular techniques are available. Endovascular approaches are the mainstay of elective treatment of aneurysms and are suitable for many ruptured aneurysms. Open procedures are generally reserved for truly emergent cases or for aneurysms not amenable to endovascular repair.

Most symptomatic aneurysms, pseudoaneurysms, mycotic aneurysms, and many larger true aneurysms warrant intervention. Otherwise, indications and approach for repair vary for each anatomical subtype. Generally, endovascular therapy offers high technical success rates with significantly lower morbidity and mortality and should be considered even in ruptured cases [6] (Fig. 104.3).

#### 104.3.2.1 SAAs
Guidelines from the Society for Vascular Surgery recommend repair of SAAs larger than 3 cm. Smaller aneurysms can safely be monitored with annual imaging. Repair is also indicated for

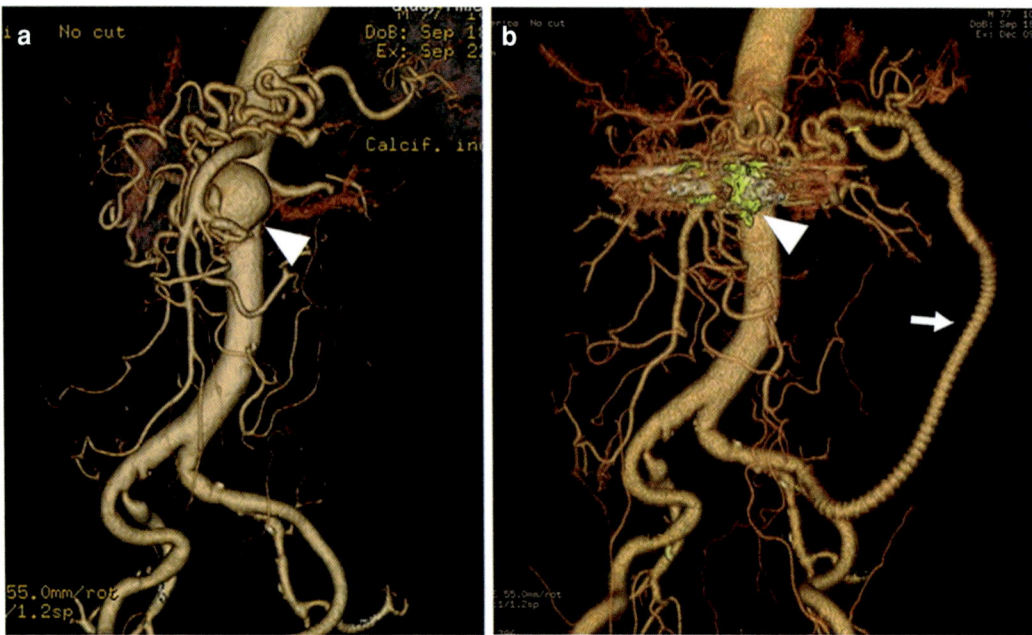

**Fig. 104.3** (a) CTA 3D reconstruction of inferior pancreaticoduodenal artery aneurysm. (b) Images after successful coil embolization [27]

symptomatic aneurysms and for those in women of childbearing age, regardless of size. Relative indications for repair include patients with portal hypertension or those undergoing consideration for liver transplantation and in aneurysms undergoing surveillance with growth above 0.5 cm in 1 year.

Repair of SAAs can be accomplished by either open or endovascular techniques. Endovascular repair is accomplished by isolation of the aneurysmal segment, either by coil embolization of the proximal and distal arterial segment, by embolization of the aneurysmal segment itself with coils or cyanoacrylate glue, or by placement of a stent graft to occlude the aneurysm sac [6] (Fig. 104.4). Hemodynamically unstable patients should be emergently taken to the operating room for laparotomy. Open repair of SAAs involves simple ligation of the aneurysm at its proximal and distal margin.

For proximal or mid-vessel lesions, collateral flow to the spleen is provided via the short gastric arteries, and ligation or embolization of the aneurysm is adequate. In aneurysms of distal splenic artery near the splenic hilum, splenectomy is typically performed due to concerns for ischemia and splenic infarction. Distal pancreatectomy may be additionally necessary for SAAs associated with pancreatitis [12].

Patients who undergo splenectomy should receive vaccinations for encapsulated bacteria (*Neisseria meningitis*, *Haemophilus influenza*, and *Streptococcus pneumonia*) 14 days postoperatively. Alternatively, these vaccinations can be administered 14 days preoperatively in planned elective cases where there is concern for splenic perfusion and function based on the characteristics of the aneurysm or other patient comorbidities.

### 104.3.2.2 HAAs

Asymptomatic HAAs larger than 2 cm or those that grow more than 0.5 cm in 1 year should be considered for repair per the Society of Vascular Surgery clinical practice guidelines. In patients with vasculitis or with positive blood cultures, HAAs should be repaired regardless of size [6].

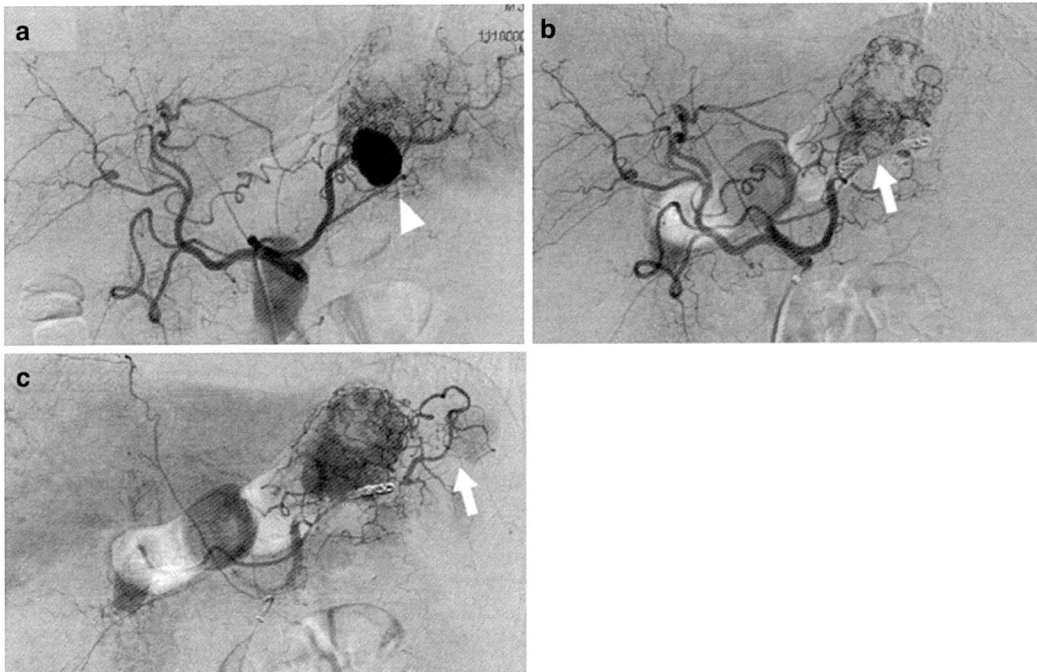

**Fig. 104.4** Endovascular coil embolization of SAA. (**a**) Angiogram demonstrating SAA. (**b**) Coil embolization of inflow and outflow to aneurysmal sac. (**c**) Delayed images demonstrating filling of spleen via collaterals [27]

The operative approach for repair of HAAs is predicated on the location of the aneurysm within the hepatic artery with respect to the liver as well as its size. Endovascular interventions are the primary treatment modality for intrahepatic HAAs when feasible. Most intrahepatic ruptured HAAs and pseudoaneurysms are amenable to endovascular techniques. Large intrahepatic aneurysms (>5 cm) should be considered for open resection of the lobe in which the aneurysm is located, as embolization may put a large segment of liver at risk of ischemia and necrosis [22, 38].

Roughly three quarters of HAAs that require laparotomy for hemorrhagic shock are extrahepatic. Repair should allow for exclusion of the aneurysm while maintaining circulation to the liver, either via resection of the aneurysm with interposition graft or by endovascular stent graft. Open surgical revascularization using autologous vein conduit is recommended if endovascular stent graft exclusion is not possible due potential occlusion of critical hepatic artery branches by the graft at the landing zones. Temporary occlusion of the hepatic artery during repair can help determine if revascularization of the hepatic artery is necessary [15, 22, 38].

### 104.3.2.3 CAAs

Repair is indicated in nonruptured CAAs greater than 2 cm in diameter. Asymptomatic aneurysms less than 2 cm can safely be monitored with annual imaging.

Before repair, the condition of the superior mesenteric, pancreaticoduodenal, and gastroduodenal arteries should be evaluated, as these vessels provide critical collateral perfusion to the liver, pancreas, and foregut in case of loss of celiac arterial flow artery [39]. Endovascular repair can be achieved via coil or glue embolization, thrombin injection, and endovascular stent grafting. Because CAAs typically involve the proximal portion of the celiac trunk, absence of a proximal landing zone may limit endovascular treatment options [40]. Open repair options for celiac artery aneurysms include aneurysmectomy, aneurysmorrhaphy, aortoiliac or aortohepatic bypass, and celiac artery ligation. In cases of rupture, ligation can be used with low risk of hepatic ischemia and is typically well tolerated. If revascularization is required, aortoiliac bypass with a prosthetic graft can be performed [41].

### 104.3.2.4 SMAAs

Repair is indicated for all SMAAs regardless of size or presence of symptoms due to risk of rupture. While the endovascular approach is preferred, endovascular repair of SMA aneurysms beyond the first few centimeters will likely occlude major branches of the vessel and can lead to bowel ischemia. In these cases, open repair should be considered. Options for open repair include simple ligation, aneurysmorrhaphy for saccular aneurysms, or interposition graft. Repair of the aneurysm may necessitate resection of part of the small bowel. Postoperatively patients should be carefully monitored for symptoms of new bowel ischemia due to graft failure or embolism to the bowel [42].

Indications for repair of the remaining visceral aneurysm subtypes are summarized in Table 104.1.

### 104.3.3 Prognosis

Prognosis for repaired VAAs is excellent. Both open and endovascular approaches achieve high rates of technical success. Regardless of type or technique, all vascular reconstruction methods require lifelong postoperative surveillance with cross-sectional imaging. Coils or other radiopaque materials used in endovascular methods may create artifact on CT imaging, leading some authors to recommend serial imaging with contrast-enhanced ultrasound or MRI [43].

Complications of VAA repair are typical of vascular repairs and reconstructions. Endovascular interventions should be monitored for recanalization, coil migration, graft occlusion, or endoleak in stent graft repairs. Interposition grafts are complicated by occlusion or bleeding [27].

**Table 104.1** Recommendations for aneurysm repair by location

| Location | Indications/recommendations |
|---|---|
| All | • Pseudoaneurysms<br>• Mycotic aneurysms<br>• Symptomatic/ruptured |
| Splenic | • Size >3 cm<br>• All sizes in women of childbearing age |
| Hepatic | • Size >2 cm<br>• Growth >0.5 cm/year |
| Celiac | • Size >2 cm<br>• Growth >0.5 cm/year |
| Superior mesenteric | • All sizes |
| Gastric/gastroepiploic | • All sizes |
| Jejunal/Ileal | • Size >2 cm |
| Colic | • All sizes |
| Gastroduodenal/pancreaticoduodenal | • All sizes |

The primary complication after endovascular repair of SAAs is splenic infarct, followed by pancreatitis. For open repair of SAAs, complications include pancreatic tail leak, abscess, or postoperative bleeding requiring splenectomy [44]. For HAAs, hepatic ischemia, abscess formation, and cholecystitis have been reported [14]. Occlusion of SMA reconstructions with clot can lead to bowel necrosis and short gut syndrome [40].

**Dos and Don'ts**
- Small SAAs and HAAs can be monitored with annual imaging.
- Visceral artery pseudoaneurysms, mycotic aneurysms, and splenic artery aneurysms in pregnant patients should be repaired regardless of symptoms or size.
- The presence of collateral flow to the organs distal to an aneurysm drives the selection of surgical technique for repair. Consider imaging to evaluate the patency of collateral vessels prior to repair.
- In patients who undergo repair of SAAs without splenectomy, still consider vaccination against encapsulated bacteria if there is concern for maintenance of collateral flow to the spleen.

**Take-Home Messages**
- VAAs are rare, and knowledge about their pathogenesis is limited.
- Most VAAs are asymptomatic until rupture.
- Ruptured VAAs carry a high mortality and are a true surgical emergency.
- Endovascular repair is generally preferred to open repair, though anatomic considerations govern the selection of surgical approach.

# References

1. Barrionuevo P, Malas MB, Nejim B, Haddad A, Morrow A, Ponce O, et al. A systematic review and meta-analysis of the management of visceral artery aneurysms. J Vasc Surg. 2020;72(1):40S–5S.
2. Panayiotopoulos YP, Assadourian R, Taylor PR. Aneurysms of the visceral and renal arteries. Ann R Coll Surg Engl. 1996;78(5):412.
3. Pitton MB, Dappa E, Jungmann F, Kloeckner R, Schotten S, Wirth GM, et al. Visceral artery aneurysms: incidence, management, and outcome analysis in a tertiary care center over one decade. Eur Radiol. 2015;25(7):2004–14.
4. Huang Y-K, Hsieh H-C, Tsai F-C, Chang S-H, Lu M-S, Ko P-J. Visceral artery aneurysm: risk factor analysis and therapeutic opinion. Eur J Vasc Endovasc Surg. 2007;33(3):293–301.
5. Grego FG, Lepidi S, Ragazzi R, Iurilli V, Stramanà R, Deriu GP. Visceral artery aneurysms: a single center experience. Cardiovasc Surg. 2003;11(1):19–25.

6. Chaer RA, Abularrage CJ, Coleman DM, Eslami MH, Kashyap VS, Rockman C, et al. The Society for Vascular Surgery clinical practice guidelines on the management of visceral aneurysms. J Vasc Surg. 2020;72(1):3S–39S.
7. Saba L, Anzidei M, Lucatelli P, Mallarini G. The multidetector computed tomography angiography (MDCTA) in the diagnosis of splenic artery aneurysm and pseudoaneurysm. Acta Radiol. 2011;52(5):488–98.
8. Agrawal GA, Johnson PT, Fishman EK. Splenic artery aneurysms and pseudoaneurysms: clinical distinctions and CT appearances. Am J Roentgenol. 2007;188(4):992–9.
9. Abbas MA, Stone WM, Fowl RJ, Gloviczki P, Oldenburg WA, Pairolero PC, et al. Splenic artery aneurysms: two decades experience at Mayo Clinic. Ann Vasc Surg. 2002;16(4):442–9.
10. Tessier DJ, Stone WM, Fowl RJ, Abbas MA, Andrews JC, Bower TC, et al. Clinical features and management of splenic artery pseudoaneurysm: case series and cumulative review of literature. J Vasc Surg. 2003;38(5):969–74.
11. Khurram R, Al-Obudi Y, Glover TE, Shah R, Khalifa M, Davies N. Splenic artery pseudoaneurysm: challenges of non-invasive and endovascular diagnosis and management. Radiol Case Rep. 2021;16(6):1395–9.
12. Messina LM, Shanley CJ. Visceral artery aneurysms. Surg Clin North Am. 1997;77(2):425–42.
13. Pulli R, Dorigo W, Troisi N, Pratesi G, Innocenti AA, Pratesi C. Surgical treatment of visceral artery aneurysms: a 25-year experience. J Vasc Surg. 2008;48(2):334–42.
14. Abbas MA, Fowl RJ, Stone WM, Panneton JM, Oldenburg WA, Bower TC, et al. Hepatic artery aneurysm: factors that predict complications. J Vasc Surg. 2003;38(1):41–5.
15. Berceli SA. Hepatic and splenic artery aneurysms. Semin Vasc Surg. 2005;18(4):196–201.
16. Fankhauser GT, Stone WM, Naidu SG, Oderich GS, Ricotta JJ, Bjarnason H, et al. The minimally invasive management of visceral artery aneurysms and pseudoaneurysms. J Vasc Surg. 2011;53(4):966–70.
17. Brocker JA, Maher JL, Smith RW. True pancreaticoduodenal aneurysms with celiac stenosis or occlusion. Am J Surg. 2012;204(5):762–8.
18. Stanley JC, Whitehouse WM, Martin S. Clinical importance and management of splanchnic artery aneurysms. J Vasc Surg. 1986;3(5):5.
19. Cordova AC, Sumpio BE. Visceral artery aneurysms and pseudoaneurysms—should they all be managed by endovascular techniques? Ann Vasc Dis. 2013;6(4):687–93.
20. Hallett JW. Splenic artery aneurysms. Semin Vasc Surg. 1995;8(4):321–6.
21. Corey MR, Ergul EA, Cambria RP, English SJ, Patel VI, Lancaster RT, et al. The natural history of splanchnic artery aneurysms and outcomes after operative intervention. J Vasc Surg. 2016;63(4):949–57.
22. Lal RB, Strohl JA, Piazza S, Aslam M, Ball D, Patel K. Hepatic artery aneurysm. J Cardiovasc Surg. 1989;30(3):509–13.
23. Stone WM, Abbas M, Cherry KJ, Fowl RJ, Gloviczki P. Superior mesenteric artery aneurysms: is presence an indication for intervention? J Vasc Surg. 2002;36(2):234–7; discussion 237.
24. Lorelli DR, Cambria RA, Seabrook GR, Towne JB. Diagnosis and management of aneurysms involving the superior mesenteric artery and its branches—a report of four cases. Vasc Endovasc Surg. 2003;37(1):59–66.
25. Shanley CJ, Shah NL, Messina LM. Uncommon splanchnic artery aneurysms: pancreaticoduodenal, gastroduodenal, superior mesenteric, inferior mesenteric, and colic. Ann Vasc Surg. 1996;10(5):506–15.
26. Stone WM, Abbas MA, Gloviczki P, Fowl RJ, Cherry KJ. Celiac arterial aneurysms: a critical reappraisal of a rare entity. Arch Surg. 2002;137(6):670–4.
27. Obara H, Kentaro M, Inoue M, Kitagawa Y. Current management strategies for visceral artery aneurysms: an overview. Surg Today. 2020;50(1):38–49.
28. Ferrero E, Viazzo A, Ferri M, Robaldo A, Piazza S, Berardi G, et al. Management and urgent repair of ruptured visceral artery aneurysms. Ann Vasc Surg. 2011;25(7):981.e7–11.
29. Barrett JM, Van Hooydonk JE, Boehm FH. Pregnancy-related rupture of arterial aneurysms. Obstet Gynecol Surv. 1982;37(9):557–66.
30. Holdsworth RJ, Gunn A. Ruptured splenic artery aneurysm in pregnancy. A review. BJOG Int J Obstet Gynaecol. 1992;99(7):595–7.
31. Carr SC, Pearce WH, Vogelzang RL, McCarthy WJ, Nemcek AA, Yao JST. Current management of visceral artery aneurysms. Surgery. 1996;120(4):627–34.
32. Case courtesy of Dr Roberto Schubert, Radiopaedia.org, rID: 14340.
33. Case courtesy of Dr Domenico Nicoletti, Radiopaedia.org, rID: 58684.
34. Case courtesy of Dr Bruno Di Muzio, Radiopaedia.org, rID: 21574.
35. Case courtesy of Dr Vincent Tatco, Radiopaedia.org, rID: 45838.
36. Chiaradia M, Novelli L, Deux J-F, Tacher V, Mayer J, You K, et al. Ruptured visceral artery aneurysms. Diagn Interv Imaging. 2015;96(7–8):797–806.
37. Hossain A, Reis ED, Dave SP, Kerstein MD, Hollier LH. Visceral artery aneurysms: experience in a tertiary-care center. Am Surg. 2001;67(5):432–7.
38. Lumsden AB, Mattar SG, Allen RC, Bacha EA. Hepatic artery aneurysms: the management of 22 patients. J Surg Res. 1996;60(2):345–50.
39. Graham LM, Stanley JC, Whitehouse WM, Zelenock GB, Wakefield TW, Cronenwett JL, et al. Celiac artery aneurysms: historic (1745–1949) versus con-

temporary (1950–1984) differences in etiology and clinical importance. J Vasc Surg. 1985;2(5):757–64.
40. Chadha M, Ahuja C. Visceral artery aneurysms: diagnosis and percutaneous management. Semin Intervent Radiol. 2009;26(3):196–206.
41. Sessa C, Tinelli G, Porcu P, Aubert A, Thony F, Magne J-L. Treatment of visceral artery aneurysms: description of a retrospective series of 42 aneurysms in 34 patients. Ann Vasc Surg. 2004;18(6):695–703.
42. Carr SC, Mahvi DM, Hoch JR, Archer CW, Turnipseed WD. Visceral artery aneurysm rupture. J Vasc Surg. 2001;33(4):806–11.
43. Hemp JH, Sabri SS. Endovascular management of visceral arterial aneurysms. Tech Vasc Interv Radiol. 2015;18(1):14–23.
44. Tulsyan N, Kashyap VS, Greenberg RK, Sarac TP, Clair DG, Pierce G, et al. The endovascular management of visceral artery aneurysms and pseudoaneurysms. J Vasc Surg. 2007;45(2):276–83.

## Further Reading

Abbas MA, Stone WM, Fowl RJ, Gloviczki P, Oldenburg WA, Pairolero PC, et al. Splenic artery aneurysms: two decades experience at Mayo Clinic. Ann Vasc Surg. 2002;16(4):442–9.

Barrionuevo P, Malas MB, Nejim B, Haddad A, Morrow A, Ponce O, et al. A systematic review and meta-analysis of the management of visceral artery aneurysms. J Vasc Surg. 2020;72(1):40S–5S.

Chaer RA, Abularrage CJ, Coleman DM, Eslami MH, Kashyap VS, Rockman C, et al. The Society for Vascular Surgery clinical practice guidelines on the management of visceral aneurysms. J Vasc Surg. 2020;72(1):3S–39S.

Corey MR, Ergul EA, Cambria RP, English SJ, Patel VI, Lancaster RT, et al. The natural history of splanchnic artery aneurysms and outcomes after operative intervention. J Vasc Surg. 2016;63(4):949–57.

# Management of Complications Occurring After Pancreas Transplantation

## 105

Fabio Vistoli, Emanuele Federico Kauffmann, Niccolò Napoli, Gabriella Amorese, and Ugo Boggi

## 105.1 Introduction

**Learning Goals**
- To understand the indications and principal technique for pancreas and kidney transplantation
- To identify the main complications after pancreas transplantation and their management
- To identify the main complications after kidney transplantation and their management

One hundred years after insulin discovery and 55 years after the first human procedure performed at the University of Minnesota, pancreas transplantation (Pthe Tx) remains the only treatment option that consistently reestablish insulin independence in beta-cell penic diabetic patients. Islet cell transplantation is an alternative and less invasive approach to replenish beta-cell reserve in diabetic patients, but achievement of insulin independence is less predictable and usually short-lived. Successful PTx dramatically improves quality of life and may prolong survival expectancy, especially in patients with end-stage diabetic nephropathy who also receive kidney transplantation. Diabetic nephropathy is indeed a major turning point in the natural history of diabetes with strong prognostic implications. Forty years after the onset of diabetes, only 10% of the patients who develop nephropathy are alive as compared to 70% of the patients without renal disease. Therefore, the presence of diabetic nephropathy dictates the need of PTx, in combination with a kidney, in most recipients, and provides the rationale for classification of PTx recipients in three categories. In selected pre-uremic diabetic patients, a PTx alone (PTA) can reverse diabetes and possibly prevent progression of either microvascular or macrovascular complications of diabetes. In patients with overt diabetic nephropathy, a renal graft is also needed to correct uremia. Ideally, the two grafts are transplanted during the same operation as a simultaneous pancreas and kidney transplantation (SPK). Finally, in post-uremic patients (i.e., in those who have already received a renal transplantation), a pancreas after kidney transplantation (PAK) may be required to prevent recurrence of diabetic nephropathy, to improve quality of life, and possibly to increase long-term survival.

F. Vistoli · E. F. Kauffmann · N. Napoli · U. Boggi (✉)
Division of General and Transplant Surgery,
University of Pisa, Pisa, Italy
e-mail: f.vistoli@med.unipi.it; emanuele.kauffmann@unipi.it; niccolo.napoli@unipi.it; u.boggi@med.unipi.it

G. Amorese
Division of Anesthesia and Intensive Care, Azienda Ospedaliera Universitaria Pisana, Pisa, Italy
e-mail: g.amorese@ao-pisa.toscana.it

In PTA and PAK, the pancreas graft is considered solitary since it is not accompanied by a kidney from the same donor that may act as a "sentinel" for pancreas rejection. Although pancreatic and renal rejection is not always concordant, solitary pancreas grafts are at higher risk of rejection. Solitary pancreatic graft is also at increased risk for vascular thrombosis. The prevalence of diabetes is high and increasing worldwide. By the year 2030, 66.5 millions of adults (8.1% of the overall population) in Europe and 53.2 millions of adults (12.1% of the overall population) in North America will have a diagnosis of diabetes. Depending on the definition of type 1 diabetes, a study demonstrated that in the United States between 740,000 and 970,000 adults suffer from type 1 diabetes. Even if SPK is currently performed also in a growing number of patients with type 2 diabetes, considering that approximately 20% of the patients with type 1 diabetes suffer from diabetic nephropathy after 20–25 years of disease, there is an enormous number of potential SPK recipients. Unfortunately, most of these patients are referred for transplantation only when SPK is no longer feasible mostly due to exceedingly high cardiovascular risk. On the other hand, some patients will never receive a SPK due to organ shortage.

## 105.2 Diagnosis and Indications to Pancreas Transplantation

SPK is feasible in patients with insulin-dependent diabetes (mostly type 1 diabetes) and end-stage renal disease (either on dialysis or with a creatinine clearance <20 mL/min). Selected patients with type 2 diabetes, and low insulin resistance, may also be suitable. PAK is an option in patients with a functioning renal graft (creatinine clearance ≥45 mL/min) to achieve insulin independence and protect the renal graft against recurrence of diabetic nephropathy. PTA is indicated in patients with unawareness hypoglycemia and is an option in patients with chronic complications of diabetes that evolve despite optimal medical therapy. Indication to any category of PTx needs to be confirmed at the end of an exhaustive workup that aims to exclude the presence of contraindications. Excluding general contraindications to transplantation, such as major psychiatric disorders, active infections, ongoing or recent malignant tumors, and so forth, high cardiovascular is the leading contraindication to all types of PTx and especially to SPK. In patients referred for PAK, specific attention should be paid to baseline level of renal graft function as the burden of potential surgical, medical, and oncologic complication could lead to premature loss of renal function. In patients referred for PTA, baseline level of native renal function is key to avoid accelerated loss of renal function that is mostly caused by the use of calcineurin inhibitors (tacrolimus or cyclosporine). In all patients, a thorough immunologic screening is required for the selection of a compatible donor, as the pancreas is particularly vulnerable to rejection. All PTx recipients are frail, because of long-standing diabetes and associated complications. Frailty makes them particularly susceptible to some complications, such as infections, and greatly increases overall risk when compared to nondiabetic recipients of other solid organs.

## 105.3 Complications Occurring After Pancreas Transplantation

All PTx categories are associated with a high rate of posttransplant complications, ranging from 15% to 43% [1], that may lead to pancreas graft loss. Early graft loss caused by a non-immunologic complication is commonly identified as "technical failure." Rates of technical failure approached 25% in the 1980s and are now around 7–9% [2] thanks to improvements in in donor and recipient selection, organ procurement and preservation, anesthesia, surgery, and perioperative care. In general, the primary complication responsible of pancreatic graft loss is technical failure, followed by acute or chronic rejection. Technical failure is understood as the loss of the graft in the first 3 months of transplant. Main reasons of early failure are vascular thrombosis (50%), pancreatitis (20%), infection (18%), fistulas (6.5%), and hemorrhage (2.4%) [3]. In PAK and PTA recipients, missed rejection is the leading cause of graft failure also in the early posttransplant period. Other common complications are infection and dehiscence of the abdominal wall [4]. The high incidence of postoperative surgical complications is explained by the predisposition of the pancreas graft to vascular thrombosis and is compounded by the high degree of complexity of PTx. Surgery has many pitfalls that may occur at any of the following steps: organ procurement, back table preparation of the graft (that includes at least arterial reconstruction), in vivo vascular reconstruction, and drainage of exocrine secretions. The proclivity of pancreatic grafts for vascular thrombosis is largely caused by the simultaneous occurrence of all predisposing factors included in the triad of Virchow. Hypercoagulability is caused by diabetes. Disturbed hemodynamics (stasis and turbulence) is the consequence of splenectomy and enterectomy that drive a low flow in a large vascular bed. Endothelial damage occurs as a consequence of the ischemia-reperfusion injury. Severity of postoperative complications requires repeat surgery in 10–20% of recipients. Relaparotomy is associated with a risk of graft loss ranging between 74% and 89%. A study clearly showed that repeat surgery reduces graft survival at one year (82–95.5% vs. 32–77%) [5]. Other risk factors for surgical complications include prolonged time in peritoneal dialysis, donor or recipient with a body mass index >28 kg/m$^2$, donor or recipient age over 45 years, cerebrovascular disease as cause of donor death, prolonged preservation time (>20 h), retransplantation, and previous abdominal surgery. Early diagnosis of postoperative complications is considered important to maximize the chances of graft rescue while reducing the risks on recipients. However, clinical signs of ongoing complications may be difficult to detect in diabetic patients who often suffer from diabetic neuropathy and are receiving high dose immunosuppression. Timely diagnosis requires a prompt radiologic evaluation, based on ultrasonography (contrast-enhanced or not) and/or contrast-enhanced CT scan. Considering that PTX creates a "new radiologic anatomy," radiologists should be specifically prepared to face this scenario [6, 7]. If the pancreas rescue is possible (in relation to patient condition, extent of the pathology, contamination of the operative field, and graft function), it is advisable to preserve the graft because in the long-term PTx improves survival, independently from occurrence of early complications (Fig. 105.1). However, in individuals receiving SPK or PAK, it is mandatory to balance the risk of impairing renal graft function with the attempt to salvage the pancreas graft as loss of renal function is associated with worse prognostic implications. If the pancreas graft is eventually lost but the renal function is preserved, the patient could be reconsidered for a PAK. Ideal timing for PAK is within 1 year of renal transplant. Pancreas graft rejection is the next, main, cause for graft loss. In the early days of PTx, 80% of SPK recipients developed an acute rejection in the first year after transplantation. Isolated rejection of the pancreas graft accounted for 27% of these episodes and was eventually followed by graft loss in up to 20% of the patients. The criteria used for the diagnosis of pancreatic graft rejection are increased serum creatinine levels (the concept of "sentinel kidney" in SPK), decreased amylasuria (PTx with exocrine bladder drainage), and high serum amylase and lipase levels that cannot be explained otherwise. Pancreatic biopsy (possibly under ultrasonography guidance) is considered today the gold standard for diagnosis of pancreatic rejection. Despite better pancreatic transplant results, infectious complications remain the primary causes of morbidity and mortality. The most frequent etiology is bacterial infection, and the urinary tract and abdominal wall are the most affected sites. Patients receiving PTx have a high risk of developing cytomegalovirus infection because of the frequent use of depleting antibodies for induction of immunosuppression. The mean incidence is 25%. Early diagnosis, especially in fungal infection, is key for success of treatment. Administration of antibiotics, antifungal agents, and antiviral agents are recommended. In a later phase, the major complications are related to the clinical picture of chronic rejection and infectious complications. Myocardial infarction and sudden death are other significant causes of mortality, related to diabetic

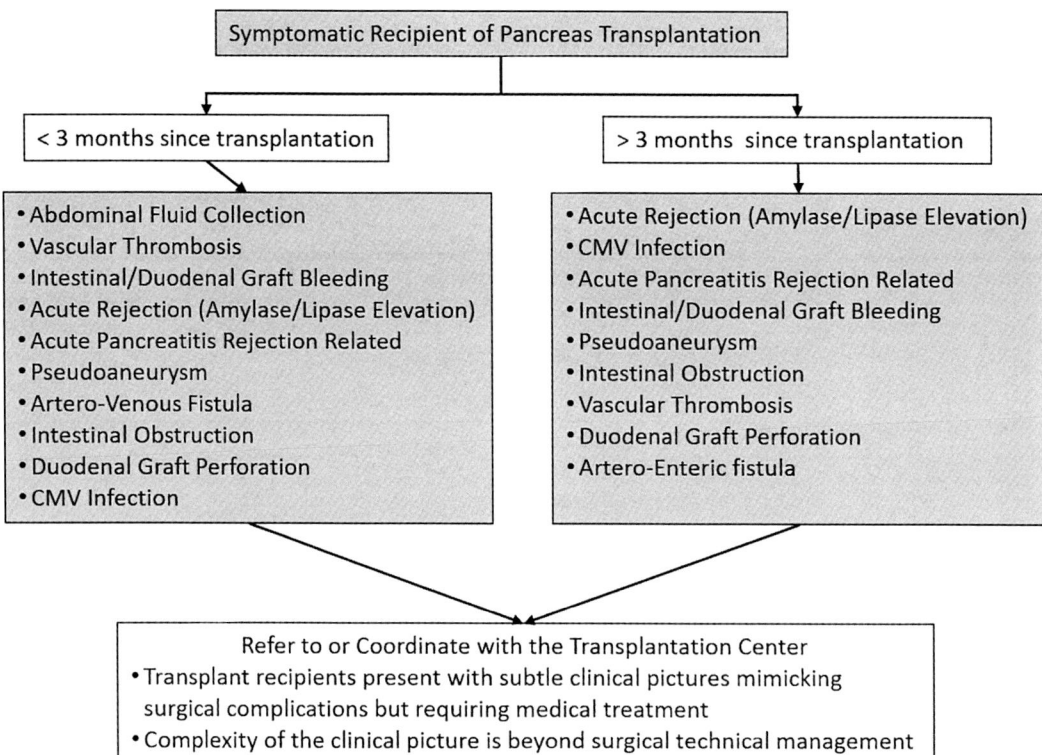

**Fig. 105.1** Main complications after pancreas transplantation. Problems are stratified according to the time from the transplant and listed in order of probability. In any circumstances it is advisable, if the clinical conditions are permissive, to refer the patient to (or at least to coordinate with) the transplant center. In most cases, the symptoms are subtle, and the management goes beyond the aspects of surgical techniques, requiring specific transplant-related skills that consider potential causes, medical, surgical, and immunological, of the complications as a whole

chronic complications (diabetic macroangiopathy and diabetic autonomic neuropathy).

## 105.4 Surgical Techniques for Pancreas (and Kidney) Transplantation

The pancreatic graft consists of the entire gland with an attached (short) duodenal segment. After sharing of vascular pedicles with the liver, the pancreas remains with two main arterial pedicles (i.e., the splenic artery and the superior mesenteric artery) and a single vein (i.e., the portal vein). Before the graft is judged suitable for transplantation, it has to be prepared at the back table. Depending on how much dissection was performed in the donor, back table procedures may require 2–3 h. During this time, a surgeon proceeds to splenectomy, removes excess tissue (such as the mesenteric root and retroperitoneal lympho-neural tissue), checks for the presence of a valid collateral circulation between the splenic artery and the superior mesenteric artery, reconstructs a single arterial pedicle as appropriate (often using a donor Y iliac graft), trims the duodenal segment, and fixes all detectable bleeding sites. PTx is mostly performed through a transperitoneal approach even when the graft will be eventually left in the retroperitoneum. Usually, a midline incision is used, as this approach permits simultaneous transplantation of pancreas and kidney and allows the surgeon to freely decide about graft position and transplant technique. The pancreas graft is typically placed along the right flank or in the right iliac fossa. The kidney is often placed in the left iliac fossa. Depending on individual circumstances, the pancreas and the kidney may be placed ipsilaterally, usually on the right side [8]. The graft may be oriented either head-up or head-down, depending on the site of vascular reconstruction and intended technique for exocrine drainage. The site for arterial inflow and venous outflow depend on graft location (and vice versa). In the most common scenario, the arterial anastomosis is created on the right common iliac artery. Venous outflow may be directed in the superior mesenteric vein (portal venous drainage) or in a tributary vein of the systemic circulation, mostly inferior vena cava or right common iliac vein (systemic venous drainage). After graft revascularization, the graft duodenum may be anastomosed to either the intestine (enteric drainage) or the bladder (bladder drainage). Therefore, according to the type of venous and exocrine drainage, PTx can be systemic-bladder, systemic-enteric, or portal-enteric drained (Fig. 105.2). The duodenal graft is generally closed at both ends with a linear suturing device, and, mainly for hemostatic purposes, the rhyme can be reinforced with a continuous and inverted suture. In case of enteric drainage, the graft duodenum may be anastomosed to the jejunum (more frequent in case of portal venous drainage), to the ileum (more frequent in case of iliac venous drainage), or to the native duodenum. A gastric drainage is also possible. Intestinal anastomosis to jejunum or ileum may be direct on a Roux-en-Y loop. Currently, bladder drainage is used rarely and mostly for solitary pancreas transplants because it permits immunologic graft surveillance by assay of urinary amylase levels and cystoscopic biopsy of the graft duodenum. An additional advantage of this technique is the possibility to pursue conservative management of some duodenal complications. However, bladder drainage is clearly non-physiologic and is associated with frequent and severe urological and metabolic complications. Chronic urinary loss of pancreatic juice, with water and sodium bicarbonate, requires chronic intake of oral sodium bicarbonate to avoid metabolic acidosis. The erosive action of pancreatic juice on the bladder carries the risk of urologic complications and predisposes to recurrent urinary infections. Urinary reflux in the ductal system of the pancreas can cause pancreatitis. Because of these complications, approximately 10–25% of patients require conversion form bladder to enteric drainage.

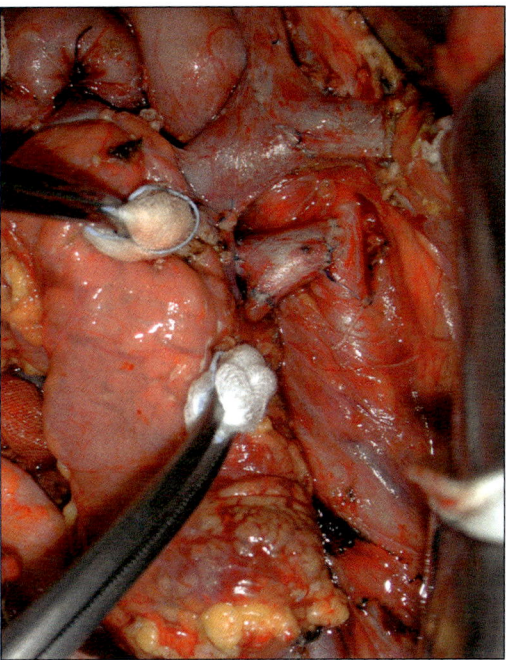

**Fig. 105.2** Portal-enteric drained pancreas transplantation. Pancreatic graft's portal vein is anastomosed in termino-lateral to the mesenteric vein just below the inferior margin of the native pancreatic head. The common branch of the arterial Y graft, used to connect superior mesenteric and splenic arteries of the pancreatic graft, is anastomosed in termino-lateral to the common iliac artery of the recipient. A Roux-en-Y jejunal loop is created in the recipient and anastomosed to the duodenal graft to drain the pancreatic exocrine secretions produced by the grafted pancreas

## 105.5 Treatment and Management of Posttransplant Complications

The main postoperative surgical complications, related to the pancreatic graft, are reported in Table 105.1. Complications may be caused by donor factors, preservation injury, long cold

**Table 105.1** Main surgical complications occurring after pancreas transplantation

| Complication | Incidence (%) |
|---|---|
| Vascular thrombosis (arterial, venous) | 3–10 |
| Pseudoaneurysm | 1–8 |
| Arteriovenous fistula | ≅1.4 |
| Arterio-enteric fistula | ≅1.4 |
| Duodenal graft complications (DGC) | ≅20 |

ischemia time, surgery in recipients, ischemia-reperfusion injury, infections, and rejection episodes.

### 105.5.1 Intestinal Complications

Intestinal complications may occur in the setting of either enteric or bladder drainage of exocrine secretions. As duodenal graft complications presenting after bladder drainage are mostly associated with urinary tract complaints and are managed by means of urologic techniques, here we address only intestinal complications occurring in patients who received an enteric drainage. Intestinal complications after PTx often involved the graft duodenum. Duodenal graft complications (DGC) occur in some 20% of PTx and may present in the early or late posttransplant period. Early complications are mostly caused by preservation injury or surgical issues. Late complications are often related to underlying infections or missed rejection episodes. Diagnosis of DGC may be difficult. To facilitate diagnosis and management of DGC has been proposed the routine use of a venting jejunostomy to permit straightforward surveillance of graft duodenum and endoscopic interventions.

#### 105.5.1.1 Duodenal Graft Perforation (DGP)

DGP is a potentially life-threatening complication. Presentation may include classical signs such as fever and abdominal pain but may also present with nonspecific complaints and less obvious clinical picture [9]. DGP can occur along the anastomotic brim or at a duodenal stump. Repair of duodenal leaks is complex. In some patients, direct closure of the breach may be sufficient. In other patients, partial or total graft duodenectomy may be required, followed by direct drainage of pancreatic exocrine secretions in the native bowel [9]. In case of severe sepsis or other reasons discouraging reconstruction, alternative options include external duct drainage [9], duct occlusion, or allograft pancreatectomy. DGP could be also treated by perforation repair and opening of a temporary venting jejunostomy. Pancreatoduodenectomy is an additional option, when concerns exist on viability of the pancreatic head [10]. Finally, in case of allograft pancreatectomy islet cell, (auto)transplantation is an option to salvage endocrine function.

#### 105.5.1.2 Intestinal Bleeding and Duodenal Graft Bleeding (DGB)

Intestinal bleeding is a relatively frequent and possibly severe complication of PTx that may be prompted or aggravated by the antiplatelet therapy that most PTx are taking as prophylaxis for cardiovascular disease. Identification of bleeding site follows standard protocols, but, especially in DGB, it is often missed as the graft duodenum can be rarely reached endoscopically, unless a duodeno-duodenostomy was performed, and hemorrhage can be intermittent. Despite most bleeding episodes resolve with discontinuation of antiplatelet therapy and conservative treatment, they typically recur and may be life-threatening so that patients should be referred to transplant centers at the first episode. Permanent treatment of DGB depends of etiology. In case of bleeding not amenable to medical treatment, either partial or total duodenectomy are an option depending on location and diffusion of the bleeding disease.

Hemodynamic stability dictates timing and type of diagnostic procedures. The early study of choice should be a CT angiogram or a systemic selective angiogram. Angiography may also permit therapeutic intervention of either permanent or temporary nature. Search for bleeding site by upper and/or lower endoscopy is often inconclusive because either intermittent hemorrhage or presence of too much blood to permit to define the source of bleeding. In case of missed diagnosis, additional tests include tagged red blood cell scan, capsule endoscopy, and double balloon enteroscopy. Mesenteric angiography is often nondiagnostic and should be pursued only when there is a strong suspicion for a nonpancreatic bleeding.

### 105.5.1.3 Intestinal Obstruction

Aherence and internal hernia can lead to reoperation, and they are more associated to intraperitoneal techniques. A rare case of intestinal occlusion reported is that of a bezoar occluding the small bowel in an SPK recipient at the level of the jejunojejunostomy of the Roux-en-Y loop used for the enteric drainage of the transplanted pancreas. In this case, early detection to pancreas graft rescue before duodenal graft rupture or the development of graft pancreatitis is important. A relaparotomy may be necessary to preserve the graft avoiding life-threatening conditions.

## 105.5.2 Abdominal Fluid Collections

Abdominal fluid collections are quite common in PTx, as a result of hematoma, lymphatic leaks, pancreatic leaks, enteric leaks, and ascites [11]. Treatment is dictated by underlying etiology, presence of symptoms, and presence of signs of infection or ongoing bleeding. In some patients, preemptive treatment may also be indicated in case of anticipated high evolution into a relevant clinical problem. Fluid collections may also be punctured to gain insights on underlying cause. Bulky perigraft fluid collections may also result in vascular compression, thus facilitating the development of vascular thrombosis. Unless urgent conditions apply, most abdominal fluid collections are treated by means of a step-up approach in which invasiveness of procedures is progressively increased in the lack of clinical/radiologic/laboratory improvement. By having said this, it is important to underscore that those clinical pictures in PTX recipients are often inconclusive, while hiding major intra-abdominal issues, so that exploratory laparotomy may be indicated to reach a reliable diagnosis. In case of extraperitoneal placement of the pancreatic graft, most perigraft fluid collections are accessible to percutaneous catheter drainage.

## 105.5.3 Vascular Complications

### 105.5.3.1 Vascular Thrombosis (VT)

VT is usually an early complication that in most patients occurs in the first month after PTx and constitutes one of the main reasons of technical failure. Late thrombosis is more typically caused by missed rejection and typically leads to graft loss. VT, in the most recent era, occurs in 3–19% of PTx [12]. Many factors are involved in pancreas graft thrombosis, and the ideal prophylaxis is not clearly established [12]. On practical grounds, most patients receive prophylaxis with either anticoagulant or anti-platelet drugs in the attempt to prevent venous thrombosis. Arterial thrombosis is less frequent and mostly associated to a technical detail. Complete thrombosis leads to graft loss. If timely detected, partial thrombosis may allow a chance for graft rescue and therefore requires surveillance by means of ultrasonography with color-Doppler that should be performed daily in the first week after PTx. Suspicious findings should be further investigated by contrast-enhanced CT-scan. Upon confirmation of partial CT, graft rescue may be attempted by increasing anticoagulation. Endovascular treatments [13] and surgical thrombectomy [14], but advantages of more aggressive treatments should be carefully balanced against their possible consequences (Fig. 105.3).

### 105.5.3.2 Pseudoaneurysm

Pseudoaneurysms (PSA) are a possible complication of PTx, are frequently of mycotic origin, and may have fatal consequences [15]. That can occur at any of the arterial anastomoses required to revascularize a pancreatic graft [12]. Non-anastomotic PSA are associated to biopsy or perigraft infected collection [16]. PSA can be incidentally discovered or present with intra-abdominal or intestinal bleeding. Bleeding is typically massive but can be intermittent. Once the diagnosis is established, PSA can be excluded

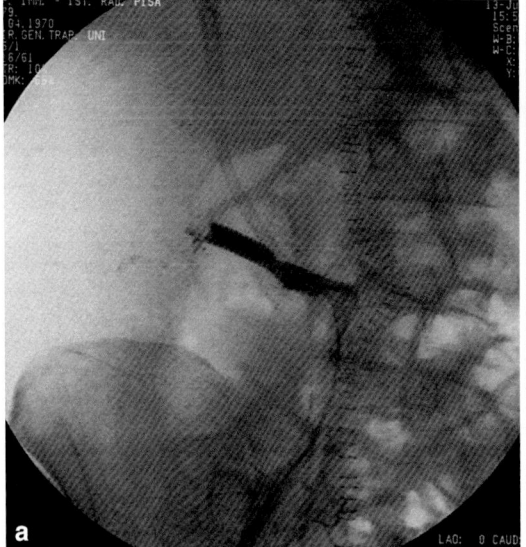 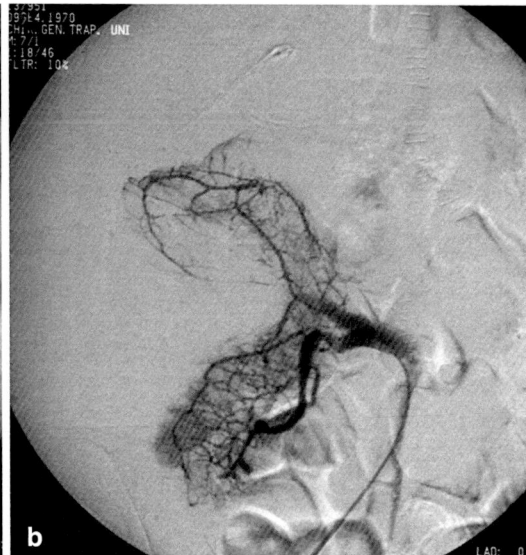

**Fig. 105.3** Arteriography images showing diagnosis and treatment results after subtotal thrombosis of a grafted pancreas. (**a**) Pretreatment arteriography showing subtotal thrombosis of the pancreas graft. Only the common iliac branch of the Y arterial graft and the mesenteric artery (anastomosed to the external iliac branch of the Y arterial graft) of the grafted pancreas graft are perfused. No parenchimography of the grafted organ is visible. (**b**) Posttreatment angiography showing the full recovery of the normal artero-venous vascularization and of the parenchimography of the pancreatic graft. The patient received a 48 h infusion of urokinase directly delivered in the common iliac branch of the Y arterial graft

by an endovascular prosthesis or embolized. However, this treatment is rarely permanent because most PSA have a mycotic etiology and bleeding is expected to recur. In many patients, permanent treatment requires allograft pancreatectomy [17] and ligation of arterial inflow. In case of insufficient collateral supply (7–21%) and distal ischemia, the limb can be revascularized by an extra-anatomical by-pass (either axillofemoral or femorofemoral) [18]. Implantation of a vascular prosthesis in the anatomic bed of the ligated/resected vascular segment is contraindicated because of the ongoing infection. Alternatively, a biologic graft can be used for in situ vascular reconstruction. The use of a bovine pericardial patch [19] was reported to prevent PSA recurrence in 98% of the patients who did not develop recurrent infection [20]. Allograft salvage is rarely feasible and should be well balanced against the consequences of recurrent PSA. Long-term aneurysm of the Y graft could present. Surgical management can be demanding and lead to graft loss. However, a careful approach allows aneurysm correction preserving pancreatic graft (Fig. 105.4).

### 105.5.3.3 Artero-Venous Fistula

Artero-venous fistula is often associated with PSA and typically occurs after a pancreas graft biopsy or as a consequence of iatrogenic injury occurred at the back table during preparation of the mesenteric root [21–23]. Small arteriovenous fistulas are incidentally discovered and can be treated conservatively. Treatment is warranted for larger shunts or in patients with hemodynamic consequences, graft disfunction, graft pancreatitis, and other local complications [21, 24]. Despite treatment, either endovascular or surgical, allograft pancreatectomy is a possible consequence of artero-venous fistula [25, 26] (Fig. 105.5).

### 105.5.3.4 Arterio-Enteric Fistula

Arterio-enteric fistula presents as life-threatening gastrointestinal bleeding in enteric-drained transplants and results from rupture of a PSA

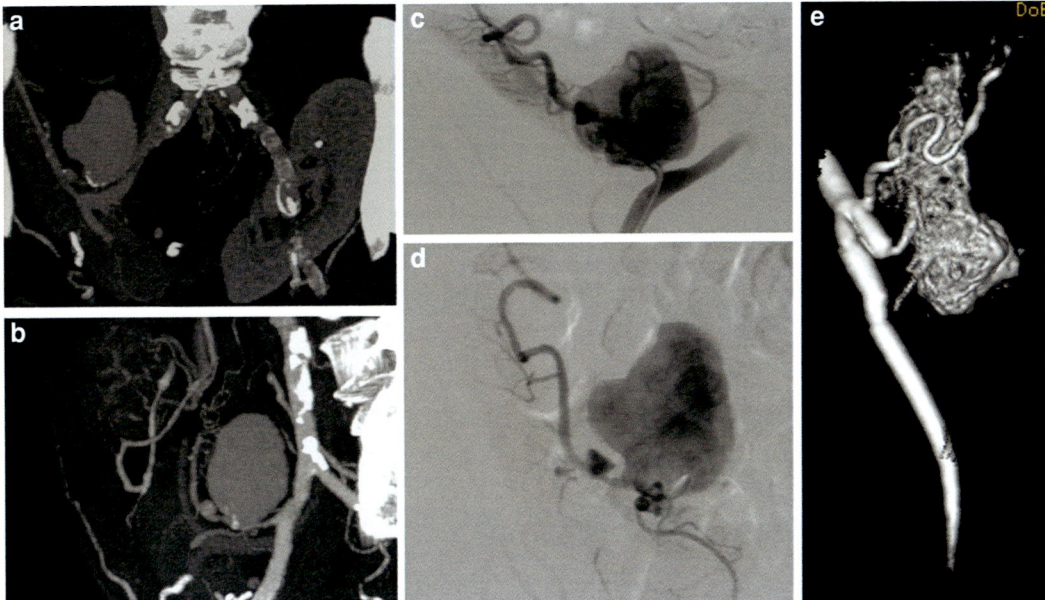

**Fig. 105.4** Arterial aneurysm of the common iliac branch of the Y graft occurred 7 years after pancreas transplantation. (**a, b**) CT scan showing the aneurysm of the common iliac branch of the Y arterial graft anastomosed to the external iliac artery of a recipient of a pancreas transplantation. (**c, d**) Arteriography showing the aneurysm and the splenic and mesenteric artery of the pancreatic graft. (**e**) Postoperative angio-RM 3D reconstruction showing postoperative results. After isolation of the aneurysm, pancreas graft was cooled on site. Then, the aneurysm was resected en bloc with the tract of the recipient's external iliac artery where the previous anastomosis was performed. The internal iliac artery was isolated, transposed, and anastomosed to the external iliac artery below the previous anastomotic tract. Pancreatic graft's splenic artery (termino-lateral) and superior mesenteric artery (termino-terminal) were anastomosed to the proximal external iliac artery stump of the recipient

into the intestine [12]. Catastrophic hemorrhage is often preceded by a "sentinel" or herald bleed that can offer the opportunity for timely diagnosis and intervention. PSAs originate from the graft splenic artery or superior mesenteric artery, the Y iliac graft, the iliac artery anastomosis, or other large recipient arteries. As already presented, PSAs have typically a bacterial of fungal etiology. Sterile PSAs are also possible and may be the consequence of complete withdrawal of immunosuppression in patients with chronic graft dysfunction/failure [27, 28].

While an endovascular approach is important to establish the diagnosis and achieve temporary hemostasis, it can rarely be the permanent treatment because intestinal fistulization creates the opportunity for ongoing infection and recurrence of bleeding. Surgery can be extremely demanding and may require a wide spectrum of procedures [23].

### 105.5.4 Complications Related to the Renal Graft

The main postoperative surgical complications, related to the kidney graft, are reported in Table 105.2.

#### 105.5.4.1 Renal Graft Thrombosis

Renal graft thrombosis can be either caused by renal vein thrombosis (0.2–3.5%) or renal artery thrombosis (0.3–3%) [29]. Long renal veins and/or multiple veins are risk factors for renal vein thrombosis. Renal artery thrombosis is caused/facilitated by severe atherosclerosis of native iliac arteries [30]. In patients with delayed graft function, and no urinary output, renal graft thrombosis can only be detected by protocol tests performed to verify graft viability (usually ultrasonography with color-Doppler). In the other patients, renal graft thrombosis presents with

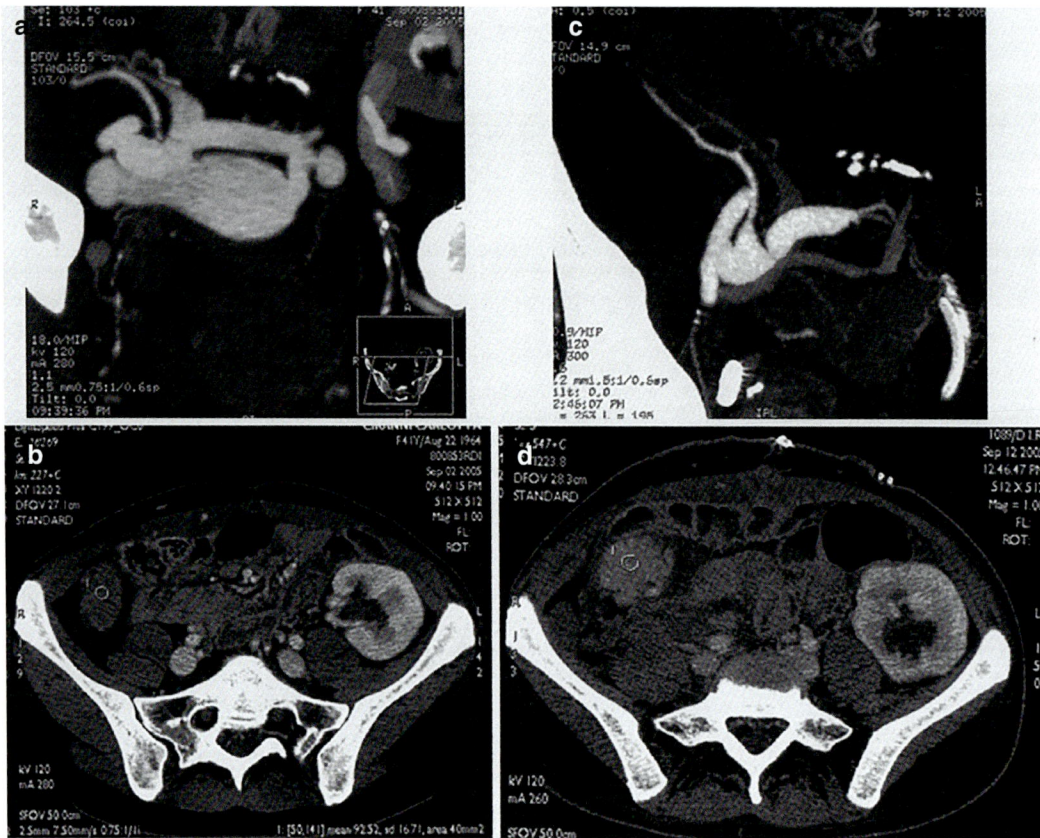

**Fig. 105.5** CT scan images showing an artero-venous fistula occurred from superior mesenteric artery and vein in the root of the mesentery of a grafted pancreas. (**a**) Preoperative CT scan 2D reconstruction of the fistula. (**b**) Preoperative CT scan image (arterial phase) showing the pancreatic graft hypoperfused due to the fistula. (**c**) Postoperative CT scan 2D reconstruction showing resolution of the fistula obtained by suture of the hole. Arterial and venous vessels of the pancreatic graft present different intensity. (**d**) Postoperative CT scan image (arterial phase) showing pancreatic graft normally perfused

**Table 105.2** Main surgical complications occurring after concomitant renal transplantation

| Complication | Incidence (%) |
| --- | --- |
| Renal vein thrombosis | 0.3–3 |
| Renal artery thrombosis | 0.2–3.5 |
| Renal graft rupture | 0.3–9.6 |
| Lymphocele | 0.6–22 |
| Vesicoureteral anastomose stenosis | 1.7 |
| Vesicoureteral anastomose leakage | 1.1 |
| Wound complication | 5 |

sudden onset oliguria or anuria that demands immediate differential diagnosis with acute rejection. Ultrasonography with color-Doppler is usually the first diagnostic test, but CT scan has a higher sensibility in defining renal artery thrombosis [29]. Graft salvage can be attempted only in patients with partial vascular thrombosis. Depending on severity, underlying cause, and vascular anatomy, graft salvage may avail of an endovascular procedure, a surgical operation, or a combination thereof.

### 105.5.4.2 Renal Graft Rupture

Spontaneous renal graft rupture is a rare complication of SPK with a reported incidence ranging between 0.3% and 9.6%. It can be caused by renal vein thrombosis, acute tubular necrosis, or acute rejection and typically occurs in the first 2–3 posttransplant weeks. Traumatic rupture is also possible at any time after transplantation. Renal graft rupture presents with sudden pain accompanied by swelling over the graft area, oliguria, or anuria with hypotension. Bleeding from the surgical incision or hematuria may also be noted. Depending on underlying cause and severity of damage, graft rescue may be attempted [31], but graft nephrectomy is required in a large proportion of patients and should be urgently performed in unstable patients [29].

### 105.5.4.3 Urological Complications (Fistula, Ureteral Stenosis)

Most urologic complications of renal transplantation involve the ureterovesical anastomosis and consist in anastomotic stenosis (1.7%), urinary leak (1.1%), and urinary reflux (0–5%). Incidence and severity of urologic complications are mostly influenced by recipient factors (such as characteristics of urinary bladder) but may also be caused/facilitated by iatrogenic injuries occurred during organ procurement or back table graft preparation, and/or surgical misadventure/poor technique at the time of transplantation. Other factors involved in the origin of urologic complications are recipient age, number of renal arteries, long preservation time, site of arterial anastomosis, occurrence of acute rejection episodes, and immunosuppressive regimen (especially early use of m-TOR inhibitors). In general, ureteric stenosis and urinary leaks are caused/facilitated by ureteral ischemia [32]. Diagnosis and treatment of urologic complications depend on timing of diagnosis, anatomy of damage, clinical conditions of the recipient, and associated predisposing factors (such voiding problems in patients with ureterovesical reflux). Permanent treatment is highly specialistic and therefore should be planned and performed at qualified transplant centers. When required by clinical conditions, most cases of uteral stenosis and urinary leak benefit from pyeloureterostomy. Placing a pyeloureterostomy in a patient with a urinary leak and therefore with a decompressed urinary tract is technically demanding and may be associated with iatrogenic graft injury.

### 105.5.4.4 Lymphocele

In kidney alone transplantation, renal grafts are placed in one iliac fossa in a retroperitoneal position. Considering that the renal graft has no left lymphatic drainage and that dissection of iliac vessels in preparation for transplantation requires division of several large lymphatics, renal transplantation creates an obvious opportunity for the onset of lymphocele. In SPK recipients, the renal graft is either left in an intraperitoneal position or is eventually placed in the retroperitoneum through an intraperitoneal approach. Communication with the peritoneal cavity offers the opportunity for reabsorption of lymphatics leaks, making lymphocele far less frequent in SPK recipients when compared to recipients of kidney-alone transplantation. Asymptomatic lymphocele requires no treatment. On the other hand, treatment is required in case of fluid collections causing a mass effect on urinary tract or iliac/renal vessels. The basic principle of treatment is drainage. Percutaneous catheter drainage is feasible in most patients but may be associated with prolonged drainage time and partial success. Intraperitoneal marsupialization is an alternative option when percutaneous catheter drainage is ineffective. Increased incidence of lymphocele has been reported during acute tubular necrosis and during acute rejection [33].

## 105.5.5 Complications Non-related to the Transplant

The main postoperative surgical complications, non-related to the transplant, are reported in Table 105.3. General surgical complications occur in approximately one-third SPK recipients and include wound infection/delayed wound healing (14.3%), postoperative bleeding (12.1%), intra-abdominal infections (7.1%), hematoma (6.6%), ileus (3.3%), and

**Table 105.3** Other surgical complications occurring after pancreas transplantation, not directly related to the pancreatic graft

| Complication | Incidence (%) |
|---|---|
| Abscess | ≅7.1 |
| Hemorrhage | 12.1 |
| Occlusion | ≅1.7–10.2 |
| Evisceration | ≅1.7 |
| Wound infection | ≅14.3 |

anastomotic insufficiency (3.3%) [34]. Wound complications are probably the most common surgical complication after a PTx, with an approximate incidence of 5%. Risk factors for wound complications include systemic factors (e.g., increased age, obesity, diabetes, and malnutrition), wound features (e.g., hematoma and dead space), and operative characteristics (e.g., poor surgical technique, lengthy operation, and intraoperative contamination). Wound infections can be divided into superficial wound infections and deep wound infections. The treatment of wound infections should follow general principles established for general surgery procedures. Immunosuppression should be adapted to permit wound healing [29]. The risk of wound complications, as well as of surgical site infections, could be reduced by minimally invasive pancreas transplantation [35–37]. Intestinal obstruction can also occur as a consequence of adhesions or internal herniation and should be treated according to standard procedures.

Postoperative bleeding is relatively frequent after PTx because most recipients are under chronic antiplatelet therapies, and anticoagulation is generally devised to reduce the risk of allograft thrombosis. Also management of bleeding follows general surgical principles. A specific issue regards management of anticoagulation. Sudden reversal of anticoagulation may be required in some patients, but attention should be paid to rebound effects that could create a prothrombotic state leading to vascular thrombosis.

## 105.6 Conclusions

In selected diabetic patients, PTx has a high therapeutic index despite being associated with frequent occurrence of severe posttransplant complications. Many of these complications are seen also in general surgical practice, while other complications are specific to PTx and are difficult to treat outside well-established transplant centers. In general, PTx recipients should be offered first aid locally and be immediately referred to qualified transplant centers for definitive care.

> **Take-Home Messages**
> - The surgeon, after pancreas transplantation, could face multiple complications.
> - Sometimes, complications after pancreas transplantation could be life-threatening because of the patient's frailty and because of the severity of the complication.
> - Complications could occur after many years after transplant also after the graft loss.
> - Prompt diagnose and management are mandatory, and these patients should be always referred to transplantation centers.

> **Dos and Don'ts**
> - In recipients of kidney and pancreas grafts, symptoms of complications could be vanishing delaying the diagnosis.
> - In case of suspicious, performing a contrast-enhanced CT scan in order to rule out a surgical complication is of main importance.
> - Do a balance between patient condition and the weight of treatment.
> - Do not limit yourself to the easier diagnose.
> - Do a balanced intervention to save the patient before organs.

> **Multiple Choice**
> 1. Extraluminal bleeding after PTx is always due to a surgical cause.
>    A. Yes
>    B. **No**
>    C. It is always intraluminal
>    D. It is a rare complication
> 2. Which is the rate of pancreatic graft loss for technical failure?
>    A. 30%
>    B. 40%
>    C. 3%
>    D. **7%**

3. Which is the most frequent surgical complication after PTx?
   A. **Duodenal graft complication**
   B. Intra-abdominal hemorrhage
   C. Vascular thrombosis
   D. Wound infection
4. In case of duodenal graft perforation?
   A. **Depending on the patient and surgical field contamination, a graft salvage could be performed.**
   B. The patient should not be operated.
   C. The graftectomy is the only way to proceed.
   D. It is always possible a salvage procedure.
5. The intestinal obstruction after PTx is?
   A. More frequent in case of extraperitoneal transplant.
   B. **More frequent in case of intraperitoneal transplant.**
   C. It is not reported.
   D. Is related to a worse prognosis.
6. Non-anastomotic pseudoaneurysm could be related to:
   A. **Biopsy**
   B. Immunosuppression
   C. Ascites
   D. Congenital malformation
7. In case of infected PSA:
   A. The endovascular treatment is always effective.
   B. The antibiotical treatment is generally effective.
   C. **The endovascular treatment sometimes is a bridge to surgery.**
   D. The graft salvage is always possible.
8. Renal graft thrombosis should be immediately excluded in case of:
   A. **Sudden onset of oliguria/anuria**
   B. Fever
   C. Pain
   D. DGF
9. Lymphocele after kidney transplantation:
   A. Should be always drained.
   B. Is a rare complication.
   C. **If asymptomatic could be not drained.**
   D. Usually lead to graft loss.
10. The frequency of ureterovesical anastomosis stenosis is:
    A. **1.7%**
    B. 10%
    C. 0.2%
    D. 3–4%

## References

1. Humar A, Kandaswamy R, Granger D, et al. Decreased surgical risk of pancreas transplantation in the modern era. Ann Surg. 2000;231:269–75.
2. Gruessner AC, Sutherland DE. Pancreas transplant outcomes for United States (US) cases as reported to the United Network of Organ Sharing (UNOS) and the International Pancreas Transplant Registry (IPTR). Clin Transpl. 2008:45–56.
3. Kandaswamy R, Stock PG, Miller J, et al. OPTN/SRTR 2019 Annual Data Report: pancreas. Am J Transplant. 2021;21(Suppl 2):138–207.
4. Humar A, Ramcharan T, Kandaswamy R, et al. Technical failures after pancreas transplants: why grafts fail and the risk factors—a multivariate analysis. Transplantation. 2004;78(8):1188–92.
5. Cornejo-Carrasco CE, Fernández-Cruz L. Re-operation in pancreas transplantation. Transplant Proc. 2014;46:3050–3.
6. Yales A, Parry C, Stephens M, Eynon A. Imaging pancreas transplants. Br J Radiol. 2013;86:20130428.
7. Neri E, Cappelli C, Boggi U, et al. Multirow CT in the follow-up of pancreas transplantation. Transplant Proc. 2004;36:507–600.
8. Boggi U, Amorese G, Marchetti P. Surgical techniques for pancreas transplantation. Curr Opin Organ Transplant. 2010;15(1):102–11.
9. Pieroni E, Napoli N, Lombardo C, et al. Duodenal graft complications requiring duodenectomy after pancreas and pancreas-kidney transplantation. Am J Transplant. 2018;18(6):1388–96.
10. Sansalone CV, Maione G, Aseni P, et al. Surgical complications are the main cause of pancreatic allograft loss in pancreas-kidney transplant recipients. Transplant Proc. 2005;37(6):2651–3.

11. O'Malley RB, Moshiri M, Osman S, et al. Imaging of pancreas transplantation and its complications. Radiol Clin N Am. 2016;54:251–26.
12. Laurencea JM, Cattral MS. Techniques of pancreas graft salvage/indications for allograft pancreatectomy. Curr Opin Organ Transplant. 2016;21:405–11.
13. Stockland AH, Willingham DL, Paz-Fumagalli R, et al. Pancreas transplant venous thrombosis: role of endovascular interventions for graft salvage. Cardiovasc Intervent Radiol. 2009;32:279–83.
14. Fernandez-Cruz L, Gilabert R, Sabater L, et al. Pancreas graft thrombosis: prompt diagnosis and immediate thrombectomy or retransplantation. Clin Transpl. 1993;7:230–23.
15. Sörelius K, Wanhainen A, Furebring M, et al. Nationwide study of the treatment of mycotic abdominal aortic aneurysms comparing open and endovascular repair. Circulation. 2016;134:1822–32.
16. Tobben PJ, Zajko AB, Sumkin JH, et al. Pseudoaneurysms complicating organ transplantation: roles of CT, duplex sonography and angiography. Radiology. 1988;169(1):65–70.
17. White SA, Shaw JA, Sutherland DE. Pancreas transplantation. Lancet. 2009;373:1808–17.
18. Gorey TF, Bulkley GB, Spees EK Jr, et al. Iliac artery ligation: the relative paucity of ischemic sequelae in renal transplant patients. Ann Surg. 1979;190:753–7.
19. Yiannoulloua P, van Dellena D, Khambalia H, et al. Successful management of a ruptured mycotic pseudoaneurysm following pancreas transplantation using bovine pericardial patch: a case report. Transplant Proc. 2014;46:2023–5.
20. McMillan WD, Leville CD, Hile CN. Bovine pericardial patch repair in infected fields. J Vasc Surg. 2012;55(6):1712–5.
21. Khan TF, Ciancio G, Burke GW III, et al. Pseudoaneurysm of the superior mesenteric artery with an arteriovenous fistula after simultaneous kidney pancreas transplantation. Clin Transpl. 1999;13(277–279):65.
22. Lowell JA, Stratta RJ, Taylor RJ, et al. Mesenteric arteriovenous fistula after vascularized pancreas transplantation resulting in graft dysfunction. Clin Transpl. 1996;10:278–81.
23. Fridell JA, Powelson JA, Kubal CA, et al. Retrieval of the pancreas allograft for whole-organ transplantation. Clin Transpl. 2014;28:1313–30.
24. Bratton CF, Hamid A, Selby JB, et al. Case report: gastrointestinal hemorrhage caused by a pancreas transplant arteriovenous fistula with large pseudoaneurysm 9 years after transplantation. Transplant Proc. 2011;43:4039–43.
25. Dalla Valle R, Capocasale E, Mazzoni MP, et al. Embolization of a ruptured pseudoaneurysm with massive hemorrhage following pancreas transplantation: a case report. Transplant Proc. 2005;37:2275–7.
26. Maupoey Ibáñez J, Boscà Robledo A, López-Andujar R. Late complications of pancreas transplant. World J Transplant. 2020;10(12):404–14.
27. Parajuli S, Odorico J, Astor BC, et al. Incidence and indications for late allograft pancreatectomy while on continued immunosuppression. Transplantation. 2017;101:2228–34.
28. Zhao J, Gao Z, Wang K. The transplantation operation and its surgical complications, understanding the complexities of kidney transplantation; 2011. Ortiz J, editor, ISBN: 978-953-307-819-9.
29. Grochowiecki T, Gałązka Z, Madej K, et al. Early complications related to the transplanted kidney after simultaneous pancreas and kidney transplantation. Transplant Proc. 2014;46(8):2815–7.
30. Shahrokh H, Rasouli H, Zargar MA, et al. Spontaneous kidney allograft rupture. Transplant Proc. 2005;37(7):3079–80.
31. Salomon L, Saporta F, Amsellem D, et al. Results of pyeloureterostomy after ureterovesical anastomosis complications in renal transplantation. Urology. 1999;53(5):908–12.
32. Lehner LJ, Hohberger A, Marschke L, et al. Analysis of risk factors and long-term outcomes in kidney transplant patients with identified lymphoceles. J Clin Med. 2020;9(9):2841.
33. Grochowiecki T, Madej K, Gałązka Z, et al. Usefulness of modified Dindo-Clavien scale to evaluate the correlation between the severity of surgical complications and complications related to the renal and pancreatic grafts after simultaneous kidney and pancreas transplantation. Transplant Proc. 2016;48(5):1677–80.
34. Boggi U, Signori S, Vistoli F, et al. Laparoscopic robot-assisted pancreas transplantation: first world experience. Transplantation. 2012;93(2):201–6.
35. Boggi U, Signori S, Vistoli F, et al. Current perspectives on laparoscopic robot-assisted pancreas and pancreas-kidney transplantation. Rev Diabet Stud. 2011;8(1):28–34.
36. Tzvetanov I, D'Amico G, Bejarano-Pineda L, et al. Robotic-assisted pancreas transplantation: where are we today? Curr Opin Organ Transplant. 2014;19(1):80–2.
37. Surowiecka-Pastewka A, Matejak-Górska M, Frączek M, et al. Endovascular interventions in vascular complications after simultaneous pancreas and kidney transplantations: a single-center experience. Ann Transplant. 2019;12(24):199–207.

## Further Reading

Boggi U, Amorese G, Marchetti P. Surgical techniques for pancreas transplantation. Curr Opin Organ Transplant. 2010;15(1):102–11.

Grochowiecki T, Gałązka Z, Madej K, et al. Early complications related to the transplanted kidney after simultaneous pancreas and kidney transplantation. Transplant Proc. 2014;46(8):2815–7.

Pieroni E, Napoli N, Lombardo C, et al. Duodenal graft complications requiring duodenectomy after pancreas and pancreas-kidney transplantation. Am J Transplant. 2018;18(6):1388–96.

Sansalone CV, Maione G, Aseni P, et al. Surgical complications are the main cause of pancreatic allograft loss in pancreas-kidney transplant recipients. Transplant Proc. 2005;37(6):2651–3.

Zhao J, Gao Z, Wang K. The transplantation operation and its surgical complications, understanding the complexities of kidney transplantation; 2011. Ortiz J, editor, ISBN: 978-953-307-819-9.

# Liver Transplant Complications Management

**106**

Rami Rhaiem, Raffaele Brustia, Linda Rached, and Daniele Sommacale

## 106.1 Introduction

> **Learning Goals**
> - To know the most frequent complications following orthotopic liver transplantation (OLT)
> - To review the most appropriate diagnostic tools for each complication
> - To understand the principle of management of complications after OLT

Nearly six decades after the first human liver transplantation (LT) performed by Professor Starzl in 1963 [1], LT has become the gold standard of care for end-stage liver disease (ESLD) and acute liver failure. Current indications primarily include end-stage cirrhosis, biliary atresia, vascular and metabolic diseases, and also, some selected malignancies like hepatocellular carcinoma (HCC) and perihilar cholangiocarcinoma [2, 3].

Despite a tremendous development of patient selection, surgical techniques, perioperative management, and immunosuppressive therapies, LT remains a complex surgery associated with multiple complications that can sometimes lead to graft failure or patient mortality. Indeed, based on data from the Scientific Registry of Transplant Recipients (SRTR) [4] and the European Liver Transplant Registry (ELTR) [5, 6], the estimated 6-month and 1-year mortality rates after LT range between 10.6% and 12.0% and between 12.7% and 18.0%, respectively. Morbidity rate of deceased donor LT in the USA reaches up to 78% [7]. These complications include surgical-specific complications, and in particular, vascular and biliary complications.

In this chapter, we will focus on the surgical complications of orthotopic LT (OLT), including arterial or venous stenosis and thrombosis, biliary strictures or leaks, and infections. We will also discuss the early detection and management of these complications, which can significantly improve the graft and patient prognosis.

R. Rhaiem · L. Rached
Department of Hepatobiliary, Pancreatic and Digestive Oncological Surgery, Robert Debré University Hospital, Reims, France

University Reims Champagne-Ardenne, Reims, France
e-mail: rrhaiem@chu-reims.fr; lrached@chu-reims.fr

R. Brustia · D. Sommacale (✉)
Department of Digestive and Hepatobiliary and Pancreatic Surgery, AP-HP, Henri-Mondor Hospital, Créteil, France

University of Paris Est, UPEC, Créteil, France
e-mail: raffale.brustia@aphp.fr; daniele.sommacale@aphp.fr

## 106.2 Arterial Complications (Table 106.1)

### 106.2.1 Hepatic Arterial Thrombosis

Hepatic arterial thrombosis (HAT) has been reported in 4–15% of adult OLT and is associated with an incidence of graft loss and mortality of 50% and 30%, respectively [8–11].

The liver inflow is ensured by both the hepatic artery (HA) and portal vein (PV). In a native liver, the sudden thrombosis or ligation of the HA is usually compensated by arterial collateral networks that quickly develop to avoid liver and biliary ischemia. In the setting of OLT, liver attachments are divided, and arterial branches are usually ligated so that all the arterial supply is dependent only on the hepatic arterial anastomosis. Thus, the sudden disruption of the arterial flow that happens with HAT is not compensated, and the graft suffers from acute ischemic injuries, which might ultimately be responsible for graft loss and mortality [9, 12].

#### 106.2.1.1 Risk Factors for HAT

Several risk factors for HAT have been identified in the literature and are usually classified as technical, donor-related, and recipient-related factors.

Small artery caliber, both technical imperfection and intraoperative difficulties, aggressive clamping, and dissection of the arterial wall have been reported as common risk factors of HAT [13, 14]. HAT are more frequent after split, living donor, and pediatric LT [10].

Arterial anatomy of both the donor and the recipient is of paramount interest in this setting. Aberrant anatomy of the donor and recipient requires, respectively, complex backtable arterial reconstruction and arterial anastomosis with small branches and thus harbors a higher risk of HAT [9]. Intraoperative arterial flow lower than 100 mL/min might predict a high risk of HAT with a positive predictive value of 97.8% [15].

In addition, during the preoperative assessment, special care must be undertaken to rule out celiac trunk atheromatous stenosis or compression by a median arcuate ligament (MAL). The presence of celiac trunk compression/stenosis harbors a higher risk of HAT [16–18].

Several other risk factors for HAT have been identified in the literature, which include: ABO incompatibility, donor-recipient mismatch for Cytomegalovirus (CMV) seropositivity, congenital/acquired coagulable state, hypotension, marginal graft, and long cold ischemic time.

In patients transplanted for HCC with pre-LT transarterial chemoembolization (TACE) as a bridge or downstaging treatment, a higher rate of HAT has been reported [19–21]. Gilbo et al. recently reported an incidence of 25 HAT over 1035 LT in a 15-year period. TACE was associated with a 6-fold increase in the likelihood of developing HAT within 90 days after LT.

Specific other risk factors of late HAT have been reported in the literature such as tobacco use, CMV seropositivity of the donor, and donor age >70 years old [22, 23].

#### 106.2.1.2 Clinical Manifestations

According to the timing of thrombosis occurrence, HAT are classified into early HAT (occurring within 1 month after LT) and delayed HAT (occurring after 1 month).

1. Early HAT

    During the first 7 days after LT, the occurrence of a very early HAT is the worst-case scenario with fulminant hepatic failure (primary graft non-function) requiring emergency active management (surgical revision and/or urgent retransplantation). Mortality rates in these cases can reach 75%, and only retransplanted patients may survive [24]. Moreover, it usually results in acute biliary ischemia, leading to sepsis, biliary leaks, and liver abscess. Early HAT may also be asymptomatic with poor clinical signs and abnormal liver function tests. For this reason, routine daily Doppler ultrasonography (D-US) is mandatory during the postoperative course of LT to increase the sensitivity of HAT detection. Even more, Nishida et al. [25] demonstrated that routine performance of D-US every 12 h after pediatric LT increases the

**Table 106.1** Vascular complications after orthotopic liver transplantation

| | Year | n | Artery | | | | Portal vein | | IVC/HV | |
| --- | --- | --- | --- | --- | --- | --- | --- | --- | --- | --- |
| | | | Stenosis | Thrombosis | Early | Late | Stenosis | Thrombosis | Stenosis | Thrombosis |
| Wozney et al. [11] | 1986 | 42 | 7 (17%) | 6 (14%) | | | 1 (2.4%) | 2 (4.7%) | 0 (0%) | 0 (0%) |
| Langnas et al. [186] | 1991 | 267 | NS | 10 (3.7%) | | | 0 (0%) | 2 (0.7%) | 0 (0%) | 1 (0.3%) |
| Settmacher et al. [187] | 2001 | 1000 | NS | NS | | | 12 (1.2%) | 10 (1%) | 11 (1.1%) | 1 (0.1%) |
| Uzochukwu et al. [188] | 2005 | 110 | 2 (1.8%) | 0 (0%) | | | 0 (0%) | 2 (1.8%) | 4 (3.6%) | 1 (0.9%) |
| Jain et al. [189] | 2005 | 834 | 17 (2%) | 31 (3.7%) | 10 (1.2%) | 21 (2.5%) | NS | NS | NS | NS |
| Silva et al. [190] | 2006 | 1257 | NS | 61 (4.8%) | 22 (1.7%) | 39 (3.1%) | NS | NS | NS | NS |
| Duffy et al. [9] | 2009 | 3912 | NS | 171 (4.4%) | | | NS | 65 (1.7%) | NS | NS |
| Wojcicky et al. [191] | 2009 | 200 | 3 (1.5%) | 5 (2.5%) | | | 2 (1%) | 0% | NS | 1 (0.5%) |
| Pareja et al. [192] | 2010 | 1674 | NS | 48 (2.8%) | 32 (1.9%) | 16 (0.9%) | NS | NS | NS | NS |
| Pérez-Saborido et al. [193] | 2011 | 240 | 4 (1.7%) | 8 (3.3%) | 4 (1.7%) | 4 (1.7%) | 1 (0.4%) | 2 (0.8%) | NS | 3 (1.2%) |

early detection of HAT and thus the indication of salvage revision arterial surgery in comparison with the standard protocol (routine D-US on postoperative day 1 and on demand thereafter). Thus, patients who experienced HAT in the 12-h D-US group had a lower rate of biliary complications and retransplantation compared to the standard protocol (respectively, 0% vs 100% and 0% vs 90.9%).

2. Late HAT

Late HAT are usually associated with a more favorable course. This may be related to the progressive onset of thrombosis, allowing collateral arterial shunts to develop. Patients may be asymptomatic, but chronic biliary ischemia can occur in recurrent cholangitis, biliary leak, liver abscess, and non-anastomotic intrahepatic biliary stenosis [13, 22, 26].

### 106.2.1.3 Diagnosis

The D-US is the first imaging technique to be performed routinely during the postoperative course of LT (even without clinical suspicion of HAT) and in case of clinical suspicion of HAT with a good specificity rate [27, 28].

Small caliber of HA, low flow in the artery, and patients with a low sonographic window are common conditions that might decrease the accuracy of US. In these situations, contrast-enhanced ultrasonography (CEUS) may be used to improve the diagnostic performance of US [29–31]. CT scan with arterial phase is a very valuable diagnostic tool with a very good accuracy even in patients with poor postoperative condition [32, 33].

Magnetic resonance imaging (MRI) has also been tested with interesting results and excellent concordance with intraoperative findings [34]. Conventional angiography is usually performed to confirm the diagnosis and to discuss the best therapeutic option.

### 106.2.1.4 Management
- HAT

    The clinical status of the patient and the timing of HAT onset are decisive criteria for management. The most severe patients are those who experience very early HAT (<7 days) with primary graft non-function, requiring immediate arterial revision and in case of failure emergency retransplantation. In extreme situations without available grafts, a temporary anhepatic phase with allograft total hepatectomy and supportive portacaval shunt has been reported as a salvage two-stage liver transplantation [35–37].

    Early HAT requires emergency revisional surgery with thrombectomy and arterial revascularization. Shortening the arterial donor artery can prevent further kinking of the arterial anastomosis with subsequent recurrent thrombosis [38].

    In some difficult cases, portal vein arterialization can allow restoration of flow after HAT [39–42]. It allows the liver, including not only hepatocytes but also the biliary tree, to have adequate blood inflow during the development of arterial collaterals. When performed as a bridge to retransplantation, the results are quite encouraging [40]. However, in the case of definitive treatment, the results are disappointing. In the Paul Brousse experience [39], three of the seven patients who underwent portal vein arterialization suffered from graft loss with one death. In addition, the major drawback of this technique is a high rate of mortality in cases of acute thrombosis of the arterioportal anastomosis and a high morbidity rate related to portal hypertension [40, 43].

    Several small series and case reports showed the use of endovascular techniques such as catheter-directed thrombolysis (CDT) or thromboaspiration and stenting with encouraging outcomes [44–47]. The results of endovascular treatment of very early HAT are acceptable but with a high risk of procedure-related complications compared to surgical revascularization [48]. In our experience (unpublished data), the results of early endovascular treatment are poor with a 30% of mortality and a 60% of retransplantation, and thus, in this setting, endovascular treatment might not be recommended as a first-line treatment for very early HAT.

In patients who experience delayed HAT, recurrent biliary septic complications are a clear indication for retransplantation. Meanwhile, sepsis management using antibiotic therapy and percutaneous drainage of the liver abscess is mandatory. In some cases, surgical resection of devitalized segments of the allograft may be discussed [49].

Nonoperative management with endovascular techniques is used in cases of late HAT with satisfactory early results. Nonetheless, several reports highlighted long-term high risk of low patency in chronic HAT with the need of further endovascular or surgical reinterventions [50–52].

- Median Arcuate Ligament (MAL)

When diagnosed preoperatively, several authors advocated for the routine release of MAL to ensure sufficient arterial blood flow after ligation of arterial collaterals of the HA during OLT [16, 17]. Czigany et al. performed a multicentric European survey to evaluate the surgical protocols of LT centers towards MAL. Only 29% preconized routine release of the ligament. Other surgical options have been reported: preservation of the GDA and HA anastomosis either to the recipient's proper HA or to a branch patch including the terminal part of the CHA and the origin of the GDA [18]; and aortohepatic bypass [18, 53]. Aortohepatic bypass has been performed as a rescue procedure after the failure of MAL release to restore a satisfactory arterial flow.

## 106.2.2 Hepatic Arterial Stenosis

Hepatic arterial stenosis/stricture (HAS) is one of the most common complications after LT. The reported incidence of HAS in the literature is 2–13% [8–10, 52, 54]. Progression of HAS may result in subsequent HAT and worst outcome. The main consequence of HAS is a chronic graft arterial ischemia with in fine the risk of allograft intrahepatic biliary stricture [55].

HAS occurs more frequently within the anastomosis, followed by the donor and then the recipient artery [10, 32].

### 106.2.2.1 Risk Factors

Microvascular rejection and microvascular injury related to hypothermic perfusion are common factors responsible for HAS. In particular, perianastomotic strictures may be related to vascular clamp injury and/or to technical issues such as twisting or kinking of the HA. HAS are more frequent after split and pediatric LT.

TACE was also associated with a higher rate of HAS [56]. However, donation after cardiac death has not been associated with a higher risk of HAS when compared to brain death donation [57].

### 106.2.2.2 Clinical Manifestations

Although asymptomatic in many patients, HAS typically presents with abnormal liver tests, liver graft dysfunction, and biliary complications.

The timing of the onset of this complication is variable. Abbasoglou et al. [58] reported a median time to diagnosis of HAS of 100 days. HAS are classified as early (<90 days after LT) or late (>90 days after LT) with comparable number of patients in each group (20 early HAS/1232 LT, 1.6% versus 19 late HAS/1232 LT, 1.5%) in the recent large cohort published by Hann et al. [55].

### 106.2.2.3 Diagnosis

D-US shows typical patterns of increased arterial resistive index (RI) in the pre-stenotic segment (RI > 0.8) associated with a low flow. The post-stenotic portion of the artery yields low RI (<0.5), a long systolic acceleration time (>0.08 s), and a tardus-parvus wave. High peak systolic velocity (>200 cm/s) at the level of the HAS is also found [32, 59].

Recently, Mohamed Afif et al. [54] developed a predictive model for HAS using both intrahepatic arterial RI and systolic acceleration time. The model showed a good discrimination performance with an AUC of 0.93% and 88.6% specificity but needs further external validation for a wider use.

D-US is useful for the diagnosis of HAS but does not allow the quantification of the stenosis. For this matter, three-dimensional reconstruction CT angiography (Fig. 106.1) is the gold standard [60] replacing diagnostic arteriogra-

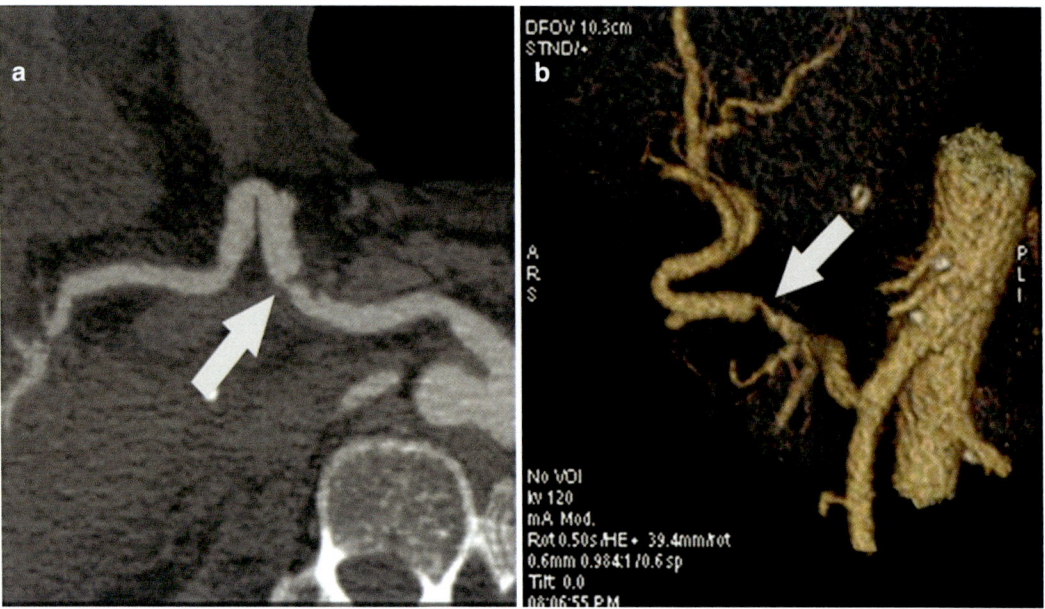

**Fig. 106.1** Computed tomography with an axial plane (**a**) and 3D reconstruction (**b**) showing a focal stenosis of the hepatic arterial anastomosis (white arrow). (Courtesy of Pr. A. Luciani)

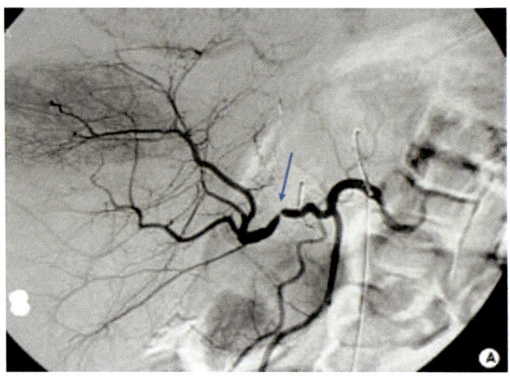

**Fig. 106.2** Conventional angiography before percutaneous angioplasty demonstrating stenosis of the hepatic artery anastomosis (blue arrow)

phy (Fig. 106.2): Critical HAS is a significant narrowing of the HA diameter >50%. MR angiography is not a reliable technique in this particular indication because of a high false-positive rate [34].

### 106.2.2.4 Management

Therapeutic options include endovascular interventional treatment, surgical revision of the arterial anastomosis, and retransplantation in severe cases with graft dysfunction, biliary septic complications, and/or associated biliary non-anastomotic strictures.

The endovascular treatment includes percutaneous transluminal angioplasty (PTA) with or without stenting. Despite conflicting results in the literature, Rostambeigi et al. [61] in their meta-analysis of case series concluded to equivalent results between PTA alone and PTA associated with stenting.

The Paul Brousse group reported their experience with endovascular treatment for critical HAS in 30 patients (>50%) [62]. Immediate success rate of PTA was 90% (27/30) with associated stenting in 24 patients. The complication rate was low (3.3%) with only one dissection of the targeted artery. The 5-year HA patency rate was 68%.

Similarly and more recently, the Beaujon group reported the long-term outcomes of 53 endovascular post-LT procedures performed mainly for HAS (52/53; 98%) [63]: Treatment included PTA alone in 18 patients and PTA associated with stenting in 34 patients. The primary success rate of procedures was 90%. After 5 years of follow-up, the HA patency rate was 81%.

These results may be improved with the development of techniques and materials. Drug-eluting stents have been introduced and used in transplanted patients to treat arterial stenosis [64]. Naidu et al. [65] compared the results of drug-eluting (DE) and bare-metal (BM) stents in 52 patients treated for HAS with PTA associated with stent placement. Patency of the HA rate was 71% after DE and 46% after BM stents. The difference was more pronounced when the authors analyzed their results in small-caliber arteries. Three-year patency of HA rates were 75% and 38%, respectively, for DE and BM stents.

Repeat endovascular treatment can be indicated in case of recurrent HAS. Sommacale et al. [66] reported their experience in 37 patients treated for HAS after OLT. Among them, 8 patients had recurrent HAS managed with 10 PTA and 94.6% patency of the HA after 66 months median follow-up.

However, it is important to know that patients with HAS may have high incidence of ischemic cholangiopathy despite efficient endovascular revascularization. Indeed, 30–40% ischemic biliary strictures rate have been reported [63, 67].

Surgical revision of the anastomotic stricture is indicated in case of failure of interventional radiology, with reported patency rates of 78% and higher complication rates than endovascular treatment [58]. Surgical options for the treatment of HAS include resection of the stricture with a new anastomosis, an aortic conduit graft, an interposition vein/artery graft, and vein patch angioplasty. Surgical revision, if indicated, aims to restore arterial flow and to prevent biliary strictures [58]. Similarly, patients with concomitant HAS and biliary complication may benefit from surgical revision with excellent long-term results. Sommacale et al. reported only one recurrence in seven patients treated with arterial revascularization and bilioenteric anastomosis after a median follow up of 76 months [68].

### 106.2.3 Hepatic Arterial Pseudoaneurysm

Hepatic arterial pseudoaneurysm (HAP) is a rare but dreadful complication of LT with an incidence of 0.3–2% [69–72].

#### 106.2.3.1 Risk Factors

HAP may be intrahepatic and/or in the extrahepatic segment of the hepatic artery. Risk factors differ according to the location of the HAP:

- Intrahepatic HAP are mainly reported after interventional procedures such as liver biopsy, percutaneous drainage, and transhepatic cholangiography [73].
- Risk factors of extrahepatic HAP are surgical or radiological endovascular manipulation of the hepatic artery/hepatic arterial anastomosis and local sepsis; the last being the most important risk factor reported in the literature [69, 73, 74]. A recent review of the literature identified 81 patients with post-LT HAP [70]: More than 77% had documented infectious complications. Bile leak, fistulizing Roux-en-Y hepaticojejunostomy, and primary sclerosing cholangitis were the most important risk factors for this complication.

HAP-related infectious complications present usually within 2 months after LT while noninfected HAP occurs later.

#### 106.2.3.2 Clinical Manifestations and Diagnosis

HAP are usually asymptomatic before complications, which are thus discovered during post-LT routine imaging surveillance (Fig. 106.3). Intrahepatic HAP may rupture with subcapsular/intraparenchymal hematoma and severe hemobilia. Rupture of extrahepatic HAP is a life-threatening complication with massive hemoperitoneum and sudden hypovolemic shock. The mortality rate can reach 50% [74].

#### 106.2.3.3 Management

Long-term antibiotic/antifungal treatments are mandatory and should be guided by microbiological findings.

Management and repair of HAP are challenging:

- For intrahepatic HAP, selective arterial embolization is an interesting option, especially for distal aneurysms. When HAP is proximal,

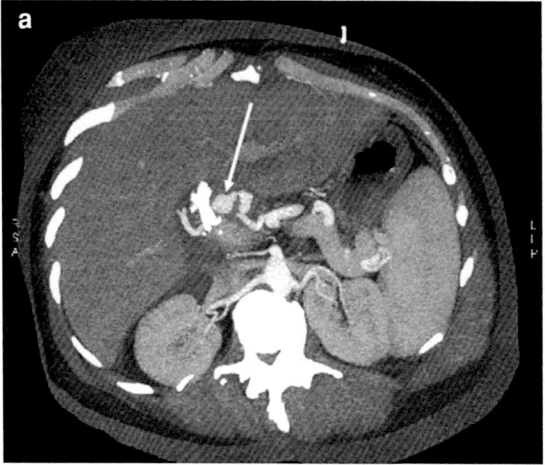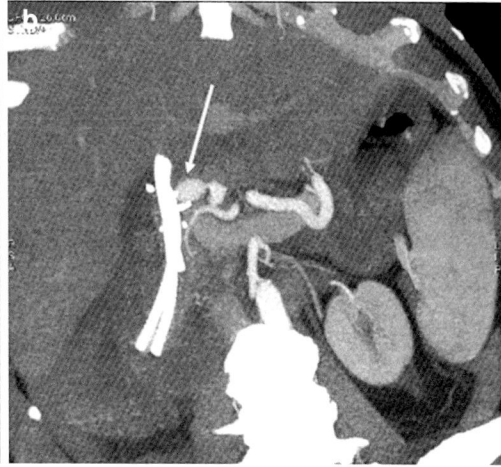

**Fig. 106.3** MIP reconstructions (**a**: axial; **b**: coronal view) showing extrahepatic pseudoaneurysm of the hepatic artery (white arrow) in patient who experienced post-LT biliary fistula already managed with the placement of biliary stents. (Courtesy of Pr. A. Luciani)

arterial vascularization of the embolized liver is compensated by the development of collateral branches through the hilar plate. In rare cases, embolization may lead to extensive biliary ischemia and in this setting, retransplantation can be required.
- For extrahepatic HAP, clinical presentation is crucial for therapeutic management. In asymptomatic or stable patients, interventional radiology with either selective embolization or stenting of the HA is the first option.

Surgery is the only available option for instable patients with ruptured extrahepatic HAP and in case of failure of interventional radiology: excision of the HAP or ligation of the hepatic artery is required. Arterial revascularization of the allograft during the same surgery is recommended but not always possible in the case of instable patients. Arterial revascularization in difficult situations can be performed using splenic artery transposition (Fig. 106.4) [75]. Surgical or endovascular treatment without hepatic artery revascularization can lead to liver failure, death, or ischemic biliary stricture in up to 70% of cases.

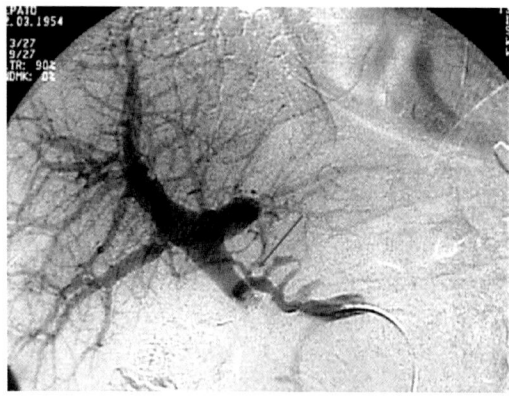

**Fig. 106.4** Conventional angiography confirming patency of a portal vein arterialization (blue arrow) with splenic artery transposition after ligation of the hepatic artery for a ruptured hepatic artery pseudoaneurysm

In the experience of the Beaujon group with the management of postop-OLT HAP, endovascular treatment achieved the best results with no mortality and 100% long-term graft survival. In the surgical group, early mortality rate and long-term graft survival were 28% and 57%, respectively, in the revascularized group, whereas higher postoperative mortality rate (80%) and no long-term graft survival were observed in the ligation group [74].

## 106.3 Portal Vein Complications

Portal vein thrombosis (PVT) and stenosis (PVS) are uncommon complications of OLT, accounting for less than 2% of cases [9, 76, 77], but with the potential for significant morbidity and mortality. Post-LT PVT reduces significantly the overall survival after OLT [9].

Portal vein anastomosis during OLT is classically an end-to-end anastomosis with a growth factor to allow a better expansion of the vein lumen after declamping [78].

## 106.3.1 Risk Factors

Non-tumoral pre-LT PVT has been considered for a long time as a relative contraindication for LT because of a higher risk of postoperative portal vein thrombosis. Numerous classifications have been proposed; Yerdel's classification being the most widely used (Fig. 106.5) [79]. A new classification has been described with a better correlation with surgical strategy [80]. Several technical modifications have been described to perform portal vein (PV) anastomosis in patients with pre-LT PVT

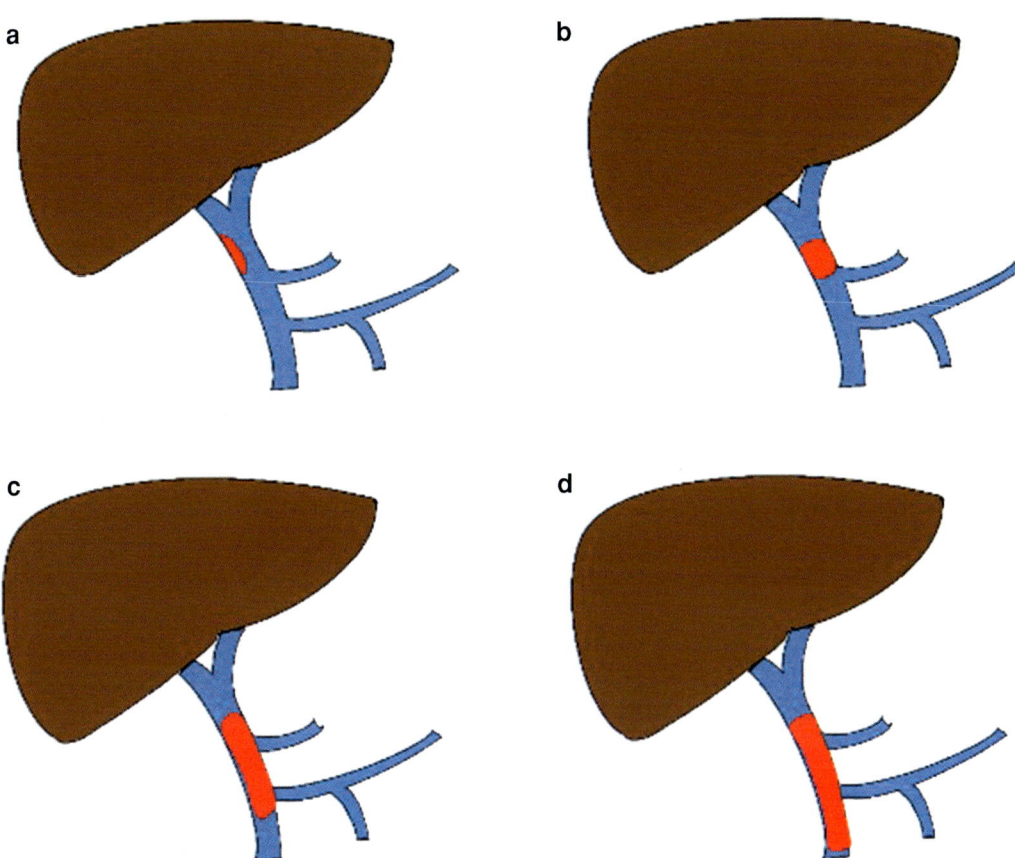

**Fig. 106.5** Classification of Yerdel for non-tumoral portal vein thrombosis. (**a**) Grade 1—Minimally or partially thrombosed portal vein (PV), in which the thrombus is mild or, at the most, confined to <50% of the vessel lumen with or without minimal extension into the superior mesenteric vein (SMV). (**b**) Grade 2—50% occlusion of the PV, including total occlusions, with or without minimal extension into the SMV. (**c**) Grade 3—Complete thrombosis of both PV and proximal SMV. Distal SMV is open. (**d**) Grade 4—Complete thrombosis of the PV and proximal as well as distal SMV

- For Yerdel's Types 1 and 2: Eversion thrombectomy or resection of the thrombosed portion of the portal vein in case of inlaid thrombosis are the standard techniques. To improve portal inflow, ligation either of portosystemic shunts [81] or of the left renal vein (in the case of large splenorenal shunts) [82] may be required.
- For Yerdel's Type 3: If the recipient's superior mesenteric vein is patent, a mesentericoportal shunt using a jump graft can be an option for portal reconstruction. The graft is chosen among a venous graft, a synthetic graft, or an arterial graft. Our preference in this indication goes to the arterial graft because of a lower risk of thrombosis secondary to low flow into the portal vein in comparison with venous grafts and because of the lack of evidence about the long-term results of synthetic grafts in the literature [83].
- For Yerdel's Type 4: Coronary-portal anastomosis in case of an enlarged coronary vein [80, 84].
- For Yerdel's Type 4: a cavoportal hemitransposition with either cavoportal (Fig. 106.6) or renoportal anastomosis. The latter technique is performed in patients with a developed shunt to the left renal vein. These techniques have the drawback of a high risk of portal hypertension and primary graft non-function, especially with the cavoportal reconstruction. In this setting, side-to-side or side-to-end anastomosis is preferable to reduce the flow from the vena cava to the portal vein [85]. Interesting long-term results of renoportal anastomosis were recently reported by Azoulay et al. with a 5-year patient and graft survival of 76% and 73%, despite 42.9% portal hypertension [86].
- In case of massive portal and mesenteric thrombosis, multivisceral transplantation can be considered [80, 87–89].

In this instance, in very selected cases, scarce series reported portal vein arterialization with anastomosis above the PVT [90–93]. The results are acceptable, but this technique cannot be recommended as a standard procedure for this indication [94].

Cheng et al. [95] reported several risk factors for intraoperative PVT in the setting of pediatric

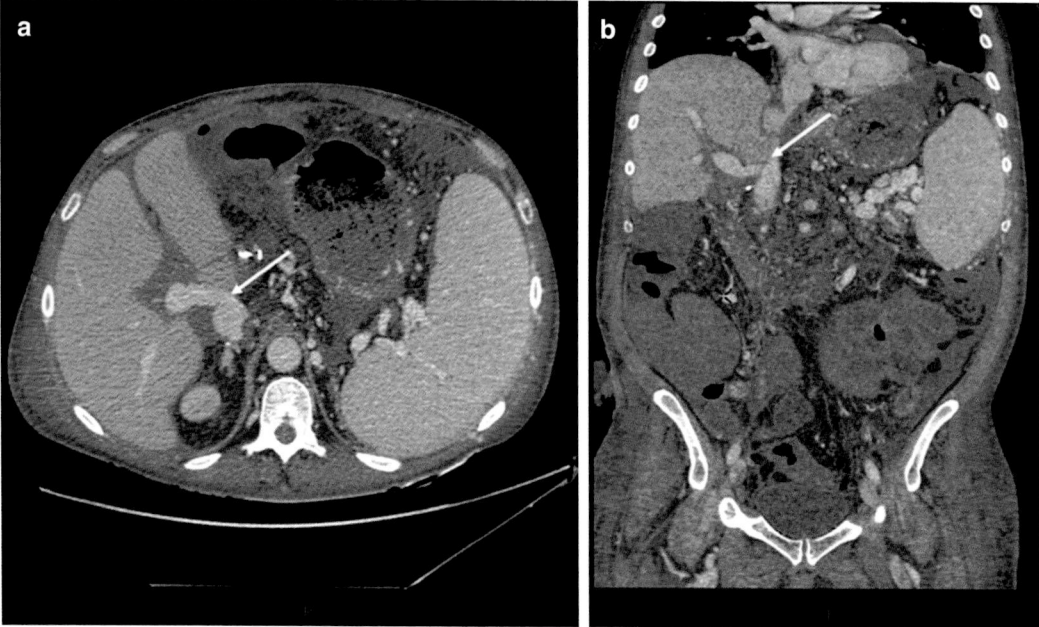

**Fig. 106.6** Postoperative computed tomography scan (**a**: axial; **b**: Coronal slices) showing portocaval hemitransposition (white arrow) for a preoperative Grade 4 portal vein thrombus

living donor LT. Among them, several risk factors are applicable to adult OLT: low portal flow, small-diameter veins (<5 mm), pre-LT PVT in the recipient, donor-recipient vessel size discrepancies, and the use of vascular grafts for reconstruction. Reyes et al. [96] recently developed a predictive index for post-LT PVT that included varices, prior variceal ligation/sclerotherapy, thrombocytopenia and overweight with a sensitivity of 78% but with a low specificity. Yerdel et al. [79] identified preoperative portal hypertension with previous treatment (TIPS, sclerotherapy, splenectomy) as an important risk factor of PVT.

Twisting and kinking of the portal vein anastomosis is a frequent technical error that may lead to PVT or stenosis.

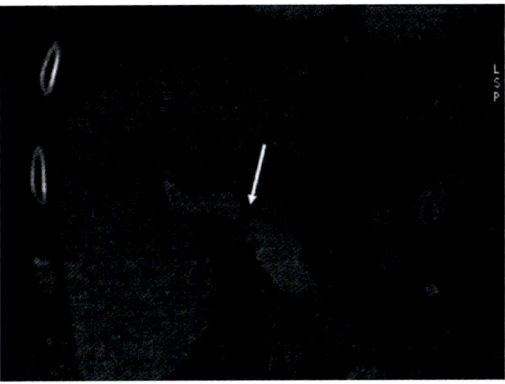

**Fig. 106.7** Coronal computed tomography scan view showing focal portal vein stenosis (white arrow). (Courtesy of Pr. A. Luciani)

### 106.3.2 Clinical Manifestations

PVT are usually symptomatic with either acute liver failure or complications of portal hypertension (ascites, splenomegaly, and variceal bleeding). However, PV stenosis (PVS) is likely asymptomatic. A chronic, non-diagnosed PVS results in portal hypertension.

### 106.3.3 Diagnosis

Diagnostic imaging is of paramount importance. In PVT, a real-time echography may demonstrate an echogenic thrombus, with Doppler US confirming either the absence or the presence of blood flow around a non-occluding thrombus [8]. In PV stenosis (PVS), US confirm a high velocity at the site of the anastomosis with a peak systolic velocity >125 cm/s at the level of the anastomosis with normal proximal flow (anastomotic-to-preanastomotic velocity ratio of 3:1) and distal turbulences [8]. The specificity of these D-US signs may reach 95–100% for PVS [97].

CT and MRI provide excellent information, with the possibility of high-quality three-dimensional reconstruction, to confirm the diagnosis of PVT/PVS: an intraluminal filling defect in the case of thrombosis and a focal stenosis in the case of PVS (Fig. 106.7) [8].

### 106.3.4 Management

Management of PVT depends on the timing of the onset of thrombosis and the severity of its clinical manifestations:

- For patients experiencing early PVT (<72 h) with fulminant liver failure, retransplantation may be the best option. Usually, surgical exploration, thrombectomy, or surgical resection with immediate portal reconstruction with or without grafting is effective to restore a normal portal flow [98, 99]. In this instance, arterialization of the portal vein may be an acceptable option in difficult situations (Fig. 106.8).
- In case of late PVT with preserved graft function, medical treatment of portal hypertension in combination with primary or secondary prevention of bleeding from oesophagal varices alone, reduces the chance of preservation of long-term graft function [9]. Successful endovascular management has been reported but mainly in case series including PTA with or without stent placement and thrombolysis [10, 98]. The transjugular approach may be associated with a transhepatic portosystemic shunt (TIPS) as an effective treatment for portal hypertension consequences [100]. Despite the high rates of complications and mortality reported in previous reports, recent reports

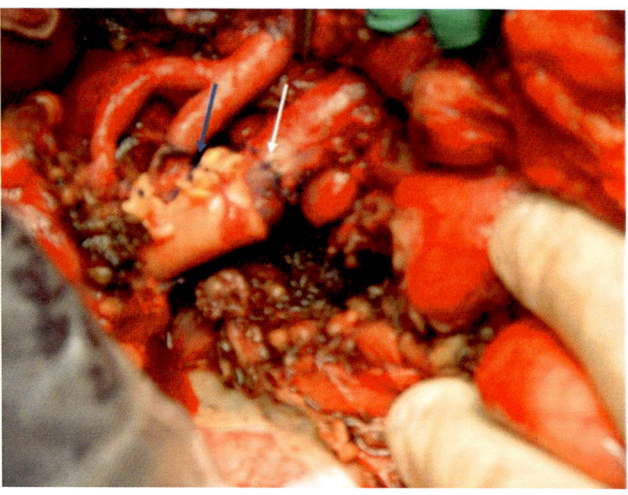

**Fig. 106.8** Intraoperative view illustrating portal vein arterialization (white arrow) after thrombosis of the portal vein anastomosis (blue arrow): end-to-side anastomosis between the right hepatic artery and the portal vein above the thrombosis

describe safer techniques of intrahepatic or transjugular approaches with more standardized protocols for thrombolytic agents [101–103].

When it comes to PVS, endovascular treatment is highly effective using PTA which is associated in some cases with stenting [104, 105]. Khan et al. [104] reported a 100% technical success rate in 23 patients, among whom 14 had LT. All patients were treated with PTA and stent placement. Portal vein patency after 1 year was 91%.

Surgical revision/reconfection of the portal anastomosis or retransplantation for PVS are rarely indicated.

## 106.4 IVC and Hepatic Vein Complications

In OLT, several options are available for the reconstruction of the inferior vena cava (IVC):

- Resection of the recipient retrohepatic IVC and reconstruction with two end-to-end anastomosis superiorly and inferiorly to the donor IVC [106].
- The "piggyback" technique with preservation of the recipient IVC and anastomosis between the donor's vena cava and the recipient's hepatic veins [107, 108]. This original technique was reported to harbor a higher risk of caval anastomosis [109].
- The three-hepatic vein technique [110] by creating a common large stoma in the recipient IVC using a venoplasty. This technique can be performed with preservation of the caval flow and offers a lower rate of outflow block and postoperative Budd-Chiari syndrome than the two-vein technique [111].
- Closure of the recipient's hepatic vein stumps and side-to-side anastomosis between donor and recipient's retrohepatic IVC [112]. The same author reported afterwards on an end-to-side anastomosis [113]. A wide cavo-cavostomy cranially to the donor inferior vena cava in a door-lock manner is performed.

This technique is easier than the original technique, with a shorter anhepatic phase and excellent outcomes with less complications [114].

Outflow complications following OLT are uncommon, with an incidence <2% [10, 115, 116].

These complications are represented by IVC/hepatic vein stenosis and/or thrombosis, which jeopardize the outflow of the allograft.

### 106.4.1 Risk Factors

Acute IVC stenosis may be related to technical issues such as suprahepatic caval kinking or difference in donor and recipient vessel caliber.

Compression by a postoperative perianastomotic hematoma can present with IVC stenosis.

Late IVC stenosis is usually caused by anastomotic stricture, IVC thrombosis, fibrosis, hyperplasia, and chronic compression by an enlarged allograft [117].

### 106.4.2 Clinical Manifestations

Clinical presentation varies depending on the location of the stenosis/thrombosis: infra-hepatic stenosis presents with lower extremity edema, and suprahepatic stenosis may be responsible of a Budd-Chiari syndrome.

### 106.4.3 Diagnosis

Increase of velocity, distension of the hepatic veins, and loss of phasicity of the hepatic venous Doppler waveform are classic signs of IVC stenosis.

Vein narrowing on CT and MRI may be associated with Budd-Chiari and portal hypertension radiological features (Fig. 106.9) [32, 59].

In case of IVC thrombosis, intraluminal thrombus may be found on US and seen on CT and MRI as intraluminal defect.

### 106.4.4 Management

Endovascular treatment with angioplasty and stent placement has been reported with excellent outcomes [118, 119]. Special care has to be taken during the confection of the caval anastomosis because in our experience mandatory intraoperative refection in the case of an ouflow block after the "piggyback" technique was associated with a 70% mortality rate (unpublished data).

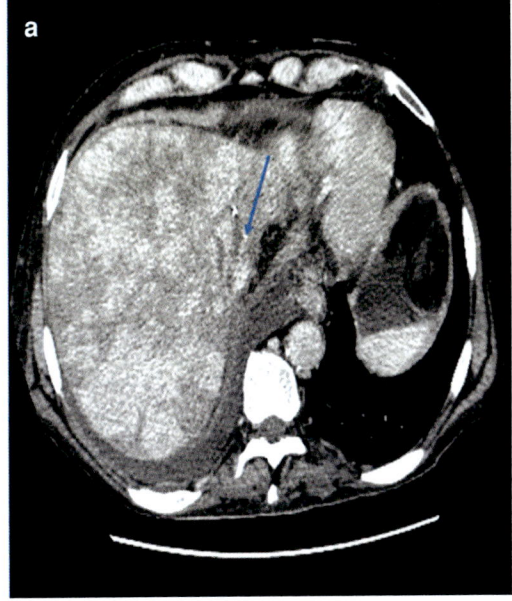
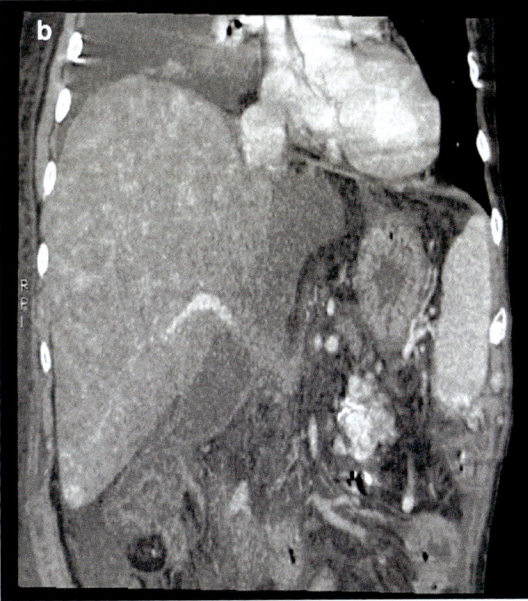

**Fig. 106.9** Acute IVC thrombosis following orthotopic liver transplantation: Computed tomography scan with axial (**a**) and coronal (**b**) slices demonstrating thrombosis of left and median hepatic veins (blue arrow) with a markedly heterogenous enhancement of liver parenchyma and ascites

## 106.5 Biliary Complications

Biliary complications (BC) are one of the most frequent and troublesome complications after OLT. They occur in up to 25% of patients [120–122]. Approximately 70% of these complications are early, occurring within the first three months post-OLT, and are related to an increase in morbidity and mortality rates [123]. There are various types of biliary complications. They are classified into early and late BC according to the timing of onset. No clear definition in the literature is available, but clearly, early complications occur within 1–3 months after LT, while late BC happen after 3 months [120, 124].

According to the lesion location, strictures and leaks are classified as anastomotic or non-anastomotic.

These complications are associated with a high rate of hospital readmissions and re-interventions and thus have a major impact on morbidity, mortality, and graft survival.

### 106.5.1 Risk Factors

Potential risk factors for BC include hepatic artery complications (stenosis or thrombosis), an advanced donor's age, prolonged ischemia time, and infections [121, 125, 126].

All patients with BC shall undergo D-US examination to rule out an arterial complication. Hepatic artery thrombosis/stenosis is a well-known cause of BC. Reduced arterial flow into the hepatic artery with splenic artery steal syndrome or stenosis of the celiac trunk may also be responsible for BC.

Among the technical risk factors, excessive tension on the anastomosis, the use of electrocautery in contact with the biliary mucosa, and extensive peribiliary dissection while harvesting the graft have to be avoided to prevent the occurrence of BC [127].

Biliary fistula is a clear risk factor for subsequent biliary stenosis after OLT.

With the increasing harvesting of deceased cardiac death donors (DCD), the rate of biliary complications, especially non-anastomotic strictures, has been reported. Initial reports from the Wisconsin University described three times more non-nastomotic stricture (NAS) with DCD-LT than with brain death donors (DBD) [128]. Pine et al. [129] reported 20% of NAS with DCD versus 0% with DBD. Similar results were observed by De Vera et al. [130] with a higher biliary complication rate and graft loss. Hypothermic-oxygenated machine perfusion (HOPE) seems to reduce the risk of BC in DCD–LT [131, 132], and more recently, dual-HOPE has been compared in a multicentric European randomized controlled trial with static cold storage in 156 DCD-LT [133]. After 6 months of follow up, the incidence of biliary NAS (primary endpoint) was 6% in the Dual-HOPE group versus 18% in the control group.

Another well-known risk factor for BC is reduced-size grafts. Indeed, BC rates reported with split LT were around 25% and after living donor LT were around 25–40% [7, 122].

The type and incidence of BC generally depend on the type of reconstruction. There are mainly two types of biliary anastomoses: a choledocho-choledochostomy or a choledochojejunostomy:

- A choledochocholedochostomy (CC) is the most common type of anastomosis in OLT. It is an end-to-end anastomosis between the recipient's common bile duct and the donor's bile duct below the bifurcation. It is preferred because it is technically easier, preserves the sphincter of Oddi as a natural barrier to prevent reflux of enteric content to the biliary tract [134], and maintains access for endoscopic procedures in the postoperative period.
- A bilioenteric anastomosis with a choledochojejunostomy (CJ) sutures the donor's bile duct to a jejunal loop in a Roux-en-Y fashion.

The anastomosis of choice is the CC anastomosis. In case of mismatch in size between the donor and recipient bile ducts or of primary biliary disease like primary sclerosing cholangitis (PSC), cholangiocarcinoma, or biliary atresia, a bilioenteric anastomosis is suitable, despite the longer operative time and greater difficulty.

In case of size mismatch, the Berlin group reported favorable outcomes with a side-to-side CC anastomosis [135]. Davidson et al. [136] performed a randomized controlled trial comparing end-to-end and side-to-side CC with comparable results between the two techniques. Paes-Barbossa et al. [137] in their meta-analyses of biliary anastomosis techniques in OLT recommended either non-drained end-to-end or drained side-to-side CC.

Also, in PSC settings, several authors reported equivalent results with duct-to-duct CC and Roux-en-Y CJ [138–140]. The meta-analysis of Wells et al. showed no significant differences in 1-year patient and graft survivals, biliary complications rate, and or recurrence [141].

Another technical factor related to BC is the placement of the trans-anastomotic T-tube, which remains very controversial. Classic arguments for T-tube placement are the decompression of the biliary anastomosis, the prevention of anastomotic strictures, and easier postoperative access for radiological diagnostic and interventional investigations. But several studies showed higher rates of infectious complications and T-tube insertion site leaks. Two recent meta-analyses found a higher rate of BC with T-tube placement [142, 143]. In France, a multicentric randomized trial (BILIDRAINT), comparing the placement of a transanatomotic T-tube and non-drained biliary anastomosis, was aborted because of a higher mortality rate in the drainage group. The Lyonnais Group described their technique with a T-tube placement and retroperitoneal tunnel to reduce the rate of biliary fistula, especially after the removal of the drain [144].

Internal biliary stent placement was also reported to reduce the risk of biliary complications. The results are conflicting, and no clear consensus can be drawn [145–148].

## 106.5.2 Diagnosis

Biliary complications are often found incidentally in asymptomatic patients with slightly elevated liver enzymes. When symptomatic, they often present with signs of cholangitis like jaundice, fever, and abdominal pain. In that case, liver function tests followed by an abdominal ultrasound with Doppler will help diagnose up to 60% of these complications. Doppler ultrasound helps visualize the biliary tree as well as the vasculature. If a T-tube is still in place, a T-tube cholangiography is a quick and easy way to explore the biliary tree. In case of suspicion of hepatic artery stenosis or thrombosis, a CT angiography is indicated. However, for BC, the imaging technique of choice is magnetic resonance cholangiopancreatography (MRCP) [149]. It is a noninvasive study that can map the biliary tree and has a high sensitivity for the diagnosis of biliary obstruction with comparable diagnostic accuracy to direct cholangiography [150, 151] and endoscopic retrograde cholangio-pancreatography (ERCP) and/or percutaneous transhepatic cholangiography (PTC) [152].

In case of high suspicion of BC, ERCP and PTC are performed mainly as a therapeutic nonsurgical approach. In patients with end-to-end CC, ERCP is required, but in patients with Roux-en-Y anastomosis, PTC is the only possible alternative. Management depends on the type of BC and will be discussed accordingly.

## 106.5.3 Biliary Leaks

Biliary leaks (BL) occur in up to 25% of OLTs and mostly during the first 3 months post OLT [120]. Table 106.2 shows the results of BL in the reports that have focused on BC rates. The type and incidence of bile leaks depend on the type of anastomosis. Leaks mainly involve the anastomotic site but can also occur at non-anastomotic sites like the cystic duct remnant or the site of T-tube insertion. Anastomotic leaks can either reflect technical problems or ischemia at the level of the anastomosis. Non-anastomotic leaks are mainly related to T-tube removal but can also be due to bile duct ischemia, as in the case of HAT.

Early anastomotic BL can be caused by ischemic lesions at the distal part of the donor bile duct, sphincter of Oddi hypertension, proximal obstruction, or most frequently unplanned T-tube removal. Non-anastomotic no-T-tube early BL

**Table 106.2** Incidence of biliary complications after orthotopic liver transplantation

| | Year | n | Leaks | | Strictures | | |
|---|---|---|---|---|---|---|---|
| | | | Anastomotic leak | T-tube leak | Anastomotic stenosis | NAS | Total |
| Lerut et al. [76] | 1987 | 393 | 15 (3.8%) | 11 (2.7%) | 20 (5%) | NS | 52 (13.2%) |
| Neuhaus et al. [194] | 1994 | 300 | 0.30% | 1.30% | 0.60% | NS | 2.30% |
| Greif et al. [123] | 1994 | 1490 | 29 (1.9%) | 18 (1.2%) | 81 (5.4%) | 12 (0.8%) | 188 (12.6%) |
| Hernandez et al. [195] | 1999 | 300 | 14 (4.7%) | 9 (3%) | 10 (3.3%) | 2 (0.67%) | 54 (18%) |
| Scatton et al. [196] | 2001 | 180 | 4 (2.2%) | 7 (3.9%) | 5 (2.8%) | 4 (2.2%) | 44 (24.5%) |
| Thethy et al. [197] | 2004 | 376 | 22 (5.8%) | 4 (1%) | 30 (8%) | 4 (1%) | 55 (14.6%) |
| Abdullah et al. [198] | 2005 | 184 | 12 (6%) | NS | 22 (12%) | 4 (2.2%) | 32 (17.4%) |
| Wójcicki et al. [199] | 2005 | 42 | 7 (16.6%) | 0 (0%) | 3 (7%) | NS | 12 (28.6%) |
| Li et al. [200] | 2007 | 84 | 2 (2.3%) | 3 (3.6%) | 8 (9.5%) | 1 (1.2%) | 16 (19%) |
| Perrakis et al. [201] | 2010 | 245 | 14 (5%) | 6/99 (6%) | 27 (11%) | 13 (5%) | 60 (24%) |
| Akamatsu et al. [125] | 2010 | 11,547 | 668/8585 (7.8%) | NS | 1314/11,547 (12%) | NS | NS |
| Król et al. [202] | 2011 | 87 | 0 (0%) | 0 (0%) | 9 (10.3%) | 5 (5.7%) | 15 (17%) |
| Gaman et al. [203] | 2013 | 471 | 57 (12%) | NS | 72 (15%) | 32 (6.8%) | 131 (28%) |
| Gastaca et al. [204] | 2014 | 743 | 15 (2%) | 24 (3.2%) | 17 (2.3%) | 2 (0.27%) | 73 (9.8%) |
| Nemes et al. [205] | 2015 | 14,411 | 8.50% | NS | 14.70% | NS | 23% |
| Coelho et al. [206] | 2017 | 153 | 7 (4.6%) | NS | 30 (19.6%) | NS | 37 (24%) |
| Song et al. [207] | 2021 | 3320 | 289 (8.9%) | NS | 284/3248 (8.7%) | NS | 723/3248 (22%) |

are mainly ischemic, and verification of the patency of the arterial anastomosis is mandatory. Late BL are mostly caused by HAT or planned T-tube removal [120, 153].

Depending on the size of the leakage and the presence or absence of symptoms, anastomotic bile leaks can be managed with conservative, surgical, or nonsurgical (endoscopic vs radiological) interventions.

With the exception of ischemia, most causes of biliary leaks can be managed by nonsurgical interventions. Indeed, ERCP followed by sphincterotomy and stent placement allows nearly 90% BL healing [125, 154]. A biliary stent has to remain in situ at least for 3 months before extraction to avoid insufficient tissue healing. Associated bilomas and fluid collections have to be managed by percutaneous drainage and antibiotic therapy. Some centers advocated the superiority of nasobiliary tube but it remains not widely used because of its low tolerance and the risk of migration [155].

In patients with Roux-en-Y reconstruction, PTC plays an important role.

Fully covered self-expandable metal stents (SEMS) have been indicated in case of failure of plastic stents [156, 157]. Luigiano et al. [158] reported a 94% success rate in 34 patients managed with SEMS. This excellent short-term result of SEMS must be balanced with the higher risk of biliary stenosis that can reach 35% [159].

Large and complex BL require surgical revision to avoid biliary septic complications and a subsequent chronic consequence on the graft.

Table 106.3 summarizes data on BC management according to the most cited series in the literature.

### 106.5.4 Biliary Strictures

Bile duct strictures (BS) can be categorized into anastomotic (AS) and non-anastomotic strictures (NAS). They have been reported in 10–15% of

**Table 106.3** Management of biliary complications after orthotopic liver transplantation

| | Year | n | Biliary stricture | | Bile leak | |
|---|---|---|---|---|---|---|
| | | | Endoscopic/percutaneous | Surgical/retransplantation | Endoscopic/percutaneous | Surgical/retransplantation |
| Pfau et al. [208] | 2000 | 260 | 8/13 (61.5%) | 5/13 (38.5%) | 26/31 (84%) | 5/31 (16%) |
| Thethy et al. [197] | 2004 | 376 | 12/34 (35%) | 22/34 (65%) | 20/22 (91%) | 2/22 (9%) |
| Abdullah et al. [198] | 2005 | 184 | 5/22 (23%) | 17/22 (77%) | 8/12 (66%) | 4/12 (33%) |
| Gunawansa et al. [209] | 2011 | 296 | 25/63 (40%) | 38/63 (60%) | 10/17 (59%) | 7/17 (41%) |
| Györi et al. [210] | 2016 | 1188 | 80/148 (54%) | 67/148 (45%) | 18/61 (29%) | 43/61 (71%) |
| Coelho et al. [206] | 2017 | 153 | 9/27 (33%) | 18/27 (67%) | 5/12 (42%) | 7/12 (58%) |

patients and mostly in the first 12 months post OLT. AS occur later than NAS. Among NAS, ischemic lesions present within the first year while immunological NAS tend to happen later [160–162]. Most cases of NAS are related to biliary ischemia as around 50% of patients presenting with NAS have HAT [160].

The major risk factors for strictures remain the donor's age, previous bile leaks, and CC type of reconstruction.

Early BS are due to technical mistakes (kinking of the biliary anastomosis secondary to excessive length of bile ducts), whereas late BS are mainly related to chronic ischemic lesions causing scarring and fibrosis of the biliary tissues.

They usually present with symptoms of acute cholangitis.

Anastomotic strictures are usually treated with endoscopic or percutaneous dilation and stenting with a high success rate. In case of failure of endoscopic/radiological techniques, surgery can be an alternative option with resection of the anastomosis and reconstruction with a Roux-en-Y choledochojejunostomy.

Non-anastomotic strictures can be located anywhere in the biliary tree, they can be extrahepatic or intrahepatic. As opposed to AS, NAS are harder to treat, and nonsurgical interventions usually fail to treat them. It often requires surgical re-intreventions. Extrahepatic NAS can be treated like AS with anastomotic resection and Roux-en-Y reconstruction, but intrahepatic strictures often require retransplantation.

### 106.5.5 Biliary Stones and Cast Syndrome

Filling defects on cholangiography are mostly a pathognomonic finding of bile duct stones (BDS), sludge, or casts. They can occur at any time after OLT. They are usually caused by increased viscosity or decreased velocity of bile flow. Any type of stricture or obstruction can favor the formation of sludge and eventually stones. Spier et al. [163] reported additional risk factors for BDS in their case-control study with 1289 LT. Incidence of BDS was 3.8%, with a significantly higher risk of BDS in patients with bile duct pathology, total cholesterol ≥200 mg/dL, and triglyceride ≥150 mg/dL. Meanwhile, the use of ursodeoxycholic acid was a protective factor against BDS.

Biliary CAST syndrome (Fig. 106.10) is defined as the presence of hardened endobiliary material, usually containing biliary epithelium debris, resulting in obstructive jaundice and cholangitis [164, 165]. Reported incidence vary between 2% and 3.6% [164]. Lemmers et al. reported Intraductal hyperintense T1 signal and a "duct-to-duct" image as specific MRI features on MRI [164].

Management is usually endoscopic with a sphincterotomy and stone extraction with or without stenting. PTC can also play a role when endoscopy is not possible. Rarely, medical treatment with ursodeoxycholic acid can be effective after BDS formation.

In CAST syndrome, despite adequate endoscopic treatment, high rates of subsequent biliary strictures were reported with the worst prognosis

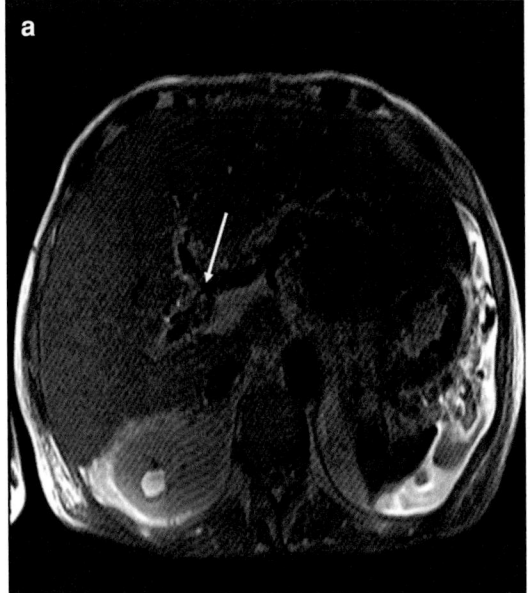

**Fig. 106.10** (a) Half-Fourier single-shot turbo spin-echo (HASTE) axial T2-weighted sequence showing enlarged intrahepatic biliary ducts with hypo-intensity endobiliary content in the hepatic duct of the right posterior sector (white arrow). (Courtesy of Pr. A. Luciani). (b) 3D T2-weighted turbo spin-echo (TSE) MRCP showing notably dilated intrahepatic ducts with diffuse heterogenous endoluminal material

in comparison to common biliary anastomotic and non-anastomotic strictures [164].

## 106.6 Other Rare Complications

Intestinal perforation after LT is a rare but dreadful complication with an incidence that can reach 5% [166].

The presence of adhesions and in particular the presence of hepatobiliary surgery history [167], the duration of the transplantation procedure, the need for reoperation, severe portal hypertension, and early PVT [168] are associated with a higher incidence of bowel perforation following OLT. LT for polycystic liver disease is also associated with a higher risk of intestinal perforation [169].

Fungal septicemia, usually from an enteric source, has been identified as a specific risk factor, occurring more frequently in patients with bowel perforation and possibly precipitating the occurrence of fulminant hepatic failure.

Diagnosis may be difficult because of the absence of specific clinical signs due to the use of immunosuppressive therapy.

Management includes active anti-fungal treatment and reintervention with reported favorable outcomes (no mortality) in early diagnosed patients [166, 170]. Fang et al. reported a 30% mortality rate in patients experiencing intestinal perforation despite adequate management.

## 106.7 Small-for-Size Syndrome

Small-for-size syndrome (SFSS) is a well-known complication of partial LT, split LT, and also living donor LT (LDLT).

To date, no universal definition is available for the SFSS. The definition of Dahm et al. [171] proposed SFS dysfunction and SFS nonfunction. These definitions are based on both the presence of small-for-size graft (SFSG) criteria and the postoperative course within the first week after LT:

- SFSG is defined as a graft-to-recipient body weight ratio (GRWR) <0.8%.
- For SFS dysfunction, for three consecutive days, two from the following three complications must be present: total bilirubin >100 µmol/L; international normalized ratio (INR) >2 and encephalopathy grade 3 or 4.

For SFS non-function, the occurrence of death or salvage retransplantation during the first 7 days after LT.

Obviously, this clinical situation requires the exclusion of all technical and nontechnical complications that might follow LT and expose primary graft non-function.

Post-LT liver biopsies showed ischemic patterns with disruption of the sinusoidal line, hepatocyte ballooning, enhanced cholestasis, and the transformation of Ito cells into fibroblasts [172–174].

In addition to graft size, several other risk factors have been identified in the literature as being associated with a poor graft outcome. Age of the donor >50 years, graft steatosis >30%, prolonged cold and warm ischemia times, ischemia/reperfusion injury, and portal graft hyperperfusion and hypertension are among the most relevant risk factors [175, 176].

Indeed, portal pressures >20 mmHg have been reported by the Kyoto group to have the worst impact on graft outcome and survival [177]. These results have been validated by subsequent partial-LT studies. This cutoff has been dropped to 15 mmHg by Ogura et al. [178]. Despite the absence of correlation between portal venous pressure and flow [179], it was obvious that portal vein hyperperfusion with a portal venous flow >270 mL/s was associated with an increased hepatic venous portal gradient (HVPG >15 mmHg) and a lower graft survival.

To overcome the negative effect of portal hypertension and hyperperfusion on graft survival, graft inflow modulation (GIM) has been applied by several teams, especially in the setting of LDLT, to prevent subsequent histological damage. Indeed, splenectomy, splenic artery ligation/embolization, and portocaval shunts have been reported to improve the postoperative course of SFSG [176, 180–182]. Somatostatin showed also promising results in experimental studies and preliminary clinical trials on the immediate modification of liver graft hemodynamics [183–185]. This successful modulation did not have a clear impact on postoperative liver function in the Troisi et al. randomized clinical trial [184]. Same authors performed a literature review of GIM techniques in partial LT with heterogenous studies consisting mainly in small series. The obvious result is an interesting decrease in morbidity rates in modulated grafts in comparison to control groups, but there is no clear correlation between the improvement in graft and patient survivals [176].

GIM has been applied intraoperatively to lower PV pressure/flow and thus increase HA flow or postoperatively as a salvage procedure in patients with obvious portal hypertension jeopardizing post-LT liver function.

Most authors applied GIM in case of PVP ≥20 mmHg after reperfusion [183–185]. With a more precise hemodynamic evaluation after reperfusion, Sainz-Barriga et al. [179] proposed GIM in case of portal graft hyperperfusion with a portal vein flow (≥360 mL/min/100 g of LW), severe portal hypertension (HVPG ≥15 mmHg), and a low hepatic artery flow (<100 mL/min). This indication prevents the portal perfusion from decreasing dramatically in patients with a high PVP but normal or low portal vein flow, which may alter liver regeneration and function.

**Dos and Don'ts**
- Well-studied graft choice, perfect surgical technique, and codified active postoperative surveillance are key parameters for good LT outcomes.
- Adequate management of LT complications is the cornerstone of a longer graft and the patient's survival.
- In very early HAT, emergency revisional surgery and/or retransplantation have to be undertaken.
- In specific indications, interventional radiology (for vascular complications)

and endoscopy (for biliary complications) present excellent outcomes which can avoid difficult revisional surgery.
- Any delay or mismanagement may result in graft loss and mortality.

**Take-Home Messages**
- Liver transplantation is the gold standard of treatment for end-stage liver disease. The main limitation is organ shortage that pushed transplantation centers to adopt newer and more difficult techniques like split LT, extending donor criteria, and harvesting in DCD and, in the same setting, when available, using LDLT.
- Fine knowledge of LT complications might allow surgeons to improve LT outcomes and reduce the risk of threatening complications.
- The continuous development of interventional techniques allowed for the safe and efficient treatments of numerous complications without requiring surgical revision, thus reducing the need for both retransplantation and the morbidity/mortality associated with revisional surgery.

**Questions and Answers**
1. **What is the timing of occurrence of early hepatic arterial thrombosis following liver transplantation?**
   A. 7 days
   B. **30 days**
   C. 60 days
   D. 90 days
2. **What is the major complication of early hepatic arterial thrombosis following liver transplantation?**
   A. Abnormal liver tests
   B. Renal failure
   C. Cholangitis
   D. **Primary graft non-function**
3. **Which is the first diagnostic exam to perform in case of clinical suspicion of hepatic arterial thrombosis following liver transplantation?**
   A. **Doppler ultrasound**
   B. CT scan with arterial phase
   C. MRI
   D. Angiography
4. **What is the first emergency treatment for early hepatic arterial thrombosis following liver transplantation?**
   A. **Arterial revisional surgery**
   B. Endovascular thrombectomy
   C. Liver retransplantation
   D. Curative anticoagulant treatment alone
5. **Among the following, what is the most dreadful complication after liver transplantation?**
   A. **Early arterial thrombosis**
   B. Portal vein thrombosis
   C. Arterial stenosis
   D. Biliary stenosis
6. **What is the first treatment for hepatic arterial stenosis following liver transplantation?**
   A. Arterial revisional surgery
   B. **Endovascular treatment**
   C. Medical treatment
   D. Retransplantation
7. **What were the results of the French multicentric randomized controlled trial (BILIDRAIN) comparing T-tube placement to non-drained biliary anastomosis?**
   A. Equivalent long-term results
   B. Higher biliary anastomotic stricture after T-tube placement
   C. **Higher mortality rate after T-tube placement**
   D. Higher biliary fistula in the non-drained group

8. **What is the incidence of hepatic arterial thrombosis after liver transplantation?**
   A. 2–5%
   B. **5–15%**
   C. 15–20%
   D. 30–40%

9. **What is the incidence of biliary stenosis after liver transplantation?**
   A. 3–5%
   B. **10–15%**
   C. 20–25%
   D. 25–30%

10. **What is the definition of a small-for-size graft?**
    A. Graft-to-recipient body weight ratio (GRWR) < 0.4%
    B. Graft-to-recipient body weight ratio (GRWR) < 0.6%
    C. **Graft-to-recipient body weight ratio (GRWR) < 0.8%**
    D. Graft-to-recipient body weight ratio (GRWR) < 1%

**Acknowledgments** Special thanks to Dr. Nicola De Angelis for his valuable contribution to the revision of the final manuscript.

# References

1. Starzl TE, Marchioro TL, Kaulla KNV, Hermann G, Brittain RS, Waddell WR. Homotransplantation of the liver in humans. Surg Gynecol Obstet. 1963;117:659–76.
2. Burra P, Samuel D, Sundaram V, Duvoux C, Petrowsky H, Terrault N, et al. Limitations of current liver donor allocation systems and the impact of newer indications for liver transplantation. J Hepatol. 2021;75: S178–90.
3. Panayotova G, Lunsford KE, Latt NL, Paterno F, Guarrera JV, Pyrsopoulos N. Expanding indications for liver transplantation in the era of liver transplant oncology. World J Gastrointest Surg. 2021;13(5): 392–405.
4. Thuluvath PJ, Guidinger MK, Fung JJ, Johnson LB, Rayhill SC, Pelletier SJ. Liver transplantation in the United States, 1999–2008. Am J Transplant. 2010;10(4):1003–19.
5. Adam R, Karam V, Delvart V, O'Grady J, Mirza D, Klempnauer J, et al. Evolution of indications and results of liver transplantation in Europe. A report from the European Liver Transplant Registry (ELTR). J Hepatol. 2012;57(3):675–88.
6. Burroughs AK, Sabin CA, Rolles K, Delvart V, Karam V, Buckels J, et al. 3-Month and 12-month mortality after first liver transplant in adults in Europe: predictive models for outcome. Lancet. 2006;367(9506):225–32.
7. Freise CE, Gillespie BW, Koffron AJ, Lok ASF, Pruett TL, Emond JC, et al. Recipient morbidity after living and deceased donor liver transplantation: findings from the A2ALL Retrospective Cohort Study. Am J Transplant. 2008;8(12):2569–79.
8. Craig EV, Heller MT. Complications of liver transplant. Abdom Radiol. 2021;46(1):43–67.
9. Duffy JP, Hong JC, Farmer DG, Ghobrial RM, Yersiz H, Hiatt JR, et al. Vascular complications of orthotopic liver transplantation: experience in more than 4,200 patients. J Am Coll Surg. 2009;208(5):896–903; discussion 903–5.
10. Piardi T, Lhuaire M, Bruno O, Memeo R, Pessaux P, Kianmanesh R, et al. Vascular complications following liver transplantation: a literature review of advances in 2015. World J Hepatol. 2016;8(1):36–57.
11. Wozney P, Zajko AB, Bron KM, Point S, Starzl TE. Vascular complications after liver transplantation. AJR Am J Roentgenol. 1986;147(4):657–63.
12. Bekker J, Ploem S, de Jong KP. Early hepatic artery thrombosis after liver transplantation: a systematic review of the incidence, outcome and risk factors. Am J Transplant. 2009;9(4):746–57.
13. Mourad MM, Liossis C, Gunson BK, Mergental H, Isaac J, Muiesan P, et al. Etiology and management of hepatic artery thrombosis after adult liver transplantation. Liver Transpl. 2014;20(6):713–23.
14. Puliti Reigada CH, de Ataide EC, de Almeida Prado Mattosinho T, Boin IFSF. Hepatic artery thrombosis after liver transplantation: five-year experience at the State University of Campinas. Transplant Proc. 2017;49(4):867–70.
15. Marín-Gómez LM, Bernal-Bellido C, Alamo-Martínez JM, Porras-López FM, Suárez-Artacho G, Serrano-Diaz-Canedo J, et al. Intraoperative hepatic artery blood flow predicts early hepatic artery thrombosis after liver transplantation. Transplant Proc. 2012;44(7):2078–81.
16. Czigany Z, Boecker J, Morales Santana DA, Bednarsch J, Meister FA, Amygdalos I, et al. Median arcuate ligament compression in orthotopic liver transplantation: results from a single-center analysis and a European Survey Study. J Clin Med. 2019;8(4):550.
17. Fukuzawa K, Schwartz ME, Katz E, Mor E, Emre S, Acarli K, et al. The arcuate ligament syndrome in liver transplantation. Transplantation. 1993;56(1):223–4.
18. Lubrano J, Scatton O, Randone B, Molinier N, Massault PP, Legmann P, et al. Median arcuate

ligament in orthotopic liver transplantation: relevance to arterial reconstruction. Transplant Proc. 2008;40(10):3532–5.
19. Gilbo N, Van Praet L, Jochmans I, Sainz-Barriga M, Verslype C, Maleux G, et al. Pre-operative transcatheter arterial chemo-embolization increases hepatic artery thrombosis after liver transplantation - a retrospective study. Transpl Int. 2018;31(1):71–81.
20. Lin T-S, Chiang Y-C, Chen C-L, Concejero AM, Cheng Y-F, Wang C-C, et al. Intimal dissection of the hepatic artery following transarterial embolization for hepatocellular carcinoma: an intraoperative problem in adult living donor liver transplantation. Liver Transpl. 2009;15(11):1553–6.
21. Panaro F, Ramos J, Gallix B, Mercier G, Herrero A, Niampa H, et al. Hepatic artery complications following liver transplantation. Does preoperative chemoembolization impact the postoperative course? Clin Transpl. 2014;28(5):598–605.
22. Gunsar F, Rolando N, Pastacaldi S, Patch D, Raimondo ML, Davidson B, et al. Late hepatic artery thrombosis after orthotopic liver transplantation. Liver Transpl. 2003;9(6):605–11.
23. Stewart ZA, Locke JE, Segev DL, Dagher NN, Singer AL, Montgomery RA, et al. Increased risk of graft loss from hepatic artery thrombosis after liver transplantation with older donors. Liver Transpl. 2009;15(12):1688–95.
24. Hong JC, Yersiz H, Farmer DG, Duffy JP, Ghobrial RM, Nonthasoot B, et al. Longterm outcomes for whole and segmental liver grafts in adult and pediatric liver transplant recipients: a 10-year comparative analysis of 2,988 cases. J Am Coll Surg. 2009;208(5):682–9; discussion 689–91.
25. Nishida S, Kato T, Levi D, Naveen M, Berney T, Vianna R, et al. Effect of protocol Doppler ultrasonography and urgent revascularization on early hepatic artery thrombosis after pediatric liver transplantation. Arch Surg. 2002;137(11):1279.
26. Gupta G, Sood P, Kumar G, Hughes C, Sturdevant M, Humar A, et al. Late hepatic artery thrombosis after liver transplant in adults associated with high mortality: Abstract# C1944. Transplantation. 2014;98:744.
27. Bhattacharjya S, Gunson BK, Mirza DF, Mayer DA, Buckels JA, McMaster P, et al. Delayed hepatic artery thrombosis in adult orthotopic liver transplantation-a 12-year experience. Transplantation. 2001;71(11):1592–6.
28. Stange BJ, Glanemann M, Nuessler NC, Settmacher U, Steinmüller T, Neuhaus P. Hepatic artery thrombosis after adult liver transplantation. Liver Transpl. 2003;9(6):612–20.
29. Hom BK, Shrestha R, Palmer SL, Katz MD, Selby RR, Asatryan Z, et al. Prospective evaluation of vascular complications after liver transplantation: comparison of conventional and microbubble contrast-enhanced US. Radiology. 2006;241(1):267–74.
30. Karmazyn B, Sağlam D, Rao G, Jennings S, Mangus R. Initial experience with contrast-enhanced ultrasound in the first week after liver transplantation in children: a useful adjunct to Doppler ultrasound. Pediatr Radiol. 2021;51:1–9.
31. Torres A, Koskinen SK, Gjertsen H, Fischler B. Contrast-enhanced ultrasound for identifying circulatory complications after liver transplants in children. Pediatr Transplant. 2019;23(1):e13327.
32. Delgado-Moraleda J-J, Ballester-Vallés C, Marti-Bonmati L. Role of imaging in the evaluation of vascular complications after liver transplantation. Insights Imaging. 2019;10(1):78.
33. Kim SY, Kim KW, Kim MJ, Shin YM, Lee M-G, Lee SG. Multidetector row CT of various hepatic artery complications after living donor liver transplantation. Abdom Imaging. 2007;32(5):635–43.
34. Glockner JF, Forauer AR, Solomon H, Varma CR, Perman WH. Three-dimensional gadolinium-enhanced MR angiography of vascular complications after liver transplantation. AJR Am J Roentgenol. 2000;174(5):1447–53.
35. Montalti R, Busani S, Masetti M, Girardis M, Di Benedetto F, Begliomini B, et al. Two-stage liver transplantation: an effective procedure in urgent conditions. Clin Transpl. 2010;24(1):122–6.
36. Ringe B, Lübbe N, Kuse E, Frei U, Pichlmayr R. Total hepatectomy and liver transplantation as two-stage procedure. Ann Surg. 1993;218(1):3–9.
37. Sanabria Mateos R, Hogan NM, Dorcaratto D, Heneghan H, Udupa V, Maguire D, et al. Total hepatectomy and liver transplantation as a two-stage procedure for fulminant hepatic failure: a safe procedure in exceptional circumstances. World J Hepatol. 2016;8(4):226–30.
38. Herrero A, Souche R, Joly E, Boisset G, Habibeh H, Bouyabrine H, et al. Early hepatic artery thrombosis after liver transplantation: what is the impact of the arterial reconstruction type? World J Surg. 2017;41(8):2101–10.
39. Bhangui P, Salloum C, Lim C, Andreani P, Ariche A, Adam R, et al. Portal vein arterialization: a salvage procedure for a totally de-arterialized liver. The Paul Brousse Hospital experience. HPB (Oxford). 2014;16(8):723–38.
40. Maggi U, Camagni S, Reggiani P, Lauro R, Sposito C, Melada E, et al. Portal vein arterialization for hepatic artery thrombosis in liver transplantation: a case report, Doppler-ultrasound aspects, and review of the literature. Transplant Proc. 2010;42(4):1369–74.
41. Tsivian M, Neri F, Prezzi D, Puviani L, Pacile V, Bertelli R, et al. Portal vein arterialization in hepatobiliary surgery and liver transplantation. Transplant Proc. 2007;39(6):1877–8.
42. Yoshiya S, Yoshizumi T, Iseda N, Takeishi K, Toshima T, Nagao Y, et al. Anastomosis of the common hepatic artery and round ligament as portal vein arterialization for hepatic artery occlusion after deceased donor liver transplantation: a case report. Transplant Proc. 2020;52(2):641–3.
43. Hidalgo E. Portal vein arterialization: 'enjoy' it responsibly. HPB. 2014;16(8):739.

44. Abdelaziz O, Hosny K, Amin A, Emadeldin S, Uemoto S, Mostafa M. Endovascular management of early hepatic artery thrombosis after living donor liver transplantation. Transpl Int. 2012;25(8):847–56.
45. Argirò R, Raso A, Vidali S, Morosetti D. Endovascular thromboaspiration with neurointerventional devices for early hepatic artery thrombosis after split liver transplant. BMJ Case Rep. 2021;14(5):e240583.
46. Gastaca M, Gomez J, Terreros I, Izquierdo J, Ruiz P, Prieto M, et al. Endovascular therapy of arterial complications within the first week after liver transplant. Transplant Proc. 2020;52(5):1464–7.
47. Li T, Sun X-D, Yu Y, Lv G-Y. Intra-arterial thrombolysis for early hepatic artery thrombosis after liver transplantation. World J Clin Cases. 2021;9(7):1592–9.
48. Abdelaziz O, Osman AMA, Hosny KA, Emad-Eldin S, Serour DK, Mostafa M. Management of early hepatic artery thrombosis following living-donor liver transplantation: feasibility, efficacy and potential risks of endovascular therapy in the first 48 hours post-transplant-a retrospective cohort study. Transpl Int. 2021;34(6):1134–49.
49. Sommacale D, Dondero F, Sauvanet A, Francoz C, Durand F, Farges O, et al. Liver resection in transplanted patients: a single-center Western experience. Transplant Proc. 2013;45(7):2726–8.
50. Hamby BA, Ramirez DE, Loss GE, Bazan HA, Smith TA, Bluth E, et al. Endovascular treatment of hepatic artery stenosis after liver transplantation. J Vasc Surg. 2013;57(4):1067–72.
51. Kogut MJ, Shin DS, Padia SA, Johnson GE, Hippe DS, Valji K. Intra-arterial thrombolysis for hepatic artery thrombosis following liver transplantation. J Vasc Interv Radiol. 2015;26(9):1317–22.
52. Maruzzelli L, Miraglia R, Caruso S, Milazzo M, Mamone G, Gruttadauria S, et al. Percutaneous endovascular treatment of hepatic artery stenosis in adult and pediatric patients after liver transplantation. Cardiovasc Intervent Radiol. 2010;33(6):1111–9.
53. Jurim O, Shaked A, Kiai K, Millis JM, Colquhoun SD, Busuttil RW. Celiac compression syndrome and liver transplantation. Ann Surg. 1993;218(1):10–2.
54. Mohamed Afif A, Anthony APM, Jamaruddin S, Su'aidi SU, Li HH, Low ASC, et al. Diagnostic accuracy of Doppler ultrasound for detecting hepatic artery stenosis after liver transplantation. Clin Radiol. 2021;76(9):708.e19–25.
55. Hann A, Seth R, Mergental H, Hartog H, Alzoubi M, Stangou A, et al. Biliary strictures are associated with both early and late hepatic artery stenosis. Transplant Direct. 2021;7(1):e643.
56. Goel A, Mehta N, Guy J, Fidelman N, Yao F, Roberts J, et al. Hepatic artery and biliary complications in liver transplant recipients undergoing pretransplant transarterial chemoembolization. Liver Transpl. 2014;20(10):1221–8.
57. Lee DD, Paz-Fumagalli R, Croome KP, Paz D, Wright L, Nguyen JH, et al. Hepatic artery stenosis after liver transplant: donation after cardiac death donor vs donation after brain death donor grafts. Clin Transpl. 2018;32(11):e13413.
58. Abbasoglu O, Levy MF, Vodapally MS, Goldstein RM, Husberg BS, Gonwa TA, et al. Hepatic artery stenosis after liver transplantation—incidence, presentation, treatment, and long term outcome. Transplantation. 1997;63(2):250–5.
59. Singh AK, Nachiappan AC, Verma HA, Uppot RN, Blake MA, Saini S, et al. Postoperative imaging in liver transplantation: what radiologists should know. Radiographics. 2010;30(2):339–51.
60. Quiroga S, Sebastià MC, Margarit C, Castells L, Boyé R, Alvarez-Castells A. Complications of orthotopic liver transplantation: spectrum of findings with helical CT. Radiographics. 2001;21(5):1085–102.
61. Rostambeigi N, Hunter D, Duval S, Chinnakotla S, Golzarian J. Stent placement versus angioplasty for hepatic artery stenosis after liver transplant: a meta-analysis of case series. Eur Radiol. 2013;23(5):1323–34.
62. Rajakannu M, Awad S, Ciacio O, Pittau G, Adam R, Cunha AS, et al. Intention-to-treat analysis of percutaneous endovascular treatment of hepatic artery stenosis after orthotopic liver transplantation. Liver Transpl. 2016;22(7):923–33.
63. Breguet R, Dondero F, Pupulim L, Goossens N, Sepulveda A, Francoz C, et al. Endovascular treatment of arterial complications after liver transplantation: long-term follow-up evaluated on Doppler ultrasound and magnetic resonance cholangiopancreatography. Cardiovasc Intervent Radiol. 2019;42(3):381–8.
64. Dalal A. Organ transplantation and drug eluting stents: perioperative challenges. World J Transplant. 2016;6(4):620–31.
65. Naidu S, Alzubaidi S, Knuttinen G, Patel I, Fleck A, Sweeney J, et al. Treatment of hepatic artery stenosis in liver transplant patients using drug-eluting versus bare-metal stents. J Clin Med. 2021;10(3):380.
66. Sommacale D, Aoyagi T, Dondero F, Sibert A, Bruno O, Fteriche S, et al. Repeat endovascular treatment of recurring hepatic artery stenoses in orthotopic liver transplantation. Transpl Int. 2013;26(6):608–15.
67. Chen G-H, Wang G-Y, Yang Y, Li H, Lu M-Q, Cai C-J, et al. Single-center experience of therapeutic management of hepatic artery stenosis after orthotopic liver transplantation. Report of 20 cases. Eur Surg Res. 2009;42(1):21–7.
68. Sommacale D, Rochas Dos Santos V, Dondero F, Francoz C, Durand F, Sibert A, et al. Simultaneous surgical repair for combined biliary and arterial stenoses after liver transplantation. Transplant Proc. 2011;43(5):1765–9.
69. Chen J, Weinstein J, Black S, Spain J, Brady PS, Dowell JD. Surgical and endovascular treatment of hepatic arterial complications following liver transplant. Clin Transpl. 2014;28(12):1305–12.
70. Harrison J, Harrison M, Doria C. Hepatic artery pseudoaneurysm following orthotopic liver transplantation: increasing clinical suspicion for a rare but lethal pathology. Ann Transplant. 2017;22:417–24.

71. St Michel DP, Goussous N, Orr NL, Barth RN, Gray SH, LaMattina JC, et al. Hepatic artery pseudoaneurysm in the liver transplant recipient: a case series. Case Rep Transplant. 2019;2019:9108903.
72. Thorat A, Lee C-F, Wu T-H, Pan K-T, Chu S-Y, Chou H-S, et al. Endovascular treatment for pseudoaneurysms arising from the hepatic artery after liver transplantation. Asian J Surg. 2017;40(3):227–31.
73. Marshall MM, Muiesan P, Srinivasan P, Kane PA, Rela M, Heaton ND, et al. Hepatic artery pseudoaneurysms following liver transplantation: incidence, presenting features and management. Clin Radiol. 2001;56(7):579–87.
74. Volpin E, Pessaux P, Sauvanet A, Sibert A, Kianmanesh R, Durand F, et al. Preservation of the arterial vascularisation after hepatic artery pseudoaneurysm following orthotopic liver transplantation: long-term results. Ann Transplant. 2014;19:346–52.
75. Logaldo D, Costantini Brancadoro E, Ballabio A, Zurleni T. Splenic artery transposition graft for hepatic artery aneurysm and occlusion. Ann Vasc Surg. 2017;42:300.e7–300.e10.
76. Lerut JP, Gordon RD, Iwatsuki S, Starzl TE. Human orthotopic liver transplantation: surgical aspects in 393 consecutive grafts. Transplant Proc. 1988;20(1 Suppl 1):603–6.
77. Marujo WC, Langnas AN, Wood RP, Stratta RJ, Li S, Shaw BW. Vascular complications following orthotopic liver transplantation: outcome and the role of urgent revascularization. Transplant Proc. 1991;23(1 Pt 2):1484–6.
78. Starzl TE, Iwatsuki S, Shaw BW. A growth factor in fine vascular anastomoses. Surg Gynecol Obstet. 1984;159(2):164–5.
79. Yerdel MA, Gunson B, Mirza D, Karayalçin K, Olliff S, Buckels J, et al. Portal vein thrombosis in adults undergoing liver transplantation: risk factors, screening, management, and outcome. Transplantation. 2000;69(9):1873–81.
80. Bhangui P, Lim C, Levesque E, Salloum C, Lahat E, Feray C, et al. Novel classification of non-malignant portal vein thrombosis: a guide to surgical decision-making during liver transplantation. J Hepatol. 2019;71(5):1038–50.
81. Gomez Gavara C, Bhangui P, Salloum C, Osseis M, Esposito F, Moussallem T, et al. Ligation versus no ligation of spontaneous portosystemic shunts during liver transplantation: audit of a prospective series of 66 consecutive patients. Liver Transpl. 2018;24(4):505–15.
82. Lee S-G, Moon D-B, Ahn C-S, Kim K-H, Hwang S, Park K-M, et al. Ligation of left renal vein for large spontaneous splenorenal shunt to prevent portal flow steal in adult living donor liver transplantation. Transpl Int. 2007;20(1):45–50.
83. Conzen KD, Pomfret EA. Liver transplant in patients with portal vein thrombosis: medical and surgical requirements. Liver Transpl. 2017;23(S1):S59–63.
84. Ghazwani S, Panaro F, Navarro F. Is portal vein thrombosis still a contraindication for liver transplantation? A single-institute's 5-year experience and literature review. TRRM. 2016;8:31–6.
85. Bhangui P, Lim C, Salloum C, Andreani P, Sebbagh M, Hoti E, et al. Caval inflow to the graft for liver transplantation in patients with diffuse portal vein thrombosis: a 12-year experience. Ann Surg. 2011;254(6):1008–16.
86. Azoulay D, Quintini C, Rayar M, Salloum C, Llado L, Diago T, et al. Renoportal anastomosis during liver transplantation in patients with portal vein thrombosis: first long-term results from a multicenter study. Ann Surg. 2021;10 https://doi.org/10.1097/SLA.0000000000004797.
87. Canovai E, Ceulemans LJ, Gilbo N, Duchateau NM, De Hertogh G, Hiele M, et al. Multivisceral transplantation for diffuse portomesenteric thrombosis: lessons learned for surgical optimization. Front Surg. 2021;8:645302.
88. Tekin A, Beduschi T, Vianna R, Mangus RS. Multivisceral transplant as an option to transplant cirrhotic patients with severe portal vein thrombosis. Int J Surg. 2020;82:115–21.
89. Vianna RM, Mangus RS, Kubal C, Fridell JA, Beduschi T, Tector AJ. Multivisceral transplantation for diffuse portomesenteric thrombosis. Ann Surg. 2012;255(6):1144–50.
90. Cheng Y, Chen Y, Jiang Y, Zhang X. Ten-year survival after portal vein arterialization in liver transplantation. Ann Palliat Med. 2019;8(5):79092–792.
91. Paloyo S, Nishida S, Fan J, Tekin A, Selvaggi G, Levi D, et al. Portal vein arterialization using an accessory right hepatic artery in liver transplantation. Liver Transpl. 2013;19(7):773–5.
92. Bonnet S, Sauvanet A, Bruno O, Sommacale D, Francoz C, Dondero F, et al. Long-term survival after portal vein arterialization for portal vein thrombosis in orthotopic liver transplantation. Gastroenterol Clin Biol. 2010;34(1):23–8.
93. Zhang K, Jiang Y, Lv L-Z, Cai Q-C, Yang F, Hu H-Z, et al. Portal vein arterialization technique for liver transplantation patients. World J Gastroenterol. 2014;20(34):12359–62.
94. Ott R, Böhner C, Müller S, Aigner T, Bussenius-Kammerer M, Yedibela S, et al. Outcome of patients with pre-existing portal vein thrombosis undergoing arterialization of the portal vein during liver transplantation. Transpl Int. 2003;16(1):15–20.
95. Cheng YF, Chen CL, Huang TL, Chen TY, Chen YS, Takatsuki M, et al. Risk factors for intraoperative portal vein thrombosis in pediatric living donor liver transplantation. Clin Transpl. 2004;18(4):390–4.
96. Reyes L, Herrero JI, Rotellar Sastre F, Páramo JA. Risk factors and impact of portal vein thrombosis in liver transplantation. Rev Esp Enferm Dig. 2019;111(6):437–44.
97. Chong WK, Beland JC, Weeks SM. Sonographic evaluation of venous obstruction in liver transplants. AJR Am J Roentgenol. 2007;188(6):515–21.

98. Feltracco P, Barbieri S, Cillo U, Zanus G, Senzolo M, Ori C. Perioperative thrombotic complications in liver transplantation. World J Gastroenterol. 2015;21(26):8004–13.
99. Jensen MK, Campbell KM, Alonso MH, Nathan JD, Ryckman FC, Tiao GM. Management and long-term consequences of portal vein thrombosis after liver transplantation in children. Liver Transpl. 2013;19(3):315–21.
100. Lodhia N, Salem R, Levitsky J. Transjugular intrahepatic portosystemic shunt with thrombectomy for the treatment of portal vein thrombosis after liver transplantation. Dig Dis Sci. 2010;55(2):529–34.
101. Lerut JP, Goffette P, Molle G, Roggen FM, Puttemans T, Brenard R, et al. Transjugular intrahepatic portosystemic shunt after adult liver transplantation: experience in eight patients. Transplantation. 1999;68(3):379–84.
102. López-Benítez R, Barragán-Campos HM, Richter GM, Sauer P, Mehrabi A, Fonouni H, et al. Interventional radiologic procedures in the treatment of complications after liver transplantation. Clin Transpl. 2009;23(Suppl 21):92–101.
103. Cherukuri R, Haskal ZJ, Naji A, Shaked A. Percutaneous thrombolysis and stent placement for the treatment of portal vein thrombosis after liver transplantation: long-term follow-up. Transplantation. 1998;65(8):1124–6.
104. Khan A, Kleive D, Aandahl EM, Fosby B, Line P-D, Dorenberg E, et al. Portal vein stent placement after hepatobiliary and pancreatic surgery. Langenbecks Arch Surg. 2020;405(5):657–64.
105. Woo DH, Laberge JM, Gordon RL, Wilson MW, Kerlan RK. Management of portal venous complications after liver transplantation. Tech Vasc Interv Radiol. 2007;10(3):233–9.
106. Starzl TE, Groth CG, Brettschneider L, Penn I, Fulginiti VA, Moon JB, et al. Orthotopic homotransplantation of the human liver. Ann Surg. 1968;168(3):392–415.
107. Calne RY, Williams R. Liver transplantation in man. I. Observations on technique and organization in five cases. Br Med J. 1968;4(5630):535–40.
108. Tzakis A, Todo S, Starzl TE. Orthotopic liver transplantation with preservation of the inferior vena cava. Ann Surg. 1989;210(5):649–52.
109. Navarro F, Le Moine MC, Fabre JM, Belghiti J, Cherqui D, Adam R, et al. Specific vascular complications of orthotopic liver transplantation with preservation of the retrohepatic vena cava: review of 1361 cases. Transplantation. 1999;68(5):646–50.
110. Tayar C, Kluger MD, Laurent A, Cherqui D. Optimizing outflow in piggyback liver transplantation without caval occlusion: the three-vein technique. Liver Transpl. 2011;17(1):88–92.
111. Nishida S, Nakamura N, Vaidya A, Levi DM, Kato T, Nery JR, et al. Piggyback technique in adult orthotopic liver transplantation: an analysis of 1067 liver transplants at a single center. HPB (Oxford). 2006;8(3):182–8.
112. Belghiti J, Panis Y, Sauvanet A, Gayet B, Fékété F. A new technique of side to side caval anastomosis during orthotopic hepatic transplantation without inferior vena caval occlusion. Surg Gynecol Obstet. 1992;175(3):270–2.
113. Belghiti J, Ettorre GM, Durand F, Sommacale D, Sauvanet A, Jerius JT, et al. Feasibility and limits of caval-flow preservation during liver transplantation. Liver Transpl. 2001;7(11):983–7.
114. Mehrabi A, Mood ZA, Fonouni H, Kashfi A, Hillebrand N, Müller SA, et al. A single-center experience of 500 liver transplants using the modified piggyback technique by Belghiti. Liver Transpl. 2009;15(5):466–74.
115. Andrews JC. Vascular complications following liver transplantation. Semin Intervent Radiol. 2004;21(4):221–33.
116. Raby N, Karani J, Thomas S, O'Grady J, Williams R. Stenoses of vascular anastomoses after hepatic transplantation: treatment with balloon angioplasty. AJR Am J Roentgenol. 1991;157(1):167–71.
117. Darcy MD. Management of venous outflow complications after liver transplantation. Tech Vasc Interv Radiol. 2007;10(3):240–5.
118. Morochnik S, Niemeyer MM, Lipnik AJ, Gaba RC. Immediate postoperative inferior vena cava stenting to improve hepatic venous outflow following orthotopic liver transplantation. Radiol Case Rep. 2021;16(2):224–9.
119. Zhang Z-Y, Jin L, Chen G, Su T-H, Zhu Z-J, Sun L-Y, et al. Balloon dilatation for treatment of hepatic venous outflow obstruction following pediatric liver transplantation. World J Gastroenterol. 2017;23(46):8227–34.
120. Boeva I, Karagyozov PI, Tishkov I. Post-liver transplant biliary complications: current knowledge and therapeutic advances. World J Hepatol. 2021;13(1):66–79.
121. Welling TH, Heidt DG, Englesbe MJ, Magee JC, Sung RS, Campbell DA, et al. Biliary complications following liver transplantation in the model for end-stage liver disease era: effect of donor, recipient, and technical factors. Liver Transpl. 2008;14(1):73–80.
122. Zimmerman MA, Baker T, Goodrich NP, Freise C, Hong JC, Kumer S, et al. Development, management, and resolution of biliary complications after living and deceased donor liver transplantation: a report from the adult-to-adult living donor liver transplantation cohort study consortium. Liver Transpl. 2013;19(3):259–67.
123. Greif F, Bronsther OL, Van Thiel DH, Casavilla A, Iwatsuki S, Tzakis A, et al. The incidence, timing, and management of biliary tract complications after orthotopic liver transplantation. Ann Surg. 1994;219(1):40–5.
124. Moser MA, Wall WJ. Management of biliary problems after liver transplantation. Liver Transpl. 2001;7(11 Suppl 1):S46–52.
125. Akamatsu N, Sugawara Y, Hashimoto D. Biliary reconstruction, its complications and management

of biliary complications after adult liver transplantation: a systematic review of the incidence, risk factors and outcome. Transpl Int. 2011;24(4):379–92.
126. Kakizoe S, Yanaga K, Starzl TE, Demetris AJ. Evaluation of protocol before transplantation and after reperfusion biopsies from human orthotopic liver allografts: considerations of preservation and early immunological injury. Hepatology. 1990;11(6):932–41.
127. Testa G, Malagò M, Broelseh CE. Complications of biliary tract in liver transplantation. World J Surg. 2001;25(10):1296–9.
128. Foley DP, Fernandez LA, Leverson G, Chin LT, Krieger N, Cooper JT, et al. Donation after cardiac death: the University of Wisconsin experience with liver transplantation. Ann Surg. 2005;242(5):724–31.
129. Pine JK, Aldouri A, Young AL, Davies MH, Attia M, Toogood GJ, et al. Liver transplantation following donation after cardiac death: an analysis using matched pairs. Liver Transpl. 2009;15(9):1072–82.
130. de Vera ME, Lopez-Solis R, Dvorchik I, Campos S, Morris W, Demetris AJ, et al. Liver transplantation using donation after cardiac death donors: long-term follow-up from a single center. Am J Transplant. 2009;9(4):773–81.
131. Guarrera JV, Henry SD, Samstein B, Odeh-Ramadan R, Kinkhabwala M, Goldstein MJ, et al. Hypothermic machine preservation in human liver transplantation: the first clinical series. Am J Transplant. 2010;10(2):372–81.
132. Muller X, Mohkam K, Mueller M, Schlegel A, Dondero F, Sepulveda A, et al. Hypothermic oxygenated perfusion versus normothermic regional perfusion in liver transplantation from controlled donation after circulatory death: first international comparative study. Ann Surg. 2020;272(5):751–8.
133. van Rijn R, Schurink IJ, de Vries Y, van den Berg AP, Cortes Cerisuelo M, Darwish Murad S, et al. Hypothermic machine perfusion in liver transplantation - a randomized trial. N Engl J Med. 2021;384(15):1391–401.
134. Sung JY, Costerton JW, Shaffer EA. Defense system in the biliary tract against bacterial infection. Dig Dis Sci. 1992;37(5):689–96.
135. Neuhaus P, Blumhardt G, Bechstein WO, Steffen R, Keck H. Side-to-side anastomosis of the common bile duct is the method of choice for biliary tract reconstruction after liver transplantation. Transplant Proc. 1990;22(4):1571.
136. Davidson BR, Rai R, Kurzawinski TR, Selves L, Farouk M, Dooley JS, et al. Prospective randomized trial of end-to-end versus side-to-side biliary reconstruction after orthotopic liver transplantation. Br J Surg. 1999;86(4):447–52.
137. Paes-Barbosa FC, Massarollo PC, Bernardo WM, Ferreira FG, Barbosa FK, Raslan M, et al. Systematic review and meta-analysis of biliary reconstruction techniques in orthotopic deceased donor liver transplantation. J Hepatobiliary Pancreat Sci. 2011;18(4):525–36.
138. Distante V, Farouk M, Kurzawinski TR, Ahmed SW, Burroughs AK, Davidson BR, et al. Duct-to-duct biliary reconstruction following liver transplantation for primary sclerosing cholangitis. Transpl Int. 1996;9(2):126–30.
139. Esfeh JM, Eghtesad B, Hodgkinson P, Diago T, Fujiki M, Hashimoto K, et al. Duct-to-duct biliary reconstruction in patients with primary sclerosing cholangitis undergoing liver transplantation. HPB (Oxford). 2011;13(9):651–5.
140. Heffron TG, Smallwood GA, Ramcharan T, Davis L, Connor K, Martinez E, et al. Duct-to-duct biliary anastomosis for patients with sclerosing cholangitis undergoing liver transplantation. Transplant Proc. 2003;35(8):3006–7.
141. Wells MM, Croome KP, Boyce E, Chandok N. Roux-en-Y choledochojejunostomy versus duct-to-duct biliary anastomosis in liver transplantation for primary sclerosing cholangitis: a meta-analysis. Transplant Proc. 2013;45(6):2263–71.
142. Song S, Lu T, Yang W, Gong S, Lei C, Yang J, et al. T-tube or no T-tube for biliary tract reconstruction in orthotopic liver transplantation: an updated systematic review and meta-analysis. Expert Rev Gastroenterol Hepatol. 2021;15:1201–13.
143. Zhao J-Z, Qiao L-L, Du Z-Q, Zhang J, Wang M-Z, Wang T, et al. T-tube vs no T-tube for biliary tract reconstruction in adult orthotopic liver transplantation: an updated systematic review and meta-analysis. World J Gastroenterol. 2021;27(14):1507–23.
144. Navez J, Mohkam K, Darnis B, Cazauran J-B, Ducerf C, Mabrut J-Y. Biliary duct-to-duct reconstruction with a tunneled retroperitoneal T-tube during liver transplantation: a novel approach to decrease biliary leaks after T-tube removal. J Gastrointest Surg. 2017;21(4):723–30.
145. Bawa SM, Mathew A, Krishnan H, Minford E, Talbot D, Mirza DF, et al. Biliary reconstruction with or without an internal biliary stent in orthotopic liver transplantation: a prospective randomised trial. Transpl Int. 1998;11:S245–7.
146. Mathur AK, Nadig SN, Kingman S, Lee D, Kinkade K, Sonnenday CJ, et al. Internal biliary stenting during orthotopic liver transplantation: anastomotic complications, post-transplant biliary interventions, and survival. Clin Transpl. 2015;29(4):327–35.
147. Sw J, Ds K, Yd Y, So S. Clinical outcome of internal stent for biliary anastomosis in liver transplantation. Transplant Proc. 2014;46(3):856–60.
148. Yoon YC, Etesami K, Kaur N, Emamaullee J, Kim J, Zielsdorf S, et al. Biliary internal stents and biliary complications in adult liver transplantation. Transplant Proc. 2021;53(1):171–6.
149. Roos FJM, Poley J-W, Polak WG, Metselaar HJ. Biliary complications after liver transplantation; recent developments in etiology, diagnosis and endoscopic treatment. Best Pract Res Clin Gastroenterol. 2017;31(2):227–35.
150. Kitazono MT, Qayyum A, Yeh BM, Chard PS, Ostroff JW, Coakley FV. Magnetic resonance chol-

150. angiography of biliary strictures after liver transplantation: a prospective double-blind study. J Magn Reson Imaging. 2007;25(6):1168–73.
151. Seale MK, Catalano OA, Saini S, Hahn PF, Sahani DV. Hepatobiliary-specific MR contrast agents: role in imaging the liver and biliary tree. Radiographics. 2009;29(6):1725–48.
152. Boraschi P, Donati F, Gigoni R, Volpi A, Salemi S, Filipponi F, et al. MR cholangiography in orthotopic liver transplantation: sensitivity and specificity in detecting biliary complications. Clin Transpl. 2010;24(4):E82–7.
153. Scanga AE, Kowdley KV. Management of biliary complications following orthotopic liver transplantation. Curr Gastroenterol Rep. 2007;9(1):31–8.
154. Dumonceau J-M, Tringali A, Blero D, Devière J, Laugiers R, Heresbach D, et al. Biliary stenting: indications, choice of stents and results: European Society of Gastrointestinal Endoscopy (ESGE) clinical guideline. Endoscopy. 2012;44(3):277–98.
155. Oh D-W, Lee SK, Song TJ, Park DH, Lee SS, Seo D-W, et al. Endoscopic management of bile leakage after liver transplantation. Gut Liver. 2015;9(3):417–23.
156. Ayoub WS, Esquivel CO, Martin P. Biliary complications following liver transplantation. Dig Dis Sci. 2010;55(6):1540–6.
157. Irani S, Baron TH, Law R, Akbar A, Ross AS, Gluck M, et al. Endoscopic treatment of nonstricture-related benign biliary diseases using covered self-expandable metal stents. Endoscopy. 2015;47(4):315–21.
158. Luigiano C, Bassi M, Ferrara F, Fabbri C, Ghersi S, Morace C, et al. Placement of a new fully covered self-expanding metal stent for postoperative biliary strictures and leaks not responding to plastic stenting. Surg Laparosc Endosc Percutan Tech. 2013;23(2):159–62.
159. Phillips MS, Bonatti H, Sauer BG, Smith L, Javaid M, Kahaleh M, et al. Elevated stricture rate following the use of fully covered self-expandable metal biliary stents for biliary leaks following liver transplantation. Endoscopy. 2011;43(6):512–7.
160. Ito T, Botros M, Aziz A, Guorgui JG, Agopian VG, Farmer DG, et al. Nonanastomotic biliary strictures after liver transplantation. Am Surg. 2020;86(10):1363–7.
161. Keane MG, Devlin J, Harrison P, Masadeh M, Arain MA, Joshi D. Diagnosis and management of benign biliary strictures post liver transplantation in adults. Transplant Rev (Orlando). 2021;35(1):100593.
162. Verdonk RC, Buis CI, van der Jagt EJ, Gouw ASH, Limburg AJ, Slooff MJH, et al. Nonanastomotic biliary strictures after liver transplantation, Part 2: Management, outcome, and risk factors for disease progression. Liver Transpl. 2007;13(5):725–32.
163. Spier BJ, Pfau PR, Lorenze KR, Knechtle SJ, Said A. Risk factors and outcomes in post–liver transplantation bile duct stones and casts: a case-control study. Liver Transpl. 2008;14(10):1461–5.
164. Lemmers A, Pezzullo M, Hadefi A, Dept S, Germanova D, Gustot T, et al. Biliary cast syndrome after liver transplantation: a cholangiographic evolution study. J Gastroenterol Hepatol. 2021;36(5):1366–77.
165. Mir FF, Jonnalagadda SS. Bile cast syndrome: diagnosis and management, a case series. Endosc Int Open. 2017;5(5):E321–3.
166. Lin J, Wang J, Yue P, Zhang X, Lang R, Wang Y, et al. Treatment and outcome of intestinal perforation after liver transplant surgery in adults: a single-center experience. Ther Clin Risk Manag. 2017;13:675–8.
167. Fang C, Yan S, Liu J, Zheng S. Gastrointestinal perforation after liver transplantation. Surg Pract. 2016;20(1):8–12.
168. Soubrane O, Meteini ME, Devictor D, Bernard O, Houssin D. Risk and prognostic factors of gut perforation after orthotopic liver transplantation for biliary atresia. Liver Transpl Surg. 1995;1(1):2–9.
169. Aussilhou B, Dokmak S, Dondero F, Joly D, Durand F, Soubrane O, et al. Traitement de la Polykystose Hépatique. Mise au point. Journal de Chirurgie Viscérale. 2018;155(6):485–96.
170. Yanagi Y, Matsuura T, Hayashida M, Takahashi Y, Yoshimaru K, Esumi G, et al. Bowel perforation after liver transplantation for biliary atresia: a retrospective study of care in the transition from children to adulthood. Pediatr Surg Int. 2017;33(2):155–63.
171. Dahm F, Georgiev P, Clavien P-A. Small-for-size syndrome after partial liver transplantation: definition, mechanisms of disease and clinical implications. Am J Transplant. 2005;5(11):2605–10.
172. Demetris AJ, Kelly DM, Eghtesad B, Fontes P, Wallis Marsh J, Tom K, et al. Pathophysiologic observations and histopathologic recognition of the portal hyperperfusion or small-for-size syndrome. Am J Surg Pathol. 2006;30(8):986–93.
173. Emond JC, Renz JF, Ferrell LD, Rosenthal P, Lim RC, Roberts JP, et al. Functional analysis of grafts from living donors. Implications for the treatment of older recipients. Ann Surg. 1996;224(4):544–54.
174. Troisi R, Praet M, de Hemptinne B. Small-for-size syndrome: what is the problem? Liver Transpl. 2003;9(9):S1.
175. Masuda Y, Yoshizawa K, Ohno Y, Mita A, Shimizu A, Soejima Y. Small-for-size syndrome in liver transplantation: definition, pathophysiology and management. Hepatobiliary Pancreat Dis Int. 2020;19(4):334–41.
176. Troisi RI, Berardi G, Tomassini F, Sainz-Barriga M. Graft inflow modulation in adult-to-adult living donor liver transplantation: a systematic review. Transplant Rev (Orlando). 2017;31(2):127–35.
177. Ito T, Kiuchi T, Yamamoto H, Oike F, Ogura Y, Fujimoto Y, et al. Changes in portal venous pressure in the early phase after living donor liver transplantation: pathogenesis and clinical implications. Transplantation. 2003;75(8):1313–7.

178. Ogura Y, Hori T, Moghazy WME, Yoshizawa A, Oike F, Mori A, et al. Portal pressure <15 mm Hg is a key for successful adult living donor liver transplantation utilizing smaller grafts than before. Liver Transpl. 2010;16(6):718–28.
179. Sainz-Barriga M, Scudeller L, Costa MG, de Hemptinne B, Troisi RI. Lack of a correlation between portal vein flow and pressure: toward a shared interpretation of hemodynamic stress governing inflow modulation in liver transplantation. Liver Transpl. 2011;17(7):836–48.
180. Elshawy M, Toshima T, Asayama Y, Kubo Y, Ikeda S, Ikegami T, et al. Post-transplant inflow modulation for early allograft dysfunction after living donor liver transplantation. Surg Case Rep. 2020;6(1):164.
181. Soin AS, Yadav SK, Saha SK, Rastogi A, Bhangui P, Srinivasan T, et al. Is portal inflow modulation always necessary for successful utilization of small volume living donor liver grafts? Liver Transpl. 2019;25(12):1811–21.
182. Troisi R, Ricciardi S, Smeets P, Petrovic M, Van Maele G, Colle I, et al. Effects of hemi-portocaval shunts for inflow modulation on the outcome of small-for-size grafts in living donor liver transplantation. Am J Transplant. 2005;5(6):1397–404.
183. Hessheimer AJ, Escobar B, Muñoz J, Flores E, Gracia-Sancho J, Taurá P, et al. Somatostatin therapy protects porcine livers in small-for-size liver transplantation. Am J Transplant. 2014;14(8):1806–16.
184. Troisi RI, Vanlander A, Giglio MC, Van Limmen J, Scudeller L, Heyse B, et al. Somatostatin as inflow modulator in liver-transplant recipients with severe portal hypertension: a randomized trial. Ann Surg. 2019;269(6):1025–33.
185. Xu X, Man K, Zheng SS, Liang TB, Lee TK, Ng KT, et al. Attenuation of acute phase shear stress by somatostatin improves small-for-size liver graft survival. Liver Transpl. 2006;12(4):621–7.
186. Langnas AN, Marujo W, Stratta RJ, Wood RP, Shaw BW. Vascular complications after orthotopic liver transplantation. Am J Surg. 1991;161(1):76–82; discussion 82–3.
187. Settmacher U, Stange B, Haase R, Heise M, Steinmüller T, Bechstein WO, et al. Arterial complications after liver transplantation. Transpl Int. 2000;13(5):372–8.
188. Uzochukwu LN, Bluth EI, Smetherman DH, Troxclair LA, Loss GE, Cohen A, et al. Early postoperative hepatic sonography as a predictor of vascular and biliary complications in adult orthotopic liver transplant patients. AJR Am J Roentgenol. 2005;185(6):1558–70.
189. Jain A, Costa G, Marsh W, Fontes P, Devera M, Mazariegos G, et al. Thrombotic and nonthrombotic hepatic artery complications in adults and children following primary liver transplantation with long-term follow-up in 1000 consecutive patients. Transpl Int. 2006;19(1):27–37.
190. Silva MA, Jambulingam PS, Gunson BK, Mayer D, Buckels JAC, Mirza DF, et al. Hepatic artery thrombosis following orthotopic liver transplantation: a 10-year experience from a single centre in the United Kingdom. Liver Transpl. 2006;12(1):146–51.
191. Wojcicki M, Post M, Pakosz-Golanowska M, Zeair S, Lubikowski J, Jarosz K, et al. Vascular complications following adult piggyback liver transplantation with end-to-side cavo-cavostomy: a single-center experience. Transplant Proc. 2009;41(8):3131–4.
192. Pareja E, Cortes M, Navarro R, Sanjuan F, López R, Mir J. Vascular complications after orthotopic liver transplantation: hepatic artery thrombosis. Transplant Proc. 2010;42(8):2970–2.
193. Pérez-Saborido B, Pacheco-Sánchez D, Barrera-Rebollo A, Asensio-Díaz E, Pinto-Fuentes P, Sarmentero-Prieto JC, et al. Incidence, management, and results of vascular complications after liver transplantation. Transplant Proc. 2011;43(3):749–50.
194. Neuhaus P, Blumhardt G, Bechstein WO, Steffen R, Platz KP, Keck H. Technique and results of biliary reconstruction using side-to-side choledochocholedochostomy in 300 orthotopic liver transplants. Ann Surg. 1994;219(4):426–34.
195. Hernandez Q, Ramirez P, Munitiz V, Piñero A, Robles R, Sanchez-Bueno F, et al. Incidence and management of biliary tract complications following 300 consecutive orthotopic liver transplants. Transplant Proc. 1999;31(6):2407–8.
196. Scatton O, Meunier B, Cherqui D, Boillot O, Sauvanet A, Boudjema K, et al. Randomized trial of choledochocholedochostomy with or without a T tube in orthotopic liver transplantation. Ann Surg. 2001;233(3):432–7.
197. Thethy S, Thomson BN, Pleass H, Wigmore SJ, Madhavan K, Akyol M, et al. Management of biliary tract complications after orthotopic liver transplantation. Clin Transpl. 2004;18(6):647–53.
198. Abdullah K, Abdeldayem H, Hali WO, Hemsi B, Sarrag I, Abdulkareem A. Incidence and management of biliary complications after orthotopic liver transplantation: ten years' experience at King Fahad National Guard Hospital. Transplant Proc. 2005;37(7):3179–81.
199. Wójcicki M, Lubikowski J, Zeair S, Gasińska M, Butkiewicz J, Czupryńska M, et al. Biliary complications following adult liver transplantation with routine use of external biliary drainage. Ann Transplant. 2005;10(3):21–5.
200. Li T, Chen Z-S, Zeng F-J, Ming C-S, Zhang W-J, Liu D-G, et al. Impact of early biliary complications in liver transplantation in the presence or absence of a T-tube: a Chinese transplant centre experience. Postgrad Med J. 2007;83(976):120–3.
201. Perrakis A, Förtsch T, Schellerer V, Hohenberger W, Müller V. Biliary tract complications after orthotopic liver transplantation: still the "Achilles heel"? Transplant Proc. 2010;42(10):4154–7.
202. Król R, Karkoszka H, Ziaja J, Pawlicki J, Stańczyk A, Badura J, et al. Biliary complications after orthotopic liver transplantation: a 5-year experience. Transplant Proc. 2011;43(8):3035–8.

203. Gámán G, Gelley F, Doros A, Zádori G, Görög D, Fehérvári I, et al. Biliary complications after orthotopic liver transplantation: the Hungarian experience. Transplant Proc. 2013;45(10):3695–7.
204. Gastaca M, Matarranz A, Martinez L, Valdivieso A, Ruiz P, Ventoso A, et al. Risk factors for biliary complications after orthotopic liver transplantation with T-tube: a single-center cohort of 743 transplants. Transplant Proc. 2014;46(9):3097–9.
205. Nemes B, Gámán G, Doros A. Biliary complications after liver transplantation. Expert Rev Gastroenterol Hepatol. 2015;9(4):447–66.
206. Coelho JCU, Leite LO, Molena A, De Freitas ACT, Matias JEF. Biliary complications after liver transplantation. Arq Bras Cir Dig. 2017;30(2):127–31.
207. Song S, Lu T, Yang W, Gong S, Lei C, Yang J, et al. T-tube or no T-tube for biliary tract reconstruction in orthotopic liver transplantation: an updated systematic review and meta-analysis. Expert Rev Gastroenterol Hepatol. 2021;27:1507–23.
208. Pfau PR, Kochman ML, Lewis JD, Long WB, Lucey MR, Olthoff K, et al. Endoscopic management of postoperative biliary complications in orthotopic liver transplantation. Gastrointest Endosc. 2000;52(1):55–63.
209. Gunawansa N, McCall JL, Holden A, Plank L, Munn SR. Biliary complications following orthotopic liver transplantation: a 10-year audit. HPB (Oxford). 2011;13(6):391–9.
210. Györi GP, Schwarzer R, Püspök A, Schöfl R, Silberhumer GR, Langer FB, et al. Endoscopic versus surgical management of biliary complications - outcome analysis after 1188 orthotopic liver transplantations. Dig Liver Dis. 2016;48(11):1323–9.

## Further Reading

Adam R, Karam V, Delvart V, O'Grady J, Mirza D, Klempnauer J, et al. Evolution of indications and results of liver transplantation in Europe. A report from the European Liver Transplant Registry (ELTR). J Hepatol. 2012;57(3):675–88.

Bekker J, Ploem S, de Jong KP. Early hepatic artery thrombosis after liver transplantation: a systematic review of the incidence, outcome and risk factors. Am J Transplant. 2009;9(4):746–57.

Dahm F, Georgiev P, Clavien P-A. Small-for-size syndrome after partial liver transplantation: definition, mechanisms of disease and clinical implications. Am J Transplant. 2005;5(11):2605–10.

Duffy JP, Hong JC, Farmer DG, Ghobrial RM, Yersiz H, Hiatt JR, et al. Vascular complications of orthotopic liver transplantation: experience in more than 4,200 patients. J Am Coll Surg. 2009;208(5):896–903; discussion 903–5.

Sainz-Barriga M, Scudeller L, Costa MG, de Hemptinne B, Troisi RI. Lack of a correlation between portal vein flow and pressure: toward a shared interpretation of hemodynamic stress governing inflow modulation in liver transplantation. Liver Transpl. 2011;17(7):836–48.

# Part V

# Extremities

# Emergency Vascular Access to Extremities

## 107

Frank Plani

**Learning Goals**
- Learn how to manage bleeding vascular injuries in emergency settings
- Learn the right incision for each injury
- Learn how to perform emergency vascular control

## 107.1 Introduction

### 107.1.1 Early Lessons

Physicians have dealt with bleeding vessels since antiquity, at least since the ancient Greeks and Romans [1].

They knew that partially transected vessels continue to bleed more than totally transected ones, the beneficial effects of digital compression, and the difference between arterial and venous bleeding.

Tourniquets have been used since Alexander the Great, although modern forms only appeared in the late seventeenth and eighteenth centuries [2, 3].

The principles of vascular exposure appeared much later, at the end of the nineteenth century, after the description of wound management, exposure, vascular control, perfect repair, and the need for asepsis and haemostasis on completion [1].

Ligation rather than repair remained the mainstay of vascular injury management for most of the first half of the twentieth century, and it was only in 1959, after the lessons learned in the Korean War, that over 80% of arterial injuries were repaired [4–7].

In the Vietnam War, the emphasis was on combined orthopaedic and vascular injuries, massive soft tissue injuries, and the need for relooks [1].

It is clear from the above lessons that most advances in vascular surgery have occurred in times of war, while at present one can best learn from rotating through large urban units with extensive penetrating trauma exposure and simulation courses [8].

### 107.1.2 Factors in Vascular Exposure

A number of factors affect decision-making in emergency vascular exposure and may require alternative approaches and compromises on sterility and the time and place of surgery.

F. Plani (✉)
Department of Surgery, Trauma Directorate, Chris Hani Baragwanath Academic Hospital and NetCare Alberton Hospital Level 1 Trauma Centre, University of the Witwatersrand, Johannesburg, South Africa

Trauma Division, Department of Surgery, University of the Witwatersrand, Johannesburg, South Africa

© The Author(s), under exclusive license to Springer Nature Switzerland AG 2023
F. Coccolini, F. Catena (eds.), *Textbook of Emergency General Surgery*,
https://doi.org/10.1007/978-3-031-22599-4_107

Obvious examples are the following:

1. The need for direct compression on exsanguinating vessels, by an unsterile assistant.
2. The need for exposure around Foley catheters inserted into penetrating wounds, where one does not want to puncture the balloons [9, 10].
3. High-placed tourniquets over the planned incision line, including junctional tourniquets, which would interfere with the exposure of iliac vessels or supra- and infraclavicular incisions [11, 12].
4. The need to enter one or two extra cavities, with the consequent blood and heat loss from the inability to control proximal extremity bleeding.
5. The need for adaptation of exposure and coordination in staged vascular and orthopaedic repairs [13].
6. Considerations for placement and closure of incisions in patients requiring vacuum-assisted closure and relooks in vascular damage control.

Early prehospital applications of tourniquets, in particular, have consistently shown to have significant survival advantage when compared to applications of the tourniquet in the emergency department (ED) after the patient had developed shock (90% vs. 10%) [3].

Indeed, many more emergency operations for bleeding or ischemia have been taking place as surgeons became familiar with damage control principles and injuries are managed in a staged fashion with temporary vascular shunts and vacuum dressings [2].

### 107.1.3 Preoperative Preparation and Adequate Exposure

Exposure of extremity vascular injuries must consider all eventualities in terms of proximal and distal control, assessment of the results of the surgery, and the need for harvesting of vascular conduits.

In practical terms, this will entail scrubbing and draping the chest, homolateral neck, entire upper limb for potential sternotomy or anterolateral thoracotomy in suspected injuries to the subclavian arteries and other upper limb junctional structures, chest and abdomen for iliac/lower limb junctional injuries, neck and upper limb for suspected axillary, brachial, and bifurcation injuries, lower abdomen and entire lower limb for femoral and lower injuries, and both groins for possible saphenous vein grafts in all cases [14].

Heat and blood loss need to be prevented and managed in extensive proximal control incisions.

Feet and/or hands should be kept visible within plastic bags in all cases to assess for return of circulation and peripheral perfusion.

### 107.1.4 Penetrating Trauma and Open Wounds

Penetrating trauma, degloving injuries, and mangled limb situations may generate large, contaminated wounds where exposure for vascular control would normally be affected.

In these cases, the recommendation would be for two changes to standard practice to be considered:

1. To scrub and debride tissues extensively after the vascular emergency has been dealt with.
2. To avoid opening vessels for embolectomies and instrumentation in areas where there will be doubtful tissue cover after debridement and to rather choose other segments, usually more proximal, for such procedures, such as approaching the external iliac artery extraperitoneally for control and instrumentation rather than a common femoral artery where all the soft tissues in the groin have been degloved [15].

## 107.2 Upper Extremity Injuries

### 107.2.1 General Considerations

Upper extremity trauma constitutes about 30–40% of acute vascular injuries in recent conflicts.

Very proximal injuries to the upper extremities and junctional injuries are often life-threatening emergencies and are not very commonly encountered outside of military situations or with very high levels of penetrating interpersonal violence [2, 16].

Brachial and distal injuries are much more common, and although by and large easily compressible and fully controlled by tourniquet use, the fact that the patient can still walk around and has clearly lost function of one arm makes self-help more difficult to achieve, and they can also lead to exsanguination if not controlled early. Since the brachial artery and the distal vessels are very superficial and the upper limb is thinner than the lower limb, even seemingly safe posterolateral injuries can reach the brachial artery [17].

When it comes to blunt trauma, subclavian artery injuries are sometimes associated with clavicular fractures, while brachial arteries are sometimes injured in very distal humeral fractures and elbow dislocations.

All arteries from the third portion of the subclavian artery downwards can be approached with an infraclavicular incision, followed by a medial arm incision, and a lazy S that crosses the antecubital fossa from medial to lateral and ends medial to the thenar eminence [18].

## 107.2.2 Anatomy

### 107.2.2.1 Great Vessels and Junctional Area

The anatomical structures that might be affected by injuries to the proximal portions of vessels supplying the upper extremity include the aerodigestive tract, the chest wall, and the respiratory system (Fig. 107.1).

It is in fact common to be in doubt on whether a massive haemothorax is caused by injuries to the subclavian and axillary vessels, the heart, the lungs, or the intercostal arteries [18].

Irrespective of the origin of the bleeding, these patients will usually be intubated, have intercostal drains inserted, and have Foley catheters inserted into bleeding wounds of the neck and proximal upper limbs [19, 20].

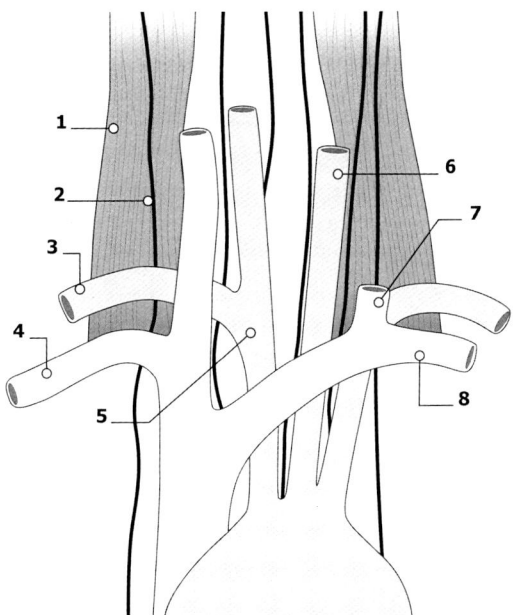

**Fig. 107.1** Structures encountered in exposure of the thoracic inlet vessels: 1: anterior scalene muscle; 2: phrenic nerve; 3: right subclavian artery; 4: right subclavian vein; 5: brachiocephalic trunk; 6: left common carotid artery; 7: left internal jugular vein; 8: left subclavian vein. (Illustration by M. Torres/Fiverr)

### 107.2.2.2 Subclavian Arteries

**Origin**

The right subclavian artery emanates from the brachio-cephalic trunk (innominate artery) behind the costo-clavicular joint and will divide into subclavian and common carotid arteries after about 3–5 cm.

The right vagus nerve crosses in front of the first part of the subclavian artery and then dips into the mediastinum behind the right innominate vein.

The right recurrent laryngeal nerve comes off the right vagus nerve, loops around the inferior border of the subclavian artery, and ascends medially in the neck between the trachea and the oesophagus.

The left subclavian artery originates as the last branch of the aortic arch, a couple of centimetres beyond the left carotid artery, and travels upwards into the neck, although the extent of the subclavian arteries above the level of the clavicle varies. Initially it is found very posteriorly, against the posterior rib cage and the fourth thoracic vertebra, but it may be more anterior and easy to mistake for the left carotid artery [21].

It is usually difficult to isolate it from a median sternotomy, although not impossible, after looping and retracting the brachiocephalic trunk and the left common carotid to the right. Both subclavian arteries become the axillary arteries at the outer border of the first rib.

In a congenital anomaly, the so-called 'bovine arch', found in up to 10% of patients, both the carotid arteries and the right subclavian artery originate from the innominate artery.

**Portions and Branches**

The anterior scalene, which is found anterior to the subclavian arteries, divides the subclavian arteries into three portions (Fig. 107.2).

First part: Branches: vertebral artery and internal mammary artery opposite each other, one going up and the other down, followed by the thyrocervical trunk (cervico-dorsal trunk).

It is crossed by the phrenic (uniquely, from lateral to medial) and vagus nerves. On the left, it is also crossed by the thoracic duct, which drains into the origin of the left innominate vein.

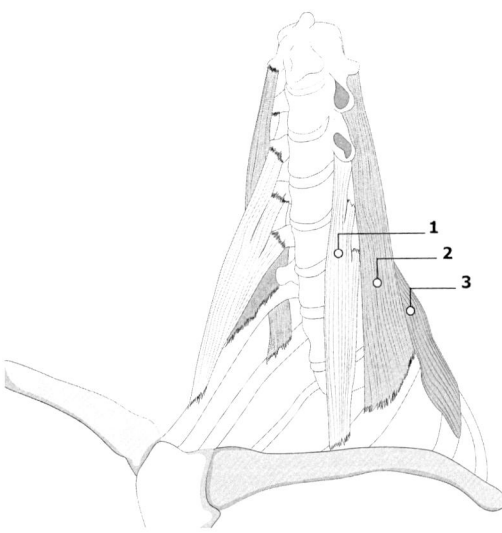

**Fig. 107.2** The scalene muscles. 1: Anterior scalene; 2: middle scalene; 3: posterior scalene. (Illustration by M. Torres/Fiverr)

Second part: Behind the scalenus anterior; only gives off one branch, the costo-cervical trunk, and sometimes the dorsal scapular artery; this last branch sometimes comes off the third part of the artery instead.

The third part is surrounded by the trunks and then the cords of the brachial plexus.

The first part extends from its origin to the medial border of the scalenus anterior muscle, the second part lies behind this muscle, and the third part extends from its lateral border to the outer aspect of the first rib where it becomes the axillary artery [22].

### 107.2.2.3 Subclavian Veins

The subclavian vein is a very feared vessel, because of its thick wall and tight adherence to the underside of the clavicle. It can however be compressed with direct pressure above and below the clavicle. It is superficial to the scalenus anterior but is otherwise mostly just above the subclavian arteries.

**Origin**

The subclavian veins are the continuation of the axillary veins beyond the lateral border of the first rib, and as the name implies, they are found under the clavicles. They join the internal jugular veins on the medial side of the anterior scalene muscles to form the innominate or brachiocephalic veins, lying in front of the anterior scalene muscles. The two innominate veins then join at the level of the inferior aspect of the costal cartilage of the first rib to form the superior vena cava.

While their more superficial position places them at a higher risk of injury than the subclavian arteries, they can be more easily exposed just by detaching the sternal and clavicular heads of the sternocleidomastoid muscles.

### 107.2.2.4 Axillary Arteries

**Origin**

The subclavian arteries become the axillary arteries at the lateral border of the first rib and then become brachial arteries at the lateral border of the teres major muscle.

## Portions and Branches

Axillary arteries are divided into three parts by the pectoralis minor muscle, medial, behind, and lateral.

*Branches*: *First part*: superior thoracic artery.
*Second part*: thoracoacromial and lateral thoracic artery.
*Third part*: subscapular and the anterior and posterior humeral circumflex (Fig. 107.3).

The cords of the brachial plexus are posterior at first, then surround the artery, and then become the named nerves at the level of the distal axillary artery and proximal brachial artery [23].

### 107.2.2.5 Brachial Arteries

#### Origin

The axillary artery becomes the brachial arteries at the inferior border of the teres major muscle until its bifurcation in the terminal branches of the radial and ulnar arteries just beyond the antecubital fossa.

The brachial artery has a mainly subcutaneous course.

Of note, the ulnar artery supplies mainly the anterior, or flexor compartment, of the forearm while the radial artery supplies mainly the posterior, or extensor compartment.

It is found medial to the humerus between the biceps and the triceps muscles and surrounded by the median nerve medially and the ulnar and radial nerves more laterally.

#### Branches

Profunda brachii artery, arising postero-medially, the superior ulnar collateral artery, and the inferior ulnar collateral artery. The profunda brachii artery is particularly important it supplies collateral circulation between the axillary artery and the forearm.

### 107.2.2.6 Radial and Ulnar Arteries

#### Origin

After the brachial artery crosses the antecubital fossa, it bifurcates into the radial and ulnar arteries. The radial artery is the more superficial and therefore more readily felt, but the ulnar artery is thicker.

#### Branches

Branches of ulnar artery: Anterior and posterior ulnar recurrent arteries, and the common interosseous artery, followed by the terminal branch, the superficial palmar artery. Branch of the radial artery: Radial recurrent artery.

## 107.2.3 Exposure

### 107.2.3.1 Great Vessels, Junctional Area, and Proximal Subclavian Arteries

#### Incisions

Median Sternotomy
The median sternotomy is the incision of choice when having to obtain proximal control of the junctional area vessels and subclavian vessels.

It allows for exposure of the aortic arch and all its branches, the innominate veins and the proximal subclavian arteries, and the common carotids, access to both hemithoraces and internal cardiac massage. At a push, it allows for aortic cross clamping, although it is not comfortable and often requires pushing the heart to the right when you least want to do that [23].

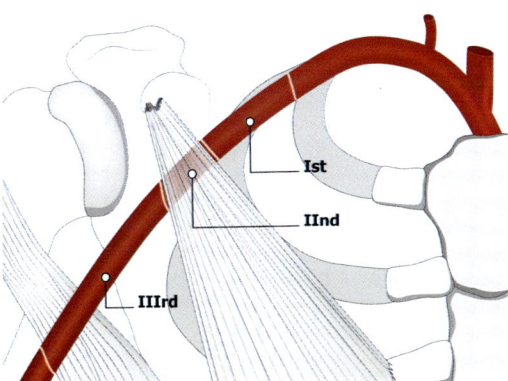

**Fig. 107.3** Parts of the axillary artery in relation to the pectoralis minor muscle and the origin of the brachial artery beyond the teres major muscle. (Illustration by M. Torres/Fiverr)

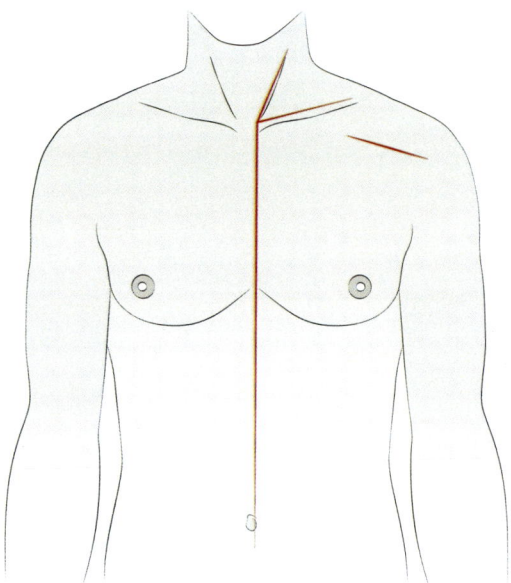

**Fig. 107.4** Midline sternotomy with extension into a neck exploration, supraclavicular exploration, and infraclavicular exposure. (Illustration by M. Torres/Fiverr)

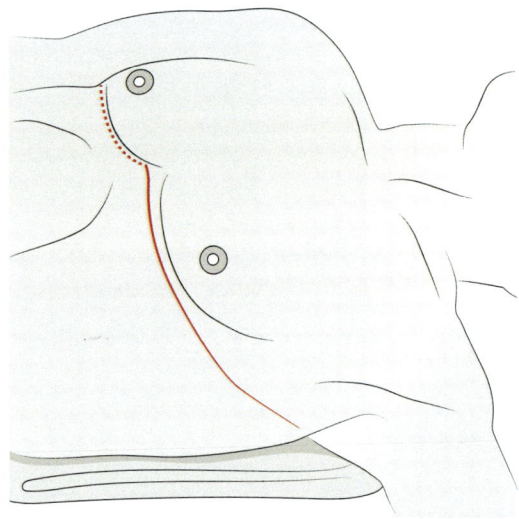

**Fig. 107.5** Left anterolateral thoracotomy and extension across the sternum into a partial clamshell incision. (Illustration by M. Torres/Fiverr)

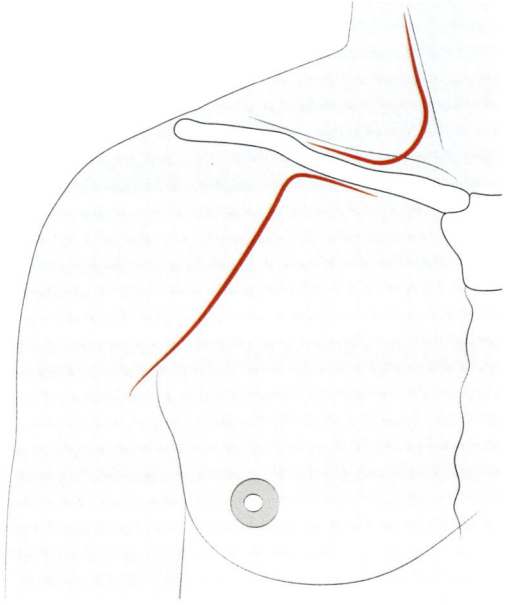

**Fig. 107.6** Supraclavicular exposure extended into a right-sided neck exploration and a separate infraclavicular incision. (Illustration by M. Torres/Fiverr)

It can be extended into the neck for access to the neck vessels and as a supraclavicular extension for the proximal right subclavian artery and mid-portion subclavian vessels on both sides (Fig. 107.4).

### Anterolateral Thoracotomy

If the patient is peri-arrest or has been arrested, however, an anterolateral thoracotomy in the fourth or fifth intercostal space can be done in seconds using a blade and a pair of scissors, can be extended to a clamshell equally fast, and allows for easier aortic cross clamping and equally easy internal cardiac massage. One can only cross clamp the proximal left subclavian artery from this incision, and therefore a median sternotomy may need to be added for proximal control of the other junctional arteries (Fig. 107.5).

### Supraclavicular Incision

The skin and the platysma are incised in the same direction, just above the proximal clavicle.

As soon as the clavicular head of the SCM is identified, it is divided, and the same would apply to the sternal head as well, if injuries to the subclavian and internal jugular veins are suspected: superior retraction of both heads of the SCM muscle will expose the venous bifurcation (Fig. 107.6).

Then take the fat off the next muscle, the scalenus anterior, and retract it and dissect it superiorly and laterally, and it will expose the scalenus anterior, with the vagus and the phrenic nerve coursing across it. It must be noted that the phrenic nerve crosses from lateral to medial, unlike all other cranial nerves.

There are two ways of mobilizing the scalenus anterior: piecemeal and by sharp dissection, the latter only possible after the phrenic nerve has been identified and retracted out of the way.

In order to identify the subclavian artery at this point, it is wise to expose the more superficial internal jugular vein, and the subclavian artery will be found between its lateral border and the clavicle, under which it then dips [21].

If one needs more proximal exposure, one can divide the strap muscles, and identify the first part of the subclavian arteries.

This incision has been described as part of a trapdoor incision, with a partial sternotomy and third intercostal incision, but is rarely needed for proximal left subclavian exposure.

### Infraclavicular Incision

If a proximal subclavian artery can be excluded preoperatively, exposure will start with a supraclavicular incision from the sterno-clavicular joint laterally, ideally after placing a sandbag or a vacolitre longitudinally between the patient's shoulders to facilitate this exposure. This will be adequate for proximal control of the retroclavicular and more distal subclavian arteries even with a large peri-clavicular haematoma.

It would then continue with division of the pectoral and subclavius muscles from the clavicle, and possible dislocation of the sternoclavicular joint, division of the clavicle in its midpoint, taking care not to injure the tightly adherent subclavian vein, or even a subperiosteal claviculectomy.

This step may be omitted if proximal control could be obtained by remotely inserted balloon vascular control (Fig. 107.7).

Having obtained proximal control, the subclavian artery can be approached with a subclavicular incision in the delto-pectoral groove, about 2 cm below the clavicle, an incision that could then be extended in a highly protocolized fashion all the way to the carpal tunnel and beyond.

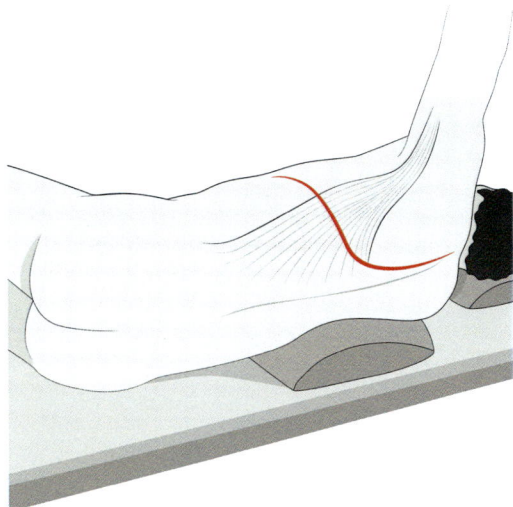

**Fig. 107.7** Left posterolateral thoracotomy. (Illustration by M. Torres/Fiverr)

### 107.2.3.2 Subclavian Veins

These are the classic patients with major venous bleeding, often controlled with a Foley catheter or manual compression all the way to the operating room. With ongoing bleeding, the exposure of choice is a median sternotomy with a neck or supraclavicular incision. In the latter case, subclavicular compression will also reduce the backflow [18].

### Incisions and Control

After making the median sternotomy incision and after the division or excision of the thymus and exposure of the arch, one will start compressing and tensing the innominate veins and follow the vein from there. Immediately after, one will expose the presumably not injures internal jugular vein and follow it to its origin and junction with the subclavian vein. The origin of the subclavian vein will then be apparent, and, in a very proximal injury, complete division of both heads of the sternocleidomastoid muscle from the sternum and from the clavicle will expose the anterior surface of the junction and allow for repair. If the injury is more distal, the innominate and internal jugular veins should be looped and controlled while achieving distal control by direct pressure, and the course of the vein can be followed from medial to lateral and gently eased from the underside of the clavicle.

### 107.2.3.3 Axillary Artery and Proximal Brachial Artery

#### Incisions

The axillary arteries run under both pectoralis muscles. Pectoralis major can be divided, split along its fibres, or if greater exposure is needed, its tendon can be divided close to its humeral origin.

The pectoralis minor can then be divided close to its insertion on the acromion process to expose the second part of the axillary artery. The body habitus of patients will determine the extent of the incisions, both in morbidly obese patients and even more so in very muscled patients [18].

The third part continues laterally, becoming the brachial artery as it crosses the lower edge of the teres major muscle. The axillary and brachial arteries can then be exposed quite superficially, between the biceps, which are then retracted superiorly, and the triceps, which are then retracted inferiorly. The anatomical landmarks are quite easy to follow since the bellies of the triceps and biceps are easily palpated and kept apart to expose the neurovascular bundle.

For injuries below the clavicle, the point of proximal control is the distal subclavian or proximal axillary artery immediately below the edge of the clavicle. The proximal third of the axillary artery is above and behind the vein and in front of the cords of the brachial plexus.

### 107.2.3.4 Distal Brachial Artery and Bifurcation

#### Incisions

The distal brachial artery can be exposed medially above the ante-cubital fossa, taking the median nerve as the landmark anywhere along the arm. In the pulseless limb, the median nerve can be easily confused for the artery if one is not aware of their surgical anatomy. Another point of confusion may be that the artery in young people can become almost cordlike, especially after a tourniquet or handling tissues, and the best option is to follow it up to an unexposed area, where its structure becomes obvious.

Distal control can usually be obtained at the distal end of the wound, but in very proximal injuries and exceptionally large upper limbs, a distally placed tourniquet can allow for easier distal control.

This is particularly useful in very angled and comminuted open fractures, where initial manual compression and subsequent vessel retrieval at surgery can be difficult [22].

The exposure of the brachial artery is straightforward, by feeling the pulsation against the humerus, with the artery being medial, while the median nerve stays more superior and lateral.

The artery then becomes more anterior and travels in front of the biceps tendon just above the elbow, but then dips below the bicipital aponeurosis [24].

This must then be divided to identify and have access to the bifurcation, which is very unpredictable in location. The universal recommendation of being on the artery and following it down, cutting upwards from the artery, will allow one to incise the biceps aponeurosis and discover the bifurcation from within.

### 107.2.3.5 Radial and Ulnar Arteries

#### Incisions

Proximal control will be easily obtained with a pneumatic tourniquet, or, once in the operating theatre, by exposing and controlling the brachial artery above the elbow.

The incision for exposure of the terminal arteries of the upper limb is generally the same as for a fasciotomy, which is in fact very frequently required after radial and ulnar injuries.

It is a lazy S incision, ending past the carpal tunnel and going around the thenar eminence at the base of the thumb (Fig. 107.8).

To have direct access to the radial artery, one can follow the medial border, or brachioradialis, and the artery will be between it and the radius. At the wrist, one would make a longitudinal incision just lateral to the pulse.

The ulnar artery is a lot deeper, under pronator teres and staying within the muscles of the flexor compartment, only becoming palpable close to the wrist.

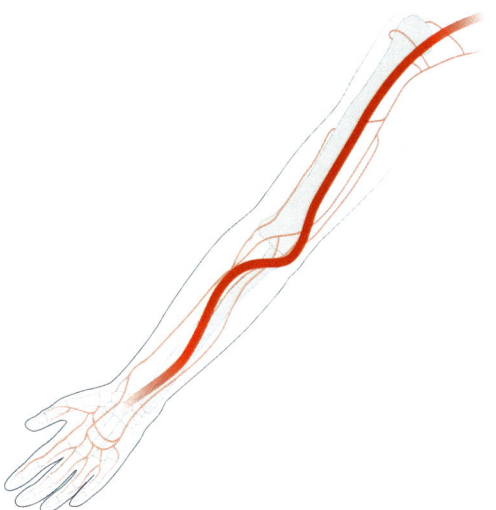

**Fig. 107.8** Full vascular exposure of the upper limb with one incision over axillary artery, brachial artery, over the ante-cubital fossa to the lateral side and lazy S to the palm of the hand. (Illustration by M. Torres/Fiverr)

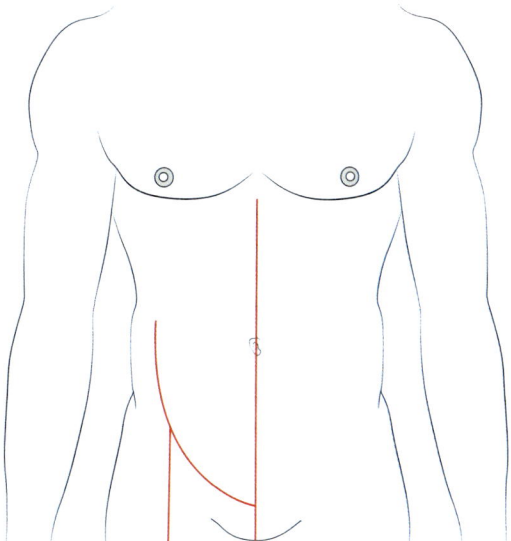

**Fig. 107.9** Incisions for proximal control of lower extremity vascular injuries: midline laparotomy, Rutherford-Morrison incision for extraperitoneal iliac artery access and vertical groin incision starting above the groin crease. (Illustration by M. Torres/Fiverr)

It can be exposed directly by making a medial incision and separating the flexor muscles and retracting them superolaterally, directly between the flexor carpi ulnaris and the flexor digitorum superficialis. But it is a lot safer to make a fasciotomy incision and access it under vision from its origin.

At the wrist, one can expose it with a longitudinal incision, staying medial to the artery to avoid the ulnar nerve, which runs more laterally [23].

## 107.3 Lower Extremities

### 107.3.1 General Considerations

#### 107.3.1.1 The Junctional Area and Iliac Vessels

A presentation on the exposure of extremity vascular injuries of the lower extremities must start with the profoundly serious abdominal junctional area, comprising the lower abdomen and the groins, which could affect the iliac vessels and their branches, as well as the common and proximal superficial and profunda femoral vessels [25].

This is the area most talked about in the context of improvised explosive devices in military settings, rockfalls in the mining, and heavy construction and industrial sectors, and pelvic fractures from bicycle and motorcycle crashes in traffic settings.

It is the area for which junctional tourniquets and resuscitative endovascular balloon occlusion of the aorta (REBOAs) were developed to be used in prehospital and emergency department situations [26, 27] (Fig. 107.9).

In terms of surgical management, it is the area which often requires aortic cross clamping, above the bifurcation and sometimes in the chest, and, in less dramatic circumstances, leads to indecision on whether to do a full laparotomy, a low midline laparotomy, a Rutherford-Morrison (hockey stick) incision with extraperitoneal control, or, in the case of an inadequate groin incision, on whether to split the inguinal ligament and obtain control of the external iliac vessels in that fashion [25].

#### 107.3.1.2 Femoral and Popliteal Vessels

Vascular injuries below the groin cause compressible bleeding, although often with difficulty, especially in obese and very muscled patients and in the presence of fractures, resulting in the success of tourniquets in only about ¾ of patients. That is why proximal vascular control is essential before exposing the wounds [27].

Injuries to the femoral and popliteal regions are more common than iliac vessel injuries in civilian practice and comprise about 25% of all extremity vascular injuries. They are the injuries that prompted the reintroduction of the tourniquet by many medical military services and emergency medical services and led to the Stop the Bleed® campaign by the American College of Surgeons Committee on Trauma (ACS COT). The devastating effect of uncontrolled extremity bleeding, mainly in the lower limbs, is illustrated by the fact that in a study among the US Armed Forces, considering those who died of combat wounds from 2001 to 2009, nearly 41% had potentially survivable injuries if haemorrhage had been controlled in a more prompt and effective manner [28, 29].

Pneumatic tourniquets have been used for orthopaedic and reconstructive surgery for a long time and need no introduction. They should replace the prehospital windlass tourniquets the patient is coming into the hospital with as soon as possible, for ease of use and to minimize local trauma on the segments where they are applied [2].

Popliteal injuries are exceedingly difficult to access, and are often diagnosed late, especially in blunt trauma following falls and knee dislocations, and this leads to frequent amputations. Furthermore, the most direct approach, the posterior approach with a prone patient, is unsuitable in most acute trauma situations.

Therefore, popliteal vessels are challenging to approach and treat. It is the least accessible vessel in the lower extremity, and the collateral flow around the knee is not sufficient to sustain viability of the lower leg if flow of the popliteal artery is interrupted [30].

#### 107.3.1.3 Tibio-Peroneal Vessels

The tibial arteries appear to be the most injured extremity vessels, up to 36% of the total, due to penetrating trauma from gunshots in 37% of cases and traffic-related accidents in 26% of cases [31].

**Anatomy**

Iliac Arteries

Origin

The common iliac artery originates near the fourth lumbar vertebra at the aortic bifurcation.

It then enters the pelvis, where it ends at the pelvic brim, where it splits into the internal and external iliac arteries.

The external iliac arteries are protected by the walls of the pelvis and then rise to become the common femoral arteries underneath the inguinal ligaments. The bifurcation and the origins of the external and internal iliac arteries are very easily accessible in the extraperitoneal prevesical space, where they can be readily looped to control pelvic and lower extremity bleeding [28].

The external iliac artery then travels down and runs laterally along the medial border of the iliopsoas muscle and then between the symphysis pubis and the anterior superior iliac spine before going underneath the inguinal ligament to enter the thigh as the common femoral artery.

Branches

Just before the inguinal ligament, it gives off two major branches: the inferior epigastric artery and the deep circumflex iliac artery, both of which have an important role in perfusing the inferior abdominal wall.

The deep circumflex iliac artery forms an important anastomosis with the ascending branch of the lateral circumflex femoral artery.

The internal iliac artery is about 3 cm long and disappears medially into the pelvic cavity, where it splits into anterior and posterior divisions [25].

The anterior division has several visceral branches for the bladder, rectum, and reproductive organs, the obturator artery, and the internal pudendal artery, while the posterior division has a number of branches supplying the pelvic walls and buttocks.

## Common, Superficial, and Deep Femoral Artery

### Origin

The common femoral artery lies in the femoral triangle, medial to the femoral nerve and lateral to the femoral vein for just about 3 or 4 cm from the inguinal ligament (Poupart's ligament) to its bifurcation into the profunda femoral artery which sets off postero-laterally into the muscles of the thigh and the superficial femoral artery which continues anteromedially in the sub-sartorial (Hunter's) canal and becomes the popliteal artery.

The walls of this canal are as follows: Sartorius muscle anteriorly, vastus medialis laterally, adductor longus, and magnus posteromedially. It becomes the popliteal artery as it passes through the adductor magnus into the popliteal canal.

The femoral vein changes from being medial to posterior in relation to the artery at the distal femoral and popliteal artery levels and then becomes more lateral just above the knee. One of its branches, the lateral circumflex femoral vein, crosses the origin of the artery and should be ligated and divided before exploring the profunda femoris artery.

The greater saphenous vein is the most medial vascular structure, which then drains into the common femoral vein near the femoral triangle.

## Popliteal Artery

### Origin

The popliteal vessels and the two terminal branches of the sciatic nerve, the tibial and common peroneal nerves, are found in the popliteal fossa, a subcutaneous structure bound by the following muscles: the semimembranosus and semitendinosus, the biceps femoris superiorly, and the two heads of the gastrocnemius inferiorly. Its floor consists of the knee joint capsule, the distal femur between the two condyles, the proximal tibia, and the popliteus muscle. The popliteal artery and the popliteal vein travel in remarkably close proximity, and very often they are both injured [32].

### Branches

The popliteal artery gives off important genicular branches above and below the knee, which play an important role in providing alternative blood supply to the surrounding tissues. The popliteal artery should nevertheless be considered an end artery since this collateral circulation is inadequate in acute settings.

It then bifurcates and becomes the tibio-peroneal trunk after giving off the anterior tibial artery a few centimetres below the knee, roughly at the level of the tibial plateau and where the soleus muscles attach to the tibia.

The tibio-peroneal trunk itself bifurcates after 2 or 3 cm into the lateral peroneal and the posterior tibial artery, which continues all the way under the soleus and gastrocnemius behind the medial malleolus to the foot in a postero-medial fashion [31].

The anterior tibial artery travels close to the front of the interosseous membrane, pierces the upper part of the interosseous membrane within the anterior compartment of the leg, and becomes the dorsalis pedis artery in the foot.

In about 5% of cases, the popliteal artery ends in a trifurcation of the anterior tibial, posterior tibial, and lateral peroneal arteries.

## Exposure

### General Considerations

#### Groin Incisions

A groin incision is the baseline incision for the exposure of lower extremity injuries in trauma, except for extremely peripheral vessels, and it will often be extended up or down if more proximal or distal vessels are injured. It is important to remember that the groin crease does not correspond in position to the inguinal ligament, being about 3 cm lower than the inguinal ligament.

Even injuries to suspected or confirmed popliteal arteries might have to start with a groin exposure to be able to have proximal control of the profunda femoris as well as the superficial femoral arteries. With suspected iliac injuries, the type of proximal incision or extension may be debatable, but the femoral vessels will have to be secured at the groin.

As mentioned in the introduction, torrential, incontrollable bleeding can occur even with relatively peripheral vessels such as the popliteal artery and vein, and for this reason, exposure should be from the nipple to the knees and below, if a sudden, unexpected aortic cross clamping and internal cardiac massage become necessary.

Other Incisions

The contralateral groin is often also prepared for saphenous vein harvesting or for endovascular techniques.

Preparations should be made for the position the patient will be mainly operated in, namely, supine for iliac, common, and proximal superficial femoral injuries, with slight flexion for distal femoral injuries, and flexion and medial rotation for popliteal injuries and injuries beyond the bifurcation. Very rarely in acute trauma will a posterior approach to the popliteal fossa be considered [25].

Adaptations of positions and incisions may be needed with patients with orthopaedic damage control external fixators, although stabilized limbs are always preferable and all external fixators are anterior or lateral.

### 107.3.1.4 Common Iliac Vessels

The common iliac vessels are intra-abdominal structures, best exposed after controlling the aorta above the bifurcation with a left medial visceral rotation or a direct approach to the anterior aspect of the aorta above the bifurcation. Distal control once inside the peritoneal cavity is obtained by exposing the distal common iliacs and the origin of the external and internal iliacs on the medial aspect of the pelvis after mobilization of the bladder and access to the Retzius space. This allows for easy, immediate control against the bony pelvis prior to mobilization and looping of the vessels.

Junctional tourniquets have been developed primarily for prehospital and military uses in devastating lower limb injuries, and their in-hospital use is still unproven, but they could have a place in obtaining proximal control at the distal aortic and bifurcation levels [10].

### 107.3.1.5 External Iliac Vessels

**Laparotomy for Other Reasons**

As mentioned above, external iliac vessels can be controlled from within the abdomen, if one is already doing a laparotomy for other causes, or common iliac vessel exposure is needed initially, such as for severe pelvic bleeding requiring clamping or ligating the internal iliac arteries. Access to them is either by incising the peritoneum over them or, for more distal injuries, extraperitoneally in the Retzius space.

In an unstable patient with suspected external iliac vessel injuries, the sequence will still be to do a laparotomy, expose the aorta at the bifurcation, loop both common iliac arteries, obtain control of the external and internal iliacs of the injured side, and then see if the injury can be repaired through the laparotomy incision or if a groin incision is needed for distal control and anastomosis [19].

**Primary Exposure of External Iliac Vessels**

The primary reason for exposing uninjured external iliac vessels is to effect proximal control in case of very high common femoral artery injuries, just below the inguinal ligament.

While direct pressure is applied by an assistant to the bleeding femoral vessels, a J-shaped, hockey-stick, Rutherford-Morrison, renal transplant incision is carried out [25].

The easiest is to start the incision as a muscle splitting Gridiron incision, separating the external and internal obliques, then identify the peritoneum, and turn it into a muscle cutting incision progressively sweeping the peritoneum medially until the pulsation of the iliac vessels sitting on the ileo-psoas muscle can be felt [24].

One must avoid entering the peritoneal cavity lest the field be obscured by bowel loops, and that being the case, the easiest is then to open it widely, place a swab over the bowel loops, and retract them with a broad retractor such as a Kelly or a Deaver. At risk may be also the ureter, IVC, iliac veins, sympathetic fibres, etc. In the case of iliac veins, it is always prudent to loop the iliac arteries before placing instruments away from the vein [27].

At that stage, one can control the vessels and proceed to the groin incision, or, in case of inadequate haemostasis, divide the inguinal ligament from proximal to distal, staying just on top of the vessels and cutting away from them.

The alternative to the Rutherford-Morison incision is to divide the inguinal ligament in the line of the vessels from a groin incision, which may be expedient if one has fewer assistants but may interfere with the application of direct pressure.

### 107.3.1.6 Exposure of Femoral Vessels at the Groin

**Incision**
The groin incision is used to access injuries to femoral vessels that are not actively exsanguinating and popliteal and trifurcation injuries.

In some cases, injuries to superficial femoral and distal vessels that are not actively bleeding can be addressed directly by obtaining proximal and distal control in the vicinity of the injured segment itself.

The classical groin incision starts at the midpoint of the inguinal ligament, roughly halfway between the pubic tubercle and the anterior iliac spine, and is about 10 cm long, over the course of the superficial femoral artery, with a slightly medial direction towards the medial femoral condyle.

It is important to start above the inguinal skinfold; otherwise, one may start dissecting onto the superficial femoral artery and miss the origin of the profunda initially [24].

One should try and preserve some important collateral vessels, namely, the circumflex iliac artery coming off the common femoral artery and the deep femoral vein, unless profunda femoris artery exposure is needed, in which case it should be divided and ligated.

In case the homolateral saphenous vein needs to be utilized, one should rather create a lazy S incision, so as to have good access to the femoral vessels and the saphenous vein as well.

**Further Exposure**
After incising skin, subcutaneous tissue, and fascia, the scissors opening of the common femoral sheath is affected and continues to stay in the middle of the anterior aspect of the artery to avoid transecting collaterals, until enough space has been created to safely pass a loop around the artery. The same procedure will be used in following the superficial femoral artery distally. There is usually only one small vein crossing over the anterior aspect of the common femoral artery, under the inguinal ligament, and that can be divided to avoid damaging it with proximal retraction [28].

This dissection will allow for the sequential exposure and looping of the common, superficial, and then profunda femoral arteries, the origin of which will be exposed by medial retraction on the loops above and below its origin. The very proximal profunda femoris artery can be repaired after division of the circumflex vein that drapes around its origin.

The vessel loops around the common and superficial femoral arteries are retracted upwards and medially to expose the profunda femoris artery, and a vessel loop is placed around it.

## 107.3.1.7 Exposure of the Distal Superficial Femoral Artery and Popliteal Vessels Above the Knee

### Incision
Positioning: It is crucial to have the bent knee externally rotated and supported on a sandbag or equivalent.

Incision: The incision is made over the sartorius muscle, which is then retracted posteriorly, to expose the supra-genicular popliteal artery as it comes out of the adductor canal (Fig. 107.10).

### Further Exposure
The superficial femoral artery in the adductor canal: After incising subcutaneous tissue and the adductor aponeurosis, the adductor longus is kept medial, or inferior, in the incision, while the sartorius and vastus medialis muscles are retracted

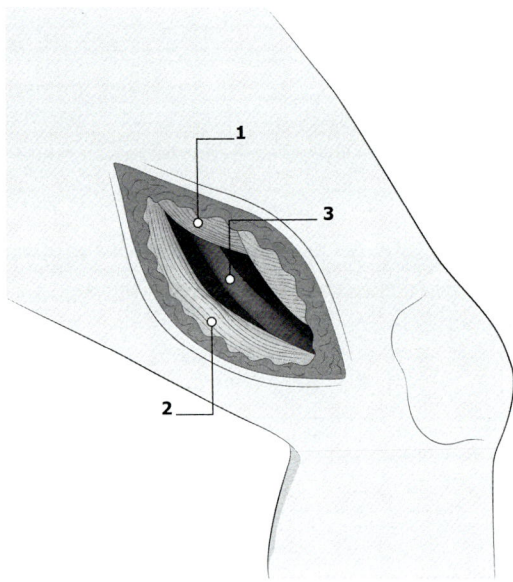

**Fig. 107.11** Supragenicular exposure of proximal popliteal artery; 1: tendon of adductor magnus; 2: sartorius muscle; 3: popliteal artery. (Illustration by M. Torres/Fiverr)

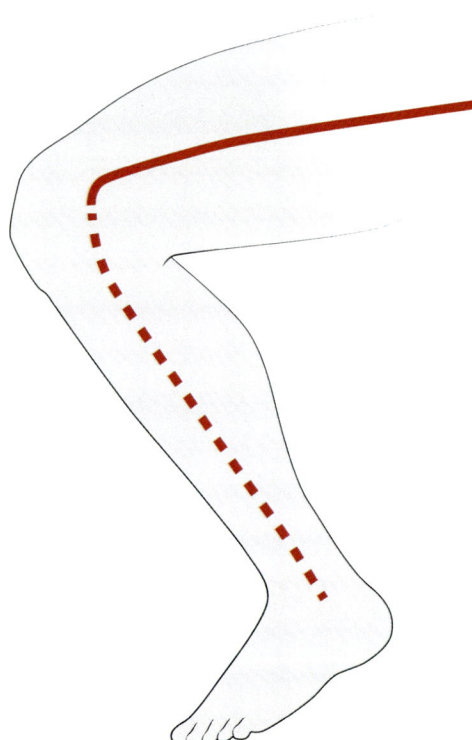

**Fig. 107.10** Supragenicular incision extended across the knee. (Illustration by M. Torres/Fiverr)

laterally, or superiorly, in the line of incision (Fig. 107.11).

Lower down, on the other hand, the popliteal artery is in a fixed position between the adductor tendon proximally and the gastrocnemius distally. It will be best exposed by retracting the sartorius posteriorly, while dividing the pes anserinus after retracting it anteriorly.

## 107.3.1.8 Exposure of the Popliteal Vessels Below the Knee

Positioning: In this case, the sandbag should be placed above the knee under the bent and externally rotated knee joint to open the space between the posterior border of the tibia and the soleus and gastrocnemius [30].

### Incision
The incision is the same as the proximal part of a medial lower leg fasciotomy, postero-medial, about 4 cm behind the tibia, and it ensures that the greater saphenous vein is kept in the anterior wound flap. Unlike in elective vascular sur-

gery, it is not uncommon that supra-genicular and infra-genicular incisions must be joined together, not only in order to expose bleeding from collaterals and veins but also when the limb is very swollen because of haematoma, a delay in surgery, or significant venous injuries, in which case a lower leg fasciotomy may not be enough. In those cases, the gracilis, semimembranosus, and semitendinosus, the adductor magnus, and the medial head of the gastrocnemius may need to be divided close to their bony insertions to allow for the swelling to be unhindered. This will need to be addressed due to morbidity and medial knee instability, despite later attempts at reconstruction, but there is often no choice. Just dividing the gastrocnemius however will have surprisingly little effect on future recovery (Fig. 107.12).

## Posterior Approach

If exposure of the whole length of the popliteal artery is required, it is better to turn the patient prone and make a lazy S posterior incision over the popliteal fossa, starting from the postero-medial thigh, then going across from medial to lateral right behind the knee, and then continuing laterally down the leg, more posterior than a lateral fasciotomy incision (Fig. 107.13).

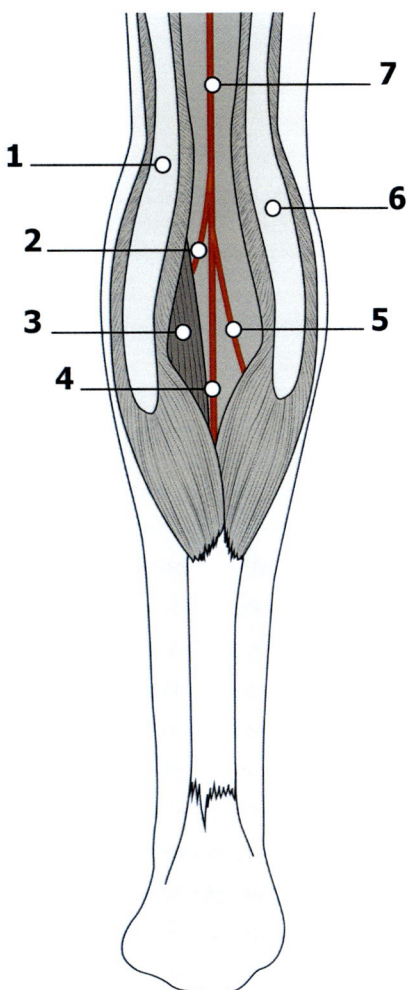

**Fig. 107.13** Posterior view of popliteal vessels. 1: Lateral head of gastrocnemius; 2: anetrior tibial artery; 3: soleus muscle; 4: peroneal artery; 5: posterior tibial artery; 6: medial head of gastrocnemius; 7: popliteal artery. (Illustration by M. Torres/Fiverr)

### 107.3.1.9 Exposure of the Tibial and Peroneal Vessels

As mentioned above, the incision is likely to be a continuation of an incision made to access vessels in the groin or the thigh, or part of a medial fasciotomy incision, behind the medial edge of the tibia and just behind the greater saphenous vein.

### Exposure of the Bifurcation and Trifurcation

Exposure of the popliteal artery will continue up to the bifurcation, with loops around the popliteal

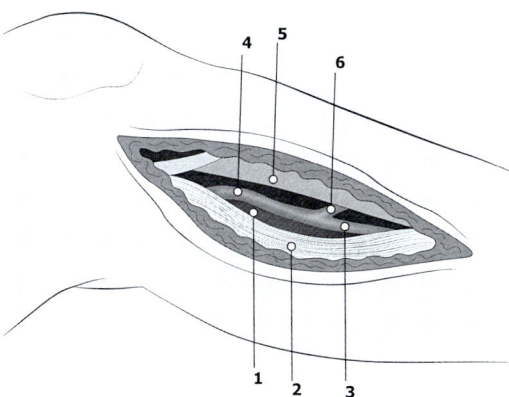

**Fig. 107.12** Exposure of the infragenicular distal popliteal artery and bifurcation of the anterior tiboial artery and tibio-peroneal trunk. 1: Popliteal vein; 2: gastrocnemius muscle; 3: tibioperoneal trunk; 4: distal popliteal artery; 5: tibia; 6: anterior tibial artery. (Illustration by M. Torres/Fiverr)

artery and its terminal division into the anterior tibial artery and the tibio-peroneal trunk. The first structure encountered is the popliteal vein, while the tibial nerve is safely protected, being posteromedial to the artery [33].

At this level, it is especially useful to separate the soleus muscle from the tibia with a combination of scissors and non-toothed forceps to help with piecemeal exposure of the two end vessels while retracting the gastrocnemius posteriorly.

### Exposure of Anterior Tibial Artery

A dedicated exposure of the anterior tibial artery is exceedingly rare as an emergency procedure, since an injury to this artery, lying as it does in the depths of the extensor muscles in the anterior compartment, is likely to be associated with a mangled limb and treated as such.

In case of isolated injuries, the best approach will be through a longitudinal incision over the anterior compartment or as part of a lateral fasciotomy incision.

Proximally, the proximal fibula may need to be excised, while distally, the artery will be found lying on the interosseous membrane between the tibialis anterior and extensor digitorum longus muscles.

> **Dos and Don'ts**
>
> **Dos**
> - Resuscitate patients before thinking of vascular exposure.
> - Prepare for proximal control.
> - Use proximal and distal tourniquets if there is massive venous bleeding as well.
> - Prepare for injuries at various levels and plan for the best exposure at each level.
> - Use magnification even for large vessels.
> - Divide muscles and insertions as needed.
> - Prepare for fasciotomy in all cases of delays and combined arterial and venous injuries.
> - Be prepared to divide the inguinal ligament, if necessary, and repair it later.
> - Continue to use a tourniquet for proximal control while obtaining distal control and exposure if major tissue destruction occurs.
> - Make a big incision for the popliteal artery bifurcation and be prepared to expose a good length of the tibia to have a good tibio-peroneal trunk exposure.
>
> **Don'ts**
> - Do not sacrifice control for sterility: unscrubbed assistants compressing a vessel are better than exsanguination.
> - Do not hope to be able to obtain anatomical control with a big haematoma; instead, do more proximal control.
> - Do not rely on tunnelling grafts under the clavicles and across the knees in the presence of massive haematomas; a socked patient will be much more swollen the next morning and will have a compartment syndrome.
> - Do not open vessels for instrumentation where there is poor tissue cover: it will break down, and so will the suture line on the vessel.
> - Do not think that a trapdoor incision gives you good access to the proximal subclavian artery; it might end up being a full sternotomy and cause major muscle damage to the pectorals and serratus anterior if it is too high.
> - Do not explore lateral arm wounds from a lateral approach; there can be injuries to the brachial artery.
> - Do not explore a bleeding lateral thigh wound from a lateral approach; it is much better to obtain control of the profunda femoris at the groin first.
> - Do not make your groin incision below the inguinal skin fold; you will probably end up with the superficial femoral artery.
> - Do not use a posterior approach to the popliteal artery in an acute setting with an unstable patient.

### Take-Home Messages
- Exposure of proximal extremity vessels can be very demanding in an acute setting and difficult to master without practicing in high penetrating trauma units, and one should try to attend cadaver-based vascular access courses or spend time in units with high loads of penetrating trauma.
- When in doubt, obtain very proximal control, such as aortic control, followed by distal control, and then move to less proximal control in phases.
- Opt for a long incision rather than risking compartment syndrome or ongoing peri-genicular arterial and venous bleeding around the knee.
- Always plan fasciotomy incisions. When exploring actively bleeding vessels, you are likely to need one.

### Multiple Choice Questions
1. In exposing common iliac vessels
   A. **One must avoid entering the peritoneal cavity**
   B. Peritoneal cavity must always be entered
   C. Use laparoscopy
   D. Start distally in perform incision
2. Proximal vascular control:
   A. Very proximal control is useless
   B. **Proximal control must always be attempt**
   C. It is more important distal control
   D. It is important but without aortic clamping
3. Fasciotomy
   A. It is useless
   B. **It is useful for limb compartment syndrome**
   C. Can be performed into the abdomen
   D. Must be performed always bilaterally

### References

1. Rich NM, Walker AJ. Chapter 1: The vascular injury legacy. In: Rasmussen T, Tai N, editors. Rich's vascular trauma. 3rd ed. Amsterdam: Elsevier; 2015.
2. Kragh JF Jr, Walters TJ, Baer DG, Fox CJ, Wade CE, Salinas J, Holcomb JB. Survival with emergency tourniquet use to stop bleeding in major limb trauma. Ann Surg. 2009;249(1):1–7.
3. Boulger E, Carlbom A. Chapter 1.5.2: Tourniquets. In: Velmahos GC, Degiannis E, Doll D, editors. Penetrating trauma. 2nd ed. Berlin: Springer; 2017.
4. Jahnke EJ Jr, Seeley SF. Acute vascular injuries in the Korean War: an analysis of 77 consecutive cases. Ann Surg. 1953;138(2):158–77.
5. Hughes CW. The primary repair of wounds of major arteries; an analysis of experience in Korea in 1953. Ann Surg. 1955;141(3):297–303.
6. Inui FK, Shannon J, Howard JM. Arterial injuries in the Korean conflict: experiences with 111 consecutive injuries. Surgery. 1955;37(5):850–7.
7. Spencer FC, Grewe RV. The management of arterial injuries in battle casualties. Ann Surg. 1955;141(3):304–13.
8. Shackelford S, Garofalo E, Shalin V, Pugh K, Chen H, Pasley J, Bowyer M, et al. Development and validation of trauma surgical skills metrics: preliminary assessment of performance after training. J Trauma Acute Care Surg. 2015;79(1):105–10.
9. Du Toit DF. Chapter 34: Penetrating trauma to the subclavian vessels. In: Velmahos GC, Degiannis E, Doll D, editors. Penetrating trauma. 2nd ed. Berlin: Springer; 2017.
10. Evans C, Chaplin T, Zelt D. Management of major vascular injuries: neck, extremities, and other things that bleed. Emerg Med Clin N Am. 2018;36:181–202.
11. CRoC® Combat Ready Clamp - Combat Medical Systems. https://combatmedical.com/product/croc-combatready-clamp.
12. Stigall K, Blough PE, Rall JM, Kauvar DS. Conversion of the abdominal aortic and junctional tourniquet (AAJT) to infrarenal resuscitative endovascular balloon occlusion of the aorta (REBOA) is practical in a swine hemorrhage model. J Spec Oper Med. 2021;21(1):30–6.
13. Martin MJ, Salim A. Chapter 64: Peripheral arterial injuries from penetrating trauma. In: Velmahos GC, Degiannis E, Doll D, editors. Penetrating trauma. 2nd ed. Berlin: Springer; 2017.
14. Feliciano DV. Pitfalls in the management of peripheral vascular injuries. Trauma Surg Acute Care Open. 2017;2:1–8.
15. Monteiro T, Pereira B, Chiara O, Weber D, Ansaloni L, Bendinelli C, Coccolini F, et al. WSES position paper on vascular emergency surgery. World J Emerg Surg. 2015;10:49.

16. Smith S, White J, Wanis KN, Beckett A, McAlister VC, Hilsden R. The effectiveness of junctional tourniquets: a systematic review and meta-analysis. J Trauma Acute Care Surg. 2018;86(3):532–9.
17. Waller CJ, Cogbill TH, Kallies KJ, Fox CJ, Harrison PB, et al. Contemporary management of subclavian and axillary artery injuries—a Western Trauma Association multicenter review. J Trauma Acute Care Surg. 2017;83(6):1023–31.
18. Baker AC, Clouse WD. Chapter 14: Upper extremity and junctional zone injuries. In: Rasmussen T, Tai N, editors. Rich's vascular trauma. 3rd ed. Amsterdam: Elsevier; 2015.
19. Jordan R, Obmann M, Song B, Nikam S, Mariner D, et al. Hybrid approach to complex vascular injury secondary to blast induced scapulothoracic dissociation. Trauma Case Rep. 2019;23:100236.
20. Sise MJ. Chapter 2: Diagnosis and early management. In: Rasmussen T, Tai N, editors. Rich's vascular trauma. 3rd ed. Amsterdam: Elsevier; 2015.
21. Salim A, Olufajo O, Martin MJ. Chapter 65: Axillary and brachial vessels. In: Velmahos GC, Degiannis E, Doll D, editors. Penetrating trauma. 2nd ed. Berlin: Springer; 2017.
22. Wahlberg E, Goldstone J. Chapter 2: Vascular injury of the thoracic outlet area. In: Wahlberg E, et al., editors. Emergency vascular surgery: a practical guide. 2nd ed. Berlin: Springer; 2017.
23. Wahlberg E, Goldstone J. Chapter 3: Vascular injuries in the upper extremities. In: Wahlberg E, et al., editors. Emergency vascular surgery: a practical guide. 2nd ed. Berlin: Springer; 2017.
24. Talving P, Benjamin ER. Chapter 32: Upper extremity: brachial artery injury. In: Demetriades D, Inaba K, Velmahos G, editors. Atlas of surgical techniques in trauma. Cambridge: Cambridge University Press; 2015.
25. Kumar NG, Knipp BS, Gillespie DL. Chapter 15: Lower extremity vascular trauma. In: Rasmussen T, Tai N, editors. Rich's vascular trauma. 3rd ed. Amsterdam: Elsevier; 2015.
26. Ivatury R, Maier RV, Di Saverio S, Leppaniemi A, Coccolini F, et al. American Association for the Surgery of Trauma–World Society of Emergency Surgery guidelines on diagnosis and management of peripheral vascular injuries. J Trauma Acute Care Surg. 2020;89:1183–96.
27. Bekdache O, Paradis T, Razek T, et al. Intermittent use of resuscitative endovascular balloon occlusion of the aorta in penetrating gunshot wound of the lower extremity. Can J Surg. 2019;62(6):E9–E12.
28. Martin MJ, McClelland JM, Salim A, King DR. Chapter 66: Femoral vessels. Chapter 67: Popliteal vessels. In: Velmahos GC, Degiannis E, Doll D, editors. Penetrating trauma. 2nd ed. Berlin: Springer; 2017.
29. Velmahos G, Gelbard R. Chapter 35: Femoral artery injuries. In: Demetriades D, Inaba K, Velmahos G, editors. Atlas of surgical techniques in trauma. Cambridge: Cambridge University Press; 2015.
30. Wahlberg E, Goldstone J. Chapter 9: Vascular injuries in the legs. In: Wahlberg E, et al., editors. Emergency vascular surgery: a practical guide. 2nd ed. Berlin: Springer; 2017.
31. Franz RW, Shah KJ, Halaharvi D, et al. A 5-year review of management of lower extremity arterial injuries at an urban level I trauma center. J Vasc Surg. 2011;53(6):1604–10.
32. Demetriades D, Inaba K, Velmahos G. Chapter 36: Popliteal artery. In: Talving P, Nash N, editors. Atlas of surgical techniques in trauma. Cambridge: Cambridge University Press; 2015.
33. Sandhu J, La Punzina C, Kothuru R. Case report: Triple vessel injury with single penetrating trauma to the lower extremity requiring popliteal to posterior tibial artery bypass. Trauma Case Rep. 2018;15:32–5.

## Further Reading

Demetriades D, Inaba K, Velmahos G. Atlas of surgical techniques in trauma. Cambridge: Cambridge University Press; 2015.

Kobayashi L, Coimbra R, Reva V, Moore EE, Ivatury R, Maier RV, Di Saverio S, Leppaniemi A, Coccolini F, et al. American Association for the Surgery of Trauma–World Society of Emergency Surgery guidelines on diagnosis and management of peripheral vascular injuries. J Trauma Acute Care Surg. 2020;89: 1183–96.

Rasmussen T, Tai N, editors. Rich's vascular trauma. 3rd ed. Amsterdam: Elsevier; 2015.

Velmahos GC, Degiannis E, Doll D, editors. Penetrating trauma. 2nd ed. Berlin: Springer; 2017.

Wahlberg E, Goldstone J. Emergency vascular surgery: a practical guide. 2nd ed. Berlin: Springer; 2017.

# Extremity Vascular Injuries

# 108

Viktor A. Reva and
Adenauer Marinho de Oliveira Góes Junior

## 108.1 Introduction

Vascular injuries (VI) represent a significant challenge for emergency physicians and trauma surgeons. Injury pattern, severity of the patient's condition, prehospital care, availability of resources, and personal skills all impact the outcome. Extremity VIs (EVIs) can have two devastating consequences: exsanguination and ischemia, which are responsible for the greatest possible mortality and morbidity. The sooner a bleeder is recognized and appropriate pre- and in-hospital care is provided, the better are the chances of survival. Penetrating EVIs lead to hemorrhage, which may be easily compressible, while blunt EVIs can lead to threatened ischemia that—if not timely addressed—becomes irreversible. Expeditious patient transfer to a surgical facility, rapid hemorrhage control, and limb reperfusion have been demonstrated to be of paramount importance for patient's survival and limb salvage.

There are different treatment strategies: total vascular care, in the form of definitive vascular reconstruction, and vascular damage control. Also, within these strategies, there are different treatment options. While open vascular techniques and their short- and long-term outcomes are well investigated and proven, endovascular and hybrid options are rapidly developing, which opens up a new era in VI management. This era, however, is yet to be based on the "life over limb" principle.

> **Learning Goals**
> - Vascular injuries to the extremities represent the majority of vascular injuries in civilian and military settings, and are responsible for high mortality and morbidity due to exsanguination and limb ischemia.
> - A broad spectrum of interventions can be applied to address a vascular lesion, depending on the morphology of the injury, the patient's physiology, and the availability of resources. Open surgery remains the first-line option, but endovascular and hybrid techniques also have huge potential.
> - Temporary shunting represents a viable vascular damage control option for hemodynamic instability, severe soft tissue loss, orthopedic injuries, and austere environments.

V. A. Reva (✉)
Department of War Surgery, Kirov Military Medical Academy, Saint-Petersburg, Russian Federation

A. Marinho de Oliveira Góes Junior
Federal University of Pará (UFPA) and University Center of Pará State (CESUPA), Belém, PA, Brazil

### 108.1.1 Epidemiology

Modern studies demonstrate a stable or slightly increased rate of civilian VIs from 1.6% to 5.9% [1–4], while the rate of combat-related VIs in a modern war is approximately five times higher than in previous conflicts, accounting for 6.6–17.6% of all trauma admissions [5–7]. EVIs account for 45–80% of all VIs [2, 3, 8, 9].

Patients of all ages and sexes are at risk of suffering vascular trauma (VT); however, it predominates among young men [10, 11]. In geriatric and pediatric populations, VT is relatively rare [1–3]. Males are subject to VT in 70–80% of cases [1–3, 9]. In adults, lower extremities are injured more often than upper extremities [2, 9], which has been especially highlighted in a military cohort of patients [5, 7].

Lower (LEVI) and upper (UEVI) EVIs present differently in patients due to some morphological differences, e.g., larger muscles, fewer collaterals, and tighter compartments. Hemorrhage from LE arterial injury (LEAI) is more difficult to control, and patients with LEAIs are more critically ill upon hospital admission and have significantly higher perioperative complication rates, including a need for major limb amputation, compared to patients with UEAIs (7.8% vs. 1.3%) [12]. However, the rates of associated venous, nerve, and orthopedic injuries are similar between LEVI and UEVI [12].

Two thirds of UEAIs are distal (mostly radial and ulnar) and one third are proximal (mostly brachial) [13]. A National Trauma Data Bank (NTDB) analysis has demonstrated the most common LEAIs to be in the popliteal (35.5%) and superficial femoral arteries (SFA) (27.8%), followed by the common femoral artery (CFA) (18.4%) and tibial arteries (21.2%) [14]. A femoral artery is also the most frequently injured vessel in combat [15, 16].

Approximately every tenth patient with EVI has more than one AI [13, 17]. Concomitant vein and nerve injury, respectively, is present in every fourth and tenth LEAI patient [14]. In children, UEAIs, e.g., brachial, radial, and ulnar artery injuries, are the most common, and UEVIs are more frequently associated with nerve injuries [1].

### 108.1.2 Etiology

Civilian VIs are almost evenly split between blunt and penetrating injuries [1, 3, 8, 9]. Penetrating injuries are encountered less frequently in the pediatric population [1, 18]. In military settings, depending on the nature of conflict, either explosions or gunshot injuries are predominant, while the former can reach 70–73% of vascular-related injuries in modern warfare [6, 7].

Among adult penetrating injuries, gunshot wounds and stab wounds account for the majority of VT cases in civilian practice. In children younger than 6 years, falls and road traffic accidents are the most common causes of blunt trauma, while glass cuts are the most common cause of penetrating injuries [11, 19].

Blunt trauma is usually complex and occurs secondarily to either fractures or dislocations [20, 21]. Every fourth or fifth patient with UEAI or LEAI has a simultaneous orthopedic injury [14, 17]. Popliteal artery injury, below-knee multiple arterial injuries, associated two-bone fractures, and great tissue loss have been shown to be significant risk factors with regard to outcome [22, 23]. In the pediatric population, isolated VT is more common, so children have less severe injuries compared to adults [1].

### 108.1.3 Classification

VIs can be arterial, venous, or combined. Venous injuries are mainly related to vein rupture or thrombosis. To stratify arterial injuries, some classifications have been proposed. The American Association for the Surgery of Trauma classification, which divides VIs according to the caliber of the injured vessel, is valid but has limited practical utilization. Some other classifications are presumed to have greater practicability in terms of: (a) localization of a bleeder, (b) vascular patency, and (c) level of limb ischemia.

Markov et al. proposed that VIs should be categorized as "noncompressible" or "compressible" [8], which has a great impact on treatment strategy. EVIs are amenable to tourniquet placement in order to obtain temporary hemostasis ("compressible") [8, 11], but subclavian/axillary and common femoral vessels, classified as "junctional" injuries, are not amenable and therefore carry a higher risk of exsanguination being "noncompressible."

According to the W. Biffl classification of cerebrovascular injuries, peripheral AIs can be stratified in the same way as occlusive and nonocclusive injuries, depending on vascular patency and vessel wall integrity [24]. Nonocclusive injuries are presented as an intimal irregularity/tear (Grade I—with <25% narrowing), a dissection/intramural hematoma (Grade II—with >25% narrowing), or a partial transection with pseudoaneurysm (PSA) formation (Grade III). Occlusive injuries are typically presented as a vessel thrombotic occlusion (where the vessel wall is preserved, Grade IV) or complete transection (Grade V).

Specifically regarding extremity injuries, a few classifications of limb ischemia have been proposed in the literature. In 1971, Russian military surgeon Vadim Kornilov mooted the idea that sensory and motor deficit is partly due to the ischemia in a vascularly injured extremity and not due to primary nerve damage [25]. He proposed a simplified grading index of limb ischemia, with a division into compensated (viable), uncompensated (threatened), and irreversible ischemia for extremity arterial injuries (Table 108.1). The Rutherford classification was created in 1986 as a standard to analyze and report on acute ischemic events in patients with occlusive peripheral arterial disease [26]. "Threatened ischemia" was further stratified into marginally threatened and immediately threatened ischemia bordering on the irreversible. Understanding level of ischemia is crucial to further appropriate treatment.

**Table 108.1** Defining level of limb ischemia (according to V. Kornilov and R. Rutherford) based on simple diagnostic tests

| Distal pulses | Doppler signal | Movements by affected extremity | Level of ischemia |
|---|---|---|---|
| No/weak | Yes | Active | Viable |
| No | No | Passive | Threatened |
| No | No | Neither active nor passive | Irreversible |

## 108.1.4 Pathophysiology

Severe exsanguination is the leading cause of low survival among patients with VIs. A pathophysiological circle known as the "lethal triad" or, most recently, the "lethal diamond," which includes coagulopathy, hypothermia, acidosis, and hypocalcemia, triggered in response to severe blood loss, represents the most typical and dangerous pathophysiological state in trauma. Ongoing hemorrhage results in acute traumatic coagulopathy, hypothermia, and poor oxygen delivery, which provoke global tissue hypoperfusion that leads to acidosis, coagulopathy, etc. To interrupt the lethal circle by controlling hemorrhage and adequately restoring circulation, there are two main treatment strategies known as vascular damage control and damage control resuscitation.

Another pathophysiological aspect of EVIs is ischemia-reperfusion injury. Level of ischemia and the limb salvage prognosis are influenced by efficiency of collateral circulation, grade and level of arterial injury, and extent of soft tissue damage rather than time from injury. Although increased delay in revascularization of an injured artery is associated with poor outcomes [19, 27], time from injury or time of ischemia itself does not determine treatment strategy. Duration of total (tourniquet) and warm (no flow in a major artery) ischemia is ubiquitously considered to be limited to 2–6 h, respectively (correlates to rhabdomyolysis). It has been demonstrated that there are negative associations between the duration of ischemia and the rate of complications and/or limb salvage. A tourniquet dwell time of >60 min, however, was found to be associated with more rhabdomyolysis, wound infection, and neurologic compromise without an increase in the amputation rate [28]. A recent NTDB analysis of patients with LEAIs who had undergone vascular repair within 60 min post-injury demonstrated a significantly lower amputation rate of 6% compared to patients operated on within 1–3 h (11.7%) and 3–6 h (13.4%), respectively [27]. Thus, expedited reperfusion is required to improve morbidity and patient recovery.

## 108.2 Diagnosis

Signs of EVIs have long been described as "hard signs" and "soft signs" [11, 29, 30]. The hard signs are overt and reliably defined major arterial injuries, while the soft signs generate an index of suspicion for possible arterial or/and venous injury. It has been demonstrated that almost 100% of patients (with rare exceptions) presenting with hard signs on admission have a confirmed major EVI [29]. Hard, soft, and no signs of VIs were encountered in 5.5%, 11.5%, and 83% of patients with extremity trauma, respectively [29]. Recently, some authors have proposed a strategy of using hemorrhagic (arterial transection) and ischemic (arterial occlusion) signs instead [31].

### 108.2.1 Clinical Presentation and Physical Examination

All trauma victims should be accessed by the ATLS protocol, and signs of vascular injury are to be searched for during the primary survey, secondary survey and radiographic evaluation of the injured limb, if indicated [11].

EVI diagnosis is primarily based on simple clinical signs: limb temperature assessment, capillary refill, and sensory and motor loss. The AAST-WSES guidelines have updated and uniform information regarding hard and soft signs [11]. Hard signs include pulsatile hemorrhage, expanding/pulsating hematoma, loss of distal pulses, and bruit/thrill, while soft signs include non-pulsatile hemorrhage, non-expanding hematoma, diminished pulse, history of hemorrhage/hypotension, previously applied tourniquet, neurologic deficit, and wound proximity to named vessels. As a general rule, patients presenting hard signs or with hemodynamic instability should be transported directly to the operating room without additional diagnostic imaging. In well-organized trauma systems, computed tomography (CTA) or on-table angiography can be considered.

In the setting of hemodynamic stability, diagnostic uncertainty (soft signs of VI), or suspicion of concomitant injuries, imaging should be considered. Diagnosis goes from simple to complex. It is of paramount importance to state that the presence of normal distal pulses does not exclude a proximal arterial injury; and, on the other hand, that diminished and even absent pulses may be due to arterial spasm, especially in children [11, 30]. However, patients suffering from low-energy trauma and revealing no signs of VI may be safely discharged. Follow-up in an outpatient setting is advised due to the risk of late presentation of small vascular injuries [11, 30]. In high-energy trauma, additional imaging may help to reveal occult injuries (Fig. 108.1).

The ankle-brachial pressure index (ABPI), or arterial index (if arterial pressure is measured on both upper/lower limbs), is simple, noninvasive, inexpensive, and easy to perform and should be considered as part of the physical examination of all patients presenting "soft signs." An ABPI >0.9 practically excludes an AI, while an ABPI <0.9 warrants further investigation [11, 32] (Fig. 108.1). An exception is made for patients sustaining multilevel injuries to the same limb, like multiple penetrating injuries or more than one fracture, since in those cases physical examination may not be able to determine the site of the VI [30, 32]. Of note, abnormal pulse examination in patients who had suffered a knee dislocation had a sensitivity and a specificity of only 79% and 91%, respectively, in the detection of AI [33]. Thus, a high degree of suspicion must be maintained, and post-reduction imaging is recommended to reliably exclude a popliteal AI.

In the case of associated orthopedic injuries, traction to the extremity and limb realignment are recommended before measuring the ABPI to avoid false-negative results. The location of a wound may preclude placing a blood pressure cuff, and ABPI may also not be accurate in the presence of atherosclerotic lesions. These indices are focused on major arteries, but injuries to the deep brachial/femoral artery, or peroneal arteries, are not detected because no direct flow from these arteries is measured distally. Minor luminal injuries (that do not affect flow), such as small intimal flaps, may not be detected. The indices do not detect venous injuries and are also less sensitive in hypotensive and/or hypothermic patients,

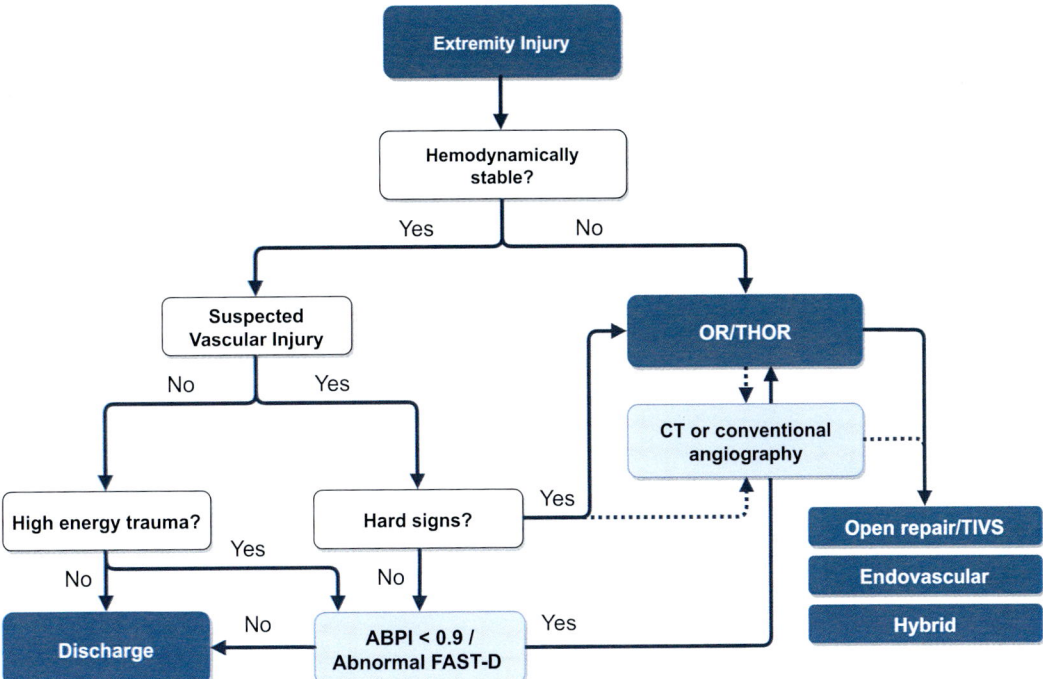

**Fig. 108.1** Algorithm for diagnosis and treatment of extremity vascular injuries. *ABPI* ankle-brachial pressure index, *CT* computed tomography, *FAST-D* Focused Assessment with Sonography for Trauma—Doppler protocol, *OR* operation room, *TIVS* temporary intravascular shunting, *THOR* trauma hybrid operation room

and should therefore be used with caution in those patients [11].

## 108.2.2 Laboratory and Imaging Tests

Laboratory markers of EVIs are nonspecific and relate to blood loss and hypoperfusion. Basic blood tests, such as lactate (>4 mmol/L), pH (<7.25), base deficit (>6 mmol/L), hemoglobin (<11.0 g/dL), and the international normalized ratio (>1.5), as well as abnormal viscoelastic tests (tromboelastography/metry), are regarded as independent predictors of poor outcome. A high level of serum creatinine, urea, or myoglobin is a sign of severe reperfusion injury.

Imaging tests include doppler or duplex ultrasonography (DUS), conventional (CA), and CTA. Historically, CA has been the gold-standard method for investigating vascular trauma. However, arterial puncture itself can lead to puncture-site hemorrhage, hematoma, thrombosis, distal embolism, and even nerve iatrogenic injuries, with a total complication rate that reaches 9% [11].

Recently, noninvasive radiology techniques have evolved and are being widely used in trauma surgery. DUS and CTA are contemporary imaging modalities that have different roles, characteristics, and also availability.

### 108.2.2.1 Doppler Ultrasound (DUS)

Ultrasound imaging has become a first-line screening tool in the diagnosis of suspected EVIs. The DUS method is noninvasive and free of radiation exposure, and it has demonstrated as high as 97% diagnostic accuracy with regard to VI [30]. Although operator-dependent, in skilled hands, 2D imaging may be useful in revealing a PSA, an intimal flap, or a partial/complete arterial thrombus, while color DUS may demonstrate a diminished or even absent flow in the true and false lumens (arterial dissection) or the filling of the PSA.

In addition to 2D and color DUS, spectral Doppler waveforms are of paramount importance.

Normal arterial waveforms in the resting limbs typically show a triphasic pattern, while biphasic, monophasic, or even no-flow are expected in patients with a proximal arterial lesion (stenosis, dissection, or occlusion); if normal triphasic flow is detected distally from the traumatized limb segment, a severe AI may be ruled out [34]. This approach called D-FAST (focused goal-directed Doppler procedure) has been proposed as a triage tool in both prehospital and in-hospital settings. In positive cases (absent, monophasic, or biphasic waveforms at the dorsalis pedis/posterior tibial arteries), further imaging is required [11].

Besides professional experience, other factors such as a more rigid arterial wall, chronic stenosis/occlusion, or collateral circulation related to atherosclerotic lesion and arterial hypo/hypertension can jeopardize DUS interpretation. For these reasons, the specificity of DUS in detecting a severe AI is not guaranteed, and further investigations should be considered when a non-triphasic flow is observed.

Another aspect assessed with DUS is flow velocity. Normal arterial peak systolic velocities (PSVs) are around 100 cm/s in proximal arterial segments (e.g., CFA), while distal segments show a PSV of about 50 cm/s (e.g., tibial arteries). Thus, low flow PSV or even absent flow is to be expected in severe arterial injuries.

### 108.2.2.2 Computed Tomography Angiography (CTA)

CTA has supplanted CA as the gold-standard imaging modality for VT evaluation. CTA's sensitivity and specificity in identifying UEVI and LEVI are high, exceeding 90% [11]. The advantages of CTA include low risk, low cost, high accuracy, speed, and availability. In addition, it provides additional information on associated soft tissue or bone injuries, which can be used as anatomic landmarks for surgical access planning. Compared to CA, CTA generates multipurpose images that require postprocessing to reduce the amount of information provided to the vascular structures. Axial and multiplanar reformatted images are usually accompanied by maximum intensity projections and a form of 3D volume rendering. The goal of these additional images is to provide overviews of the vasculature that are partially comparable to angiography.

Examination should be preferably performed with a 64-slice multidetector scanner, but 16-slice scanners can provide acceptable image quality [11, 35]. For upper extremity CTA, venous access should preferably be placed in the non-injured arm, and ideally, the injured extremity should be raised above the head, decreasing beam hardening from the torso. For a lower extremity CTA, the patient's legs should be secured to the table, and both limbs should be included in the field of view, since the inclusion of the contralateral extremity may be useful as a reference during the interpretation of findings on the injured side, such as those that raise suspicion of an arteriovenous fistula (AVF).

CTA signs of injury can be classified as direct or indirect. Direct signs relate to the vessel wall and often indicate significant VT that may require either open or endovascular repair and include occlusion, thrombosis, intimal dissection, spasm, external compression, PSA, active arterial hemorrhage, and AVF. Indirect signs represent findings within the perivascular soft tissues, such as perivascular hematoma, a projectile tract near a neurovascular bundle, and shrapnel at a distance of <5 mm from a vessel. The presence of VT indirect signs should raise suspicion of an occult injury [11].

CTA may become nondiagnostic with poor timing of contrast material injection, which may be seen in multiple injury patients with circulatory compromise or multilevel VT. The main limitation to utilizing CTA is hemodynamic instability. However, the development of trauma hybrid operation rooms (THORs), which represent a combination of an operation room (OR), angio suite, and CT, in many centers worldwide, alleviates this disadvantage. In a standard trauma OR, when additional imaging is required, CA is an alternate option.

### 108.2.2.3 Conventional Angiography

The role of CA cannot be overestimated. If CTA is not readily available, and multiple artifacts caused by metal fragments related to ballistic injury are present, the patient is hemodynami-

# 108 Extremity Vascular Injuries

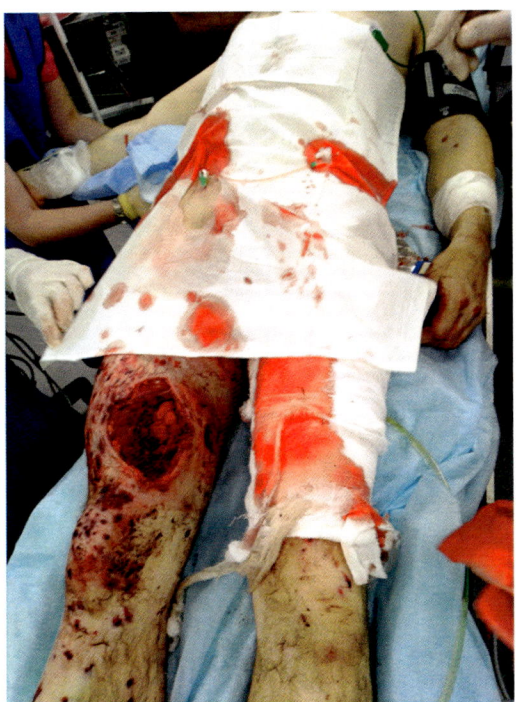

**Fig. 108.2** Early arterial access for pre-, intra-, and postoperative angiography as an additional tool for treatment of gunshot femoral artery and vein injury. A 6-Fr antegrade femoral sheath is inserted in the right leg

cally unstable, and CA can be performed in an OR. There are some indications for angiography: ABPI <0.9 when additional imaging is required, multiple extremity injury, and multiple orthopedic injury (fractures, dislocations) in the case of suspected VI [11] (Fig. 108.1).

Performing angiography in an angio suite may delay open intervention, exacerbate ischemia, and thereby negatively impact morbidity. It can be performed on-table by using a single arterial puncture technique or with a catheter (a sheath) placed proximally in a targeted artery (Fig. 108.2).

> **Differential Diagnosis**
> Some "classical" signs of limb ischemia, such as pain, paresthesia, and paresis, can be seen in the case of neurogenic trauma. In multiple (especially complex pelvic-extremity orthopedic) injuries with at least some "P" clinical signs, a VI should be suspected until proven otherwise. Peripheral flow can also be compromised in elderly people in severe shock. A bilateral pulse check and DUS provide the information necessary to exclude limb-threatening injuries.
>
> A delayed mass in a zone of recent penetrating injury should be differentiated from an abscess. Diagnostic puncture or even incision to evacuate the mass can result in catastrophic hemorrhage. Physical examination and DUS can reliably rule out a PSA formation.

## 108.3 Treatment

There are four main current options to treat EVIs: nonoperative management (NOM), open surgery, endovascular surgery (interventional radiology), and hybrid surgery (Table 108.2). The latter is a combination of open and endovascular techniques.

### 108.3.1 Medical Treatment

Up until the mid-twentieth century, treatment provided for EVIs resulted in high primary and secondary amputation rates. Today, however, there are few indications for NOM (Table 108.2). A majority of patients suffering from injuries to segments containing paired arteries (lower leg, lower arm) have been demonstrated to be successfully managed without arterial reconstruction, provided there is no ongoing hemorrhage and distal ischemia. Injury to branch vessels (deep femoral artery, circumflex artery, etc.) can be managed either conservatively (no hemorrhage or/and expanding hematoma) or endovascularly.

Overall, NOM can be considered in selected stable patients with minor EVIs without active hemorrhage or signs of distal ischemia [11]. Patients subject to NOM should be monitored closely, and any change in clinical examination

**Table 108.2** Different approaches to extremity vascular injury management according to different treatment strategies

| Strategy | NOM | Open | Endovascular | Hybrid |
|---|---|---|---|---|
| Definitive vascular procedure | • <5 mm intimal disruption<br>• Adherent intimal flaps<br>• Intact distal circulation<br>• No active hemorrhage | Arterial reconstruction (repair, end-to-end anastomosis, autologous vein OR PTFE grafting) | Recanalization and stent/stent-graft implantation | Balloon occlusion of the injury zone OR proximal control followed by open repair |
| Vascular damage control | • Tourniquet<br>• Local hemostatic agent<br>• Observation in minor VIs | Temporary intravascular shunting<br>Ligation | Endovascular temporary shunting (Emergency stenting) | Direct site endovascular repair<br>Extracorporeal arterial shunting |

*NOM* nonoperative management, *PTFE* polytetrafluoroethylene, *VI* vascular injury

should be followed by immediate repeat imaging, and open or endovascular intervention.

### 108.3.1.1 Endovascular Treatment

Even though open repair remains the gold standard for the vast majority of EVIs, endovascular techniques and tools are evolving. The increased use of endovascular techniques to treat arterial trauma, particularly stent-grafts for limb revascularization, has been well documented in the literature [36]. The PROspective Observational Vascular Injury Trial (PROOVIT) registry, however, demonstrates that endovascular techniques are used least frequently in EVIs [9].

Endovascular options are divided into "occlusive" (for minor, branch vessels) and "opening" (for major VIs) procedures. Choosing an appropriate treatment strategy depends on the localization of the injury, degree of vessel wall injury, severity of condition, and resources (Fig. 108.3).

Embolization with a variety of materials is an option for management of bleeding from minor arteries, while in-line flow can be restored using covered stents. A typical scenario for EVI is embolization of DFA branches after a penetrating injury or a severe femur fracture. While no crossing of the lesion is typically required for embolization (except in cases when "back door" embolization is necessary), the inability to recanalize a VI makes stent-graft placement impossible. However, some experimental studies have demonstrated the potential of emergency stent/stent-graft placement in occlusive arterial injuries—a method of temporary endovascular shunting [37]. Alternate techniques of through-and-through recanalization may be used to achieve intraluminal guidewire positioning in difficult cases [38, 39].

There is an increased use of endovascular interventions to treat axillo-subclavian AIs due to difficult accessibility; endoluminal stent-grafting can be the first-line treatment irrespective of the patient's status [38] (Fig. 108.4). In most centers, however, endovascular repairs are more frequently used for subclavian than for axillary AI [40].

SFA injuries may also be managed primarily by stent-graft placement. Short-term outcomes show that SFA injuries treated by open repair are associated with a higher fasciotomy rate, but no differences in mortality and cost were found compared to endovascular repair. However, long-term outcomes are still not well investigated [36].

Associated complications of stenting procedures include in-stent occlusion, deformation and kinking, loss of vessel branches after stent-graft placement, and intimal hyperplasia. Worth noting is that extremities (especially the popliteal artery) are subjected to hyperflexion and extension, which makes endovascular stent-graft placement controversial regarding its long-term effect. It requires prolonged dual antiplatelet therapy, which might be contraindicated in severe multiple injuries. For these reasons, stent-graft place-

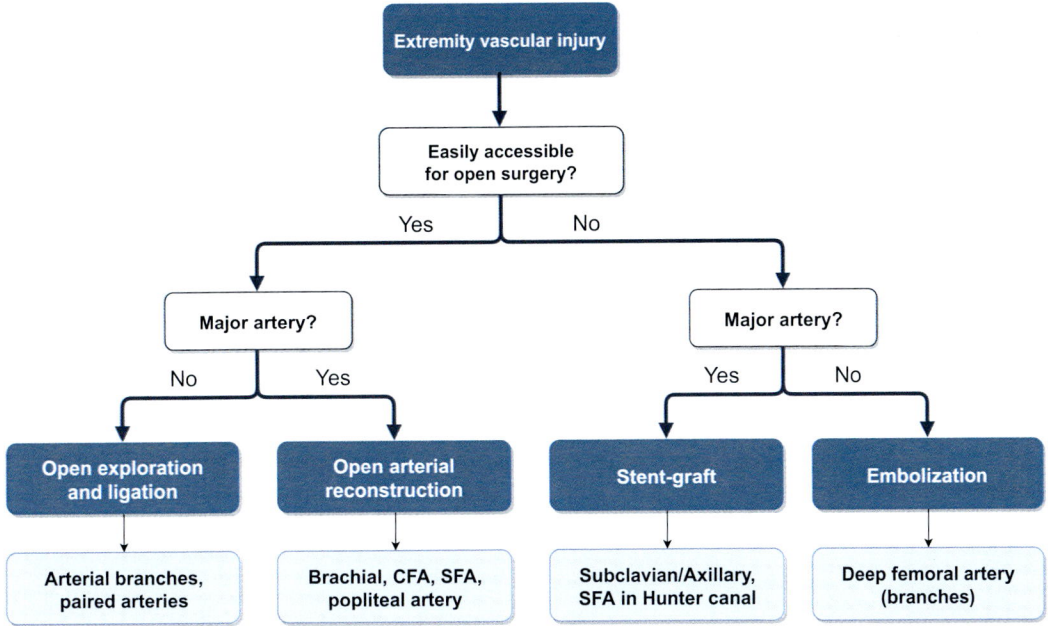

**Fig. 108.3** Algorithm for choosing an appropriate endovascular method to treat extremity vascular injuries. *CFA* common femoral artery, *SFA* superficial femoral artery

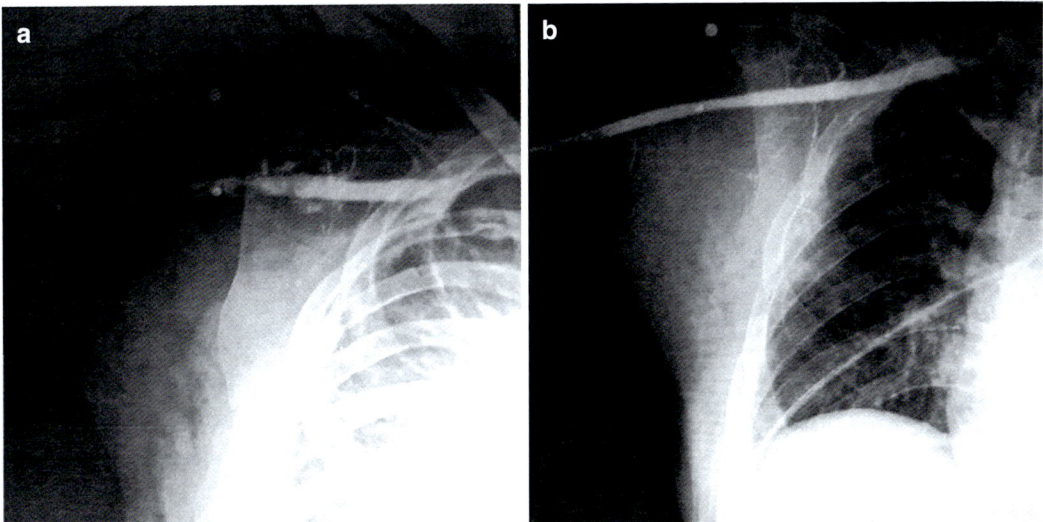

**Fig. 108.4** An axillary artery gunshot injury with lateral injury and thrombosis (**a**). A self-expanded covered stent implanted in a zone of injury with return of normal limb perfusion (**b**)

ment can also be used as a bridging technique until the patient is stable enough to undergo definitive complex arterial reconstruction [39].

Pediatric patients are also not the best candidates for endovascular trauma treatment. As well as an increased propensity for vasospasm, the use of endovascular techniques is often not possible due to vessel size and is often discouraged given children's increased lifespan and likelihood of further vessel growth.

Endovascular therapy is frequently adequate for the subacute phase of trauma, like treating

AVF and PSAs, and for small vascular injuries, frequently undiagnosed on physical examination and only detected on CTA. Endovascular techniques have a huge potential for treatment not only of acute/subacute VIs but also of hemodynamically unstable patients within the concept of endovascular resuscitation, trauma, and bleeding management (EVTM) [41].

Endovascular interventions can be performed in traditional operating rooms ("semi-hybrid" rooms equipped with a good-quality C-arm), angiography suites, and the increasingly common THORs. The unique environment, alongside the development of dedicated endovascular trauma services, allows for better streamlining of the multidisciplinary care of the complex trauma patient.

Hybrid and semi-hybrid rooms provide unique opportunities for the implementation of hybrid (open + endovascular) procedures. A method of direct site endovascular repair has recently been proposed, where a special stent-graft is inserted into the injured vessel immediately after open exploration [42]. The method can also be used as a damage control option.

### 108.3.1.2 Anticoagulation

The use of perioperative systemic anticoagulation for EVIs is still controversial. Multiple studies have shown that anticoagulation given to patients with traumatic VIs without absolute contraindication has not been reported to increase the rate of bleeding complications [11]. It has been found that, although the use of intraoperative anticoagulation does not significantly change intraoperative blood loss or overall bleeding complications, it also fails to demonstrate any improvement in rates of reoperation or limb salvage. Further, others have suggested a relation between prolonged hospital stay and increased blood product use [11].

Comparative analysis of patients given heparin and aspirin and receiving no anticoagulant/antiplatelet agents has found no statistically significant difference in the rates of bleeding, compartment syndrome, or mortality.

Overall, while systemic anticoagulation for VIs does not definitively increase bleeding risk, it also does not seem to improve outcomes, and its routine use is not recommended [11]. Local use of anticoagulants during surgery is, however, justified.

## 108.3.2 Surgical Treatment

### 108.3.2.1 General Considerations

The management of bleeding EVIs should begin in the prehospital scenario. The Hartford consensus postulates that no one should die from uncontrolled hemorrhage. Multiple studies have demonstrated that a tourniquet is rapid, safe, and effective and is a lifesaving method for hemorrhage control.

Previous recommendations on tourniquet use vary. However, recent studies have emphasized that waiting until trauma center arrival to apply a tourniquet is associated with lower BP, an increased need for plasma transfusions, a higher rate of transfusion within the first hours, and a greater than 4.5-fold increase in mortality. A tourniquet should be used when extremity hemorrhage presents a threat to life. In these cases, it should be applied as soon as significant bleeding is noted or suspected, and application should not be delayed [11] (Fig. 108.5).

Within the current paradigm, a majority of patients with EVIs undergo open surgical treatment. Once a VI is diagnosed, open exposure is performed: (a) to achieve proximal and distal arterial control (pre-clamping systemic anticoagulation if not contraindicated), (b) to carefully assess a VI zone (e.g., exclude through-and-through injury, inspect for intimal tear, etc.), (c) to prepare vascular ends for reconstructive surgery (e.g., thrombectomy, achieving antegrade and retrograde flow, flushing with heparinized saline), (d) to perform the appropriate type of arterial repair (e.g., lateral suture, end-to-end anastomosis, autologous vein or Dacron/polytetrafluoroethylene (PTFE)) grafting or temporary shunting), followed by skin closure and distal limb perfusion evaluation.

Before incision, appropriate prepping and draping have to be performed: on the upper part of the body, from the mandible to mid-abdomen

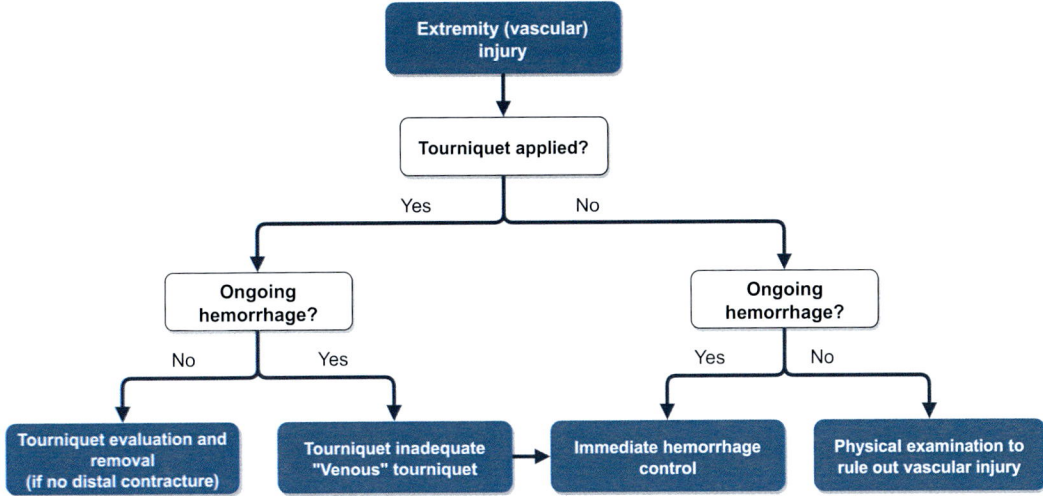

**Fig. 108.5** Decision-making algorithm for hemorrhage control in suspected extremity vascular injury

in the case of UEVI, and on the lower part, below the costal margin, including bilateral groins and lower legs to facilitate great saphenous vein (GSV) harvest for possible complex reconstruction, in the case of LEVI.

The majority of AIs can be repaired primarily with lateral sutures or resectioned with end-to-end anastomoses, but autologous vein grafting is an alternate option if the gap between arterial ends exceeds 2 cm, which is required in 20–30% of cases. For small-caliber arteries, the distal segment of the GSV is typically harvested as a conduit, while a proximal GSV fits better for the reconstruction of large-caliber arteries. The longer segment of the vein is harvested and reversed prior to reconstruction. A standard vascular instrumental set and some specialized instruments are used for revascularization (Table 108.3).

Although the GSV remains the best vascular conduit for complex arterial reconstruction, prosthetic grafts are an alternate option in cases of: (a) large caliber vessels, (b) low energetic trauma with minimal risk of infection, (c) a well-vascularized area of injury, (d) no available vein to harvest, or (e) no time or personnel for harvesting the vein. Among prosthetic grafts, PTFE has proven superior to Dacron because it maintains structural integrity even in the face of staphylococcal infection with a low incidence of anastomotic disruption [11].

**Table 108.3** Surgical and endovascular toolbox for extremity vascular injuries

*Open surgery*
Magnifying surgical glasses (2.5–3.5×)
Fogarty catheter 3-Fr and 4-Fr
Cardiovascular Prolene suture 5.0 and 6.0
Vessel loops
Rummel tourniquets
Prosthetic grafts (PTFE, Dacron); 6 and 8 mm in diameters
Temporary shunts (Pruitt shunt; Javid shunt; plastic tubes, e.g., IV lines and nasogastric tubes)
*Basic specialized instruments*
Scalpel No.11
Pots scissors
Volkman retractors
DeBakey tweezers
Vascular clamps
*Endovascular and hybrid surgery*
Imaging system (angio suite, mobile fluoroscopic unit [C-arm] with vascular package)
Contrast injection system (optional)
Mobile radiolucent table (optimally with floating deck)
Puncture needles 18 gauge
Micropuncture sets
Sheaths (5–8 Fr, 11–25 cm long)
Diagnostic and interventional (hydrophilic and non-hydrophilic) 0.035″ wires of different types and lengths
Diagnostic catheters 5 Fr of different types (BERN, MP, Contralateral, Cobra, Pigtail)
Interventional catheters (guiding catheters) of different types

(continued)

**Table 108.3** (continued)

| |
|---|
| Covered self-expandable stent-grafts (6–8–10 mm in diameter, 4–6–8 cm long) |
| Self-expanding bare metal stents (6–8–10 mm in diameter, 4–6–8 cm long) |
| Dilatation (balloon) catheters (different sizes) |
| Coils (3–5–7–9 mm in diameter) |
| Liquid embolization substances (Onyx, PHIL, glue) |
| Endovascular snare 6–10 mm |
| Inflation devices |
| Torque devices |
| Contrast media |

Careful debridement, minimal blood loss, and minimized operative trauma, covering the zone of anastomosis with viable tissues, and short-term wound drainage help prevent infectious complications.

### 108.3.2.2 Vascular Damage Control

Complex arterial reconstruction may be time-consuming, lead to additional blood loss and morbidity, worsen the patient's condition, and even lead to death. An alternate abbreviated strategy titled "vascular damage control" can be implemented in three main types: upon "common" indications—due to severe trauma and unstable hemodynamics (type I); upon "local" indications—performed intraoperatively due to severe soft tissue loss, orthopedic trauma, or/and severe limb ischemia (type II); upon "tactical" indications—where there are no appropriate skills for definitive reconstruction and no available resources, e.g., combat environments, rural hospitals, etc. (type III).

A high incidence of associated orthopedic injuries creates a logistical and clinical challenge for management and complicates the function of the affected extremity. Prolonged ischemia can worsen outcomes, and surgical strategy depends on the degree of limb ischemia. Limb perfusion is the first priority in threatened ischemia, so temporary or definitive (reconstruction) blood flow restoration has to be performed first. By contrast, in viable ischemia, orthopedic intervention can precede vascular surgery. Intraoperative temporary intravascular shunting (TIVS) (where open exposure > TIVS > external fixation > definitive reconstruction) is an important tool for any arterial injury associated with orthopedic trauma.

A variety of temporary shunts are available on the market. For large caliber arteries, a Javid or Sundt shunt might be an option, while for small caliber arteries, a Pruitt shunt (8–10 Fr) is preferable as it can be simply inserted into the vessels and is self-fixing to the vessel wall by inflating balloons that require no additional securing (Fig. 108.6). Instead, any plastic or silicone tube (e.g., intravenous line, nasogastric tube or even chest tube) can be inserted into the injured artery with a patency reaching 12–24 h.

### 108.3.2.3 Compartment Pressure Monitoring and Release

Prolonged ischemia results in skeletal-muscle injury followed by swelling. Inside strict compartments, e.g., the lower leg, the forearm, rarely the thigh or buttock, ischemia leads to the elevation of intracompartmental pressure (ICP), additional compression of injured muscles, exacerbation of perfusion, and, thus, secondary injury and necrosis. Monitoring and early release of the leg/arm compartments is crucial for reconstructed vascular patency, and a better clinical and functional outcome.

Clinical and instrumental monitoring of an ischemic limb allows for a timely diagnosis and an early decision on compartment release. Classical signs of progressive ischemia, e.g., the six "Ps"—pain, pallor, paresthesia, paresis, pulselessness, and poikilothermia—are good markers and can indicate a need for fasciotomy. Sometimes, however, clinical findings are controversial, and ICP measurement is required. Special or hand-made devices (manometer—three-way stopcock—needle) can be used for pressure monitoring (Fig. 108.7). If ICP exceeds 30 mmHg or perfusion pressure (calculated as the difference between diastolic blood pressure and ICP) is less than 30 mmHg, then wide compartmental release (fasciotomy) should be performed.

Overall, main indications for wide fasciotomy include prolonged (threatened) limb ischemia (typically >4–6 h of warm ischemia or 1–1.5 h of tourniquet ischemia), concomitant major vein injury, and severe soft tissue and/or orthopedic injury. If there is any doubt regarding elevated ICP, a fasciotomy is advocated.

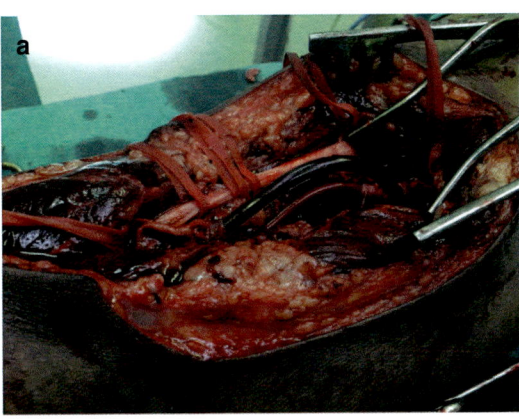
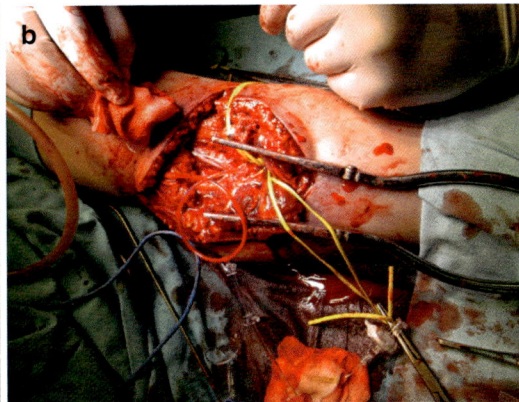

**Fig. 108.6** Temporary intraoperative intravascular shunting: (**a**) both artery and vein by plastic tubes, (**b**) brachial artery by a Pruitt shunt

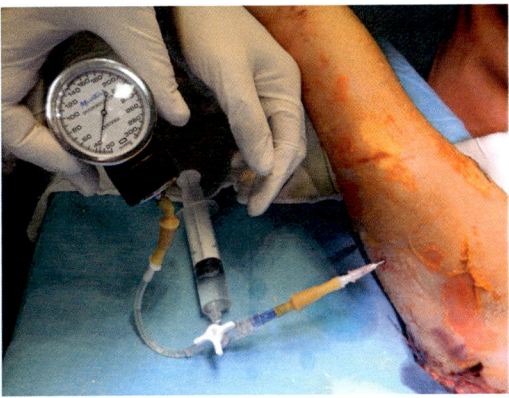

**Fig. 108.7** A hand-made device for intracompartmental pressure monitoring, consisting of a manometer, a syringe, and a needle connected by a three-way stopcock. The manometer demonstrates the intracompartmental pressure is exceeding 30 mmHg, which necessitates fasciotomy

If performed early, fasciotomies are associated with a shorter length of stay, lower rates of infectious complications, and lower amputation rates (Fig. 108.8a).

As significantly elevated ICP can compromise vascular anastomosis, in some cases, a fasciotomy can be performed even before arterial reconstruction [43]. Double- or single-incision four-compartment fasciotomy is performed to release lower leg compartments. The former is faster and more reliable in releasing four compartments, but carries a risk of skin necrosis between incisions. The latter may be longer and carry the risks of iatrogenic injury. For forearm fasciotomy, a long palmar incision, extended by carpal tunnel decompression, is typically performed (Fig. 108.8b).

### 108.3.2.4 Upper Extremity Vascular Injuries

**Axillary**

Axillary artery injuries are encountered in less than 5% of VIs and may often be missed on initial evaluation. Although rare, high mortality and limb disability (3–33%) are reported. Morbidity tends to be higher in blunt trauma, where isolated axillary AIs are associated with shoulder dislocations and proximal humerus fractures and carry a higher morbidity due to associated neurologic, orthopedic, and soft tissue injuries [40].

Open surgery is the standard management procedure, while endovascular techniques have been rarely described in the literature relative to the subclavian artery. This is likely due to the high flexibility of the axillary region, which can affect the long-term outcome. Surgical access is typically performed in the axillary fossa, and the infra- or supraclavicular approach is used for proximal arterial control.

**Brachial and Radial/Ulnar**

A lower margin of the teres major muscle marks the change in name from axillary to brachial artery. The latter is the second-most frequently injured artery among all EVIs, accounting for

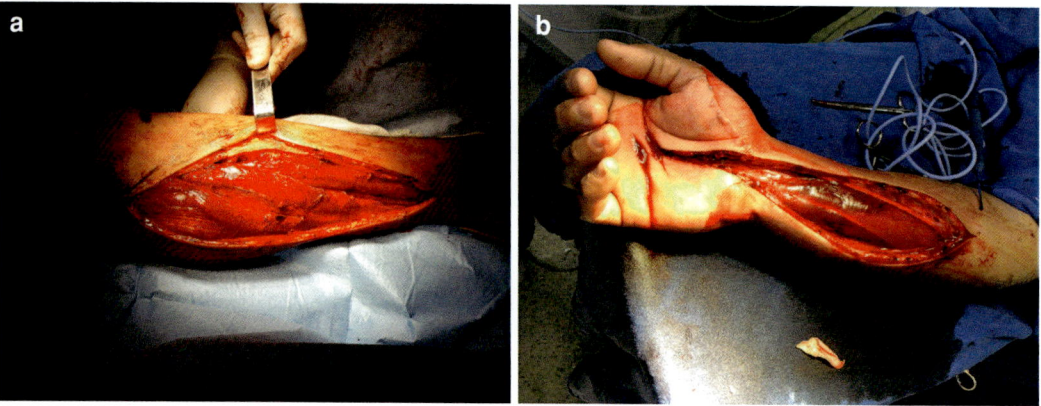

**Fig. 108.8** Wide lower leg (**a**) and forearm (**b**) fasciotomy to release compartment syndrome

approximately 25–33% [44]. Hemorrhage from the brachial artery is easily compressible, and the survival rate reaches 95–100%. Due to rich collateral circulation, morbidity is low (1–4% amputations) even when delayed restoration of perfusion is achieved or in the presence of occluded repairs [44]. Isolated radial and ulnar injuries with an intact palmar arch confirmed by DUS after occlusion of the injured vessel can be ligated with extremely low rates of distal ischemia and amputation [11].

The main collateral in the upper arm is the deep brachial artery, so outcome is influenced by localization of the injury, above or below this branch: the risk of amputation is twice as high after ligation of the "common brachial" artery when compared to the "superficial brachial" artery.

The brachial artery lies superficially, and is therefore not well protected against wound infection. It is of small caliber and tends to spasm, which increases the risk of thrombotic complications after arterial repair. Any stenosis or tension after lateral or circular suture increases the risk of early thrombosis.

Brachial vessels can be rapidly exposed via a longitudinal incision along the medial groove of the biceps and triceps muscles. Extension of this incision obliquely across the antecubital fossa and onto the volar forearm can be used to access the proximal radial and ulnar arteries. The same incision on a forearm is used for wide fasciotomy if required.

### 108.3.2.5 Lower Extremity Vascular Injuries

#### Femoral

The femoral artery is most frequently injured, and depending on the localization of the injury zone, mortality and morbidity may differ [43].

Access to the femoral vessel can be obtained by a vertical groin incision, generous enough to expose the bifurcation of the CFA. In cases of a high CFA injury, the inguinal ligament may require dissection, and obtaining proximal control through a "hockey stick" incision with retroperitoneal dissection and control of the external iliac artery may be necessary. A large hematoma in the inguinal area precludes straightforward access to the CFA, and inguinal oblique access above the inguinal crease is a better option for proximal control. Exposure of the proximal SFA is obtained through a longitudinal incision on the medial thigh, as the midportion of the vessel is located posterior to the Sartorius muscle, which is retracted posteriorly to gain complete exploration [11].

#### Popliteal

Popliteal artery injuries account for only 0.2% of all traumatic injuries. These limb-threatening injuries are among the most complex and deserve special consideration. They give rise to the highest rates of amputation among all EVIs (29–72% in military and 12–50% in civilian practice), and even if limb salvage is obtained, significant disability due to associated injuries may ensue [11, 43].

Knee dislocations and around-the-knee fracture dislocations are insidious injuries that can lead to an occult popliteal artery injury. Upon primary examination, no diminished pulse can be detected, but delayed arterial thrombosis results in rapid progression of ischemia, so CTA or even CA is recommended [30].

The popliteal artery is divided into three segments: supra- (P1), retro- (P2), and infrageniculari (P3). P1 and P3 segments can be approached through a medial incision, external rotation of the injured limb and elevation and flexing of the knee. The artery is in a fixed position, at the adductor tendon proximally and the gastrocnemius distally. The incision is made medially using the posterior edge of the femur; using this anatomical landmark helps avoid injury to the GSV. Division of the medial head of the gastrocnemius muscle and the semimembranosus and semitendinosus tendons is often required to provide a complete view of the P1 (no further tendon suturing required). To expose P3, the incision is extended along the posterior margin of the tibia. Division of the soleus may be required to isolate the tibioperoneal trunk [11]. If the P2 segment requires an extended surgical approach, the above and below the knee medial incisions can be merged, and the medial muscles of insertion (pes anserinus: mm. sartorius, gracilis, semitendinosus) can be divided, exposing the popliteal vessels along all their length.

When preoperative imaging is available, the surgical approach can be pre-planned. A transverse line should be traced above the upper border of the patella, which is proximal, as the posterior "S" access will provide a comfortable exposure. In cases where a more proximal dissection is anticipated, medial access is probably the wisest choice. Popliteal artery injury frequently necessitates lower leg fasciotomy [43].

### Arteries Below the Knee

The lower leg contains three main arteries: the anterior tibial artery, the posterior tibial artery, and the peroneal artery (the latter two coming from the tibioperoneal trunk). In general, the longer the vessels leading to the foot remain patent, the greater is the chance of limb salvage. It has been shown that no amputations occurred in patients with two or more patent vessels to the foot, whereas there was a 68.2% amputation rate documented for patients with no patent vessels, and a 16.0% rate for those with only one patent vessel [11].

It is generally accepted that, if no significant ischemia is present, an injury to one of the three main arteries can be managed by simple ligation, or NOM if no hemostasis is necessary.

#### 108.3.2.6 Venous Injuries

Optimal management of venous injuries to an extremity is still unclear. Before the Vietnam War, vein ligation was routine, with the belief that venous repair would lead to deep venous thrombosis, clot propagation, and subsequent pulmonary embolism. However, the latter half of the twentieth century saw a shift toward more frequent venous repair. There is still much debate in the literature as to whether ligation or reconstruction should be the method of choice for venous injuries to an extremity [11].

While some venous injury series reported that the majority of patients (63%) were treated with ligation without significant differences in postoperative thromboembolic complications compared to those who received venous repair, other studies found that, although mortality was unchanged, ligation was significantly associated with increase in the fasciotomy rate (44.6% vs. 33.5%), secondary amputation (6.1% vs. 3.4%), and hospital length of stay [11].

Proponents of routine ligation claim that many venous repairs evolve into thromboses, that venous stasis after ligation is mitigated by collaterals, and that, even though injured veins are frequently ligated, multiple studies have demonstrated no permanent sequelae, including with regard to the amputation rate.

Conversely, those in favor of repair report acceptable patency rates and a theoretical reduction in venous hypertension after repair. Some authors have stated that, even though thrombosis after venous repair has been reported in up to 39–80% of cases, recanalization is frequently documented. They argue that even short-term patency may allow time for the recruitment of venous collaterals to prevent venous stasis symptoms. Further, reports from surgical teams and experimental work suggest that maintaining the limb outflow has a protective effect over and above the repair/shunt performed on a simultaneous AI [11].

There is general agreement that adverse outcomes appear to be common after popliteal vein injuries, suggesting that particular care should be paid to them and that an attempt at popliteal vein repair should be made if possible [11].

In summary, when the venous injury is amenable to being managed by simple repair, such as lateral venorrhaphy, the vein should be repaired. If more complex techniques are required, it is of paramount importance to take into account the patient's physiological status and concomitant injuries. However, if there is a "damage control" scenario, more complex repairs for injured peripheral veins should not be undertaken. If possible, a venous TIVS should be installed, particularly if a concomitant arterial TIVS is required (Fig. 108.6a). If shunting is not required/possible, the vein should be ligated. Fasciotomy should be considered after major vein ligation or TIVS.

### 108.3.3 Prognoses, Outcomes, and Complications

Ideal circumstances: a patient suffering from EVI, rapidly delivered to a trauma center without ongoing hemorrhage, suspected of and diagnosed with a vascular lesion, has undergone fast and precise open/endovascular/hybrid repair and fasciotomy (if indicated) and has the highest chance for survival and limb function recovery.

Overall, the rate of amputation remains high. Patients who sustained EVIs demonstrated to have an amputation rate of 1–11% for UEVI and LEVI, respectively, with a higher amputation rate for blunt trauma and for lower extremities [1, 12, 22, 27]. The numbers are comparable to those for the military (excluding blast injuries) and the pediatric population [1, 7, 15, 16].

Regardless of extremity, blunt VT is associated with a significantly higher amputation rate (6.7% vs. 1.3%) and mortality (4.8% vs. 3.8%) compared to penetrating trauma [12]. EVIs are associated with a significant risk of death. LEAI was independently associated with a twofold increase in mortality for both blunt and penetrating injuries [12]. Popliteal and femoral artery injuries are exposed to the highest risk of amputation, reaching 28–37% [45, 46] and even 70% for late presentations [47]. In shank and around-the-knee injuries, the more patent vessels to the foot remain, the greater is the chance of limb salvage [48].

Severe blunt extremity injury represents a significant challenge to providing optimal care for saving a limb and its function. Many scores have been proposed to decide whether a severely injured limb should be salvaged or amputated. For instance, in 1990, Johansen et al. developed the Mangled Extremity Severity Score (MESS). A MESS of $\geq 7$ has been used as a cutoff point for predicting the need for early amputation, but has not proven reliable in predicting limb salvage in adults [11, 49].

The Popliteal Scoring Assessment for Vascular Extremity Injuries in Trauma (POPSAVEIT) score offers a simpler and more practical approach to stratifying penetrating and blunt popliteal trauma cases regarding limb salvage probability. The identified risk factors for limb amputation probability in this study were systolic blood pressure <90 mmHg (1 point), associated orthopedic injury (2 points), and a lack of preoperative pedal Doppler signals (2 points) or lack of palpable pedal pulses, if Doppler unavailable (1 point). A POPSAVEIT score $\geq 3$ is associated with higher limb amputation risk [50].

Main early complications include hemorrhage and progressive ischemia due to shunt thrombosis or occult dissection. While in the hospital, extremity hemorrhage can be easily compressed, bridging to surgery; marginally threatened ischemia can lead to amputation.

Delayed complications can manifest as a PSA or AVF/aneurysm. The time interval between the primary injury and manifestation of clinical symptoms may take 10 years or even more. A PSA is a pulsatile hematoma (typically

2–3 weeks after injury) that communicates with an artery through a disruption in the arterial wall. Unlike a true aneurysm, which is bounded by the arterial walls, a PSA is bounded by surrounding tissues (Fig. 108.9). An AVF typically occurs after a penetrating mechanism simultaneously injures the adjacent artery and vein, creating an abnormal communication between them.

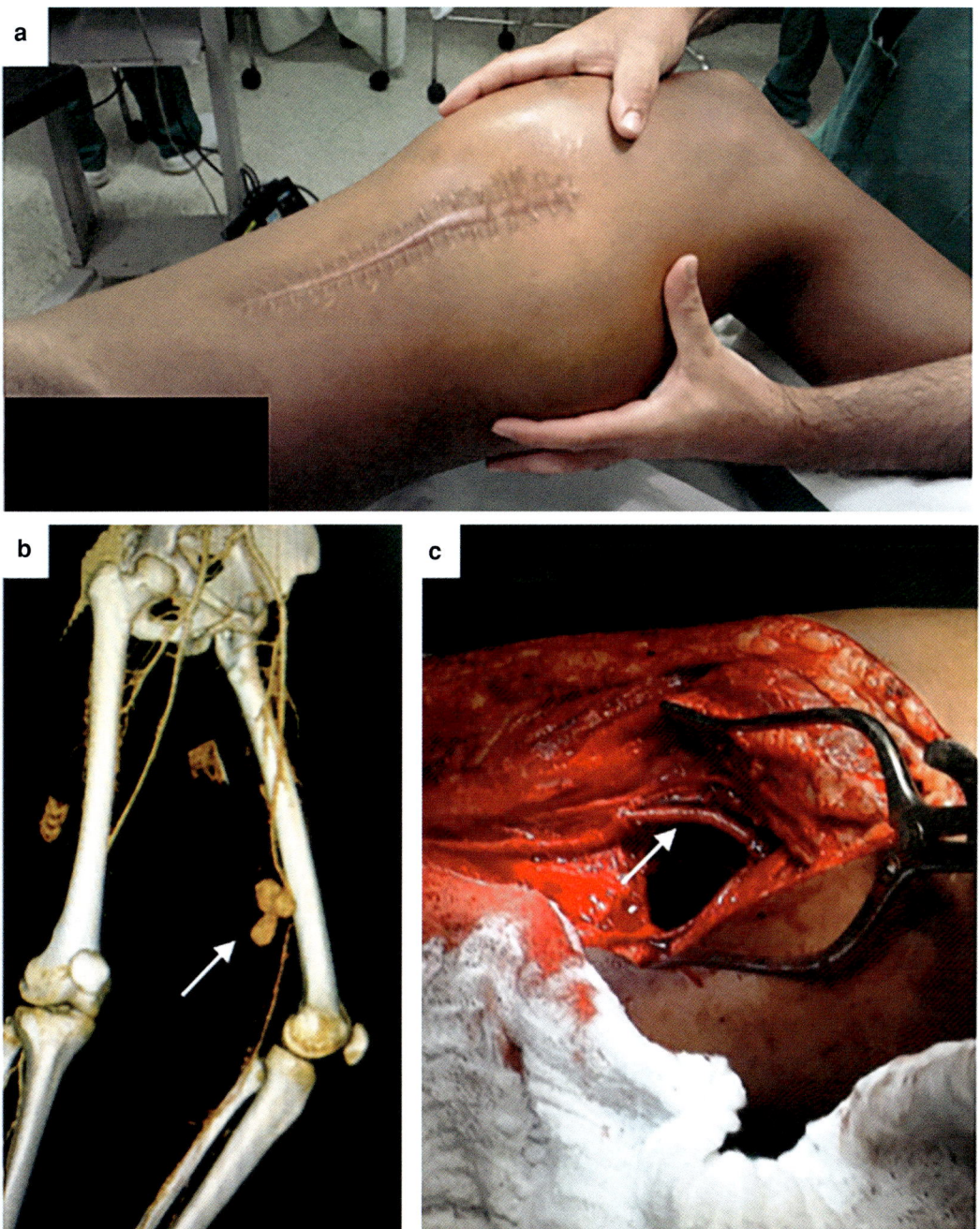

**Fig. 108.9** A superficial femoral artery pseudoaneurysm after a gunshot injury to a thigh: (**a**) diagnosed by computed tomography angiography; (**b**) aneurysm indicated by arrow. (**c**) Scheduled arterial reconstruction being performed with autologous vein grafting

These late presentations of peripheral injuries may lead to progressive swelling, having pressure effects on the surrounding structures, and even life- and limb-threatening complications, such as thromboembolism, compartment syndrome, limb ischemia, and rupture leading to catastrophic bleeding. Both PSA and AVF are clinically suspected by the mechanism of the previously sustained trauma, pulsatile mass, and thrill and murmur, even though these last two signs are more intense in AF fistulas.

Diagnosis can be reliably confirmed by DUS and CTA. Nowadays, CA is usually performed as a component of endovascular treatment via therapeutic embolization or stent-graft deployment. Open surgical treatment may consist of resectioning and end-to-end anastomosis or reconstruction with autogenous venous grafting. For selected cases, excision with ligation of the involved vessels can be performed, depending on the territory and collateral circulation.

> **Dos and Don'ts**
>
> **Dos**
> - Stop external hemorrhage first.
> - Have a high (indexed) suspicion of vascular injury in cases of penetrating or high-energy blunt trauma.
> - Proceed with additional diagnostic tests if in doubt. Duplex ultrasonography and CT angiography are good choices.
> - Repeatedly check peripheral pulses 24 h after reconstruction.
> - Consider using objective scores as a screening tool to make a decision about limb salvage or amputation.
> - Always think of increasing the role of endovascular interventions in trauma.
> - Consider temporary proximal balloon occlusion instead of open extended exposure and clamping.
> - Temporary shunting is a good option for temporary restoration of limb perfusion.
> - Monitor for compartment syndrome and liberally use fasciotomy if indicated.
>
> **Don'ts**
> - Do not explore enlarging/pulsating hematoma without proximal arterial control in virgin territory.
> - Do not release a tourniquet if signs of irreversible ischemia have developed. Proceed with amputation.
> - Do not try to suture vessels when antegrade and retrograde flow is not achieved.
> - Do not do vascular repair with tension; consider autologous vein grafting if in doubt.
> - Do not fix orthopedic fractures before restoring perfusion in threatened ischemia.

> **Take-Home Messages**
> - Peripheral vascular injuries represent the majority of vascular injuries and lead to high mortality and morbidity due to exsanguination and limb ischemia.
> - A simple-to-complex diagnostic approach—structured physical examination, Doppler ultrasonography, and computed tomography angiography—minimizes the risk of missing vascular injuries.
> - Degree of limb ischemia and hemodynamic stability are key factors in defining a treatment strategy.
> - Open surgery remains the gold standard for the treatment of peripheral vascular injuries, but endovascular and hybrid techniques have huge potential.
> - Temporary shunting is a viable option for unstable patients, for severe orthopedic/soft tissue trauma, and in case of limited resources.

## Ten Questions

1. A patient arrives on your shift 6 h after sustaining a shot wound to the right thigh. There is gushing bleeding and no distal pulses; blood pressure is 60/40 mmHg, and heart rate is 140 bpm. During surgical exploration, a partial transection of the femoral artery and vein is found. Your best choice is to perform:
   A. Arterial bypass and venous ligation.
   B. Arterial bypass, venous ligation and leg fasciotomies.
   C. **Arterial and venous temporary shunts, and leg fasciotomies**.
   D. Arterial and venous temporary shunts.

2. A patient has sustained a stab wound to the external side of the thigh. He presents to the hospital with a pulsatile hematoma and normal distal pulses; his blood pressure is 110/70 mmHg, and his heart rate is 110 bpm. An angio-CT confirms a profunda femoral artery's branch pseudoaneurysm. Your best choice is to perform:
   A. Open surgical exploration and ligation.
   B. Open surgical exploration and bypass.
   C. Endovascular treatment by stent-graft deployment.
   D. **Endovascular treatment by coil embolization**.

3. You are treating a patient who was a victim of a stab wound to the left axilla 40 min ago. The patient arrives with pulsatile bleeding and a diminished (but palpable) radial pulse. Temporary hemostasis is obtained at the ER by placing a Foley catheter through the wound; there are no other injuries, and the patient is still hemodynamically stable. A strategy that should be considered prior to exploring the injury site is to:
   A. **Perform an angiography using a femoral approach and place a balloon catheter on the distal subclavian artery for proximal vascular control**.
   B. Perform a transbrachial retrograde artery cannulation for proximal vascular control.
   C. Perform forearm fasciotomy due to the high risk of compartmental syndrome.
   D. Perform an angio-CT.

4. Key in deciding between a limb salvage attempt by vascular reconstruction or a primary limb amputation is/are:
   A. Time elapsed from injury.
   B. **Degree of limb ischemia and hemodynamic stability**.
   C. The presence of associated arterial and venous injuries.
   D. The presence of associated bone fractures.

5. A good candidate for nonoperative treatment would be a patient presenting:
   A. A brachial pseudoaneurysm detected by angio-CT.
   B. An arteriovenous fistula between femoral vessels found on a conventional angiography.
   C. **An anterior tibial artery occlusion detected by angio-CT on a patient sustaining a tibial fracture**.
   D. A biphasic pedal waveform on Doppler examination after a knee dislocation.

6. A patient suffering from a gunshot wound to a mid-upper arm is admitted to your hospital 3 h after the injury with a tourniquet applied at the scene. Neither active nor passive movements by the affected limb are noted. An optimal strategy would be:
   A. Immediate tourniquet removal and vascular exposure.
   B. Tourniquet removal followed by angio-CT to evaluate a zone of injury.

C. Subclavian artery access for proximal arterial control, followed by tourniquet removal and vascular reconstruction.
D. **Early amputation below the tourniquet**.

7. After stent-graft placement into a superficial femoral artery in a patient having associated traumatic brain injury with intracranial hematoma, the following anticoagulation therapy is required:
   A. **No anticoagulation**.
   B. Dual antiplatelet therapy.
   C. Unfractioned heparin under control of activated partial thromboplastin time.
   D. Low-molecular weight heparin if no decompressive craniotomy required.

8. A military surgeon with limited vascular experience and expertise is taking a casualty with a deeply ischemic leg into an operation room. Your advice for him would be:
   A. Perform fasciotomy first.
   B. Harvest the great saphenous vein and perform definitive arterial reconstruction.
   C. **Achieve proximal control, put in a shunt, and evacuate the patient**.
   D. Administer systemic heparin and evacuate the patient.

9. After completion of vascular reconstruction, you see that distal pulses are weak. The next step would be:
   A. **Check and correct anastomosis**.
   B. Leave it. It is due to a temporary spasm.
   C. Transport the patient to a tertiary trauma center.
   D. Perform angiography and stent-grafting.

10. An unstable patient with pelvic fractures has an associated external iliac artery occlusion with severe limb ischemia. In addition to orthopedic surgery, you would perform:
    A. Nonoperative management.
    B. Laparotomy for proximal control, open exposure, and complex arterial reconstruction.
    C. **Femoral-femoral bypass**.
    D. Contralateral femoral access, recanalization of the lesion followed by stent-graft implantation.

# References

1. Barmparas G, Inaba K, Talving P, David J-S, Lam L, Plurad D, et al. Pediatric vs adult vascular trauma: a National Trauma Databank review. J Pediatr Surg. 2010;45(7):1404–12.
2. Branco BC, DuBose JJ, Zhan LX, Hughes JD, Goshima KR, Rhee P, et al. Trends and outcomes of endovascular therapy in the management of civilian vascular injuries. J Vasc Surg. 2014;60(5):1297–307, 1307.e1.
3. Konstantinidis A, Inaba K, Dubose J, Barmparas G, Lam L, Plurad D, et al. Vascular trauma in geriatric patients: a national trauma databank review. J Trauma. 2011;71(4):909–16.
4. Perkins ZB, De'Ath HD, Aylwin C, Brohi K, Walsh M, Tai NRM. Epidemiology and outcome of vascular trauma at a British Major Trauma Centre. Eur J Vasc Endovasc Surg. 2012;44(2):203–9.
5. Rasmussen TE, Clouse WD, Jenkins DH, Peck MA, Eliason JL, Smith DL. The use of temporary vascular shunts as a damage control adjunct in the management of wartime vascular injury. J Trauma. 2006;61(1):8–12; discussion 12–5.
6. White JM, Stannard A, Burkhardt GE, Eastridge BJ, Blackbourne LH, Rasmussen TE. The epidemiology of vascular injury in the wars in Iraq and Afghanistan. Ann Surg. 2011;253(6):1184–9.
7. Patel JA, White JM, White PW, Rich NM, Rasmussen TE. A contemporary, 7-year analysis of vascular injury from the war in Afghanistan. J Vasc Surg. 2018;68(6):1872–9.

8. Markov NP, DuBose JJ, Scott D, Propper BW, Clouse WD, Thompson B, et al. Anatomic distribution and mortality of arterial injury in the wars in Afghanistan and Iraq with comparison to a civilian benchmark. J Vasc Surg. 2012;56(3):728–36.
9. DuBose JJ, Savage SA, Fabian TC, Menaker J, Scalea T, Holcomb JB, et al. The American Association for the Surgery of Trauma PROspective Observational Vascular Injury Treatment (PROOVIT) registry: multicenter data on modern vascular injury diagnosis, management, and outcomes. J Trauma Acute Care Surg. 2015;78(2):215–22; discussion 222–3.
10. Góes Junior AMO, Simões Neto JFA, Abib SCV, de Andrade MC, Ferraz TC. Vascular trauma in the Amazon: updating the challenge. Rev Col Bras Cir. 2018;45(4):e1844.
11. Kobayashi L, Coimbra R, Goes AMO, Reva V, Santorelli J, Moore EE, et al. American Association for the Surgery of Trauma-World Society of Emergency Surgery guidelines on diagnosis and management of peripheral vascular injuries. J Trauma Acute Care Surg. 2020;89(6):1183–96.
12. Tan T-W, Joglar FL, Hamburg NM, Eberhardt RT, Shaw PM, Rybin D, et al. Limb outcome and mortality in lower and upper extremity arterial injury: a comparison using the National Trauma Data Bank. Vasc Endovasc Surg. 2011;45(7):592–7.
13. Franz RW, Skytta CK, Shah KJ, Hartman JF, Wright ML. A five-year review of management of upper-extremity arterial injuries at an urban level I trauma center. Ann Vasc Surg. 2012;26(5):655–64.
14. Kauvar DS, Sarfati MR, Kraiss LW. National trauma databank analysis of mortality and limb loss in isolated lower extremity vascular trauma. J Vasc Surg. 2011;53(6):1598–603.
15. Brusov PG, Nikolenko VK. Experience of treating gunshot wounds of large vessels in Afghanistan. World J Surg. 2005;29(Suppl 1):S25–9.
16. Woodward EB, Clouse WD, Eliason JL, Peck MA, Bowser AN, Cox MW, et al. Penetrating femoropopliteal injury during modern warfare: experience of the Balad Vascular Registry. J Vasc Surg. 2008;47(6):1259–64; discussion 1264–5.
17. Franz RW, Shah KJ, Halaharvi D, Franz ET, Hartman JF, Wright ML. A 5-year review of management of lower extremity arterial injuries at an urban level I trauma center. J Vasc Surg. 2011;53(6):1604–10.
18. Branco BC, Naik-Mathuria B, Montero-Baker M, Gilani R, West CA, Mills JL, et al. Increasing use of endovascular therapy in pediatric arterial trauma. J Vasc Surg. 2017;66(4):1175–1183.e1.
19. Jaipuria J, Sagar S, Singhal M, Bagdia A, Gupta A, Kumar S, et al. Paediatric extremity vascular injuries - experience from a large urban trauma centre in India. Injury. 2014;45(1):176–82.
20. Sciarretta JD, Macedo FIB, Otero CA, Figueroa JN, Pizano LR, Namias N. Management of traumatic popliteal vascular injuries in a level I trauma center: a 6-year experience. Int J Surg Lond Engl. 2015;18:136–41.
21. Rozycki GS, Tremblay LN, Feliciano DV, McClelland WB. Blunt vascular trauma in the extremity: diagnosis, management, and outcome. J Trauma. 2003;55(5):814–24.
22. Topal AE, Eren MN, Celik Y. Lower extremity arterial injuries over a six-year period: outcomes, risk factors, and management. Vasc Health Risk Manag. 2010;3(6):1103–10.
23. Liang NL, Alarcon LH, Jeyabalan G, Avgerinos ED, Makaroun MS, Chaer RA. Contemporary outcomes of civilian lower extremity arterial trauma. J Vasc Surg. 2016;64(3):731–6.
24. Biffl WL, Moore EE, Offner PJ, Brega KE, Franciose RJ, Burch JM. Blunt carotid arterial injuries: implications of a new grading scale. J Trauma. 1999;47(5):845–53.
25. Kornilov V. Surgical approach and techniques in major vascular trauma at staged military care. Leningrad: Kirov Military Medical Academy; 1971.
26. Rutherford RB, Baker JD, Ernst C, Johnston KW, Porter JM, Ahn S, et al. Recommended standards for reports dealing with lower extremity ischemia: revised version. J Vasc Surg. 1997;26(3):517–38.
27. Alarhayem AQ, Cohn SM, Cantu-Nunez O, Eastridge BJ, Rasmussen TE. Impact of time to repair on outcomes in patients with lower extremity arterial injuries. J Vasc Surg. 2019;69(5):1519–23.
28. Kauvar DS, Miller D, Walters TJ. Tourniquet use is not associated with limb loss following military lower extremity arterial trauma. J Trauma Acute Care Surg. 2018;85(3):495–9.
29. Inaba K, Branco BC, Reddy S, Park JJ, Green D, Plurad D, et al. Prospective evaluation of multidetector computed tomography for extremity vascular trauma. J Trauma. 2011;70(4):808–15.
30. deSouza IS, Benabbas R, McKee S, Zangbar B, Jain A, Paladino L, et al. Accuracy of physical examination, ankle-brachial index, and ultrasonography in the diagnosis of arterial injury in patients with penetrating extremity trauma: a systematic review and meta-analysis. Acad Emerg Med. 2017;24(8):994–1017.
31. Romagnoli AN, DuBose J, Dua A, Betzold R, Bee T, Fabian T, et al. Hard signs gone soft: a critical evaluation of presenting signs of extremity vascular injury. J Trauma Acute Care Surg. 2021;90(1):1–10.
32. Levy BA, Zlowodzki MP, Graves M, Cole PA. Screening for extremity arterial injury with the arterial pressure index. Am J Emerg Med. 2005;23(5):689–95.
33. Barnes CJ, Pietrobon R, Higgins LD. Does the pulse examination in patients with traumatic knee dislocation predict a surgical arterial injury? A meta-analysis. J Trauma. 2002;53(6):1109–14.
34. Montorfano MA, Montorfano LM, Perez Quirante F, Rodríguez F, Vera L, Neri L. The FAST D protocol: a simple method to rule out traumatic vascular injuries of the lower extremities. Crit Ultrasound J. 2017;9(1):8.
35. Callcut RA, Mell MW. Modern advances in vascular trauma. Surg Clin North Am. 2013;93(4):941–61, ix.

36. Degmetich S, Brenner M, Firek M, Zakhary B, Coimbra BC, Coimbra R. Endovascular repair is a feasible option for superficial femoral artery injuries: a comparative effectiveness analysis. Eur J Trauma Emerg Surg. 2022;48(1):321–8.
37. Reva VA, Madurska M, Samokhvalov I, Denisov A, Telickiy S, Seleznev A, et al. The role of endovascular stents in an experimental model of traumatic arterial occlusion – the temporary endo-shunt. J Endovasc Resusc Trauma Manag 2020 Apr 7 [cited 2021 Apr 30];4(1). https://journal.jevtm.com/index.php/jevtm/article/view/116.
38. DuBose JJ, Rajani R, Gilani R, Arthurs ZA, Morrison JJ, Clouse WD, et al. Endovascular management of axillo-subclavian arterial injury: a review of published experience. Injury. 2012;43(11):1785–92.
39. Rohlffs F, Larena-Avellaneda AA, Petersen JP, Debus ES, Kölbel T. Through-and-through wire technique for endovascular damage control in traumatic proximal axillary artery transection. Vascular. 2015;23(1):99–101.
40. Angus LDG, Gerber N, Munnangi S, Wallace R, Singh S, Digiacomo J. Management and outcomes of isolated axillary artery injury: a five-year national trauma data bank analysis. Ann Vasc Surg. 2020;65:113–23.
41. Hörer T. Resuscitative endovascular balloon occlusion of the aorta (REBOA) and endovascular resuscitation and trauma management (EVTM): a paradigm shift regarding hemodynamic instability. Eur J Trauma Emerg Surg. 2018;44(4):487–9.
42. Davidson AJ, Neff LP, DuBose JJ, Sampson JB, Abbot CM, Williams TK. Direct-site endovascular repair (DSER): a novel approach to vascular trauma. J Trauma Acute Care Surg. 2016;81(5 Suppl 2 Proceedings of the 2015 Military Health System Research Symposium):S138–43.
43. Pereira BMT, Chiara O, Ramponi F, Weber DG, Cimbanassi S, De Simone B, et al. WSES position paper on vascular emergency surgery. World J Emerg Surg. 2015;10:49.
44. Asensio JA, Kessler JJ, Miljkovic SS, Kotaru TR, Dabestani PJ, Kalamchi LD, et al. Brachial artery injuries operative management and predictors of outcome. Ann Vasc Surg. 2020;69:146–57.
45. Lang NW, Joestl JB, Platzer P. Characteristics and clinical outcome in patients after popliteal artery injury. J Vasc Surg. 2015;61(6):1495–500.
46. Ratnayake A, Samarasinghe B, Bala M. Outcomes of popliteal vascular injuries at Sri Lankan war-front military hospital: case series of 44 cases. Injury. 2014;45(5):879–84.
47. Gopinathan NR, Santhanam SS, Saibaba B, Dhillon MS. Epidemiology of lower limb musculoskeletal trauma with associated vascular injuries in a tertiary care institute in India. Indian J Orthop. 2017;51(2):199–204.
48. Branco BC, Linnebur M, Boutrous ML, Leake SS, Inaba K, Charlton-Ouw KM, et al. The predictive value of multidetector CTA on outcomes in patients with below-the-knee vascular injury. Injury. 2015;46(8):1520–6.
49. Asensio JA, Dabestani PJ, Miljkovic SS, Kotaru TR, Kessler JJ, Kalamchi LD, et al. Popliteal artery injuries. Less ischemic time may lead to improved outcomes. Injury. 2020;51(11):2524–31.
50. O'Banion LA, Dirks R, Farooqui E, Saldana-Ruiz N, Yoon WJ, Pozolo C, et al. Popliteal scoring assessment for vascular extremity injuries in trauma study. J Vasc Surg. 2021;74(3):804–813.e3.

## Further Reading

Hörer T, Rasmussen TE, DuBose JJ, White JM, editors. Endovascular resuscitation and trauma management – EVTM. Springer; 2020. 442 p

Kobayashi L, Coimbra R, Goes AMO, Reva V, Santorelli J, Moore EE, et al. American Association for the Surgery of Trauma-World Society of Emergency Surgery guidelines on diagnosis and management of peripheral vascular injuries. J Trauma Acute Care Surg. 2020;89(6):1183–96.

Pereira BMT, Chiara O, Ramponi F, Weber DG, Cimbanassi S, De Simone B, et al. WSES position paper on vascular emergency surgery. World J Emerg Surg. 2015;10:49.

Rasmussen TE, Tai NRM, editors. Rich's vascular trauma. 3rd ed. Elsevier; 2016. 368 p

Trio Tryck AB. Top Stent: the art of endovascular hybrid trauma and bleeding management. Orebro University Hospital; 2017. 220 p

# Extremities Trauma 109

Ingo Marzi, Cora Rebecca Schindler, and Philipp Störmann

## 109.1 Introduction

The extent of extremity trauma ranges from minor injuries that can be difficult to diagnose to complex fractures and extensive soft tissue damage. They can become a vital threat whether the injury occurs as an isolated trauma or in the context of multiple injuries. Many fractures and soft tissue injuries require time-critical interventions to the ensure rescue of the extremity and the best functional outcome. Efficient therapy is essential to redress functional deficit and pain and to regain mobility and quality of life as soon as possible.

> **Learning Goals**
> - Assessment and management of extremity trauma in acute care
> - Surgical emergency indications and procedures
> - Handling of extremity trauma in multiple injured patients

Extremity trauma is defined as an injury to one or more functional components (bones, nerves, vessels, soft tissue) of the limb. In Anglo-American terminology, a severe limb injury occurs when three of the four functional components are affected and the preservation of the functional limb is at risk [1, 2].

### 109.1.1 Epidemiology

Extremity trauma is common, with an annual incidence of 981 per 100,000 per year. In Germany, due to extremity injuries, in 2019, 861,973 patients were hospitalized [3]. Traffic, work, and domestic accidents, as well as falls, sport-related accidents, and violence, are the leading causes of extremity trauma. High-impact injuries and sports accidents are more likely to affect healthy, physically active adults. The most common isolated injuries are fractures of the distal forearm and lower leg in 20- to 60-year-olds (incidence 17–25%) [4]. The prevalence of extremity injuries in patients with multiple trauma exceeds 50% and mainly involves the femur (16.5%) and the tibia (12.6%), followed by radius fractures (9.9%) [2, 5].

Due to demographic change, the incidence of fractures increases after the age of 65, largely related to comorbidities (e.g., cardiovascular disease, gait instability, or osteoporosis) [6]. The leading accident mechanism in patients older

I. Marzi (✉) · C. R. Schindler · P. Störmann
Department of Trauma-, Hand and Reconstructive Surgery, University Hospital Frankfurt,
Frankfurt am Main, Germany
e-mail: marzi@trauma.uni-frankfurt.de;
ingo.marzi@kgu.de; cora.schindler@kgu.de;
philipp.stoermann@kgu.de

© The Author(s), under exclusive license to Springer Nature Switzerland AG 2023
F. Coccolini, F. Catena (eds.), *Textbook of Emergency General Surgery*,
https://doi.org/10.1007/978-3-031-22599-4_109

than 65 years of age is a fall from lower height, which is closely related to isolated limb fractures, particularly of the (proximal) femur, humerus, and radius [7].

Amputation injuries are rare (0.2–1%) and mainly occur on fingers and the distal lower extremity in patients between 20 and 40 years of age in work (68%) and traffic accidents (18%) [8]. However, direct vessel injuries and bleeding from muscle and soft tissue damage might result in an acute, life-threatening hemorrhage.

### 109.1.2 Classification

The *Arbeitsgemeinschaft für Osteosynthesefragen* (AO) classification of the long tubular bones was published in 1987 by *Müller* et al. and later supplemented by the AO. It represents the international standard for the classification of fractures. Diagnostic imaging is required for exact AO classification. The affected bone, location within the bone, fracture type, and joint involvement result in an alphanumeric code that classifies the complexity and severity of the fracture [9]. In addition, a module for soft tissue injury classification has been developed. To date, modern fracture treatment and guideline development are largely based on the 2018 version of the AO Fracture and Dislocation Compendium, among others [10].

The classification according to *Tscherne* and *Oestern* is a standardized grading of soft tissue injuries based on severity in open and closed fractures or dislocations (Table 109.1) [11]. The *Gustilo-Anderson* classification (Table 109.2) is used internationally to classify open fractures and focuses on a more precise description of soft tissue conditions. Using the subtypes, a more accurate assessment of the risk of complications can be made [12]. Both classifications are used for diagnostic and treatment management as well as for estimating the risk of complications and the chances of recovery.

The Abbreviated Injury Scale (AIS) was introduced in 1969 by the Association for the Advancement of Automotive Medicine. It evaluates the severity of injuries in terms of their lethality risk. Due to its complexity, the AIS is used less in clinical practice than in science and quality assessment. It also provides the basis for scoring multiple injuries using the Injury Severity Score (ISS) or the New Injury Severity Score (NISS) [13]. The consensus of international publications defines an severe extremity trauma with AIS $\geq 3$ points [5].

**Table 109.1** Oestern and Tscherne Classification for closed fractures

| | |
|---|---|
| Grade 0 | Indirect injury with simple fracture pattern Minor soft tissue damage |
| Grade I | Simple to moderate fracture pattern Superficial skin abrasion and contusion |
| Grade II | Moderate to severe fracture pattern Deep (contaminated) abrasion, direct muscle/skin contusion impending compartment syndrome |
| Grade III | Severe fracture type Extensive skin and muscle contusion, severe contamination, subcutaneous décollement Rupture of major blood vessel or nerve Decompensated compartment syndrome |

Tscherne H, Oestern HJ: Pathophysiology and classification of soft tissue injuries associated with fractures. In: Fractures with soft tissue injuries. Tscherne H, Gotzen L.: Berlin; Springer Verlag (1984), S. 1–9

### 109.1.3 Pathophysiology

In extremity trauma, the integrity of all four functional components of the limb (bones, nerves, vessels, soft tissue) can be compromised. Traumatic fractures are caused by a direct or indirect force that exceeds the elasticity of the bone. Traumatic joint dislocation (luxation) is a complete displacement of the joint surface and often associated with the rupture of ligaments and the capsule of the joint. Luxation fractures are defined as simultaneous dislocation and fracture at a joint, as often occures in the ankle, for example. Fractures and luxations can be either closed, without injury to the overlying skin, or open (see Tables 109.1 and 109.2) [14]. In open fractures, pathogenic bacteria can enter the wound and bone from outside, so that these injuries have an increased risk of wound infection and osteitis [15]. Depending on the location of the injury, there may be relevant blood loss of up

**Table 109.2** Gustilo-Anderson classification for open fractures

|  | Type I | Type II | Type III | Type IIIB | Type IIIC |
|---|---|---|---|---|---|
| Energy impact | Low | Moderate | High | | |
| Wound size | <1 cm | 1–10 cm | >10 cm | | |
| Soft tissue damage | Minimal | Moderate | Extensive | | |
| Contamination | Clean | Minimal/moderate | Extensive | | |
| Fracture pattern | Single fracture with minimal comminution | Simple/minimal segmental fracture | Severe comminution and segmental fracture | | |
| Periosteal stripping | No | No | No | Yes | |
| Local skin coverage | Adequate soft tissue cover | | Adequate | Inadequate soft tissue cover—requiring tissue flap | |
| Neurovascular injury | No | | No | No | Requiring vascular surgery/amputation |

Gustilo RB, Anderson JT. Prevention of infection in the treatment of one thousand and twenty-five open fractures of long bones: Retrospective and prospective analyses. J Bone Joint Surg Am. 1976;58:453–8

to 2000 mL caused by a vascular rupture in the soft tissues or the fracture itself [14, 16].

Example of blood loss (up to):

- Femur: 2000 mL
- Tibia: 1000 mL
- Humerus: 800 mL
- Forearm: 400 mL

Isolated (direct) and concomitant (e.g., humerus fracture) peripheral nerve injuries are a significant cause of morbidity and disability but affect only about 2% of all trauma patients [17].

Décollement is a severe soft tissue damage caused by tangential shear injury of the epidermis, dermis, and possibly subcutis (e.g., in collision or run-over injuries). The uninjured epidermis is detached from its physical base over a substantial area, along with the dermis, subcutis, and supplying blood vessels [18]. Detached flaps of skin and soft tissue are at high risk of necrosis and severe infections.

Acute compartment syndrome most commonly occurs after a closed fracture of long tubular bones (p.e. tibia, Femur) or crush injury to the extremity. In fractures or after reperfusion following ischaemia, the volume within the myofascial compartment increases due to the accumulation of blood and other tissue fluids, the volume within the myofascial compartment increases due to the accumulation of blood and other tissue fluids. The increase in volume leads to increased pressure within the inelastic muscle fascia or compartment. This pressure on the capillary bed and thin-walled venous system leads to ischaemia, severe pain and nerve paralysis. This pressure on the capillary bed and thin-walled venous system can lead to irreversible ischaemic and mechanical damage to the myoneural tissue within the affected compartment [19].

## 109.2 Diagnosis

### 109.2.1 Clinical Presentation

The clinical presentation depends on the type and severity of the injury. Blood loss in closed injuries is often underestimated; it can be up to 2000 mL (femur). First and foremost, attention to symptoms that signal a threat to vital functions should be obtained (shock signs, state of consciousness). Isolated trauma to an extremity should be directly addressed and focused on for diagnosis. If the patient suffers from multiple injuries, the basic principle is that the most threatening injuries and disturbances of the patient's vital functions must be recognized and treated quickly. The first diagnostic phase ("primary survey") is prioritized (ABCDE algorithm, ATLS®) with the goal of identifying potentially fatal injuries [20, 21]. In the secondary survey, all relevant injuries and diseases are diagnosed, and additional imaging techniques (for example, X-ray, computed tomography (CT)) are used [14].

The following points are particularly important for the clinical examination:

- Mechanism of accident (low- vs. high-energy trauma)
- General condition of the patient (e.g., signs of shock or bleeding)
- Isolated or multiple injuries (primary survey/ABCDE algorithm)
- Pain (localization and intensity)
- Malposition or unstable limb/joint
- Soft tissue damage (i.e., hematoma, wounds, open fractures)
- Peripheral pulses, sensibility, and motor function (e.g., skin color, temperature, paresthesia)
- Indirect fracture signs (e.g., contusion mark, swelling)
- Signs of compartment syndrome (intense pain, tightness of muscle, tingling/burning sensation)

Depending on the suspected diagnosis, there are plenty of specific clinical examinations of the limb function (e.g., "Jobe test" for suspected rupture of the supraspinatus tendon) (see handbooks of orthopaedic trauma).

## 109.2.2 Tests

### 109.2.2.1 Radiological Examination

Following clinical examination, radiological imaging is the standard procedure in the diagnostics of extremity injuries. Conventional radiography (always min. two planes) is both inexpensive and sensitive and therefore the method of choice. Other imaging techniques, such as computed tomography (CT) and magnetic resonance imaging (MRI), are used secondarily, e.g., to validate a suspected fracture, to balance injury severity, or to evaluate a soft tissue injury, e.g., vessels, nerves, or ligaments. Above all, they are used for further therapy and surgery planning. Sonography is easily available and efficient. It plays a role primarily in the acute diagnosis of soft tissue injuries (e.g. haematoma, ligaments), but can also be used for fracture imaging if necessary [22]. Radiological vascular imaging should be indicated generously, if necessary, as part of the imaging, especially for dislocations of large joints (knee) and extensive soft tissue injuries (grade II + III according to *Oestern and Tscherne*, grade III + IV according to *Gustillo-Anderson*) [23].

In addition, there are various apparative tools such as Doppler sonography to verify peripheral blood flow or intramuscular pressure (IMP) measurement to monitor impending compartment syndrome [19, 23].

### 109.2.2.2 Laboratory Tests

Blood tests should be performed, especially in cases of severe extremity injuries. First and foremost, parameters that indicate hemorrhage or ischemia (hemoglobin, hematocrit, lactate, coagulation parameters, electrolytes) should be monitored. Specific markers such as creatine kinase, myoglobin, D-dimers, creatinine, and uric acid provide additional indication of the severity of injury and may be important in preventing secondary damage (rhabdomyolysis, "crush kidney"). Urine tests (sediment, pH) can complement the findings.

> **Differential Diagnosis**
> The differential diagnoses of extremity trauma, such as contusion vs. fracture or soft tissue injury vs. open fracture, can be easily and quickly ruled out by imaging techniques (X-ray). A CT (CT angio for vascular injury) or MRI (ligaments, musculature) can provide definitive information. If there is any doubt about the relevance of a vascular/nerve lesion, surgical exploration must be performed. Important in the diagnosis and treatment of extremity injuries, especially multiple injuries, is the rapid and correct assessment of the injury severity and need for treatment to avoid an acute life-threatening situation or consequential damage because of misalignment, ischemia or nerve lesions.

## 109.3 Treatment

The treatment intentions for extremity injuries are to regain organ function to maintain mobility, quality of life, and return to work. Generally, treatment depends on the severity and location of the injury as well as the presence of associated injuries.

### 109.3.1 Surgical Treatment

#### 109.3.1.1 Factures and Luxation

Early repositioning and immobilization of the fracture are essential to avoid secondary damage to surrounding tissues such as cartilage, nerves, and vessels and to prevent complications. Initial testing of peripheral perfusion, motor function, and sensitivity is crucial. To decompress potentially compromised soft tissues, repositioning is usually performed with longitudinal traction of the limb and axial alignment. Except for ankle and distal radius fractures, adjacent joints should be included in immobilization whenever possible. The aim is to achieve a physiologically neutral position.

Luxations are also often accompanied by severe injury to the stabilizing ligaments (e.g., rupture of radial and ulnar collateral ligaments after elbow dislocation) with a persistent re-dislocation tendency that can only be fixed by surgical reconstruction. Special care should be taken with knee dislocations, which are often associated with severe nerve and vascular damage and require surgical intervention with vascular reconstruction. Talus dislocation fractures are rare but severe injuries. Because of its physiologic reduced blood flow, a relevant perfusion deficit is rapidly present, making salvage of the talus often difficult.

After repositioning and splinting, re-evaluation of peripheral circulation, motor function, and sensibility is obligatory.

Stable fractures can be primarily splinted and surgically treated in the course of consolidation of the soft tissues (5–7 days) by osteosynthesis.

The type of surgical treatment and the priority of care depend largely on the general condition of the patient and the soft tissue condition of the extremity. It ranges from early total care (ETC) with primary definitive treatment to damage control surgery (DCS; Fig. 109.1) with primary stabilization of the limb by an external fixator. For severely dislocated, unstable, or open fractures in grade III, surgical reduction and stabilization are required to prevent major bleeding and soft tissue or joint damage caused by perfusion deficit and compartment syndrome. The gold standard in DCS treatment is the use of an external fixator. In this case, the definitive osteosynthesis can be performed after the consolidation of the affected soft tissue after 5–7 days [24–27].

Open wounds and fractures should be covered sterilely until surgery to reduce the risk of wound infection and subsequent osteomyelitis. Bleeding can be stopped by elevation of the limb and compression. The bleeding vessel must be compressed proximally by applying a pressure pad and bandage. Tourniquets that completely cut off the blood flow are only used in exceptional life-threatening situations such as massive blood loss in multiple trauma. They are applied as proximal as necessary and as distal as possible. Caution: they can cause bruising and severe soft tissue damage.

Major open soft tissue injuries should be consistently debrided and temporarily covered, e.g., with vacuum seals.

Cave: Closed soft tissue injuries are frequent underestimated. Especially in the case of décollement or covered vascular ruptures, they can be associated with massive blood loss and severe damage to surrounding tissues. That may lead to hemodynamic instability or secondary necrosis with increased risk of infections.

#### 109.3.1.2 Amputation

A distinction is made between major and minor amputations. These primarily relate to the muscle mass contained within the amputate, which is most sensitive to anoxemia (the period between the complete interruption of blood flow and restoration of the first arterial vessel anastomosis). The duration of anoxemia affects primary healing as well as subsequent regained functionality of the replanted limb. For macro-replantations, the

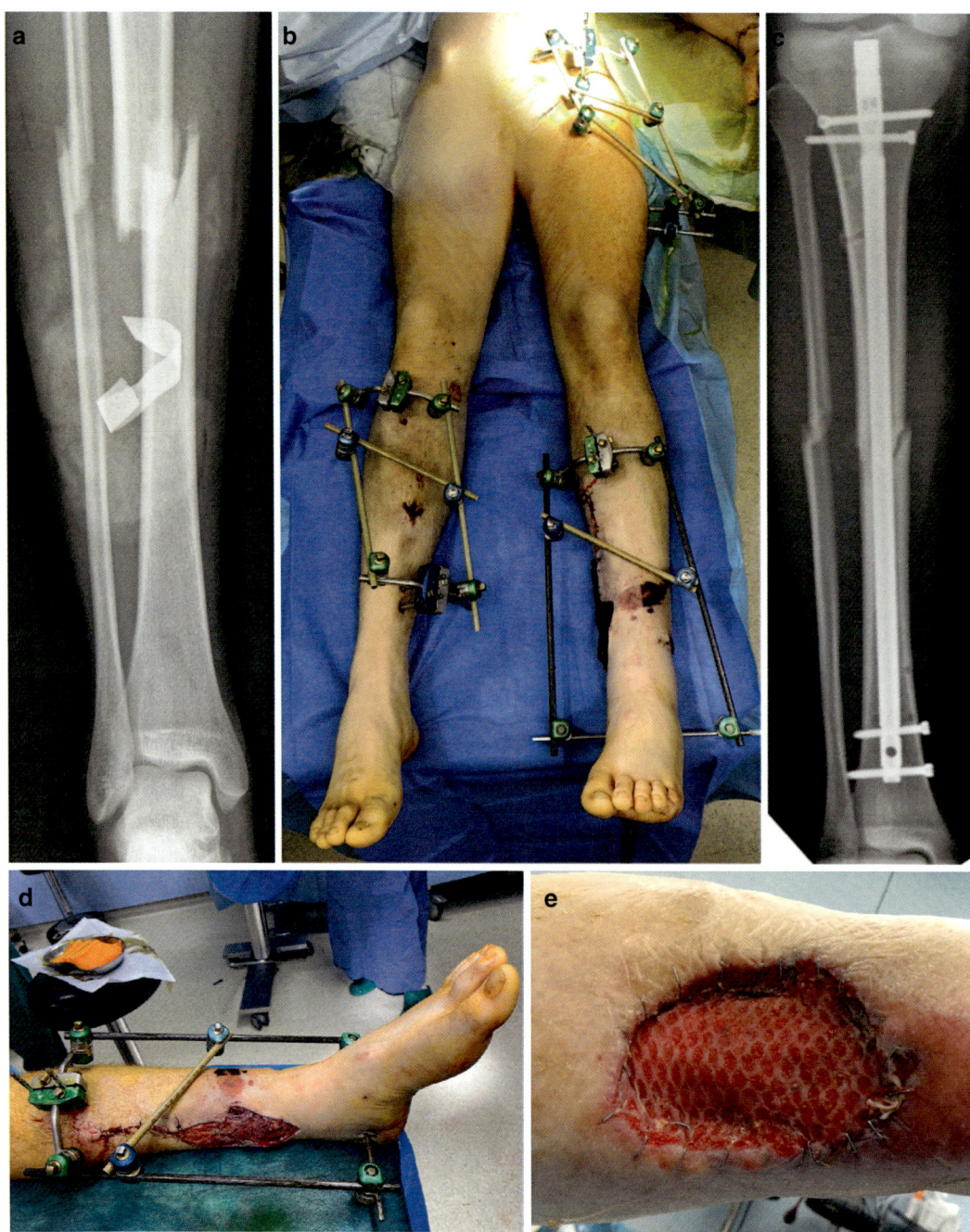

**Fig. 109.1** Twenty-six-year-old motorcyclist crashed into a car and suffered multiple extremities trauma (**a**–**e**). After primary survey with central venous cannulation, invasive blood pressure monitoring, volume therapy, single shot antibiotics and a booster tetanus vaccination the patient was immediately taken to the OR for Damage Control Surgery. Stabilization of the unstable and open fractures (**a**) was performed by external fixators (**b**). After vital stabilization and soft tissue consolidation, successive definitive treatment of the extremity injuries was initiated, e.g. intramedullary stabilisazion of the tibia (**c**). The soft tissue defects like 3° open tibia fracture (**d**) were treated with vacuum seals and finally covered by plastic surgery with skin grafting (**e**)

maximum tolerable anoxemia period is assumed to be 4–6 h. Proximal major amputations may lead to ischemia-reperfusion syndrome, which may be life-threatening for the patient. In addition, the mechanisms of injury leading to proximal amputations are usually characterized by high impact. For all replantations, clear-cut replantations might be possible in stable patients, but crush and pull-out injuries are usually not possible to replant; both for minor and major amputations. For micro-replantations, the anoxemia interval is approximately 15 h. Minor amputations include all amputations of the hand and foot up to just proximal to the wrist or ankle. The thumb is an urgent indication for replantation due to its crucial functional importance.

In incomplete amputations, preoperative cooling should be avoided to preserve residual blood flow. Immobilization by splinting is indicated to avoid tearing of the tissue section [28, 29].

### 109.3.1.3 Extremities Trauma in Multiple Injured Patients

In polytrauma, the treatment of life-threatening injuries and efficient stabilization of the patient in the first hours after trauma are the priorities ("treat first what kills first"). The priority and timing of treatment are based on the severity of the injury and its importance to the patient's overall condition. Treatment of unstable and open fractures with an external fixator (DCS) is the method of choice [16, 24, 25, 30].

The timing of secondary care for the extremities in polytrauma should be carefully considered. In the first days after trauma, major surgical procedures, e.g., femur nailing, can cause a "second hit" (inflammatory immune response) [24]. To avoid missed injuries, a second survey is mandatory.

### 109.3.2 Medical Treatment

It is important to provide the injured patient with adequate analgesia to avoid pain, stress, and the development of chronic regional pain syndrome (CRPS).

If there are signs of major bleeding, the principles of acute shock therapy must be applied, with at least two large-lumen venous lines, volume therapy, coagulation stabilization, and circulatory support medications, if necessary.

In the presence of an open fracture, the Eastern Association for the Surgery of Trauma Guidelines (EAST Guidelines) recommend the early parenteral application of a first-generation cephalosporin (e.g., cefazolin) for osteomyelitis prophylaxis, since bacteria from the primary wound are often multisensitive. For soft tissue injuries in Gustilo grades I and II, antibiotic prophylaxis should be discontinued after 24 h. Soft tissue injuries in Gustilo grade III should be treated for at least 72 h. Tetanus protection must also be checked and refreshed if necessary.

### 109.3.3 Prognosis

Common complications after extremity trauma include functional deficits due to axial and rotational malalignment, vascular or nerve injury, early arthrosis, deficient wound healing or infection, and subsequent pseudarthrosis (non-union) [31, 32].

Prolonged immobility can lead to osteopenia and may result in fracture healing disorders or internal complications such as pneumonia, urinary tract infection, and thrombosis [22].

Large wounds, decollements, and open fractures carry a high risk of posttraumatic infections with serious sequelae such as wound healing disorders, soft tissue defects, or osteomyelitis, which may result in prolonged and complicated surgical treatment, including amputation. Often, removal of the implants, long-term antibiotic therapy, or even plastic surgery (flap) is necessary [33].

> **Dos and Don'ts**
> **Dos**
> - "Treat first what kills first".
> - Immobilize injured limbs.
> - Dress wounds and open sterile fractures.

- Replace dislocated joints and fractures immediately.
- Perform compartment monitoring for indicated injury patterns.
- Provide immediate care for extremity injuries with disruption of peripheral circulation, sensitivity, or motor function and open fractures.

**Don'ts**
- Don't lose valuable time in emergency care by focusing on less important injuries.
- Don't perform intramedullary osteosynthesis on large bones immediately after blunt chest trauma.
- Don't forget the second and tertiary surveys.

**Take-Home Messages**
- Treat first what kills first—in the case of multiple trauma.
- Prevent missed injuries: The primary survey is always followed by a second survey.
- Do not underestimate the potential loss of blood from closed extremity injuries.
- Take note of the recovery time after multiple trauma before secondary care of extremity injuries ("second hit").
- Unrelenting pain, maximum swelling, ischemia, and loss of sensation are signs of compartment syndrome.
- Dislocations and grossly dislocated fractures must always be immediately reduced and provisionally stabilized.
- Evaluation of peripheral blood flow, motor function, and sensitivity is mandatory before and after fracture/joint repositioning.
- Disruption of peripheral circulation, sensitivity, and motor function and open fractures require immediate care.
- Vascular injuries with peripheral loss of blood flow are an immediate surgical indication for primary vascular reconstruction.

**Multiple Choice Questions**
1. In ABC
   A. Extremities are A
   B. Extremities are B
   C. Extremities are C
   D. **They are not present**
2. Compartment syndrome
   A. Is characterized by the restless pain
   B. **The 5 P**
   C. Only swelling
   D. Only fever
3. Vascular reconstructions
   A. Must be performed after bone synthesis
   B. **Must be performed as soon as possible**
   C. Are not necessary
   D. Are performed by the orthopedic surgeon

## References

1. Kloen P, Prasarn ML, Helfet DL. Management of the mangled extremity. Strategies Trauma Limb Reconstr. 2012;7(2):57–66.
2. Hardy BM, King KL, Enninghorst N, Balogh ZJ. Trends in polytrauma incidence among major trauma admissions. Eur J Trauma Emerg Surg. 2022; https://doi.org/10.1007/s00068-022-02200-w.
3. Gesundheitsberichterstattung des Bundes. Diagnosedaten der Krankenhäuser ab 2000 ICD10: S40–99. 2021. https://www.gbe-bund.de/gbe/!pkg_olap_tables.prc_set_page?p_uid=gast & p_aid=83165696 & p_sprache=D & p_help=2 & p_indnr=550 & p_ansnr=83835938 & p_version=3 & D.001=1000001 & D.946=14456 & D.011=44302.
4. Meisinger C, Wildner M, Stieber J, Heier M, Sangha O, Döring A. Epidemiologie der extremitätenfrakturen. Orthopade. 2002;31(1):92–9.
5. Bläsius FM, Horst K, Hildebrand F. Inzidenz, präklinisches Management und Klassifikation schwerer Extremitätenverletzung. Notfall + Rettungsmedizin. 2020;23(6):404–11, https://doi.org/10.1007/s00068-022-02200-w.
6. de Laet CEDH, Pols HAP. Fractures in the elderly: epidemiology and demography. Best Pract Res Clin Endocrinol Metab. 2000;14(2):171–9.
7. Woolf AD. Preventing fractures in elderly people. BMJ. 2003;327(7406):89–95.
8. Friedel R. Die komplexe Handverletzung und Mikroamputationsverletzungen. In: Towfigh H, Hierner R, Langer M, Friedel R, editors. Handchirurgie. Berlin: Springer Berlin Heidelberg; 2011.

9. Müller ME, Koch P, Nazarian S, Schatzker J. The comprehensive classification of fractures of long bones. Berlin: Springer Berlin Heidelberg; 1990.
10. Meinberg E, Agel J, Roberts C, Karam M, Kellam J. Fracture and Dislocation Classification Compendium—2018. J Orthop Trauma. 2018;32(1):S1–S170.
11. Oestern H-J, Tscherne H. 148. Klassifizierung der Frakturen mit Weichteilschaden Langenbecks Arch Chir. 1982;358(1).
12. Kim PH, Leopold SS. Gustilo-Anderson classification. Clin Orthop Relat Res. 2012;470(11):3270–4.
13. Baker SP, O'Neill B, Haddon W, William BL. The Injury Severity Score. J Trauma Injury Infect Crit Care. 1974;14(3):187–96.
14. Wohlrath B, Schweigkofler U, Hoffmann R. Präklinische Versorgung von Extremitätenfrakturen und Luxationen. Notfallmedizin up2date. 2015;10(01):61–72.
15. Newton EJ. Acute complications of extremity trauma. Emerg Med Clin North Am. 2007;25:751–61.
16. Fenwick A, Pfann M, Mayr J, Antonovska I, Wiedl A, Feldmann M, Nuber S, Förch S, Mayr E. Anticoagulants and fracture morphology have a significant influence on total blood loss after proximal femur fractures. Eur J Trauma Emerg Surg. 2023;49(1):173–9. https://doi.org/10.1007/s00068-022-02090-y.
17. Taylor CA, Braza D, Rice JB, Dillingham T. The incidence of peripheral nerve injury in extremity trauma. Am J Phys Med Rehabil. 2008;87(5):381–5.
18. Metter D. Das Decollement als Anfahrverletzung. Zeitschrift für Rechtsmedizin. 1980;85(3):211–9.
19. Schmidt AH. Acute compartment syndrome. Orthop Clin N Am. 2016;47(3):517–25.
20. Polytrauma Guideline Update Group. Level 3 guideline on the treatment of patients with severe/multiple injuries : AWMF Register-Nr. 012/019. Eur J Trauma Emerg Surg. 2018;44(Suppl 1):3–271. https://doi.org/10.1007/s00068-018-0922-y.
21. Ull C, Jansen O, Seybold D, Königshausen M, Schildhauer TA, Gessmann J. Differences between primary and secondary definitive osteosynthesis for fractures of the lower leg with concomitant acute compartment syndrome. Eur J Trauma Emerg Surg. 2020;46(5):1167–73. https://doi.org/10.1007/s00068-019-01089-2.
22. Regel G, Bayeff-Filloff M. Diagnostik und sofortige Therapiemaßnahmen bei Verletzungen der Extremitäten. Der Unfallchirurg. 2004;107(10):919–26.
23. Gümbel D, Naundorf M, Napp M, Ekkernkamp A, Seifert J. Diagnostik und Management peripherer Gefäßverletzungen. Der Unfallchirurg. 2014;117(5):445–460.
24. Marzi I, Rose S. In: Marzi I, Rose S, editors. Praxisbuch polytrauma. 1st ed. Köln: Dt. Ärzteverlag; 2012.
25. Volpin G, Pfeifer R, Saveski J, Hasani I, Cohen M, Pape HC. Damage control orthopaedics in polytraumatized patients - current concepts. J Clin Orthop Trauma. 2021;12(1):72–82.
26. Scherer J, Coimbra R, Mariani D, Leenen L, Komadina R, Peralta R, Fattori L, Marzi I, Wendt K, Gaarder C, Pape HC, Pfeifer R. Standards of fracture care in polytrauma: results of a Europe-wide survey by the ESTES polytrauma section. Eur J Trauma Emerg Surg. 2022; https://doi.org/10.1007/s00068-022-02126-3.
27. Pfeifer R, Kalbas Y, Coimbra R, Leenen L, Komadina R, Hildebrand F, Halvachizadeh S, Akhtar M, Peralta R, Fattori L, Mariani D, Hasler RM, Lefering R, Marzi I, Pitance F, Osterhoff G, Volpin G, Weil Y, Wendt K, Pape HC. Indications and interventions of damage control orthopedic surgeries: an expert opinion survey. Eur J Trauma Emerg Surg. 2021;47(6):2081–92. https://doi.org/10.1007/s00068-020-01386-1.
28. Busch K, Gohritz A, Vogt P. Amputation und Replantation an der Hand. Orthopädie und Unfallchirurgie up2date. 2008;3(2):115–32.
29. Barzen K, Koch DA, Schweigkofler U, Hoffmann R. Management schwerer Weichteil- und Amputationsverletzungen. Notfallmedizin up2date. 2021;16(02):199–217.
30. Bouillon B, Pieper D, Flohé S, Eikermann M, Prengel P, Ruchholtz S, et al. Level 3 guideline on the treatment of patients with severe/multiple injuries. Eur J Trauma Emerg Surg. 2018;44:1–269.
31. von Laer L. Schicksal und klinische Bedeutung des posttraumatischen Rotationsfehlers nach Oberschenkelschaftfrakturen im Wachstumsalter. In: Blauth W, Ulrich H-W, editors. Spätergebnisse in der Orthopädie. Berlin: Springer; 1986.
32. Schmidt HGK, Hadler D, Wurm M, Juergens C. Therapie der Infekt-/Defekt-Pseudarthrosen der unteren Extremitäten. Trauma und Berufskrankheit. 2003;5:s318–27.
33. Gerlach U-J, Grimme C, Schoop R. Akute posttraumatische Osteitis. Trauma und Berufskrankheit. 2009;11(S2):203–6.

## Further Reading

Meinberg EG, Agel J, Roberts CS, Karam MD, Kellam JF. Fracture and Dislocation Classification Compendium-2018. J Orthop Trauma. 2018;32(Suppl 1):S1–S170. https://doi.org/10.1097/BOT.0000000000001063. PMID: 29256945

Pape HC, Sander R, Borelli J Jr. The Poly-Traumatized patient with fractures. Berlin: Springer; 2011.

Pasquale MD, Frykberg ER, Tinkoff GH, ACS Committee on Trauma; Ad Hoc Committee on Outcomes. Management of complex extremity trauma. Bull Am Coll Surg. 2006;91(6):36–8. PMID: 18551956

WHO and International Association for the Surgery of Trauma and Surgical Intensive Care, Guidelines for essential trauma care. ISBN 92 4 154640 9.

# Extremity Compartment Syndrome

# 110

Dominik A. Jakob, Elizabeth R. Benjamin, and Demetrios Demetriades

## 110.1 Introduction

**Learning Goals**
- Identify patients at risk for extremity CS.
- Learn the early and late signs of CS and how to perform the appropriate investigations for definitive diagnosis.
- Familiarity with the anatomy of the extremity muscle compartments and the technique of a decompressive fasciotomy.

### 110.1.1 Epidemiology

Young males are at a higher risk for extremity CS due to their increased muscle mass. After extremity trauma, approximately 1% of patients require fasciotomy. The incidence of CS requiring fasciotomy varies widely by the mechanism and type of injury, reaching up to 42% in patients who sustained a combined arterial and venous injury [1]. The lower leg is the most common site for compartment syndrome, followed by the forearm, thigh, arm, foot, and buttocks, in this order [2–6].

### 110.1.2 Etiology

Extremity CS is most common after severe trauma, with approximately 75% of cases associated with long bone fractures. The most common fractures causing limb compartment syndrome are tibial shaft (40%) and forearm (18%) fractures [7]. Other common etiologies include vascular injuries, particularly combined arterial and venous injuries, soft tissue crush injuries, and circumferential burns [8]. Iatrogenic causes include external compression by tight bandages or casts, accidental extravasation of fluids in the soft tissues, and excessive crystalloid fluid resuscitation. In rare occasions, prolonged general anesthesia in morbidly obese patients may cause compartment syndrome in the buttocks. Prolonged extremity compression in unconscious patients, often after narcotic overdose or alcohol intoxication, is another cause of CS observed with increasing frequency. In rare cases, excessive physical exercise, such as long-distance running, particularly by untrained people, may cause CS. Medical conditions such as bleeding diathesis or pharma-

**Table 110.1** Risk factors for compartment syndrome

| |
|---|
| *SEVERE TRAUMA* |
| Long bone fractures |
| Injury to vascular structures |
| Crush injury |
| *SPONTANEOUS HEMORRHAGE, HEMATOMA* |
| Hereditary bleeding disorder |
| Pharmacological anticoagulation |
| *EDEMA - INCREASED PERMEABILITY* |
| Circumferential burns |
| Accidental fluid extravasation in soft tissue, excessive crystalloid fluid resuscitation |
| SIRS |
| Others: thrombosis, tourniquet use |
| *OTHERS* |
| External compression by splints or casts, myositis, rhabdomyolysis, soft tissue infection, excessive physical exercise |

cological anticoagulation may cause spontaneous bleeding in a muscle compartment and result in CS. Common risk factors for extremity CS are summarized in Table 110.1.

### 110.1.3 Classification

Extremity compartment syndromes can be separated into acute and chronic [9]. The present chapter focuses on acute extremity CS. Chronic extremity compartment syndrome is characterized by a recurrent exercise-induced increase in compartment pressure with transient neurologic symptoms and pain. Typically, the symptoms resolve with rest.

CS can be classified as primary (direct limb-related injury) and secondary (non-limb-related injury), such as after massive crystalloid fluid resuscitation [10]. Alternatively, extremity CS is divided into early, when tissue pressure elevation lasts for less than 4 h, and late, if it lasts for more than 4 h [11]. Ischemia lasting longer than 4–6 h causes irreversible damage to the muscles and nerves.

### 110.1.4 Pathophysiology

The normal muscle compartment pressure is less than 8 mmHg. Increase in pressure to >20–25 mmHg results in tissue perfusion impairment, and at >30–40 mmHg, the ischemia is considered critical and an emergency fasciotomy should be considered. An alternative to the absolute compartment pressure is the perfusion pressure (diastolic pressure minus the compartment pressure). A perfusion pressure of <30 mmHg indicates severe tissue hypoperfusion and is considered an indication of an emergency fasciotomy [12].

Nerve ischemia lasting for more than 4 h and muscle ischemia for more than 6 h can cause irreversible damage, and for this reason, early intervention is essential [13–15]. Depending on the severity and duration of the ischemia, the patient may develop true muscle necrosis, chronic muscle contracture, sensory deficit, paralysis, and, in severe cases, loss of limb. Volkmann contracture in the upper extremity and foot drop in the lower extremity are specific clinical patterns for this terminal state.

In addition to local complications, the ischemic muscle damage causes myoglobinemia and myoglobinuria, which can result in acute kidney injury. Myoglobin has a direct toxic effect on the renal tubular epithelium and can cause tubular occlusion due to precipitation. Myoglobin levels are rarely measured, and a common practice is the measurement of creatine phosphokinase (CPK) levels. CPK levels >5000 units/L in adults, especially in elderly or severely injured patients, and >3000 units/L in children, were found to be an independent risk factor for acute kidney injury [16, 17]. Young males are significantly more likely to have CPK levels >5000 units/L because of the greater muscle mass in this group. Other laboratory changes include hyperkalemia and hypocalcemia, which are a potentially dangerous cardiotoxic combination.

### 110.1.5 Surgical Anatomy

Extremity fascial compartments contain muscles, nerves, and blood vessels.

**Upper Extremity**
The upper extremity fascial compartments include two in the upper arm, three in the forearm, and ten in the hand.

- The upper arm contains a relatively large anterior and posterior compartment, separated medially by the brachial artery and median nerve. The anterior compartment contains the biceps, the brachialis and coracobrachialis, and the musculocutaneous nerve. The posterior compartment contains the triceps and the radial nerve.
- The forearm is separated into three muscle compartments: the anterior or flexor compartment, which contains the muscles responsible for wrist flexion and pronation of the forearm. These muscles are innervated by the median and ulnar nerves and receive blood supply mainly from the ulnar artery. The posterior or extensor compartment, which contains the muscles responsible for wrist extension, is innervated by the radial nerve, and the blood supply is provided mainly by the radial artery. The mobile wad is a group of three muscles on the radial aspect of the forearm that act as flexors at the elbow joint. These muscles are often grouped together with the dorsal compartment. The blood supply is provided by the radial artery and the innervation by branches of the radial nerve.
- The hand includes ten separate osteofascial compartments. The transverse carpal ligament, over the carpal tunnel, is a strong and broad ligament. The tunnel contains the median nerve and the finger flexor tendons.

**Lower Extremity**

The lower extremity fascial compartments include three gluteal, three thigh, four calf, and nine of the foot.

- The buttock includes the muscle compartments of the gluteus maximus, the gluteus medius/minimus, and the extension of the fascia lata of the thigh into the gluteal region. The sciatic nerve is the only major neurovascular structure in the compartments of the buttock.
- The thigh consists of three compartments. The anterior compartment contains the quadriceps femoris and sartorius muscles, as well as the femoral vessels and femoral nerve. The posterior compartment contains the biceps femoris, semitendinosus, and semimembranosus muscles, as well as the sciatic nerve. The medial compartment contains the adductor muscle group and the gracilis muscle.
- The lower leg has four compartments: the anterior, lateral, superficial posterior and deep posterior. The anterior and lateral compartments are the most common sites of extremity compartment syndrome. The anterior compartment contains the anterior tibial artery and the deep peroneal nerve. The lateral compartment contains the superficial peroneal nerve. The superficial posterior compartment contains the sural nerve. The deep posterior compartment contains the posterior tibial artery and the tibial nerve.
- The foot contains a total of nine muscle compartments.

## 110.2 Diagnosis

The diagnosis of CS is based on a combination of clinical examination, CPK level, and direct measurement of compartment pressures.

### 110.2.1 Clinical Presentation

The diagnosis of extremity CS requires a high index of suspicion combined with knowledge of the underlying risk factors. The "six Ps" (pain, paresthesia, pallor, poikilothermia, pulselessness, and paralysis) are signs and symptoms classically described in the extremity CS. Pain out of proportion, often not responding to analgesia, is the most common and earliest clinical finding. Usually, pain can be exacerbated by a passive stretch of the involved muscle. Another relatively early sign is paresthesia, which indicates hypoxia in nerve tissue within a compartment. Altered sensation between the first and second toe, for example, could indicate a deep peroneal nerve ischemia from an anterior compartment syndrome of the lower leg. The involved compartment often feels tense to palpation. However, this finding is operator-dependent and often lacks reproducibility. Pulselessness, pallor, and paralysis are late symptoms, and in their presence, the prognosis is often poor.

Overall, the positive predictive value of the clinical findings is low, and the specificity and negative predictive value are high [18]. These findings suggest that the clinical features of compartment syndrome are more useful in their absence in excluding the diagnosis than they are when present in confirming the diagnosis. Although clinical suspicion is important, the diagnosis of CS in the trauma population is often difficult. Trauma patients are frequently altered or require intubation, sedation, or paralysis, making a reliable and reproducible assessment of the extremity difficult. The diagnosis of extremity CS in very young children is particularly challenging because escalating pain may not be easily identified, and the clinical diagnosis should be based on three As: anxiety, agitation, and increasing analgesic requirement [19].

## 110.2.2 Investigations

Given the poor positive predictive value of clinical examination and the difficulties inherent in the trauma population, a low threshold to perform direct compartment pressure measurements should be encouraged. Direct measurement of muscle compartment pressures is the most objective test for definitive diagnosis and should always be performed in suspected cases.

There are no specific diagnostic laboratory tests. However, elevated CPK levels in high-risk patients should raise the suspicion of a compartment syndrome. Myoglobinuria can develop within 4 h of the onset of extremity CS. The urine is dark, brownish, or red when viewed macroscopically, but hematuria is absent on microscopic urine analysis.

An abnormal $SaO_2$ in the affected toes and fingers is a late finding of extremity CS and is not appropriate to detect early stages.

Multiple techniques for direct compartment pressure measurement have been described [20–22]. Direct compartment pressures may be obtained with a variety of commercial devices or using a simple arterial line setup with an 18-gauge needle. It is recommended to measure the pressure in all compartments of the suspected region.

A commonly used commercial device for direct measurement of the compartment pressure is the hand-held Stryker® intracompartmental pressure system. For pressure measurement, the needle is connected to the diaphragm chamber and the diaphragm to the prefilled syringe. The assembled system is then inserted into the opened Stryker device. The flap is closed and the device turned on. The zero button is pressed, and when the display shows zero, the needle is inserted perpendicularly through the skin into the muscle (Fig. 110.1). After a slow injection of 0.3 mL into the compartment and a waiting time of a few seconds to reach equilibrium, the pressure can be read on the display.

In general, a side port needle, as provided with the above device, is more accurate at measuring the compartment pressure, as regular needles may obstruct when entering the soft tissue and falsify the measurement. In the absence of this device, however, an arterial line transducer with an 18-gauge needle can be used with good results, as long as the needle is flushed after introduction into the muscle compartment.

A muscle compartment pressure >30–40 mmHg or a perfusion pressure <30 mmHg is indicative of compartment syndrome and should prompt consideration of decompressive fasciotomy.

### 110.2.2.1 Instructions for Measurement of the Different Anatomical Compartments

**Arm:** The arm is kept in a neutral position because flexion or extension at the elbow can affect compartment pressure. The needle is inserted perpendicular to the skin in the middle third of the anterior and the posterior arm, respectively.

**Forearm**: The forearm is kept in a neutral position before measuring the compartment pressure. For measurement of the pressure in the flexor compartment, the needle is inserted perpendicular to the skin into the middle third of the flexor surface of the forearm. For the dor-

# 110 Extremity Compartment Syndrome

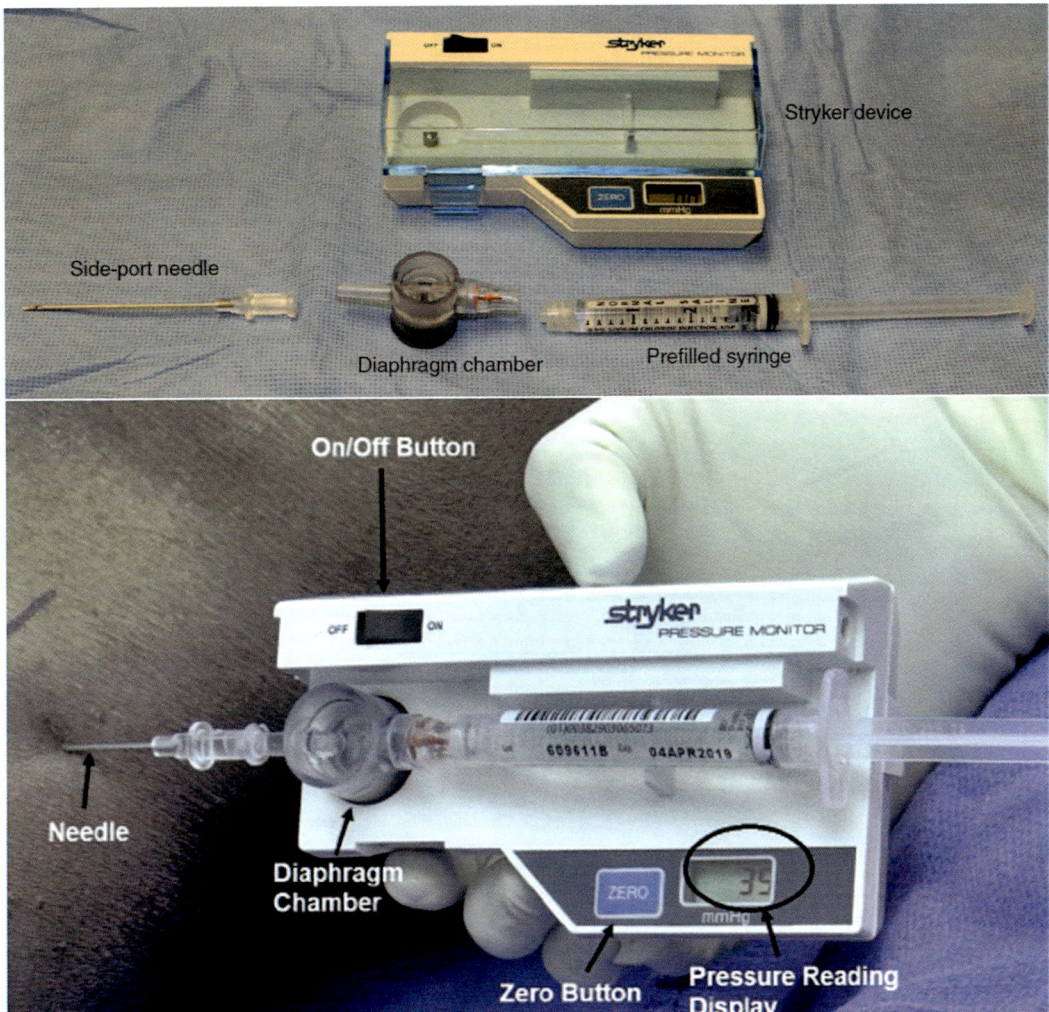

**Fig. 110.1** The Stryker system is a commercially available system to measure extremity compartment pressures. It includes the device base, a side-port needle, a prefilled syringe, and a diaphragm chamber (top). (With permission, Atlas of Surgical Techniques in Trauma, eds Demetriades, Inaba, Velmahos, Cambridge University Press, 2015). The assembled system is placed into the Stryker® device and the system turned on. The zero button is pressed, and the system should show "00." The needle is then inserted perpendicularly through the skin into the muscle. After a slow injection of 0.3 mL into the compartment and a waiting time of a few seconds to reach equilibrium, the pressure can be read on the display (bottom). (With permission, Color Atlas of Emergency Trauma, third edition, eds Demetriades, Chudnofsky, Benjamin, Cambridge University Press, 2021)

sal (extensor), the needle is inserted perpendicular to the skin into the middle third of the extensor surface of the forearm.

**Buttock**: The compartment pressures in the buttock are best measured with the patient in the prone or lateral position. The needle is inserted into the gluteus maximus, in the lateral upper quadrant, to avoid injury to the sciatic nerve. For measurement of the pressure in the gluteus medius muscle compartment, the needle is inserted deeper.

**Thigh**: The medial muscle compartment of the thigh rarely develops compartment syndrome. For this reason and because of the risk of vascular injuries, there is no need for routine pressure measurements in this compartment. For anterior compartment pressure measurements of the thigh, the needle is inserted perpendicularly into the skin, in the middle third of the anterior thigh. For posterior compartment pressures of the thigh, the needle is inserted in the middle third of the posterior thigh.

**Lower leg**: For measurement of the anterior compartment pressure of the lower leg, the needle is inserted perpendicular to the skin approximately two fingerbreadths lateral to the anterior border of the tibia. For the lateral compartment, the entry point is approximately one fingerbreadth anterior to the line joining the head of the fibula and the lateral malleolus. For measurement of the superficial posterior compartment pressure, the needle is inserted in the middle of the calf, at the junction of the upper and middle thirds of the leg. For the deep posterior compartment, the needle is inserted about one fingerbreadth posterior to the medial border of the tibia, at the junction of the upper and middle third of the leg.

> **Differential Diagnosis**
> The diagnosis of extremity CS is often delayed or missed, with potentially serious medical and medicolegal implications. In trauma patients, the intractable pain of CS may be incorrectly attributed to the primary injury and the swelling associated with the hematoma around the fracture or in the soft tissues. In patients with major venous ligation and extremity swelling, the differential diagnosis should include deep venous thrombosis and extremity CS.

## 110.3 Treatment

### 110.3.1 Medical Treatment

In cases at risk for extremity CS or those with moderately increased compartment pressures, administration of mannitol may reduce the risk of CS and the need for fasciotomy [23]. In these cases, the authors recommend 0.5 g/kg of Mannitol administered over 20 min, provided that the patient is hemodynamically stable. Mannitol is contraindicated in the setting of hemorrhagic shock or hemodynamic instability.

In patients with delayed diagnosis and elevated CPK levels, in addition to decompressive fasciotomy, intensive fluid resuscitation to achieve a minimum urine output of 1 mL/kg/h and maintaining slightly alkaline urine may reduce the risk of acute kidney injury. Administration of mannitol in patients with very high levels of CPK may be beneficial in preventing acute kidney injury.

### 110.3.2 Surgical Treatment

#### 110.3.2.1 General Operative Principles

Decompressive fasciotomy should be performed emergently in all patients with extremity CS. The role of routine prophylactic fasciotomy in patients at risk for CS is controversial. We do not advocate routine prophylactic fasciotomies if the patient can be monitored closely in a hospital environment because of the local complications associated with the procedure [24]. However, in austere environments where close monitoring is not possible, prophylactic fasciotomies should be considered.

Good anatomic knowledge of the extremity muscle compartments is essential to perform adequate decompression and avoid neurovascular injuries.

The skin incisions should be generous to provide adequate decompression of the muscle compartments. Similarly, all fasciae should be opened along their entire length. The fasciotomy skin incisions should always be left open. All nonviable muscles should be excised because of the risk of necrosis and infection, which may lead to the loss of limb. Muscle not contracting to electrocautery stimulation is not viable and should be removed. The questionably viable muscle may be preserved and reevaluated at a second-look operation. After hemostasis is achieved, the extremity wounds should be dressed with gauze dampened with sterile normal saline with gentle compression for hemostatic purposes. Application of a negative pressure system (VAC) should be avoided at the initial stage because of the increased risk of bleeding. A second-look operation should take place within 24 h of the index operation and perform further muscle debridement, as needed. Negative pressure systems at this stage are recommended because they reduce tissue edema, prevent skin retraction, and facilitate primary skin closure.

### 110.3.2.2 Upper Extremity Fasciotomy

For the upper arm, the two muscle compartments can be released through a single lateral skin incision, extending from just below the deltoid insertion to the lateral condyle (Fig. 110.2, left). The skin flaps are mobilized anteriorly and posteriorly at the fascial level. The intermuscular septum between the anterior and posterior compartments is identified, and each compartment is incised longitudinally (Fig. 110.2 right).

The forearm compartments can be released with two incisions. A volar incision decompresses the volar compartment and the mobile wad. The dorsal incision decompresses the dorsal compartment. There are various approaches to volar fasciotomy described. We recommend the "lazy S" incision, which should begin 2–3 cm proximal to the antecubital fossa between the biceps and triceps and end along the ulnar edge proximal to the wrist, passing the radial border in the midforearm. The incision is then carried to the midwrist and then curved up onto the hand medial to the thenar eminence (Fig. 110.3). After

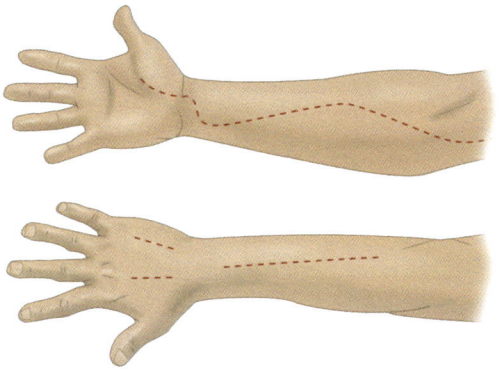

**Fig. 110.3** The forearm is decompressed using a serpentine incision on the volar surface crossing the flexor retinaculum, a longitudinal incision on the dorsal surface, and two additional incisions on the dorsal hand. (With permission, Atlas of Surgical Techniques in Trauma, eds Demetriades, Inaba, Velmahos, Cambridge University Press, 2015)

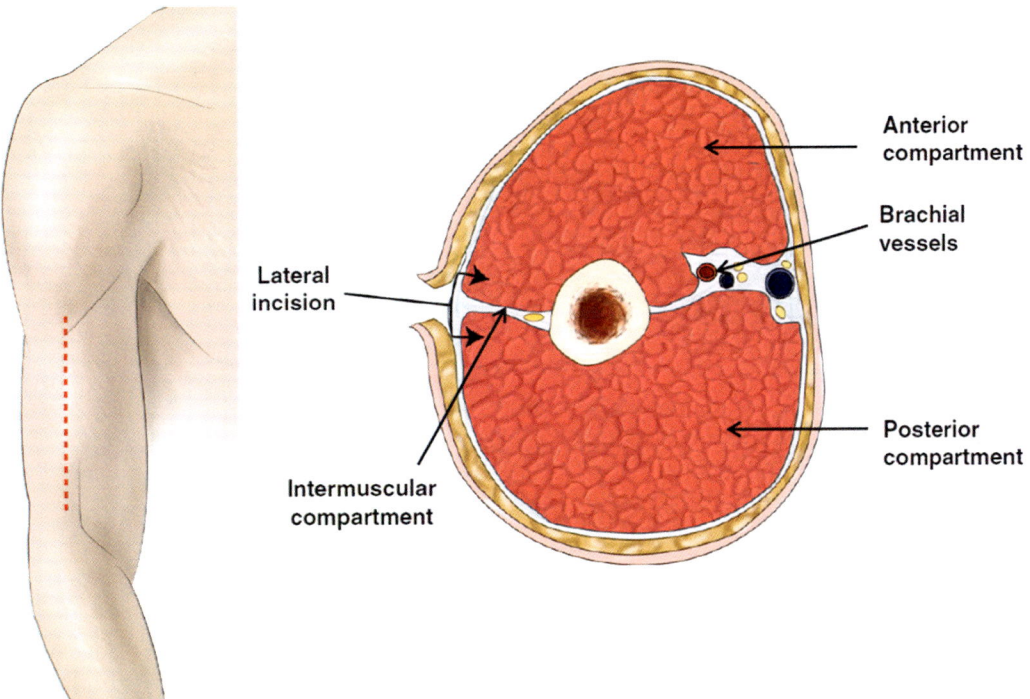

**Fig. 110.2** The upper arm fasciotomy can be achieved through a single lateral incision (**left**). This incision is used to access the anterior and posterior compartments (**right**). (With permission, Atlas of Surgical Techniques in Trauma, eds Demetriades, Inaba, Velmahos, Cambridge University Press, 2015)

the skin incision, the subcutaneous tissue is dissected down to the muscular fascia, and the flexor muscle bellies are exposed and opened with scissors. Wide epimysiotomy (sectioning of the muscle sheath) is required over all muscle bellies of the volar forearm. An important component of the volar fasciotomy is the release of the carpal tunnel. The palmar fascia is incised to expose the transverse carpal ligament (flexor retinaculum), which has to be completely divided in order to fully decompress the carpal tunnel. The underlying median nerve, which is located directly deep in the divided flexor retinaculum, must be protected.

The dorsal compartment of the forearm is released by a longitudinal incision that begins 2 cm distal to the lateral epicondyle of the humerus and continues to the midwrist (Fig. 110.3). After exposure of the extensor muscle compartment, they are opened longitudinally.

The hand's oseofascial compartments can be released with carpal tunnel release (described above) and two dorsal incisions, which are made on the dorsum of the hand over the second and fourth metacarpal spaces (Fig. 110.3). On either side of each tendon, the compartments are opened with longitudinal slits in the fascia. To access and divide the fascia, the extensor tendon can be retracted.

### 110.3.2.3 Lower Extremity Fasciotomies

Fasciotomies of the buttocks are performed with the patient in the prone or lateral decubitus position. Decompression can either be done with a traditional question-mark incision or via a midaxial longitudinal incision.

The question mark incision starts lateral to the posterior superior iliac spine, courses laterally in a curvilinear fashion along the iliac crest toward the greater trochanter, then swings back medially along the inferior border of the buttock and extends over the midline of the posterior upper thigh (Fig. 110.4, top). The fascia of the gluteus maximus underlying the incision is encountered and released. To access the gluteus medius and minimus compartments, the gluteus maximus muscle needs to be split in a muscle-sparing fashion. The inferior part of the question mark incision is used to release the tensor fascia lata compartment.

Similar to the question mark incision, the midaxial longitudinal incision begins just lateral to the posterior superior iliac spine but then extends posterolaterally toward the lateral thigh (Fig. 110.4, bottom). At the greater trochanter, the incision proceeds inferiorly along the lateral aspect of the thigh. The access to the muscle compartments is identical to the description above for the question mark incision.

For thigh fasciotomies, the patient is placed in a supine position and prepped from the iliac crest to the foot. A lateral incision is performed to release the anterior and posterior thigh compartments. The medial compartment is rarely affected but could be decompressed by a medial incision. The incision starts just distal of the greater trochanter and continues in a linear way to a few cm proximal to the lateral femoral condyle (Fig. 110.5, top). The underlying fascia lata is encountered and divided with a longitudinal incision to decompress the anterior compartment. The posterior compartment is accessed after mobilization of a skin flap and incision of the fascia posterior to the intercompartmental septum. As an alternative, the posterior compartment can be accessed via the anterior compartment and the incision of the intercompartmental septum (Fig. 110.5, bottom).

For the lower leg fasciotomy, the compartments can be released using a two-incision approach. The lateral incision decompresses the anterior and lateral compartments, and the medial incision decompresses the superficial and deep posterior compartments.

The lateral incision is placed longitudinally, approximately two fingerbreadths anterior to the fibula. The incision starts two fingerbreadths below the fibular head and continues to two fingerbreadths above the lateral malleolus (Fig. 110.6, top). The skin and subcutaneous tissue are divided, and skin flaps are created to expose the underlying fascia covering the anterior and lateral compartments. For the anterior compartment decompression, a longitudinal incision is performed anterior to the septum, and

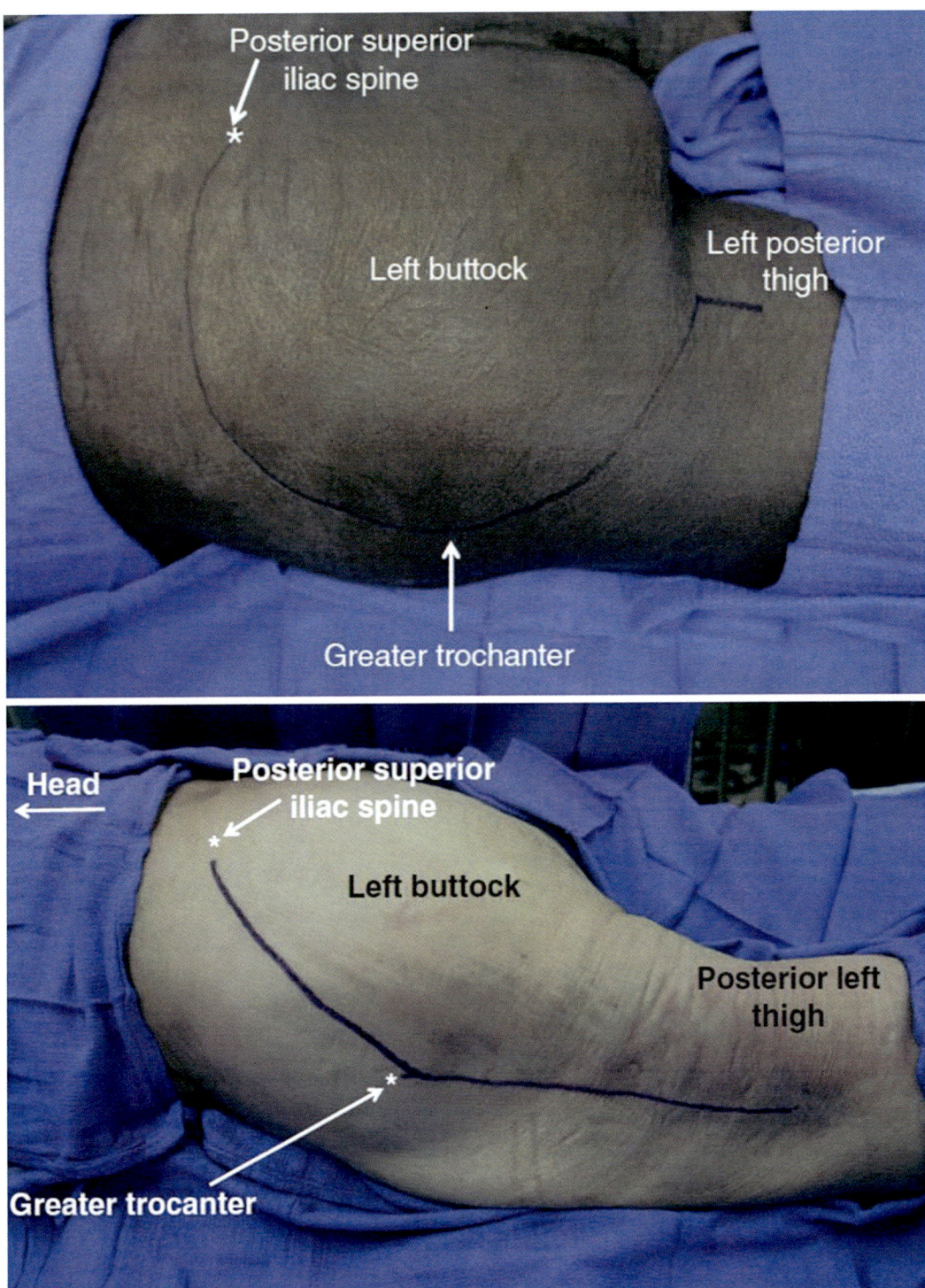

**Fig. 110.4** The buttock compartments can be released using the question mark (top) or midaxial longitudinal incision (bottom). (With permission, Atlas of Surgical Techniques in Trauma, eds Demetriades, Inaba, Velmahos, Cambridge University Press, 2015)

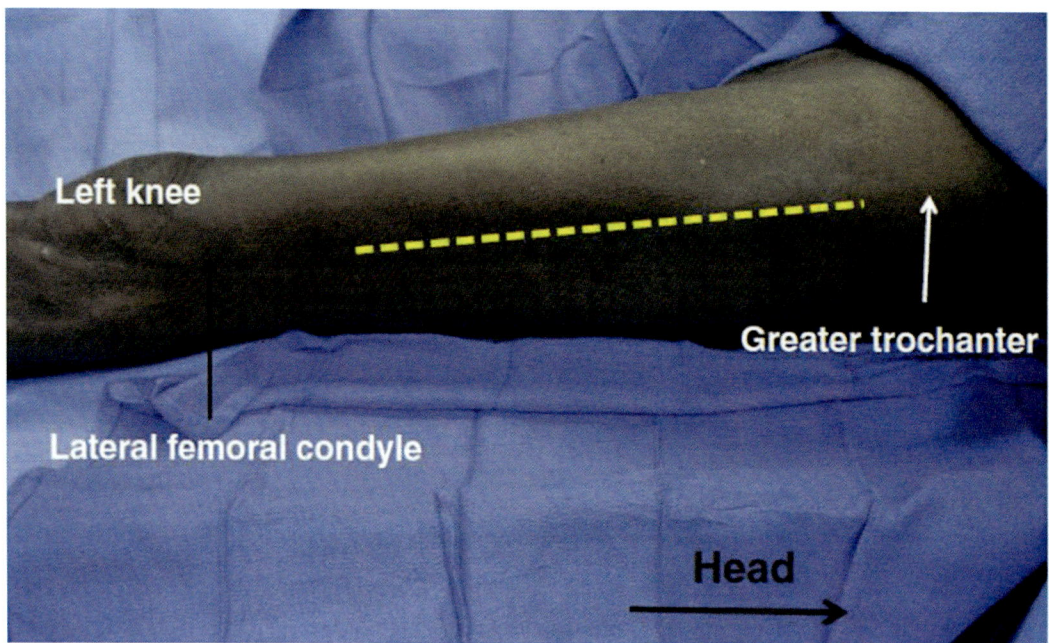

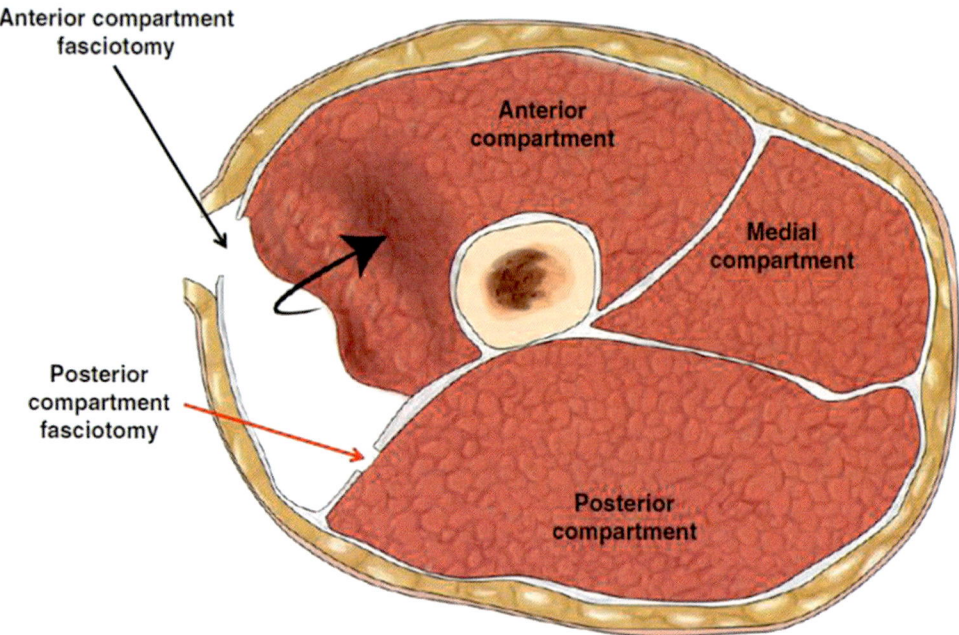

**Fig. 110.5** The anterior and posterior compartments of the thigh are decompressed through a lateral incision (top). The anterior compartment is released directly, and the posterior compartment can be released directly through the development of a skin flap or by incising the intramuscular septum via the anterior compartment (bottom). (With permission, Atlas of Surgical Techniques in Trauma, eds Demetriades, Inaba, Velmahos, Cambridge University Press, 2015)

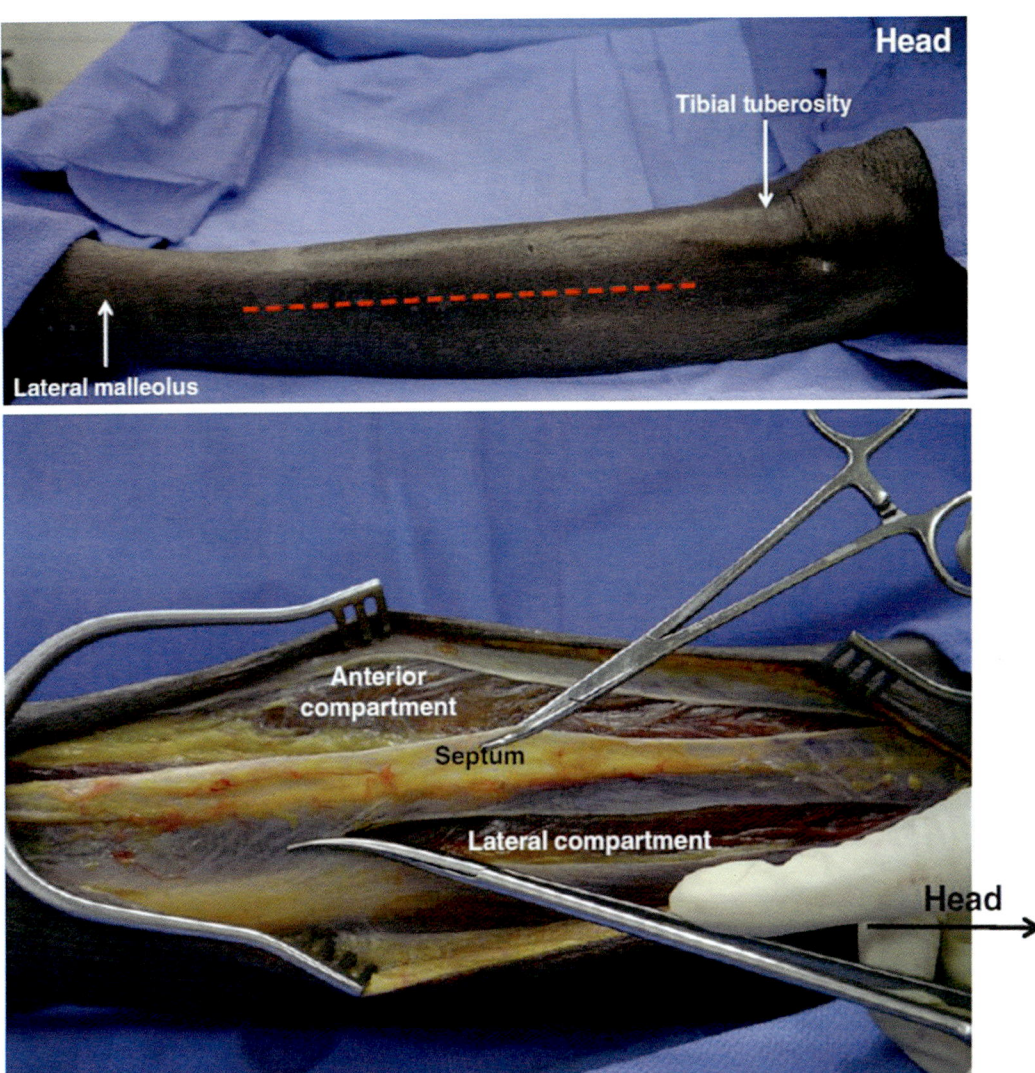

**Fig. 110.6** The anterior and lateral compartments of the lower leg are decompressed through a lateral incision, which starts two fingerbreadths below the fibular head and ends two fingerbreadths above the lateral malleolus, in a line approximately two fingerbreadths anterior to the fibula (top). After exposure of the fascia, the septum, which separates the anterior and lateral compartments, is identified. Posterior to the septum, the lateral compartment is decompressed with long scissors (bottom). (With permission, Atlas of Surgical Techniques in Trauma, eds Demetriades, Inaba, Velmahos, Cambridge University Press, 2015)

the fascia is opened using long scissors, with the tips pointed toward the tibia tuberosity superiorly and the big toe inferiorly. For the lateral compartment decompression, a longitudinal incision is performed posterior to the septum, and the fascia is opened using long scissors, with the tips pointed toward the head of the fibula superiorly and the lateral malleolus inferiorly (Fig. 110.6, bottom).

The posterior lower leg compartments can be exposed through a medial incision, placed two fingerbreadths medial to the tibial edge. The incision starts two fingerbreadths below the medial aspect of the knee and extends two fingerbreadths

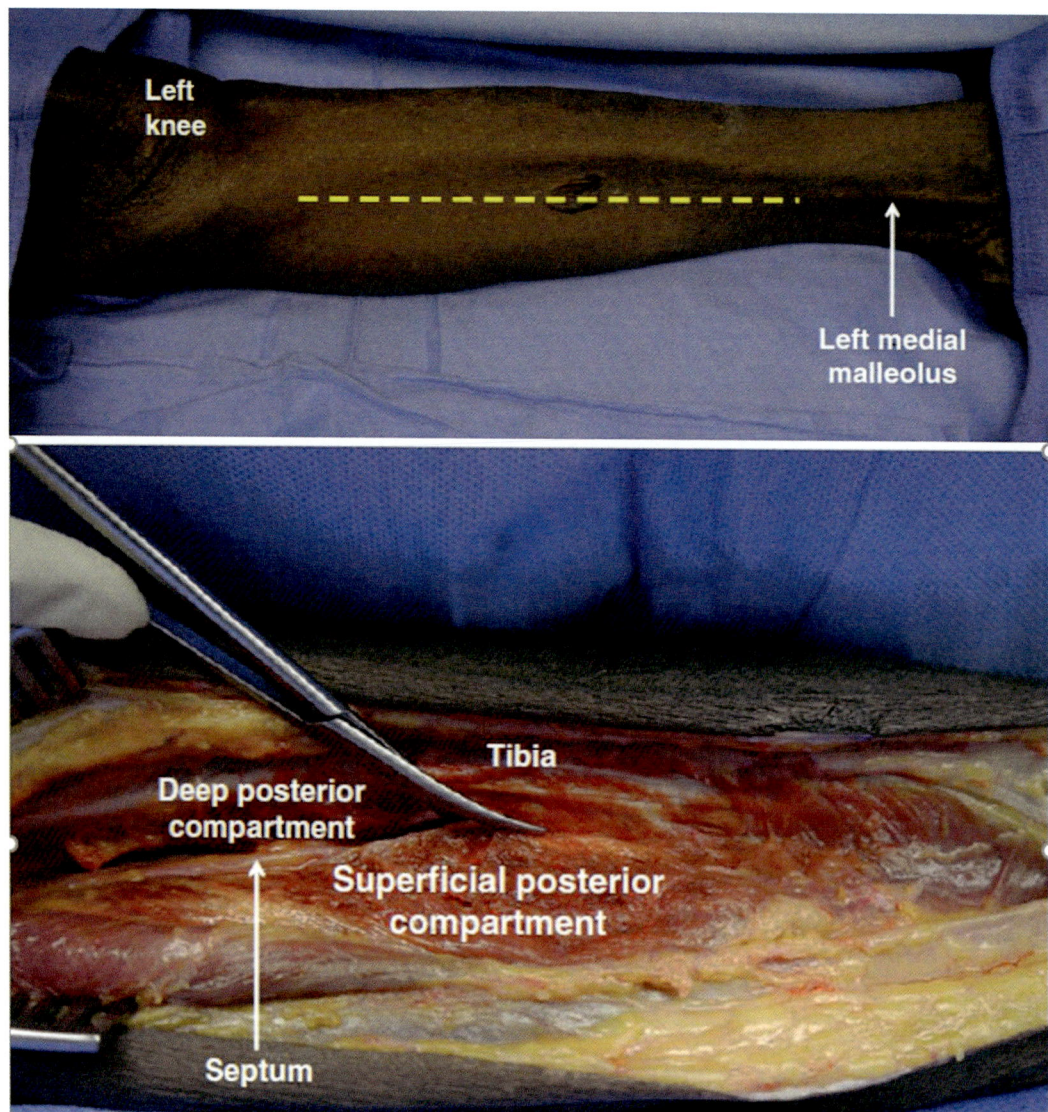

**Fig. 110.7** The medial incision starts two fingerbreadths below the medial aspect of the knee and ends two fingerbreadths above the medial malleolus, in a line approximately two fingerbreadths medial to the tibia (top). The superficial compartment is released with a fascial incision, made about two fingerbreadths posterior to the tibia. The deep posterior compartment is best decompressed with a facial incision just behind the edge of the tibia (bottom). (With permission, Atlas of Surgical Techniques in Trauma, eds Demetriades, Inaba, Velmahos, Cambridge University Press, 2015)

above the medial malleolus (Fig. 110.7, top). The saphenous vein should be preserved. The superficial posterior compartment is encountered first and released by fascial incision. The deep posterior compartment is accessed by dividing the soleus from the posterior edge of the tibia along the shaft (Fig. 110.7, bottom). The identification of the posterior neurovascular bundle and the posterior surface of the tibia ensures the proper release of the deep compartment.

The foot compartments can be accessed and released by three incisions: a medial incision, which extends from a point below the medial malleolus to the metatarsophalangeal joint, and two dorsal incisions over the second and fourth metatarsal shafts. Ensure an adequate skin bridge between the two dorsal incisions to avoid necrosis. After the raising of the skin flaps, each of the interosseous compartments can be released. Avoid injuries to the neurovascular bundle when performing the medial incision.

### 110.3.3 Prognosis

Prognosis of the affected extremity depends on numerous factors, including associated soft tissue, neurovascular, and bony injuries, the duration and severity of ischemia, comorbidities, and most importantly time to fasciotomy. In general, early diagnosis with decompressive fasciotomy within 4 h of the onset of ischemia is associated with good functional outcomes. Delays of >4–6 h are associated with a high incidence of poor functional outcomes and limb loss.

> **Dos and Don'ts**
> **Dos**
> - Have a high index of suspicion for extremity CS in high-risk patients.
> - If in doubt about the clinical diagnosis, measure the pressures in all compartments of the involved anatomical area.
> - Know the anatomy of the extremity compartments.
> - During decompressive fasciotomy, perform a generous skin incision and a long fasciotomy. Explore all compartments!
> - Excise nonviable muscle (not contracting on cautery stimulation).
> - Perform liberal prophylactic fasciotomy in austere environments and whenever close monitoring is not possible or reliable.
>
> **Don'ts**
> - Do not cover the fingers or toes with dressings in high-risk patients.
> - Do not escalate the dose of strong analgesics, before you rule out a CS in high-risk patients.
> - Do not rely exclusively on clinical examination to rule out the diagnosis of CS. Clinical examination is often unreliable.
> - Do not perform routine prophylactic fasciotomy if the patient can be closely monitored and reevaluated.

> **Take-Home Messages**
> - Delayed or missed extremity CS is common; therefore, a high index of suspicion, consideration of underlying risk factors, serial clinical examinations, pressure measurements, and serial CK levels are key factors to ensure early diagnosis and timely fasciotomy in extremity CS.
> - Clinical examination alone is often not reliable in diagnosing early-onset extremity CS. Compartment pressures should be always measured if the clinical examination is inconclusive.
> - Compartment pressures >30–40 mmHg or perfusion pressures <30 mmHg should prompt an emergency fasciotomy.
> - Anatomical knowledge of the extremity compartments is essential for compartment pressure measurements, adequate decompressive fasciotomy, and prevention of iatrogenic injuries to the neurovascular bundle.

> **Multiple Choice Questions**
> 1. Which of the following is true?
>    A. Extremity muscle compartments can tolerate only 12 h of ischemia before muscle necrosis occurs.
>    B. Physical exam is the primary method of diagnosing extremity CS in the obtunded patient as compartment pressures and CPK levels are unreliable.

C. Mannitol is well tolerated in hypotensive patients as a treatment for extremity CS.
D. Absolute compartment pressures greater than 30 mmHg or perfusion pressures less than 30 mmHg are concerning for extremity CS.

Correct Answer: D

2. What anatomical area is most commonly affected by an extremity CS?
   A. Hand
   B. Forearm
   C. Thigh
   D. Lower leg

Correct Answer: D

3. We suspect a lower leg CS. Which compartment is most likely to be affected?
   A. Anterior or lateral compartment
   B. Deep posterior compartment
   C. Superficial posterior compartment
   D. All compartments are equally affected

Correct Answer: A

4. What is the earliest and most reliable clinical sign in a conscious and alert patient?
   A. Pallor
   B. Pain out of proportion
   C. Pulselessness extremity
   D. Poikilothermia

Correct Answer: B

5. What is the next step in a clinically suspected extremity CS?
   A. Immediately proceed with fasciotomy
   B. Intracompartmental pressure measurement in all potentially affected muscle compartments
   C. Observation
   D. Elevation of the affected limb

Correct Answer: B

6. Which of the following is false?
   A. A medial thigh incision is always required when performing a thigh fasciotomy, as the medial thigh compartment has a high incidence of CS.
   B. The anterior and lateral compartments of the lower leg are most commonly affected by CS.
   C. Entry into the deep posterior compartment is confirmed with visualization of the neurovascular bundle on the posterior aspect of the tibia.
   D. The serpentine volar incision of the forearm is insufficient to decompress all compartments of the forearm in the setting of CS.

Correct Answer: A

7. What answer is correct about the fasciotomy of the thigh?
   A. Medial thigh incision is rarely needed because all muscle compartments (including the medial compartment) are accessible through a lateral incision.
   B. When performing a lateral incision to decompress a thigh CS, the saphenous vein is at risk.
   C. Medial incision has always to be performed when decompressing a CS of the thigh.
   D. Medial thigh incision is rarely needed because the medial muscle compartment is rarely affected.

Correct Answer: D

8. Extremity compartment syndrome is more likely to develop in which group of trauma patients:
   A. Young male patients.
   B. Elderly female patients.
   C. Elderly male patients.
   D. Age does not matter.

Correct Answer: A

9. The deep posterior compartment of the lower leg is the most commonly missed or incompletely released compartment. What is an easy way to identify this compartment after performing a medial incision?
   A. Identification of the posterior tibial neurovascular bundle just behind the medial edge of the tibia.

B. Identification of the saphenous vein.
C. Identification of the superficial peroneal nerve.
D. Identification of the anterior intermuscular septum of the lower leg.

Correct Answer: A

10. What is the most important factor defining the outcome of an extremity CS?
    A. Adequate crystalloid-sparing resuscitation
    B. Maintaining the mean arterial pressure
    C. Early diagnosis with timely fasciotomy
    D. Comorbidities of the patient

Correct Answer: C

## References

1. Branco BC, Inaba K, Barmparas G, Schnuriger B, Lustenberger T, Talving P, et al. Incidence and predictors for the need for fasciotomy after extremity trauma: a 10-year review in a mature level I trauma centre. Injury. 2011;42(10):1157–63. https://doi.org/10.1016/j.injury.2010.07.243.
2. Kistler JM, Ilyas AM, Thoder JJ. Forearm compartment syndrome: evaluation and management. Hand Clin. 2018;34(1):53–60. https://doi.org/10.1016/j.hcl.2017.09.006.
3. Ojike NI, Roberts CS, Giannoudis PV. Compartment syndrome of the thigh: a systematic review. Injury. 2010;41(2):133–6. https://doi.org/10.1016/j.injury.2009.03.016.
4. Maeckelbergh L, Colen S, Anne L. Upper arm compartment syndrome: a case report and review of the literature. Orthop Surg. 2013;5(3):229–32. https://doi.org/10.1111/os.12054.
5. Henson JT, Roberts CS, Giannoudis PV. Gluteal compartment syndrome. Acta Orthop Belg. 2009;75(2):147–52.
6. Lutter C, Schoffl V, Hotfiel T, Simon M, Maffulli N. Compartment syndrome of the foot: an evidence-based review. J Foot Ankle Surg. 2019;58(4):632–40. https://doi.org/10.1053/j.jfas.2018.12.026.
7. Kostler W, Strohm PC, Sudkamp NP. Acute compartment syndrome of the limb. Injury. 2004;35(12):1221–7. https://doi.org/10.1016/j.injury.2004.04.009.
8. McQueen MM, Gaston P, Court-Brown CM. Acute compartment syndrome. Who is at risk? J Bone Joint Surg Br. 2000;82(2):200–3. https://doi.org/10.1302/0301-620x.82b2.9799.
9. McLaughlin N, Heard H, Kelham S. Acute and chronic compartment syndromes: know when to act fast. JAAPA. 2014;27(6):23–6. https://doi.org/10.1097/01.JAA.0000446999.10176.13.
10. Tremblay LN, Feliciano DV, Rozycki GS. Secondary extremity compartment syndrome. J Trauma. 2002;53(5):833–7. https://doi.org/10.1097/00005373-200211000-00005.
11. Whitesides TE, Heckman MM. Acute compartment syndrome: update on diagnosis and treatment. J Am Acad Orthop Surg. 1996;4(4):209–18. https://doi.org/10.5435/00124635-199607000-00005.
12. Whitesides TE, Haney TC, Morimoto K, Harada H. Tissue pressure measurements as a determinant for the need of fasciotomy. Clin Orthop Relat Res. 1975;113:43–51. https://doi.org/10.1097/00003086-197511000-00007.
13. Hartsock LA, O'Farrell D, Seaber AV, Urbaniak JR. Effect of increased compartment pressure on the microcirculation of skeletal muscle. Microsurgery. 1998;18(2):67–71. https://doi.org/10.1002/(sici)1098-2752(1998)18:2<67::aid-micr1>3.0.co;2-r.
14. Elliott KG, Johnstone AJ. Diagnosing acute compartment syndrome. J Bone Joint Surg Br. 2003;85(5):625–32.
15. Donaldson J, Haddad B, Khan WS. The pathophysiology, diagnosis and current management of acute compartment syndrome. Open Orthop J. 2014;8:185–93. https://doi.org/10.2174/1874325001408010185.
16. Byerly S, Benjamin E, Biswas S, Cho J, Wang E, Wong MD, et al. Peak creatinine kinase level is a key adjunct in the evaluation of critically ill trauma patients. Am J Surg. 2017;214(2):201–6. https://doi.org/10.1016/j.amjsurg.2016.11.034.
17. Talving P, Karamanos E, Skiada D, Lam L, Teixeira PG, Inaba K, et al. Relationship of creatine kinase elevation and acute kidney injury in pediatric trauma patients. J Trauma Acute Care Surg. 2013;74(3):912–6. https://doi.org/10.1097/TA.0b013e318278954e.
18. Ulmer T. The clinical diagnosis of compartment syndrome of the lower leg: are clinical findings predictive of the disorder? J Orthop Trauma. 2002;16(8):572–7. https://doi.org/10.1097/00005131-200209000-00006.
19. Bae DS, Kadiyala RK, Waters PM. Acute compartment syndrome in children: contemporary diagnosis, treatment, and outcome. J Pediatr Orthop. 2001;21(5):680–8.
20. Rorabeck CH, Castle GS, Hardie R, Logan J. Compartmental pressure measurements: an experimental investigation using the slit catheter. J Trauma. 1981;21(6):446–9.

21. Willy C, Gerngross H, Sterk J. Measurement of intracompartmental pressure with use of a new electronic transducer-tipped catheter system. J Bone Joint Surg Am. 1999;81(2):158–68. https://doi.org/10.2106/00004623-199902000-00003.
22. Mubarak SJ, Owen CA. Double-incision fasciotomy of the leg for decompression in compartment syndromes. J Bone Joint Surg Am. 1977;59(2):184–7.
23. Hutton M, Rhodes RS, Chapman G. The lowering of postischemic compartment pressures with mannitol. J Surg Res. 1982;32(3):239–42. https://doi.org/10.1016/0022-4804(82)90097-x.
24. Velmahos GC, Theodorou D, Demetriades D, Chan L, Berne TV, Asensio J, et al. Complications and nonclosure rates of fasciotomy for trauma and related risk factors. World J Surg. 1997;21(3):247–52; discussion 53. https://doi.org/10.1007/s002689900224.

## Further Reading

Demetriades D, Chudnofsky CR, Benjamin ER, editors. Color atlas of emergency trauma. 3rd ed. Cambridge University Press; 2021.

Demetriades D, Velmahos G, Inaba K, editors. Atlas of surgical techniques in trauma. 2nd ed. Cambridge University Press; 2019.

von Keudell AG, Weaver MJ, Appleton PT, Bae DS, Dyer GSM, Heng M, et al. Diagnosis and treatment of acute extremity compartment syndrome. Lancet. 2015;386(10000):1299–310. https://doi.org/10.1016/S0140-6736(15)00277-9.

# Fasciitis 111

Yutaka Harima, Norio Sato, and Kaoru Koike

## 111.1 Introduction

NF is a rare but life-threatening infection of soft tissue. NF commonly occurs in subcutaneous tissue and the superficial fascia of the extremities, rapidly spreads throughout the body, and causes sepsis and multiple organ failure. The mortality rate of NF is not low, and delayed diagnosis and treatment can cause patient death. However, it is difficult to diagnose the patient as having NF in the early stages. You need to become able to diagnose earlier and treat more appropriately. In this chapter, we describe NF, especially its diagnosis and treatment.

> **Learning Goals**
> - You become able to understand that early diagnosis and early treatment are important.
> - You become able to explain how to diagnose NF.
> - You become able to understand and perform surgical treatment for NF.

Y. Harima · N. Sato (✉)
Ehime University Hospital, Ehime, Japan
e-mail: drnori@m.ehime-u.ac.jp

K. Koike
Kyoto Medical Center, Kyoto, Japan
e-mail: kkoike@kuhp.kyoto-u.ac.jp

### 111.1.1 Epidemiology

The incidence of NF has been reported to range between 0.3 and 5 cases per 100,000 people per year [1–4], though this varies by country and region.

### 111.1.2 Etiology

NF occurs by a bacterial infection in the subcutaneous tissue and superficial fascia. NF also occurs in the trunk, head, and neck, but often in the extremities [5]. The risk factors are reported to be increasing age, diabetes mellitus, alcoholism, malnutrition, peripheral vascular disease, heart disease, renal failure, cancer, immune system impairment, chronic skin infection, IV drug abuse, and post-operation [5–7]. NF generally develops in patients after either penetrating trauma or non-penetrating trauma (muscle strain, sprain, or contusion), a mucosal breach (mucosal tear), or a skin breach (varicella lesions, insect bites, or injection drugs).

### 111.1.3 Classification

NF is classified into four categories according to etiology and microbiology [8] (Table 111.1). Type I infection is polymicrobial infection involving aerobic and anaerobic bacteria. It is

**Table 111.1** Classification of NF based on etiology and microbiology

| Type | Etiology | Microorganisms |
|---|---|---|
| I | Polymicrobial Synergistic Often bowel flora-derived | Mixed anaerobes and aerobes E. coli Pseudomonas spp. Bacteroides spp. |
| II | Often monomicrobial Skin- or throat-derived | Group A β-hemolytic streptococcus (GAS) Occasionally with Staphylococcus aureus |
| III | Gram-negative Often marine-related organisms | Vibrio spp. mainly Pasteurella multocida Haemophilus influenzae Klebsiella spp. Aeromonas spp. |
| IV | Fungal Usually trauma-associated Immunocompetent patients | Candida spp. in immunocompromised patients Zygomycetes in immunocompetent patients |

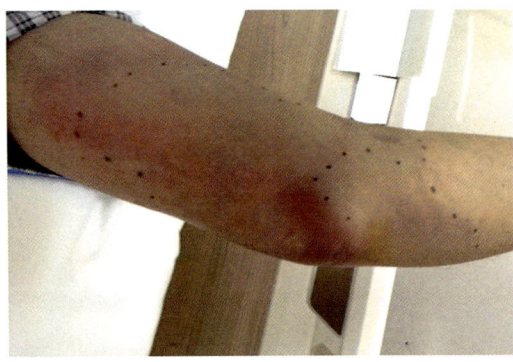

**Fig. 111.1** The patient had felt sick since 4 days ago, and erythema appeared in his left upper extremity 1 day ago. Because swelling and pain also appeared, he visited us. Cellulitis was suspected initially. However, the LRINEC score was 6, and symptoms were getting worse. We diagnosed as NF. We made a skin incision and collected a specimen. Group A streptococcus was found in the specimen. We amputated his left upper extremity on the same day

more likely to occur in elderly people and people with underlying illnesses. Type II infection is monomicrobial infection. Causative bacteria are Gram-positive bacteria including group A *streptococcus* and methicillin-resistant *Staphylococcus aureus* (MRSA). Type II infection can occur in young people and healthy people. Type III infection is infection caused by *Vibrio vulnificus* and *Aeromonas hydrophila*. Type IV infection is fungal infection. It is more likely to occur in immunocompromised patients.

### 111.1.4 Pathophysiology

It is suggested that there are two processes for how NF occurs [6]. One is that infection initially occurs in subcutaneous tissues with a portal of bacterial entry. Bacteria invade subcutaneous tissues through wounds after penetrating trauma or breaches of skin and mucosa, and infection extends to deep tissues. The other is that infection spontaneously occurs in deep tissues without a portal of bacterial entry. Infection occurs in deep tissues after non-penetrating trauma or without trauma and extends to superficial tissues.

Only mild erythema is initially observed on the skin (Fig. 111.1). Within a few days, the inflammation worsens, the skin turns dusky and purplish, and bullae appear. Patients often get bacteremia, and metastatic infections may be observed. The skin becomes ischemic, and tissues rapidly become gangrenous [6, 9]. As a result, patients die.

## 111.2 Diagnosis

### 111.2.1 Clinical Presentation

The main clinical presentations of NF are reported to be soft tissue edema (75%), erythema (72%), severe pain (72%), tenderness (68%), fever (60%), skin bullae, and necrosis (38%) [10]. But patients may initially complain of malaise, myalgias, diarrhea, and anorexia [6]. Some patients have no cutaneous findings in the early stages. As a result, the diagnosis may be incorrect or delayed.

In the case of occurring initially in the deep tissues by group A *streptococcus*, the patient may complain of severe pain that does not match the cutaneous findings. It is said to increase pain and can be a clue for diagnosis. However, it may be absent or weakened in patients taking painkillers [6].

Patients get worse in a few days, and tachycardia, leukocytosis, acidosis, and hyperglycemia begin to be observed. When these symptoms have been observed, patients may already be septic.

### 111.2.2 Test

Chin-Ho Wong et al. reported that the Laboratory Risk Indicator for Necrotizing Fasciitis (LRINEC) score is useful to detect NF in its early stage [11]. You check the total white blood cell count, hemoglobin, sodium, glucose, serum creatinine, and C-reactive protein in the laboratory findings (Table 111.2). When the LRINEC score is 6 or 7, NF is suspected, but other soft tissue infections are also possible. When the LRINEC score is 8 or greater, there is a 75% risk of NF. However, the LRINEC score is low sensitive, and you can't rule out NF even if the LRINEC score is low [12].

In radiography, computed tomography (CT), and magnetic resonance imaging (MRI), soft tissue swelling in patients with group A streptococcal infection and gas in the tissues of patients with Type I infection or gas gangrene will be found [6]. However, these findings may also be found in other soft tissue infections and are not specific to NF. CT may show the involvement of the fascia and its lack of enhancement [13]. MRI may show hyperintensity and thickening of intermuscular fascia on T2-weighted images [14]. Though CT and MRI are sensitive, it takes time to perform both. Bedside ultrasound may also show subcutaneous tissue thickening with fluid accumulation and subcutaneous gas in the affected area [15]. It can be performed simply and quickly and may be useful for early diagnosis, but its sensitivity is relatively low.

The most useful test is to remove the affected tissues surgically (Flowchart 111.1). Some studies suggested that frozen section soft tissue biopsy is useful for the early diagnosis of NF [16, 17]. However, a frozen section may not contain lesions, and it is less reliable than removing tissues surgically. When you have removed tissues surgically, you can perform debridement or amputation at the same time. The obtained specimens are used for Gram's staining and culture, which are crucial for identifying causative bacteria and giving antibiotic treatment [6].

**Table 111.2** LRINRC score

|  | Value | Score |
|---|---|---|
| CRP (mg/L) | <150 | 0 |
|  | ≥150 | 4 |
| WBC (/mm) | <15 | 0 |
|  | 15–25 | 1 |
|  | ≥25 | 2 |
| Hb (g/dL) | ≥13.5 | 0 |
|  | 11–13.5 | 1 |
|  | <11 | 2 |
| Sodium (mmol/L) | ≥135 | 0 |
|  | <135 | 2 |
| Creatinine (mg/dL) | <1.6 | 0 |
|  | ≥1.6 | 2 |
| Glucose (mg/dL) | <180 | 0 |
|  | ≥180 | 1 |

> **Differential Diagnosis**
> Though it is difficult to distinguish NF from other soft tissue infections such as cellulitis, the LRINEC score is helpful for diagnosis. When symptoms are progressing rapidly, NF is more likely. Clinical presentations that distinguish NF from cellulitis are reported to be pain out of proportion, recent surgery, hypotension, diarrhea, altered mental status, erythema progressing beyond marked margins, skin fluctuance, hemorrhagic bullae, and skin necrosis [18]. Gas gangrene is necrotizing soft tissue infection as well as NF. It occurs in muscle tissues by gas-producing bacteria, such as *Clostridium* species.

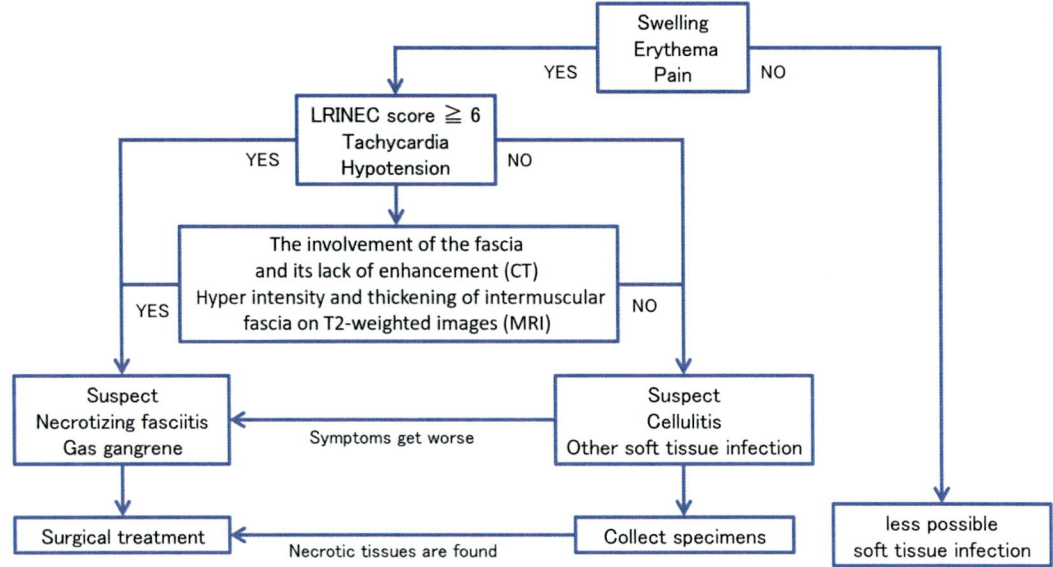

**Flowchart 111.1** Algorithm of diagnosis

## 111.3 Treatment

### 111.3.1 Surgical Treatment

You should not hesitate to perform surgery because surgical treatment is most important in the treatment of NF. When you have suspected NF, you should perform surgery as possible as early. Some studies suggested that early surgery decreases the mortality of NF [19, 20]. In surgery, you identify the extent of infection, evaluate the need for debridement or amputation of an extremity, and perform debridement or amputation of an extremity if necessary (Fig. 111.2). You can also obtain specimens for Gram's staining and culture. It is important to remove infected or necrotic tissues as widely and appropriately as possible in the first surgery [10, 21, 22].

The next day, you should re-examine the surgical site and evaluate the need for additional surgical removal. If necessary, you should remove infected or necrotic tissues additionally. You should evaluate the affected area and surgically remove bad tissues many times until you have performed complete elimination of infected or necrotic tissues [10, 23].

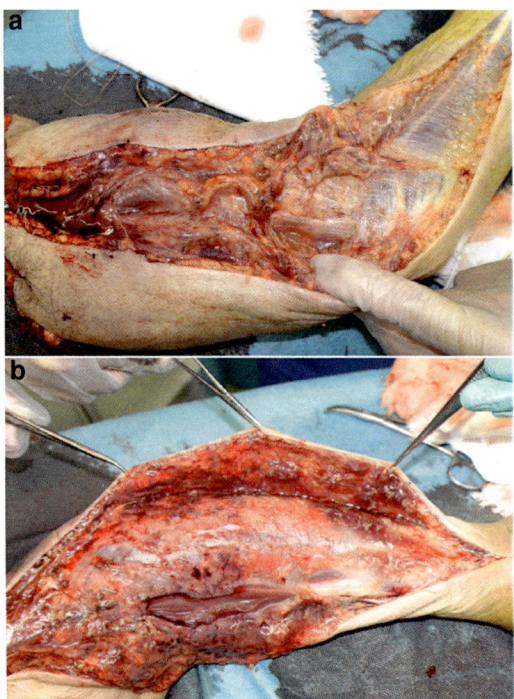

**Fig. 111.2** Left shoulder disarticulation was performed. Subcutaneous tissue and fascia inside the left upper arm looked necrotic (**a**). Fascia outside the left upper arm and in forearm extension side also looked necrotic (**b**). Because the affected area extended to the chest, we performed left pectoralis major fascia resection additionally

After you have controlled the infection of the affected area and removed all infected or necrotic tissues completely, you close the wound. However, you can't often perform primary closure because soft tissues and skin have been widely removed. You need to reconstruct the soft tissues and close the wound with muscle flaps and skin grafts.

Some studies suggested that negative pressure wound therapy (NPWT) is effective for reconstructing soft tissues [24, 25]. NPWT improves the local wound environment through contraction of the wound, stabilization of the wound environment, removal of extracellular fluid, and micro-deformation at the foam-wound interface. Additionally, NPWT speeds wound healing and increases blood flow around wounds. As a result, NPWT can reduce the time to wound closure [26].

### 111.3.2 Medical Treatment

Infectious Diseases Society of America (ISDA) recommends that you start empiric antibiotic treatment broadly in consideration of both polymicrobial (mixed aerobic and anaerobic bacteria) and monomicrobial (group A *streptococcus*, community-acquired MRSA) infections [21]. You should treat with vancomycin, linezolid, or daptomycin plus piperacillin-tazobactam or a carbapenem, or plus ceftriaxone and metronidazole, or plus fluoroquinolone and metronidazole, as empiric therapy. You should change antibiotics appropriately when you have detected the sensitivity of causative bacteria (Table 111.3). You should treat with clindamycin plus penicillin when the causative bacteria are group A *streptococcus*. Streptococcal toxin and cytokine production can be suppressed by clindamycin, but there are group A *Streptococcus* that are resistant to clindamycin. Therefore, you should use penicillin too. You should continue antibiotic treatment until you have found no necrotic tissues and the patient has got better and had no fever for 2–3 days [21].

The efficacy of intravenous immune globulin (IVIG) in streptococcal toxic shock syndrome has been studied because it is considered that IVIG may be beneficial to patients by neutralizing streptococcal toxin [21]. Some studies sug-

**Table 111.3** Antibiotic treatment

| Type of infection | First-line antibiotic agent | Adult dosage |
|---|---|---|
| Mixed infections | Piperacillin-tazobactam plus vancomycin | 3.37 g every 6–8 h |
| | | 30 mg/kg/day in 2 divided doses |
| | Imipenem-cilastatin | 1 g every 6–8 h |
| | Meropenem | 1 g every 8 h |
| | Ertapenem | 1 g daily |
| | Cefotaxime plus metronidazole or clindamycin | 2 g every 6 h |
| | | 500 mg every 6 h |
| | | 600–900 mg every 8 h |
| *Streptococcus* | Penicillin plus clindamycin | 2–4 million units every 4-6 h |
| | | 600–900 mg every 8 h |
| *Staphylococcus aureus* | Nafcillin | 1–2 g every 4 h |
| | Oxacillin | 1–2 g every 4 h |
| | Cefazolin | 1 g every 8 h |
| | Vancomycin (for resistant strains) | 30 mg/kg/day in 2 divided doses |
| | Clindamycin | 600–900 mg every 8 h |
| *Clostridium* species | Clindamycin plus penicillin | 600–900 mg every 8 h |
| | | 2–4 million units every 4–6 h |
| *Aeromonas hydrophila* | Doxycycline plus ciprofloxacin or ceftriaxone | 100 mg every 12 h |
| | | 500 mg every 12 h |
| | | 1–2 g every 24 h |
| *Vibrio vulnificus* | Doxycycline plus ceftriaxone or cefotaxime | 100 mg every 12 h |
| | | 1 g 4 times daily |
| | | 2 g 3 times daily |

gested that IVIG has benefits, but the sample size was not enough in one study [27]. In the other study, more patients were undergoing surgery and receiving clindamycin in the IVIG group than in the control group [28]. In a recent study, IVIG did not improve mortality and hospital length of stay in NF [29].

Some studies suggested that hyperbaric oxygen therapy (HBOT) significantly decreases the mortality of NF [30, 31]. But other studies suggested that HBOT has no benefit [32, 33]. Because HBOT needs time to perform, it may interfere with surgical treatment, and its benefit is controversial.

### 111.3.3 Prognosis

The mortality of NF has been reported to be 20–30% [3, 34, 35], even if appropriate treatment has been performed. The longer it takes to diagnose and treat, the higher the mortality is. When you have not performed debridement or amputation early and appropriately, the result is treatment failure and a poor prognosis. As NF progresses, it causes sepsis and multiple organ failure. Therefore, patients need not only surgical and antibiotic treatment but also systemic treatment according to their symptoms.

> **Dos and Don'ts**
> - Do not miss the timing for performing surgery.
> - Do not hesitate to perform debridement and amputation of an extremity.
> - Remove infected and necrotic tissues appropriately and repeatedly.
> - Check Gram's staining and culture, and choose antibiotics appropriately.

> **Take-Home Messages**
> - It is important to diagnose and treat NF as soon as possible.
> - Obtaining specimens from the affected area surgically is most useful in the diagnosis.
> - You must repeat this step to remove infected and necrotic tissues until they are not found.

> **Questions**
> 1. Which are the causative bacteria when healthy people get necrotizing fasciitis?
>    A. Mixed bacteria
>    B. Group A *streptococcus*
>    C. *Vibrio vulnificus*
>    D. Fungus
> 2. Which are the causative bacteria when people with diabetes mellitus get necrotizing fasciitis?
>    A. Mixed bacteria
>    B. Group A *streptococcus*
>    C. *Vibrio vulnificus*
>    D. Fungus
> 3. Choose one of the following that is not a skin finding of necrotizing fasciitis.
>    A. Tenderness
>    B. Edema
>    C. Itch
>    D. Erythema
> 4. Which test is most useful for necrotizing fasciitis?
>    A. Blood test
>    B. Blood culture
>    C. Diagnostic resection
>    D. Radiograph

5. The blood tests performed on the patient suspected of having necrotizing fasciitis are the following. Total white cell count is 18/mm. Hemoglobin is 12.0 g/dL. Sodium is 136 mmol/L. Creatinine is 1.7 mg/dL. Glucose is 160 mg/dL. C-reactive protein is 160 mg/L. How much is the LRINEC score?
   A. 5
   B. 6
   C. 7
   D. 8

6. Which of the following may not be visible on CT in patients with necrotizing fasciitis?
   A. Soft tissue swelling
   B. Involvement of the fascia
   C. Gas in the tissues
   D. Enhancement of the fascia

7. Which treatment is most important for necrotizing fasciitis?
   A. Antibiotic treatment
   B. Fluid infusion
   C. Incisional drainage
   D. Debridement or amputation of an extremity

8. To what extent should you remove tissues from the patient when you perform surgery for the patient with necrotizing fasciitis?
   A. To remove the affected tissues once
   B. To amputate an affected extremity
   C. To remove infected or necrotic tissues many times
   D. To collect the affected tissues

9. Which is not appropriate as empiric therapy for necrotizing fasciitis?
   A. Daptomycin plus piperacillin-tazobactam
   B. Vancomycin plus carbapenem
   C. Linezolid plus metronidazole
   D. Vancomycin plus piperacillin-tazobactam

10. How high is the mortality rate of necrotizing fasciitis?
    A. 5–10%
    B. 20–30%
    C. 40–50%
    D. 70–80%

**Answer:** 1. B; 2. A; 3. C; 4. C; 5. D; 6. D; 7. D; 8. C; 9. C; 10. B

## References

1. Glass G, Sheil F, Ruston J, Butler P. Necrotising soft tissue infection in a UK metropolitan population. Ann R Coll Surg Engl. 2015;97(1):46–51.
2. Naseer U, Steinbakk M, Blystad H, Caugant DA. Epidemiology of invasive group A streptococcal infections in Norway 2010–2014: a retrospective cohort study. Eur J Clin Microbiol Infect Dis. 2016;35(10):1639–48.
3. Nelson GE, Pondo T, Toews KA, Farley MM, Lindegren ML, Lynfield R, et al. Epidemiology of invasive group A Streptococcal infections in the United States, 2005–2012. Clin Infect Dis. 2016;63(4):478–86.
4. Bocking N, Matsumoto C-L, Loewen K, Teatero S, Marchand-Austin A, Gordon J, et al. High incidence of invasive group A Streptococcal infections in remote indigenous communities in Northwestern Ontario, Canada. Open Forum Infect Dis. 2017;4(1):ofw243.
5. Lancerotto L, Tocco I, Salmaso R, Vindigni V, Bassetto F. Necrotizing fasciitis: classification, diagnosis, and management. J Trauma Acute Care Surg. 2012;72(3):560–6.
6. Stevens DL, Bryant AE. Necrotizing soft-tissue infections. N Engl J Med. 2017;377(23):2253–65.
7. Hua C, Bosc R, Sbidian E, De Prost N, Hughes C, Jabre P, et al. Interventions for necrotizing soft tissue infections in adults. Cochrane Database Syst Rev. 2018;5(5):CD011680.
8. Morgan MS. Diagnosis and management of necrotising fasciitis: a multiparametric approach. J Hosp Infect. 2010;75(4):249–57.
9. Fais P, Viero A, Viel G, Giordano R, Raniero D, Kusstatscher S, et al. Necrotizing fasciitis: case series and review of the literature on clinical and medico-legal diagnostic challenges. Int J Legal Med. 2018;132(5):1357–66.
10. McHenry CR, Piotrowski JJ, Petrinic D, Malangoni MA. Determinants of mortality for necrotizing soft-tissue infections. Ann Surg. 1995;221(5):558–63; discussion 563–5.

11. Wong CH, Khin LW, Heng KS, Tan KC, Low CO. The LRINEC (Laboratory Risk Indicator for Necrotizing Fasciitis) score: a tool for distinguishing necrotizing fasciitis from other soft tissue infections. Crit Care Med. 2004;32(7):1535–41.
12. Fernando SM, Tran A, Cheng W, Rochwerg B, Kyeremanteng K, Seely AJE, et al. Necrotizing soft tissue infection: diagnostic accuracy of physical examination, imaging, and LRINEC score: a systematic review and meta-analysis. Ann Surg. 2019;269(1):58–65.
13. Carbonetti F, Cremona A, Carusi V, Guidi M, Iannicelli E, Di Girolamo M, et al. The role of contrast enhanced computed tomography in the diagnosis of necrotizing fasciitis and comparison with the laboratory risk indicator for necrotizing fasciitis (LRINEC). Radiol Med. 2016;121(2):106–21.
14. Kim K-T, Kim YJ, Won Lee J, Kim YJ, Park S-W, Lim MK, et al. Can necrotizing infectious fasciitis be differentiated from nonnecrotizing infectious fasciitis with MR imaging? Radiology. 2011;259(3):816–24.
15. Magalhães L, Martins SRP, Nogué R. The role of point-of-care ultrasound in the diagnosis and management of necrotizing soft tissue infections. Ultrasound J. 2020;12(1):3.
16. Majeski J, Majeski E. Necrotizing fasciitis: improved survival with early recognition by tissue biopsy and aggressive surgical treatment. South Med J. 1997;90(11):1065–8.
17. Nawijn F, Hietbrink F, Van Dijk MR. Getting it right the first time: frozen sections for diagnosing necrotizing soft tissue infections. World J Surg. 2021;45(1):148–59.
18. Alayed KA, Tan C, Daneman N. Red flags for necrotizing fasciitis: a case control study. Int J Infect Dis. 2015;36:15–20.
19. Bucca K, Spencer R, Orford N, Cattigan C, Athan E, McDonald A. Early diagnosis and treatment of necrotizing fasciitis can improve survival: an observational intensive care unit cohort study. ANZ J Surg. 2013;83(5):365–70.
20. Nawijn F, Smeeing DPJ, Houwert RM, Leenen LPH, Hietbrink F. Time is of the essence when treating necrotizing soft tissue infections: a systematic review and meta-analysis. World J Emerg Surg. 2020;15(1):4.
21. Stevens DL, Bisno AL, Chambers HF, Dellinger EP, Goldstein EJ, Gorbach SL, et al. Practice guidelines for the diagnosis and management of skin and soft tissue infections: 2014 update by the infectious diseases society of America. Clin Infect Dis. 2014;59(2):147–59.
22. Sartelli M, Guirao X, Hardcastle TC, Kluger Y, Boermeester MA, Rasa K, et al. 2018 WSES/SIS-E consensus conference: recommendations for the management of skin and soft-tissue infections. World J Emerg Surg. 2018;13:58.
23. Goldstein EJC, Anaya DA, Dellinger EP. Necrotizing soft-tissue infection: diagnosis and management. Clin Infect Dis. 2007;44(5):705–10.
24. Baharestani MM. Negative pressure wound therapy in the adjunctive management of necrotizing fasciitis: examining clinical outcomes. Ostomy Wound Manage. 2008;54(4):44–50.
25. Lee J, Jung H, Kwon H, Jung S-N. Extended negative pressure wound therapy-assisted dermatotraction for the closure of large open fasciotomy wounds in necrotizing fasciitis patients. World J Emerg Surg. 2014;9(1):29.
26. Orgill DP, Manders EK, Sumpio BE, Lee RC, Attinger CE, Gurtner GC, et al. The mechanisms of action of vacuum assisted closure: more to learn. Surgery. 2009;146(1):40–51.
27. Darenberg J, Ihendyane N, Sjolin J, Aufwerber E, Haidl S, Follin P, et al. Intravenous immunoglobulin G therapy in streptococcal toxic shock syndrome: a European randomized, double-blind, placebo-controlled trial. Clin Infect Dis. 2003;37(3):333–40.
28. Kaul R, McGeer A, Norrby-Teglund A, Kotb M, Schwartz B, O'Rourke K, et al. Intravenous immunoglobulin therapy for streptococcal toxic shock syndrome—a comparative observational study. Clin Infect Dis. 1999;28(4):800–7.
29. Kadri SS, Swihart BJ, Bonne SL, Hohmann SF, Hennessy LV, Louras P, et al. Impact of intravenous immunoglobulin on survival in necrotizing fasciitis with vasopressor-dependent shock: a propensity-score matched analysis from 130 US hospitals. Clin Infect Dis. 2017;64(7):877–85.
30. Shaw JJ, Psoinos C, Emhoff TA, Shah SA, Santry HP. Not just full of hot air: hyperbaric oxygen therapy increases survival in cases of necrotizing soft tissue infections. Surg Infect. 2014;15(3):328–35.
31. Devaney B, Frawley G, Frawley L, Pilcher DV. Necrotising soft tissue infections: the effect of hyperbaric oxygen on mortality. Anaesth Intensive Care. 2015;43(6):685–92.
32. Wang C. Hyperbaric oxygen for treating wounds. Arch Surg. 2003;138(3):272.
33. Willy C, Rieger H, Vogt D. Hyperbaric oxygen therapy for necrotizing soft tissue infections: contra. Chirurg. 2012;83(11):960–72.
34. Jabbour G, El-Menyar A, Peralta R, Shaikh N, Abdelrahman H, Mudali IN, et al. Pattern and predictors of mortality in necrotizing fasciitis patients in a single tertiary hospital. World J Emerg Surg. 2016;11(1):40.
35. Van Stigt SFL, De Vries J, Bijker JB, Mollen RMHG, Hekma EJ, Lemson SM, et al. Review of 58 patients with necrotizing fasciitis in the Netherlands. World J Emerg Surg. 2016;11(1):21.

## Further Reading

Hua C, Bosc R, Sbidian E, De Prost N, Hughes C, Jabre P, et al. Interventions for necrotizing soft tissue infections in adults. Cochrane Database Syst Rev. 2018;5:CD011680.

Morgan MS. Diagnosis and management of necrotising fasciitis: a multiparametric approach. J Hosp Infect. 2010;75(4):249–57.

Sartelli M, Guirao X, Hardcastle TC, Kluger Y, Boermeester MA, Rasa K, et al. 2018 WSES/SIS-E consensus conference: recommendations for the management of skin and soft-tissue infections. World J Emerg Surg. 2018;13:58.

Stevens DL, Bryant AE. Necrotizing soft-tissue infections. N Engl J Med. 2017;377(23):2253–65.

Stevens DL, Bisno AL, Chambers HF, Dellinger EP, Goldstein EJ, Gorbach SL, et al. Practice guidelines for the diagnosis and management of skin and soft tissue infections: 2014 update by the infectious diseases society of America. Clin Infect Dis. 2014;59(2):147–59.

# Bone Infections

## 112

Luigi Branca Vergano and Mauro Monesi

## 112.1 Introduction

> **Learning Goals**
> - To identify different groups of osteomyelitis: children's osteomyelitis, spontaneous osteomyelitis, diabetic foot osteomyelitis, pressure ulcer osteomyelitis, periprosthetic joint infections, fracture-related infections, and osteomyelitis.
> - To know and choose the most adequate diagnostic tools to better recognize the different types of osteomyelitis.
> - To understand the general treatment options (medical and surgical) for the different groups of osteomyelitis and then tailor the therapy to each patient.

Cierny defined osteomyelitis as "infected dead bone enveloped with compromised soft tissue"; this definition, although concise, is very clear: it highlights that the problem does concern not only the bone but also the surrounding tissues [1].

L. Branca Vergano (✉)
Orthopaedic and Trauma Department, Santa Chiara Hospital, APSS Trento, Trento, Italy
e-mail: luigi.brancavergano@apss.tn.it

M. Monesi
Orthopaedic and Trauma Department, Bufalini Hospital, AUSL Romagna, Cesena, FC, Italy

There are many groups (or families) of osteomyelitis: even though they may have some common characteristics (clinical appearance, laboratory and imaging features, treatment options, etc.), some important differences can be detected among the various groups. To better understand and underscore these differences, each paragraph in this chapter will divide osteomyelitis didactically, as you can see in Table 112.1, into seven types: osteomyelitis in children (CO), spontaneous (or subacute) osteomyelitis in adults (SO), osteomyelitis in the diabetic foot (DFO), osteomyelitis in pressure ulcer lesions (PUO), osteomyelitis in periprosthetic joint infection (PJI), fracture-related infections and osteomyelitis (FRIO) [2–7].

The general features of each group will be discussed, with particular emphasis on the most frequent family of osteomyelitis (FRIO); an exhaustive description and treatment of every group is beyond the scope of this book, and readers can study the area of interest in more depth with the books and papers listed at the end of the chapter.

### 112.1.1 Epidemiology

The epidemiology of osteomyelitis varies significantly in the different groups, and there can be considerable differences between different world regions.

In high-income countries, CO occurs in about 2–13 out of 100,000 children per year, while, in

**Table 112.1** Groups of osteomyelitis

| Group of osteomyelitis | Main features |
|---|---|
| Osteomyelitis in children (CO) | Typical of children with open physis; often the result of hematogenous seeding of bacteria to the metaphyseal region of the bone |
| Spontaneous (or subacute) osteomyelitis in adults (SO) | Hematogenous infection of bone, characterized by an insidious course, with paucity of systemic symptoms |
| Osteomyelitis in diabetic foot (DFO) | Frequent complication of diabetic foot ulcers, with deep penetration of the infections and involvement of long and short bones of the foot |
| Osteomyelitis in pressure ulcers lesions (PUO) | Patients with neurological diseases are prone to develop pressure ulcers due to their immobility. If left untreated, these ulcers can extend to the bone |
| Osteomyelitis in periprosthetic joint infection (PJI) | In case of untreated infection of a prosthesis (hip, knee, shoulder, etc.), the bone can be potentially involved, with consequent mobilization of the implant and spread of the infection to the entire bone segment |
| Fracture-related infections and osteomyelitis (FRIO) | Consequence of a musculoskeletal trauma that involves the bone. This scenario is complicated by the fracture and by the possible presence of hardware (plates, screws, nails, etc.) |

low-income countries, it is much more common (43–200/100,000). In high-income countries, the incidence of acute and subacute hematogenous osteomyelitis in children has been declining in recent years: this is the result of reduced virulence of responsible pathogens, together with increased host resistance and increasing availability and effectiveness of antibiotics. In low-income countries, especially in Sub-Saharan Africa, a large proportion of the pediatric population resides in rural areas and faces poverty and malnutrition, creating a milieu where chronic osteomyelitis can arise. Moreover, the high incidence of sickle cell disease (a well-recognized risk factor for osteomyelitis) worsens the scenario [8, 9].

The exact incidence of SO is unknown. Hematogenous osteomyelitis is rare in individuals beyond their teens, occurring only in immunocompromised hosts. The most common site of SO is the spine, with an approximate incidence of 2.2 out of 100,000 per year. Recent studies suggest that the incidence of spinal infections is now increasing in relation to increased use of vascular devices and a rise in intravenous drug abuse. Pyogenic spondylodiscitis (infection affecting the vertebral body and the intervertebral disc) is twice as common in men, and it most commonly occurs in adults over 50 years of age [3, 10].

The global prevalence of diabetic foot varies from 3% in Oceania to 13% in North America, with a global average of 6.4%. The annual incidence of diabetic foot ulcers in diabetic patients is about 2–5%, and the lifetime risk ranges from 15% to 20%. DFO occurs from 10–15% of moderately infected ulcers to 50% in severely infected ones. DFO can affect any bone but most frequently the forefoot (90%), followed by the midfoot (5%) and the hindfoot (5%) [11].

As a result of pressure in combination with shear associated with immobility, pressure ulcers mostly occur in para- or tetraplegic patients after spinal cord injuries, or in geriatric or intensive care settings. PUO can be a complication of a chronic sacral pressure ulcer, but it is not as common as one would imagine. Contrary to the perception that exposed bone must contain osteomyelitis, in several case series in which bone biopsies were conducted, the histological evidence of osteomyelitis was reported in a minority of such patients. In stage 4 pressure ulcer lesions, deep-seated infections, including contiguous osteomyelitis, have been reported in 17–32% of these cases [12, 13].

After joint replacement, PJIs occur in 0.3–1.7% of hip, 0.5–2% of knee, 1–3.9% of shoulder, and 2–9% of ankle prosthesis. The annual incidence of periprosthetic joint infections has been slightly increasing in recent years; the greatest risk period is during the first 2 years, in which 60–70% of infections occur. The involvement of a peri-implant bone by the infection can be avoided with a thorough and timely intervention, impeding the involvement of the entire bone segment [6, 14].

Infection associated with orthopedic internal fixation devices occurs in 1–2% of cases after closed fractures and in up to 25–30% after open fractures (2–4% for grades I and II; between 4% and 52% for grade III fractures according to the Gustilo-Anderson classification). In general, the increasing use of internal fixation and the emergence of antibiotic-resistant microorganisms have exacerbated this problem, while many specific factors have been identified as increasing the risk of infection: medical comorbidities, smoking, location of the fracture (tibia), polytrauma, penetrating, blast, and combat injuries, compartment syndrome, irradiation-related fractures, pathological fractures, pelvic fractures requiring arterial embolization, and nonunions [15–17].

### 112.1.2 Etiology

Local and systemic factors of the patient can influence the onset, the spread, and the persistence of the infection, as well as the type of bacteria that colonize and infect the patient. Some well-recognized systemic risk factors for the development of a bone infection are nicotine and alcohol abuse, drug use, obesity, diabetes mellitus, malignant diseases, and allergies to components of implanted hardware (chrome and nickel). On the other hand, local risk factors are hypoperfusion of a body region (e.g., traumatized limb or artery occlusive disease, etc.), venous stasis and chronic lymphedema, radiogenic fibrosis, and severe scarring due to previous surgery. Furthermore, only placing a surgical implant weakens immune defense: in fact, theoretically, 100,000,000 germs are required to cause an infection in a bone, but only 10,000–100,000 germs are required in the presence of an internal device [1, 16].

The most common organism isolated in CO is *Staphylococcus aureus* (60% of cases in children between the ages of 1 month and 5 years), with methicillin-resistant *Staphylococcus aureus* (MRSA) increasing in prevalence in recent years. The second most common organism is *Streptococcus*; group B *Streptococcus* is prevalent in the first 2 months of life. Less frequent are gram-negative organisms like *Escherichia coli*, *Proteus*, *Pseudomonas*, and *Brucella*. Salmonella isolation is common in developing countries and often associated with sickle cell disease [8, 9].

The most common site of infection in SO is the spine, followed by long bones and the pelvis. As in CO, *Staphylococcus aureus* is the most common cause. Hematogenous seeding of gram-negative organisms may result from intra-abdominal infections or urinary tract infections. *Pseudomonas aeruginosa* and *Serratia marcescens* are found more frequently in intravenous drug abusers (Fig. 112.1), *Salmonella* and *Propionibacterium* in patients with sickle cell disease, and *Klebsiella pneumoniae* in diabetes mellitus patients. The last organism is frequent in long-bone osteomyelitis, mimicking a bone tumor lesion. While, in the past, *Mycobacterium tuberculosis* was considered to be the most common cause of spinal infections (50% of the cases), in recent times the microbiology of spinal infections has changed: nowadays, the most common cause is *Staphylococcus aureus*, followed by *Streptococcus*, *Enterococcus*, and *E. coli* [3, 9, 18].

*Staphylococcus aureus* is the most commonly involved organism in DFO (50% of the cases), with an increasing rate of infection by MRSA in recent years, followed by *Staphylococcus epidermidis*, *Streptococcus*, and Enterobacteriaceae. Among gram-negative bacteria, *E. coli*, *Klebsiella pneumoniae*, and *Proteus* are the most common isolated microorganisms. Most of the time, DFO is sustained by polymicrobial flora, reflecting soft tissue infections in diabetic patients [11].

PUO is frequently sustained by mixed flora (*Staphylococcus aureus*, *Streptococcus*, *Pseudomonas* above all); the common and wide use of antibiotics in this particular population may affect culture results. Furthermore, in many

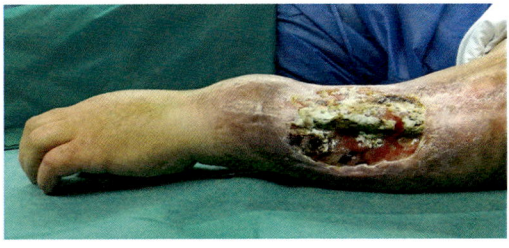

**Fig. 112.1** Chronic osteomyelitis of the left forearm (Cierny-Mader type IV) in a 38-year-old drug abuser; large soft tissue defect and necrotic ulna can be seen

studies about PUO, anaerobic cultures were not routinely utilized [5, 12].

In acute PJIs, characterized by draining and dehiscence of the wound, *Staphylococcus* species are the most commonly reported; again, with the increasing rate of isolation of MRSA, that represents a major risk for implant failure and acute mobilization. Other microorganisms involved in acute PJIs are *Enterococcus* and gram-negative bacilli. Chronic PJIs are either exogenously or—rarely—hematogenously acquired. They are typically caused by microorganisms of low virulence, including coagulase-negative staphylococci and anaerobic bacteria such as *Propionibacterium acnes*. These infections are often diagnosed with considerable delay; their clinical features are chronic joint effusion, pain due to inflammation, or implant loosening. Even in PJIs, polymicrobial flora is common [11, 14].

In FRIO, an organism can reach the fracture site at the time of injury (direct contamination in an open fracture), during treatment (hospital-acquired infections), or via the hematogenous route. The timing of the manifestation of infection (early vs. late) has been associated with specific pathogens, even though strong evidence is lacking. Nosocomial contamination has been demonstrated to be the most common source of lower limb FRIO. *Staphylococcus* species are the most commonly responsible, both in early and late infections; in some areas, MRSA is now more frequent than methicillin-susceptible. Enterobacteriaceae are the second most common species in early (within 2 weeks) post-operative infections. Coagulase negative staphylococci, streptococci, and anaerobes, on the other side, are often found in late infections; in these infections, also lower virulence skin flora, such as *Corynebacterium* and *Propionibacterium*, are increasingly identified. Polymicrobial infections are present in up to 30% of the cases. In recent years, some "problematic" bacteria, which are multiresistant and extremely difficult to treat, have been increasing in FRIO: methicillin-resistant *Staphylococcus epidermidis* (MRSE), *Acinetobacter baumannii*, highly resistant enterococci, and extended-spectrum betalactamase (ESBL)-producing pseudomonas. In clinically obvious FRIO, negative culture can be obtained; the most common reason is the prior use of antimicrobials. Other common factors include insufficient microbiological testing, an inadequate quantity of specimens, failure to obtain representative samples, or the fact that some infections could be sustained by organisms that cannot be cultured [1, 15–17].

Table 112.2 summarizes the most frequently isolated organisms from the different types of osteomyelitis.

## 112.1.3 Classification

The Cierny-Mader classification of adult osteomyelitis was published 35 years ago; it still represents a valid method to identify the clinical stage of osteomyelitis to aid in treatment planning and to act as a prognostic indicator. The Cierny-Mader classification can be used for all groups of osteomyelitis; for PJIs and FRIO, some specific classifications will be discussed separately. The Cierny-Mader classification consists in 12 clinical stages, combining three host classes (A-host, B-host, and C-host) and four anatomic variants (types I, II, III, and IV). The anatomic type determines the surgical approach, whereas the host class regulates the selection of therapeutic options. The clinical stage of osteomyelitis, together with the anatomic site of the infection, will direct treatment: palliative or curative, simple or complex, limb-sparing or radical (amputation) [16, 18, 19].

Healthy patients are designated as A-hosts; patients with comorbidities affecting their response to stress, trauma, or infection are classified as B-hosts. The rate of treatment failure is higher in B-hosts, both for general pathologies (immunodeficiency, metabolic disease, etc.) and for regional problems (wound healing deficiencies, arteriopathy, etc.). Host optimization (treatment and correction of the altered metabolic status due to comorbidities) can improve B-host outcomes, bringing them close to those for A-hosts. If the risks of a potential treatment outweigh the benefits, the patient is classified as C-host: the cure for these patients is palliative.

**Table 112.2** Most frequently isolated microorganisms in different types of osteomyelitis

| Type of osteomyelitis | Acute (or early) infections | Chronic (or late) infections |
|---|---|---|
| Children osteomyelitis | Staphylococcus aureus, Streptococcus (group B); Salmonella (in sickle cell patients) | |
| Spontaneous osteomyelitis | Staphylococcus aureus; Pseudomonas aeruginosa and Serratia marcescens (drug abusers); Salmonella and Propionibacterium (in sickle cell patients); Klebsiella pneumoniae (in diabetics) | |
| Spine spontaneous osteomyelitis | Staphylococcus aureus, Streptococcus, Enterococcus and Escherichia coli; Mycobacterium tuberculosis (developing countries) | |
| Diabetic foot osteomyelitis | Polymicrobial infections: Staphylococcus aureus (MRSA), Staphylococcus epidermidis, Streptococcus, Escherichia coli, Klebsiella pneumoniae, Proteus | |
| Pressure ulcer osteomyelitis | Polymicrobial infections: Staphylococcus aureus, Streptococcus, Pseudomonas | |
| Periprosthetic joint infections | Staphylococcus aureus, Staphylococcus epidermidis, Streptococcus, Enterococcus spp., Escherichia coli, Pseudomonas aeruginosa | Coagulase-negative staphylococci, anaerobic bacteria (Propionibacterium acnes) |
| Fracture-related infections | Staphylococcus aureus (MRSA), Enterobacteriaceae | Coagulase-negative staphylococci, streptococci and anaerobic bacteria; increasing "difficult" organisms: methicillin-resistant Staphylococcus epidermidis (MRSE), Acinetobacter baumanii, extended-spectrum betalactamase (ESBL)-producing Pseudomonas |

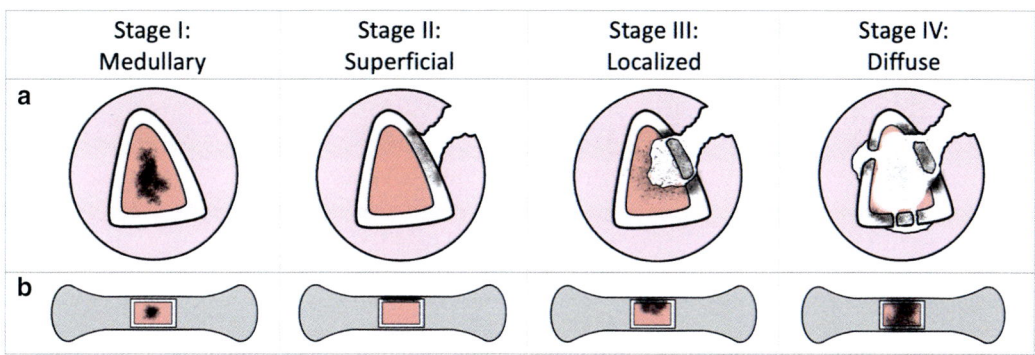

**Fig. 112.2** Cierny-Mader classification. (**a**) Transversal plane vision. (**b**) Coronal plane vision. (Reproduced with permission from the paper *Developments in antibiotic-eluting scaffolds for the treatment of osteomyelitis*, Appl. Sci. 2020, 10(7), 2244; by MDPI (Multidisciplinary Digital Publishing Institute))

The anatomic types (or stages) of osteomyelitis increase in complexity from stage I to stage IV (Fig. 112.2).

- Stage I: medullary osteomyelitis. The nidus is confined to the endosteum as dense scar, infarcted marrow, and dead bone. Soft-tissue involvement is usually reactive and responsive to removal of the nidus or to a short course of antibiotics. It can be diaphyseal or metaphyseal.
- Stage II: superficial osteomyelitis. The nidus is an exposed bony surface, at the base of a

chronic, open wound. The medullary contents are not involved.
- Stage III: localized osteomyelitis. This is characterized by a full-thickness, cortical sequestrum (dead bone). After debridement of the sequestrum, the bony segment will still be stable.
- Stage IV: diffuse osteomyelitis. This is an infection that combines the characteristics of stage I, II, and III osteomyelitis with the additional feature of instability of the bone. In fact, these lesions are either intrinsically unstable or become unstable after complete debridement.

Other methods of characterization (rather than "classification") exist that divide osteomyelitis into categories and are useful in describing this pathology [20]:

- Hematogenous (derived from or transported by blood) osteomyelitis or secondary to a contiguous focus of infection.
- Acute or chronic osteomyelitis (the exact period of time that differentiates these categories can vary in different scenarios—see below).

The most important PJI classification is based on the time since the primary onset of the symptoms. This directly suggests the maturation stage of the biofilm (see Sect. 112.1.4) and is crucial in choosing the optimal treatment strategy [21, 22].

- Acute PJI. The clinical symptoms are acute pain, fever, a red and swollen joint, and a wound problem (discharge, dehiscence). The symptoms typically appear within 3–4 weeks after prosthetic implantation. The infection is generally acquired during surgery or hospitalization. The causative organisms are high-virulence bacteria; the biofilm is considered still immature.
- Chronic PJI. The symptoms appear 3–4 weeks after the operation. They are often long-lasting and not severe: pain, sinus tract, malfunction, and mobilization of the implant. The organisms involved are low-virulence bacteria, acquired during hospitalization or—rarely—via hematogenous route. The biofilm is mature and strictly adherent to the implant.

Also for FRIO, a chronological classification is widely accepted. It is based on the time between internal fixation and the diagnosis of infection [16, 17].

- Early infections (within 2 weeks after implantation). They are the most common and are associated with virulent organisms (*Staphylococcus aureus*, *Streptococcus pyogenes*, aerobic gram-negative bacilli). As mentioned for PJIs, organisms at an early stage are susceptible to antibiotics, which are associated with less biofilm and bone sequestrum formation.
- Delayed infections (3–10 weeks after implantation). They are associated with low- or moderate-virulent organisms, usually skin flora such as *Staphylococcus aureus* or *Staphylococcus epidermidis*. The infection can severely interfere with fracture healing; it is hard to eradicate due to the presence of biofilm, sequestra, and microbial resistance.
- Late infections (>10 weeks after implantation) are commonly associated with delayed diagnosis. Typical organisms are *Staphylococcus aureus*, *Staphylococcus epidermidis*, and *Pseudomonas aeruginosa*. The clinical features, suggested treatment, and general prognosis are similar to those of delayed infections.

A more specific classification was described by Romanò, who divides FRIO into three types [23]:

- Type I infections: the implant is stable and there is progressive callus formation. These cases may be treated nonoperatively, with antibiotics, and can reach complete fracture union.
- Type II infections: there is stable osteosynthesis but poor or absent callus formation/progression. Stability of the implant should be maintained with hardware retention. Infection

is controlled surgically (debridement) and with drugs. Bone healing can be stimulated with physical stimulation, biological factors, or mechanical strategy (implementation of fixation).
- Type III infections: the implant is grossly unstable, and callus formation is absent. Hardware removal is required, and other strategies of fixation are needed, together with infection surgical treatment.

### 112.1.4 Pathophysiology

CO is considered a spontaneous osteomyelitis, but a blunt trauma can precede the onset of symptoms in more than 60% of the cases, and in some studies, in 15% of the cases, an entry point is suspected. From bloodstream, organisms settle in the juxta epiphyseal areas (metaphysis or epiphysis of long bones, especially around the knee). An anatomical factor that could explain this localization is the peculiar vascular architecture in the metaphysis, which prompts stagnation of blood flow, thrombosis, and the multiplication of bacteria. Afterwards, from the metaphysis, the infection can spread to the epiphysis through the joint or, in children in their first year of life, through direct vascular anastomosis. In acute infections, pus is formed within the metaphysis and tracks through the Haversian system to the cortex, elevating the periosteum and forming a subperiosteal abscess ("acute osteoperiostitis"). The rising pressure, vascular stasis, infective thrombosis, and periosteal stripping compromise the blood supply, and portions of cortical bone become necrotic (sequestra). The pus either reenters the bone at another level or discharges out into the soft tissues and through the skin (sinus tract or fistula). The periosteum responds to infection by laying down new bone: in chronic cases, this involucrum surrounds the dead and infected bone [9, 24].

In SO, infection usually begins in the diaphysis and may spread to the entire medullary canal. The vertebrae are the most common site of infection in adults, but hematogenous osteomyelitis also occurs in the long bones and pelvis. Patients affected by sickle cell disease are at high risk for SO; because of their shape, the erythrocytes are more likely to become trapped in small, slow-flowing vessels, leading to occlusion, bone necrosis, and consequent superinfection. In acute SO, cortical erosion by pus can lead to a soft tissue abscess and then form a sinus tract to the skin. Otherwise, the pus can erode the joint capsule, causing septic arthritis. As in CO, in chronic cases, dead bone (sequestrum) can be enveloped by sclerotic and poorly vascularized bone covered by a thickened periosteum, scarred muscle, and subcutaneous tissue (involucrum). Antibiotics and the host's innate immune system cannot reach the avascular area inside the involucrum. In vertebral SO, the microorganisms gain access to the spine via Batson's venous plexus, which anastomoses with both the systemic veins and the portal venous system. The bacteria settle on the vertebral end plate and then spread to the intervertebral disc and to contiguous vertebral bodies through intermetaphyseal anastomoses (spondylodiscitis). As the infection continues, progressive bone and disc destruction occurs (Fig. 112.3). If not treated, the infection can reach the spinal canal, causing epidural abscess [18, 25, 26].

DFO is usually a contiguity infection, the consequence of a soft tissue infection that spreads into the bone, involving the cortex first and then the marrow. A large variety of bacteria may colonize diabetic foot ulcers; these bacteria can subsequently infect the subcutaneous tissue and then the deepest tissues (fascia, muscles, tendons, joints, and, finally, bone), causing necrosis and gangrene [11, 18].

In PUO, the bone infection is generally restricted to the superficial layer of the cortical bone, even in ulcers that have been present for months or years. The bone reacts to pressure ulcers with reactive fibrosis, medullary edema, and reactive bone formation, and it is often impossible to distinguish this paraphysiologic reaction from PUO; only histopathology is diriment in such cases [12].

PJI and FRIO recognize similar pathophysiology, because of the bacteria's behavior in the early and late phases. At inoculation, bacteria

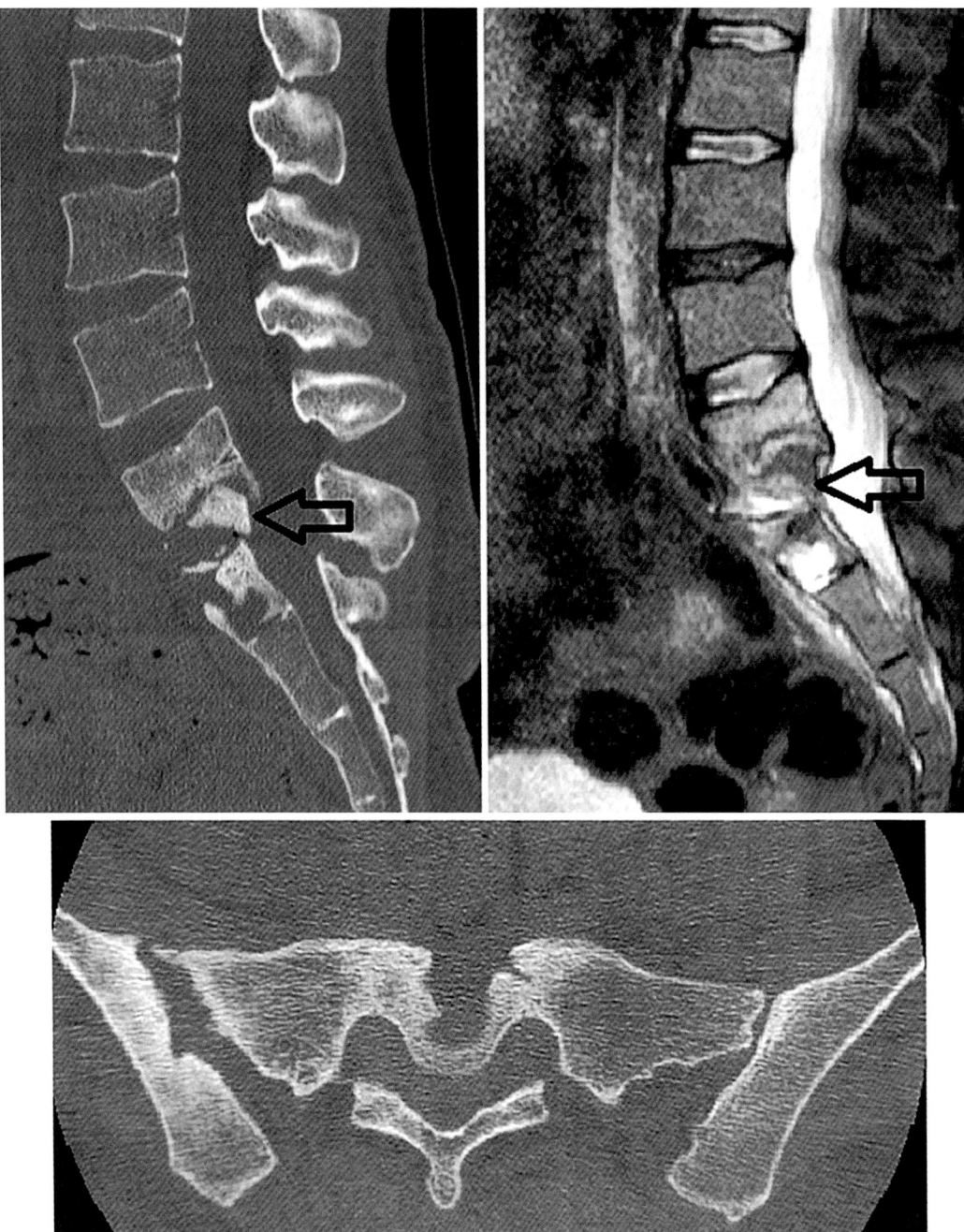

**Fig. 112.3** CT and MR imaging of spontaneous spondylodiscitis in a drug abuser. Complete destruction of L5 body (black arrows) can be noted in sagittal cuts; the axial CT cut evidences lysis of S1 and involvement of the right sacroiliac joint

are in planktonic form and susceptible to host defenses and antibiotics; soon, bacteria initiate infection in the soft tissue and replicate rapidly. In the following 1–2 weeks, bacteria produce a biofilm consisting of extracellular polysaccharides. This biofilm incorporates cells (sessile state of bacteria) and extracellular products and strictly adheres to implant surfaces. Biofilm-bound organisms are resistant to phagocytosis, and the exopolysaccharide matrix hinders the penetration of antibiotics and antibodies. Macrophages and granulocytes accumulate around implants, but they are functionally defective; their products can damage the surrounding tissues. Surface-associated material from staphylococci induces leukocyte production of TNF-a, IL-I, and IL-6. These cytokines hyperactivate osteoclasts, and excessive bone is reabsorbed from infected areas adjacent to the implant and the fracture, leading to mechanical failure, instability, nonunion, and persistence of infection. Although the mechanism is still unknown, it is believed that increased soft tissue irritation, difficulty in revascularization, hematoma, and evolving dead space resulting from excess motion of the fracture and/or implant are all factors favorable to the persistence of infection. Bacteria can survive in a sessile state for decades; at any time, they can transfer from this state to a planktonic state and overgrow the body like metastases [1, 6, 16, 17, 19].

## 112.2 Diagnosis

### 112.2.1 Clinical Presentation

In osteomyelitis, the clinician might typically expect signs and symptoms peculiar to infection: fever, malaise, pain, swelling, redness, and warmth in the affected bone segment; impaired movement of the adjacent joints; and difficulty in weight bearing and walking. However, this is not the rule, and in some cases, even only one of these symptoms should be a warning signal of a potential bone infection. The clinical presentation of osteomyelitis has some characteristic features in the different groups of bone infections, as described below.

CO is located mainly in the lower limbs (70%), and, secondarily, in the upper limbs (20%) and other bones. The femur and tibia are involved in about 60% of all locations. Acute cases occur in all age groups, with a small peak in incidence among prepubertal boys. Children this age are particularly involved in strenuous physical activity and prone to traumatic and microtraumatic injury, potential genesis of CO. In general, children look ill and have a high temperature; local tenderness and swelling can be found in the superficial bone segment. Sometimes cellulitis in a child can be a sign of osteomyelitis. Infants may have a "pseudoparalysis" of the affected limb, and at this age, the simultaneous involvement of multiple bones is not uncommon [8, 9, 24].

The clinical diagnosis of SO is still difficult; as a matter of fact, the acute phase is often missed (apart from those cases with impairment of general status and clear local signs), while signs and symptoms in subacute cases are extremely nonspecific. Particularly, in spine osteomyelitis, an early diagnosis is mandatory before serious complications occur; unfortunately, many patients do not seek medical attention until their symptoms become severe and debilitating. Deep boring back pain, unrelieved by rest or position, is the most common symptom of pyogenic vertebral osteomyelitis. The lumbar region is affected in approximately 45% of patients, followed by the thoracic spine (35%) and the cervical spine (20%). In the final stages, motor and sensory defects can occur as a consequence of the spinal canal spreading of the infection [2, 9, 18, 26].

Diabetic patients may show an ingrown toenail, cellulitis, deep space infection, or perforating foot ulcer. Infected wounds usually show purulent secretions or other signs of inflammation (swelling, erythema, blood serum secretion, or simply blood with or without bone fragments); however, DFO can occur without any local sign of inflammation. The potential for bone involvement should be suspected in all patients with diabetic foot ulcers and clinical signs of infection, in chronic wounds, and in case of ulcer recurrence. The clinical diagnosis of DFO is even more challenging in case of concomitant vascular pathologies or peripheral neuropathies. There are two clinical signs considered to be predictive of DFO. The first is the width and depth of the foot ulcer: deep ulcers (>3 mm) are more easily associated with an underlying osteomyelitis than superficial ulcers. The second is the "probe-to-bone test" (PTB), which is performed by probing the ulcer area with a sterile blunt probe. If the probe reaches the bone surface, the PTB is considered positive [11, 18].

The most severe pressure ulcers (so-called stage IV) usually affect the tissue overlying the sacrum, ischial bones, and femoral heads, and therefore PUO is typically found in these locations. The diagnosis of osteomyelitis can be puzzling because it is not easy to differentiate a PUO from simple microbial colonization of the ulcer or from noninfectious pressure-related bone changes underneath an ulcer. Moreover, patients with spinal cord injury are very often unable to report local pain, and the subjective symptoms can be completely absent. Systemic symptoms (like fever) seem to be more likely correlated with soft tissue infection rather than with the extent of bone involvement [5, 12].

There are well-known risk factors associated with PJIs: obesity, diabetes, rheumatoid arthritis, immunosuppressive medications, and malignancy. The clinical manifestation of acute PJIs can vary depending on the virulence of the microorganisms, the host immune response, the soft tissue structure surrounding the joint, and the joint involved. The most common signs or symptoms are pain, joint swelling or effusion, erythema or warmth around the joint, fever, wound dehiscence, drainage, or the presence of a sinus tract communicating with the arthroplasty. In contrast, chronic PJIs can be clinically undistinguishable from aseptic failure of the prosthetic implant: patients report chronic pain and deterioration of implant function. A sinus tract is present in only a few chronic cases [6, 22].

The risk of FRIO is correlated with the extent of the bone and soft tissue injury, with previous or current surgery at the same site, and with history of skin or deep infections. Signs and symptoms of FRIO are strictly similar to those of PJIs. In acute cases, fever, chills, and night sweats characterize the general status, while warmth, redness, swelling, and pus drainage reflect the local situation. In chronic FRIO, all the local and systemic symptoms described may be lacking, so that the only sign of suspicion is the nonunion of the fracture. In this case, a clinical differentiation from an aseptic nonunion is impossible, and further exams are deemed necessary (Fig. 112.4) [7, 27].

### 112.2.2 Tests

When bone infection is suspected, a complete blood count is useful for evaluating leukocytosis, which is quite common in acute osteomyelitis before therapy. The leukocyte count rarely exceeds 15,000/µL acutely and is usually normal in chronic osteomyelitis. Conversely, anemia is commonly observed in chronic cases. In metastatic and some metabolic bone diseases, alkaline phosphatase (ALP), calcium, and phosphate are elevated, but they are usually within normal limits in osteomyelitis. The erythrocyte sedimentation rate (ESR) and C-reactive protein (CRP) are often elevated; however, they both lack specificity. In cases of proven osteomyelitis, both tests may be used for follow-up and assessing response to therapy [1].

Diagnosis of osteomyelitis is based on the isolation of the pathogen from the bone lesion or from blood cultures. In case of hematogenous osteomyelitis, positive blood cultures could eliminate the need for a bone biopsy (if there is strong radiographic evidence of osteomyelitis). Bone and tissue samples (at least five every debridement) are more effective than swabs in detecting contaminant organisms. If a bone biopsy cannot be obtained, the culture of purulent material is an option that is not definitive and must be interpreted with caution. We strongly point out that wound swabs are obsolete. Superficial swabs are neither sensitive nor specific in wounds and sinus tracts because contamination and colonization from skin flora are common; the primary pathogen or secondary pathogen(s) can be missed in polymicrobial infections. Even heavy growth of a common pathogen is not indicative of its involvement. If orthopedic implants, foreign bodies, and/or sequestra are removed during debridement, sonication (a low-frequency ultrasound procedure used to detach biofilm-bound organisms) is essential to isolate bacteria [1, 8, 16, 19].

Histopathology of acute osteomyelitis consists of inflammatory exudates composed of fibrin, polymorphonuclear leucocytes, and macrophages in the acute stage. In chronic cases, fibrosis of the marrow with a chronic inflammatory infiltrate and plasma cell predominance can

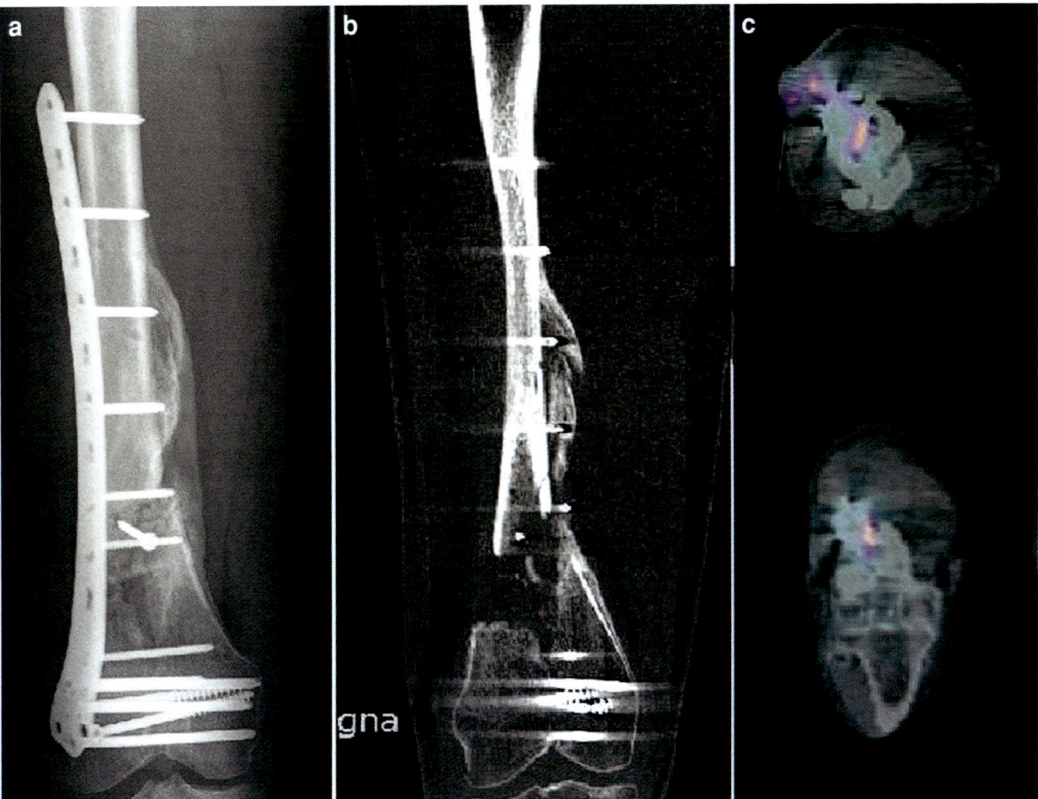

**Fig. 112.4** Septic nonunion of the right femur after distal femur plating of an open fracture. (**a**) X-ray, apparently normal. (**b**) CT showing a large bone defect in the metaphyseal region. (**c**) FDG-PET revealing infection, with glucose hypercaptation at the level of the bone defect

be observed, along with fragments of necrotic bone with multinucleated giant cells. New technologies, such as mass spectrometry, pulsed field gel electrophoresis, and DNA pyrosequencing, are showing promising results in detecting and characterizing pathogens. These techniques can be applied to all pathogen classes and species, and can detect any organism regardless of its culturability, prior antimicrobial treatment, or metabolic state [2].

In SO, the diagnosis can often be made only after careful study of the histopathologic features of the lesions. In PUO, the challenge is to distinguish between colonizing and invasive bacteria, as both originate from the commensal cutaneous flora; even histological analysis of bone biopsies sometimes cannot securely diagnose a bone infection. In PJIs, synovial fluid can be easily obtained; it is not indicative of bone involvement from the infection, but if it is positive for bacteria, an in-depth study with other diagnostic tools is strongly recommended. After fixation of a fracture, CRP usually peaks on the second postoperative day and normalizes after 2–3 weeks. A persistently raised CRP beyond 4–7 days after surgery should lead the physician to rule out an infection. In FRIO, when the implant must be removed, it is necessary to collect at least five tissue samples from around the infected implant, prior to its removal. After that, prolonged enrichment broth cultures (from 5 to 14 days) are required, as well as the sonication of the implant [2, 6, 13, 28].

Conventional radiograms are always the first diagnostic step of bone infection. The earliest changes (that lag at least 10–14 days after the onset of the infection) include swelling of the soft tissue, periosteal thickening or elevation, and focal osteopenia. In order for the radiographs to show lytic changes, at least 50–75% of the bone matrix must have been destroyed. In chronic osteomyelitis, sequestra, involocra, and cloacae (an open involucrum with drainage of purulent and necrotic material) can be observed. Some particular cases of chronic bone infections are Brodie abscess (lytic lesion in oval configuration, surrounded by thick reactive sclerosis) and Garrè's sclerosing osteomyelitis (subperiosteal bone apposition in the mandible, typical of children and young adults) [18, 19].

Ultrasonography is useful in the diagnosis of fluid collections, periosteal involvement, or abnormalities in the surrounding soft tissues and may provide guidance for diagnostic aspiration, surgical drainage, and tissue biopsy. In CO, ultrasonography enabled an immediate positive diagnosis in case of the pathognomic aspect of subperiosteal abscess [16, 18].

Computed tomography (CT) is a useful method to detect early osseous erosion or, in the advanced stages, to document the presence of sequestra, involocra, foreign bodies, and gas formation (the last one is a sign of severe osteomyelitis or of the presence of a sinus tract). However, this procedure has low sensitivity and sensibility, and its limitations are the impossibility to show bone marrow edema and the streak artifact when metallic implants are present [16, 18].

Magnetic resonance imaging (MRI) is the most sensitive and specific imaging modality for the detection of bone infections, providing anatomic details and accurate information on the extent of the infectious process in bone and soft tissues (Fig. 112.5). In the early phases of osteomyelitis, MRI shows localized marrow abnormalities (edema and hyperemia) with decreased intensity on T1-weighted images and increased intensity on T2-weighted images. In subsequent phases, it reveals the presence of sinus tracts and can differentiate between a bone or soft-tissue infection. Its limitations are the presence of metal implants in the region of interest (focal artifacts) and the low specificity in differentiating infection from neoplasm [19, 28].

Bone scintigraphy provides a nonspecific but sensitive detection of osseous disease; particularly, a technetium-labelled diphosphonates scan demonstrates increased isotope accumulation in areas of increased blood flow and reactive new bone formation. On the contrary, a indium-111-labelled white blood cell scan is more specific in identifying infections, can be used to help diagnose and localize osteomyelitis, and is useful in evaluating the response to treatment [18].

18F-fluorodeoxyglucose positron emission tomography (FDG-PET) was primarily used for detecting hypermetabolic malignancies. However, PET has been discovered to be useful in infections where glucose metabolism is also increased; it has a sensitivity of nearly 100% and a specificity of above 90%. Information gathered from PET/CT scans is three-dimensional, thus allowing for a precise anatomical location of the infection; furthermore, the images are minimally distorted by metal artifacts, resulting in images that are extremely useful in diagnosing infections in fractures with hardware in situ (Fig. 112.4) [16].

Table 112.3 shows the principal findings of the different imaging techniques, with their pros and cons.

Some peculiar features in the process of imaging the different groups of osteomyelitis are listed below.

In spine osteomyelitis, there are no radiographic changes in the first 2–3 weeks. After this period, X-rays show a loss of disc height and paravertebral soft tissue shadow; this is followed by a loss of cortical integrity of the end plate with progressive vertebral destruction. The degree of bone destruction is best imaged on a CT scan. At the final stage, the infections can lead to spinal deformity (typically kyphosis). MRI, with and without gadolinium contrast enhancement, has become the gold standard in identifying spinal infections and assessing the neural elements (Fig. 112.3); enhancement of the vertebral body, disc space, or epidural space is a key sign of infection [9].

The role of imaging to diagnose PUO is poorly defined and limited by the variable specificity of

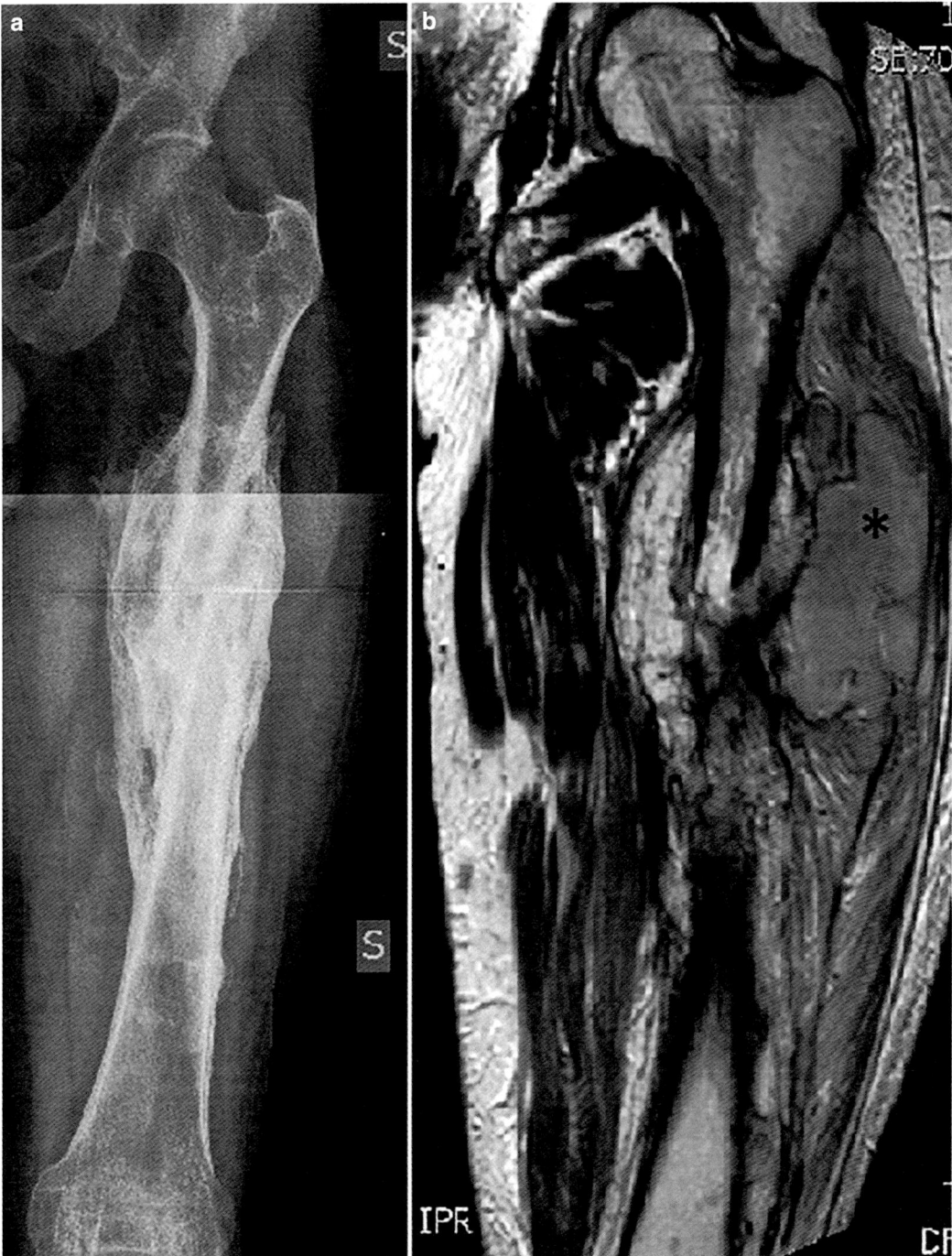

**Fig. 112.5** Reactivation of chronic osteomyelitis of the left femur, as the outcome of an open fracture previously treated with external fixation. (**a**) X-ray showing a healed fracture, intense periosteal reaction with multiple thick layers. (**b**) MRI showing fluid collection (asterisk) in the soft tissues, derived from the medullary canal

**Table 112.3** Imaging of osteomyelitis: findings, pros and cons

| Diagnostic imaging technique | Findings in osteomyelitis | Pros and cons |
|---|---|---|
| X-rays | Early stages: periosteal thickening or elevation, focal osteopenia<br>Advanced stages: osteolysis, sequestra, involocra, cloacae | Pros: simple exam, wide availability<br>Cons: poor sensitivity and specificity |
| Sonography | Fluid collections, periosteal involvement, or abnormalities in the surrounding soft tissues | Pros: guidance for diagnostic aspiration and surgical drainage of abscess<br>Cons: operator-dependent |
| Computer tomography (CT) | Early stages: osseous erosion<br>Advanced stages: sequestra, involocra, foreign bodies, and gas formation | Pros: three-dimensional images<br>Cons: poor sensitivity and specificity, streak artefact with metallic implants |
| Magnetic resonance imaging (MRI) | Early stages: bone marrow abnormality (edema and hyperemia)<br>Late stages: precise localization and extent of infection in bone and soft tissues | Pros: accurate, high sensitivity and specificity<br>Cons: artefact with metallic implant |
| Bone scintigraphy (technetium-labelled diphosphonates) | Isotope accumulation in areas of reactive new bone formation | Pros: high sensitivity<br>Cons: low specificity (increased specificity with Indium-111–labelled white blood cell) |
| 18F-fluorodeoxyglucose positron emission tomography (FDG-PET) | Glucose uptake in areas of active infections | Pros: high sensitivity and specificity. Three-dimensional images, precise anatomical location of infection. Minimal artefact with metal implants |

the different imaging techniques. MRI may have utility in assessing the depth of associated soft tissue involvement and providing guidance for surgical management [12].

Bone scintigraphy with indium-labelled white blood cells is highly sensitive and specific in diagnosing PJIs, while three-phase bone scintigraphy with technetium-labelled diphosphonates has high sensitivity. The latter exam shows uptake of the isotope in the area of bone remodeling but lacks specificity due to a positive result even in aseptic loosening of the prosthesis. FDG-PET does not appear to be superior to the aforementioned exams in diagnosing PJIs [6].

Diagnostic imaging for FRIO, especially FDG-PET, is useful to acquire more certainty regarding the presence or absence of infection, to visualize the anatomic details of the disease, and to establish the degree of fracture healing and implant stability. An important addition in recent times is the possibility of hybrid imaging (single photon emission CT [SPECT]/CT, PET/CT, PET/MRI), which allows for better anatomic details of the bone involved [29].

### Differential Diagnosis

Differential diagnosis between SO and benign or malignant neoplasms (above all, osteoid osteoma, Ewing sarcoma, osteosarcoma, metastatic tumors, non-ossifying fibroma, chondromyxoid fibroma, and giant cell tumor) is difficult based solely on radiographs; MRI can give more information but has been reported as nonspecific and variable, depending on the anatomic location, cause, and duration. Culture can be negative in SO; in some cases, biopsy and histology are needed for a secure diagnosis [2, 30].

In the presence of a prosthesis, aseptic loosening or an allergy to implant material should be ruled out. Bone scintigraphy and, if possible, microbiologic analysis of samples are necessary to distinguish the different scenarios.

In case of nonunion after fixation of a fracture, infection should always be ruled out, regardless of negative clinical and macroscopic signs of osteomyelitis. CRP and a blood exam can be normal even in an infected nonunion. FDG-PET is extremely useful in differentiating the two entities; in case of persistent suspicion of an infection, a biopsy for culture and histology should be done before revision surgery.

## 112.3 Treatment

Treatment of osteomyelitis can be medical (mainly by administration of antibiotics, together with pharmacological correction of other comorbidities) and surgical (debridement, bone resection, implant removal or substitution, or amputation in recalcitrant and life-threating infections). Most cases require a balanced combination of the two strategies to achieve the final result: the goal of the treatment can be eradication or simply control of the infection, aimed, at least, at improving the patient's quality of life. Thus, therapy of bone infections requires a multidisciplinary approach: both surgical and medical specialists should be involved in tailoring the specific treatment to the patient. While there are some basic concepts valid for every type of bone infection, some distinctive features of treatment for the different groups of osteomyelitis will be discussed separately.

In early cases of CO (less than 48 h from onset), the infection can often be treated and completely resolved with intravenous antibiotics. However, if the child does not improve with medical treatment, surgery is indicated: the objective of the operation is to release the pressure inside the bone, thus preventing the formation of a subperiosteal abscess [9].

In SO, medical treatment alone cannot usually control the infection, and, with the sole use of antibiotics, a high rate of recurrence of infection is reported. Only in spondylodiscitis do the majority of cases (nearly 90%) respond to non-operative treatment, together with rest and spinal immobilization with a spinal brace. In case of failure of pharmacological therapy, surgery is recommended [2].

In DFO, the goal of treatment is to suppress the infection and maintain limb integrity; unfortunately, recurrent or new bone infections occur in most patients, and resection or major amputation is very often needed [18].

Patients affected by PUO that are treated with a combined approach consisting of antibiotic treatment and surgery are less likely to be readmitted to the hospital compared with those patients who received either antibiotic or surgical therapy [5].

Debridement, antibiotics, irrigation, and implant retention (DAIR) is an option to temporarily alleviate symptoms in case of PJIs in old and frail patients. On the contrary, in patients fit to undergo major surgery, one-stage or two-stage revisions can be planned [14, 31].

When analyzing studies about FRIO, it is clear that there is enormous heterogeneity in treatment protocols. Treatment strategies are strongly influenced by the presence of union, by the mechanical stability of the implant, and by the time interval between fixation and infection. However, the common cornerstones of treatment are extensive and multiple debridements, dead space management, and soft tissue coverage. The final goal is to eradicate infection and lead fracture to union. It must be noted that, in this group of osteomyelitis, prevention of infection is mandatory, with adequate antisepsis, careful handling of bone and soft tissues, and accurate debridement of open fractures [7, 17, 32].

### 112.3.1 Medical Treatment

Conservative therapy, even without the administration of antibiotics, is only indicated for "host C" patients with chronic osteomyelitis without local or systemic signs of inflammation. In such cases, complete recovery is not pursued. In selected patients, brief courses of antibiotics, in case of exacerbation of symptoms, may be administered. Sometimes, chronic suppressive oral antibiotics are needed to control the infection; ideal drugs should have good bioavailability, low toxicity, and adequate bone penetration. Prolonged antibiotic treatment can lead to adverse drug reactions such as allergy, cutaneous rash, antibiotic-associated colitis, bone marrow suppression, leukopenia, thrombocytopenia, and drug fever [1, 33, 34].

However, it should be kept in mind that, as a rule, antibiotic therapy is a purely adjuvant therapy, with the highest effectiveness found after radical surgical debridement. For this reason, following debridement and the collection of samples for microbiological and histopathological analysis, in all the other patients ("host A" and "host B"), intravenous empirical antimicrobial therapy is started and should be broad-spectrum and cover the organisms most frequently isolated in infections. Therapy should be tailored according to local epidemiology of resistance rates, antibiotic formularies, and risk factors for the individual patient [17].

Another nonsurgical tool for treating bone infections is hyperbaric oxygen. This therapy provides oxygen to promote collagen production, angiogenesis, and healing in an ischemic or infected wound. Although results obtained in clinical trials are encouraging, the real effectiveness of hyperbaric oxygen is still debated [18].

As mentioned before, some early cases of CO can be effectively treated with intravenous antibiotics alone, without any surgery. Usually, the contaminant organism is isolated from the bloodstream. In the case of empiric therapy, clindamycin and first-generation cephalosporins are the primary choices [8].

In SO, the duration of treatment is 4–6 weeks. Trials of longer courses of intravenous or oral antibiotics (6 months or more) do not suggest any improvement compared with 6 weeks of therapy. Although research has shown that oral and parenteral therapies achieve similar success rates, clinicians are accustomed to considering the use of intravenous antibiotics during hospitalization, followed by oral antibiotics for the rest of the necessary period. Some authors suggest that, after accurate debridement, short-term antibiotic treatment regimens (2 weeks) might offer similar rates of infection eradication while avoiding the risk of renal and hepatic damage associated with prolonged antibiotic use. Furthermore, a short-term antibiotic regimen lowers the risk of bacterial antibiotic resistance [18].

In DFO, the duration of antibiotic therapy is not completely defined. Usually, 4–6 weeks are deemed adequate after debridement surgery, and at least 3 months in the case of antibiotic therapy alone [11].

Numerous case series in the literature have failed to identify a relationship between healing of PUO and whether antibiotics were administered or not, whether they were administered intravenously or orally, or the duration of antibiotic administration. Thus, a prolonged course (more than 6 weeks) of antibiotics is not suggested to treat sacral osteomyelitis [21].

Pharmacological treatment of PJIs and FRIO can be divided into three stages: empirical treatment, specifically targeted treatment, and the occasional need for long-term suppression. In the selection of antibiotics, bacterial susceptibility, bone penetration, and side effects should be considered. In case of implant retention, antibiotic therapy with sufficient anti-biofilm activity is required; rifampin has been demonstrated to have anti-Staphylococcal biofilm activity in vitro. A major limitation of rifampin, however, is the propensity for bacteria to develop resistance, which is why it should always be administered with a second antibiotic. In the context of gram-negative infections from retained implants, fluoroquinolones have demonstrated sufficient anti-biofilm activity and are frequently used. Although arbitrary, the duration of intravenous antibiotics is typically 6 weeks following implant removal and 12 weeks following retention. Recent evidence suggests that switching the route from intravenous to oral with an antibiotic with high oral bioavailability within 1 week is safe and effective. Examples of antibiotics with high oral bioavailability are rifampin, fluoroquinolones, clindamycin, cotrimoxazole, and tetracyclines [31, 32].

### 112.3.2 Surgical Treatment

CO, in acute cases that evolve into abscessualization, should be treated as soon as possible. The surgical approach is directly onto the abscess. The periosteum is incised and the pus evacuated. High-volume saline is used to wash the cavity. Several samples are taken for culture and sensibility. Some authors suggest decompressing the metaphysis by drilling one to three cortical holes, while others do not recommend any procedures on the bone. The skin is closed on suction drains (or with drains for continuous irrigation), and the limb is immobilized in a plaster cast [9, 24].

In SO, radical debridement is key to a successful treatment: all necrotic tissue must be excised. It is better to remove a little more than a little less. Soft tissues are resected to supple, well-perfused margins; nonviable muscle is identified by its dark color, mushy consistency, failure to contract when pinched with forceps or electrocautery, and the absence of bleeding when cut. The sinus tract, if present, is excised with the surrounding tissues. Then, the bone is excised until the exposed surfaces bleed uniformly. The necrotic bone does not bleed and is more yellowish than viable white bone. All foreign bodies and sequestra are removed. Biopsies are taken and sent for histologic and microbiological examination (including samples to detect fungi and mycobacterial species). Inadequate debridement is the main cause of recurrence. Whenever possible, the wound is closed following debridement. In the case of primary closure of the wound, all dead space must be eliminated by living tissue (transpositions, acute shortening to contact, etc.) and/or by implants containing antimicrobial agents (antibiotic beads or spacers). In the latter case, the high concentration of local antibiotics in a closed space will allow for work in a theoretically sterile field in the second-stage surgery. If necessary, a local or distance flap should be performed. A flap does not lead to revascularization of the bone, but is a safe soft tissue closure with good vascularization that is also valid to deliver antibiotics locally from the bloodstream [1, 19, 28]. Negative-pressure assisted closure has not proven to be beneficial. Some technical notes should be pointed out for each type of Cierny-Mader stage osteomyelitis [35]:

1. Type I. The excision of the nidus is necessary to eradicate the infection. The approach can be direct (through a cortical window) or indirect (reaming through the canal in long bones). The dead space remaining after debridement is usually limited and confined to the medullary canal. Usually, the bone does not require protection from an insufficiency fracture following treatment.
2. Type II. In these cases, there is a soft-tissue defect, so preoperative planning must focus on restoration of the soft-tissue envelope. Surgical treatment begins with the resection of soft tissues to viable margins and then the resection of infected bone. Local transpositions and free flaps are the most common methods to restore and reconstruct soft-tissue defects.
3. Type III. A thorough debridement commonly leads to a composite defect, involving both bone and soft tissue. If the bone excision interrupts the continuity of the segment or poses a risk for fragility fracture, stabilization is needed: osseous transfer, internal fixation with an antibiotics depot, and external fixation are some options. If, after bone resection, a significant amount of dead space remains, reconstruction can be postponed after antibiotics spacer positioning for some weeks. Soft-tissue defects are addressed as discussed for type-II lesions.
4. Type IV. After debridement, an unstable bony segment is typical. Nearly all treatment protocols call for a staged reconstruction. Alternatively, soft-tissue restoration and bony reconstruction can take place simultaneously in the form of a vascularized bone graft with a skin paddle, a bone transport, or various combinations of shortening and lengthening with external fixation.

When localized to the spine, SO requires surgery in any of the following situations: significant bone destruction causing spinal instability, neurological deficits, and sepsis caused by a spine infection unresponsive to antibiotics. The goals of surgery are debridement of infected tissues, restoration of spinal stability (with bone graft and/or metal instrumentation), and recovery or, at least, limitation of the degree of neurological impairment with decompression of the spinal canal [26].

Treatment of DFO is not standardized and should be evaluated on a case-by-case basis. Surgical treatment can be conservative (only the infected bone and the nonviable soft tissues are removed) or radical (amputation). Conservative surgery associated with prolonged antibiotic therapy may be effective in many cases. A partial amputation (such as removal of a ray or a metatarsal head), in association to a peripheral neuropathy, can increase biomechanical impairments of the foot, thus promoting reulceration or new ulcerations in different areas. On the contrary, aggressive therapy—amputation—is a mandatory and usually definitive treatment under certain circumstances [11, 18].

In PUO involving the ischium or the sacrum, the most commonly accepted surgical strategy consists of a two-stage operation. The first step is debridement of infected and devitalized tissue, with multiple bone biopsies for microbiological documentation, followed by negative pressure therapy. After improvement of local situation and normalization of laboratory exams, the reconstructive surgery is performed using a regional myo- or fascio-cutaneous flap [13, 36].

Debridement, antibiotics, and implant retention (DAIR) in PJIs could be performed in early postoperative infections (within 3 months of prosthesis implantation) or in late hematogenous infections with less than 3 weeks of symptoms, even with less favorable positive outcomes in the latter case. During DAIR, it is fundamental to remove and substitute the mobile parts of the prosthesis (head, glenosphere, polyethylene, or metallic liner) to reduce the bacterial load. In late PJIs, the solution is often the substitution of the implant with one-stage or two-stage procedures. In the latter choice, an antibiotic spacer must be positioned between the two stages, waiting for the complete eradication of the infection. Other surgical options are prosthesis removal without reimplantation (i.e., the Girdlestone procedure for the hip) or followed by joint fusion (arthrodesis) and amputation in nonresponsive, life-threatening cases [6, 31, 37].

The characterizing aspect of treating FRIO is that the problems to solve are the infection and the healing of the fracture. There are two main surgical strategies to treat fracture-related infections: the first one consists of DAIR (point 1, below), while the second one consists of debridement, implant removal, or exchange (point 2, below) [27].

1. Fracture union can occur even in the presence of infection; usually, the healing process is slower but possible. With this assumption, DAIR is a feasible option. A thorough preoperative assessment of the patient and of the bony segment involved is mandatory; subsequently, the intra-operative assessment of fracture stability and the evaluation of bone and/or soft tissue defects following adequate debridement are the cornerstones of DAIR. Acute/early infections, with an immature biofilm, a stable implant, minimal interfragmentary motion between the bony fragments, and adequate soft tissue coverage are necessary conditions for the final success of this technique.

2. In the case of infected nonunion, the surgical management is much more complicated. An aggressive and thorough debridement is essential to remove all nonviable or necrotic tissue; the internal fixation device must be removed (Fig. 112.6). Wound lavage is performed using a large amount of normal saline. After these procedures, the result is a combination of soft tissue and bone defects with an unstable fracture; further orthopedic and/or plastic reconstructive approaches are required. In the context of a two-stage implant exchange, local antibiotic delivery and management of the dead space can be dealt with using an antibiotic-impregnated spacer (cement beads and chains or cement intramedullary rods). Antibiotics used in cement must be heat stable and should not interfere with the structural integrity of the cement itself. The fracture can be stabilized with an external fixator. After complete recovery from the infection, the cement is removed and a new internal fixation device is positioned; a bone graft is added, with the possibility of using biodegradable

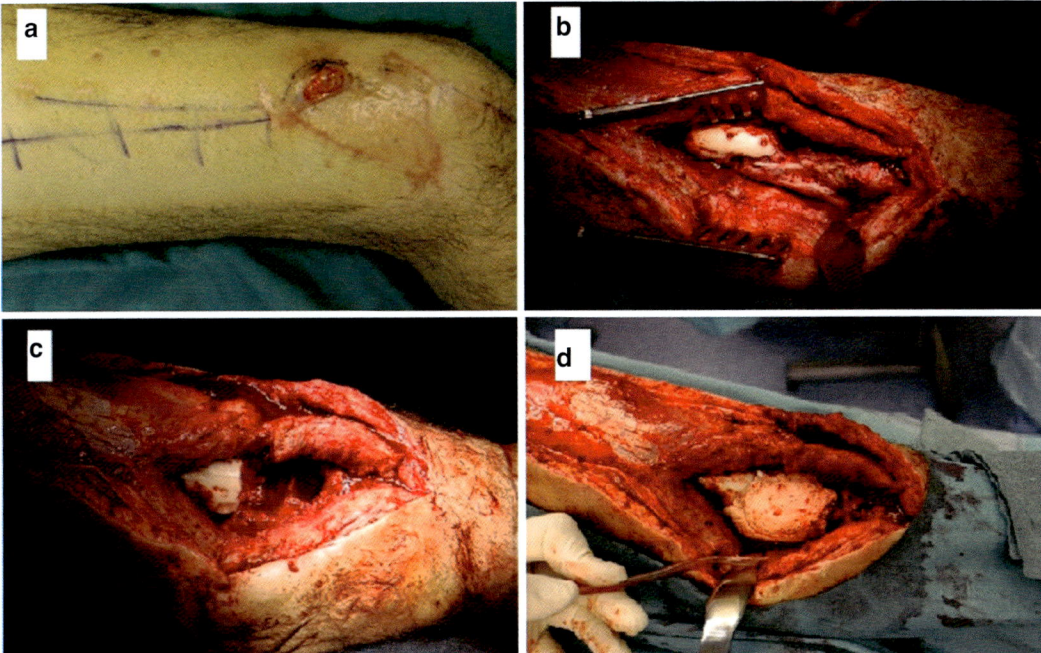

**Fig. 112.6** Clinical appearance of osteomyelitis in a septic nonunion of the right femur. (**a**) Sinus tract on the lateral aspect of the thigh. (**b**) Nonunion with sclerotic and necrotic bone. (**c**) Debridement and bone resection until viable and bleeding tissue is obtained. (**d**) Management of the dead space with antibiotic-loaded cement

ceramics or bioactive glass as adjunctive bactericide agents. If persistent infection is suspected, the spacer should be replaced by another antibiotic spacer after 4–8 weeks; as a matter of fact, after this period of time, antibiotic delivery is minimal and biofilm can form on the spacer itself. When using antibiotic cement to fill the dead space (the Masquelet technique), a pseudo-membrane encloses this spacer; in the second operation, this pseudo-membrane is the optimal environment to receive a bone graft because of its vascularity and richness in growth factors. Another option, if one-stage surgery is chosen, is the use of an external fixator as definitive treatment. The most widely used fixator is a circular frame (Ilizarov external fixator), which has many advantages: it is useful for large segmental defects (>6 cm), especially when realignment of deformities is also desired, it provides good fixation in cancellous bone, it is particularly useful in the periarticular region, and it allows for various strategies of shortening and lengthening of the bone without a need for cement or bone graft. The Ilizarov frame, on the other hand, has some disadvantages and limits: it may require more time to reach union, it is often poorly tolerated by patients, there is a risk of pin-tract infections, and it is sometimes technically very demanding. In massive bone defects, free vascularized bone transfers are another option, feasible only in specialized centers [1, 10, 17, 38].

Amputation is still a reliable measure for gaining control over an infection. In a septic emergency, this remains the procedure of choice ("life before limb"), or it is very often the final stage of a long unsuccessful treatment.

### 112.3.3 Prognosis

It is difficult to define the prognosis of bone infections because of the extreme variability among the different groups of osteomyelitis and, within each group, the different features of the specific infection and the heterogeneity of the patients involved.

Cases of acute CO in developed countries are rarely fatal (<1/1000); unfavorable outcomes may however occur, since sequelae rates vary regionally and depend on many factors such as antibiotic resistance, economic conditions, and access to healthcare [8].

"Osteomyelitis never heals" was a common statement in the past about SO; nowadays, the prognosis has radically changed, with success rates reported from 65% to 95% in different studies, with success intended as complete eradication of the infection without any recurrence of the disease [1].

DFO is associated with a high percentage of recurrence, despite a long antibiotic therapy. The prognosis depends on many factors, including vascular blood supply and the presence of neuropathy. The rate of infection recurrence is approximately 30% [11].

In the presence of PJIs, the DAIR approach has resulted in successful infection eradication in up to 85% of the cases, while the two-stage strategy is effective in 88–100% of the cases [22].

Although 20% of the patients with FRIO require multiple debridements, using both medical and surgical interventions, complete healing from infection may range from 69% to 94% of the cases. Treatment failure and recurrence of disease can ultimately lead to major amputation of the affected limb (3–8%) [27].

Persistence and extension of the infection can lead, in acute osteomyelitis, to complications such as sepsis, with the necessity for amputation of the infected limb, or, in chronic osteomyelitis, to difficulty ambulating, loss of strength, and pain.

In about 1% of chronic bone infections, malignant transformation can be observed in chronic draining sinuses. The most common neoplasm is squamous cell carcinoma (Marjolin's ulcer); its incidence is very low in developed countries, but it remains a major problem in countries with poor healthcare. It is a rare and late complication, developing 20–40 years after a chronic bone infection. Malignant transformation begins in the skin or epithelium of the fistula and infiltrates the adjacent tissues, including the bone. The increase in fistulous drainage or exophytic growth of an ulcer or mass can be warning signs of malignant transformation. The histopathological mechanism of cancerization is still unknown. When malignant transformation is diagnosed, it is essential to stage the neoplastic disease and assess the presence of distant metastases [39, 40].

> **Dos and Don'ts**
> 
> **Dos**
> - During surgical debridement, remove a little more than a little less.
> - Collect at least five tissue samples for microbiological culture.
> - Consider that a nonunion is always at risk of being a septic nonunion.
> 
> **Don'ts**
> - Take samples with swabs from a wound or fistula.
> - Delay surgery, waiting for culture results, in acute osteomyelitis.
> - Generalize treatment strategies when dealing with different types of bone infections.

> **Take-Home Messages**
> - CO must be treated immediately with administration of antibiotics and should be operated in case of complications.
> - SO, including spine infections, needs prompt diagnosis with adequate imaging to avoid persistence and evolution into chronic osteomyelitis.
> - DFO is at high risk of recrudescence and chronicization; it is sometimes wiser to adopt an aggressive treatment, even if it requires radical procedures.
> - In case of PJIs, DAIR is recommended only in early infections; in late ones, a two-stage procedure, concluding with

prosthesis reimplantation, ensures excellent results.
- The keys to treating FRIO are debridements, dead space management, and soft tissue coverage, aside from adequate duration of targeted antibiotic therapy.

**Questions**
**The correct answer is the one marked with ***

1. The bone site most frequently involved in spontaneous osteomyelitis is:
   A. spine *
   B. pelvis and proximal femur
   C. proximal and distal tibia
   D. ribs and sternum
2. Isolation of methicillin-resistant *Staphylococcus aureus*
   A. is extremely rare in children's osteomyelitis
   B. is always less frequent than methicillin-sensible *St. aureus* in all types of osteomyelitis
   C. is increasing in prevalence in all types of osteomyelitis *
   D. is isolated only in acute bone infections
3. The most useful classification for fracture-related infections and osteomyelitis is
   A. Cierny-Mader classification
   B. chronological classification (early, delayed, and late infections)
   C. Romanò classification (that analyzes the stability of the implant and the healing status of the fracture)
   D. all the listed classifications are equally important, because they describe different aspects and features of the problem *
4. Which of the following diseases is more correlated with spontaneous osteomyelitis, especially in low-income countries?
   A. Sickle cell disease *
   B. Chronic obstructive pulmonary disease
   C. Cirrhosis of the liver
   D. Malaria
5. Osteomyelitis in pressure ulcer lesions is quite uncommon and should be differentiated from
   A. microbial colonization of the ulcer
   B. superficial infection of the ulcer
   C. noninfectious pressure-related bone changes underneath an ulcer
   D. all of them *
6. The earliest changes visible on standard X-rays in case of osteomyelitis are
   A. sequestra, involucra, and cloacae
   B. diffuse bone lysis
   C. swelling of the soft tissue, periosteal thickening or elevation, and focal osteopenia *
   D. pathological fracture
7. In case of suspected nonunion of a fracture, the most specific and sensible exam is
   A. MR with gadolinium
   B. 18F-fluorodeoxyglucose positron emission tomography (FDG-PET) *
   C. Bone scintigraphy
   D. Angio-TC
8. Intravenous antibiotics alone, without any surgery, can completely eradicate
   A. some children osteomyelitis *
   B. bone infection correlated to intramedullary nailing
   C. chronic femoral shaft infections
   D. antibiotics alone are always ineffective in eradicating osteomyelitis
9. Radical debridement for spontaneous osteomyelitis
   A. is unnecessary in tibial bone infections

B. should never remove too much bone because of the risk of segment instability
　　C. consists in bone and soft tissues wide resection, till obtaining viable and bleeding tissues *
　　D. is always followed by fixation of the bone segment
10. In case of sinus drain over a suspected humerus osteomyelitis:
　　A. samples from the fistula are taken with swabs and sent for microbiological examination
　　B. the first exam is an X-ray with barium-base contrast (fistulogram)
　　C. diagnostic exams together with lab tests should guide to the appropriate diagnosis and treatment *
　　D. gentamicin-coated nail is an option for definitive treatment

# References

1. Hogan A, Heppert VG, Suda AJ. Osteomyelitis. Arch Orthop Trauma Surg. 2013;133(9):1183–96. https://doi.org/10.1007/s00402-013-1785-7. Epub 2013 Jun 16. PMID: 23771127
2. Shih HN, Shih LY, Wong YC. Diagnosis and treatment of subacute osteomyelitis. J Trauma. 2005;58(1):83–7. https://doi.org/10.1097/01.ta.0000114065.25023.85. PMID: 15674155
3. Huang PY, Wu PK, Chen CF, Lee FT, Wu HT, Liu CL, Chen TH, Chen WM. Osteomyelitis of the femur mimicking bone tumors: a review of 10 cases. World J Surg Oncol. 2013;11:283. https://doi.org/10.1186/1477-7819-11-283. PMID: 24148903; PMCID: PMC3874770
4. Graeber A, Cecava ND. Vertebral osteomyelitis. 2020 Jul 21. In: StatPearls [Internet]. Treasure Island, FL: StatPearls Publishing; 2020. PMID: 30335289.
5. Bodavula P, Liang SY, Wu J, VanTassell P, Marschall J. Pressure ulcer-related pelvic osteomyelitis: a neglected disease? Open Forum Infect Dis. 2015;2(3):ofv112. https://doi.org/10.1093/ofid/ofv112. PMID: 26322317; PMCID: PMC4551477
6. Tande AJ, Patel R. Prosthetic joint infection. Clin Microbiol Rev. 2014;27(2):302–45. https://doi.org/10.1128/CMR.00111-13. PMID: 24696437; PMCID: PMC3993098
7. Bezstarosti H, Van Lieshout EMM, Voskamp LW, Kortram K, Obremskey W, McNally MA, Metsemakers WJ, Verhofstad MHJ. Insights into treatment and outcome of fracture-related infection: a systematic literature review. Arch Orthop Trauma Surg. 2019;139(1):61–72. https://doi.org/10.1007/s00402-018-3048-0. Epub 2018 Oct 20. PMID: 30343322; PMCID: PMC6342870
8. Peltola H, Pääkkönen M. Acute osteomyelitis in children. N Engl J Med. 2014;370(4):352–60. https://doi.org/10.1056/NEJMra1213956. PMID: 24450893
9. Ray PS, Simonis RB. Management of acute and chronic osteomyelitis. Hosp Med. 2002;63(7):401–7. https://doi.org/10.12968/hosp.2002.63.7.1983. PMID: 12187599
10. Egol KA, Singh JR, Nwosu U. Functional outcome in patients treated for chronic posttraumatic osteomyelitis. Bull NYU Hosp Jt Dis. 2009;67(4):313–7. PMID: 20001930
11. Giurato L, Meloni M, Izzo V, Uccioli L. Osteomyelitis in diabetic foot: a comprehensive overview. World J Diabetes. 2017;8(4):135–42. https://doi.org/10.4239/wjd.v8.i4.135. PMID: 28465790; PMCID: PMC5394733
12. Wong D, Holtom P, Spellberg B. Osteomyelitis complicating sacral pressure ulcers: whether or not to treat with antibiotic therapy. Clin Infect Dis. 2019;68(2):338–42. https://doi.org/10.1093/cid/ciy559. PMID: 29986022; PMCID: PMC6594415
13. Andrianasolo J, Ferry T, Boucher F, Chateau J, Shipkov H, Daoud F, Braun E, Triffault-Fillit C, Perpoint T, Laurent F, Mojallal AA, Chidiac C, Valour F, Lyon BJI Study Group. Pressure ulcer-related pelvic osteomyelitis: evaluation of a two-stage surgical strategy (debridement, negative pressure therapy and flap coverage) with prolonged antimicrobial therapy. BMC Infect Dis. 2018;18(1):166. https://doi.org/10.1186/s12879-018-3076-y. PMID: 29636030; PMCID: PMC5894174
14. Zimmerli W. Clinical presentation and treatment of orthopaedic implant-associated infection. J Intern Med. 2014;276(2):111–9. https://doi.org/10.1111/joim.12233. PMID: 24605880
15. Kuehl R, Tschudin-Sutter S, Morgenstern M, Dangel M, Egli A, Nowakowski A, Suhm N, Theilacker C, Widmer AF. Time-dependent differences in management and microbiology of orthopaedic internal fixation-associated infections: an observational prospective study with 229 patients. Clin Microbiol Infect. 2019;25(1):76–81. https://doi.org/10.1016/j.cmi.2018.03.040. Epub 2018 Apr 10. PMID: 29649599
16. Fang C, Wong TM, Lau TW, To KK, Wong SS, Leung F. Infection after fracture osteosynthesis - Part I. J Orthop Surg (Hong Kong). 2017;25(1):2309499017692712. https://doi.org/10.1177/2309499017692712. PMID: 28215118
17. Foster AL, Moriarty TF, Trampuz A, Jaiprakash A, Burch MA, Crawford R, Paterson DL, Metsemakers WJ, Schuetz M, Richards RG. Fracture-related infection: current methods for prevention and treatment. Expert Rev Anti-Infect Ther. 2020;18(4):307–21.

https://doi.org/10.1080/14787210.2020.1729740. Epub 2020 Feb 19. PMID: 32049563
18. Calhoun JH, Manring MM. Adult osteomyelitis. Infect Dis Clin N Am. 2005;19(4):765–86. https://doi.org/10.1016/j.idc.2005.07.009. PMID: 16297731
19. Cierny G III. Surgical treatment of osteomyelitis. Plast Reconstr Surg. 2011;127(Suppl 1):190S–204S. https://doi.org/10.1097/PRS.0b013e3182025070. PMID: 21200291
20. Ayoade F, Li DD, Mabrouk A, Todd JR. Prosthetic Joint Infection. 2020 Sep 27. In: StatPearls [Internet]. Treasure Island (FL): StatPearls Publishing; 2020. PMID: 28846340.
21. Arvieux C, Common H. New diagnostic tools for prosthetic joint infection. Orthop Traumatol Surg Res. 2019;105(1S):S23–30. https://doi.org/10.1016/j.otsr.2018.04.029. Epub 2018 Jul 26. PMID: 30056239
22. Izakovicova P, Borens O, Trampuz A. Periprosthetic joint infection: current concepts and outlook. EFORT Open Rev. 2019;4(7):482–94. https://doi.org/10.1302/2058-5241.4.180092. PMID: 31423332; PMCID: PMC6667982
23. Romanò CL, Romanò D, Logoluso N, Drago L. Bone and joint infections in adults: a comprehensive classification proposal. Eur Orthop Traumatol. 2011;1(6):207–17. https://doi.org/10.1007/s12570-011-0056-8. Epub 2011 Apr 14. PMID: 21837262; PMCID: PMC3150792
24. Labbé JL, Peres O, Leclair O, Goulon R, Scemama P, Jourdel F, Menager C, Duparc B, Lacassin F. Acute osteomyelitis in children: the pathogenesis revisited? Orthop Traumatol Surg Res. 2010;96(3):268–75. https://doi.org/10.1016/j.otsr.2009.12.012. PMID: 20488146
25. Al Farii H, Zhou S, Albers A. Management of osteomyelitis in sickle cell disease: review article. J Am Acad Orthop Surg Glob Res Rev. 2020;4(9):e2000002–10. https://doi.org/10.5435/JAAOSGlobal-D-20-00002. PMID: 32890008; PMCID: PMC7470010
26. Tsantes AG, Papadopoulos DV, Vrioni G, Sioutis S, Sapkas G, Benzakour A, Benzakour T, Angelini A, Ruggieri P, Mavrogenis AF, World Association Against Infection In Orthopedics And Trauma W A I O T Study Group On Bone And Joint Infection Definitions. Spinal infections: an update. Microorganisms. 2020;8(4):476. https://doi.org/10.3390/microorganisms8040476. PMID: 32230730; PMCID: PMC7232330
27. Metsemakers WJ, Kortram K, Morgenstern M, Moriarty TF, Meex I, Kuehl R, Nijs S, Richards RG, Raschke M, Borens O, Kates SL, Zalavras C, Giannoudis PV, Verhofstad MHJ. Definition of infection after fracture fixation: a systematic review of randomized controlled trials to evaluate current practice. Injury. 2018;49(3):497–504. https://doi.org/10.1016/j.injury.2017.02.010. Epub 2017 Feb 20. PMID: 28245906
28. Mouzopoulos G, Kanakaris NK, Kontakis G, Obakponovwe O, Townsend R, Giannoudis PV. Management of bone infections in adults: the surgeon's and microbiologist's perspectives. Injury. 2011;42(Suppl 5):S18–23. https://doi.org/10.1016/S0020-1383(11)70128-0. PMID: 22196905
29. Govaert GAM, Kuehl R, Atkins BL, Trampuz A, Morgenstern M, Obremskey WT, Verhofstad MHJ, McNally MA, Metsemakers WJ, Fracture-Related Infection (FRI) Consensus Group. Diagnosing fracture-related infection: current concepts and recommendations. J Orthop Trauma. 2020;34(1):8–17. https://doi.org/10.1097/BOT.0000000000001614. PMID: 31855973; PMCID: PMC6903359
30. Dhanoa A, Singh VA. Subacute osteomyelitis masquerading as primary bone sarcoma: report of six cases. Surg Infect. 2010;11(5):475–8. https://doi.org/10.1089/sur.2009.011. PMID: 20858161
31. Sousa R, Abreu MA. Treatment of prosthetic joint infection with debridement, antibiotics and irrigation with implant retention - a narrative review. J Bone Jt Infect. 2018;3(3):108–17. https://doi.org/10.7150/jbji.24285. PMID: 30013891; PMCID: PMC6043472
32. Fang C, Wong TM, To KK, Wong SS, Lau TW, Leung F. Infection after fracture osteosynthesis - Part II. J Orthop Surg. 2017; https://doi.org/10.1177/2309499017692714.
33. Wang X, Fang L, Wang S, Chen Y, Ma H, Zhao H, Xie Z. Antibiotic treatment regimens for bone infection after debridement: a study of 902 cases. BMC Musculoskelet Disord. 2020;21(1):215. https://doi.org/10.1186/s12891-020-03214-4. PMID: 32264852; PMCID: PMC7140329
34. McNally M, Govaert G, Dudareva M, Morgenstern M, Metsemakers WJ. Definition and diagnosis of fracture-related infection. EFORT Open Rev. 2020;5(10):614–9. https://doi.org/10.1302/2058-5241.5.190072. PMID: 33204503; PMCID: PMC7608516
35. Parsons B, Strauss E. Surgical management of chronic osteomyelitis. Am J Surg. 2004;188(1A Suppl):57–66. https://doi.org/10.1016/S0002-9610(03)00292-7. PMID: 15223504
36. Dudareva M, Ferguson J, Riley N, Stubbs D, Atkins B, McNally M. Osteomyelitis of the pelvic bones: a multidisciplinary approach to treatment. J Bone Jt Infect. 2017;2(4):184–93. https://doi.org/10.7150/jbji.21692. PMID: 29119077; PMCID: PMC5671931
37. Mahmoud SS, Sukeik M, Alazzawi S, Shaath M, Sabri O. Salvage procedures for management of prosthetic joint infection after hip and knee replacements. Open Orthop J. 2016;10:600–14. https://doi.org/10.2174/1874325001610010600. PMID: 28144373; PMCID: PMC5226968
38. Winkler H. Treatment of chronic orthopaedic infection. EFORT Open Rev. 2017;2(5):110–6. https://doi.org/10.1302/2058-5241.2.160063. PMID: 28630748; PMCID: PMC5467682
39. Li Q, Cui H, Dong J, He Y, Zhou D, Zhang P, Liu P. Squamous cell carcinoma resulting from chronic osteomyelitis: a retrospective study of 8 cases. Int

J Clin Exp Pathol. 2015;8(9):10178–84. PMID: 26617726; PMCID: PMC4637541
40. Cappello JC, Donick II. Squamous cell carcinoma as a complication of chronic osteomyelitis. J Foot Surg. 1981;20(3):136–41. PMID: 7276451

## Further Reading

Bezstarosti H, Van Lieshout EMM, Voskamp LW, Kortram K, Obremskey W, McNally MA, Metsemakers WJ, Verhofstad MHJ. Insights into treatment and outcome of fracture-related infection: a systematic literature review. Arch Orthop Trauma Surg. 2019;139(1):61–72. https://doi.org/10.1007/s00402-018-3048-0. Epub 2018 Oct 20. PMID: 30343322; PMCID: PMC6342870

Cierny G III. Surgical treatment of osteomyelitis. Plast Reconstr Surg. 2011;127(Suppl 1):190S–204S. https://doi.org/10.1097/PRS.0b013e3182025070. PMID: 21200291

Giurato L, Meloni M, Izzo V, Uccioli L. Osteomyelitis in diabetic foot: a comprehensive overview. World J Diabetes. 2017;8(4):135–42. https://doi.org/10.4239/wjd.v8.i4.135. PMID: 28465790; PMCID: PMC5394733

Peltola H, Pääkkönen M. Acute osteomyelitis in children. N Engl J Med. 2014;370(4):352–60. https://doi.org/10.1056/NEJMra1213956. PMID: 24450893

Sousa R, Abreu MA. Treatment of prosthetic joint infection with debridement, antibiotics and irrigation with implant retention - a narrative review. J Bone Jt Infect. 2018;3(3):108–17. https://doi.org/10.7150/jbji.24285. PMID: 30013891; PMCID: PMC6043472

# Part VI

# Soft Tissues

# Necrotizing Soft Tissue Infection

Ashley A. Holly, Therese M. Duane, and Morgan Collom

> **Learning Goals**
> - Be able to identify the early and late signs and symptoms of NSTI.
> - Understand the different pathophysiology of each of the four classes of NSTI.
> - Be able to choose appropriate antimicrobial therapy based on the causative organism.

## 113.1 Introduction

Necrotizing soft tissue infections are quite rare. Most practicing physicians will see one case of NSTI during their career, making it a challenge for most physicians to be able to recognize the early signs and symptoms of this disease and act promptly. On average, there are only 500–1500 cases of NSTI reported each year, with an incidence of 0.4 per 100,000 individuals in the United States, as reported by the Centers for Disease Control and Prevention. NSTI tends to occur at higher rates in patients with advanced age, obesity, diabetes, alcoholism, immunosuppression, and other chronic conditions. However, it is important to note that up to 20% of cases occur in patients without any predisposing conditions or risk factors. Additionally, there are geographical and regional differences in etiology and microbiology at the national and regional levels [1].

## 113.2 Etiology

NSTIs are caused when bacteria penetrate the skin's protective barrier and enter the subcutaneous space. The low blood supply to this area creates a hypoxic environment with little immunologic response, which is an ideal environment for bacteria to rapidly multiply. The most common situations in which bacteria are able to penetrate the skin are through traumatic wounds, incisions, diabetic foot ulcers, decubitus ulcers, the perineum, and a perforated viscus. NSTI can occur at any site on the body, but the most common locations are the perineum, genitalia, abdomen, and extremities. One factor that has contributed to making NSTIs difficult to diagnose is that many NSTIs have had different names over time based on location. Examples of this are Fournier's gangrene, necrotizing fasciitis, clostridial myonecrosis, synergistic necrotizing cellulitis, and gas gangrene.

---

Morgan Collom has died before the publication of this book.

A. A. Holly (✉) · T. M. Duane
Texas Health Resource, Fort Worth, TX, USA

M. Collom (Deceased)
Medical City Plano, Plano, TX, USA

## 113.3 Classification

Necrotizing soft tissue infections are classified into four different types based on the pathogen of origin. This classification system was first described by Giuliano and colleagues [2]. Type I infections are polymicrobial infections, type II are monomicrobial infections, type III are marine infections and type IV are fungal infections.

### 113.3.1 Type I Infections

The most common NSTIs are the type I class of infections, which are polymicrobial and represent approximately 75% of all NSTIs. Hence, initial treatment should begin with broad-spectrum antibiotic treatment. On average, four organisms are cultured from a single infection. These polymicrobial infections are often comprised of gram-positive cocci, gram-negative rods, and anaerobes. From these, the most common gram-positive organisms are *Staphylococcus aureus*, *Streptococcus pyogenes*, and *Enterococcus species*. The most common gram-negative rod isolate is *Escherichia coli*. Lastly, the most common isolated anaerobes have been *Bacteroides* and *Peptostreptococcus* [2].

Type I infections also tend to occur in older patients with more medical comorbidities. These infections are more commonly located in the perineum and have occurred as a result of a perforated viscus, diabetic foot ulcers, or decubitus ulcers. Polymicrobial infections are less lethal than some monomicrobial infections but can still cause extensive local damage.

### 113.3.2 Type II Infections

Type II NSTIs tend to be much more aggressive and virulent than the more common polymicrobial infections. They often present much more acutely with a higher potential for local aggressive spread. Signs of systemic toxicity, as well as toxic shock, are more likely. Type II infections tend to occur in younger, healthier patients with a history of trauma, IV drug use, or surgery. The most likely pathogens in this group include group A β-hemolytic streptococci (GAS), *Clostridium* species, and community-acquired methicillin-resistant *Staphylococcus aureus* (CA-MRSA).

The species most frequently associated with type II NSTIs is *Streptococcus pyogenes* [1]. These rapidly progressive NSTIs are associated with a high mortality rate [3–6]. Pathogenic strains produce multiple exotoxins and virulence factors, causing life-threatening infections in otherwise healthy individuals [3, 4, 7]. The exotoxins commonly released include hemolysins, fibrinolysins, hyaluronidases, antiphagocytic M proteins, leukocidins, and streptolysins O and S. These exotoxins cause damage by preventing phagocytosis and bacterial clearance, damaging neutrophils, and breaking down hyaluronic acid and other connective tissues.

Clostridium infections (gas gangrene) are quite rare and are typically associated with traumatic wounds, puncture wounds, and IV drug use. These infections can quickly progress from injury to systemic toxicity and death in just a few hours. Many *Clostridia* species are endemic to the soil; however, with the rise of IV drug use, there has also been a rise in the prevalence of *Clostridia* species isolated from this patient population [8]. There are two main exotoxins that are responsible for the rapid destructive spread and systemic toxicity associated with these infections, which are α-toxin and θ-toxin. Clostridium reproduces every 8 min, which produces α-toxin (phosphorylase C) and θ-toxin (perfringolysin). Early on, these toxins are potent platelet agonists, which can lead to platelet aggregation, thrombus formation, and ultimately ischemia. As the toxins are absorbed locally, they can cause neutrophil dysfunction and death. As the infection progresses and the toxins are absorbed systemically, they can cause intravascular hemolysis, increase vascular permeability, and directly inhibit myocardial contractility.

Community-acquired methicillin-resistant *Staphylococcus aureus* (CA-MRSA) NSTIs are on the rise. CA-MRSA infections tend to affect healthy patients outside of the hospital. They are common in prisoners, contact sports team members, military personnel, IV drug users, institutional residents, and individuals who attend child and adult daycare. The main virulence factor that CA-MRSA produces is a coagulase that causes tissue destruction and invasion. In addition, it has the ability to produce Panton-Valentine leucocidin, which is a white blood cell and dermonecrotic toxin.

### 113.3.3 Type III Infections

Type III NSTI infections are caused by gram-negative marine organisms such as *Vibrio vulnificus* and *Aeromonas* species. *Vibrio vulnificus* is the most common and is found predominantly in warm coastal waters, including the southern United States [9–11]. Infection can occur through an open wound or a break in the skin while being exposed to seawater or seafood harboring the bacteria. Less commonly, the infection is acquired through the ingestion of colonized oysters, which results in hematogenous spread in patients with cirrhosis. Type III infections tend to follow a similar progression as type II infections. They can present with hemorrhagic bullae, ecchymosis, and cellulitis [11]. However, significant systemic toxicity, including multiorgan failure and cardiovascular collapse, can occur rapidly and early.

### 113.3.4 Type IV Infections

Fungal NSTIs are the rarest of all NSTIs and also carry a high mortality rate. There are only a handful of reported cases. It appears that the risks of systemic fungal infections are similar to the risks associated with fungal NSTIs, which include primary immunosuppression, poorly controlled diabetes, obesity and chronic alcoholism. The most common isolated fungus from a polymicrobial NSTI is *Candida* spp., while the most common monomicrobial fungal NSTI is due to mucormycosis [12].

## 113.4 Diagnosis

### 113.4.1 History

A thorough history and physical examination are the most critical components in establishing a diagnosis of NSTI as the diagnosis is heavily reliant on clinical gestalt rather than diagnostic testing. A clinical diagnosis of NSTI continues to remain a challenge for most physicians due to the rarity of the disease as well as the early symptoms mimicking much more common conditions such as cellulitis and erysipelas. There are several comorbidities that may predispose a patient to develop an NSTI, which include obesity, diabetes, liver and kidney failure, alcoholism, immunosuppression, and vasculopathy. However, up to a fifth of patients with NSTI lack a single comorbidity. The source of the injury is often ambiguous as well. Only a small proportion of patients will present with a history of trauma, IV drug use, surgical incision, or a puncture wound. The majority of patients without a clear source of injury usually present with an infected perineum, diabetic foot ulcer, decubitus ulcer, or seeding in the soft tissue from a perforated viscus. It seems the most important component of a patient's history and physical exam is the chronology of the disease. The signs and symptoms of NSTI progress much more rapidly compared to those of cellulitis or an abscess.

### 113.4.2 Clinical Characteristics

There are no pathognomonic symptoms for NST's and clinical presentation can vary depending on the microbiological pathogen, anatomical location, and depth of infection. Early in the disease process, the most common symptoms are erythema, warmth, tenderness, swelling, skin hypersensitivity, pain out of proportion to the exam, and pain beyond the margin of erythema and fever. The majority of these symptoms are nonspecific and common in many other conditions, making early diagnosis difficult. The two most important early symptoms, which should alert the physician of a possible NSTI, are pain out of proportion to the exam and tenderness beyond the area of erythema. Both of these symptoms may point to a rapidly progressive infection that has spread deep into the subcutaneous tissue and muscles while only causing early skin changes. As the infection progresses, later symptoms can develop, which include bullae, violaceous erythema, necrotic tissue, crepitus, cutaneous anesthesia, and shock. Once these later signs and symptoms develop, the prognosis is poor.

### 113.4.3 Diagnostic Tools

There is no specific diagnostic study that can confirm or rule out an NSTI. A diagnosis must be based on clinical suspicion with the assistance of a few diagnostic studies when appropriate. When clinical suspicion is high for NSTI, delay in diagnostic studies should be avoided as the time to treatment is critical.

### 113.4.4 Laboratory

Laboratory values tend to be nonspecific and can only help aid in diagnosis. In patients with NSTI, it is not uncommon to see leukocytosis, leukopenia, or bandemia. Other common lab abnormalities can include elevations in creatinine, BUN, lactic acid, creatine phosphokinase, hyponatremia, and coagulopathy. A study by Wall and colleagues found that a WBC count >15,400 cells/mm$^3$ or a serum sodium level <135 mmol/L had a negative predictive value of 99% and a sensitivity of 90%. These lab values lack specificity and only have a positive predictive value of 26%, which can rule out NSTI, but not confirm it [13, 14].

Currently, the most widely adopted diagnostic tool is the Laboratory Risk Indicator for Necrotizing Fasciitis (LRINEC), established by Wong and colleagues [15] (Table 113.1). LRINEC is a set of six independent variables, with each variable given a specific number toward a final score. These final scores are broken down into three categories: low risk, intermediate risk, and high risk (Table 113.2). Scores greater than 6 correspond to a PPV of 92% and an NPV of 96%. LRINEC scores are to be used as an adjunct to help risk stratify patients with suspected NSTI. Although this score is widely used, it has never been validated.

**Table 113.1** LRINEC score system

| LRINEC variable | Value | Score |
|---|---|---|
| WBC (cells/mm$^3$) | <15 | 0 |
|  | 15–25 | 1 |
|  | >25 | 2 |
| Sodium (mmol/L) | >135 | 0 |
|  | <135 | 2 |
| Creatinine (mg/dL) | <1.6 | 0 |
|  | >1.6 | 2 |
| Hemoglobin (g/dL) | >13.5 | 0 |
|  | 11–13.5 | 1 |
|  | <11 | 2 |
| Glucose (mg/dL) | <180 | 0 |
|  | >180 | 1 |
| C-reactive protein (mg/L) | <150 | 0 |
|  | >150 | 4 |
| Sum of points | Risk category | Necrotizing fasciitis probability |
| <5 | Low | <50% |
| 6–7 | Intermediate | 50–75% |
| >8 | High | >75% |

[15]

New data looking at biomarkers showed that Ficolin-2, a pattern recognition molecule, could be used to predict short-term mortality (<28 days). Hansen et al. concluded that a low Ficolin-2 level on admission (<1.9 μg/mL) was independently associated with higher short-term mortality [17]. Another biomarker, Pentraxin-3 (PTX-3), is a marker of inflammation similar to CRP. Elevation in the levels of PTX-3 was shown to correlate with increased disease severity and mortality in a prospective study by Hansen et al. [18]. This study was not able to establish an independent association of morbidity and mortality but shows a potential role in the future pending further analysis.

### 113.4.5 Imaging

Due to the rapid lethality of NSTI, imaging studies should be utilized cautiously and not delay the time to treatment. If imaging can be obtained quickly in a stable patient, a plain radiograph is the gold standard, followed by computed tomog-

**Table 113.2** Antimicrobial therapy options for NSTI

| Agent | Dose | Remarks |
|---|---|---|
| *Classic empiric agents* | | |
| Vancomycin (MRSA) | 15 mg/kg IV q12h | Often more readily available and lower in cost |
| Penicillin (gram-positive) | 2–4 MU IV q4–6h | |
| Gentamicin (gram-negative) | 5–7 mg/kg IV q24h | |
| Clindamycin | 600–900 mg IV q8h | |
| *Other empiric agents* | | |
| Tigecycline | 100 mg IV then 50 mg IV q12h | MRSA, gram-positive, gram-negative, anaerobic |
| Clindamycin | 600–900 mg IV q8h | |
| Ceftaroline | 600 mg q12h | MRSA, gram-positive, gram-negative, anaerobic |
| Metronidazole | 500 mg IV q6–8h | |
| Clindamycin | 600–900 mg IV q8h | |
| Vancomycin | 15 mg/kg IV q12h | |
| Clindamycin | 600–900 mg IV q8h | |
| PLUS one of the following: | | |
| Imipenem/cilastatin | 1 g IV q6–8h | |
| Meropenem | 1 g IV q8h | |
| Ertapenem | 1 g IV q24h | |
| Cefotaxime | 2 g IV q6h | |
| Vancomycin | 15 mg/kg IV q12h | |
| Clindamycin | 600–900 mg IV q8h | |
| Metronidazole | 500 mg IV q6–8h | |
| PLUS one of the following: | | |
| Piperacillin/tazobactam | 3.375 g IV q6h | |
| Ciprofloxacin | 400 mg IV q12h | |

| Pathogen specific | | |
|---|---|---|
| Agent | Dose | Remarks |
| *Group A Streptococcal* | | |
| Penicillin + Clindamycin | 2–4 MU IV q4–6h / 600–900 mg IV q8h | In severe cases, PCN should be combined with clindamycin or macrolide to avoid treatment failure |
| *Clostridial* | | |
| Penicillin + Clindamycin | 2–4 MU IV q4–6h / 600–900 mg IV q8h | In severe cases, PCN should be combined with clindamycin to avoid treatment failures and neutralize toxins |
| *CA-MRSA* | | |
| Vancomycin | 15 mg/kg IV q12h | Agent of choice, Risk AKI |
| Linezolid | 600 mg IV q12h | Inhibit toxin production |
| Daptomycin | 4 mg/kg IV q24h | Second choice, bactericidal |
| Ceftaroline | 600 mg IV q12h | Bactericidal MRSA and VISA |
| Quinupristin/Dalfopristin | 7.5 mg/kg IV q8h | Effective against VRSA |
| *Vibrio* | | |
| Cefotaxime + Minocycline | 2 g IV q6h / 200 mg IV then 100 mg IV q12h | Combination most effective |

[16]

raphy per current recommendations from the American College of Radiology. A plain radiograph may demonstrate subcutaneous emphysema or air tracking in the soft tissue. This finding is highly specific for a clostridial NSTI, but not sensitive for any of the remaining types of NSTI. Computed tomography is only slightly more sensitive than a plain radiograph, but is nonspecific and may demonstrate air tracking, fascial separation, fascial thickening, and possible deep abscess formation. Ultrasound and magnetic resonance imaging have no role [19].

### 113.4.6 Macroscopic/Microscopic

Macroscopic diagnosis is typically performed intraoperatively. Common macroscopic findings of an NSTI are weeping of "dishwater" or hemorrhagic fluid from facial planes, a lack of bleeding, noncontractile muscle, grey necrotic tissue, and a positive "finger test." This test is positive when the surgeon is able to use his finger to dissect through tissue that is normally strong and adherent. Macroscopic findings are helpful in guiding the extent of the excision and debridement. To achieve a microscopic diagnosis, a biopsy must be taken of the deep fascia and muscle. Ideally, the biopsy specimen should reveal liquefaction necrosis, thrombosed blood vessels, and PMN infiltrates. Microscopic diagnosis is impractical and typically unnecessary as macroscopic findings are generally considered adequate for diagnosis.

> **Differential Diagnosis**
> - Complicated soft tissue infection
> - Non-necrotizing cellulitis
> - Abscess

## 113.5 Medical Treatment

### 113.5.1 Antibiotic Therapy

Broad-spectrum antimicrobial therapy should begin immediately after NSTI is suspected. Most NSTI are polymicrobial, and empiric antibiotic therapy should cover gram-positive, gram-negative, anaerobes, and MRSA, considering local microbiological susceptibility [20, 21].

Even NSTIs that are commonly monomicrobial (e.g., extremity infections due to trauma or IV drug use) should be treated broadly until proper identification of the pathogen is achieved through cultures and sensitivities. In addition, the adjuvant uses of an antimicrobial with ribosomal synthesis inhibitory properties (e.g., clindamycin, linezolid) should be considered to reduce the production of certain toxins (e.g., alpha-toxin, super antigen M protein).

Table 113.2 summarizes the recommendations for empiric therapy as well as pathogen-specific therapy.

### 113.5.1.1 Duration

Empiric antibiotic treatment should be continued until cultures and sensitivities can guide the de-escalation of antibiotic coverage. Discontinuation of antibiotic therapy can be considered once the patient is hemodynamically stable, the WBC has normalized, and all debridement has been completed. In general, a shorter course (e.g., <7 days) of antibiotics is adequate and has similar clinical outcomes compared to a more prolonged course [22].

### 113.5.2 Surgical Treatment

The mainstay treatment for NSTI is immediate and adequate surgical debridement of all devitalized and necrotic tissue (Fig. 113.1). Multiple studies have concluded that there is a seven- to ninefold increase in mortality if surgical debridement is delayed or inadequate [23]. The adequacy of debridement is difficult to define, therefore making this determination subjective and dependent on each surgeon's experience and judgement.

One expected pitfall is not making the incision wide enough. Surgeons who lack experience treating NSTI tend to make incisions that are too small. Although excessively wide and aggressive incisions and debridement can have their own set of complications, patients with incisions and debridement that are too small tend to have a worse outcome. It is recommended that the initial incision extends outside the area of initial induration and cellulitis. This incision should be carried down through the subcutaneous tissue until the deeper muscle layers are reached. Thorough exploration of the tissue and fascial planes must occur to guide the extent of debridement. All necrotic and devitalized tissue must be excised. As previously mentioned, this tissue is often necrotic in color and is easily dissected with a positive "finger test." Murky grey or "dirty dishwater" fluid may be encountered from the fascial planes as well. Excision should be carried out until healthy tissue is reached. This healthy tissue should exhibit brisk bleeding, and the muscle should show visible contractility upon stimula-

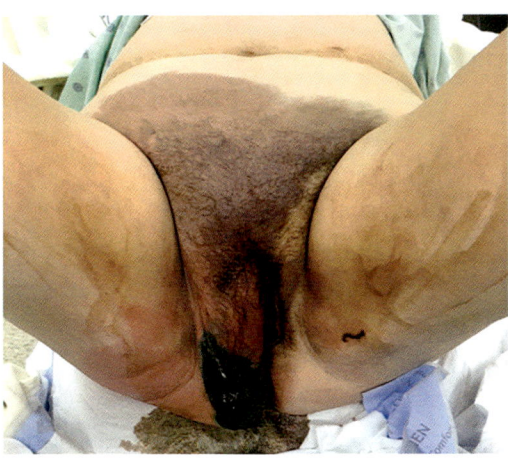 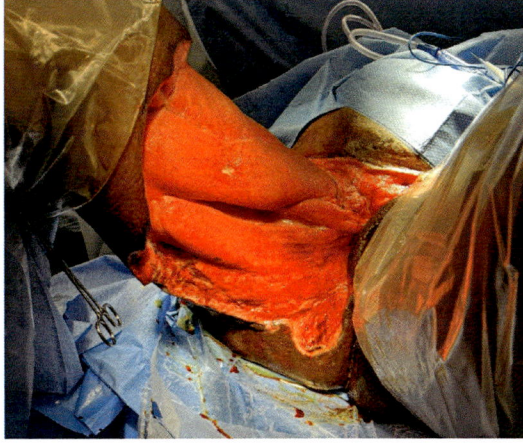

**Fig. 113.1** Perineal necrotizing soft tissue infection prior to debridment procedures. Treatment of patient with aggressive excision and debridement [33, 34]

tion with electrocautery. It is also important to send the tissue to microbiology for Gram stain and culture to help guide and de-escalate aggressive initial antibiotic therapy.

Frequent reevaluation is a mainstay of therapy. It is usual practice to return to the operating room within 24 h of the initial debridement. This recommendation is based on several retrospective reviews [23–25]. Recently, a prospective study was conducted by Okoye et al. comparing the timing of repeat debridement and its effects on the morbidity and mortality of patients [26]. This multivalent analysis of 64 patients with NSTI determined that patients who underwent early repeat debridement had significantly better morbidity and mortality compared to the group that underwent delayed debridement. A retrospective cohort study by Chang et al. supported these findings. Their study showed that patients with an LRINEC score >8 who had a primary amputation had a mortality benefit compared to those who had a delayed amputation [27].

Wound care after surgical debridement has traditionally been done with the use of wet-to-dry dressings to facilitate mechanical debridement. While this method of wound care is still adequate, the use of negative pressure wound therapy systems has become increasingly common. The use of negative pressure wound systems has demonstrated advantages to traditional wound therapy with decreased length of stay and decreased time to heal [28, 29]. It is also easier for patients to manage, with the dressing change occurring every 3–4 days rather than changing the wet-to-dry dressings one to two times a day. Skin grafting and reconstructive procedures can be performed once the patient has been stabilized and the infection has been fully treated.

#### 113.5.2.1 Support

The last aspect of treatment is intense physiologic support. Close hemodynamic monitoring in an intensive care unit with the use of invasive monitoring (e.g., arterial and central venous lines) is highly recommended. Many of these patients will require aggressive fluid resuscitation and ionotropic support. Blood products should also be made readily available. Serial laboratory values should be taken to monitor blood glucose, renal function, and electrolyte shifts. Lastly, early enteral nutritional support is recommended as patients are in a high catabolic state and have high caloric and protein requirements.

### 113.5.3 Adjunctive Therapy

#### 113.5.3.1 Hyperbaric Oxygen

Hyperbaric oxygen may be used as an adjunct to therapy but should never replace or delay surgical and antimicrobial therapies. HBO theoretically works by increasing the supply of oxygen to the wound, which should promote healing and inhibit bacterial growth. However, there is no high-level evidence to support the use of HBO in the treatment of NSTI.

### 113.5.4 IVIG

What does IVIG stand for? The goal of IVIG therapy is to decrease the circulating amount of bacterial exotoxin, which is responsible for causing systemic toxicity. IVIG accomplishes this by binding to the bacterial exotoxin. The use of IVIG in the treatment of streptococcal toxic shock syndrome has revealed improved outcomes, according to Linnér and colleagues [30]. However, the use of IVIG in the treatment of streptococcal TSS in patients with NSTI has not been able to show any statistically significant survival benefit. This was further echoed by the INSTINCT trial by Madsen et al. in 2017. This blinded randomized controlled trial involving patients in the ICU with NSTI was unable to find any difference in the physical component summary between the group that received IVIG and the group that received the placebo [31].

## 113.6 Prognosis

There have only been modest improvements in mortality since 1871, with an average mortality rate of 25%. Disfigurement and disability are common complications due to the extensive surgical debridement that must occur to control infection. Plastic surgery and reconstructive surgeries following the resolution of the infection may be necessary to lessen this disfigurement [32].

Patients who underwent extensive debridement of one or more of their limbs may develop contractures during the healing process. Complications such as pneumonia, urinary tract infections, catheter-related bloodstream infections, and secondary soft tissue infections are common. During debridement of Fournier's gangrene, more specific complications can occur, which include impotence, decreased sperm count, and motility. Fecal incontinence may occur when debridement involves the perianal or perirectal region, making it a difficult location to heal with constant fecal contamination. Diverting loop colostomy is often performed in these specific situations to allow for non-contaminated wound care and adequate wound healing.

**Dos and Don'ts**
- Do not postpone lifesaving treatment.
- When NSTI is suspected, start broad-spectrum antibiotics immediately.
- Do not delay wide surgical debridement of all devitalized skin and soft tissue.
- Delay is associated with a seven- to ninefold increased risk of mortality if surgical debridement is delayed or inadequate.
- Do return to the operating room within 24 h for re-evaluation of the adequacy of debridement.

**Take-Home Messages**
- NSTI are usually polymicrobial.
- Early diagnosis remains difficult.
- The mortality rate remains at 25%.
- Initial antibiotic therapy should always be broad-spectrum with aggressive de-escalation.
- Early surgical treatment is a mainstay of therapy.

**Questions**
1. A 23-year-old male with a history of intravenous drug use presents to the emergency department with a tender, erythematous, swollen left arm with a small amount of drainage. He is mildly tachycardic. Which of the following imaging studies would be the least helpful in making a diagnosis of NSTI?
   A. MRI
   B. CT
   C. Ultrasound
   D. Plain XR
2. A 45-year-old obese female with a history of diabetes presents to the ED with complaints of swelling, pain, and foul-smelling drainage from her groin. Her heart rate is 125 bpm. She is febrile at

39 °C and slightly hypotensive at 90/50. What is this patient's LRINEC score based on the lab values below? What is her associated risk?

Sodium: 128 mEq/L. Glucose: 170 mg/dL. Creatinine: 1.3 mg/dL. WBC count: 17,000/mm³. Hemoglobin: 10.5 g/dL. C-reactive protein: 152

3. A 58-year-old male is POD #1 from an exploratory laparotomy. On examination, his wound is very tender, indurated, and has begun to weep slightly. You suspect a possible NSTI. What organism is most likely the cause of infection?
   A. CA-MRSA
   B. Streptococcus pyogenes
   C. Clostridium perfringens
   D. Escherichia coli

4. Which of the following is NOT a risk factor for the development of NSTI?
   A. IV drug use
   B. Diabetes
   C. Obesity
   D. Alcoholism
   E. None of the above

5. Match the organism to the correct antibiotic regimen.
   1. Clostridium species      A. Doxycycline, cefotaxime
   2. CA-MRSA                  B. Vancomycin, penicillin, gentamicin, clindamycin
   3. Vibrio species           C. Penicillin, clindamycin
   4. Polymicrobial            D. Linezolid

Answers

1. C.
2. 10. High Risk.
3. B.
4. E.
5. 1: C; 2: D; 3: A; 4: B.

## References

1. Kao LS, Lew DF, Arab SN, et al. Local variations in the epidemiology, microbiology, and outcome of necrotizing soft-tissue infections: a multicenter study. Am J Surg. 2011;202(2):139–45. [PubMed: 21545997]
2. Elliot DC, Kufera JA, Myers RA. Necrotizizng soft tissue infections: risk factors for mortality and strategies of management. Ann Surg. 1996;224:672–83.
3. Kiska DL, Thiede B, Caracciolo J, Jordan M, Johnson D, Kaplan EL, et al. Invasive group A streptococcal infections in North Carolina: epidemiology, clinical features, and genetic and serotype analysis of causative organisms. J Infect Dis. 1997;176(4):992–1000.
4. Eriksson BK, Andersson J, Holm SE, Norgren M. Epidemiological and clinical aspects of invasive group A streptococcal infections and the streptococcal toxic shock syndrome. Clin Infect Dis. 1998;27(6):1428–36.
5. Eriksson BK, Norgren M, McGregor K, Spratt BG, Normark BH. Group A streptococcal infections in Sweden: a comparative study of invasive and noninvasive infections and analysis of dominant T28 emm28 isolates. Clin Infect Dis. 2003;37(9):1189–93.
6. Darenberg J, Luca-Harari B, Jasir A, Sandgren A, Pettersson H, Schalen C, et al. Molecular and clinical characteristics of invasive group A streptococcal infection in Sweden. Clin Infect Dis. 2007;45(4):450–8.
7. Nichols RL, Florman S. Clinical presentations of soft-tissue infections and surgical site infections. Clin Infect Dis. 2001;33(Suppl 2):S84–93.
8. Bryant AE, Stevens DL. Clostridial myonecrosis: new insights in pathogenesis and management. Curr Infect Dis Rep. 2010;12(5):383–91. [PubMed: 21308521]
9. Vinh DC, Embil JM. Rapidly progressive soft tissue infections. Lancet Infect Dis. 2005;5(8):501–13.
10. Blake PA, Merson MH, Weaver RE, Hollis DG, Heublein PC. Disease caused by a marine Vibrio. Clinical characteristics and epidemiology. N Engl J Med. 1979;300(1):1–5.
11. Klontz KC, Lieb S, Schreiber M, Janowski HT, Baldy LM, Gunn RA. Syndromes of Vibrio vulnificus infections. Clinical and epidemiologic features in Florida cases, 1981–1987. Ann Intern Med. 1988;109(4):318–23.
12. Bartram L, Aaron JA. Fingal nectrotizing skin and soft tissue infections. Curr Fungal Infect Rep. 2019;13:146–56.
13. Wall D, Kleain S, Black S, de Virgilio C. A simple model to help distinguish necrotizing from non-necrotizing soft-tissue infections. J Am Coll Surg. 2000;191(3):227–31. [PubMed: 10989895]
14. Wall D, de Virgilio C, Black S, Klein S. Objective criteria may assist in distinguishing necrotizing fasciitis from nonnecrotizing sift-tissue infections. Am J Surg. 2000;179(1):17–21.

15. Wong CH, Khin LW, Heng KS, Tan KC, Low CO. The LRINEC (Laboratory Risk Indicator for Necrotizing Fasciitis) score: a tool for distinguishing necrotizing fasciitis from other soft tissue infections. Crit Care Med. 2004;32(7):1535–41.
16. Duane TM, Huston JM, Collom M, Beyer A, Parli S, Buckman S, Shapiro M, McDonald A, Diaz J, Tessier JM, Sanders J. Surgical Infection Society 2020 updated guidelines on the management of complicated skin and soft tissue infections. Surg Infect. 2021; https://doi.org/10.1089/sur.2020.436. PMID: 33646051
17. Hansen MB, Rasmussen LS, Pilely K, Hellemann D, Hein E, Madsen MB, et al. The lectin complement pathway in patients with necrotizing soft tissue infection. J Innate Immun. 2016;8(5):507–16.
18. Hansen MB, Rasmussen LS, Garred P, Bidstrup D, Madsen MB, Hyldegaard O. Pentraxin-3 as a marker of disease severity and risk of death in patients with necrotizing soft tissue infections: a nationwide, prospective, observational study. Crit Care. 2016;20:40.
19. Hakkarainen TW, Kopari NM, Pham TN, Evans HL. Necrotizing soft tissue infections: review and current concepts in treatment, systems of care, and outcomes. Curr Probl Surg. 2014;51(8):344–62.
20. May AK, Stafford RE, Bulger EM, Heffernan D, Guillamondegui O, Bochicchio G, et al. Treatment of complicated skin and soft tissue infections. Surg Infect. 2009;10(5):467–99.
21. Tessier JM, Sanders J, Sartelli M, Ulrych J, De Simone B, Grabowski J, et al. Necrotizing soft tissue infections: a focused review of pathophysiology, diagnosis, operative management, antimicrobial therapy, and pediatrics. Surg Infect. 2020;21(2):81–93.
22. Lauerman MH, Kolesnik O, Sethuraman K, Rabinowitz R, Joshi M, Clark E, et al. Less is more? Antibiotic duration and outcomes in Fournier's gangrene. J Trauma Acute Care Surg. 2017;83(3):443–8.
23. Bilton BD, Zibari GB, McMillan RW, Aultman DF, Dunn G, McDonald JC. Aggressive surgical management of necrotizing fasciitis serves to decrease mortality: a retrospective study. Am Surg. 1998;64(5):397–400; discussion 400–1.
24. McHenry CR, Piotrowski JJ, Petrinic D, Malangoni MA. Determinants of mortality for necrotizing soft-tissue infections. Ann Surg. 1995;221(5):558–63; discussion 63–5.
25. Green RJ, Dafoe DC, Raffin TA. Necrotizing fasciitis. Chest. 1996;110(1):219–29.
26. Okoye O, Talving P, Lam L, Smith J, Teixeira PG, Inaba K, et al. Timing of redebridement after initial source control impacts survival in necrotizing soft tissue infection. Am Surg. 2013;79(10):1081–5.
27. Chang CP, Hsiao CT, Lin CN, Fann WC. Risk factors for mortality in the late amputation of necrotizing fasciitis: a retrospective study. World J Emerg Surg. 2018;13:45.
28. Pan A, Cauda R, Concia E, Esposito S, Sganga G, Stefani S, et al. Consensus document on controversial issues in the treatment of complicated skin and skin-structure infections. Int J Infect Dis. 2010;14(Suppl 4):S39–53.
29. Endorf FW, Cancio LC, Klein MB. Necrotizing soft-tissue infections: clinical guidelines. J Burn Care Res. 2009;30(5):769–75.
30. Linner A, Darenberg J, Sjolin J, Henriques-Normark B, Norrby-Teglund A. Clinical efficacy of polyspecific intravenous immunoglobulin therapy in patients with streptococcal toxic shock syndrome: a comparative observational study. Clin Infect Dis. 2014;59(6):851–7.
31. Madsen MB, Hjortrup PB, Hansen MB, Lange T, Norrby-Teglund A, Hyldegaard O, et al. Immunoglobulin G for patients with necrotising soft tissue infection (INSTINCT): a randomised, blinded, placebo-controlled trial. Intensive Care Med. 2017;43(11):1585–93.
32. Elliott DC, Kufera JA, Myers RA. Necrotizing soft tissue infections. Risk factors for mortality and strategies for management. Ann Surg. 1996;224(5):672–83.
33. Holly A. Advanced necrotizing soft tissue infection in a female patient. JPEG. 2016.
34. Holly A. Photograph of appropriate level of debridement down to healthy tissue. Authors personal collection. 2021.

## Further Reading

Duane TM, Huston JM, Collom M, Beyer A, Parli S, Buckman S, Shapiro M, McDonald A, Diaz J, Tessier JM, Sanders J. Surgical Infection Society 2020 updated guidelines on the management of complicated skin and soft tissue infections. Surg Infect. 2021; https://doi.org/10.1089/sur.2020.436. Epub ahead of print

Endorf FW, Cancio LC, Klein MB. Necrotizing soft-tissue infections: clinical guidelines. J Burn Care Res. 2009;30(5):769–75.

Sartelli M, Guirao X, Hardcastle TC, et al. 2018 WSES/SIS-E consensus conference: recommendations for the management of skin and soft-tissue infections. World J Emerg Surg. 2018;13:58.

# Cutaneous and Subcutaneous Abscesses

## 114

Jan Ulrych

## 114.1 Introduction

> **Learning Goals**
> - Knowledge of current epidemiology and microbial aetiology of cutaneous and subcutaneous abscesses (including the increased emergence of community-acquired MRSA).
> - Recognition of skin abscess symptoms (it is most often a clinical diagnosis) and implementation of microbiological examination and ultrasound imaging in the diagnostic process.
> - Selection of the appropriate therapeutic management and knowledge of the principles of surgery and antimicrobial therapy of skin abscess.

Abscess and cellulitis are the most common types of pyogenic skin and soft tissue infections in surgery. Pyogenic skin and soft tissue infection is characterised by the production of purulent exudate. Cutaneous and subcutaneous abscesses are defined as a localised collection of pus within the dermis or subcutaneous space. Cellulitis is interstitial purulent inflammation spreading diffusely in the dermis and subcutaneous tissue. Both forms of exudative purulent inflammation are caused by pyogenic (pus-producing) bacteria.

Although most abscesses are due to bacterial infection, sterile abscesses can occur in some patients. A sterile abscess is caused by the injection of various irritants, particularly oil-based drugs that may not be fully absorbed and cause local irritation. A sterile abscess is a subcutaneous, hard, solid lesion that can mimic scar tissue.

### 114.1.1 Epidemiology

Cutaneous and subcutaneous abscesses are common worldwide. In recent years, cutaneous and subcutaneous abscesses have become much more frequent in some geographic regions. In the United States, emergency department visits for skin abscesses were more than doubled over the 10-year study period (from 1.2 million in 1996 to 3.28 million in 2005; $p < 0.01$) [1]. An ongoing rise in the incidence of outpatient visits for skin infections was demonstrated in the period 2000–2013. However, this dramatic incidence rise was followed by a plateau in the incidence of purulent skin and soft tissue infections during 2013–2015 in the USA [2]. Beside the increase in outpatient visits for abscess/cellulitis, the significant increase in the trend of skin and soft

J. Ulrych (✉)
First Department of Surgery, Department of Abdominal, Thoracic Surgery and Traumatology, First Faculty of Medicine, Charles University and General University Hospital, Prague, Czech Republic
e-mail: Jan.Ulrych@vfn.cz

tissue infection-associated hospitalization was reported in the United States [3, 4]. In Europe, the epidemiology of cutaneous abscess is not so dramatic. Nevertheless, in period 1991–2006 hospital admission rates increased threefold for abscesses/cellulitis in the United Kingdom [5]. Skin and soft tissue infections represent a significant burden to the health care system worldwide.

Regarding age as a risk factor, the incidence rate of abscess and cellulitis is higher in persons 65 years of age and older and in children less than 5 years of age [6]. Regarding sex and susceptibility to skin infection, a search of electronic health records revealed an increased odds ratio of 2.4 for skin and soft tissue infection caused by *Staphylococcus aureus* in males versus females [7].

Skin abscesses may occur in healthy individuals without any predisposing conditions. However, some predisposing factors associated with a higher risk of skin abscess is usually identified in many patients (Table 114.1).

### 114.1.2 Aetiology

Abscess is caused by bacteria that enter and infect the cutaneous and subcutaneous tissue through breaks in the skin, such as minor skin trauma, burns and insect bites, or hair follicles. Therefore, the microbial aetiology of abscesses often comes from indigenous bacteria flora colonising the skin of healthy individuals (Gram-positive cocci). However, skin abscesses can be caused by a wide spectrum of exogenous bacteria infiltrating the skin and soft tissue during the trauma as well. Cutaneous and subcutaneous abscesses are usually monomicrobial, but they can be caused by more than one pathogen.

In many cases of skin and soft tissue infections, the microbial aetiology remains unknown because many episodes of skin and soft tissue infections are not usually cultured. Ray et al. reported in a retrospective population-based study that only 23% of skin and soft tissue infection episodes were cultured, and a potentially clinically relevant pathogen was isolated in only 54% of those episodes [6]. Most culture-positive abscesses are caused by *Staphylococcus aureus* (80%), followed by *Streptococcus pyogenes* and beta-hemolytic streptococci (10–20%). Gram-negative bacilli and anaerobes (including *Escherichia coli*, *Pseudomonas aeruginosa*, *Bacteroides* spp., etc.) are more common in patients with skin abscess located in the axillary, perioral, perirectal, perineal, and vulvovaginal body areas, and anaerobes are cultured more frequently among intravenous drug users [8]. We can conclude that *Staphylococcus aureus* is the most common cause of cutaneous and subcutaneous abscesses. *Staphylococcus aureus* was responsible for the dramatic increase in the incidence of abscess during recent years in the USA and worldwide.

From clinically relevant multi-drug-resistant pathogens, the major pathogen involved in cutaneous and subcutaneous abscesses is methicillin-resistant *Staphylococcus aureus* (MRSA). MRSA was first discovered in the 1960s and rocognised as a characteristic healthcare-associated pathogen. However, since the 1990s, MRSA has been reported as a microbial aetiology of community-onset infections, primarily skin and soft tissue infections. These MRSA strains are called community-acquired MRSA (CA-MRSA). CA-MRSA strains have a different phenotypic characteristic and a distinct genetic background compared to the traditional healthcare-associated MRSA strains. CA-MRSA isolates tend to be resistant to fewer antibiotics and to produce different toxins (Panton-Valentine leucocidin, etc.) responsible for the enhanced pathogenicity. In the United States, CA-MRSA has become a major microbial aetiology of skin and soft tissue infections. In Pennsylvania, the

**Table 114.1** Predisposing factors for cutaneous and subcutaneous abscesses

| Risk factors | Examples |
|---|---|
| Trauma and skin barrier disruption | Abrasion, penetrating wound, pressure ulcer, insect bite, drug injection, radiation therapy |
| Skin inflammation | Eczema, psoriasis, varicella |
| Oedema | Due to venous insufficiency, impaired lymphatic drainage |
| Obesity | |
| Immunodeficiency | Diabetes mellitus, HIV, immunosuppression therapy |

annual incidence of CA-MRSA increased by 34% from 2005 to 2009 [9]. Ray et al. also reported increase in MRSA-associated skin and soft tissue infections between 1998 and 2009; moreover, the proportion of CA-MRSA isolates increased steadily from 6% in 1998 to 46% in 2009 [6]. Notwithstanding the results of previous studies, other authors have reported a recent decline in MRSA-associated skin and soft tissue infections among children and adults in some regions of the USA [10]. However, CA-MRSA remains the most important pathogen related to community-onset abscess and cellulitis in the United States.

Epidemiology of MRSA in community-acquired skin and soft tissue infections varies significantly in Europe compared to the USA. A prospective multicentre European study has demonstrated that the overall MRSA prevalence rate in community-onset skin and soft tissue infections was 15.1%, ranging from 0% in the United Kingdom to 29% in Italy [11]. Moreover, the predominant clone USA300 CA-MRSA was absent among community-infected patients in Europe [11]. Ultimately, MRSA prevalence for purulent skin and soft tissue infections in Europe is much lower in comparison to the United States.

### 114.1.3 Classification

Standard classification of cutaneous and subcutaneous abscesses distinguishes simple superficial abscesses from complex abscesses. Superficial simple abscesses are usually well-circumscribed and uniloculated. These abscesses should not have an extension into deeper tissues. Complex abscesses are characterised by their specific location (perineal, perianal, axillary), the pathogens involved (polymicrobial, resistant pathogens), and patient characteristics (e.g., immunodeficiency). Complex abscesses are typically well circumscribed too; however, they are often located in deep soft tissue and may be multiloculated. If managed incorrectly, these complex abscesses can develop into more complicated soft-tissue infections.

In the context of classification, it should be mentioned the different forms of skin abscesses associated with distinct features and different diagnostic-therapeutic management: abscesses in injecting drug users, abscesses associated with animal and human bites, perianal and perirectal abscesses, and abscesses developing in damaged skin.

Cutaneous/subcutaneous abscesses are the most frequently reported infections in people who inject drugs (past-month prevalence 6.1–32.0%, and lifetime prevalence 6.2–68.6%) [12]. The most common skin involved corresponds to injection sites: the upper extremities (antecubital fossae), lower extremities, and groin. Specific risk factors were identified: injecting once or more a day, reusing needles and syringes, practising subcutaneous or intramuscular injection, taking four or more attempts (skin punctures) to achieve an injection, and comorbidities [13]. In injecting drug users, two main bacteria sources can be determined: the drug user himself/herself (oropharynx, skin, anus) and the environment (contaminated needles, syringes, and injectable drugs). Compared with the general population, cutaneous/subcutaneous abscesses in injection drug users are less likely to involve *Staphylococcus aureus*, including MRSA, and more likely to involve streptococci and anaerobes (polymicrobial infection) [8]. Foreign bodies, such as broken needles, could be located inside the abscess cavity. Surgeons should be careful and not explore abscess cavity with fingers for risk of injury. Abscess may be confused with pseudoaneurysm, hematoma, cellulitis, or thrombosed vein. Surgeons should keep differential diagnoses in mind, and ultrasonography should be performed before surgery.

Animal and human bites are associated with significant risk of skin and soft tissue infection. The risk of infection depends on the type of bite. High risk of bite wound infection was reported in cases of cat bites, dog bites, and human bites. The microbial pathogens are part of the normal oral flora of biting animals. There is a wide and diverse spectrum of bacteria in each animal [14]. Despite the poor state of the evidence regarding universal antibiotic prophylaxis, most experts recommend early antibiotic treatment for 3–5 days for fresh, deep wounds and wounds in critical body areas (hands, feet, areas near joints, face, genitals), and for persons at high risk of infection [15]. If the patient is more than 24 h after the bite and there are no clinical symptoms of infection, antibiotics should not be administered.

Infections developing in damaged skin (burns, pressure ulcers, diabetic foot) are more frequently associated with cellulitis than with abscess. Damaged skin predisposes to bacterial colonisation followed by invasive infection of surrounding vital tissue. Only incision and drainage of purulent content do not result in the resolution of infection. Surgical debridement is necessary to remove all necrotic tissue. Increased susceptibility to bacterial infection is caused by a disrupted skin barrier and a decreased blood supply to surrounding tissue. Unfortunately, treatment outcomes are not satisfying in most cases due to the comorbidities.

Perianal and perirectal abscesses are complex abscesses in nature. However, characteristics of perianal and perirectal abscesses are so different compared to common cutaneous and subcutaneous abscesses that this topic is usually incorporated as a separate chapter in the section on benign anorectal disease.

### 114.1.4 Pathophysiology

The pyogenic cutaneous/subcutaneous abscess is caused by a localised host acute inflammatory response to bacterial infection. The skin, which contains several layers of keratinocytes, serves as a mechanical barrier to prevent the entry of bacteria into deeper tissue. Even a minor trauma to the skin enables entry of pathogenic bacteria into the underlying tissue and initiates an inflammatory response. A crucial role in initiating the immune response is played by keratinocytes and antigen-presenting cells in the skin (Langerhans cells, dendritic cells). These host cells produce antimicrobial peptides against bacteria ($\beta$-defensins) and release proinflammatory cytokines that contribute to the fast influx of polymorphonuclear leukocytes (PMNs). PMNs remove invading bacteria through a process called phagocytosis and kill bacteria by an oxygen-dependent bactericidal mechanism. However, *Staphylococcus aureus* produces many virulence factors, and some of these factors may protect from the antibacterial activity of PMNs or directly alter PMN function (affect PMN recruitment, alter phagocytosis, and cause host cell lysis—cytolytic toxins including Panton-Valentine leucocidin, etc.). Both bacteria and PMNs contribute to local tissue damage and the formation of cutaneous/subcutaneous abscesses. The centre of the abscess contains an acute inflammatory exudate composed of many viable and necrotic PMNs, tissue debris, fibrin, and bacteria. Maturation of the abscess is accompanied by the proliferation of fibroblasts, tissue repair at the abscess margin, and formation of a fibrous capsule at the periphery of the abscess. Abscess formation is a host protective mechanism used to contain and eliminate the invading pathogens.

## 114.2 Diagnosis

Cutaneous/subcutaneous abscess is most often a clinical diagnosis readily identified by the patient's history and physical examination alone. Therefore, the diagnosis of cutaneous and subcutaneous abscess is usually based on clinical manifestations. Laboratory tests (including blood count, bacteria culture, and antimicrobial susceptibility testing) and radiographic imaging are not routinely required.

### 114.2.1 Clinical Manifestation

Cutaneous and subcutaneous abscesses are associated with characteristic clinical manifestations in the involved skin area. The patient suffers from the pain. Traditional local manifestations of abscesses include warmth, redness, and swelling. The characteristic morphologic feature of the cutaneous/subcutaneous abscess is fluctuant lesion. It means palpable motion caused by movement of the pus inside the abscess. Abscess may manifest without cellulitis, or it can be associated with surrounding cellulitis. In case of advanced cellulitis, identifying the exact location of the abscess may be difficult. Sometimes there are swollen lymph nodes—regional lymphadenopathy. Symptoms of systemic toxicity (fever, shivering fit, fatigue) are unusual. Late clinical manifestations include abscess perforation. Abscesses eventually burst and spontaneously drain yellow pus.

On the opposite side, sterile abscesses may be cool, skin-coloured, and painless.

### 114.2.2 Laboratory Tests and Imaging

Laboratory tests used in patients with skin and soft tissue infections include a blood tests and microbiological examination.

Laboratory inflammatory biomarkers (leukocytes, C-reactive protein) support the clinical suspicion of infection. However, laboratory blood tests are not routinely required for making diagnosis in patients with uncomplicated superficial skin abscesses and for patients without comorbidities.

The bacterial aetiology of a skin abscess is difficult to establish based on clinical manifestation alone; therefore, microbiological examination may be warranted. Routine bacterial cultures and antimicrobial susceptibility testing are not necessary in healthy patients who are not going to receive antibiotics after abscess drainage. Microbiological examination is required for patients treated with antibiotics or for patients who meet one of the risk criteria listed in Table 114.2. Microbiological examination includes Gram staining, bacteria culture, and antimicrobial susceptibility testing. Results of microbiological examination may be altered during the pre-analytic period; therefore, the surgeon should know how to perform the right sampling technique, and how to ensure appropriate specimen storage and transportation. Swabbing is not the best technique for specimen collection because only small volume of specimen is obtained. Biological material should be collected into a sterile test tube or injection syringe with a combi-stopper. For microbiological examination of an abscess, it is recommended to collect 2–5 mL of pus, as well as a sample of the abscess wall [16]. The abscess wall samples are recommended based on the fact, that microbiological examination of pus alone may not reveal the causative pathogen because bacteria in the pus are often destroyed by leukocytes.

Radiographic examination is not the cornerstone for skin abscess diagnosis; however, ultrasound imaging may be helpful in cases in which the diagnosis is uncertain. Physicians' clinical assessment for abscess may be limited (in obese patients) or equivocal in cases with extensive overlying and surrounding cellulitis (abscess is not correctly recognised in 30–50%). Use of bedside ultrasonography performed by an experienced person could potentially improve diagnostic accuracy and lead to improved management decisions. Ultrasound imaging may help to confirm the fluid collection, determine its size, and detect loculations and foreign bodies in the abscess cavity. An abscess is represented by a hypoechoic or anechoic area of fluid collection. Based on the systematic review of the literature, the sensitivity and specificity of ultrasound imaging for cutaneous/subcutaneous abscess diagnosis ranged from 89% to 98% and 64% to 88%, respectively [17]. The sensitivity and specificity of the clinical assessment ranged from 75% to 90% and 55% to 83%, respectively; these differences did not reach statistical significance [17]. Ultrasonography rarely changes therapy management when the surgeon is sure regarding the diagnosis of a skin abscess. However, ultrasonography may change drainage decisions in approximately 25% of cases if the surgeon is not sure regarding the presence or absence of an abscess [18]. We can conclude that ultrasonography is helpful in cases of equivocal clinical manifestations of an abscess. X-ray examination is not

**Table 114.2** Criteria for microbiological examination in patients with skin abscess

Severe local infection (extensive surrounding cellulitis)
Systemic signs of infection (fever)
History of recurrent or multiple abscesses
Failure of initial antibiotic treatment
Extremes of age (young infants or the elderly)
Immunocompromised patients
Regions where *S. aureus* antibiotic susceptibility is unknown or rapidly changing

a reliable imaging method for the diagnosis of cutaneous/subcutaneous abscess, but it can be useful for detection of a foreign body in the abscess. Computed tomography can be used to assess large complex abscess location and proximity to critical structures such as blood vessels or nerves if it is necessary for surgery dicision.

> **Differential Diagnosis**
> Cutaneous and subcutaneous abscesses can be confused with many non-infectious and infectious illnesses or skin pathologies. A cutaneous/subcutaneous abscess should be distinguished from the following skin lesions: epidermoid cysts, vascular malformation, lymphadenopathy, bursitis, folliculitis, furuncles and carbuncles, pilonidal disease, and hidradenitis suppurativa.
>
> In the context of differential diagnosis, it is crucial to differentiate the skin abscesses from other bacterial skin and soft tissue infections—erysipelas and cellulitis. Erysipelas is a superficial skin infection involving the upper dermis. A clinical feature of erysipelas is a raised, sharply demarcated erythematous lesion. Most erysipelas is caused by *Streptococcus pyogenes*. Cellulitis is an infection of the deep dermis and subcutaneous tissue, and it is characterised by a poorly defined erythematous lesion with induration. Sometimes there may be a skin abscess surrounded by erythema and induration; therefore, the recognition of purulent cellulitis is very important.

## 114.3 Therapy

In the United States, most cutaneous and subcutaneous abscesses are often managed within emergency departments or primary care offices under local anaesthesia. Patients with complex abscesses, those with significant comorbidities, and those who are systemically unwell usually need surgery under general anaesthesia. In Europe, current practice in the management of cutaneous and subcutaneous abscesses is a little bit different. Most patients are managed by the surgical team rather than in the emergency department, and most patients are managed under general anaesthesia, so they must stay in the hospital [19].

Treatment of cutaneous and subcutaneous abscesses is based on surgery, and eventually antibiotic therapy is required. A superficial simple abscess is usually treated by surgery alone. Complex complicated abscesses require both surgery and antibiotic therapy simultaneously.

### 114.3.1 Surgery

The principle of surgery treatment is "source control". Incision and drainage is the standard treatment for cutaneous and subcutaneous abscesses. More surgery techniques for the drainage of skin abscesses have been proposed. Conventional incision and drainage is usually recommended as the surgical technique of the choice. In simple cutaneous/subcutaneous abscesses, this technique involves making a linear incision through the total length of the abscess, followed by blunt dissection and the spontaneous drainage. A large, complex complicated abscess may be drained with multiple incisions rather than a long, single incision. Conventional incision and drainage technique ensures a high treatment success rate; however, it is a more painful procedure, and long incision may result in a poor cosmetic outcome. In recent years, a new surgery technique called "the loop drainage technique" was developed as an alternative to the conventional incision and drainage. This loop drainage technique involves making two small stab incisions at each pole of the abscess and tying a loop drain on the top of the skin. This technique allows for continued drainage of the abscess cavity associated with no need to repack the wound, less pain, and a better cosmetic outcome. The existing literature data suggest that the loop drainage technique has a little bit lower failure rate than conventional incision and drainage (8.3% and 14.2%, respectively) [20]. Another surgical technique used in the treatment of cutaneous/subcutaneous abscesses is needle aspiration. In the last decade, it was questioned whether needle aspiration was a feasible treatment option for cutaneous and subcutaneous abscesses. In a randomised controlled trial, the overall treatment failure rate for conventional incision and drainage compared to ultrasound-guided needle aspiration was 20% and 74%, respectively [21]. Treatment failure of ultrasound-guided needle aspiration is unacceptably high; therefore, currently, needle aspiration is not recommended for cutaneous and subcutaneous abscess management. Increased viscosity of the purulent material and compartmentalization of the abscess cavity are the two most important limitations of needle aspiration.

Ultrasonography is not only a diagnostic tool but also can be helpful for identifying the right place for incision prior to surgery. In patients with clinically apparent abscesses on physical examination, incision and drainage without ultrasonography is a reasonable option. Ultrasound-guided abscess incision is preferred for skin abscesses hidden in severe cellulitis.

There is a strong consensus on surgery technique, but evidence-based recommendations regarding incision timing, irrigation, packing, pain management, etc. are still lacking. Timing of incision is a crucial factor because premature incision before abscess demarcation is not curative and may be harmful. On the other hand, delayed incision can cause local destructive progression and spontaneous abscess perforation. In cases of immature abscesses associated with surrounding cellulitis, antibiotics and local application of heat can help in treatment. Antibiotics can result in significant improvement in symptoms and a rapid resolution of the surrounding cellulitis. Applying heat to the abscess can help it shrink. The most effective way to apply heat is to put a warm compress on the affected skin. However, this therapy is not a substitute for surgery and should not be continued for more than 36 h. Reassessment of the local clinical manifestation is necessary within this period. After surgical incision, an abscess cavity should be explored to remove pus, necrotic tissue, and foreign bodies. Irrigation is frequently used as a standard part of conventional abscess drainage despite a lack of data demonstrating the benefit of reducing the bacterial load in abscesses through irrigation. No consensus exists on the type and volume of fluid. The abscess cavity is usually irrigated repetitively with saline solution until all visible pus is removed. The abscess cavity should be left open to allow further pus to drain away. Moreover, further pus drainage can be facilitated by the placement of a Penrose drain or tube drain. The packing should prevent premature abscess cavity closure and allow ongoing drainage, and periodic packing replacement should provide debridement. However, these theoretic benefits have never been verified, and the role of packing remains unclear. Based on the results of the cross-sectional survey, wound packing is still common practice in the United Kingdom [19]. If packing is used, the surgeon should avoid overpacking the wound because this may cause increased pain without improving drainage. Simply covering with a sterile dressing is usually the easiest and most effective treatment. Healing by secondary intention is the traditional approach to cutaneous and subcutaneous abscess management. In recent years, some authors have reported that primary closure with sutures has similar failure and recurrence rates compared to healing by secondary intention [22]. Primary closure may be considered in some cases, but it has not been recommended routinely yet, and primary closure of abscess cavities is rarely used in routine practice [23].

### 114.3.2 Antibiotic Therapy

Based on recommendations in previous and recent international guidelines (IDSA 2014, WSES/SIS 2018), patients with uncomplicated simple cutaneous/subcutaneous abscesses do not need antibiotics after successful surgical incision and drainage [15, 24]. However, systemic antibiotics should be given to all patients with complex skin abscesses and abscesses associated with specific risk factors (symptoms of systemic infection, immunocompromised patients, large and multiple abscesses, extremes of age, lack of response to incision and drainage, abscesses with significant cellulitis, MRSA aetiology). Two randomised trials and a systematic literature review demonstrated that the use of systemic antibiotics for cutaneous and subcutaneous abscesses after incision and drainage resulted in an increased rate of clinical cure [25–27]. Moreover, the benefit of antibiotic therapy was proven even in patients with small abscesses (<2 cm). Providing critical appraisal, it should be mentioned that in both randomised trials, the study group had a high MRSA prevalence (45% and 49%) [25, 26]. Currently, the benefit of systemic antibiotics for the therapy of skin abscesses in populations with low MRSA prevalence is a matter of debate.

Antimicrobial therapy should begin promptly and be guided by the severity of the abscess's clinical manifestations and its clinical response to antibiotics. Outpatient management including oral antibiotics for 5 days is indicated in patients with a mild infection. Patients with complicated and severe infections require parenteral antimicrobial therapy with extended administration for 7–14 days. An intravenous-to-oral therapy switch should be considered when criteria for clinical stability have been reached. This approach reduces the length of stay in the hospital.

Initial antimicrobial therapy is empiric in nature and guided by presumed microbial pathogens. Empiric antimicrobial therapy should be tailored to culture and susceptibility results when available. In general, antimicrobial therapy for patients with cutaneous and subcutaneous abscesses who warrant antibiotics should cover Gram-positive cocci, especially *Staphylococcus aureus*. Empiric antibiotic therapy for MRSA is recommended for patients at risk for CA-MRSA. Antibiotics directed against MRSA should be considered based on local epidemiology (hospitals with more than 20% of MRSA in all invasive hospital isolates or a geographic region with a high prevalence of MRSA in the community), specific risk factors for MRSA (Table 114.3), and clinical condition of patient [15]. Antibiotics recommended for MRSA infections—oral options (clindamycin, trimethoprim and sulfamethoxazole, doxycycline, linezolid) and intravenous options (clindamycin, vancomycin, teicoplanin, tigecycline, linezolid). Empiric broad-spectrum antibiotics with coverage of Gram-positive, Gram-negative, and anaerobic bacteria are recommended for complex abscesses, abscesses in injecting drug users, and abscesses developing in damaged skin.

Despite the antimicrobial therapy recommendation reported in the international guidelines, regional microbial epidemiology and local incidence of resistant bacteria should also be considered when choosing antibiotics.

**Table 114.3** Populations at increased risk for CA-MRSA

| Risk factors for CA-MRSA |
|---|
| • Children <2 years old |
| • Athletes (mainly contact-sport participants) |
| • Injection drug users |
| • Homosexual males |
| • Military personnel |
| • Inmates of correctional facilities, residential homes, or shelters |
| • Vets, pet owners, and pig farmers |
| • Patients with post-flu-like illness and/or severe pneumonia |
| • History of colonisation or recent infection with CA-MRSA |
| • History of antibiotic consumption in the previous year, particularly quinolones, or macrolides |

Note: Accepted from Sartelli et al. [15]

**Dos and Don'ts**
- Drain the superficial simple skin abscess through a linear incision and the complex skin abscess by multiple incisions.
- Do not use routinely ultrasound-guided needle aspiration for treatment of cutaneous and subcutaneous abscesses.
- If the clinical manifestation of a skin abscess is not characteristic, use ultrasound for the identification of the pus collection and perform an ultrasound-guided abscess incision.
- Do not administer routinely antibiotics in patients with superficial simple abscesses after successful incision and drainage.
- Consider antibiotics in the treatment of complex abscesses. Consider empiric

antimicrobial therapy for MRSA based on local epidemiology and for patients at high risk for CA-MRSA.
- Administer empiric broad-spectrum antibiotics with coverage of Gram-positive, Gram-negative, and anaerobic bacteria for complex abscesses in perineal, perianal, and axillary body regions and for abscesses in injecting drug users, and for abscesses developing in damaged skin.

### 114.3.3 Prognosis

Even without treatment, simple cutaneous and subcutaneous abscesses in healthy people rarely result in death and are associated with a favourable prognosis. Complex abscesses can develop into more complicated skin and soft-tissue infections, causing systemic toxicity. If these complex abscesses are managed correctly, favourable outcomes are reported as well. A significantly worse prognosis is related to community-onset abscesses in injecting drug users. Lewer et al. documented 50-fold increased risk of severe bacterial skin infections in injecting drug users when compared to the general population [28]. Most injecting drug users usually undertake self-care as their first response to a worsening infection and take more days to seek medical attention. Delayed healthcare seeking potentially exacerbates infection severity, which in turn increases poorer health outcomes and complications [13].

#### Take-Home Messages
- *Staphylococcus aureus* is the most frequent causative pathogen responsible for community-onset cutaneous and subcutaneous abscesses; the emergence of CA-MRSA is responsible for increase in the incidence and severity of skin and soft tissue infection in some geographic regions (USA).
- If the surgeon is not sure regarding the presence/absence of a skin abscess, ultrasonography may change drainage decisions in approximately 25% of all cases; moreover, ultrasound can also be helpful for identifying the right place for incision prior to surgery.
- Incision and drainage is the standard treatment for cutaneous and subcutaneous abscesses; ultrasound-guided needle aspiration is not recommended.
- Empiric antibiotic therapy for MRSA should be considered based on local epidemiology and for patients at high risk for CA-MRSA.
- Despite favourable prognosis of cutaneous and subcutaneous abscesses in the general population, worse outcomes are reported in community-onset skin abscesses in injecting drug users.

#### Questions
1. **What is the clinical feature of cutaneous and subcutaneous abscesses?**
   A. Painful, erythematous, oedematous, fluctuant, nodular lesion
   B. Painful, erythematous, oedematous, gently raised, sharply demarcated lesion
   C. Painful, erythematous, oedematous, poorly defined lesion with induration
   D. None of the answers is correct
2. **The major pathogen involved in cutaneous and subcutaneous abscesses is:**
   A. *Streptococcus pyogenes*
   B. *Staphylococcus epidermidis*
   C. *Staphylococcus aureus*
   D. *Clostridium perfringens*
3. **Which of the following sentences regarding complex abscesses is true?**
   A. Complex abscesses are characterised by their specific location, the pathogens involved, and patient characteristics.

B. Complex abscesses are usually of MRSA origin.
   C. Intravenous antibiotic therapy alone is the method of choice for the treatment of complex abscesses.
   D. Complex abscesses are associated with poor outcomes even if they are managed correctly.
4. **Athletes (mainly contact-sport participants), military personnel, and prisoners are at increased risk for cutaneous and subcutaneous abscesses caused by:**
   A. methicillin-resistant *Staphylococcus aureus* (MRSA)
   B. vancomycin-resistant *Enterococcus faecalis* (VRE)
   C. extended-spectrum β-lactamase producing *Escherichia coli*
   D. extended-spectrum β-lactamase producing *Klebsiella pneumoniae*
5. **Which of the following sentences regarding the indication for the microbiological examination of cutaneous and subcutaneous abscesses is correct?**
   A. Gram staining, bacteria culture, and antimicrobial susceptibility testing are indicated in all patients with cutaneous and subcutaneous abscesses.
   B. Routine Gram staining, bacteria cultures, and antimicrobial susceptibility testing are not necessary in healthy patients who are not going to receive antibiotics after abscess incision and drainage.
   C. Gram staining, bacteria culture, and antimicrobial susceptibility testing are indicated only in patients with skin abscesses with a diameter >8 cm.
   D. Gram staining, bacteria culture, and antimicrobial susceptibility testing are indicated based on the surgeon's judgment.
6. **Which of the following sentences regarding cutaneous and subcutaneous abscesses in injecting drug users is not true?**
   A. The most common locations of abscesses are the antecubital fossae and groin.
   B. Abscesses in injecting drug users are less often caused by *Staphylococcus aureus* (including MRSA) and more often caused by streptococci and anaerobes compared to abscesses in the general population.
   C. More attempts (skin punctures) to achieve an injection of a drug are not a significant risk factor for skin abscess in injecting drug users.
   D. It is recommended to do ultrasound imaging to exclude pseudoaneurysm before surgery for a groin abscess in injecting drug users.
7. **Principle of diagnosis. Which of the following sentences is correct?**
   A. Diagnosis of cutaneous and subcutaneous abscesses is usually clinical.
   B. Ultrasound imaging is necessary for the correct diagnosis of a skin abscess in nearly all cases.
   C. X-ray examination is used routinely in most patients with skin abscesses to exclude bone trauma.
   D. All these answers are true.
8. **A previously healthy 35-year-old man comes to the emergency department because of a 2-day history of worsening pain in his left forearm. He has no history of trauma. He has no known allergies, and his temperature is 37.8 °C. The dorsal forearm is swollen and tender with erythema (10 × 5 cm) that has poorly defined borders. During the palpation examination, you are not sure about the fluctuation in the centre of this ery-**

thematous lesion. Which of the following diagnostic-therapeutic management approaches do you prefer?
A. Watch-and-wait strategy
B. Start with antibiotic therapy and reassess local clinical manifestations in the next 48 h
C. Use ultrasound imaging for confirmation/exclusion of fluid (pus) collection
D. Perform a probatory surgical incision in the centre of the erythematous lesion

9. A 45-year-old woman comes to the emergency department with a 1-day history of painful resistance in the posterior part of her right thigh. Physical examination reveals the erythematous fluctuant nodular lesion with a diameter of 2 × 3 cm. Her temperature is 37.5 °C. She has no history of diabetes mellitus and other comorbidities. What is the most appropriate next therapeutic management?
A. Antibiotic therapy alone
B. Surgical incision and drainage alone
C. Surgical incision and antibiotic therapy together
D. Ultrasound-guided needle aspiration alone

10. A 75-year-old man comes to the emergency department with a 3-day history of redness and swelling in the right side of the abdominal wall lateral to the umbilicus. Examination shows an area of diffuse erythema with a diameter of 8 × 10 cm. It is warm and tender to touch, and you can palpate a fluctuant centre lesion. The patient says that he administered the subcutaneous injection (low-molecular-weight heparin) a few days before the onset of this lesion.

He is obese. He has type 2 diabetes mellitus and coronary heart disease. He appears ill, and his temperature is 38.7 °C. You indicate surgical drainage and antibiotic therapy. Which of the next antibiotics are you going to choose?
A. Penicillin
B. Amoxycillin/clavulanic acid
C. Cefazolin
D. Clindamycin

## References

1. Taira BR, Singer AJ, Thode HC Jr, Lee CC. National epidemiology of cutaneous abscesses: 1996 to 2005. Am J Emerg Med. 2009;27(3):289–92.
2. Fritz SA, Shapiro DJ, Hersh AL. National trends in incidence of purulent skin and soft tissue infections in patients presenting to ambulatory and emergency department settings, 2000–2015. Clin Infect Dis. 2020;70(12):2715–8.
3. Hersh AL, Chambers HF, Maselli JH, Gonzales R. National trends in ambulatory visits and antibiotic prescribing for skin and soft-tissue infections. Arch Intern Med. 2008;168(14):1585–91.
4. Suaya JA, Mera RM, Cassidy A, O'Hara P, Amrine-Madsen H, Burstin S, et al. Incidence and cost of hospitalizations associated with Staphylococcus aureus skin and soft tissue infections in the United States from 2001 through 2009. BMC Infect Dis. 2014;14:296.
5. Hayward A, Knott F, Petersen I, Livermore DM, Duckworth G, Islam A, et al. Increasing hospitalizations and general practice prescriptions for community-onset staphylococcal disease, England. Emerg Infect Dis. 2008;14(5):720–6.
6. Ray GT, Suaya JA, Baxter R. Incidence, microbiology, and patient characteristics of skin and soft-tissue infections in a U.S. population: a retrospective population-based study. BMC Infect Dis. 2013;13:252.
7. Castleman MJ, Pokhrel S, Triplett KD, Kusewitt DF, Elmore BO, Joyner JA, et al. Innate sex bias of Staphylococcus aureus skin infection is driven by α-hemolysin. J Immunol. 2018;200(2):657–68.
8. Jenkins TC, Knepper BC, Jason Moore S, Saveli CC, Pawlowski SW, Perlman DM, et al. Microbiology and initial antibiotic therapy for injection drug users and non-injection drug users with cutaneous abscesses in the era of community-associated methicillin-resistant Staphylococcus aureus. Acad Emerg Med. 2015;22(8):993–7.

9. Casey JA, Cosgrove SE, Stewart WF, Pollak J, Schwartz BS. A population-based study of the epidemiology and clinical features of methicillin-resistant Staphylococcus aureus infection in Pennsylvania, 2001–2010. Epidemiol Infect. 2013;141(6):1166–79.
10. Acree ME, Morgan E, David MZ. S. aureus infections in Chicago, 2006–2014: increase in CA MSSA and decrease in MRSA incidence. Infect Control Hosp Epidemiol. 2017;38(10):1226–34.
11. Bouchiat C, Curtis S, Spiliopoulou I, Bes M, Cocuzza C, Codita I, et al. ESCMID Study Group on Staphylococci and Staphylococcal Infections (ESGS). MRSA infections among patients in the emergency department: a European multicentre study. J Antimicrob Chemother. 2017;72(2):372–5.
12. Larney S, Peacock A, Mathers BM, Hickman M, Degenhardt L. A systematic review of injecting-related injury and disease among people who inject drugs. Drug Alcohol Depend. 2017;171:39–49.
13. Wright T, Hope V, Ciccarone D, Lewer D, Scott J, Harris M. Prevalence and severity of abscesses and cellulitis, and their associations with other health outcomes, in a community-based study of people who inject drugs in London, UK. PLoS One. 2020;15(7):e0235350.
14. Abrahamian FM, Goldstein EJ. Microbiology of animal bite wound infections. Clin Microbiol Rev. 2011;24(2):231–46.
15. Sartelli M, Guirao X, Hardcastle TC, Kluger Y, Boermeester MA, Raşa K, et al. 2018 WSES/SIS-E consensus conference: recommendations for the management of skin and soft-tissue infections. World J Emerg Surg. 2018;13:58.
16. Miller JM, Binnicker MJ, Campbell S, Carroll KC, Chapin KC, Gilligan PH, et al. A guide to utilization of the microbiology laboratory for diagnosis of infectious diseases: 2018 update by the Infectious Diseases Society of America and the American Society for Microbiology. Clin Infect Dis. 2018;67(6):e1–e94.
17. Alsaawi A, Alrajhi K, Alshehri A, Ababtain A, Alsolamy S. Ultrasonography for the diagnosis of patients with clinically suspected skin and soft tissue infections: a systematic review of the literature. Eur J Emerg Med. 2017;24(3):162–9.
18. Mower WR, Crisp JG, Krishnadasan A, Moran GJ, Abrahamian FM, Lovecchio F, et al. Effect of initial bedside ultrasonography on emergency department skin and soft tissue infection management. Ann Emerg Med. 2019;74(3):372–80.
19. Thomas O, Ramsay A, Yiasemidou M, Hardie C, Ashmore D, Macklin C, et al. The surgical management of cutaneous abscesses: a UK cross-sectional survey. Ann Med Surg (Lond). 2020;60:654–9.
20. Gottlieb M, Schmitz G, Peksa GD. Comparison of the loop technique with incision and drainage for skin and soft tissue abscesses: a systematic review and meta-analysis. Acad Emerg Med. 2021;28(3):346–54.
21. Gaspari RJ, Resop D, Mendoza M, Kang T, Blehar D. A randomized controlled trial of incision and drainage versus ultrasonographically guided needle aspiration for skin abscesses and the effect of methicillin-resistant Staphylococcus aureus. Ann Emerg Med. 2011;57(5):483–91.e1.
22. Singer AJ, Taira BR, Chale S, Bhat R, Kennedy D, Schmitz G. Primary versus secondary closure of cutaneous abscesses in the emergency department: a randomized controlled trial. Acad Emerg Med. 2013;20(1):27–32.
23. Schmitz G, Goodwin T, Singer A, Kessler CS, Bruner D, Larrabee H, et al. The treatment of cutaneous abscesses: comparison of emergency medicine providers' practice patterns. West J Emerg Med. 2013;14(1):23–8.
24. Stevens DL, Bisno AL, Chambers HF, Dellinger EP, Goldstein EJ, Gorbach SL, et al. Practice guidelines for the diagnosis and management of skin and soft tissue infections: 2014 update by the Infectious Diseases Society of America. Clin Infect Dis. 2014;59(2):147–59.
25. Daum RS, Miller LG, Immergluck L, Fritz S, Creech CB, Young D, et al. A placebo-controlled trial of antibiotics for smaller skin abscesses. N Engl J Med. 2017;376(26):2545–55.
26. Talan DA, Moran GJ, Krishnadasan A, Abrahamian FM, Lovecchio F, Karras DJ, et al. Subgroup analysis of antibiotic treatment for skin abscesses. Ann Emerg Med. 2018;71(1):21–30.
27. Gottlieb M, DeMott JM, Hallock M, Peksa GD. Systemic antibiotics for the treatment of skin and soft tissue abscesses: a systematic review and meta-analysis. Ann Emerg Med. 2019;73(1):8–16.
28. Lewer D, Hope VD, Harris M, Kelleher M, Jewell A, Pritchard M, et al. Incidence and treatment costs of severe bacterial infections among people who inject heroin: a cohort study in South London, England. Drug Alcohol Depend. 2020;212:108057.

# Further Reading

Esposito S, Bassetti M, Concia E, De Simone G, De Rosa FG, Grossi P, et al. Italian Society of Infectious and Tropical Diseases. Diagnosis and management of skin and soft-tissue infections (SSTI). A literature review and consensus statement: an update. J Chemother. 2017;29(4):197–214.

Sartelli M, Guirao X, Hardcastle TC, Kluger Y, Boermeester MA, Raşa K, et al. 2018 WSES/SIS-E consensus conference: recommendations for the management of skin and soft-tissue infections. World J Emerg Surg. 2018;13:58.

Stevens DL, Bisno AL, Chambers HF, Dellinger EP, Goldstein EJ, Gorbach SL, et al. Practice guidelines for the diagnosis and management of skin and soft tissue infections: 2014 update by the Infectious Diseases Society of America. Clin Infect Dis. 2014;59(2):147–59.

# Surgical Site Infections

### 115

A. Walker and M. Wilson

> **Learning Goals**
> - Appreciate the high burden of morbidity caused by SSI and the need for effective auditing practices.
> - Know the likely causative organisms for SSI and how they interfere with normal wound healing.
> - Recognise patients at high risk for developing SSIs, and consider perioperative and surgical strategies to minimise their occurrence.

## 115.1 Introduction

Surgical site infection (SSI) is one of the most common postoperative complications in both elective and emergency surgery, occurring in at least 5% of all patients and significantly higher following emergency surgery. An estimated 110,800 SSI occurred in the USA in 2015 [1], with each SSI estimated to increase hospital inpatient stay by 6 days on average and be a major contributor to patient morbidity and mortality [2, 3]. With the annual volume of major surgical procedures estimated to exceed 234.2 million cases worldwide [4], SSI are likely to represent an underestimated burden for both patients and healthcare providers. SSIs are also a major risk factor for the development of wound dehiscence and incisional hernias (IH), resulting in further increased morbidity to patients and cost to healthcare resources [5].

In contrast to the increased burden of wound complications and SSI associated with emergency surgery, there is a relative paucity of evidence available compared to the elective setting. Pragmatic hurdles, including difficulties in patient recruitment and a lack of follow-up for these patients, contribute to this problem. Here we offer guidance based on the existing body of emergency surgery research, with additional guidance and opinion derived from the elective laparotomy setting.

### 115.1.1 Epidemiology

The reported incidence of SSI after surgery varies widely, due to not only geographic and health-economic factors but also variation in SSI surveillance practices and case definitions [6]. In the USA, an estimated 110,800 SSI occurred in 2015; however, the true incidence is most likely

A. Walker (✉)
Forth Valley Royal Hospital, Larbert, Scotland, UK

University of Edinburgh, Edinburgh, Scotland, UK
e-mail: Alex.walker@ed.ac.uk

M. Wilson
Forth Valley Royal Hospital, Larbert, Scotland, UK
e-mail: michael.wilson3@nhs.scot

significantly higher as most infections may be diagnosed after discharge from the hospital [7, 8] and hence escape standard auditing practices.

In England in 2019–2020, the national SSI Surveillance Service (SSISS) collecting data on open surgical procedures from 17 surgical categories identified hip and knee replacement surgery as carrying the lowest SSI risk (0.5% for both), whereas bile duct, liver, or pancreatic surgery as well as large bowel surgery carried the highest risk of SSI (9.1% and 8.3%, respectively), with the median time to infection varying from 6 days for cholecystectomy to 22 days for knee replacement [9]. The breakdown of SSI by anatomical plane reveals large differences between procedures; 75% of SSI for bile duct, liver, and pancreatic surgery were organ/space SSIs, whereas these accounted for 32% of SSI in large bowel surgery and 22% in hip replacement.

Rates of SSI vary by geographical location and, in particular, by the country's Human Development Index (HDI). This is partly explained by low- and middle-HDI countries having correspondingly higher rates of emergency surgery than high-HDI countries, as well as increased proportions of contaminated and dirty surgery. In addition, low-HDI countries carry a higher risk of SSI independent of the acuity of care and degree of contamination [8].

The additional cost burden of each SSI is estimated to lie between $10,443 and $25,546 US dollars per infection in the USA [10]. The presence of multi-drug-resistant organisms can increase the cost further, with MRSA SSI adding a mean weighted $13,901 cost to a hospital stay in the USA [11] and up to 12-fold increased rates of mortality.

### 115.1.2 Aetiology and Risk Factors

Surgical wound class is a major risk factor for SSI, as the bacterial inoculum both in the affected tissues and in the incision will inevitably be high. The risk of SSI increases with each class of wound contamination (Table 115.1).

Risk factors for SSI are categorised into patient- and procedure-related risk factors (Table 115.2). Although the scope for modifying or optimising risk factors is often limited in the context of emergency surgery, it is nonetheless important to identify these in order to inform the peri- and intra-operative decision-making, obtain informed consent, and implement risk-reduction strategies for SSI.

Although the exact mechanism of action for these risk factors is often unclear, most patient-related risk factors are likely to be related to the impairment of innate host defences, acting both on the clearance of infectious organisms and impairing the wound healing process.

**Table 115.2** Risk factors for surgical site infection

| Patient factors | Surgical factors |
| --- | --- |
| • Higher ASA[a] | • Emergency surgery |
| • Age | • Wound class |
| • Diabetes | • Site of surgery (gastroduodenal, small- and large-bowel) |
| • Obesity (BMI ≥ 30 kg/m$^2$) | |
| • Poor nutritional status | • Prolonged operation time |
| • Smoking history | • Need for intraoperative blood transfusion |
| • Alcohol excess | • Break in sterile technique |
| • High-dose or long-term steroid treatment | |

[a] *ASA* American Society of Anaesthesiologists physical status classification system

**Table 115.1** Wound classification by degree of contamination

| Clean | Clean-contaminated | Contaminated | Dirty |
| --- | --- | --- | --- |
| • Elective | • Urgent/emergency care that is otherwise clean | • Non-purulent inflammation | • Purulent inflammation |
| • No trauma | • Elective opening of hollow viscera, minimal spillage | • Gross spillage from GI tract | • Pre-operative perforation of hollow viscera |
| • Hollow viscera not entered | • Not encountered infected bile or urine | • Encounter with infected bile or urine | • Penetrating trauma >4 h |
| • E.g. hernia repair, lipoma cision | • Minor break in sterile technique | • Major break in sterile technique | |
| | | • Penetrating trauma <4 h | |
| | | • Chronic open wound to be grafted or covered | |

### 115.1.3 Classification

SSIs can be categorised by the anatomical plane affected: skin and subcutaneous tissue (superficial incisional SSI), musculofascial planes (deep incisional SSI), and organs or deep space, including the peritoneum and pleura (organ or space SSI) (Fig. 115.1). For incisional SSI, the anatomical plane refers to the deepest layer affected. Intraperitoneal organ/deep space SSI will tend to occur in dependent areas: the pelvis, hepatorenal recess (Morrison's pouch), and splenorenal space.

### 115.1.4 Pathophysiology

#### 115.1.4.1 Physiology of Wound Healing

The process of surgical wound healing begins at the moment the tissue is incised and is characterised by four overlapping and interconnected phases: *haemostasis*, *inflammation*, *proliferation*, and *remodelling*.

From the time of incision, blood components initiate *haemostasis* at the wound edge. This includes platelet aggregation and the release of products such as platelet-derived growth factor (PDGF) and tissue growth factor beta (TGF-β).

Within 48 h of incision, polymorphonuclear neutrophils (PMNs) infiltrate the wound and scavenge necrotic tissue and debris during the initial phase of *inflammation*. PMNs are short-lived and soon die by apoptosis, a process driven in part by infiltrating wound macrophages which characterise the late period of tissue *inflammation* [12]. These macrophages continue to debride the wound by phagocytosis of cellular debris and apoptotic bodies whilst also releasing cytokines including tissue necrosis factor alpha (TNF-α) and TGF-β, eventually leading to the recruitment and activation of fibroblasts [13].

*Proliferation* is driven by both macrophages and fibroblasts starting between days 2 and 5 after tissue incision; the local release of chemokines drives angiogenesis, and fibroblasts secrete fibrillar material into the wound, providing an initial disorganised extracellular matrix (ECM).

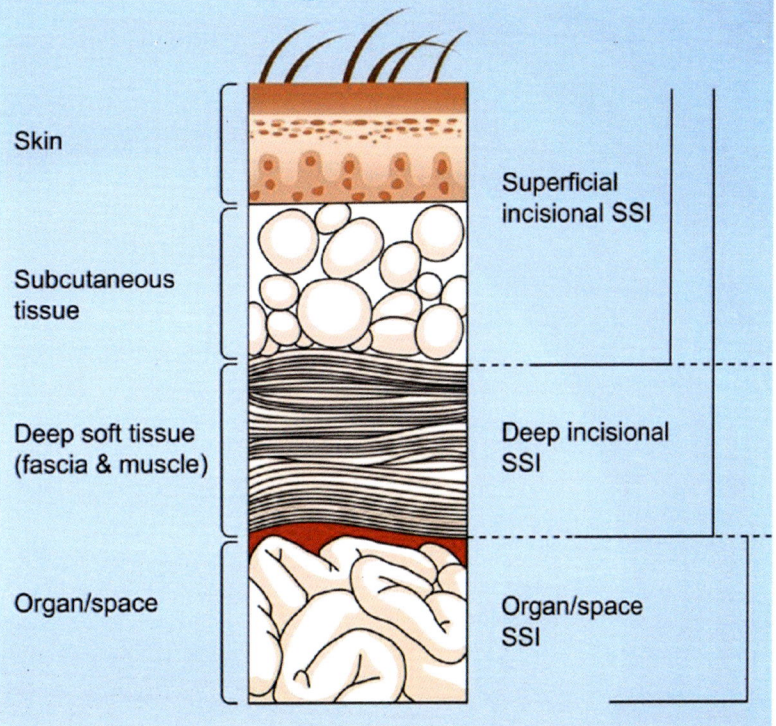

**Fig. 115.1** Classification of surgical site infections by anatomical plane. (Reproduced from [52])

Fibroblasts also take on a contractile phenotype to become myofibroblasts, which contract the ECM and bring together the wound edges, narrowing the superficial gap for re-epithelialisation.

The final phase of wound healing is *remodelling*, whereby a balance of ECM resorption and deposition occurs and replaces the disorganised and weak early ECM with mature scar tissue. Collagen content increases during this stage with a relative decrease in type III collagen [14]. The process can take up to one year to complete, and the tensile strength can reach up to 80% of the original uninjured tissue strength.

Bacteria disrupt the normal wound healing process through a variety of mechanisms. Through direct effects as well as the secretion of endotoxins, they disturb and prolong the inflammatory phase of healing, increase the level of tissue matrix metalloproteinases, and reduce protease inhibitors, leading to poor wound healing or tissue degradation. Bacteria can also move beyond local tissue infection to invasive infection in adjacent tissue.

### 115.1.4.2 Pathogens in SSI

Causative organisms for SSIs vary depending on the type of surgery and the infected anatomical plane. Organisms usually originate from the patient's endogenous flora; however, they can also be from exogenous sources where a break in sterile conditions occurs. Infections are frequently polymicrobial. Enterobacterales (enteric Gram-negative bacilli), a third of which are *E. coli*, are the most common causative organisms, accounting for up to 29.6% of superficial SSIs and 26.2% of deep incisional or organ/space SSIs. This proportion increases in colonic surgery, where Enterobacterales account for 48.5% of superficial SSIs and 55.7% of deep or organ/space SSIs. *Staphylococcus aureus* is the second most prevalent causative organism for SSIs and can include both methicillin-sensitive and resistant strains depending on regional prevalence, with coagulase-negative staphylococci (CoNS) and *Pseudomonas* spp. being the next most common organisms (Table 115.3).

Drug-resistant organisms are a significant and worsening global concern. A recent prospective study in Saudi Arabia reported that up to 27.7% of Gram-positive and 16.1% of Gram-negative SSI are caused by resistant organisms, and the GlobalSurg collaborative has also identified a high proportion of antimicrobial resistance in SSI, particularly in low-HDI countries (35.9% resistant strains compared with 16.6% in high-HDI countries) [8]. MRSA and vancomycin-resistant *Enterococcus* (VRE) are the most common resistant pathogens encountered worldwide; however, carbapenem and cephalosporin resistance in Enterobacterales organisms and multi-drug-resistant (MDR) organisms, including *E. coli*, are also encountered and present an established threat to modern-day medicine.

**Table 115.3** Most common causative organisms for SSI

| | |
|---|---|
| Enterobacterales | *Escherichia coli* |
| | *Klebsiella* spp. |
| | *Enterobacter* spp. |
| | *Proteus* spp. |
| Gram-positive cocci | *Staphyloccus aureus* |
| | *Enterococcus* spp. |
| | Coagulase-negative staphylococci |
| | *Streptococcus* spp. |
| Non-fermenting gram-negative bacteria | *Pseudomonas* spp. |
| | *Acinetobacter* spp. |
| Fungi | *Candida* spp. |
| Anaerobic bacilli | *Bacteroides* spp. |
| Unknown/no identified pathogen | |

## 115.2 Diagnosis

### 115.2.1 Risk Prediction

Multiple tools have been devised to predict the risk of SSI for patients, with the intention of targeting risk-reduction strategies for high-risk patients and for monitoring SSI rates across healthcare networks. An inherent difficulty for SSI risk prediction tools is the need to balance a simple tool based on routinely collected data with the wide variety of SSI incidence for different categories of surgical procedures and across multiple risk factors. Initial attempts at devising a universal SSI risk prediction tool have now been superseded by procedure-specific algorithms; however, predictive ability overall remains poor [15, 16].

An example of an SSI risk prediction model is the CDC National Healthcare Safety Network (NHSN) risk index (Table 115.4), which uses three variables accounting for patient- and procedure-specific risk factors. An NHSN risk index of 2–3 has been shown to significantly increase the risk of SSI across a number of surgical procedures, and high-risk patients are up to four times more likely to develop an SSI [9].

### 115.2.2 Diagnostic Criteria

Surgical site infections (SSIs) occur at the operative site within 30 days of surgery, or within 90 days of surgery where foreign bodies, including prostheses and mesh, are used. A diagnosis of SSI usually requires purulent discharge from the wound or evidence of a collection or an inflammatory process (*rubor, calor, dolor, tumor*) with breakdown in tissue apposition. The most commonly adopted definition and classification for SSI is that by the Centers for Disease Control and Prevention (CDC) (Table 115.5) [1].

## 115.3 Prevention and Treatment

### 115.3.1 SSI Prevention

Prevention is better than cure, and in the case of SSI, a range of peri- and intra-operative strategies have been shown to reduce the incidence of infection [17]. These strategies can broadly be divided into peri-operative care and surgical strategies.

#### 115.3.1.1 Peri-operative Care

**Pre-operative Antibiotics**
Antibiotics should be given when there is a confirmed or high suspicion of infection. Antibiotics

**Table 115.4** NHSN risk index. Low risk = 0–1, high risk = 2–3

| NHSN criteria | Points |
| --- | --- |
| ASA score ≥ 3 | 1 |
| Operation duration ≥ 'T-time'[a] | 1 |
| Contaminated or dirty wound | 1 |

[a] T-time defined as ≥75th percentile for that operation

**Table 115.5** Criteria for SSI, adapted from the Centre for Disease Control and Prevention

|  | Superficial incisional SSI[a] | Deep incisional SSI | Organ/space SSI |
| --- | --- | --- | --- |
| Time frame | Within 30 days | Within 30 days or 90 days if implants used | Within 30 days or 90 days if implants used |
| Anatomical plane | Skin and subcutaneous tissue | Deep soft tissues (e.g. musculofascial layer) | Deeper to the relevant musculofascial plane, in a recognised site of organ/space SSI |
| Infection criteria | • Purulent discharge from wound<br>• Positive microbiology from a suspected SSI<br>• Localised pain or tenderness, swelling, erythema, or heat<br>AND<br>Superficial incision is deliberately opened[b]<br>• Clinical diagnosis by an experienced practitioner | • Purulent discharge from the deep wound<br>• Localised pain, tenderness or fever (>38 °C)<br>AND<br>Deep layer spontaneously dehisces or is deliberately opened or aspirated<br>AND<br>Positive microbiology<br>• Abscess or evidence of deep incisional infection detected on gross anatomical or histopathological examination, or imaging | • Purulent discharge from a drain placed into the organ/space (during or after the procedure)<br>• Positive microbiology from a suspected SSI<br>• Organ/space abscess or evidence of infection detected on gross anatomical or histopathological examination, or imaging |

[a] Includes laparoscopic port sites
[b] Cellulitis does not meet criteria for SSI diagnosis

should be administered through the parenteral route, and the timing of administration, where practicable, should aim to achieve the highest target site concentration at the time of incision. This is broadly accepted to be within 30–60 min of incision for most antibiotics or 2 h for vancomycin and fluoroquinolones [18]. Antibiotic choice should be dictated by the type of surgery involved and the most likely pathogens encountered during that surgery whilst also taking into account local hospital guidelines and antimicrobial resistance patterns..

Intra-operative re-dosing during surgery should be considered for extended surgery or for estimated blood losses of over 1500 mL. The specific dose frequency of antibiotics will depend on the antibiotic's particular pharmacokinetics. For example, beta-lactam agents exhibit antimicrobial activity when their target tissue concentration remains above the bacterial minimal inhibition concentration (MIC), hence making them suitable for higher frequency dosage or continuous infusion. In contrast, peak serum concentration is more closely associated with efficacy for aminoglycosides, and re-dosing is therefore not necessary during surgery [17, 19].

### Peri-operative Normothermia

Hypothermia is an independent risk factor for mortality in major trauma patients and forms part of the physiological "lethal triad" along with acidosis and coagulopathy [20]. Core body temperature is normally kept within a narrow homeostatic range. However, in the emergency setting, particularly in the context of major trauma, patients are prone to hypothermia due to a combination of environmental exposure, heat loss from open wounds and surgical incisions, and homeostatic derangements caused by anaesthesia.

The benefit of normothermia during surgery also applies to SSI; during major elective and emergency surgery, maintaining normothermia has been shown to decrease the rate of SSI. In a series of 200 patients undergoing elective colorectal surgery, Kurz et al. [21] reported a decrease in SSI from 19% to 6% for patients where normothermia was maintained through a combination of forced air and fluid warming.

### Glycaemic Control

Diabetes is a recognised risk factor for poor wound healing and SSI [8]. Moreover, acute hyperglycaemia has also been shown to have deleterious effects on the physiological wound healing process and to contribute to increased rates of SSI. The immune system, neutrophils, in particular, shows an impaired inflammatory response in the presence of hyperglycaemia, characterised by delayed migration/chemotaxis and defective phagocytosis. Keratinocyte migration and proliferation are hampered by the hyperglycaemic environment, in turn preventing re-epithelialisation from taking place [22]. Hyperglycaemia also enhances the deleterious effects of hypoxia on wound healing through a variety of mechanisms.

Retrospective cohort studies of surgical patients have shown pre- and postoperative hyperglycaemia (above 10.0 mmol/L) to be significant predictors of SSI. The intensity of glycaemic control should be cautious; the NICE-SUGAR trial collaboration has shown that "tight" glycaemic control (4.5–6.0 mmol/L) is overall deleterious with increased incidence of severe hypoglycaemia. A conventional glucose target of 10.0 mmol/L or less is an adequate target perioperatively and in particular for postoperative ICU patients [23].

### Supplemental Oxygen

Increased oxygen delivery to tissues was thought to reduce the rate of SSI by improving tissue healing. Although early studies suggested a benefit for supplemental oxygen (usually 80%), more recent large RCTs and meta-analyses have shown no clear benefit for supplemental oxygen and have raised the possibility of long-term harm [24, 25]. Definitive evidence is still lacking, in particular data for emergency surgery.

### 115.3.1.2 Surgical Strategies

### Skin Preparation and Optimal Incision

The midline incision remains the most common method of laparotomy in emergency surgery. It offers quick and adequate access to the abdominal cavity and avoids the need to enter musculofascial planes such as the rectus sheath, which may be relevant for contaminated or dirty wounds. Although it leads to higher incisional hernia rates than the paramedian incision, the latter is more time-consuming to perform, which may be disadvantageous in emergency surgery [26]. There is no difference in the rate of SSI between different types of access [27], although caution should be used when wound contamination is anticipated.

Hair at the surgical site has not been shown to increase the risk of SSI; it should not be removed unless necessary, in which case clippers should be used rather than shaving [28]. The debate over skin scrubbing solution is ongoing; however, evidence favours alcohol-based solutions over aqueous agents, and chlorhexidine may be superior to povidone-iodine [29].

**Wound Protectors**

Wound protector devices, or "wound retractors", consist of a semi-flexible ring connected to an impervious membrane, used to protect wound edges and improve surgical exposure during laparotomy. The semi-flexible ring is introduced intraperitoneally with the membrane forming a drape over the wound edge. The membrane either hangs freely outside the abdominal cavity ("single ring") or is connected to a second rigid ring providing a frame for support and retracting the wound edge (the "double-ring" design, Fig. 115.2). Wound protectors are thought to reduce the SSI rate by acting as a physical barrier and preventing the incursion of pathogens into the skin and subcutaneous tissue protected by the device. They also provide haemostasis to the wound edge, and by controlling humidification and preventing environmental exposure to the wound edge, they may contribute to local temperature control.

Evidence from several meta-analyses supports the use of wound protector devices, in particular double-ring designs. There is a pooled risk reduction of 30% and up to 70% with the use of dual-ring wound protector designs for overall SSI and superficial SSI. The benefit of reducing SSI applies both to clean-contaminated and contaminated wounds, with an unclear benefit for dirty wounds [30, 31].

It should be noted, however, that the largest randomised controlled trial investigating the role of wound protectors (the ROSSINI Trial, $n = 760$), which was conducted across elective and emergency settings and included in both meta-analyses, did not show a benefit of wound protector devices. In this study, the overall postoperative SSI rate was 25.0%, with no significant difference between wound protector and control groups [32].

**Fascial Closure**

Interrupted or Continuous Sutures
The evidence base for fascial closure technique is heterogenous, in part due to the wide variety of interrupted closure methods reported in the lit-

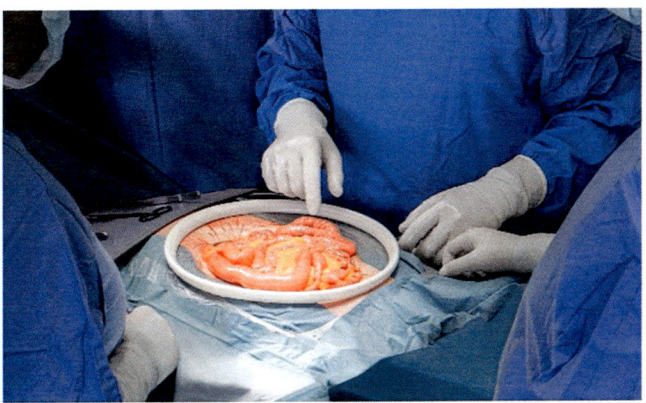 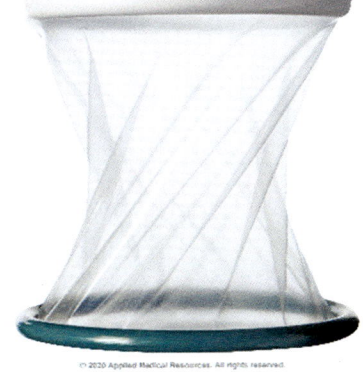

**Fig. 115.2** Double-ring wound protectors reduce the incidence of SSI

erature. However a systematic review and meta-analysis by van't Riet et al. concluded there is no significant difference between interrupted and continuous sutures in terms of SSI or incisional hernias. The continuous fascial closure technique is significantly faster, which makes it more appropriate in the context of emergency surgery [33]. A suture length-to-wound length ratio (SL/WL) of 4/1 or higher reduces the incisional hernia rate [34], and animal models have shown that this ratio provides a high rate of collagen deposition as long as excessive pulling along the suture line with consequent tissue ischaemia is avoided [14].

### Absorbable or Non-absorbable Sutures

As discussed above, the early stages of wound healing are characterised by an inflammatory response with progressive deposition and strengthening of the extracellular matrix, which can take up to a year to reach its maximal tensile strength. This long remodelling phase and the overall reduction in tensile strength mean incisional hernias can take between months and years to develop [35], leading some surgeons to advocate closure with non-absorbable sutures. However, the use of non-absorbable sutures such as polypropylene is associated with increased postoperative pain and the development of stitch sinus infections in the longer term.

### Coated Sutures

The potential for suture material to act as a foreign body and contribute to SSIs is well known, and monofilament sutures such as polydioxanone or polypropylene have a lower bacterial burden than multifilament sutures such as polyglactin 910. The use of antiseptic suture coating ("Plus sutures") further reduces bacterial counts and has the added benefits of localised action, low acute toxicity and altered resistance patterns. Triclosan is the most commonly used coating; however, other coatings including chlorhexidine-based coatings are also available [36, 37].

In a meta-analysis by Daoud [38] including 4800 patients from 15 randomised controlled trials, triclosan-coated polyglactin 910 braided sutures were shown to reduce the risk of SSI by up to 30% versus uncoated polyglactin 910. This included clean, clean-contaminated, and contaminated wounds. A cost analysis by Leaper et al. [39] suggests an overall cost saving of between £63 and £470 per surgical procedure.

Evidence for the use of coated sutures for dirty wounds is still relatively sparse; although its clinical effectiveness for polyglactin 910 is clear [40], in contrast there is conflicting evidence for coated polydioxanone sutures. A well-conducted trial by Justinger et al. [41] including clean-contaminated and contaminated wounds has shown a reduction in SSI using loop-coated polydioxanone suture closure across all categories of wound contamination; however, the result from a meta-analysis including mostly elective surgeries remains equivocal [42]. The FALCON trial, run by the GlobalSurg collaborative, is due to report results and may shed further evidence on the effectiveness of antiseptic-coated sutures in both elective and emergency settings.

## Skin Closure

### Wound Washout and Topical Antibiotics

Skin and subcutaneous tissue washout using saline, povidone-iodine, or antibiotic solution is widely practised and assumed to reduce the rate of SSI. It is thought to work by dilution of local pathogens and physical removal of devitalised tissue, with advocates suggesting it should be vigorous enough to remove debris but careful to avoid further trauma to the wound edge.

A Cochrane meta-analysis of surgical wound washout found that studies were highly heterogenous but suggested a possible benefit for both povidone-iodine wound treatment and wound washout with pressurised saline. Both of these findings were of low certainty given the heterogenous studies and risks of publication bias [43].

### Staples or Sutures

The most common methods of skin closure after emergency surgery are disposable skin staples, interrupted non-dissolvable sutures, and continuous subcuticular dissolvable sutures. Although there is a paucity of evidence from emergency general surgery to favour one strategy over another, current evidence suggests that continuous subcuticular suturing decreases the rate of superficial wound infection as opposed to interrupted sutures [44]. Similarly, skin staples have been shown to increase superficial wound infection in both orthopaedic and obstetric surgery [45, 46].

Evidence from emergency abdominal surgery is lacking to support either strategy of skin closure; however, studies of skin closure during elective abdominal surgery show no difference in the rate of superficial skin dehiscence or SSI between subcuticular and stapled skin closure [47, 48]. It should be noted, however, that continuous subcuticular skin closure can add up to 30 min of operative time. Although stapled skin closure is not recommended as routine for the closure of emergency surgery, in some circumstances including prolonged operative time or ahead of a planned re-look laparotomy, closure with staples is a reasonable recourse.

Negative Pressure Wound Therapy (NPWT)
NPWT uses a suction pump to provide continuous or intermittent negative pressure to the wound (Fig. 115.3). This promotes blood flow and oxygenation to the wound, as well as controlling wound exudate to help promote granulation and wound healing. NPWT has been used for over 25 years and applied to various wound types, in particular diabetic, vascular, and pressure ulcers, burns, and donor sites.

The use of NPWT in traumatic wounds remains contentious: although a Cochrane review including a heterogenous population of surgical patients concluded NPWT can reduce SSI [49], a separate review assessing its use in open traumatic fracture wound closures suggests with moderate certainty that NPWT does not improve wound healing and does not provide a cost-effective treatment modality [50].

The use of NPWT has more recently been used for prophylactic surgical wound management. A meta-analysis by Hyldig et al. [51] showed that amongst a mixed group of scheduled and unscheduled operations, incisional NPWT had a lower incidence of SSI and seroma formation (relative risks of 0.54 and 0.48, respectively), with a non-significant reduction in wound dehiscence. A number of trials are assessing the use of NPWT in obese women undergoing planned or emergency C-sections, and it is possible that the amount of subcutaneous fat and patient BMI are factors that may allow surgeons to target the use of NPWT to high-risk patients.

## 115.3.2 Treatment of SSI

Although a large proportion of SSIs present in the early postoperative period, they may take between weeks and months to present, including after discharge from hospital. It is therefore advisable to have an established institutional SSI surveillance mechanism in place, particularly for high-risk patients.

The broad principles of SSI management involve drainage of infection, debridement of tissue, and the early institution of antibiotics.

### 115.3.2.1 Incisional SSI
Most incisional SSI will be associated with fluid or purulent collections, and it is advisable to drain this fluid or pus to prevent worsening local or invasive infection and promote wound healing. For superficial incisional SSI, a partial opening

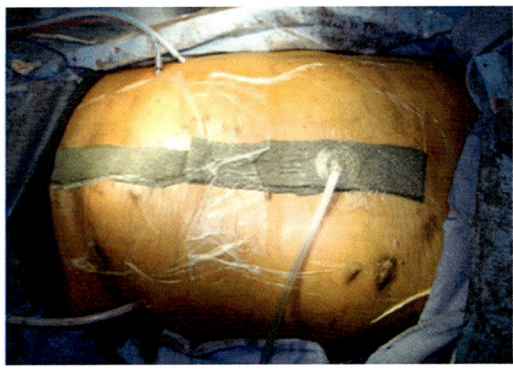

**Fig. 115.3** NPWT should be considered for wounds at high risk of SSI. (Reproduced from [53])

may be made to drain the wound, with localised removal of involved clips or sutures. Where an infection is extensive or there is concern about deep incisional SSI or wound dehiscence, the wound and fascial layer should be probed as a defect in the musculofascial layer will usually require formal operative reintervention and repair. Early treatment with antibiotics is usually required for incisional SSI, using empirical broad-spectrum antibiotics or guided by wound sampling. However, for small and limited superficial incisional SSI, drainage of pus and the use of antiseptics with appropriate interactive moist dressings may be sufficient to control the infection.

Where early measures have failed to control the infection, the portion of skin over the infected wound segment should be opened for wound debridement, at which point it may be allowed to heal by secondary intention or with the use of NPWT, or in very selected cases by delayed primary closure.

### 115.3.2.2 Deep-Space SSI

Deep-space SSI may present with a failure to progress or acute deterioration and a new onset of sepsis in the postoperative phase. A high index of suspicion is required, and radiological imaging will usually confirm the diagnosis. Deep-space SSI may lead to severe and life-threatening infection, and the initial response to resuscitation and broad-spectrum antibiotics will guide the decision to proceed with further radiologically guided drainage or operative management.

Empirical broad-spectrum antibiotics should be used in the first instance, guided by sensitivities from peripheral blood cultures or aspirates when these become available. The use of percutaneous drainage of abscesses greater than 4 cm in diameter should be considered and will often depend on the precise abscess location and local availability of interventional radiology.

In the unusual circumstance where the above measures fail to adequately resolve the deep-space SSI, surgical management should be considered.

> **Dos and Don'ts**
> - DO have a range of closure methods available to decrease the risk of SSI.
> - DO remove dressings and inspect the postoperative wound when patients are at high risk of SSI.
> - DO obtain microbiology samples from SSIs to guide antibiotic choice.
> - DON'T leave the closure of high-risk surgical wounds to inexperienced surgeons.
> - DON'T continue prophylactic antibiotics unless infection is suspected or confirmed.
> - DON'T assume your SSI outcomes are low unless you can show this through a rigorous audit.

> **Take-Home Messages**
> - Surgical site infection carries significant morbidity and mortality.
> - Targeted therapies and bundles should be initiated for patients at high risk of SSI.
> - Treatment of SSI relies on the drainage of infection, debridement of tissues, and appropriate antibiotic stewardship.
> - Institutions should have audit structures in place to monitor the incidence of SSI.

> **Questions**
> 1. Three days after an emergency Hartmann's resection, a patient develops pain, redness, and swelling around the caudal aspect of their laparotomy wound. The skin remains epithelialized; however, a fluctuant mass is felt. Which of the following is true:
>    A. This does not constitute an SSI as there is no break in the skin.

B. **Skin incision should be performed to drain the collection.**
   C. There is no value in obtaining microbiology samples as skin flora are the only possible pathogens.
   D. If an SSI is suspected, the entire length of the wound needs to be opened.
2. With regards to tissue healing:
   A. Wound hypothermia improves wound healing by decreasing metabolic demand on inflammatory cells.
   B. Bacterial pathogens cause an increase in protease inhibitors in the infected wound.
   C. After the tissue remodelling phase, injured tissue reaches a tensile strength equal or superior to that of uninjured tissue.
   D. **Cellular wound debridement by macrophages occurs during the inflammatory phase of healing.**
3. An emergency right hemicolectomy is performed on a 76-year-old man with an obstructing colorectal tumour. They suffer from insulin-controlled type 2 diabetes and mild chronic kidney disease, and their ASA score is 3. There is no perforation or inflammation present during surgery; however, the operation is prolonged due to bleeding and the patient requires an intraoperative blood transfusion. With regards to their risk of SSI.
   A. Their CDC NHSN risk score is 1 and they have a low risk of SSI.
   B. Their CDC NHSN risk score is 1 and they have a high risk of SSI.
   C. Their CDC NHSN risk score is 2 and they have a low risk of SSI.
   D. **Their CDC NHSN risk score is 2 and they have a high risk of SSI.**
4. A haemodynamically unstable patient with blunt abdominal injury undergoes an exploratory laparotomy. Which perioperative strategies should NOT be implemented to reduce SSI risk:
   A. Maintain normothermia through a combination of forced air and warmed intravenous fluids and blood products.
   B. **Maintaining tight glycaemic control to between 4.5 and 6.0 mmol/L.**
   C. Consider re-dosing of antibiotics if blood loss over 1.5 L is confirmed during surgery.
   D. Aggressive fluid and blood resuscitation to maintain tissue perfusion.
5. With regards to antiseptic-coated (Plus) sutures:
   A. Triclosan is a novel suture coating with a poorly understood safety profile.
   B. **The use of triclosan-coated polyglycatin 910 reduces the rate of SSI as compared to uncoated polyclycatin 910.**
   C. Triclosan only has a narrow spectrum of activity against Gram positive bacteria derived from skin flora.
   D. Cost-benefit studies have failed to show a cost savings effect for the use of Plus sutures.
6. Which of the following is NOT a recognised surgical strategy for reducing SSI:
   A. **Interrupted fascia sutures rather than continuous suturing.**
   B. Use of single-ring wound protectors.
   C. Use of clippers where hair removal is required.
   D. Fascia closure with Plus sutures.
7. Surgical site infections.
   A. Are an uncommon complication of emergency surgery.
   B. Always present within 14 days of surgery.

C. Occur most commonly in clean-contaminated wounds.
D. **Are a risk factor for incisional hernias.**

8. Regarding pathogens in SSI.
   A. Positive microbiology is mandatory for a diagnosis of SSI.
   B. **Infections are frequently polymicrobial.**
   C. Antimicrobial resistance is uncommon in SSIs.
   D. Fungal infections do not cause SSIs.

9. Negative pressure wound therapy.
   A. Should not be applied in patient with excessive subcutaneous tissue.
   B. Is only used to treat established SSIs.
   C. **Promotes blood flow and oxygenation to the wound.**
   D. Has a clear evidence base supporting its use in traumatic wounds.

10. After emergency laparotomy, a decision is made to close the fascia with loop polydioxanone. Each suture length is 150 cm. If the laparotomy wound measures 40 cm, what is the minimum number of sutures required for adequate wound closure?
    A. 1
    B. **2**
    C. 3
    D. 4

# References

1. National Healthcare Safety Network. Surgical site infection event (SSI). Centres Dis Control Prev. 2021;(January):1–39.
2. Kirkland KB, Briggs JP, Trivette SL, Wilkinson WE, Sexton DJ, Kirkland KB, Briggs JP, Trivette SL, Wilkinson WE, Sexton DJ. The impact of surgical-site infections in the 1990s: attributable mortality, excess length of hospitalization, and extra costs. Infect Control Hosp Epidemiol. 1999;20(11):725–30.
3. Badia JM, Casey AL, Petrosillo N, Hudson PM, Mitchell SA, Crosby C. Impact of surgical site infection on healthcare costs and patient outcomes: a systematic review in six European countries. J Hosp Infect. 2017;96(1):1–15. https://doi.org/10.1016/j.jhin.2017.03.004.
4. Weiser TG, Regenbogen SE, Thompson KD, Haynes AB, Lipsitz SR, Berry WR, et al. An estimation of the global volume of surgery: a modelling strategy based on available data. Lancet. 2008;372(9633):139–44.
5. van Ramshorst GH, Eker HH, van der Voet JA, Jeekel J, Lange JF. Long-term outcome study in patients with abdominal wound dehiscence: a comparative study on quality of life, body image, and incisional hernia. J Gastrointest Surg. 2013;17(8):1477–84.
6. Meijerink H, Lamagni T, Eriksen HM, Elgohari S, Harrington P, Kacelnik O. Is it valid to compare surgical site infections rates between countries? Insights from a study of English and Norwegian Surveillance Systems. Infect Control Hosp Epidemiol. 2017;38(2):162–71.
7. El-Saed A, Balkhy HH, Alshamrani MM, Aljohani S, Alsaedi A, Al Nasser W, et al. High contribution and impact of resistant gram negative pathogens causing surgical site infections at a multi-hospital healthcare system in Saudi Arabia, 2007–2016. BMC Infect Dis. 2020;20(1):1–9.
8. Bhangu A, Ademuyiwa AO, Aguilera ML, Alexander P, Al-Saqqa SW, Borda-Luque G, et al. Surgical site infection after gastrointestinal surgery in high-income, middle-income, and low-income countries: a prospective, international, multicentre cohort study. Lancet Infect Dis. 2018;18(5):516–25.
9. Elgohari S, S. Thelwall, T. Lamagni et al. Surveillance of surgical site infections in NHS hospitals in England. Public Heal Engl. 2014;(April 2019):29.
10. Scott RDI. The direct medical costs of healthcare-associated infections in U.S. hospitals and the benefits of prevention. 2009.
11. Engemann JJ, Carmeli Y, Cosgrove SE, Fowler VG, Bronstein MZ, Trivette SL, et al. Adverse clinical and economic outcomes attributable to methicillin resistance among patients with Staphylococcus aureus surgical site infection. Clin Infect Dis. 2003;36(5):592–8.
12. Meszaros AJ, Reichner JS, Albina JE. Macrophage-induced neutrophil apoptosis. J Immunol. 2000;165(1):435–41.
13. Leibovich SJ, Ross R. A macrophage dependent factor that stimulates the proliferation of fibroblasts in vitro. Am J Pathol. 1976;84(3):501–14.
14. Höer JJ, Junge K, Schachtrupp A, Klinge U, Schumpelick V. Influence of laparotomy closure technique on collagen synthesis in the incisional region. Hernia. 2002;6(3):93–8.
15. Grant R, Aupee M, Buchs NC, Cooper K, Eisenring MC, Lamagni T, et al. Performance of surgical site infection risk prediction models in colorectal surgery: external validity assessment from three European national surveillance networks. Infect Control Hosp Epidemiol. 2019;40(9):983–90.
16. Mu Y, Edwards JR, Horan TC, Berrios-Torres SI, Fridkin SK. Improving risk-adjusted measures of

surgical site infection for the national healthcare safety network. Infect Control Hosp Epidemiol. 2011;32(10):970–86.
17. De Simone B, Sartelli M, Coccolini F, Ball CG, Brambillasca P, Chiarugi M, et al. Intraoperative surgical site infection control and prevention: a position paper and future addendum to WSES intra-abdominal infections guidelines. World J Emerg Surg. 2020;15(1):1–23.
18. Hawn MT, Richman JS, Vick CC, Deierhoi RJ, Graham LA, Henderson WG, et al. Timing of surgical antibiotic prophylaxis and the risk of surgical site infection. JAMA Surg. 2013;148(7):649–57.
19. Pea F, Viale P. Bench-to-bedside review: appropriate antibiotic therapy in severe sepsis and septic shock - does the dose matter? Crit Care. 2009;13:1–13.
20. Shafi S, Elliott A, Gentilello L. Is hypothermia simply a marker of shock and injury severity or an independent risk factor for mortality in trauma patients? Analysis of a large national trauma registry. J Trauma. 2005;59(5):1081–5.
21. Kurz A, Sessler D, Lenhardt R. Perioperative normothermia to reduce the incidence of surgical-wound infection and shorten hospitalization. Study of Wound Infection and Temperature Group. N Engl J Med. 1996;334(19):1209–15.
22. Lan CCE, Wu CS, Kuo HY, Huang SM, Chen GS. Hyperglycaemic conditions hamper keratinocyte locomotion via sequential inhibition of distinct pathways: new insights on poor wound closure in patients with diabetes. Br J Dermatol. 2009;160(6):1206–14.
23. The NICE-SUGAR Study Investigators. Intensive versus conventional glucose control in critically ill patients. N Engl J Med. 2009;360(13):1283–97.
24. Cohen B, Schacham YN, Ruetzler K, Ahuja S, Yang D, Mascha EJ, et al. Effect of intraoperative hyperoxia on the incidence of surgical site infections: a meta-analysis. Br J Anaesth. 2018;120(6):1176–86. https://doi.org/10.1016/j.bja.2018.02.027.
25. Henneberg SW, Simonsen I. Effect of high perioperative oxygen fraction. JAMA. 2009;302(14):1543–50.
26. Cox PJ. Towards no incisional hernias: lateral paramedian versus midline incisions. J R Soc Med. 1986;79(December):711–2.
27. Bickenbach KA, Karanicolas PJ, Ammori JB, Jayaraman S, Winter JM, Fields RC, et al. Up and down or side to side? A systematic review and meta-analysis examining the impact of incision on outcomes after abdominal surgery. Am J Surg. 2013;206(3):400–9. https://doi.org/10.1016/j.amjsurg.2012.11.008.
28. Tanner J, Norrie P, Melen K, Tanner J, Norrie P, Melen K. Preoperative hair removal to reduce surgical site infection. Cochrane Database Syst Rev. 2011;(11):CD004122.
29. Sidhwa F, Itani KMF. Skin preparation before surgery. Surg Infect. 2015;16(1):14–23.
30. Kang S II, Oh HK, Kim MH, Kim MJ, Kim DW, Kim HJ, et al. Systematic review and meta-analysis of randomized controlled trials of the clinical effectiveness of impervious plastic wound protectors in reducing surgical site infections in patients undergoing abdominal surgery. Surgery. 2018;164(5):939–45.
31. Sajid MS, Rathore MA, Sains P, Singh KK. A systematic review of clinical effectiveness of wound edge protector devices in reducing surgical site infections in patients undergoing abdominal surgery. Updat Surg. 2017;69(1):21–8.
32. Pinkney TD, Calvert M, Bartlett DC, Gheorghe A, Redman V, Dowswell G, et al. Impact of wound edge protection devices on surgical site infection after laparotomy: multicentre randomized controlled trial (ROSSINI Trial). BMJ. 2013;347(7919):1–13. https://doi.org/10.1136/bmj.f4305.
33. van't Riet M, Steyerberg EW, Nellensteyn J, Bonjer HJ, Jeekel J. Meta-analysis of techniques for closure of midline abdominal incisions. Br J Surg. 2002;89:1530–356.
34. Israelsson LA, Millbourn D. Closing midline abdominal incisions. Langenbecks Arch Surg. 2012;397(8):1201–7.
35. Fink C, Baumann P, Wente MN, Knebel P, Bruckner T, Ulrich A, et al. Incisional hernia rate 3 years after midline laparotomy. Br J Surg. 2014;101(2):51–4.
36. Obermeier A, Schneider J, Wehner S, Matl FD, Schieker M, Von Eisenhart-Rothe R, et al. Novel high efficient coatings for anti-microbial surgical sutures using chlorhexidine in fatty acid slow-release carrier systems. PLoS One. 2014;9(7):e101426.
37. Tae BS, Park JH, Kim JK, Ku JH, Kwak C, Kim HH, et al. Comparison of intraoperative handling and wound healing between (NEOSORB® plus) and coated polyglactin 910 suture (NEOSORB®): a prospective, single-blind, randomized controlled trial. BMC Surg. 2018;18(1):1–10.
38. Daoud FC, Edmiston CE, Leaper D. Meta-analysis of prevention of surgical site infections following incision closure with triclosan-coated sutures: robustness to new evidence. Surg Infect. 2014;15(3):165–81.
39. Leaper DJ, Edmiston CE, Holy CE. Meta-analysis of the potential economic impact following introduction of absorbable antimicrobial sutures. Br J Surg. 2017;104(2):e134–44.
40. Leaper D, Wilson P, Assadian O, Edmiston C, Kiernan M, Miller A, et al. The role of antimicrobial sutures in preventing surgical site infection. Ann R Coll Surg Engl. 2017;99(6):439–43.
41. Justinger C, Slotta JE, Ningel S, Gräber S, Kollmar O, Schilling MK. Surgical-site infection after abdominal wall closure with triclosan-impregnated polydioxanone sutures: results of a randomized clinical pathway facilitated trial (NCT00998907). Surgery. 2013;154(3):589–95.
42. Henriksen NA, Deerenberg EB, Venclauskas L, Fortelny RH, Garcia-Alamino JM, Miserez M, et al. Triclosan-coated sutures and surgical site infection in abdominal surgery: the TRISTAN review, meta-analysis and trial sequential analysis. Hernia. 2017;21(6):833–41.

43. Norman G, Atkinson RA, Smith TA, Rowlands C, Rithalia AD, Crosbie EJ, et al. Intracavity lavage and wound irrigation for prevention of surgical site infection. Cochrane Database Syst Rev. 2017;2017(10):CD012234.
44. Gurusamy KS, Davidson BR. Continuous versus interrupted skin sutures for non-obstetric surgery. Cochrane Database Syst Rev. 2013;2013(2):CD010365.
45. Tuuli MG, Rampersad RM, Carbone JF, Stamilio D, Macones GA, Odibo AO. Staples compared with subcuticular suture for skin closure after cesarean delivery: a systematic review and meta-analysis. Obstet Gynecol. 2011;117(3):682–90.
46. Smith TO, Sexton D, Mann C, Donell S. Sutures versus staples for skin closure in orthopaedic surgery: meta-analysis. BMJ. 2010;340(7749):747.
47. Imamura K, Adachi K, Sasaki R, Monma S, Shioiri S, Seyama Y, et al. Randomized comparison of subcuticular sutures versus staples for skin closure after open abdominal surgery: a multicenter open-label randomized controlled trial. J Gastrointest Surg. 2016;20(12):2083–92. https://doi.org/10.1007/s11605-016-3283-z.
48. Tsujinaka T, Yamamoto K, Fujita J, Endo S, Kawada J, Nakahira S, et al. Subcuticular sutures versus staples for skin closure after open gastrointestinal surgery: a phase 3, multicentre, open-label, randomised controlled trial. Lancet. 2013;382(9898):1105–12. https://doi.org/10.1016/S0140-6736(13)61780-8.
49. Norman G, Goh EL, Dumville JC, Shi C, Liu Z, Chiverton L, et al. Negative pressure wound therapy for surgical wounds healing by primary closure. Cochrane Database Syst Rev. 2020;5:CD009261.
50. Papes D. Negative pressure wound therapy for open fractures. JAMA. 2018;320(16):1709.
51. Hyldig N, Birke-Sorensen H, Kruse M, Vinter C, Joergensen JS, Sorensen JA, et al. Meta-analysis of negative-pressure wound therapy for closed surgical incisions. Br J Surg. 2016;103(5):477–86.
52. Condon R, Sherertz R, Gaynes RP, Martone WJ, Jarvis WR, Emori TG, et al. CDC definitions of nosocomial surgical site infections, 1992: a modification of CDC definitions of surgical wound infections. Infect Control Hosp Epidemiol. 1992;13(10):606–8.
53. Gassman A, Mehta A, Bucholdz E, Abthani A, Guerra O, Maclin MM Jr, et al. Positive outcomes with negative pressure therapy over primarily closed large abdominal wall reconstruction reduces surgical site infection rates. Hernia. 2015;19:273–8.

## Further Reading

Bhangu A, Ademuyiwa AO, Aguilera ML, Alexander P, Al-Saqqa SW, Borda-Luque G, Costas-Chavarri A, Drake TM, Ntirenganya F, Fitzgerald JE, Fergusson SJ. Surgical site infection after gastrointestinal surgery in high-income, middle-income, and low-income countries: a prospective, international, multicentre cohort study. Lancet Infect Dis. 2018;18(5):516–25.

De Simone B, Sartelli M, Coccolini F, Ball CG, Brambillasca P, Chiarugi M, Campanile FC, Nita G, Corbella D, Leppaniemi A, Boschini E. Intraoperative surgical site infection control and prevention: a position paper and future addendum to WSES intra-abdominal infections guidelines. World J Emerg Surg. 2020;15(1):10.

UK, NICE Guideline Updates Team. Surgical site infections: prevention and treatment. 2019.